WORLD HEALTH ORGANIZATION

INTERNATIONAL AGENCY FOR RESEARCH ON CANCER

N-NITROSO COMPOUNDS: OCCURRENCE, BIOLOGICAL EFFECTS AND RELEVANCE TO HUMAN CANCER

Proceedings of the VIIIth International Symposium
on *N*-Nitroso Compounds held in Banff, Canada,
5–9 September 1983

EDITORS

I.K. O' NEILL, R.C. VON BORSTEL, C.T. MILLER,
J. LONG & H. BARTSCH

IARC Scientific Publications No. 57

INTERNATIONAL AGENCY FOR RESEARCH ON CANCER
LYON
1984

The International Agency for Research on Cancer (IARC) was established in 1965 by the World Health Assembly, as an independently financed organization within the framework of the World Health Organization. The headquarters of the Agency are at Lyon, France.

The Agency conducts a programme of research concentrating particularly on the epidemiology of cancer and the study of potential carcinogens in the human environment. Its field studies are supplemented by biological and chemical research carried out in the Agency's laboratories in Lyon and, through collaborative research agreements, in national research institutions in many countries. The Agency also conducts a programme for the education and training of personnel for cancer research.

The publications of the Agency are intended to contribute to the dissemination of authoritative information on different aspects of cancer research.

Oxford University Press, Walton Street, Oxford OX2 6DP

London   New York   Toronto
Delhi   Bombay   Calcutta   Madras   Karachi
Kuala Lumpur   Singapore   Hong Kong   Tokyo
Nairobi   Dar es Salaam   Cape Town
Melbourne   Auckland

and associated companies in
Beirut   Berlin   Ibadan   Mexico City   Nicosia

Oxford is a trade mark of Oxford University Press

Published in the United States
by Oxford University Press, New York

ISBN 0 19 723055 5
ISBN 92 832 1157 x (Publisher)
© International Agency for Research on Cancer 1984

PRINTED IN SWITZERLAND

CONTENTS

ORGANIZERS OF THE EIGHTH INTERNATIONAL MEETING ON N-NITROSO COMPOUNDS: OCCURRENCE, BIOLOGICAL EFFECTS AND RELEVANCE TO HUMAN CANCER

Canadian Executive Committee

R.C. von Borstel, University of Alberta, Edmonton (*Co-chairperson*)
C.T. Miller, Environment Canada (*Co-chairperson*)
J.E. Long, Health and Welfare Canada (*Co-chairperson*)
M.C. Archer, Ontario Cancer Research Institute
C. Chappel, F.D.C. Consultants Inc.
N.W. Choi, University of Manitoba
P.G. Scholefield, National Cancer Institute of Canada
N.P Sen, Health and Welfare Canada
H. F. Stich, British Columbia Cancer Research Centre
D. Williams, Health and Welfare Canada

Organizing Secretariat of the International Agency for Research on Cancer, Lyon, France

H. Bartsch
I.K. O'Neill
M. Castegnaro
Y. Granjard
E. Heseltine

The meeting was co-sponsored by the following six Canadian organizations:

Agriculture Canada
Alberta Heritage Foundation for Medical Research
Consumer and Corporate Affairs Canada
Environment Canada
Health and Welfare Canada
University of Alberta, Edmonton

Contributors

GeneBioChem
Hoffmann-La Roche
Swiss Bank Corporation (Greifengasse Branch, Basel)
Thermo Electron

FOREWORD

This volume, published as the proceedings of the Eighth International Meeting on *N*-Nitroso Compounds held in Banff, Alberta, Canada, focuses solely on *N*-nitroso compounds and their precursors, as did previous publications in this series. Many of the contributions confirm the widespread occurrence of *N*-nitroso compounds in the human environment and the fact that they can be formed endogenously in man from normal dietary constituents. Although they are clearly established as animal carcinogens, a causal relation between *N*-nitroso compounds and human cancer has not yet been rigorously established. At this meeting, for the first time, epidemiological evidence was presented to show such an association: oral cancer was linked with snuff dipping, and *N*-nitrosamines are the only carcinogens that have been detected in snuff, at levels exceeding by two orders of magnitude those in other consumer products. These data indicate that *N*-nitrosamine levels found in our environment may be sufficient to cause oral cancer in man and raise even more strongly the suspicion that they may be involved in other human cancers as well.

Because of their ubiquitous occurrence and their potent carcinogenicity (in 40 animal species), the endeavours of many research institutions, including this Agency, to identify sources of *N*-nitroso compounds in our environment and to find means for preventing exposure to them seem to be fully justified. In fact, there are many ways in which *N*-nitrosamine levels in food and in manufactured products can be lowered and many ways in which in-vivo nitrosation and potentiating risk factors, for example micronutrient deficiencies, may be reduced. Such preventive measures can clearly be implemented today, as pointed out in the closing remarks of Peter Magee who, together with M. Barnes, discovered in 1956 the carcinogenicity of *N*-nitrosodimethylamine in rats.

N-Nitroso compounds have also served as very valuable tools in basic cancer research, and many presentations in these proceedings contribute to our understanding of the cellular and molecular mechanisms by which *N*-nitroso compounds induce cancer.

I would like to thank the Programme Committee and all the members of the Canadian Executive Committee, in particular Drs R.C. Von Borstel, C.T. Miller and J.E. Long, who worked together to organize a meeting of such high quality. I express my deep gratitude to the co-sponsors of the meeting – the Alberta Heritage Foundation for Medical Research, the University of Alberta, Edmonton, and the four Departments of the Federal Canadian Government, Agriculture, Consumer and Corporate Affairs, Environment, Health and Welfare, as well as to the industrial companies that provided financial support. The highly efficient organization and management of the meeting at the Banff Conference Center by Mrs C. Hardie and her staff deserve particular acknowledgement.

Lorenzo Tomatis, M.D.
Director,
International Agency
for Research on Cancer,
Lyon, France

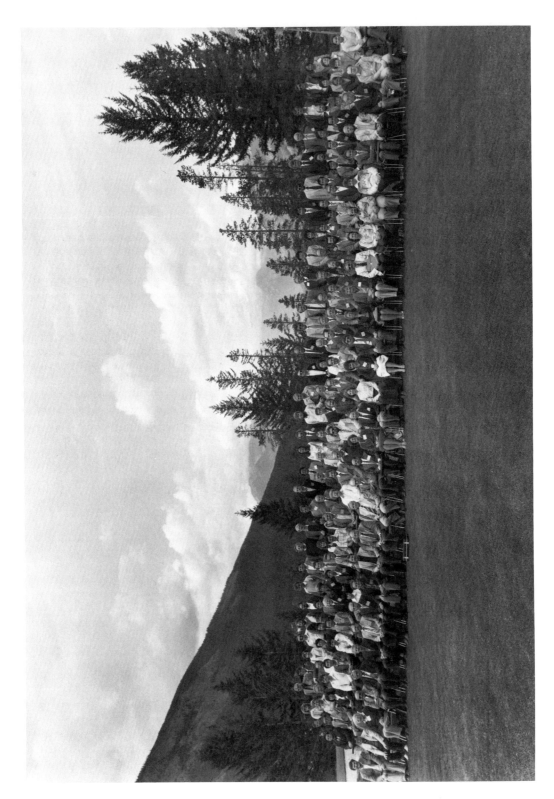

INTRODUCTION

The present volume, published as the Proceedings of the Eighth International Meeting on *N*-Nitroso Compounds[1], reflects in its title the increasing interest being generated to assess the relevance of these compounds to human cancer. The overview preceding the contributions to these proceedings was prepared from the reports of those chairing the sessions and is intended to highlight new and important developments and approaches. An attempt has been made to systematize the nomenclature of the *N*-nitroso compounds (p. 991) to ensure that chemists and biologists are referring to the same substances. In order to increase the usefulness of this large volume, *subject* and *author* indexes have been included at the end of this volume.

The editors wish to thank the chairpersons and the organizers for their contributions during the meeting, and the Programme and Executive Committee, whose guidance and assistance were invaluable.

The Editors

Lyon, 30 January 1984

---

[1]   Ninth Meeting to be held on 1–5 September 1986 in Vienna, Austria, following the 14th International Cancer Congress in Budapest (21–27 August 1986)

N-NITROSO COMPOUNDS: OCCURRENCE, BIOLOGICAL EFFECTS AND RELEVANCE TO HUMAN CANCER - AN OVERVIEW [1]

In this review of the contributions presented in this volume, emphasis is placed on three aspects:

(i) new and important developments of methods and approaches that could help in understanding of basic mechanisms of carcinogenesis and suggestions for such studies on humans in situations in which exposure to *N*-nitroso compounds, or their precursors, is known to be or to have been high and in which methods exist for monitoring such exposure;

(ii) significant advances in laboratory methods that could be applied to an integrated laboratory and epidemiological approach; and

(iii) deficiencies in present knowledge and inadequacies of available methods, with suggestions for possible future directions of research to fill these gaps.

1. *Occurrence and formation of* N-*nitroso compounds*

New data on precursors of *N*-nitroso compounds (NOC) and on their occurrence were reported. The general population can be exposed *via* foodstuffs both to preformed NOC and to their precursors; the latter react with nitrosating agents to yield NOC and other reactive intermediates. As examples, tyramine and 1-methyl-1,2,3,4-tetrahydro-β-carboline-3-carboxylic acid, present in soya sauce, were mentioned as precursors that give rise to mutagenic compounds after nitrosation (p. 17). Elevated levels of both dimethylamine and *N*-nitroso-dimethylamine (NDMA) have been found in the intestines of patients with chronic renal failure (p. 161). *N*-Nitrosation of peptides has been studied in order to elucidate conditions under which polypeptides and proteins present in the gastric juice or mucosa might be converted to *N*-nitroso derivatives of biological significance (p. 7). Polyunsaturated lipids were found to be capable of serving as *N*-nitrosating agents in mouse skin after exposure to nitrogen dioxide, raising the possibility that similar reactions might be responsible for *N*-nitrosamine formation in other tissues (p. 283). Intravenous or oral administration to human subjects of nitrate (p. 193) including ammonium nitrate given to prevent formation of renal stones reproducibly increased endogenous formation of *N*-nitrosoproline (NPRO). A background of endogenously formed NPRO is unaffected by ingestion of ascorbate or α-tocopherol (p. 223), two known inhibitors of *N*-nitrosation reactions.

---

[1] This overview was prepared by a committee composed of M.C. Archer, H. Bartsch (Secretary), P. Bogovski, M. Börszönyi, B.C. Challis, P. Correa, E. Heseltine (Technical Editor), T. Kawabata, L. Keefer, P. Kleihues, W. Lijinsky, P.N. Magee, A.B. Miller, C.T. Miller, I.K. O'Neill (Rapporteur), A.E. Pegg, R. Preussmann, R.A. Scanlan, N. Sen, S.R. Tannenbaum and R.C. von Borstel

[2] Figures in parentheses refer to page numbers in this volume.

Thus, humans can synthesize NOC endogenously; good evidence for the occurrence of these reactions comes from studies in which proline (p. 223), piperazine (p. 171) and aminopyrine (p.179) were used as nitrosatable amines. The extent of the nitrosation reaction was shown to be linked to (dietary) intake of nitrite and nitrate; however, smoking (p. 811) and in-vivo oxidation of ammonia (p. 241) are also contributing factors; induced inflammation enhanced the rate of nitrate synthesis by oxidation of ammonia (p. 247) and related substrates. The role of bacteria-mediated nitrosation has been investigated further (p. 275), and an *Escherichia coli* strain has been shown to catalyse *N*-nitrosamine formation from nitrite and an amine.

Many *N*-nitrosation inhibitors, such as ascorbic acid and α-tocopherol, have been characterized and used to advantage in lowering exposure to NOC (p. 223). Dietary phenolics (p. 213) appear to play a complex role, causing either increased or decreased endogenous formation of NOC such as NPRO, depending on factors such as pH and rate of production of saliva and the ratio of concentrations of precursor nitrite and amine.

Several new findings on the chemistry of formation and decomposition of NOC were described, including photolysis in non-aqueous media (p. 365). Formation and inhibition were also demonstrated to occur in emulsions (p. 347). Nitrite-ester mediated NOC formation from nitrite and amines was reported (pp. 311, 353). Progress has been made in the safe destruction of carcinogenic *N*-nitrosamides (p. 387).

2. *Analytical advances and identification of new NOC*

Significant progress has been made in developing high-performance liquid chromatographic (HPLC) and gas-liquid chromatographic (GLC) methods for analysing nitrosamides, by (i) post-column HPLC chemical denitrosation of the nitrosamides followed by chemi-luminescence detection of the liberated NO, and (ii) modification of the Thermal Energy Analyzer pyrolysis conditions to enable detection of nitrosamides after separation by GLC (p. 121).

New developments and improvement of methods for the analysis of non-volatile NOC were presented (p. 138). Although progress has been made, more research will be required before the nature of most non-volatile NOC in foods and biological fluids can be elucidated.

For example, samples of canned cured meat and Chinese cabbage were found to contain apparently high concentrations of total NOC (p. 25), as determined by the method of Walters *et al.* Future work should be directed toward establishing that all NOC respond on a molar basis in this procedure, so that all NOC exposures can be quantified individually.

N-Nitrosothiazolidine 4-carboxylic acid (NTCA) and *N*-nitroso-2-methylthiazolidine 4-carboxylic acid (NMTCA) (*cis* and *trans* isomers) (pp. 77, 87) were isolated and identified in human urine for the first time. Future research should attempt to establish the origin and the biological significance of these two compounds. As the easily nitrosatable amino precursors, thiazolidine 4-carboxylic acid and its 2-methyl derivative, are formed readily by reaction of formaldehyde or acetaldehyde with cysteine *in vitro* and *in vivo* (p. 77), measurement of NTCA and NMTCA in urine may provide a further index for endogenous nitrosation in the human body and may also allow monitoring of exposure of human subjects to precursors like formaldehyde, acetaldehyde, nitrate and nitrite.

3. *DNA repair, macromolecular adducts and biological effects*

A DNA repair protein which removes alkyl groups from the O^6-position of guanine in DNA was described (p. 575); this protein was studied in human lymphocytes (p. 561), in various human organs and in rat liver and brain at various stages of fetal and post-natal development

(p. 571). Its concentration depends on both organ and species, the highest amounts being found in human liver (p. 575). Attempts have been made to relate low rate of DNA repair and high rate of cellular replication with cancer risk in rodent organs with different susceptibilities to induction of cancer by N-nitrosoalkylureas (p. 571).

The production of monoclonal antibodies (p. 589) of high specificity and affinity for alkylated deoxynucleosides and their use for quantitating these adducts (i.e., for monitoring human exposure to alkylating agents) by radioimmunoassay or immunofluorescence techniques was described. Another approach for exposure monitoring (p. 589) involved measurement of the formation of deuterated 7-methylguanine and S-methylcysteine in rats exposed to deuterated aminopyrine, a drug which yields NDMA *in vivo* upon nitrosation.

The results of a number of bioassays in which the same NOC were given to rats and hamsters were summarized (p. 617). The striking difference in target organs in which tumours occurred is difficult to explain on the basis of the known pathways for activation or DNA repair in these species and suggests an influence of other, presently unknown, factors possibly related to gene expression in cells at the time of interaction with the carcinogens.

The organ specificity of N-methyl-N'-nitro-N-nitrosoguanidine (MNNG) (p. 603) for the glandular cells of the stomach in rodents did correlate, however, with the high concentration of thiols in those cells, which facilitate decomposition of the carcinogen (p. 603). N-Nitroso-methylbenzylamine (NMBzA) was shown to be activated to a methylating agent in the target cells of rodents in which it induces tumours (p. 595), i.e., the oesophagus, lung and liver. NMBzA was also reported to be metabolized by oesophageal microsomes from humans (p. 473) but at a lower rate than by those from rats.

Data on the metabolism and genetic and carcinogenic activities of a variety of N-nitrosamines (p. 401) and N-nitramines (p. 485) were presented. Carcinogenic NOC previously reported to be non-mutagenic gave positive responses in a yeast test system (p. 721). Tumours were induced by N-nitrosodiethylamine (NDEA) in the liver, kidney, oral cavity and trachea of pythons, bringing the number of animal species in which N-nitroso compounds produce tumours up to 40 (p. 677).

The analysis of a large BIBRA/UK government study on dose and time relationships for N-nitrosamine carcinogenesis in rats was presented (p. 627). Two years of chronic treatment with NDMA and NDEA led to a clearly measurable cancer risk at a dose of 10 μg/kg body weight per day.

The underlying chemistry by which chemotherapeutic N-nitrosoalkylureas interact with DNA was described (p. 689); the formation of DNA adducts might be predicted on the basis of stereo-electronic control. It was shown in experimental systems that the antineoplastic activities of certain new nitrosoureas can be dissociated, at least partially, from their carcinogenicity (p. 695).

4. *Metabolism and modifying factors*

NDMA has been shown to be hydroxylated by a specific cytochrome P-450 isozyme which is inducible, for example, by pyrazole and acetone but not by phenobarbital (p. 423). Metabolic activation of N-nitrosamines can take place not only by oxidation at the carbon atom in the position α to the N-nitroso group, but also at the β- or ω-carbon atoms (p. 401); such reactions have important consequences for the metabolic fate and organotropic effects of N-nitrosodialkylamines.

A β-nitrosaminoaldehyde has been synthesized as a model compound, and the aldehyde group has been shown to be highly electrophilic (p. 429). As a consequence, such compounds can form reactive diazonium ions without metabolic activation. The nitrosaminoaldehyde was also active as a transnitrosating agent. These reactions may explain the biological activity of

N-nitrosamines such as N-nitrosodiethanolamine (NDELA), which can be oxidized to a monoaldehyde.

Various chemicals, e.g., ethanol, disulfiram (p. 519) (used as an anti-alcoholism drug in humans), certain isothiocyanates (p. 797), phenols (p. 213), coumarins and indoles of natural origin (p. 797), were shown to have marked effects on the pharmacokinetics and metabolism of N-nitrosamines, influencing in turn their carcinogenic effects in experimental animals, both qualitatively (target organ) and quantitatively (incidence). Similarly, in rats on a zinc-deficient diet, NDMA did not produce the expected tumours of the liver and kidneys, but tumours were induced in the forestomach (p. 543).

Ethanol, in small quantities, was shown to alter the distribution and metabolism of small oral doses of NDMA and NDEA in rats, increasing by several-fold the alkylation of DNA in organs that are particularly susceptible to their carcinogenic effect (p. 501) (i.e., the kidney for NDMA and the oesophagus for NDEA). As demonstrated with NDMA, this effect is the result of prevention of first-pass clearance in the liver of the N-nitrosamine. There is suggestive evidence that this also happens in humans, since a relatively high level of N-nitrosamines has been observed in human blood after ingestion of high nitrate meals with alcohol. Therefore, the influence of alcohol consumption on human cancer may be mediated through an effect on the pharmacokinetics of N-nitrosamines derived from diet, from tobacco smoke and from endogenous synthesis (pp. 501, 867).

5. NOC in tobacco carcinogenesis

(a) Formation and analysis of NOC in tobacco products

That NOC occur in fermented tobacco and tobacco smoke is now established (p. 743), and this is the greatest and most widespread source of human exposure presently known (except for some occupational exposures). Eleven volatile and two non-volatile N-nitrosamines, including four volatile tobacco-specific nitrosamines (TSNA), have been detected (p. 743). The concentrations of TSNA are high in tobacco smoke and even higher in snuff and chewing tobacco (p. 743). The concentration of NOC, especially TSNA, was shown to be related to the nitrate content of tobacco products (p. 878). Levels of volatile N-nitrosamines are considerably higher in sidestream smoke than in mainstream smoke (p. 743). There was greater endogenous nitrosation in smokers than in non-smokers (pp. 811, 819).

(b) Carcinogenicity and metabolic activation of TSNA

4-(N-Methyl-N-nitrosamino)-1-(3-pyridyl)-1-butanone (NNK) has been shown to be a potent carcinogen (p. 763) which can cross the placental barrier in animals (p. 787). A metabolite of NNK can be reconverted to the parent compound, thus leading to prolonged exposure to NNK (p. 805). In metabolic studies *in vitro* and in experimental animals, NNK and N-nitrosonornicotine (NNN) were shown to be readily converted into electrophiles that can interact with DNA (p. 805).

(c) Epidemiological studies and tobacco NOC

Epidemiological data on types of tobacco that determine the risk of developing cancer at sites such as the lung, larynx and bladder were reviewed. No important difference in risk due to the method of curing tobacco was noted (p. 867).

The correlation between oral cancer and chewing of betel quid (often containing tobacco) observed in India and other south-east Asian countries is well established (p. 851). In studies to identify the etiological agents involved, it was shown that nitrosation of arecoline, a betel-nut alkaloid, leads to the formation of three NOC, of which N-nitroso-N-methylpropionitrile was carcinogenic to experimental animals (p. 859). This carcinogen and other products arising from nitrosation of betel-nut constituents should be investigated further to establish whether they play a role in oral cancer produced in betel-quid chewers.

An association between human cancer and tobacco chewing and snuff dipping has been confirmed in some southern states of the USA (p. 837); tumours usually arise at the site in the mouth where the tobacco product is retained. Since these non-combusted tobacco products have not yet been shown to contain carcinogens other than TSNA (in relatively high concentrations), a direct correlation between N-nitrosamine exposure and human cancer must be assumed in this specific case, although the role of alcohol has not been fully examined.

6. *Epidemiological studies and combined laboratory/epidemiology investigations to link NOC and their precursors with human cancers*

A number of epidemiological studies were performed to investigate possible links between adverse biological effects in humans and presumed exposure to NOC and their precursors; however, in no case were NOC clearly identified as the agents responsible, nor was the exposure quantified. Such data are still suggestive and indicate that further investigations must be performed using approaches that allow a more precise estimate of human exposure to NOC. Some evidence was presented linking presumed exposure to NOC or precursors with the development of cerebral tumours (p. 887). The consumption by parents of large amounts of Icelandic smoked mutton was suggested to induce diabetes in their male progeny (p. 911). This diabetogenic effect was also produced experimentally in male offspring of mice fed with Icelandic smoked mutton after mating. High (mg/kg) levels of N-nitrosothiazolidine and NTCA were detected in smoked meat products, including Icelandic mutton (p. 911). In a follow-up study on patients who had undergone gastric surgery or who had been treated for pernicious anaemia (situations in which it has been hypothesized that abnormally large amounts of NOC are produced), an excess incidence of gastric cancer over that expected was found (p. 895). A higher concentration of nitrate in saliva was found (p. 921) in subjects living in a high-risk area for cholangiocarcinoma in Thailand than in those living in a low-risk area. However, these findings need further confirmation.

Several industrial processes were described in which occupational exposure to high concentrations of volatile N-nitrosamines may occur (p. 938). Exposure to NDELA can be monitored biologically in the urine of workers (p. 943). Only a small number of studies are in progress in which the role of occupational exposure to N-nitrosamines is being assessed; more such epidemiological investigations are warranted.

The excretion of nitrosated amino acids was compared in subjects suffering from chronic atrophic gastritis (at high risk for gastric cancer) and in healthy controls (p. 957). Following ingestion of nitrate and proline, urinary NPRO levels in the patients were dependent on gastric pH, showing maximal yields at around pH 2. Healthy controls excreted no apparent excess of NPRO. Urinary NPRO was not correlated with total intragastric NOC in any study subject, but smokers excreted more total N-nitrosamino acids in their urine than non-smokers. These data indicate that endogenous nitrosation does occur in the human stomach; however, its relation to the induction of upper gastrointestinal cancer remains to be proven.

The effects of H2 blockers on intragastric nitrosation was examined in healthy volunteers and in duodenal ulcer patients who ingested proline. The concentration of NPRO excreted in the urine was not affected by treatment with ranitidine, but that of NTCA was significantly increased (p. 971).

Hypochlorhydric subjects showed a significant reduction in mean total NOC concentration in gastric juice after four weeks' treatment with ascorbic acid; the total rose again one month after discontinuing treatment. Mean gastric concentrations of nitrite and of nitrate-reducing organisms were also lowered by ascorbic acid treatment. There was a significant reduction in total NOC during ascorbic acid treatment in patients with partial gastrectomy but not in those suffering from pernicious anaemia or atrophic gastritis.

A high concentration of nitrite was detectable, especially one hour after ingestion of nitrate, in the gastric juice of subjects with chronic atrophic gastritis and in those who had undergone partial gastrectomy.

The etiological factors that may be involved in the causation of oesophageal cancer in certain provinces of Northern China were summarized (p. 948), providing evidence that NOC and their precursors are probably involved. The excretion of urinary N-nitrosamino acids by inhabitants living in high-risk (Linxian) and low-risk (Fanxian) areas for oesophageal cancer was compared. Linxian subjects excreted significantly more nitrate and N-nitrosamino acids (NPRO, NTCA, NMTCA) than those living in Fanxian. When Linxian subjects were given ascorbic acid (3 × 100 mg after each meal), the level of urinary N-nitrosamino acids was reduced to those found in Fanxian. Ascorbic acid, an efficient inhibitor of endogenous nitrosation, should now be examined in intervention trials.

7. *Conclusions*

In view of the evidence that has been accumulated and presented at this meeting on the possible role of NOC in the causation of human cancer, a causal association, although not yet rigorously established, must be assumed. On the grounds of biochemical and histopathological data, there is also little reason to believe that humans are resistant to the carcinogenic action of NOC. Therefore, preventive measures against the induction of cancer in humans by NOC should be devised and implemented (p. 987): (i) a reduction in exposure to NOC, e.g., by limiting the use of tobacco products; (ii) use of inhibitors of the nitrosation reaction, like ascorbic acid, to reduce exposure to NOC, in particular those formed in the mammalian body; and (iii) selective inhibition of the metabolic activation of N-nitrosamines, although this difficult approach has not yet been fully explored.

LIST OF PRESENTATIONS

ENVIRONMENTAL OCCURRENCE OF *N*-NITROSO COMPOUNDS AND NITROSATABLE PRECURSORS

NEW *N*-NITROSO COMPOUNDS AND IMPROVED METHODS OF ANALYSIS

FORMATION OF N-NITROSO COMPOUNDS. CATALYSIS, INHIBITION AND MECHANISMS

MODIFIERS OF METABOLISM AND CARCINOGENICITY
OF *N*-NITROSO COMPOUNDS

DNA REPAIR AND DETECTION OF ALKYLATED MACROMOLECULES

BIOLOGICAL EFFECTS: CARCINOGENICITY AND MUTAGENICITY

CARCINOGENIC EFFECTS RELATED TO TOBACCO AND BETEL QUID

EPIDEMIOLOGY AND COMBINED LABORATORY/EPIDEMIOLOGY STUDIES

KEYNOTE ADDRESS AND CLOSING REMARKS

ENVIRONMENTAL OCCURRENCE OF *N*-NITROSO COMPOUNDS AND NITROSATABLE PRECURSORS

OCCURRENCE AND EXPOSURE TO *N*-NITROSO COMPOUNDS AND PRECURSORS

R. PREUSSMANN

Institute of Toxicology and Chemotherapy, German Cancer Research Center, 6900 Heidelberg, FRG

INTRODUCTION

Reliable knowledge about potential human health risks due to exposure to environmental *N*-nitroso compounds is of relatively recent origin. After the formation of carcinogenic nitrosamines in tobbaco smoke (from nitrogen oxides and tobacco amines) was first suggested (Druckrey & Preussmann, 1962), Ender and his colleagues (1964) provided the first evidence of the occurrence of *N*-nitrosodimethylamine (NDMA) in nitrite-treated fish-meal (Sakshaug *et al.*, 1965), and Sander (1967) was the first to provide unequivocal proof of endogenous nitrosamine formation from precursors, after an earlier negative result in an animal experiment (Druckrey *et al.*, 1963). Using nonspecific detection methods, many of the early results on the environmental occurrence of nitrosamines were unreliable, and the methods used were of low sensitivity. The development of a nitrosamine-specific, highly-sensitive chemiluminescence detector (Thermal Energy Analyzer, TEA) by D. Fine and his colleagues (1975) was therefore a landmark in the field of determination of environmental *N*-nitroso compounds. Applications of that reliable method for trace analysis provided unequivocal evidence of the environmental occurrence of these potent carcinogens.

Present knowledge of human exposure to nitrosamines shows a rather complex pattern, which is summarized in Figure 1. The overall exposure can be subdivided into exposure to preformed *N*-nitroso compounds (exogenous exposure, subdivided into 'life-style' and occupational exposure) and into exposure by in-vivo formation of such compounds from precursors, e.g., nitrosatable amino compounds and nitrosating agents (endogenous exposure).

The following short review cannot go into detail, but concentrates on more general aspects, indicates any progress in preventive measures to avoid human exposure (a field in which considerable success has been achieved) and, finally, indicates needs for further research on environmental *N*-nitroso compounds.

Many aspects of the problem are illuminated by several recent reviews, such as those on analysis (Preussmann *et al.*, 1983), on environmental occurrence (Eisenbrand, 1981; National Research Council, 1981; Scanlan & Tannenbaum, 1981; Preussmann & Eisenbrand, 1984; Preussmann, 1984), on precursors (WHO, 1977; National Research Council, 1981; Hartmann, 1982) and on carcinogenesis (IARC, 1978; Preussmann & Stewart, 1984). The proceedings of the biannual International Meetings on Environmental *N*-Nitroso Compounds, published by IARC (Walker *et al.*, 1978, 1980; Bartsch *et al.*, 1982), contain indispensable material on all aspects of the problem.

Fig. 1. Environmental N-nitroso compounds and human exposure

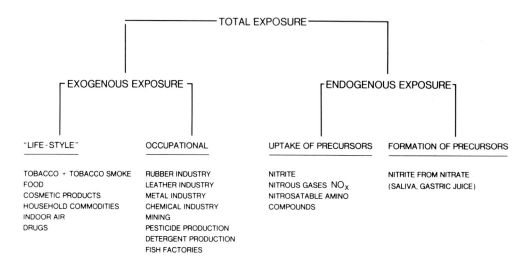

EXOGENOUS EXPOSURE

It must be emphasized at once that only 'volatile' N-nitrosamines are usually referred to when speaking of exposure to preformed N-nitrosamines in the human environment. With the exception of N-nitrosodiethanolamine (NDELA), some N-nitrosamino acids and the tobacco-specific N-nitrosamines (TSNA), no systematic study of human exposure to non-volatile N-nitroso compounds is available, owing to the lack of generally applicable and specific trace analytical methods for this group of compounds.

Life-style exposure

Tobacco and tobacco smoke: Practically all available data on the occurrence of N-nitroso compounds in tobacco and tobacco smoke come from the pioneering work of Hoffmann, Brunnenmann, Hecht and their colleagues (see reviews by Hoffmann *et al.,* 1982a,b; Hecht *et al.,* 1983). From this work, it is evident that tobacco and its smoke are responsible for the highest non-occupational nitrosamine exposure known. Since this important topic is a major point of discussion at the present meeting, only some representative data will be given here (Tables 1 and 2).

These tables and other available data illustrate the following important facts:
- The nitrate concentration in tobacco is of crucial importance for nitrosamine yields in tobacco smoke.
- The concentrations of volatile nitrosamines in side-stream smoke are consistently higher than those in main-stream smoke. (The relevance of this to passive smoking remains to be established).
- TSNA arise from nitrosation of tobacco alkaloids either during tobacco processing or during burning.
- NDELA contamination of tobacco and its smoke results from the use of the diethanolamine salt of maleic hydrazide.

Table 1. Volatile N-nitrosamines (NDMA, N-nitrosodimethylamine; NEMA, N-nitrosoethylmethylamine; NDEA, N-nitrosodiethylamine; NPYR, N-nitrosopyrrolidine) in tobacco smoke (μg/cigarette)

	NDMA		NEMA		NDEA		NPYR	
	MS[a]	SS[b]	MS	SS	MS	SS	MS	SS
Commercial cigarettes (USA)	6–65	680–1 040	0.4–8	9–30	1–8	8–73	5–33	205–390
French cigarettes	4–29		0.5–3		0.1–0.6		11–25	
Low-nitrate experimental cig. tes	10–20		0.1–1.2		2–3		3–6	
High-nitrate experimental cig. tes	76–97		5–9		3–5		32–52	
Small cigars	43	1 770	0.4	75	1	29	5	612

[a] Mainstream smoke
[b] Sidestream smoke

Table 2. Tobacco-specific nitrosamines[a] and N-nitrosodiethanolamine (NDELA) in tobacco and tobacco smoke

	Tobacco (mg/kg)				Mainstream smoke (ng/cigarette)			
	NNN	NNK	NAT	NDELA	NNN	NNK	NAT	NDELA
Commercial cig. (USA)	1.4–1.7	0.7	1.3–1.6	115–199	0.24–0.31	0.1–0.15	0.3–0.4	24–36
French cigarettes	2.7–11.9	0.5–1.1	1.5–2.0	–	0.5–3.2	0.1–0.4	0.2–0.6	
Low-nitrate experimental cig.	0.2–0.6	0.1–0.4	0.4–0.6	–	0.4–0.6	0.16–0.4	0.4–0.5	
High-nitrate experimental cig.	7	3.2	–	–	3.7	0.32	4.6	
Small cigars	45	35	13	419	5.5	4.2	1.7	68
Columbian cigars (5.7 g)	11	1	3	108	3.2	1.9	1.9	10

[a] NNN, N-nitrosonornicotine; NNK, N-4-(methylnitrosamino)-1-(3-pyridyl)-1-butanone; NAT, N-nitrosoanatabine

Table 3. N-Nitrosamines[a] in snuff (µg/kg)

	NDMA	NPYR	NMOR	NDELA	NNN	NNK	NAT	NAD
Snuff (USA) 4 different brands	2–215	2–360	24–690	290–3 300	2 200–33 000	600–8 300	1 700–40 000	100–1 900
Snuff (USA)	2	2	31	600	830	210	240	10
Snuff (Sweden) 5 different brands	2–60	2–210	2–44	225–390	2 000–6 100	600–1 700	900–2 400	40–140
Snuff (Bavaria)					6 100–6 700	1 500	1 900–4 900	
Snuff (Denmark)					4 500	1 400–7 000	2 700–6 200	

[a] NDMA, N-nitrosodimethylamine; NPYR, n-nitrosopyrrolidine; NMOR, N-nitrosomorpholine; NNN, N-nitrosonornicotine; NNK, N-4-(methylnitrosamino)-1-(3-pyridyl)-1-butanone; NAT, N′-nitrosoanatabine; NAD, nicotinamide adenine dinucleotide

– TSNA and other nitrosamines are the only known carcinogens in snuff, and their high concentration (Table 3) might be responsible for the increased risk of oral cancer in snuff dippers. *N*-nitrosomorpholine (NMOR) in snuff probably arises from morpholine used in preparing wax-layers in cardboard snuff containers.
– The high concentrations of nitrosatable amines in tobacco and smoke might also constitute a considerable additional risk factor by providing precursors for endogenous nitrosation.

From the available data, the exposure of smokers to total nitrosamines may be estimated by summation of all eight nitrosamines presently identified (National Research Council, 1981). Thus, a smoker of 20 cigarettes/day inhales between 16 µg (US commercial cigarettes) and 86 µg (French non-filter cigarettes) per day. Hoffmann and his colleagues (1982a,b) have shown that volatile nitrosamines in tobacco smoke can be removed selectively by cellulose acetate filters and that filters considerably reduce TSNA in smoke as well. Avoidance of tobacco ribs and stems, rich in nitrate, is another method for reducing nitrosamine concentrations in tobacco smoke. There can be no doubt that nitrosamine levels in snuff (Table 3) can also be lowered. Of course, the most effective measure to prevent tobacco-related diseases is to stop smoking.

Food: Very thorough and representative data are available for volatile nitrosamines in food. It has been shown that beer, and not nitrite-cured meat products or cheeses, as expected earlier, was the mainsource of the nitrosamine burden in food. Using the average per-caput consumption of different food products and their average nitrosamine content, our own results (Preussmann *et al.*, 1979; Spiegelhalder *et al.*, 1980), based on almost 3000 food samples analysed, are given in Table 4. They demonstrate that the total *N*-nitrosodimethylamine (NDMA) intake was 1.1 µg/person per day in 1979 and that 64% of that intake resulted from the consumption of beer. Stephany and Schuller (1980) calculated the same total intake from their studies of Dutch food, while Gough *et al.* (1978) obtained an estimate of 0.53 µg/day from their survey of about 300 samples. This is in good agreement with the other data, since the British study did not include beer as a source of NDMA. The corresponding data from Japan, estimated by Maki *et al.* (1980), are somewhat higher (Table 5).

Table 4. Average daily intake of *N*-nitrosamines by male persons calculated from average per-cap. consumption (Ernährungsbericht, 1976) in the Federal Republic of Germany

Food	*N*-Nitrosamine[a]	Daily intake per capita (µg)	Fraction of total intake (NDMA) (%)
Beer[b]	NDMA	0.7	64
Meat and meat products	NDMA	0.1	10
	NPYR	0.1	
	NPIP	0.01	
Cheese	NDMA	0.01	1
Others	NDMA	0.2	25
	NPYR	0.03	
TOTAL	NDMA	1.1	100
	NPYR	0.1–0.15	

[a] NDMA, *N*-nitrosodimethylamine; NPYR, *n*-nitrosopyrrolidine; NPIP, *N*-nitrosopiperidine
[b] NDMA content is corrected for the proportion of sales of different types of beer

Table 5. Estimated daily intake of volatile nitrosamines from Japanese food (Maki *et al.*, 1980)

	Consumption (g/day/person)	Average concentration (µg/kg)	Intake (µg/day)
Cured meats	12	0.5	0.006
Broiled dried fish	54	30	1.62
Canned and fish products	5	5	0.025
Dairy products, eggs and chicken	76	0.7	0.53
Food seasoning	6	0.2	0.001
Oil and fats	18	0.9	0.016
Beer	30	1.6	0.05
Sake	19	0	0
Tsukemono, miso and *shogu*	27	0.3	0.008
Rice	234	0	0
		Total	2.256

Considerable reductions in exposure have been achieved in two areas. The *n*-nitrosopyrrolidine (NPYR) contamination of fried bacon was reduced from levels of 20–1 000 µg/kg in 1971–1972 to average levels of 5–15 µg/kg in 1977 (Havery *et al.*, 1978) by improved production methods, mainly by reducing levels of added and residual nitrite and adding nitrosation inhibitors, such as ascorbic acid, to the curing mixture. In the Federal Republic of Germany, the permitted concentration of nitrite in curing salt mixtures was recently reduced by 20%, and the use of nitrate has been severely restricted.

The reasons for the NDMA contamination of beer have been elucidated (Preussmann *et al.*, 1981) and have led to technological changes, such as the use of indirectly-heated kilns for malt-drying, the use of low NO_x-burners in directly-heated kilns and the use of SO_2 as a scavenger of nitrogen oxides. Consequently, the NDMA content of beer has been reduced to concentrations below 0.5 µg/kg in the Federal Republic of Germany (Preussmann *et al.*, 1981; Fromberger & Allmann, 1983), the USA (Havery *et al.*, 1981), Canada (Sen *et al.*, 1982) and The Netherlands (Ellen & Schuller, 1983). This considerable reduction of NDMA contamination of beer changed the average overall intake of volatile nitrosamines from food in the Federal Republic of Germany from 1.1 µg/day in 1979 to about 0.5–0.6 µg/day in 1981. Evidently, one major unsolved problem in this area (as in others) is the potential occurrence of non-volatile carcinogenic *N*-nitroso compounds.

Cosmetics: Di- and triethanolamine and some of their salts and amides are used on a large scale as emulsifiers in many cosmetic formulations. Nitrosamine contamination of such products many result either from the use of contaminated amines (Spiegelhalder *et al.*, 1978) or *via* nitrosation in the product with NO_x, nitrite or the bactericide 2-bromo-2-nitro-1,3-propanediol (bronopol). NDELA has been found in 27 out 29 cosmetics in a wide range of concentrations, from below 1 to 48 000 µg/kg (Fan *et al.*, 1977). Our own unpublished results confirm the occurrence of volatile nitrosamines and NDELA in many commercially-available cosmetics. Another study found 20–4113 µg/kg NDELA in cosmetic products (Klein *et al.*, 1981). *N*-Nitrosomethyl-dodecylamine, -tetradecylamine and -octadecylamine were found (Hecht *et al.*, 1982; Morrison *et al.*, 1983) in low concentrations (10–873 µg/kg) in cosmetics formulated with dimethylalkylamine oxides as nonionic detergents. NDELA is easily absorbed through human skin (Edwards *et al.*, 1979), but human exposure from this source is difficult to quantifiy.

Preventive measures could include the elimination of nitrosating agents as inhibitors of bacterial growth, blocking of nitrosamine formation by inhibitors (e.g., α-tocopherol) and elimination of easily-nitrosatable amines or the use of 'safe' amines (e.g., amines that yield non-carcinogenic or weakly carcinogenic N-nitroso compounds) (Spiegelhalder et al., 1982; Keefer & Hansen, 1982).

Indoor air: While available results indicate that airborne nitrosamines are not a general problem in outdoor atmospheres, the situation might be different for indoor air, where break-down of nitrosamines by ultra-violet photolysis is eliminated. Brunnenmann and Hoffmann (1978) found concentrations of NDMA in the range of 0.01–0.13 µg/L in highly smoke-polluted indoor environments, attributable largely to side-stream smoke, leading to exposures of 5–200 µg/h. Further systematic studies of side-stream smoke are necessary in order to reach an estimation of nitrosamine exposures in passive smoking. Nitrosamines have occasionally been found in low concentrations in kitchens (Sen et al., 1976) and in the air inside new automobiles (Rounbehler et al., 1980).

Drugs and pesticides: Both of these classes of products may contain nitrosatable amino groups and can therefore be contaminated with nitrosamines. We have found NDMA in amounts varying from 1–370 µg/kg in the easily-nitrosatable analgesic drug, aminopyrine (Eisenbrand et al., 1979), which was subsequently taken off the market. Low amounts of nitrosamines have also been found in other drugs (Krull et al., 1979).

Nitrosamine impurities and contamination in pesticides have been throughly investigated (Cohen & Bachman, 1978; Bontoyan et al., 1979) and, in general, have been largely eliminated or substantially reduced by the prevention of nitrosation reactions or the destruction of nitrosamine impurities (Probst, 1981).

Household commodities: Dishwashing liquids and surface cleaners formulated with laurylamine oxides were found to be contaminated with N-nitrosomethyldodecylamine (112–661 µg/kg) and N-nitrosomethyltetradecylamine (46–151 µg/kg) (Morrison & Hecht 1982). Rubber materials and manufactured rubber products have been shown to contain volatile nitrosamines (Ireland et al., 1980). Of particular concern are rubber nipples for babies' bottles (Preussmann et al., 1981; Havery & Fazio, 1982): all samples analysed were contaminated with various volatile nitrosamines at concentrations of 1–280 µg/kg. Nitrosamines from this source can migrate into milk or saliva. Reduction of the amount of chemical amine accelerators and stabilizers, used as precursors during vulcanization, have significantly reduced the nitrosamine contamination.

OCCUPATIONAL EXPOSURE

The largest known human exposures to exogenous N-nitrosamines occur in the work place. Several occupational settings have been shown to involve high exposure; the most important are listed in Figure 1. The best data available concern the rubber and tyre industry (Fajen et al., 1979; McGlothlin et al., 1981; Preussmann et al., 1981; Spiegelhalder & Preussmann, 1983), where airborne nitrosamines are formed from nitrosating agents used (N-nitrosodiphenylamine, NDPhA), nitrogen oxides from indoor combustion processes and from amine precursors used as accelerators and stabilizers for vulcanization. From our own data, a daily exposure of between 15 and 150 µg nitrosamines (NDMA and NMOR) can be estimated for workers in the rubber industry.

Elimination of NDPhA, reduction of airborne nitrogen oxide levels and the use of smaller amounts of amine accelerators, as well as their substitution by non-nitrosatable chemicals, lead to a considerable reduction of nitrosamine concentrations in air, often by as much as two orders of magnitude. In principle, similar reductions can also be achieved in other areas of occupational exposure by partial or total elimination of precursors. The paper of Dr. Spiegelhalder in these proceedings (see p.) gives more details concerning occupational nitrosamine exposure, possibilities for biological monitoring (especially for exposure to NDELA in machine shops using cutting fluids) and possibilities for associating nitrosamine exposure with certain occupational cancers. However, it is very likely that all areas of potential occupational exposure to nitrosamines have not yet been identified, and systematic pilot studies should be carried out wherever amines and nitrosating agents are used together.

ENDOGENOUS NITROSAMINE FORMATION FROM PRECURSORS

Intensive experimental investigations have established clearly that N-nitroso compounds can be formed *in vivo* by reaction of nitrosatable amines or amides and nitrosating agents, especially nitrite, particularly in the acid pH of the stomach. Evidence for endogenous formation from precursors which, *per se,* are not carcinogenic, has been obtained by means of several experimental approaches:
- combined administration of nitrosatable amino compounds with nitrite (induces tumours of the same type and at the same site as does the corresponding nitrosamine),
- determinations of DNA alkylation patterns (similar alkylation patterns are obtained with preformed nitrosamines),
- determination of acute toxic effects (found to be similar),
- analytical determination of nitrosamines formed *in vivo,*
- formation *in vitro* under simulated stomach conditions (pH, temperature), often using human gastric juice.

In such model experiments, high or very high doses of amines and (particularly) nitrite have always been used. Such experiments, therefore, demonstrate only the possibility of in-vivo formation of nitroso compounds. However, such conditions are quite unrealistic when compared with human exposure under normal conditions. Nitrite concentrations used in combined feeding studies are usually one to two orders of magnitude higher than the average concentration of nitrite in human saliva. However, there can be no doubt that nitrosation can also occur in humans, as has been shown by the nitrosation of proline at high nitrate exposure (Ohshima & Bartsch, 1981), as well as by subjects on a low-nitrate diet (Wagner *et al.,* 1982). We have recently shown that amidopyrine nitrosation in humans forms NDMA which was detected by monitoring its excretion in urine (Spiegelhalder *et al.,* p.). In-vivo formation of nitrosamines from inhaled nitrogen oxides has also been investigated (Iqbal *et al.,* 1980; Mirvish, 1982).

Quantification of endogenous nitrosation is almost impossible at present, in view of the many complex factors involved, especially the chemistry of nitrosation, the effects of catalysts and inhibitors and, above all, our present inability to identify important amine precursors relevant to nitrosation in humans. However, the NPRO method of Ohshima and Bartsch (1981) has recently been employed to predict the carcinogenic effects of endogenous nitrosation, using a dose-response study of endogenous N-nitrosoproline formation in rats and a deduced kinetic model (Ohshima *et al.,* 1983).

Nitrate and nitrite as precursors

Nitrite is a normal constituent of human saliva, where its concentration depends largely on the nitrate intake in food and water (Spiegelhalder *et al.,* 1976; Tannenbaum *et al.,* 1976). Dietary nitrate, after absorption from the gut, is rapidly distributed in the body *via* the blood stream and re-excreted into the oral cavity *via* the salivary glands. The oral microflora reduce nitrate to nitrite, about 5% of an ingested dose of nitrate being converted to nitrite in 24 h (Spiegelhalder *et al.*, 1976; Stephany & Schuller, 1980). The most important source of human nitrate intake is vegetable (Table 6), followed by drinking-water. From data on food consumption from several countries (The Netherlands, Sweden, USA and FRG), a mean daily intake of 90 mg nitrate and about 4 mg nitrite can be estimated with very large variations, depending mainly upon individual consumption habits.

Extensive compilations are available concerning nitrate concentrations in human food (Selenka & Brand-Grimm, 1976; National Research Council, 1981). Table 7 gives a list of those vegetables that have particularly high average nitrate contents. In such nitrate-accumulating plants, however, concentrations up to 10 000 mg/kg have been reported, usually as a consequence of excessive use of nitrogen fertilizers.

In order to eliminate such extremely high nitrate burdens, The Netherlands and Switzerland have recently enforced regulations forbidding the sale of vegetables with nitrate concentrations above 4 000 mg/kg. This first step in the right direction should be followed by other countries, and the limit might possibly be set at 2 000 mg/kg. A recent workshop in Bad Honnef, Federal Republic of Germany, clearly indicated that such upper limits can be respected, even in nitrate-accumulating plants, using adequate fertilization schemes.

Table 6.   Average nitrate and nitrite intake from food in the Federal Republic of Germany (Selenka & Brand-Grimm, 1979)

Product	Nitrate		Nitrite	
	(mg/day)	(%)	(mg/day)	(%)
Vegetables	35.7	72.4	0.3	16.9
Meat and meat products	9.1	18.5	0.9	54.6
Bread and similar products	2.7	5.5	0.5	27.3
Fruits	1.5	2.9	–	–
Cheese	0.3	0.7	0.02	1.2

Table 7.   Average concentration of nitrate in some nitrate-accumulating and other vegetables in the 1970s (National Research Council, 1981)

Vegetable	Nitrate concentra-tion (mg/kg)
Beet	2 300
Celery	2 300
Endive	1 300
Lettuce	2 800
Radish	2 100
Spinach	1 900
Cabbage	420
Cucumber	180
Potato	120
Tomato	60

Nitrogen oxides as precursors

The inhalation of nitrogen oxides (NO and NO_2) with air might lead to substantial exposure to these nitrosating agents and be responsible for 'enhanced' nitrate excretion in urine (Witter *et al.*, 1979). It might also give rise to endogenous nitrosation (Mirvish, 1982).

Natural background concentrations of NO_2 are usually in the range of $0.4–10\ \mu g/m^3$. Urban areas typically show $20–90\ \mu g/m^3$, with highest monthly means of $60–110$, highest daily means of $130–400$ and highest hourly means of $240–850\ \mu g/m^3$ (WHO, 1977). Exposure from indoor sources, such as domestic gas-fired appliances, may be considerable, and levels of up to $2\ 000$ $\mu g\ NO_2/m^3$ have been measured. Tobacco smoke has been reported to contain $100–135$ mg NO and $150–225$ mg NO_2/m^3, with considerable fluctuation, depending on the conditions of combustion (WHO, 1972). The National Research Council (1981) has estimated that 0.5 mg NO per cigarette is an average exposure for smokers.

Nitrosatable amino compounds as precursors

Among the diverse groups of amino compounds, secondary amines and alkyl amides react readily with nitrosating agents to form *N*-nitroso compounds, while primary, tertiary and quaternary amines react slowly, according to more complex nitrosation mechanisms. The well-known fast reactions of weakly-basic amines and the slow reactions of strongly-basic amines should always be kept in mind.

Although there are many scattered reports concerning the occurrence of amine precursors in the human environment, no systematic study, using reliable analytical techniques, is available to enable estimation of the exposure of humans to these compounds. Even more important, we do not know the chemical structures of the amine precursors potentially relevant to endogenous nitrosation in humans.

A short summary of present knowledge is given in a review by the National Research Council (1981), which lists foods (see also Maja, 1978), drugs, cosmetics, agricultural chemicals (including pesticides) and tobacco as major sources of amine precursors. It also mentions the endogenous production of secondary amines; e.g., from bacterial decomposition of amino acids.

One can certainly agree with the conclusion of the above review, that 'sufficient quantities of amines are present in humans to participate in nitrosation reactions under appropriate conditions'. However, this is clearly not sufficient for satisfactory risk evaluation.

Unfortunately, as well, there are almost no studies available concerning the nitrosation of peptides, their chemistry and their carcinogenic potential. This is particularly regrettable, since Challis *et al.* (1982) have postulated that the nitrosation of peptide bonds can occur under conditions prevailing in the stomach and that such structures might play a role in human gastric cancer.

FUTURE RESEARCH

I consider that the following areas deserve intensive research efforts in the near future:
(1) development of 'simple', sensitive and specific analytical methods for non-volatile *N*-nitroso compounds (including unstable nitrosamides) and their application to different environmental media; evaluation of the toxicological relevance of the foregoing compounds;
(2) elucidation of the role of nitrosamines in tobacco- and tobacco smoke-related cancer;
(3) systematic studies on occupational exposure to nitrosamines to obtain an adequate data base for further epidemiological studies; further identification of potential high-risk groups;

(4) systematic studies to evaluate the potential of urinary metabolites of nitrosamines for the biological monitoring of exposure (e.g., TSNA);

(5) identification of relevant amine precursors in endogenous nitrosation (to allow quantification of this risk factor) and clarification of the role of high nitrate exposures;

(6) investigations of nitrosated peptides and evaluation of their carcinogenic potential.

REFERENCES

Bartsch, H., O'Neill, I.K., Castegnaro, M., Okada, M., eds (1982) *N-Nitroso Compounds: Occurrence and Biological Effects (IARC Scientific Publications No. 41)*, Lyon, International Agency for Research on Cancer

Bontoyan, W.R., Law, M.W. & Wright, D.P. (1979) Nitrosamines in agricultural and home-use pesticides. *J. Agric. Food. Chem., 27,* 631–634

Brunnenmann, K.D. & Hoffmann, D. (1978) *Chemical studies on tobacco smoke. LIX, Analysis of volatile nitrosamines in tobacco smoke and polluted indoor environments*. In: Walker, E.A., Castegnaro, M., Griciute, L., Lyle, R.E., eds, *Environmental Aspects of* N-*nitroso Compounds (IARC Scientific Publications No. 19)*, Lyon, International Agency for Research on Cancer, pp. 343–356

Challis, B.C., Lomas, S.J., Rzepa, H.S., Bavin, P.M.G., Darkin, D.W., Viney, N.J. & Moore, P.J. (1982) *A kinetic model for the formation of gastric* N-*nitroso compounds*. In: Magee, P.N., ed., *Nitrosamines and Humans Cancer, (Banbury Report No. 12)*, Cold Spring Harbor, NY Cold Spring Harbor Laboratory, pp. 243–256

Cohen, J.B. & Bachman, J.D. (1978) *Measurement of environmental nitrosamines*. In: Walker, E.A., Castegnaro, M., Griciute, L., Lyle, R.E., eds, *Environmental Aspects of* N-*nitroso Compounds (IARC Scientific Publications No. 19)*, Lyon, International Agency for Research on Cancer, pp. 357–372

Druckrey, H. & Preussmann, R. (1962) Zur Entstehung carcinogener Nitrosamine am Beispiel des Tabakrauches. *Naturwissenschaften, 49,* 498

Druckrey, H., Steinhoff, D., Beuthner, H. & Klärner, P. (1963) Prüfung von Nitrit auf chronisch toxische Wirkung an Ratten. *Arzneimittel-Forsch., 13,* 320–323

Edwards, G.S., Peng, M., Fine, D.J., Spiegelhalder, B. & Kann, J. (1979) Detection of *N*-nitrosodiethanolamine in human urine following application of contaminated cosmetics. *Toxicol. Lett., 4,* 217–222

Eisenbrand, G. (1981) *N-Nitrosoverbindungen in Nahrung und Umwelt*. Wiss. Verlagsgesellschaft Stuttgart, Federal Republic of Germany

Eisenbrand, G., Spiegelhalder, B., Kann, J., Klein, R. & Preussmann, R. (1979) Carcinogenic *N*-nitrosodimethylamine as a contamination in drugs containing 4-dimethylamino-2,3-dimethyl-1-phenyl-3-pyrazolin-5-on (amidopyrine, aminophenazone). *Arzneimittel-Forsch., 19,* 867–868

Ellen, G. & Schuller, P.N. (1983) *N-Nitrosamine investigations in the Netherlands: Highlights from the last 10 years*. In: Preussmann, R., ed., *Das Nitrosamine-Problem*, Weinheim, Verlag Chemie, pp. 81–92

Ender, F., Havre, G., Helgebostad, A., Koppang, N., Madsen, R. & Ceh, L. (1969) Isolation and identification of a hepatoxic factor in herring meal produced from sodium nitrite preserved herring. *Naturwissenschaften, 51,* 637–638

Fajen, J.M., Carson, G.A., Rounbehler, D.P., Fan, T.Y., Vita, R., Goff, U. Wolf, M.H., Edwards, G.S., Fine, D.H., Reinhold, V. & Viemann, K. (1979) *N*-Nitrosamines in the rubber and tire industry. *Science, 205,* 1262–1264

Fan, T.Y., Goff, U., Song, L., Fine, D.H., Arsenault, P. & Bieman, K. (1977) *N*-Nitrosodiethanolamine in cosmetics, lotions and shampoos. *Food Cosmet. Toxicol., 15,* 423–430

Fine, D.H. & Rounbehler, D.P. (1975) Trace analysis of volatile *N*-nitroso compounds by combined gas chromatography and thermal energy analysis. *J. Chromatogr., 109,* 271–279

Fromberger, R. & Allmann, H. (1983) *Ergebnisse der Lebensmittelüberwachung in der Bundesrepublik Deutschland*. In: Preussmann, R., ed., *Das Nitrosamine-Problem*, Weinheim, Verlag Chemie, pp. 57–63

Gough, T.A., Webb, K.S. & Coleman, R.F. (1978) Estimate of the volatile nitrosamine content of UK food. *Nature, 272,* 161–163

Hartman, P.E. (1982) *Nitrates and nitrites: Ingestion, pharmacodynamics and toxicology*. In: de Serres, F.J. & Hollaender, A., eds, *Chemical Mutagens*, Vol. 7, New York, Plenum Press, pp. 211–294

Havery, D.S. & Fazio, T. (1982) Estimation of volatile N-nitrosamines in rubber nipples for babies bottles. *Food Chem. Toxicol., 20*, 939–944

Havery, D.C., Fazio, T. & Howard, J.W. (1978) Trends in levels of n-nitrosopyrrolidine in fried bacon. *J. Assoc. off. anal. Chem., 61*, 1379–1382

Havery, D.C., Hotchkiss, J.H. & Fazio, T. (1981) Nitrosamines in malt and malt beverages. *J. Food Sci., 46*, 501–505

Hecht, S.S., Morrison, J.B. & Wenninger, J.A. (1982) N-nitroso-N-methyldodecylamine and N-nitroso-N-methyltetradecylamine in hair-care products. *Food Chem. Toxicol., 20*, 165–170

Hecht, S.S., Castonguay, A., Rivenson, A., Mu, B. & Hoffmann, D. (1983) Tobacco specific nitrosamines: Carcinogenicity, metabolism and possible role in human cancer. *J. environm. Sci. Health, C1*, 1–54

Hoffmann, D., Adams, J.D., Brunnenmann, K.D. & Hecht, S.S. (1982a) *Formation, occurrence and carcinogenicity of N-nitrosamines in tobacco products.* In: Scanlan, R.A. & Tannenbaum, S.R. eds, N-*Nitroso compounds, (ACS Ser., No. 174)* American Chemical Society, Washington DC, pp. 247–273

Hoffmann, D., Brunnemann, K.D., Adams, J.D., Rivenson, A. & Hecht, S.S. (1982b) N-*Nitrosamines in tobacco carcinogenesis.* In: Magee, P.N., ed., *Nitrosamines and Human Cancer (Banbury Report No. 12),* Cold Spring Harbor, NY, Cold Spring Harbor Laboratory, pp. 211–226

IARC (1978) *IARC Monographs on the Evaluation of the Carcinogenic Risk of Chemicals to Humans,* Vol. 17, *Some N-Nitroso Compounds,* Lyon, France

Iqbal, Z.M., Dahm, K. & Epstein, S.S. (1980) Role of nitrogen dioxide in the biosynthesis of nitrosamines in mice. *Science, 207*, 1475–1477

Ireland, C.B., Hytrek, F.P. & Lasoski, B.A. (1980) Aqueous extraction of N-nitrosamines from elastomers. *Am. ind. Hyg. Assoc. J., 41*, 895–900

Keefer, L. & Hansen, T.J. (1982) *Primary amine use and other strategies for preventing human exposure to N-nitroso compounds: application to cutting fluids.* In: Bartsch, H., O'Neill, I.K., Castegnaro, M. & Okada, M., eds, N-*Nitroso Compounds: Occurrence and Biological Effects (IARC Scientific Publications No. 41),* Lyon, International Agency for Research on Cancer, pp. 245–258

Klein, D., Girard, A.M., DeSmedt, J., Fellion, Y. & Derby, G. (1982) Analyse de la nitrosodiethanolamine dans les produits de l'industrie cosmetique. *Food Cosmet. Toxicol., 19*, 233–235

Krull, I.S., Goff, U., Silvergleid, A. & Fine, D. (1980) N-Nitroso compound contamination in prescription and non-prescription drugs. *Arzneimittel Forsch., 29*, 870–874

Maja, J.A. (1978) Amines in food. *Crit. Rev. Food Sci. Nutr., 10*, 373–403

Maki, T., Tamura, Y., Shimamura, Y. & Navi, Y. (1980) Estimate of volatile nitrosamines in Japanese food. *Bull. environ. Contam. Toxicol., 25*, 257–261

McGlothlin, J.D., Wilcox, T.C., Fajen, J.M. & Edwards, G.S. (1981) *A health hazard evaluation of nitrosamines in a tire manufacturing plant.* In: American Chemical Society, *(ACS Symp. Ser. No. 149),* Washington, D.C., pp. 283–299

Mirvish, S.S. (1982) In-vivo *formation of N-nitroso compounds. Formation from nitrite and nitrogen dioxide, and relation to gastric cancer.* In: Magee, P.N., ed., *Nitrosamines and Human Cancer. (Banbury Report No. 12),* Cold Spring Harbor, Cold Spring Harbor Laboratory, NY, pp. 227–236

Morrison, J.B. & Hecht, S.S. (1982) N-nitrosomethyldodecylamine and N-nitroso-N-methyltetradecylamine in household dishwashing liquids. *Food Chem. Toxicol., 21*, 69–73

National Research Council (1981) *The Health Effects of Nitrate, Nitrite and N-Nitroso Compounds,* Part 1, Washington DC, National Academy Press

Ohshima, H. & Bartsch, H. (1981) Quantitative estimation of endogenous nitrosation in humans be monitoring N-nitrosoproline excreted in urine. *Cancer Res., 41*, 3658–3662

Ohshima, H., Mahon, G.A.T., Wahrendorf, J. & Bartsch, H. (1983) A dose-response study of N-nitrosoproline formation in rats and a deduced kinetic model for predicting carcinogenic effects caused by endogenous nitrosation. *Cancer Res. 43*, 5072–5076

Preussmann, R. (1984) Carcinogenic N-nitroso compounds and their environmental significance. *Naturwissenschaften, 71*, 25–30

Preussmann, R. & Eisenbrand, G. (1984) N-*Nitroso carcinogens in the environment.* In: Searle, C.E., ed., *Chemical Carcinogens,* 2nd ed., *(ACS Monograph Ser. no. 173)* Washington DC (in press)

Preussmann, R. & Stewart, B.W. (1984) N-*Nitroso carcinogens.* In: Searle, C.E., ed., *Chemical Carcinogens,* 2nd ed., *(ACS Monograph Ser. No. 173),* Washington DC (in press)

Preussmann, R., Eisenbrand, G. & Spiegelhalder, B. (1979) *Occurrence and formation of* N-*nitroso compounds in the environment and* in vivo. In: Emmelot, P. & Krieg, E., eds, *Environmental Carcinogenesis*, Amsterdam, Elsevier/North Holland, pp. 51–72

Preussmann, R., Spiegelhalder, B. & Eisenbrand, G. (1981) *Reduction of human exposure to environmental* N-*nitroso compounds*. In: Scanlan, R.A. & Tannenbaum, S.R., eds, *N-Nitroso Compounds (ACS Symp. Ser. No. 174)*, Washington, DC, American Chemical Society, pp. 217–228

Preussmann, R., I.K. O'Neill, G. Eisenbrand, B. Spiegelhalder, H. Bartsch, eds (1983) *Environmental Carcinogens: Selected Methods of Analysis*, Vol. 6, N-*Nitroso Compounds*, Lyon, International Agency for Research on Cancer

Probst, G.W. (1981) *Reduction of nitrosamine inpurities in pesticide fomulation*. In: Scanlan, R.A. & Tannenbaum, S.R., eds, N-*Nitroso Compounds (ACS Symp. Ser., No. 174)* Washington DC, American Chemical Society, pp. 363–382

Rounbehler, D.P., Reisch, J. & Fine, D.H. (1980) Nitrosamines in new motor-cars. *Food Cosmet. Toxicol., 18*, 147–151

Sakshaug, J., Sognen, E., Hansen, M.A. & Koppang, N. (1965) Dimethylnitrosamine: Its hepatotoxic effect in sheep and its occurrence in toxic batches of herring meal, *Nature, 206*, 1261–1262

Sander, J. (1967) Kann Nitrit in der menschlichen Nahrung Ursache einer Krebsentstehung durch Nitrosamine sein? *Arch. Hyg. Bakteriol., 151*, 22–28

Scanlan, R.A. & Tannenbaum, S.R., eds (1981) N-*Nitroso Compounds (ACS Symp. Ser. No. 174)*, Washington DC, American Chemical Society

Selenka, F. & Brand-Grimm, D. (1978) Nitrate and nitrite in human food. Calculation of daily intake and its range. *Zentralbl. Bakteriol. hyg. Abt. I (Orig. B), 161*, 1–20

Sen, N.P., Seaman, S. & Miles, W.F. (1976) Dimethylnitrosamine and nitrosopyrrolidine in fumes produced during the frying of bacon. *Food Cosmet. Toxicol., 14*, 167–170

Sen, N.P., Seaman, S. & Tessier, L. (1982) Comparison of two analytical methods for determination of dimethylnitrosamine in beer and ale, and some recent results. *J. Food Saf., 4*, 243–250

Spiegelhalder, B. & Preussmann, R. (1982) *Nitrosamines in rubber*. In: Bartsch, H., O'Neill, I.K., Castegnaro, M. & Okada, M., eds, N-*Nitroso Compounds: Occurrence and Biological Effects (IARC Scientific Publications No. 41)*, Lyon, International Agency for Research on Cancer, pp. 231–244

Spiegelhalder, B. & Preussmann, R. (1983) Occupational nitrosamine exposure. I. Rubber and tire industry. *Carcinogenesis, 4*, 1147–1152

Spiegelhalder, B., Eisenbrand, G. & Preussmann, R. (1976) Influence of dietary nitrate on nitrite content of human saliva: Possible relevance to in-vivo formation of N-nitroso compounds. *Food Cosmet. Toxicol., 14*, 545–548

Spiegelhalder, B., Eisenbrand, G. & Preussmann, R. (1978) Contamination of amines with N-nitrosamines. *Angew. Chem., Int. Ed., 17*, 367–368

Spiegelhalder, B., Eisenbrand, G. & Preussmann, R. (1980) Volatile nitrosamines in food. *Oncology, 37*, 211–216

Stephany, R.W. & Schuller, D.G. (1980) Daily dietary intakes of nitrite, nitrate and volatile N-nitrosamines in The Netherlands using the duplicate sampling technique. *Oncology, 37*, 203–210

Tannenbaum, S.R., Weisman, M. & Fett, D. (1976) The effect of nitrate intake on nitrite formation in human saliva. *Food Cosmet. Toxicol., 14*, 549–552

Wagner, D.A., Shuker, D.E., Hasic, G. & Tannenbaum, S.R. (1982) *Endogenous nitrosoproline synthesis in humans*. In: Magee, P.N., ed., *Nitrosamines and Human Cancer (Banbury Report No. 12)* Cold Spring Harbor, NY, Cold Spring Harbor Laboratory, pp. 319–344

Walker, E.A., Castegnaro, M., Griciute, L., Lyle, R.E., eds (1978) *Environmental Aspects of* N-*Nitroso Compounds (IARC Scientific Publications No. 19)*, Lyon, International Agency for Research on Cancer

Walker, E.A., Gricute, L., Castegnaro, M. & Börzsönyi, M., eds (1980) N-*Nitroso Compounds: Analysis, Formation and Occurrence (IARC Scientific Publications No. 31)*, Lyon, International Agency for Research on Cancer

Witter, J.P., Gatley, S.J. & Balish, E. (1979) Distribution of nitrogen-14 from labelled nitrate ($^{13}NO_3$) in humans and rats. *Science, 205*, 1335–1337

WHO (1977) *Environmental Health Criteria, 4,Oxides of Nitrogen*, Geneva

PRESENCE OF 1-METHYL-1,2,3,4-TETRAHYDRO-β-CARBOLINE-3-CARBOXYLIC ACIDS AND TYRAMINE AS PRECURSORS OF MUTAGENS IN SOYA SAUCE AFTER NITRITE TREATMENT

K. WAKABAYASHI, M. NAGAO, M. OCHIAI, M. TSUDA, Z. YAMAIZUMI, H. SAITÔ & T. SUGIMURA

National Cancer Center Research Institute, 1–1, Tsukiji 5 chome, Chuo-ku, Tokyo 104, Japan

SUMMARY

Soya sauce showed marked direct-acting mutagenicity toward *Salmonella typhimurium* TA100 after nitrite treatment. Three precursors showing mutagenicity after nitrite treatment were isolated from soya sauce. Their structures were determined to be (–)-(1S,3S)-1-methyl-1,2,3,4-tetrahydro-β-carboline-3-carboxylic acid [(–)-(1S,3S)-MTCA], its stereoisomer (–)-(1R,3S)-MTCA and tyramine. The numbers of revertants of TA100 induced by 1 mg each of (–)-(1S,3S)-MTCA, (–)-(1R,3S)-MTCA and tyramine, after nitrite treatment, were 17 400, 13 000 and 3 900, respectively, without $S9$ mix. The amounts of MTCA isomers and tyramine in various Japanese soya sauces showing mutagenicity after nitrite treatment were 82–678 and 17–2 250 µg/mL, respectively. Most soya sauces produced in the USA showed weaker mutagenicity than those produced in Japan and contained lower, if not undetectable, amounts of the three precursors of mutagens. The mutagenicity of MTCA isomers and tyramine accounted for 16–61 and 1–35%, respectively, of the mutagenicity of the soya sauces after nitrite treatment. The mutagen(s) produced from (–)-(1S,3S)-MTCA with nitrite was a minor product(s), the major product being the non-mutagen, (–)-(1S,3S)-1-methyl-2-nitroso-1,2,3,4-tetrahydro-β-carboline-3-carboxylic acid [(–)-(1S,3S)-MNTCA], but the mutagen 4-(2-aminoethyl)-6-diazo-2,4-cyclohexadienone, produced from tyramine with nitrite, was one of the major products.

INTRODUCTION

Epidemiological studies have indicated a correlation of gastric cancer with nitrate ingestion (Hartman, 1983). Carcinogenic N-nitroso compounds are formed when nitrite and secondary amines are given to experimental animals (Sander & Bürkle, 1969). Direct-acting N-nitroso compounds, such as N-nitroso-N-methyl-N'-nitroguanidine (Sugimura & Fujimura, 1967) and N-nitroso-N-methyl-N'-acetylurea (Druckrey *et al.*, 1970), are known to induce cancer in the glandular stomach of rodents. Direct-acting mutagenic N-nitroso compounds produced by the nitrosation reaction in the acidic conditions of the stomach are therefore suspected to be causes of human gastric cancer.

Gastric cancer is a major form of cancer in Japan (Hirayama, 1979). Both mortality from gastric cancer and nitrate ingestion *per caput* are much higher in Japan than in Europe or the USA (Hartman, 1983). These findings suggest that some nitrosatable precursors of mutagen-carcinogens present in Japanese foods are associated with the development of human gastric cancer. Japanese fish show direct-acting mutagenicity after nitrite treatment and induce tumours of the glandular stomach in rats when given by gavage (Weisburger *et al.,* 1980). Piacek-Llanes and Tannenbaum (1982) reported that nitrite-treated fava beans yielded a direct-acting mutagen. However, the structures of the mutagens (or their precursors) produced by nitrite treatment of Japanese fish and fava beans have not been elucidated.

Recently, we found that soya sauce, bean paste and fish sauce were mutagenic toward *Salmonella typhimurium* TA100, without S9 mix after nitrite treatment (Wakabayashi *et al.,* 1983). Of these foods, soya sauce showed the highest mutagenicity. This paper reports the isolation of three precursors of mutagens from Japanese soya sauce, as well as their identification and quantification. The mutagens produced from these precursors and nitrite are discussed.

MATERIAL AND METHODS

Materials

Soya sauces were purchased at markets in Tokyo, Japan (A–G, Table 1), Honolulu, Hawaii (I–K) and Madison, WI, USA (H, L and M).

Mutation assay

The preincubation method was adopted for the mutation test (Sugimura & Nagao, 1980). Revertants induced by the sample without nitrite treatment were subtracted from those induced by the sample with nitrite treatment, and the result was taken to be the mutagenic activity of the nitrite-treated sample.

Nitrite treatment

Soya sauce: A mixture of 1 mL each of soya sauce and 0.1 mol/L sodium nitrite was adjusted to pH 3.0 with 6N hydrochloric acid and incubated in the dark for 1 h at 37 °C. The nitrosating reaction was quenched by addition of 1 mL of 0.1 mol/L ammonium sulfamate. The mixture was then sterilized by passage through a Millex-HA filter (0.45 µm) and tested for mutagenicity.

Products of various stages of isolation: Samples were taken at each step of purification and diluted to 1 mL with water. To this solution, 0.6 mL of 80 mmol/L citrate-phosphate buffer (pH 3.0) and 0.2 mL of 0.5 mol/L sodium nitrite were added. When necessary, 6N hydrochloric acid were added to the mixture to adjust the pH to 3.0. To decompose excess nitrite in the incubation mixture, 0.2 mL of 0.5 mol/L ammonium sulfamate was added. The incubation conditions were the same as for soya sauce.

Authentic compounds: (–)-(1S,3S)- and (–)-(1R,3S)-1-methyl-1,2,3,4-tetrahydro-β-carboline-3-carboxylic acids (MTCAs) were synthesized by the method of Brossi *et al.* (1973). Tyramine hydrochloride was obtained from Sigma Chemical Co. (St. Louis, MO, USA). Samples of 2 mg each of (–)-(1S,3S)-MTCA and (–)-(1R,3S)-MTCA and of 4 mg tyramine hydrochloride were dissolved in 1 mL water and treated with nitrite at pH 3.0, as described above. To separate the mutagen formed from tyramine and nitrite, 5 mmol/L tyramine hydrochloride were incubated with 50 mmol/L sodium nitrite in 500 mmol/L hydrochloric acid-potassium chloride buffer (pH 1.0) for 1 h in the dark. The nitrosating reaction was stopped by adding $\frac{1}{10}$ volume of 0.5 mol/L ammonium sulfamate.

Isolation of precursors of mutagens

A sample of 80 mL of soya sauce was diluted 17-fold with water and loaded onto a charcoal column (4.0 × 16 cm). The column was washed with 2 L water, then eluted with 2 L methanol, followed by 2 L 80% methanol containing 1N acetic acid, then 2 L of methanol. These three eluates, which contained 71% of the mutagenic activity of the nitrite-treated soya sauce, were combined and evaporated. The residue (3 364 mg) was dissolved in 90 mL water and applied to an Amberlite XAD-7 column (4.0 × 19.3 cm). The column was washed with 1.25 L water, with 1.25 L methanol. The water and methanol eluates contained 14 and 31%, respectively, of the mutagenic activity of the original nitrite-treated material.

The methanol fraction was evaporated and the residue (266 mg) was separated, in portions, by high-performance liquid chromatography (HPLC) on an LS-110 styrene column (21.5 × 600 mm, Toyo Soda, Tokyo) and then on an LS-410 octadecyl silyl column (21.5 × 300 mm, Toyo Soda). The columns were washed with 50% methanol and 20% methanol, respectively, at a flow rate of 6 mL/min. Eluted material was monitored at 270 nm. Two active fractions were obtained from the LS-410 column in the elution volumes, 450–480 mL and 540–576 mL, respectively. These two fractions were evaporated, and the residues were each found to contain a single component – compound I and compound II, respectively. Compounds I and II were subjected to structural and biological characterization. From 80 mL of soya sauce, 19.4 and 4.2 mg of compounds I and II, respectively, were obtained.

The precursor present in the water effluent from the XAD-7 column was isolated as follows. The evaporated residue (2 540 mg) was dissolved in 10 mL water, and half of the solution was applied to a CM-Sephadex C-25 (Na$^+$ form) column (1.5 × 18.4 cm). The column was washed successively with 163 mL each of water, 0.1N acetic acid and water, then with 326 mL of 0.1N ammonium hydroxide. Most of the mutagenic activity was recovered in the eluate with 0.1N ammonium hydroxide. The ammonium hydroxide fraction was evaporated, and the residue (176.5 mg) was dissolved in 2 mL of water and loaded onto a Sephadex G-10 column (1.5 × 30.0 cm). The column was eluted successively with 260 mL of water and 210 mL of 30 mmol/L sodium chloride. Mutagenic activity was found in the sodium chloride eluate in the 23.4–55.8 mL elution volume. The active fractions were desalted by passage through a charcoal column (1.0 × 11 cm), onto which the active component was adsorbed. The column was washed with 100 mL water, then successively with 100 mL each of methanol, 80% methanol containing 1N acetic acid and methanol. The last three eluates were combined and evaporated, and the residue (47.5 mg) was further separated by HPLC. The HPLC conditions were as follows: column, LS-410 (21.5 × 300 mm); flow rate, 6 mL/min; eluant, 20% methanol containing 0.05% acetic acid; detection, 273 nm. Compound III was isolated in the 102–120 mL elution volume, its yield from 80 mL of soya sauce being 47.4 mg.

Spectral measurements

^{1}H-Nuclear magnetic resonance spectra were measured in a Bruker CSP-300 apparatus. Mass spectra were obtained with a JEOL 01SG-2 apparatus, and ultra-violet spectra with a Hitachi 320 spectrophotometer. Optical rotations were determined with a JASCO DIP-181 digital polarimeter.

Quantification of precursors of mutagens in various kinds of soya sauce

(–)-(1S,3S)- and (–)-(1R,3S)-MTCA: A sample of 50 μL soya sauce was applied to a thin-layer, silica gel, 60 F$_{254}$ plate (5 × 10 cm, Merck). The plate was developed with chloroform : methanol (2 : 8, v/v), and the region of R$_f$: 0.25–0.75 was scraped off and extracted three times with 5 mL ethyl acetate : methanol (1 : 1, v/v). The pooled extracts were evaporated to dryness. The residue was dissolved in 1.5 mL 20% methanol and passed through

a Millipore FH filter (0.50 μm) to remove insoluble material. The filtrate was evaporated, and the residue was dissolved in 200 μL 20% methanol and analysed by HPLC, with 20% methanol as eluant. The HPLC conditions were as follows: column, LS-410 (4 × 300 mm); flow rate, 1 mL/min; detection, 270 nm. The recoveries of (–)-(1*S*,3*S*)- and (–)-(1*R*,3*S*)-MTCA, added to soya sauce, were 97% and 83%, respectively.

Tyramine: A sample of 100 μL soya sauce was diluted 100-fold with water and applied to a CM-Sephadex C-25 (Na$^+$ form) column (1.0 × 2.0 cm). The column was washed with 20 mL water, then material was eluted with 20 mL of 0.5N ammonium hydroxide. The eluate was evaporated to dryness, and the residue was dissolved in 200 μL 1.5N acetic acid and analysed by HPLC, with 5% methanol containing 0.05% acetic acid as eluate. The conditions of HPLC were the same as for the quantification of MTCA isomers. The recovery of tyramine added to soya sauce was 91.2%.

Isolation of mutagens formed from (–)-(1S,3S)-MTCA and tyramine by nitrite treatment

A sample of 2 mg synthetic (–)-(1*S*,3*S*)-MTCA was treated with nitrite at pH 3.0, and the reaction mixture was extracted twice with 2 mL ethyl acetate. The ethyl acetate layers were combined and evaporated, and the residue was dissolved in methanol. This methanol solution was subjected to HPLC on an LS-310 silica gel column (21.5 × 300 mm, Toyo Soda), using methanol at a flow rate of 6 mL/min. The eluate was monitored at 270 nm, and an aliquot of each fraction was subjected to the mutagenicity test.

Nitrite-treated tyramine solution was injected directly onto the LS-410 column (21.5 × 300 mm) for HPLC, using 20% methanol containing 0.1% acetic acid at a flow rate of 5 mL/min, and the eluate was monitored at 270 nm. An aliquot of each fraction was assayed for mutagenicity.

RESULTS

Mutagenicities of soya sauces after nitrite treatment

The mutagenicities of various kinds of soya sauce after nitrite treatment are shown in Table 1. All of the soya sauces produced in Japan, except G, showed strong mutagenicity; 1-mL

Table 1. Mutagenicities of various kinds of soya sauces after nitrite treatment (Wakabayashi *et al.*, 1983)

Soya sauce	Place of production	Revertants per mL [a]
A	Japan, Chiba	25 200
B	Japan, Chiba	18 300
C	Japan, Chiba	24 300
D	Japan, Mie	9 600
E	Japan, Chiba	22 200
F	Japan, Chiba	24 900
G	Japan, Aichi	2 700
H	Japan, Mie	17 300
I	USA, Hawaii	4 100
J	USA, Hawaii	0
K	USA, Hawaii	2 300
L	USA, Ohio	6 100
M	USA, Wisconsin	26 600

[a] Mutagenicity was assayed on *Salmonella typhimurium* TA100 without S9 mix.

Fig. 1. Structures of compounds I, II and III: I, (–)-(1S,3S)-1-methyl-1,2,3,4-tetrahydro-β-carboline-3-carboxylic acid (MTCA); II, (–)-(1R,3S)-MTCA; III, tyramine

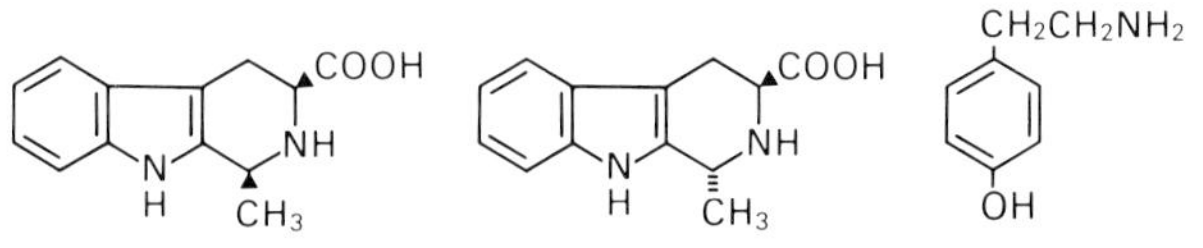

samples of these soya sauces, after nitrite treatment, induced 9 600–25 200 revertants of TA100 in the absence of S9 mix. All the soya sauces produced in the USA showed weak mutagenicity, except M, which resembled the Japanese soya sauces. Soya sauce J, which is made by acid hydrolysis of soya beans, was not mutagenic.

Identification of precursors of mutagens in soya sauce

Three precursors (compounds I, II and III) of mutagens were isolated from soya sauce A, as described above. Compounds I and II were identified as (–)-(1S,3S)-MTCA and (–)-(1R,3S)-MTCA, respectively, by comparison of their mass, ultra-violet and ^{1}H-nuclear magnetic resonance spectra and optical rotations, with those of synthetic compounds (Brossi *et al.*, 1973). The structures of these compounds are shown in Figure 1; Compound III was found to be tyramine by comparison of its physical properties with those of the authentic compound.

Mutagenicities of authentic samples of (–)-(1S,3S)-MTCA and (–)-(1R,3S)-MTCA, and tyramine after nitrite treatment

The mutagenic activities of (–)-(1S,3S)-MTCA after nitrite treatment toward TA100 and TA98, in the absence of S9 mix, were 17 400 and 1 400 revertants per mg, respectively. One mg of (–)-(1R,3S)-MTCA with nitrite induced 13 000 and 2 400 revertants of TA100 and TA98, respectively, without S9 mix. Addition of S9 mix greatly reduced the mutagenicities of these compounds.

After nitrite treatment, 1 mg tyramine induced 3 900 and 2 500 revertants of TA100 and TA98, respectively, without S9 mix. Addition of the metabolic system did not affect the mutagenicity of tyramine as much as it did that of the MTCA isomers: in the presence of S9 mix, 1 mg nitrite-treated tyramine induced 2 300 revertants of TA100 and 3 100 of TA98. Without nitrite treatment, the MTCA isomers and tyramine were not mutagenic toward TA100 or TA98, with or without S9 mix.

Amounts of (–)-(1S,3S)-MTCA and (–)-(1R,3S)-MTCA and tyramine in soya sauce

The total amounts of (–)-(1S,3S)- plus (–)-(1R,3S)-MTCA and of tyramine in various kinds of soya sauce are shown in Table 2. The mutagenicities of authentic samples of the three precursors, after nitrite treatment, are also shown as percentages of the mutagenicities of the nitrite-treated soya sauce.

Soya sauces A–F, H and M, which showed strong mutagenicity, contained larger amounts of MTCA isomers, whereas soya sauces G, I and K, which showed weak mutagenicity, contained smaller amounts of these precursors. Moreover, soya sauce J, which was not

Table 2.   Amounts of (−)-(1*S*,3*S*)- plus (−)-(1*R*,3*S*)-1-methyl-1,2,3,4-
tetrahydro-β-carboline-3-carboxylic acids (MTCA), and tyramine in
various kinds of soya sauce

Soya sauce	Amount (μg/mL)		% Mutagenicity due to	
	MTCA	Tyramine	MTCA[a]	Tyramine
A	668	1 040	44	16
B	678	930	61	20
C	378	960	26	15
D	95	18	16	1
E	604	1 100	45	19
F	521	2 250	34	35
G	82	17	50	2
H	275	660	26	15
I	55	14	22	1
J	<4[b]	<2[b]		
K	34	<2[b]	24	0
L	<4[b]	<2[b]	0	0
M	711	1 180	44	17

[a] Ratio of (−)-(1*S*,3*S*)-:(−)-(1*R*, 3*S*)-MTCA about 4 in each case
[b] Minimum amount detectable by high-performance liquid
chromatography

mutagenic, did not contain MTCA isomers. However, soya sauce L, which is a Chinese-style soya sauce, was mutagenic but contained no MTCA. The mutagenicity attributable to (–)-(1*S*,3*S*)- and (–)-(1*R*,3*S*)-MTCA amounted to up to 61% of the total mutagenicities of the various soya sauces tested.

Soya sauces A–C, E, F, H and M contained large amounts (660–2 250 μg/mL) of tyramine, but soya sauces D, G and I contained little and soya sauces J–L contained no detectable tyramine. At most, 35% of the mutagenicity of soya sauce could be attributed to tyramine.

Mutagens produced with nitrite from (–)-(1S,3S)-MTCA and tyramine

The mutagen(s) produced from (–)-(1*S*,3*S*)-MTCA and nitrite was extracted with ethyl acetate, and about 90% of the mutagenicity was recovered in the organic solvent layer. After HPLC, the ethyl acetate fraction gave more than two peaks (ultra-violet absorption) and no detectable MTCA. Material in these ultra-violet absorption peaks exhibited no mutagenicity, but a mutagenic component which showed no ultraviolet absorption was eluted as a single peak on the HPLC, just before those showing ultra-violet absorption. The main material with ultra-violet absorption, but no mutagenicity, was found to be a compound with a mono-nitroso substitution at the *N*-2 position – (–)-(1*S*,3*S*)-MNTCA – by comparison of its physical properties with those of authentic (–)-(1*S*,3*S*)-MNTCA.

When nitrite-treated tyramine was subjected to HPLC, two major ultra-violet peaks with retention times of 23 and 38 min were recovered, in addition to unchanged tyramine. Mutagenic activity was found only in the peak with a retention time of 23 min, and the mutagen in this peak was determined to be 4-(2-aminoethyl)-6-diazo-2,4-cyclohexadienone by various spectral analyses (Ochiai *et al.*, 1984). The recovery of mutagenic activity in this fraction was 92% of that in the nitrite-treated tyramine.

DISCUSSION

Soya sauce is a very common seasoning in Japan, and its annual consumption by Japanese is about 10 L *per caput*. Therefore, the daily intakes of MTCA isomers and tyramine from soya sauces A–G would be about 2–18 and 0.5–60 mg, respectively, per person. These three compounds could be formed by processes involving enzymatic reactions during production of soya sauce. MTCA isomers may be produced by condensation of L-tryptophan and acetaldehyde, which are produced by enzymatic reactions, while tyramine could be formed by decarboxylation of tyrosine by the action of tyrosine decarboxylase. These three precursors of mutagens were not detected in soya sauce J, which is made by acid hydrolysis of soya beans. The differences in the contents of MTCA isomers and tyramine in various soya sauces is presumably due to differences in the microbes used and processes involved in production of the soya sauces.

The mutagen(s) produced from (–)-(1S,3S)-MTCA and nitrite was a minor product(s). The major product, which was non-mutagenic, was identified as (–)-(1S,3S)-MNTCA, and, after nitrite treatment, more than 80% of (–)-(1S,3S)-MTCA was recovered as (–)-(1S,3S)-MNTCA. Therefore, the specific mutagenic activity of the mutagen(s) produced from (–)-(1S,3S)-MTCA by treatment with nitrite must be greater than that of N-methyl-N-nitrosourea, which is 47 per μg. Determination of the structure of this mutagen is in progress.

In contrast, the mutagen obtained by treatment of tyramine with nitrite was isolated by HPLC as one of the major products, and it was found to be 4-(2-aminoethyl)-6-diazo-2,4-cyclohexadienone on the basis of various spectral measurements. About 30% of the tyramine was recovered as a mutagenic compound after nitrite treatment. The specific mutagenic activity of this compound was 112 per μg.

MTCA isomers and tyramine are present in various foods and beverages as well as in soya sauce. For instance, MTCA is present in Japanese *sake* and tyramine in cheese, beer and soya bean paste. However, the amounts of MTCA isomers and tyramine in these materials are smaller than those in soya sauce, except in the case of some cheddar cheeses, which contain amounts of tyramine comparable to those in soya sauce (Blackwell & Mabbitt, 1965; Sato *et al.*, 1975; Yamamoto *et al.*, 1980). Therefore, carcinogenicity tests on soya sauce, MTCA isomers and tyramine in the presence of nitrite are very important. These carcinogenicity tests are being carried out in this laboratory.

ACKNOWLEDGEMENTS

This study was supported in part by Grants-in-Aid for Cancer Research from the Ministry of Health and Welfare, the Ministry of Education, Science and Culture of Japan, the Haraguchi Memorial Cancer Research Fund and the Princess Takamatsu Cancer Research Fund.

REFERENCES

Blackwell, B. & Mabbitt, L.A. (1965) Tyramine in cheese related to hypertensive crises after monoamine-oxidase inhibition. *Lancet, i,* 938–940

Brossi, A., Focella, A. & Teitel, S. (1973) Alkaloids in mammalian tissues. 3. Condensation of L-tryptophan and L-5-hydroxytryptophan with formaldehyde and acetaldehyde. *J. med. Chem., 16,* 418–420

Druckrey, H., Ivankovic, S. & Preussmann, R. (1970) Selektive Erzeugung von Carcinomen des Drüsenmagens bei Ratten durch orale Gabe von N-methyl-N-nitroso-N′-acetylharnstoff (AcMNH). *Z. Krebsforsch, 74,* 23–33

Hartman, P.E. (1983) Nitrate/nitrite ingestion and gastric cancer mortality. *Environ. Mutagen.*, **5**, 111–121

Hirayama, T. (1979) *The epidemiology of gastric cancer in Japan.* In: Pfeiffer, C.J., ed., *Gastric Cancer,* New York, Gerhard Witzstrock, pp. 60–82

Ochiai, M., Wakabaya, K., Nagao, M. & Sugimura, T. (1984) Tyramine is a major mutagen precursor in soy sauce, being convertible to a mutagen by nitrite. *Gann,* **75**, 1–3

Piacek-Llanes, B.G. & Tannenbaum, S.R. (1982) Formation of an activated *N*-nitroso compound in nitrite-treated fava beans (*Vicia fava*). *Carcinogenesis,* **3**, 1379–1384

Sander, J. & Bürkle, B. (1969) Induktion maligner Tumoren bei Ratten durch gleichzeitige Verfütterung von Nitrit und sekundären Aminen. *Z. Krebsforsch,* **73**, 54–66

Sato, S., Tadenuma, M., Takahashi, K. & Nakamura, N. (1975) Configuration of sake taste. VI. Rough taste components. 3. Tetrahydroharman-3-carboxylic acid. *Nippon Jozo Kyokai Zasshi,* **70**, 821–824

Sugimura, T. & Fujimura, S. (1967) Tumor production in glandular stomach of rat by *N*-methyl-*N'*-nitro-*N*-nitrosoguanidine. *Nature,* **216**, 943–944

Sugimura, T. & Nagao, M. (1980) *Modification of mutagenic activity.* In: de Serres, F.J. & Hollaender, A., eds, *Chemical Mutagens,* vol. 6, New York & London, Plenum Press, pp. 41–60

Wakabayashi, K., Ochiai, M., Saitô, H., Tsuda, M., Suwa, Y., Nagao, M. & Sugimura, T. (1983) Presence of 1-methyl-1,2,3,4-tetrahydro-β-carboline-3-carboxylic acid, a precursor of a mutagenic nitroso compound, in soy sauce. *Proc. natl Acad. Sci. USA,* **80**, 2912–2916

Weisburger, J.H., Marquardt, H., Hirota, M., Mori, H. & Williams, G.M. (1980) Induction of cancer of the glandular stomach in rats by an extract of nitrite-treated fish. *J. natl Cancer Inst.,* **64**, 163–167

Yamamoto, S., Wakabayashi, S. & Makita, M. (1980) Gas-liquid chromatographic determination of tyramine in fermented food products. *J. Agric. Food Chem.,* **28**, 790–793

ANALYSIS AND OCCURRENCE OF TOTAL *N*-NITROSO COMPOUNDS IN THE JAPANESE DIET

T. KAWABATA[1]

Department of Biomedical Research on Food, National Institute of Health, Shinagawa-ku, Tokyo, 141, Japan

M. MATSUI

Tokyo Research & Application Laboratory, Shimadzu Corporation, Chofu-shi, Tokyo 182, Japan

T. ISHIBASHI

Research Laboratory, Japan Medical Foods Association, Maesawa, Higashikurume-shi, Tokyo 203, Japan

M. HAMANO

Faculty of Home Economics, Tokyo Kaseigakuin University, Sanban-cho, Chiyoda-ku, Tokyo 102, Japan

SUMMARY

A quantitative technique for differentiating the total *N*-nitrosamides from the total *N*-nitroso compounds has been devised. The principle of this method is based on the chemiluminescence response of a nitroso compound under different denitrosating conditions. We also examined the effect of nitrite scavengers on the stability of *N*-nitroso compounds and found that both ammonium sulfamate and hydrazine sulfate can be satisfactorily used for the detection of chemiluminescence response with hydrogen bromide-acetic acid reagent. A survey of the occurrence of total *N*-nitroso compounds, total *N*-nitrosamides, volatile *N*-nitrosamines, nitrates and nitrites in the Japanese diet has been conducted. Fairly high levels of total *N*-nitroso compounds were detected in salt-fermented vegetables, the highest being 2 500 µg/kg in *hakusai-zuke* (salt-fermented Chinese cabbage), followed by 253 µg/kg in *takuan* (salt-fermented radish roots). It is noteworthy that the amounts of total *N*-nitroso compounds in these products almost coincided with those of total *N*-nitrosamides, although no appreciable amounts, or only trace quantities, of volatile nitrosamines could be detected in these vegetable products.

---

[1] Author to whom correspondence should be sent

INTRODUCTION

In this paper we give a brief account of some of our recent research on the determination and occurrence of total *N*-nitroso compounds in the Japanese diet. They concern: (1) development of a technique for differentiating the total *N*-nitrosamides (TNAd) from total *N*-nitroso compounds (TNC) and (2) a survey of TNC, TNAd, volatile *N*-nitroso compounds (VNA), nitrate and nitrite contents in various Japanese foods.

DIFFERENTIATION OF TOTAL *N*-NITROSAMIDES FROM TOTAL *N*-NITROSO COMPOUNDS

In order to develop a technique for differentiating TNAd fraction from TNC in food samples, the chemiluminescence response of various *N*-nitroso compounds after treatment with different denitrosating reagents has been examined, and the effects of various nitrite scavengers on the stability of *N*-nitroso compounds have been studied.

EXPERIMENTAL

Denitrosating reagents

The following reagents were tested: (1) 25% hydrogen bromide in glacial acetic acid (HBr/HAc), (2) concentrated hydrochloric acid (conc. HC1), (3) 10% hydrogen iodide in glacial acetic acid (HI/HAc), (4) glacial acetic acid (HAc) and (5) pretreatment with 5% potassium hydroxide solution for 5 min, followed by denitrosation with the HBr/HAc reagent.

Nitrite scavengers

(1) 2% ammonium sulfamate (the pH of the test solution was adjusted to 2 with 10% phosphoric acid), (2) 15% sodium azide (the pH of the test solution was adjusted to 4 or 7), and (3) hydrazine sulfate (the pH was adjusted to 4).

Apparatus and analytical procedures for TNC and TNAd

Determinations of TNC and TNAd were carried out using denitrosation techniques and a chemiluminescence analyser. The procedure and apparatus employed were almost the same as those described by Downes *et al.* (1976). The chemiluminescence analyser was a Thermal Energy Analyzer (TEA 502, Thermo Electron Corp., USA).

Reagents

N-Nitrosodimethylamine (NDMA) and *N*-methyl-*N'*-nitro-*N*-nitrosoguanidine (MNNG) (Wako Pure Chemicals, Tokyo); *N*-nitrosopyrrolidine (NPYR) (Aldrich, USA); *N*-nitroso-*N*-methyl-p-toluene sulfonamide (NMTS), *N*-nitrosomethylurethane (NMUT) and *N*-nitrosodiethanolamine (NDELA) (Tokyo Kasei Kogyo).

N-Nitrososarcosine (NSAR) and *N*-nitrosomorpholine (NMOR) were synthesized according to the method of Lijinsky *et al.* (1970). Other reagents used were of analytical grade and were employed without further purification, except for ethyl acetate. It was found that commercial ethyl acetate, even of analytical grade, is quite often contaminated with TEA-positive substance(s). Therefore, the solvent was purified by redistillation after washing with 2% ammonium sulfamate solution, pH 2.0.

RESULTS AND DISCUSSION

Comparison of various N-*nitroso compounds for chemiluminescence response after treatment with denitrosating reagents*

The results obtained are summarized in Table 1.

As can be seen, marked differences in the chemiluminescence response were observed with the denitrosating reagents tested. All the nitroso compounds denitrosated with the HBr/HAc reagent gave a positive chemiluminescence response. While *N*-nitrosamines, such as NDMA and NMOR, did not react with either conc. HCl or HI/HAc, *N*-nitrosamides, such as MNNG, apparently reacted with these reagents to give a positive chemiluminescence response. When simple HAc was applied, almost no response could be seen with *N*-nitroso compounds, with the exception of MNNG. It was observed that the *N*-nitrosamides tested were completely destroyed by the pretreatment with 5% potassium hydroxide. In contrast, all the *N*-nitrosamines remained intact and were denitrosated by subsequent treatment with HBr/HAc to give a positive chemiluminescence response. *N*-Nitrosamides are known to be particularly labile in alkali. On the basis of these findings, we have devised a technique for differentiating a nitrosamine from a nitrosamide by using denitrosation reactions with different denitrosating reagents. The most appropriate combination was found to be the following: (a) HBr/HAc, (b) conc. HCl and (c) pretreatment with 5% potassium hydroxide, followed by the HBr/HAc reagent (see Table 1).

Effect of nitrite scavengers on the stability of N-*nitroso compounds*

The effects of three types of nitrite scavengers, ammonium sulfamate, sodium azide and hydrazine sulfate, on the stability of nitrite, NDMA and MNNG were examined and the results are shown in Table 2.

Table 1. Effect of various denitrosating reagents on the chemiluminescence response of *N*-nitroso compounds

Test compound[a]	Denitrosating reagent	Relative chemiluminescence response[b]				
		HBr/HAc[c]	HCl[d]	HI/HAc[e]	HAc[f]	5% KOH[g] HBr/HAc
NaNO$_2$ (575.0 ng)		1.00	1.00	1.00	1.00	1.00
MNNG (1 224.0 ng)		1.02	2.08	0.65	0.66	0.00
NMUT (1 100.0 ng)		0.73	2.01	0.02	0.00	0.00
NMTS (1 785.0 ng)		0.94	2.37	0.00	0.00	0.00
NDMA (617.5 ng)		1.27	0.00	0.00	0.00	0.35
NPYR (842.5 ng)		0.56	0.00	0.00	0.00	0.87
NMOR (717.5 ng)		0.67	0.00	0.00	0.00	0.29
NSAR (983.2 ng)		0.85	0.00	0.00	0.00	0.23
NDELA (1 100.0 ng)		0.68	0.00	0.00	0.00	0.08

[a] MNNG, *N*-methyl-*N*′-nitro-*N*-nitrosoguanidine; NMUT, *N*-nitrosomethylurethane; NMTS, *N*-nitroso-*N*-methyl-*p*-toluene sulfonamide; NDMA, *N*-nitrosodimethylamine; NPYR, *N*-nitrosopyrrolidine; NMOR, *N*-nitrosomorpholine; NSAR, *N*-nitrososarcosine; NDELA, *N*-nitrosodiethanolamine
[b] Value relative to the chemiluminescence response (peak area) obtained with the sodium nitrite standard solution
[c] 25% Hydrogen bromide in glacial acetic acid
[d] Conc. hydrochloric acid
[e] 10% Hydrogen iodide in glacial acetic acid
[f] Glacial acetic acid
[g] Test solution was pretreated with 5% potassium hydroxide solution, followed by denitrosation with 25% HBr/HAc

Table 2. Effect of nitrite scavengers on the stability of nitrite and *N*-nitroso compounds

Test compound[a]	Nitrite scavenger	Residual test compound (%)			
		1 ml 2% ammonium sulfamate at pH 2	1 ml 15% sodium azide		5 mg hydrazine sulfate at pH 5
			at pH 4	at pH 7	
NaNO$_2$ (1.15 mg)		0.00	0.00	47.85	0.00
NDMA (1.23 mg)		99.54	88.26	99.21	98.73
MNNG (2.30 mg)		92.85	13.52	23.21	92.85

[a] NDMA, *N*-nitrosodimethylamine; MNNG, *N*-methyl-*N'*-nitro-*N*-nitrosoguanidine

A marked decrease in the MNNG content was observed when sodium azide was employed at pH 4 and 7; in addition, about 50% of the nitrite remained at pH 7. Bavin *et al.* (1982) have pointed out the inadequacy of sulfamic acid and sodium azide as nitrite scavengers; the former, in particular, leads to denitrosation of many *N*-nitroso compounds, and the latter gives an unexplained response at the chemiluminescence detector with HBr/HAc.

OCCURRENCE OF TOTAL *N*-NITROSO COMPOUNDS, TOTAL *N*-NITROSAMIDES, VOLATILE NITROSAMINES, NITRATES AND NITRITES IN THE JAPANESE DIET

We have already reported data for volatile nitrosamines, nitrates and nitrites in various Japanese foods (Kawabata *et al.*, 1980, 1982). We have now conducted a survey of the contents of TNC, TNAd, VNA and other related compounds in the Japanese diet.

Total N-nitroso compound and total N-*nitrosamide determinations*

A 50-g aliquot of the food sample (salt-dried fish, air-dried squid, fish sausages, cured meat products, salt-fermented vegetables, etc) was mixed with 100 mL 2% ammonium sulfamate, and the pH of the mixture was adjusted to 2 with 10% phosphoric acid. It was then homogenized in a mechanical blender for 3 min. After standing for 1 h, the homogenate was filtered through a suction filter (Toyo Roshi, No. 3), and 20-30 g sodium chloride were added to the filtrate, which was then extracted three times with 3×20 mL ethyl acetate. The combined extracts were made up with 20-30 g anhydrous sodium sulfate and were allowed to stand for 30-60 min, with occasional stirring, then filtered through a filter paper into a 50-mL volumetric flask. The volume was made up to exactly 50 mL with ethyl acetate. A 0.5-5 mL aliquot of the extract was subjected to the TNC determination using HBr/HAc. The aliquot for TNAd was treated with conc. HCl, and also with 5% potassium hydroxide followed by HBr/HAc.

Volatile nitrosamine, nitrate and nitrite determinations

VNA, nitrate and nitrite in the food sample were determined in the manner described in our previous papers (Kawabata *et al.*, 1980, 1982).

RESULTS AND DISCUSSION

Table 3 summarizes the results concerning the occurrence of TNC, TNAd, VNA (NDMA and NPYR) and nitrite in various fish products and cured meat products.

Almost no appreciable amounts, or only trace quantities, of TNC, TNAd and VNA could be detected in uncooked fish products. The VNA content (especially NDMA in dried squid samples) apparently increased upon broiling on a city gas range. The levels of TNC and TNAd in various cured-meat products were apparently higher than those in fish products. The TNC contents apparently depended on the residual nitrite contents.

Table 4 presents data on the TNC, TNAd, VNA, nitrate and nitrite contents of various salt-fermented vegetables. It is noteworthy that fairly high levels of TNC were detected in various samples, the highest level being 2 500 µg/kg in *hakusai-zuke* (salt-fermented Chinese cabbage), followed by 253 µg/kg in *takuan* (salt-fermented radish roots). In addition, the TNC values for these products almost coincided with those for TNAd. It may be noted that the chemical structure(s) and the origin or mechanism of formation of the *N*-nitroso compounds remain to be determined. It is also to be noted that no more than trace quantities of VNA could be detected in these products.

Although the causative agent(s) or factor(s) involved in human stomach cancer are not yet clear, some epidemiological data indicate that the high incidence of stomach cancer in Japan might be associated with the high intake of salted fish and salt-fermented vegetables (Sato *et al.*, 1959, 1961; Haenszel *et al.*, 1972). In this context, Japanese should pay attention to their habit of consuming fairly large amounts of vegetables, especially salt-fermented products.

REFERENCES

Bavin, P.M.G., Darkin, D.W. & Viney, N.J. (1982) *Total nitroso compounds in gastric juice*. In: Bartsch, H., O'Neill, I.K., Castegnaro, M. & Okada, M., eds, N-*Nitroso Compounds; Occurrence and Biological Effects (IARC Scientific Publications No. 41)*, Lyon, International Agency for Research on Cancer, pp. 337–344

Downes, M.J., Edwards, M.W., Elsey, T.S. & Walters, C.L. (1976) Determination of a non-volatile nitrosamine by using denitrosation and a chemiluminescence analyser. *Analyst, 101*, 742–748

Haenszel, W., Kurihara, M., Segi, M. & Lee, R.K.C. (1972) Stomach cancer among Japanese in Hawaii. *J. natl Cancer Inst., 49*, 963–988

Kawabata, T., Uibu, J., Ohshima, H., Matsui, M., Hamano, M. & Tokiwa, H. (1980) *Occurrence, formation and precursors of* N-*nitroso compounds in the Japanese diet*. In: Walker, E.A., Castegnaro, M., Griciute, L. & Börzsönyi, M., eds, N-*Nitroso Compounds: Analysis, Formation and Occurrence (IARC Scientific Publications No. 31)*, Lyon, International Agency for Research on Cancer, pp. 481–492

Kawabata, T., Matsui, M., Ishibashi, T., Hamano, M. & Ino, M. (1982) *Formation of* N-*nitroso compounds during cooking of Japanese food*. In: Bartsch, H., O'Neill, I.K., Castegnaro, M. & Okada, M., eds, N-*Nitroso Compounds: Occurrence and Biological Effects (IARC Scientific Publications No. 41)*, Lyon, International Agency for Research on Cancer, pp. 287–297

Lijinsky, W., Keefer, L. & Loo, J. (1970) The preparation and properties of some nitrosoamino acids. *Tetrahedron, 26*, 5137–5153

Sato, T., Fukuyama, T., Suzuki, T. & Takayanagi, J. (1959) Studies on the causation of gastric cancer. 2. The relation between gastric cancer mortality rate and salted food intake in several places in Japan. *Bull. Inst. public Health (Jpn), 8*, 187–198

Sato, T., Fukuyama, T., Suzuki, T., Takayanagi, J. & Sakai, Y. (1961) Studies on the causation of gastric cancer. 3. Intake of highly brined foods in several places with high mortality rate in Europe. *Bull. Inst. public Health (Jpn), 10*, 9–17

Table 3. Occurrence of total N-nitroso compounds (TNC), total N-nitrosamides (TNAd), volatile N-nitrosamines (VNA) and nitrites in the Japanese diet

Product	TNC[a] (μgNO/kg)	TNAd[a] (μgNO/kg)	VNA[b] (μg/kg) NDMA	VNA[b] (μg/kg) NPYR	nitrite[c] (mg/kg)
Fish products					
Salt-dried fish					
sardine, maruboshi iwashi (uncooked)	0.86	0.63	0.6	ND[d]	ND
sardine, maruboshi iwashi (city gas-broiled)	4.53	2.04	6.1	ND	ND
Pacific saury, samma hiraki (uncooked)	1.87	1.58	0.7	ND	ND
Pacific saury, samma hiraki (city gas-broiled)	6.74	5.42	3.3	ND	0.28
mackerel, aji hiraki (uncooked)	1.45	1.14	0.9	ND	ND
mackerel, aji hiraki (city gas-broiled)	6.61	3.62	7.4	ND	0.40
air-dried squid, hoshi surume (uncooked)	26.6	22.6	9.9	ND	ND
air-dried squid, hoshi surume (city gas-broiled)	37.7	22.5	37.5	ND	0.77
Others					
salt-fermented squid, ika shiokara	15.8	—	3.5	ND	ND
fish sausage 1	2.50	—	2.1	ND	0.07
fish sausage 2	3.39	—	2.6	ND	ND
Meat products					
Wiener sausage 1	24.8	—	—	—	—
Wiener sausage 2	32.6	—	—	—	—
Wiener sausage 3	40.0	—	2.8	ND	5.10
Wiener sausage 4	70.6	—	—	—	—
Wiener sausage (pork)	88.9	—	3.4	ND	10.5
Bologna sausage	12.1	—	2.0	ND	8.94
ham (fine quality)	5.51	—	2.0	ND	1.16
ham (standard)	6.67	—	3.5	ND	1.95
corned beef	27.5	—	2.3	ND	15.0
bacon	134.0	—	3.4	ND	3.27

[a]TNC and TNAd, detection limit, 0.5 μg NO/kg (expressed in terms of NO equivalent)
[b]VNA, detection limit, 0.1 μg/kg
[c]Nitrite, detection limit, 0.05 mg/kg
[d]ND, not detected

Table 4. Occurrence of total N-nitroso compounds (TNC), total N-nitrosamides (TNAd), volatile N-nitrosamines (VNA), nitrites and nitrates in the Japanese diet (salt-fermented vegetables)

Product	TNC[a] (μgNO/kg)	TNAd[a] (μgNO/kg)	VNA (μg/kg)[b]		nitrite[c] (mg/kg)	nitrate[c] (mg/kg)
			NDMA	NPYR		
Radish root, takuan 1	85.0	92.6	–	–	–	–
Radish root, takuan 2	252.6	266.2	ND[d]	ND	3.43	126.2
Radish root, takuan ume-zuke	110.0	102.2	tr[e]	0.5	1.73	264.3
Radish root, bettara-zuke	118.1	128.6	tr	ND	1.03	15.35
nara-zuke, oriental melon dipped in sake leese	5.52	–	tr	ND	1.96	29.35
Chinese cabbage, hakusai-zuke	2 466.8	2 325.4	ND	ND	31.0	258.5
Furnip leaves, nozawana	100.0	107.4	ND	tr	12.9	283.7
Broad-leaved mustard, takana	57.1	49.9	ND	ND	6.47	221.4
Pot herb mustard, kyona	98.0	101.8	ND	ND	14.3	265.4
fukujin-zuke, mixed fermented vegetables seasoned with soya sauce	7.74	–	ND	ND	2.59	3.70

[a] TNC and TNAd, detection limit, 0.5 μg NO/kg (expressed in terms of NO equivalent)
[b] VNA, detection limit, 0.1 μg/kg
[c] Nitrite and nitrate, detection limit, 0.05 mg/kg
[e] Tr, 0.1–0.5 μg/kg

MUTAGENICITY OF VARIOUS JAPANESE FOODSTUFFS TREATED WITH NITRITE.
II. DIRECTLY-ACTING MUTAGENS PRODUCED FROM
N-CONTAINING COMPOUNDS IN FOODSTUFFS

I. TOMITA, N. KINAE, Y. NAKAMURA & H. TAKENAKA

Shizuoka College of Pharmaceutical Sciences, 2-2-1 Oshika, Shizuoka 422, Japan

H. KANAMORI

Hiroshima Prefectural Institute of Public Health, Kanda 1 chome, Minami-ku Ushina, Hiroshima 734, Japan

H. HASHIZUME & T. YOKOYAMA

Wakayama Prefectural Institute of Public Health, Sunayama 3 chome, Wakayama 640, Japan

SUMMARY

Various Japanese foodstuffs show mutagenicity after nitrite treatment at pH 4.2. Among 13 groups of foodstuffs, classified by the 'market basket' method, the group containing fish showed the highest mutagenicity in the absence of metabolic activation. Taking the daily intake of these foodstuffs into consideration, the combination of groups V (soya bean paste), VI (juice), VIII (pickles and seaweed), IX (alcoholic beverages, coffee), X (fish) and XI (meat) represents 90% of the total mutagenic activity that may be supplied by food each day. The mutagenic activities of foodstuffs in groups VII (vegetables), VIII and IX were increased remarkably by nitrite treatment; the mutagenicity of alcoholic beverages was particularly affected by nitrite. The separation of wine, *sake* and beer into acidic, basic and neutral fractions scattered the premutagenic activities, with a large decrease in total activity. The chemical properties of the basic fraction of beer, which gave the highest mutagenicity after nitrite treatment, were examined, and two tetrahydro-β-carboline derivatives were identified.

INTRODUCTION

Foodstuffs such as fish, tea, soya bean sauce, soya bean paste, coffee, *sake* and Chinese wines (nondistilled), have been shown to be mutagenic when they are treated with nitrite (Marquardt *et al.*, 1977; Lin *et al.*, 1979; Lin & Tai, 1980; Nakamura *et al.*, 1980; Nagao *et al.*, 1981). There are many nitrosatable substances in these foodstuffs; a variety of compounds, especially amines (aliphatic and aromatic amines) and amides (*N*-alkyl, aryl or acyl urea, *N*-alkylcarbamate), are known to produce mutagens with nitrite (Endo & Takahashi, 1973; Mirvish, 1975; Kokatnur, *et al.*, 1978).

The present study was carried out to test the mutagenic activities not only of 213 individual foodstuffs but also of 89 foodstuffs divided into 13 categories according to the 'market basket' method. Alcoholic beverages (wine, *sake* and beer) were further selected to examine their reactivities with nitrite to produce mutagens. The chemical nature of the compounds in the basic fractions of beverages was examined and compared with that of substances isolated from the reaction mixture of tryptophan and aldehydes in a model aminocarbonyl reaction.

MATERIALS AND METHODS

Experimental materials

All foodstuffs tested were purchased from local shops in Shizuoka- or Wakayama-shi. Eighty-nine foodstuffs for the 'market basket' method were classified into 13 categories (Table 1) and 2.5- to 300-day portions were mixed or homogenized. Alcoholic beverages tested were all Japanese brands.

All chemicals used in this study were of analytical grade.

Preparation of samples for mutagenicity tests

Foodstuffs such as rice and vegetables were cooked normally; fish and meat were broiled on a city gas range. Solid samples were homogenized with distilled water (1–10 g in 40 mL), centrifuged at $16\,000 \times$ g at $0\,^\circ$C for 20 min and filtered through a Millipore filter (0.45 μm). Liquid samples and various seasonings were freeze-dried, and the residue was dissolved in dimethyl sulfoxide. Food samples of all groups except IV were placed in petri dishes and dried over phosphorus pentoxide in a vacuum desiccator overnight; the dried samples were powdered and extracted with methanol in a Soxhlet apparatus. Foodstuffs of group IV were treated without drying: samples (70 g) were mixed with methanol (100 mL) by shaking for 10 min; after centrifugation, the lower layer was again extracted with methanol (100 mL), and the methanol extracts were combined. The methanol was then evaporated in a rotary evaporator.

Table 1. Classification of foodstuffs

Group	Main foodstuffs	No. of foodstuffs
I	Rice, rice cakes	2
II	Cereals, breads, potatoes, seeds	13
III	Sugar, cakes, chocolate	8
IV	Fats, oils, mayonaise	5
V	Beans, soya bean paste, *tofu*	5
VI	Fruits, fruit and vegetable juices	6
VII	Vegetables	4
VIII	Vegetables (root), pickles, seaweeds	12
IX	Seasonings, alcoholic beverages, coffee, tea	7
X	Fish, fish pastes, molluscs, crustaceans	16
XI	Meat, eggs, ham, sausages	7
XII	Milk, cheese, yoghurt	3
XIII	Salad, cooked cakes containing meat	7

Alcoholic beverages were separated into acidic, basic and neutral fractions under ice-cooling as follows: freeze-dried wine, *sake* and beer (600 mL) were dissolved in water (100 mL), acidified to pH 3 by adding 10% sulfuric acid and then extracted three times with ethyl acetate (100 mL). The extracts were combined and washed three times with 2% sodium bicarbonate (100 mL) to obtain a neutral fraction. The combined sodium bicarbonate extracts were acidified to pH 3 by adding 10% sulfuric acid and extracted three times with ethyl acetate (100 mL). This extract was used as the acidic fraction. The water layer was made alkaline by the addition of solid sodium hydroxide and extracted three times with ethyl acetate to obtain the basic fraction. All the fractions obtained were evaporated to dryness in a rotary evaporator after addition of anhydrous sodium sulfate.

Mutagenicity tests

Mutagenicity tests on the individual foodstuffs were performed using *Salmonella typhimurium* TA100 and TA100 streptomycin-dependent (SM^d) strains, according to a modification of the method of Ames *et al.* (1975) (preincubation method, Yahagi *et al.*, 1977) or by the method described by T. Kada *et al.* (1983). The homogenate (1 mL of filtered homogenate for the modified Ames test and 10 mL for Kada's test) was added to 0.2 mol/L acetate buffer, pH 4.2 (1 mL) containing 0.1 mol/L sodium nitrite (1.0 mL) and incubated at 37 C for 10 min. After incubation, 0.1 mol/L ammonium sulfamate (1 mL) was added and incubated for 10 min to terminate the reaction. The mixture was filtered through a Millipore filter (0.45 μm) and 0.067 mol/L phosphate buffered saline (pH 7.4) was added. For controls, the same procedure was employed except that no sample was added.

Mutagenicity tests of food groups I–XIII were conducted using *S. typhimurium* TA100 and TA1535 with or without a 9 000 × *g* supernatant from rat liver.

The reaction with sodium nitrite was performed as follows: methanol extract (100 mg) dissolved in 0.2 mol/L acetate buffer (pH 4.0, 0.4 mL) was incubated at 37 C for 60 min with 0.3 mol/L sodium nitrite (prepared in 0.2 mol/L acetate buffer, pH 4.0, 0.3 mL); then, 0.3 mol/L ammonium sulfamate (prepared in the same buffer, pH 4.0, 0.3 mL) was added with 0.1 mL of the reaction mixture.

For mutagenicity tests of amines plus nitrite, 0.1 mol/L amines were incubated with 0.3 mol/L nitrite at 37 C for 10 min in acetate buffer (pH 4.2). After treatment with 0.3 mol/L ammonium sulfamate, 100 μL were used in the Ames test.

RESULTS

The mutagenic activities of food groups I–XIII, with and without nitrite treatment, are shown in Table 2: the activities of all groups except VI and X were increased after reaction with nitrite, regardless of metabolic activation; the mutagenic activities of groups VI and X were decreased by nitrite treatment in the presence of metabolic activation. An increase of more than 400 *his*$^+$ revertant colonies/g of foodstuffs was observed in groups V, VII, VIII, IX and XI; the increase in food groups VIII and IX (–S9) may correspond to 192 071 and 65 856 *his*$^+$ revertant colonies/day, respectively, assuming that the daily intake of these food groups are 197.4 g and 134.4 g, respectively. The mutagenic activities of nitrite-treated food groups VIII, X and XI represent 24.7%, 21.9% and 17.4% of the total activity of all the food groups.

The mutagenic activities of the individual foodstuffs, as tested in *S. typhimurium* TA100 and TA100 SM^d, are shown in Table 3. Alcoholic beverages such as *sake*, wine, whisky and beer had fairly high mutagenic activities with nitrite. Although alcoholic beverages contain spermidine (up to 4.4 μmol/L in red wine, 0–15.8 μmol/L in *sake* and –9.9 μmol/L in beer),

Table 2.   Mutagenic activities of food groups I–XIII with and without nitrite treatment

Group	Net his+ revertants/g				Daily intake (g/day)	Net his+ revertants/day .			
	– S9 mix		+ S9 mix			– S9 mix		+ S9 mix	
	– nitrite	+ nitrite	– nitrite	+ nitrite		– nitrite	+ nitrite	– nitrite	+ nitrite
I	0	3	0	1	235.0	0	705	0	235
II	0	151	0	55	146.3	0	22 046	0	8 046
III	0	173	0	91	36.7	0	6 349	365	3 340
IV	10	267	22	102	16.6	166	4 432	0	1 693
V	170	1 020	0	391	60.5	10 285	61 710	0	23 656
VI	143	498	35	17	168.0	24 024	83 664	5 880	2 856
VII	77	778	29	318	59.4	4 574	46 213	1 723	18 889
VIII	106	1 079	80	470	197.4	20 924	212 995	15 792	92 778
IX	104	594	40	440	134.4	13 978	79 834	5 376	59 138
X	1 853	2 051	1 757	1 484	92.0	170 476	188 692	161 644	136 528
XI	707	1 151	610	779	130.8	92 476	150 551	79 788	101 893
XII	12	32	4	18	96.2	1 154	3 078	385	1 732
XIII	36	184	0	90	17.3	623	3 183	0	1 557
Total						338 680	863 452	270 953	452 339

Table 3.   Mutagenic activities of foodstuffs after nitrite treatment

Food item	his^+-independent colonies in TA100 (no./g or mL)	SM-independent colonies in TA100 SM^d (no./g or mL)
Fish and shellfish		
Tuna, broiled	− 2 100	
Mackerel pike, raw	40	
Mackerel pike, broiled	− 850	
Jack mackerel, raw	− 365	
Jack mackerel, broiled	− 737	
Sardine, broiled	− 504	
Cod roe, raw	698	
Oyster, raw	694	
Beverages		
Cola	518	38
Chinese tea	1 296	
Persimmon tea	1 612	
Green tea	1 900	
Black tea	3 803	
Instant coffee	56 000	0
White rum	756	295
Beer		225
Whisky		387
Wine #1		612
Wine #2		1 025
Sake		1 557
Meats		
Soft salami ham	− 400	
Pork roast ham	1 050	
Wiener sausage, raw	1 250	
Hamburger	1 625	
Chicken cutlet	1 840	
Pork cutlet	2 220	
Pork ham, smoked	4 195	
Vegetables and cereals		
Rice bran		− 127
Taro		− 29
Yam		− 32
Peanuts		52
Ginger		8
Burdock		0
Corn		145
Soya beans		39
Soya sprouts		497
Seasonings		
Broth (small, dried sardines)	− 524	− 11
Soya sauce seasoning #1	− 151	− 6
Soya bean sauce	1 560	− 3
Broth (dried bonito)	− 299	0
Consommé	438	− 19
Worcester sauce	765	0
Soya bean soup	572	34
Soya sauce seasoning #2	765	109
Soya sauce seasoning #3	99	128
Soya bean paste	7 000	133

which is mutagenic under these experimental conditions with nitrite, the extent of its contribution to the overall mutagenic activity is only 0.03–0.26 %. Nagao *et al.* (1981) reported that some brands of whisky and brandy are mutagenic to *S. typhimurium* TA100 without metabolic activation, and the mutagenicity of nitrite-treated Chinese wine (nondistilled) has been reported by Lee & Fong (1979). In order to elucidate the chemical nature of the premutagen(s) in alcoholic beverages, we separated the freeze-dried samples of wines (six brands) and *sake* and beer (three brands of each) into three fractions: acidic, basic and neutral, as described above. The yield of residue varied: the total yield from the six brands of wine was greater than those from *sake* or beer; and the mutagenic activities tested without metabolic activation also varied greatly (Fig. 1). The three fractions of wine produced $1.5–4.2 \times 10^3$ his$^+$ revertants/100 mL, of which the acidic fraction represented 53.8–91.4% of the total activity. *Sake* and beer gave $5–10 \times 10^2$ and $1–1.5 \times 10^3$ *his*$^+$ revertants/100 mL, respectively.

On the basis of human consumption, we chose beer as the material from which to separate premutagen(s) that react with nitrite to produce mutagen(s). As shown in Figure 1, the specific

Fig. 1. Mutagenic activities of three fractions of alcoholic beverages after nitrite treatment. ▤, acidic fraction; ▨, basic fraction; ☐, neutral fraction. 1–6, wines; 7–9, *sakes*, 10–12, beers

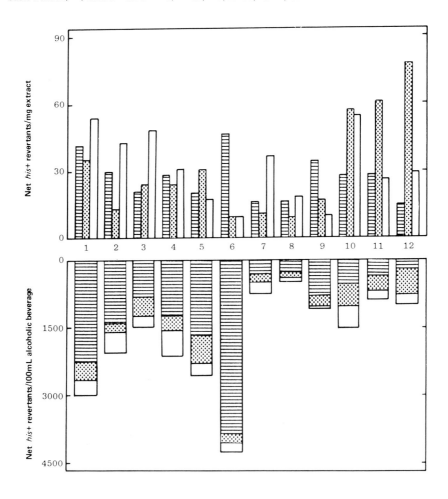

Fig. 2. Structures of mutagenic β-carboline derivatives in TLC spot A from basic fraction of beer (see text)

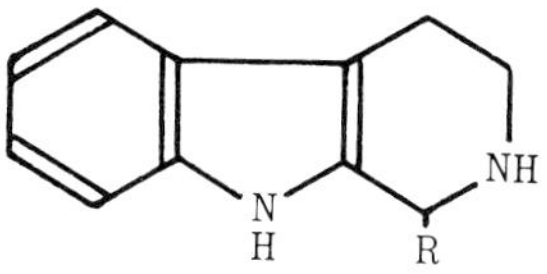

(a): R = H

(b): R = CH$_3$

mutagenic activities (net *his*[+] revertants/mg of extract), especially of the basic fraction, are fairly high (60–85 revertants/mg of the extract). A concentrate of the basic fraction of beer was therefore developed with ethyl acetate on a silica-gel plate, and the unmoved spot was extracted with methanol. When the methanol extract was developed with ethanol, two spots (A, $R_f = 0$; B, $R_f = 0.7$) were obtained. Spot A showed an ultra-violet spectrum (with a maximum at 277 nm) similar to that of 1-methyl-1,2,3,4-tetrahydro-β-carboline-3-carboxylic acid, which has been isolated from soya bean sauce (Sugimura & Sato, 1983), but its behaviour on thin-layer chromatography was different. Its chemical structure has been studied by gas-chromatographic-mass spectrometric analysis and shown to be a mixture of two β-carboline derivatives: 1,2,3,4-tetrahydro-9*H*-pyrido[3,4-b] indole (a) and its 1-methyl derivative (b) (see Fig. 2). Structural elucidation and mutagenicity data will be reported elsewhere.

DISCUSSION

A previous study (Tomita *et al.*, 1982) and the present one suggest that there are nitrite-reacting substances in foodstuffs which show mutagenicity to *S. typhimurium* TA100, TA1535 and TA100 SM^d. Nitrite-induced mutagenicities were found not only for individual foodstuffs but for all food groups tested. Since this activity was without metabolic activation, it is not due to the dimethyl- and diethylamines that are frequently found in food and beverages. Spermidine (Kokatnur *et al.*, 1978; Hotchkiss *et al.*, 1979, guanidines (Endo & Takahashi, 1973) and some amino acids, including arginine (Endo *et al.*, 1974), tryptophan and methionine (Ohta *et al.*, 1981; Ohta & Suzuki, 1983) are known to act as direct mutagens after nitrite treatment. We therefore examined the mutagenic activities of these compounds after incubation with nitrite at 37 °C for 10 min at pH 4.2 and found that spermidine and spermine show fairly high mutagenic activities to *S. typhimurium* TA100 and TA1535 (Table 4). The spermidine content of 25 foodstuffs examined, as analysed by gas chromatography, however, was 0–463 μmol/kg or L and its contribution to the observed mutagenic activities was usually calculated to be less than 1%.

Other food components that are known to produce directly-acting mutagens with nitrite include various amino carbonyl reaction products. 1-(2-Furyl)-β-carboline and its 3-carboxylic acid, which were isolated from the reaction mixture of L-tryptophan and L-ascorbic acid (Kanamori *et al.*, 1980), show increased mutagenicity in the presence of nitrite. Nondialysable melanoidins from the reaction mixtures of L-tryptophan with diacetyl, furfural or 5-hydroxy methyl furfural all show mutagenicity to *S. typhimurium* TA100 in the presence of nitrite, with activities ranging from 900–4 000 revertants/mg. The contribution of these substances to the mutagenic activities of individual foodstuffs is now being analysed.

Table 4. Increases in mutagenic activities by nitrite treatment of amines in the Ames assay without metabolic activation

Compound	Net *his*[+] revertants/µmol	
	TA1535	TA100
Agmatine	8.8	2.8
L-Arginine	–	0
Methyl guanidine	20.4	0
Sarcosine	–	0
Spermidine	244.4	144.8
Spermine	132.0	108.4
DL-Tryptophan	–	83.0

Acidic, basic and neutral fractions of alcoholic beverages also show mutagenicity after nitrite treatment. As the basic fractions of beer produced the highest activities/mg extract, the premutagenic substances therein have been separated and determined to be 1,2,3,4-tetrahydro-β-carboline and its 1-methyl derivative.

ACKNOWLEDGEMENTS

We are grateful to Dr Taijiro Matsushima (Department of Molecular Oncology, Institute of Medical Science, University of Tokyo, Tokyo) and Dr Tsuneo Kada (National Institute of Genetics, Mishima) for supplying us with *S. typhimurium* TA100 and TA100 SM[d], respectively.

This work was supported in part by Grants-in-Aid for Cancer Research from the Ministry of Health and Welfare of Japan.

REFERENCES

Ames, B.N., McCann, J. & Yamasaki, E. (1975) Methods for detecting carcinogens and mutagens with the *Salmonella*/mammalian microsome mutagenicity test. *Mutat. Res., 31,* 347–364

Endo, H. & Takahashi, K. (1973) Methylguanidine, a naturally occurring compound showing mutagenicity after nitrosation in gastric juice. *Nature, 245,* 325–326

Endo, H., Takahashi, K. & Aoyagi, H. (1974) Screening of compounds structurally and functionally related to *N*-methyl-*N'*-nitro-*N*-nitrosoguanidine, a gastric carcinogen. *Gann, 65(1),* 45–54

Hotchkiss, J.H., Scanlan, R.A., Lijinsky, W. & Andrews, A.W. (1979) Mutagenicity of nitrosamines formed from nitrosation of spermidine. *Mutat. Res., 68,* 195–199

Kada, T., Aoki, K. & Sugimura, T. (1983) Isolation of streptomicine-dependent strains from *Salmonella typhimurium* TA98 and TA100 and their use in mutagenicity tests. *Environ. Mutagenesis, 5,* 9–15

Kanamori, H., Morimoto, K., Kinae, N. & Tomita, I. (1980) The formation of the mutagenic substances in the reaction between *L*-ascorbic acid and *L*-tryptophan. *Chem. Pharm. Bull., 28(10),* 3143–3144

Kokatnur, M.G., Murray, M.L. & Correa, P. (1978) Mutagenic properties of nitrosated spermidine. *Proc. Soc exp. Biol. Med., 158,* 85–88

Lee, J.S.K. & Fong, Y.Y. (1979) Mutagenicity of Chinese alcoholic spirits. *Food Cosmet. Toxicol., 17,* 575–578

Lin, J.Y., Wang, H.I. & Yeh, Y.C. (1979) The mutagenicity of soya bean sauce. *Food Cosmet. Toxicol., 17,* 329–331

Lin, J.Y. & Tai, M.W. (1980) Mutagenicity of Chinese wine treated with nitrite. *Food Cosmet. Toxicol., 18,* 241–243

Marquardt, H., Rufino, F. & Weisburger, J.H. (1977) Mutagenic activity of nitrite-treated foods: human stomach cancer may be related to dietary factors. *Science, 196,* 1000–1001

Mirvish, S.S. (1975) Formation of *N*-nitroso compounds - chemistry, kinetics and *in vivo* occurrence. *Toxicol. appl. Pharmacol., 31,* 325–351

Nagao, M., Takahashi, Y., Wakabayashi, K. & Sugimura, T. (1981) Mutagenicity of alcoholic beverages. *Mutat. Res., 88,* 147–154

Nakamura, Y., Takenaka, H. & Tomita, I. (1980) Mutagenic activities of nitrite and its reaction products. *Mutagens Toxicol., 11,* 30–38 (in Japanese)

Ohta, T., Isa, M., Suzuki, Y., Yamahata, N., Suzuki, S. & Kurechi, T. (1981) Formation of mutagens from tryptophan by the reaction with nitrite. *Biochem. biophys. Res. Commun., 100,* 52–57

Ohta, T. & Suzuki, S. (1983) Formation of mutagens by reaction of amino acids with nitrite in acidic solution. *Agric. biol. Chem., 47,* 405–406

Sugimura, T. & Sato, S. (1983) Mutagens/carcinogens in foods. *Cancer Res.,43,* 2415–2421

Tomita, I., Nakamura, Y. & Takenaka, H. (1982) *Mutagenicity of various Japanese foodstuffs treated with nitrite.* In: Bartsch, H., O'Neill, I.K., Castegnaro, M. & Okada, M., eds, N-*Nitroso Compounds: Occurrence and Biological Effects (IARC Scientific Publications No. 41),* Lyon, International Agency for Research on Cancer, pp. 575–583

Yahagi, T., Nagao, M., Seino, Y., Matsushima, T., Sugimura, T. & Okada, M. (1977) Mutagenicities of *N*-nitrosamines on *Salmonella. Mutat. Res., 48,* 121–130

DETERMINATION OF *N*-NITROSOBIS(2-HYDROXYPROPYL)AMINE IN ENVIRONMENTAL SAMPLES

P. ISSENBERG, E.E. CONRAD[1], J.W. NIELSEN[2], D.A. KLEIN & S.E. MILLER

Eppley Institute for Research in Cancer,
University of Nebraska Medical Center, Omaha, NE, USA

SUMMARY

N-Nitrosobis(2-hydroxypropyl)amine (ND2HPA) is a potent pancreatic carcinogen in hamsters and induces gastrointestinal and respiratory tract cancer in rats. The precursor amines, diisopropanolamine (Di-PA) and triisopropanolamine (Ti-PA), are used in some manufacturing processes and in cosmetic preparations. We have found low levels of ND2HPA in commercial Ti-PA (21–270 ng/g) and in Di-PA (20–1 300 ng/g) and have demonstrated that ND2HPA is formed from Ti-PA and nitrite in a yield comparable to that observed for formation of *N*-nitrosodiethanolamine (NDELA) from triethanolamine under relatively mild conditions. After reaction for 4 h at 37 °C (10 mmol/L amine, 40 mmol/L nitrite, pH 3.0), the ND2HPA yield was 0.51%. The NDELA yield under the same conditions was 0.96%.

ND2HPA was determined by gas chromatography-thermal energy analysis (GC-TEA) and GC-high-resolution mass spectrometry (GC-MS) selected ion monitoring of the *tert*-butyldimethylsilyl (t-BDMS) ether after extraction on a Celite 560 column. The t-BDMS ethers of ND2HPA and NDELA yielded intense, structurally significant peaks at m/z 333.2030 and 305.1716, respectively. The GC-MS procedure provides sensitivity and selectivity comparable to that of GC-TEA.

INTRODUCTION

N-Nitrosobis(2-hydroxypropyl)amine (ND2HPA) is a potent pancreatic carcinogen in hamsters (Pour *et al.*, 1974) and induces tumours of the colon, respiratory tract, oesophagus and liver in rats (Lijinsky & Taylor, 1978; Pour *et al.*, 1979). ND2HPA has not been reported as an environmental contaminant, but its structural similarity to *N*-nitrosodiethanolamine (NDELA), which has been found at high levels in cosmetics (Fan *et al.*, 1977a), cutting fluids (Fan *et al.*, 1977b) and tobacco (Schmeltz *et al.*, 1977), suggests that ND2HPA could be formed from the precursor amines, diisopropanolamine (Di-PA) and triisopropanolamine (Ti-PA) under the same conditions which lead to formation of NDELA.

---

[1] Present address: Midwest Research Institute, Kansas City, MO 64112, USA
[2] Present address: The Upjohn Co., Kalamazoo, MI 49001, USA

The precursors of ND2HPA are used in some cosmetic formulations. Alkanolamines, including Di-PA and Ti-PA are used in a variety of industrial processes and commercial products, including corrosion inhibitors, detergents, gas conditioners, textiles, electroplating materials, metal cleaning and rust removal products, rubber manufacturing chemicals, fuel and lubricant additives, leather fat liquoring and tanning materials and photographic emulsions and sensitizers (Dow Chemical Co., 1981). Specific data on the amounts of Di-PA and Ti-PA used in these applications are not available.

ND2HPA was absorbed rapidly when applied to the skin of hamsters (Pour *et al.,* 1980), and a weekly cutaneous application of 50 mg induced a high incidence of pancreatic carcinomas. It is not known whether ND2HPA induces cancer of the pancreas or at other sites in humans, but there is clear potential human exposure. These studies were undertaken to develop reliable methods for quantitative determination of ND2HPA in environmental samples to allow estimation of the extent of human exposure.

MATERIALS AND METHODS

Chemicals

All chemicals used were of analytical reagent grade, except where indicated. Solvents were obtained from Burdick and Jackson (Muskegon, MI, USA; distilled in glass) and were used without additional purification. Di-PA and Ti-PA samples were purchased from Eastman Kodak Co. (Rochester, NY, USA) or were provided by Dow Chemical Co. (Midland, MI, USA).

Extraction and concentration

Samples of amines (5–10 g) were dissolved in 15–30 mL sulfamic acid solution (15% ammonium sulfamate in 12% sulfuric acid). This solution was saturated with 15–30 g ammonium sulfate, transferred to a glass column containing 25 g Celite 560 (Johns Manville Co., New York, NY, USA), sieved to remove particles smaller than 60-mesh size, and extracted with 150 mL ethyl acetate. Extracts were concentrated to 0.5 mL in a rotary evaporator (Rotavapor-RE, Büchi, Switzerland) with a water-bath temperature of 30 °C.

Derivatization

For preparation of *tert*-butyldimethylsilyl (t-BDMS) ethers, the concentrates or pure *N*-nitrosamines were transferred, in 3 mL dichloromethane, to a 5-mL Reactivial (Pierce Chemical Co., Rockford, IL, USA) and concentrated to 0.1 mL under a stream of dry nitrogen; 0.5 mL *tert*-butyldimethylchlorosilane/imidazole reagent (Applied Science Laboratories, State College, PA, USA) was added, and the solution was heated at 60 °C for 30 min. One mL of a 10% aqueous sodium hydroxide solution was added, and the mixture was extracted three times with 0.5 mL hexane. The hexane extracts, in a 3-mL Reactivial, were concentrated to 0.2 or 1 mL in a nitrogen stream.

Trimethylsilyl (TMS) ethers of ND2HPA and NDELA were prepared by adding the *N*-nitrosamine to 250 μL Tri-Sil (Pierce Chemical Co., Rockford, IL, USA). The mixture was heated at 60 °C for 30 min and injected onto the gas chromatograph column.

Gas chromatography

Quantitative determination of t-BDMS derivatives was performed using a 2 m × 2 mm i.d. glass column packed with 1% Carbowax 20 M-TPA on 100/120 mesh Chromosorb G (Johns Manville, New York, NY, USA) at 190 °C. Injector temperature was 225 °C, and helium carrier gas flow rate was 20 mL/min. The gas chromatograph (model 2200, Bendix Corp., Ronceverte, WV, USA) was connected to a Thermal Energy Analyzer (TEA, model 502, Thermo Electron Corp., Waltham, MA, USA). TEA furnace temperature was 450 °C, oxygen flow rate was 20 mL/min, and reaction chamber pressure was 0.2 torr (26.7 Pa). For combined gas chromatographic-mass spectrometric analysis (GC-MS), a 30 m × 0.32 mm i.d. fused silica capillary column coated with Durawax, DX-4 (J. & W. Scientific, Rancho Cordova, CA, USA) was operated at 140 °C. Injector temperature was 250 °C, and the split ratio was approximately 30 : 1. Linear velocity was 30 cm/sec.

Mass spectrometry

The MS9 mass spectrometer (AEI, Manchester, UK) was equipped with a solid-state electronics console (model 200, Mass Spectrometry Services, Ltd, Manchester, UK). High-resolution ($M/\Delta M = 10\,000$) spectra of reference compounds were recorded at a scan rate of 10 sec/decade and processed by a series 2 000 data system (VG Analytical, Manchester, UK).

For confirmation of identity of ND2HPA in amine samples, extracts were analysed by high-resolution selected ion monitoring (SIM) of the (M^+–57) peak of the t-BDMS derivative at m/z 333.2030. The perfluoroalkane reference peak at m/z 330.9793 and sample peaks were scanned alternately using a 200-ppm sweep width and 0.3-sec sweep time. Peak amplitudes and distances between reference and sample peaks were measured manually from the oscillograph record.

Formation of ND2HPA

Ti-PA (10 mmol/L) and nitrite (40 mmol/L) were reacted at pH 3.0 (50 mmol/L formate buffer) for 4 h at 37 °C. Triethanolamine was reacted with nitrite as a reference sample. The reaction was stopped by addition of sulfamic acid (400 mmol/L), and the mixtures were analysed by the column extraction, GC-TEA procedure.

Recovery of ND2HPA and artefact detection

ND2HPA (500 or 1 000 ng/g) was added to samples of Di-PA and Ti-PA, and the samples were analysed as described above to determine recovery of the N-nitrosamine. A solution of 5 g Ti-PA in 15 mL sulfamic acid solution was exposed to long wavelength (366 nm) ultra-violet radiation from a Model B-100A lamp (Ultra-violet Products, Inc., San Gabriel, CA, USA) for 4 h to destroy any N-nitrosamine present. This sample was analysed as described above to determine whether ND2HPA could be formed during the analytical procedure.

RESULTS

Mass spectra of t-BDMS derivatives

Mass spectra of the t-BDMS ethers of ND2HPA and NDELA are compared with spectra of TMS derivatives in Figures 1 and 2. Intense peaks corresponding to loss of a *tert*-butyl group (M^+–57) appear at m/z 333 and 305 in the spectra of the t-BDMS derivatives of ND2HPA and NDELA, respectively. The (M^+–57) peak was approximately 60% relative intensity and accounted for 11–14% of the total ion current. Composition of these ions was confirmed by accurate mass measurements.

Fig. 1. Electron impact mass spectra of (A) *N*-nitrosodiethanolamine-bis-trimethylsilylether (mw, 278) and (B) *N*-nitrosodiethanolamine-bis-*tert*-butyl-dimethylsilylether (MW 362)

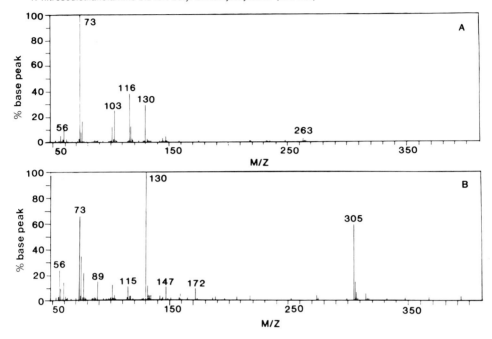

Fig. 2. Electron impact mass spectra of (A) *N*-nitrosobis(2-hydroxypropyl)amine-bis-trimethylsilylether (mw, 306) and (B) *N*-nitrosobis(2-hydroxypropyl)amine-bis-*tert*-butyldimethylsilylether (mw, 390)

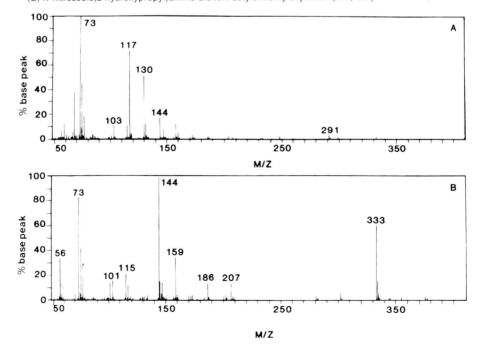

GC-TEA and GC-MS determination of ND2HPA

A GC-TEA chromatogram of a concentrate prepared from a Di-PA sample is shown in Figure 3. The ND2HPA-t-BDMS ether peak area corresponds to a concentration of 26 ng/g. ND2HPA was not detectable in the capillary column gas chromatogram when a flame-ionization detector was employed, but was readily detected employing low-resolution (M/ΔM = 1 000) SIM. Figure 4 is the SIM record for the Di-PA sample on the capillary column with monitoring of the m/z 333 ion. High-resolution SIM confirmed that this peak yielded ions at m/z 333.2 030. Concentrations measured were: GC-TEA, 26 ng/g; low-resolution SIM, 22 ng/g; high-resolution SIM, 20 ng/g.

The range of ND2HPA concentrations in Di-PA samples examined was 20–1 300 ng/g. Levels in Ti-PA were between 21 and 270 ng/g.

Fig. 3. Gas chromatographic-Thermal Energy Analyzer (TEA) chromatograms of (A) 3 ng *N*-nitrosobis(2-hydroxypropyl)amine-*tert*-butyldimethylsilylether; and (B) 2 µL of 0.2 mL concentrate prepared from diisopropanolamine containing 26 ng/g *N*-nitrosobis(2-hydroxypropyl)amine. Packed column

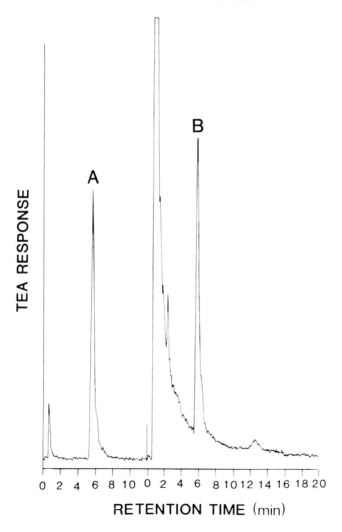

Fig. 4. Low-resolution (M/ΔM = 1 000) selected ion monitor chromatogram (m/z 333) of (A) 5 ng *N*-nitrosobis(2-hydroxypropyl)amine as *tert*-butyldimethylsilyl ether; and (B) 5 μL of 0.2 mL concentrate prepared from diisopropanolamine. Capillary column. Same sample as in Fig. 3

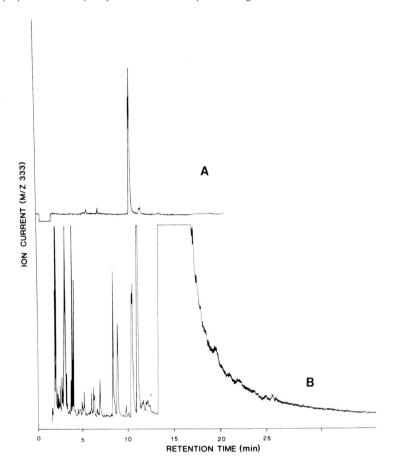

Formation of ND2HPA

The yield of ND2HPA after 4 h at 37 °C was 0.51% of the Ti-PA present. Under the same conditions, the yield of NDELA from triethanolamine was 0.96%.

Recovery of ND2HPA and artefact formation

The ND2HPA level initially determined in the Ti-PA sample was 240 ng/g. When 500 ng/g ND2HPA was added, 710 ng/g was found, indicating 96% recovery. In four samples of Di-PA to which 1 000 ng/g of ND2HPA had been added, recovery was between 83% and 99%.

No ND2HPA was detected in the Ti-PA sample exposed to ultra-violet radiation for 4 h. The initial concentration of ND2HPA in this sample was 240 ng/g. The detection limit for this experiment was approximately 70 ng/g.

DISCUSSION

We have demonstrated that ND2HPA is a trace contaminant of commercial samples of Di-PA and Ti-PA. All amine samples examined contained detectable levels of ND2HPA, the highest levels (1 300 ng/g) being found in samples that were at least five years old. Samples procured recently contained 20–25 ng/g ND2HPA. These results are consistent with those of Spiegelhalder *et al.* (1978), who found that all samples of commercial secondary amines examined by them contained trace levels of the corresponding *N*-nitrosamines. We have initiated a survey of cosmetic preparations formulated with Di-PA and Ti-PA to determine whether ND2HPA is formed at significant levels in these products. Our results suggest that ND2HPA is formed from its precursors as readily as is NDELA.

Hydroxy-*N*-nitrosamines can be determined by GC without derivatization, but minimum detection limits are at least two orders of magnitude lower when volatile derivatives are employed (Ohshima *et al.*, 1979). Mass spectra of the bis-TMS ethers of ND2HPA and NDELA contain an (M^+-15) peak, which provides structural information; however, the relative intensity of this peak is low (5–6%) but adequate if sufficient quantities of nitrosamine can be isolated (Schmeltz *et al.*, 1977). The facile loss of a *tert*-butyl group from t-BDMS ethers provides an intense (60% relative intensity) peak for routine confirmation of identity of traces of hydroxy-*N*-nitrosamines present in environmental samples. This ion contains all the heteroatoms of the original molecule and is particularly appropriate for either high- or low-resolution SIM. Use of the polar capillary GC column and high-resolution SIM obviated the need for additional clean-up of the amine samples. When packed GC columns were employed, clean-up by HPLC was required to eliminate interferences in quantitative determination of ND2HPA by high-resolution SIM. In all reference and isolated samples of ND2HPA examined, two partially resolved peaks were observed in the capillary gas chromatogram. Mass spectra of the two components were identical. We believe the two components to be diastereoisomers.

ACKNOWLEDGEMENTS

This work was supported by US Public Health Service Grant RO1 CA-29197 from the National Cancer Institute. The Thermal Energy Analyzer was lent to us by the National Cancer Institute under Contract NO1-CP33278. The mass spectrometer control console was purchased with a grant from the University of Nebraska Foundation.

REFERENCES

Dow Chemical Co. (1981) *The Alkanolamines Handbook*, Midland, MI

Fan, T.Y., Goff, U., Song, L., Fine, D.H., Arsenault, G.P. & Biemann, K. (1977a) *N*-Nitrosodiethanol-amine in cosmetics, lotions and shampoos. *Food Cosmet. Toxicol.*, **15**, 423–430

Fan, T.Y., Morrison, J., Rounbehler, D.P., Ross, R., Fine, D.H., Miles, W. & Sen, N.P. (1977b) *N*-Nitrosodiethanolamine in synthetic cutting fluids: a part-per-hundred impurity. *Science*, **196**, 70

Lijinsky, W. & Taylor, H.W. (1978) Comparative carcinogenicity of some derivatives of nitrosodi-*n*-propylamine in rats. *Ecotoxicol. environ. Saf.*, **2**, 421–426

Ohshima, H., Matsui, M. & Kawabata, T. (1979) Gas chromatographic separation of hydroxylated *N*-nitrosamines. *J. Chromatogr.*, **169**, 279–286

Pour, P., Krüger, F.W., Althoff, J., Cardesa, A. & Mohr, U. (1974) The effect of beta-oxidized nitrosamines on Syrian golden hamsters. 3. 2,2'-Dihydroxy-di-*n*-propylnitrosamine. *J. natl Cancer Inst.*, **54**, 141–146

Pour, P., Salmasi, S., Runge, R., Gingell, R., Wallcave, L., Nagel, D. & Stepan, K. (1979) Carcinogenicity of *N*-nitrosobis(2-hydroxypropyl)amine and *N*-nitrosobis(2-oxopropyl)amine in MRC rats. *J. natl Cancer Inst.,* **63**, 181–190

Pour, P., Wallcave, L., Nagel, D. & Salmasi, S. (1980) Induction of local epidermal papillomas and carcinomas by selected nitrosamines. *Cancer Lett.,* **10**, 365–373

Schmeltz, I., Abidi, S. & Hoffmann, D. (1977) Tumorigenic agents in unburned processed tobacco: *N*-nitrosodiethanolamine and 1,1-dimethylhydrazine. *Cancer Lett.,* **2**, 125–132

Spiegelhalder, B., Eisenbrand, G. & Preussmann, R. (1978) Contamination of amines with *N*-nitrosamines. *Angew. Chem. Int. Ed. Engl.,* **17**, 367–368

VOLATILE *N*-NITROSAMINES IN BABY BOTTLE RUBBER NIPPLES AND PACIFIERS. ANALYSIS, OCCURRENCE AND MIGRATION

N.P. SEN[1] & S. SEAMAN

Food Research Division, Food Directorate, Health Protection Branch, Ottawa, K1A OL2, Canada

S. CLARKSON, F. GARROD & P. LALONDE

Scientific and Laboratory Services Division, Product Safety Branch, Department of Consumer and Corporate Affairs, Ottawa K1A OC9, Canada

SUMMARY

A simple direct extraction method has been developed for rapid determination of volatile *N*-nitrosamines in rubber nipples and pacifiers. It consists of overnight extraction of the sample with dichloromethane in the presence of ascorbyl palmitate for *N*-nitrosation inhibition, filtration of the extract and rinsing of the samples with dichloromethane, concentration of the extract using a Kuderna-Danish concentrator, and final analysis by gas-liquid chromatography-Thermal Energy Analyser. The method gave excellent (80–100%) recoveries of various volatile *N*-nitrosamines that had been added to cut nipples or pacifiers at 20–80 μg/kg levels, and gave comparable or lower values than those obtained with another published method. The method is recommended for rapid screening purposes.

A survey of 30 samples of various nipples and pacifiers indicated the presence of the following *N*-nitrosamines: *N*-nitrosodimethylamine (up to 70 μg/kg), *N*-nitrosodiethylamine (up to 88 μg/kg), *N*-nitrosodi-*n*-butylamine (up to 2 796 μg/kg), *N*-nitrosopiperidine (up to 180 μg/kg), and *N*-nitrosomorpholine (up to 86 μg/kg). A more recent study, however, indicated a general decline in the levels of various volatile *N*-nitrosamines in these products. These *N*-nitrosamines were shown to migrate easily from the rubber products to liquid infant formula, orange juice and simulated human saliva.

INTRODUCTION

Our present concern about the occurrence of various *N*-nitrosamines in rubber nipples and pacifiers and their possible migration into infant formulae and saliva of infants sucking these products arose mainly from the recent findings of Spiegelhalder and Preussmann (1982).

---

[1] To whom correspondence should be sent

Earlier, Ireland *et al.* (1980) reported the occurrence of several volatile *N*-nitrosamines in a variety of rubber products such as rubber gloves, baby-bottle rubber nipples and condoms. The sources of the *N*-nitrosamines were shown to be various dialkylamine-compounding ingredients (e.g., dithiocarbamates, sulfenamides, thiuram mono- and polysulfides and thioureas) used as accelerators and stabilizers in the manufacture of the rubber products. More recently, studies in the USA (Havery & Fazio, 1982) and Japan (Ishiwata *et al.*, 1981) confirmed these findings. One interesting observation made in the US study was that even after repeated (up to seven times) sterilization of a rubber nipple, traces of *N*-nitrosamines were still found to migrate into milk that came in contact with the nipple during the sterilization process.

Various methods have been proposed to determine the levels of volatile *N*-nitrosamines in rubber nipples and pacifiers. Although they all work reasonably well and serve specific purposes, some of them are quite lengthy and time-consuming. There seems to be a need to develop a simple method that will be useful for routine analysis. The first part of our report deals with these analytical problems. In the second part, we present data on the levels of volatile *N*-nitrosamines in rubber nipples and pacifiers and on the migration of various *N*-nitrosamines from these rubber articles to infant formulae, orange juice and simulated human saliva.

EXPERIMENTAL

Determination of volatile N-nitrosamines in rubber products

Two techniques were used:

Method 1: The technique was very similar to that described by Havery and Fazio (1982) Briefly, it involved gentle shaking of the sample (cut into small pieces) with dichloromethane (DCM) in a stoppered flask overnight, followed by Soxhlet extraction of the nipple pieces with DCM for 1 h, addition of 5 mol/L sodium hydroxide to the DCM extract, isolation of the volatile *N*-nitrosamines by atmospheric distillation of the mixture at atmospheric pressure, re-extraction of the aqueous distillate with DCM, concentration of the dried DCM extract using Kuderna-Danish concentrators (both macro and micro), and final analysis by gas-liquid chromatography-Thermal Energy Analyzer (GLC-TEA). No nitrosation inhibitor was added at any stage.

GLC-TEA conditions: A 2.75 m × 3.2 mm (o.d.) Ni column was used, packed with 10% Carbowax 20 M and 5% KOH on 100/120 mesh Chromosorb WHP. Injection port (with glass injector port insert) and transfer line (from column to TEA) temperatures were 200 °C and 290 °C, respectively. The GLC oven was operated at 140 °C, and the carrier gas (Ar) flow rate was about 40 mL/min. The TEA operating conditions were similar to those described by Sen *et al.* (1983). The GLC-TEA analyses of standard *N*-nitrosamine mixtures were repeated until two successive injections gave similar results. (See note added in proof below.)

Method 2: The cut nipple pieces (≤ 2 g) were shaken gently overnight in a stoppered flask with 100 mL DCM and 100–300 mg ascorbyl palmitate. Next morning the mixture was gradually poured into an empty glass column (190 mm × 18 mm) fitted with a Teflon® stopcock and containing a loosely placed glass-wool ball at the bottom. The extract was allowed to drain from the column and filter through a coarse sintered-glass filter funnel, and the filtrate collected in a Kuderna-Danish concentrator. After all the liquid drained out of the column, the stopcock was closed, and the extraction flask was rinsed with 20 mL DCM, which was poured into the column containing the nipple pieces. The sample pieces were allowed to soak in the DCM for 10 min, and the liquid was drained out through the stopcock and filtered through sintered glass into the concentrator, as described above. The above rinsing, soaking and filtration steps were repeated once more. Finally, the combined filtrate was concentrated to 1.0 mL, as in method 1, and a 6.0-μL aliquot was analysed by GLC-TEA. For extracts that caused excessive foaming during the final concentration step (from 4 mL to 1 mL), the regular micro Snyder column was replaced with a modified column that did not contain the floating balls (Kontes Glassware, Vineland, NJ, USA, catalogue No. K-5969251, with 19/22 joints).

Determination of volatile N-nitrosamines in infant formula, orange juice and simulated saliva

The samples (except for the simulated saliva) were made alkaline and distilled at normal atmospheric pressure until about 70–80% of the aqueous starting material had been distilled. The *N*-nitrosamines in the aqueous distillate were extracted into DCM and analysed by GLC-TEA in the usual manner (Sen *et al.*, 1979). For the simulated saliva samples, the distillation step was omitted. These were made alkaline, extracted with DCM, then processed as above.

Migration studies

Migration studies were carried out by a method similar to that of Spiegelhalder and Preussmann (1982) and are described briefly in footnotes to Table 3.

Gas-liquid chromatography-high-resolution mass spectrometry (GLC-MS)

Extracts of several samples were pooled and further cleaned up by vacuum distillation ($\simeq 45\,^\circ$C) and chromatography on basic alumina, as described previously (Sen *et al.*, 1979). A 5-μL aliquot of the final concentrated extract (1.0 mL) was analysed by GLC-MS. The MS was operated in the single-ion monitoring mode for the respective molecular ions at a resolution of 5 000 (Sen *et al.*, 1979).

RESULTS AND DISCUSSION

Table 1 gives the levels of volatile *N*-nitrosamines detected in eight samples of nipples and pacifiers analysed by the two methods. As can be see, there were some major differences (e.g., in samples A_1, A_3 and J_2) between the two sets of results. In all cases, method 2 gave results that were either lower or comparable to those obtained by method 1. Halves of the same nipple or pacifier were used in the comparative studies to ensure uniformity of the samples used in the two tests (Havery & Fazio, 1982).

Several explanations, such as lower recoveries or incomplete extraction (due to omission of the Soxhlet extraction step) of the *N*-nitrosamines in method 2, could be proposed for the lower results obtained from some samples (e.g., A_1, A_3, J_2). These explanations are thought to be highly unlikely, however, because recoveries of various *N*-nitrosamines added to cut nipple pieces at 20–80 μg/kg levels were comparable (80–100%) for the two methods. Moreover, a further Soxhlet extraction of the nipple pieces from method 2 with fresh DCM failed to extract any significant quantities of *N*-nitrosamines, thus ruling out incomplete extraction. It should be mentioned that in carrying out the second Soxhlet extraction of the nipple pieces from method 2, heating was carried out in a 70 °C water bath (to avoid overheating), and about 100 mg ascorbyl palmitate were added to the DCM as a nitrosation inhibitor. Since these rubber products contain both the necessary precursors (amines and nitrosating agents) for *N*-nitrosamine formation, it is conceivable that the addition of ascorbyl palmitate in method 2 prevented or minimized artefactual formation of *N*-nitrosamines, thus explaining some of the low results obtained with this method. Additional work is needed, however, to prove this point conclusively.

Table 1. Comparison of two methods for the analysis of volatile *N*-nitrosamines in rubber nipples and pacifiers[a]

Brand	*N*-Nitrosamines[b] detected	Levels (µg/kg)	
		Method 1	Method 2
A₁	NDMA	5.6	N[c]
	NDEA	tr[d]	tr
	NDBA	tr	tr
	NPIP	53.6	44.9
A₂	NDMA	2.2	tr
	NDEA	5.6	N
	NPIP	108.0	103.7
A₃	NDEA	8.2	3.9
	NDBA	32.0	13.3
	NPIP	50.4	38.5
	unknown[e]	48.5	6.8
H₁	NDMA	6.5	4.2
J₁	NDBA	379	396
	unknown[e]	1 148	1 142
J₂	NDEA	65.9	21.1
	NDBA	938	241
	unknown[e]	701	681
K₁	NDBA	tr	N
F₁	NDMA	N	N
	NDBA	120	81.7
	NPIP	24.5	21.2

[a] All comparisons were made using halves from same nipple
[b] NDMA, *N*-nitrosodimethylamine; NDEA, *N*-nitrosodiethylamine; NDBA, *N*-nitrosodi-*n*-butylamine; NPIP, *N*-nitrosopiperidine; NPYR, *N*-nitrosopyrrolidine; NMOR, *N*-nitrosomorpholine
[c] N, negative (<1 µg/kg)
[d] tr, trace (1–2 µg/kg)
[e] Unknown with a relative retention time of 1.42 with respect to NPYR. Its concentration was estimated assuming the same molar response as that of NMOR

Ascorbyl palmitate is a well-known inhibitor of *N*-nitrosation (Sen *et al.*, 1976; Kabacoff *et al.*, 1981). Therefore, in developing the direct extraction method (method 2), it was thought that its addition would be helpful in preventing artefactual formation of *N*-nitrosamines. In order to demonstrate its usefulness, two sets of DCM extracts (one with 100 mg ascorbyl palmitate and the other without) of a rubber nipple (Brand A) were prepared by overnight extraction and the nipple pieces removed by filtration through a column, as described under method 2. Each extract was then boiled (in a 70 °C water bath) under a reflux condenser for 7 h, then directly concentrated and analysed, as described earlier. The extract prepared without ascorbyl palmitate was found to contain traces of *N*-nitrosodiethylamine and 77.8 µg/kg *N*-nitrosopiperidine whereas that from the other half of the same nipple prepared with the addition of ascorbyl palmitate contained only 46.5 µg/kg *N*-nitrosopiperidine suggesting artefactual formation of *N*-nitrosamines in the absence of ascorbyl palmitate. Although it is realized that refluxing for 7 h is not a standard analytical procedure, heating for shorter periods (e.g., 1–1.5 h during Soxhlet extraction and another 1 h during concentration) is not uncommon. Therefore, the inclusion of some ascorbyl palmitate (preferably 100 mg) in method 2 would be useful in preventing or minimizing formation of *N*-nitrosamines during the analytical process.

In comparison to method 1, method 2 is much simpler and faster. It does not employ the time-consuming Soxhlet extraction, which was shown to be unnecessary if the special rinsing procedure, the distillation and the reextraction (from aqueous distillate) steps are used. It also gave excellent (80–100%) recoveries of all the volatile N-nitrosamines listed in Table 1. The method would therefore be ideal for rapid screening purposes. Another advantage is that the same extract can be used for the analysis of nonvolatile N-nitroso compounds. Preliminary results suggest that a high-performance liquid chromatographic-TEA (HPLC-TEA) technique can be used for simultaneous analysis of vol.atile and nonvolatile N-nitroso compounds (e.g., N-nitrosodiphenylamine, N-nitrosomethylphenylamine), provided they can be separated on the HPLC column. There are two drawbacks, however. Since very little clean-up is carried out, the final extract is quite dirty, so that the glass insert in the injector port of the gas chromatograph must be replaced or cleaned quite regularly. (See note added in proof below.) The time and money saved (analysis time and materials), however, would greatly outweigh this minor disadvantage. If GLC-MS confirmation is desired, the extract can be cleaned up by low temperature vacuum distillation and chromatography on basic alumina, as reported previously (Sen *et al.*, 1979). The other disadvantage of method 2 is that it cannot be used for certain brands of pacifiers that contain too much DCM-soluble material, although it works well for most nipples and pacifiers available on the market.

Table 2 is a summary of a survey carried out between March 1982 and March 1983 on the levels of volatile N-nitrosamines detected in 30 samples of various nipples and pacifiers. Method 1 was used to obtain these results. All were positive, but both the type of N-nitrosamine detected and their levels varied widely from sample to sample. This is not surprising, because different manufacturers use different production methods (including the use of different accelerators and stabilizers). It may be noted that two samples (J and K) contained fairly high levels (up to 4 766 µg/kg, assuming the same molar response as that of N-nitrosomorpholine) on an unknown TEA-positive compound that had a relative retention time of 1.42 with respect to N-nitrosopyrrolidine and was distinguishable from N-nitrosomethylphenylamine and N-nitrosoethylphenylamine. Work on the identification of this compound is continuing.

Table 2.   Levels of volatile N-nitrosamines in baby bottle rubber nipples and pacifiers as determined by method 1 (see text for details)

Brand	No. of samples analysed	N-Nitrosamine levels (µg/kg)[a]				
		NDMA	NDEA	NDBA	NPIP	NMOR
Nipples						
A	6	N[b]–4.0	4–20[c]	N–10.4	37–146[c]	N–86.4
B	2	28–30.4[c]	N	N	N	N
C	1	N	N	4.2	N	N
D	1	0.3	1.3	N	N	N
E	1	9.4	34.4	N	N	N
F	5	N–47.7	9.2–13.3	160–341[c]	28–180[c]	N–28
G	2	N	N	332–354	N	N
H	3	23–70	N	1.6	N	N
I	1	22.3	16.3	N	N	N
J	3	N–17.2	22–88.4	938–2 796[c]	N	N
Pacifier						
K	5	N–8.6[c]	40–84[c]	N–122.6[c]	N	N–28

[a] NDMA, N-nitrosodimethylamine; NDEA, N-nitrosodiethylamine; NDBA, N-nitrosodi-n-butylamine; NPIP, N-nitrosopiperidine; NMOR, N-nitrosomorpholine
[b] N, negative (< 1 µg/kg)
[c] Confirmed by gas-liquid chromatography-high-resolution mass spectrometry

Table 3. Migration of volatile nitrosamines from various nipples and pacifiers into liquid infant formula[a], orange juice[a] and simulated human saliva[b]

Brand	Type[c]	N-Nitrosamines extracted (ng)[d]							
		NDMA		NDEA		NDBA		NPIP	
		formula	juice	formula	juice	formula	juice	formula	juice
Nipples									
A		N[e]	N	11.1	5.2	N	N	31.2	N
F		3.2	N	7.7	8.8	329	135	52.4	44
G		N	N	N	N	443	312	N	N
H		26.2	−[f]	N	−	N	−	N	−
Pacifiers		Extracted with simulated saliva							
C	PVC	<2		N		N			
E	latex	N		22.8		11.3			
F	PVC	N		N		N			
L	PVC	N		N		N			
F	latex	9.5		14.9		126			
K	latex	N		N		2 021			
L	latex	1.3		13.7		14.4			
M	latex	2.6		3.0		146			
N	latex	3.9		13.1		N			
O	latex	N		N		325			

[a] One nipple (5–9 g) was extracted for 1 h at 40 °C with 200 mL liquid infant formula or juice. Matched halves from same nipple were not used in these experiments
[b] One pacifier (1.7–13.7 g) was extracted for 24 h at 40 °C with 200 mL simulated saliva (4.2 g sodium bicarbonate, 0.5 g sodium chloride, 0.2 g potassium carbonate and 0.005 g sodium nitrite in 1 L water)
[c] PVC, polyvinylchloride polymer
[d] NDMA, N-nitrosodimethylamine; NDEA, N-nitrosodiethylamine; NDBA, N-nitrosodi-*n*-butylamine; NPIP, N-nitrosopiperidine
[e] N, negative (<2 ng)
[f] not analysed

The results of a more recent survey, carried out in July 1983, indicate a general decline in the levels of volatile *N*-nitrosamines in these products from those observed earlier (Table 2). Of 11 samples of various nipples and pacifiers analysed, only two contained > 10 µg/kg total volatile *N*-nitrosamines, and six were negative. Nine of these samples were analysed by method 2 and the remaining two by method 1.

The results (Table 3) of the migration studies suggest that significant quantities of various *N*-nitrosamines, especially *N*-nitrosodi-*n*-butylamine can migrate from these rubber products to liquid infant formula, orange juice and simulated saliva. These data are comparable to those of Spiegelhalder and Preussmann (1982) and of Havery and Fazio (1982). Moreover, any *N*-nitrosatable amine precursor that is extractable into saliva could form additional amounts of *N*-nitroso compounds *in vivo* in the stomachs of infants sucking these rubber articles (Spiegelhalder & Preussmann, 1982). Further work on migration is planned.

In summary, we have confirmed some earlier observations on the occurrence of various volatile *N*-nitrosamines in rubber nipples and pacifiers and have developed a simpler method of analysing these articles for volatile *N*-nitrosamines. It should be pointed out that method 2 measures only the volatile *N*-nitrosamines which are extractable into DCM. If one is interested in measuring the total potential for *N*-nitrosamine formation in these products, the simulated saliva extraction method of Spiegelhalder and Preussmann (1982) for *N*-nitroso compounds and their precursors should be used. Even with the latter method, it would be advisable to add small amounts of ascorbyl palmitate to the DCM extract, prior to concentration in the Kuderna-Danish concentrator.

Note added in proof: The use of Ni tubing (15 cm × 3.2 mm o.d.) packed with 1% SE-30 on Chromosorb W, high performance, 80–100 mesh, as a guard column has been found to increase column life to a great extent.

ACKNOWLEDGEMENTS

We wish to thank P.-Y. Lau of Food Research Division for carrying out the GLC-MS confirmation and R. Preussmann for providing us with *N*-nitrosomethylphenylamine and *N*-nitrosoethylphenylamine standards.

REFERENCES

Havery, D.C. & Fazio, T. (1982) Estimation of volatile *N*-nitrosamines in rubber nipples for babies' bottles. *Food Chem. Toxicol., 20,* 939–944

Ireland, C.B., Hytrek, F.P. & Lasoski, B.A. (1980) Aqueous extraction of *N*-nitrosamines from elastomers. *Am. ind. Hyg. Assoc. J., 41,* 895–900

Ishiwata, H., Kawasaki, Y., Yamamoto, M., Sasai, A., Yamada, T. & Tanimura, A. (1981) Nitrosamines in rubber nipples. *Bull. natl Inst. Hyg. Sci., 99,* 135–137

Kabacoff, B.L., Lechnir, R.J., Vielhuber, S.F. & Doublad, M.L. (1981) *Formation and inhibition of N-nitrosodiethanolamine in an anionic oil-water emulsion.* In: Scanlan, R.A. & Tannenbaum, S.R., eds, *N-Nitroso Compounds (ACS Symposium Series No. 174)*, Washington DC, American Chemical Society, pp. 149–156

Sen, N.P., Donaldson, B., Seaman, S., Iyengar, J.R. & Miles, W.F. (1976) Inhibition of nitrosamine formation in fried bacon by propyl gallate and L-ascorbyl palmitate. *J. Agric. Food. Chem., 24,* 397–401

Sen, N.P., Seaman, S. & Miles, W.F. (1979) Volatile nitrosamines in various cured meat products: Effect of cooking and recent trends. *J. Agric. Food Chem., 27,* 1354–1357

Sen, N.P., Tessier, L. & Seaman, S.W. (1983) Determination of *N*-nitrosoproline and *N*-nitrososarcosine in malt and beer. *J. Agric. Food Chem., 31,* 1033–1036

Spiegelhalder, B. & Preussmann, R. (1982) *Nitrosamines in rubber.* In: Bartsch, H., O'Neill, I.K., Castegnaro, M. & Okada, M., eds, N-*Nitroso Compounds: Occurrence and Biological Effects (IARC Scientific Publications No. 41)*, Lyon, International Agency for Research on Cancer, pp. 231–243

NEW *N*-NITROSO COMPOUNDS AND IMPROVED METHODS OF ANALYSIS

NITROSATION OF PEPTIDES

B.C. CHALLIS[1], A.R. HOPKINS & J.R. MILLIGAN

Chemistry Department, Imperial College, London SW7 2AZ, UK

R.C. MITCHELL

Smith, Kline & French Research Ltd, The Frythe, Welwyn, Herts AL6 9AR, UK

R.C. MASSEY

Ministry of Agriculture, Fisheries & Food, Haldin House, Queen St, Norwich NR2 4SX, UK

SUMMARY

The synthesis and characterization of N-(N-acetylprolyl)-N-nitroso-glycine, the first authentic N-nitrosopeptide, is described, and its stability under various conditions is reported. In acidic media, denitrosation and deamination (hydrolysis) occur concurrently, whereas in neutral and alkaline solutions, only deamination occurs.

The rates of formation and decomposition of some unprotected N-nitrosopeptides in strong acid are also reported. Conditions for the formation of such compounds in the gastric tract are discussed, together with their potential involvement in human cancer.

INTRODUCTION

Although peptides and proteins are common dietary constituents, not much is known about their interaction with nitrosating agents or the chemical and biological properties of the products. In principle, nitrosation could occur at both the terminal and peptide N-atoms, as well as at other sites in substrates containing cysteine, tryptophan, tyrosine, asparginine, glutamine, lysine and arginine moieties.

There is firm evidence that terminal N-atoms undergo nitrosation. For example, Curtius and Thompson (1906), and Curtius and Callan (1910) isolated diazo derivatives (e.g., I, Fig. 1) from the reaction of glycyl peptides with nitrite in glacial acetic acid (Fig. 1). In aqueous acid, the diazo derivative readily expels nitrogen to give the deaminated substrate (e.g., II). Rates of

---

[1] To whom requests for reprints should be addressed

CHALLIS *ET AL.*

Fig. 1. Scheme of the reaction of glycyl peptides with nitrite in glacial acetic acid

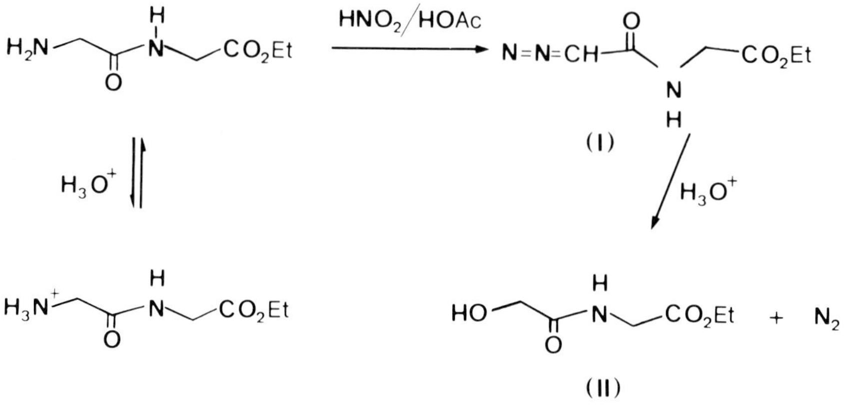

Fig. 2. Equation for the nitrosation of peptide *N*-atoms

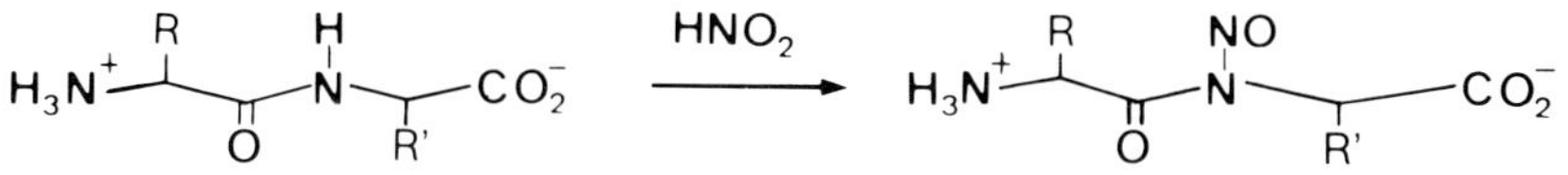

Fig. 3. Structures of *N*-nitrosopeptides (III) and *N*-(*N*-acetylprolyl)-*N*-nitrosoglycine (IV)

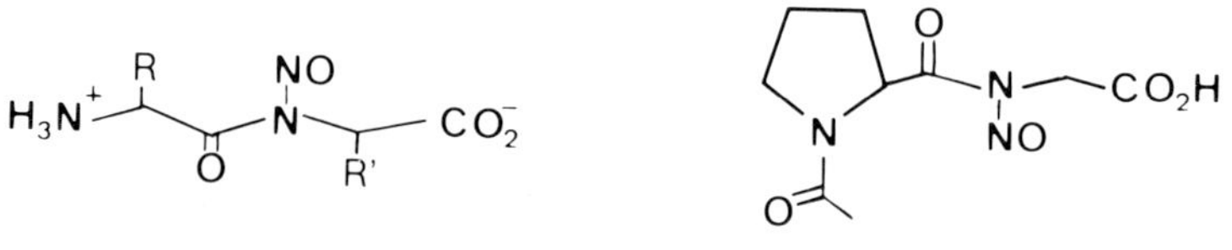

deamination of several peptides and proteins were determined by Kuroski and Hofmann (1972), who concluded that the initial nitrosation in dilute acid was brought about by dinitrogen trioxide.

There is also sound evidence that tyrosine residues in peptides and proteins undergo *C*-nitrosation. For example, several products from the reaction of pepsin (Philpot & Small, 1938) and bovine serum albumin (Knowles *et al.*, 1974) with aqueous nitrous acid probably derive from 3-nitrosotyrosine.

In contrast, evidence for the nitrosation of peptide *N*-atoms (Fig. 2) has proven elusive. The compounds observed by Pollock (1982) from reactions of dipeptides are now known to be *N*-nitrosoiminodialkanoic acids [$HO_2CCHR(HO_2CCHR')NNO$], which could form *via* an *N*-nitroso- or a diazo-peptide intermediate. Further, Bonnett and his colleagues (1975, 1979) found only tentative ^{15}N-nuclear magnetic resonance (NMR) evidence for *N*-nitrosopeptides, but they were able to isolate the *N*-nitroso derivatives as some *N*-acetylamino acid esters. The latter finding was corroborated by Chow and Polo (1980), who prepared the N-nitroso derivatives of some acylated α-amino acids in solution and showed them to decompose to several products under mild conditions.

By analogy with N-nitrosoamides, N-nitrosopeptides (III, Fig. 3) have potential for direct cellular interaction (Magee *et al.*, 1976). Thus their formation from dietary constituents in the stomach may have biological implications. Evaluation of this hypothesis requires the synthesis and examination of authentic compounds. Herein, we report on the synthesis and characterization of N-(N-acetylprolyl)-N-nitrosoglycine (IV, Fig. 3) and give preliminary information on its stability and chemical properties. Compound (IV), which was chosen to avoid complications arising from concurrent deamination or nitrosation of terminal N-atoms, appears to be the first authentic N-nitrosopeptide. We also report rates of formation and decomposition of (IV) and of several other N-nitrosopeptides (III) in aqueous acid.

MATERIALS AND METHODS

Aqueous hydrochloric acid and perchloric acid solutions were prepared by volumetric dilution of AVS and AnalaR 72% reagents, respectively, both supplied by BDH Ltd. Concentrations in the reactant solutions were checked by titration. Buffer solutions were prepared volumetrically from AnalaR grade formic acid, glacial acetic acid, potassium dihydrogen phosphate, disodium hydrogen phosphate, sodium borate and sodium hydroxide (BDH Ltd); their pH was measured both before and after reaction, with agreement to ± 0.01 units. Reagent grade hydrazine, Sulfamic acid, glycine, L-prolylglycine and L-cysteine (BDH Ltd) were used as supplied, as were glycylglycine and pentaglycine (Sigma). Other substrates were synthesized as described below.

Synthesis N-(N-acetylprolyl)-N-nitrosoglycine (IV)

N-(N-Acetylprolyl)-benzylglycinate in methylene chloride was reacted with gaseous dinitrogen tetraoxide, following White's (1955) procedure, to give the N-nitroso derivative in quantative yield as a yellow oil with the expected ultra-violet, infra-red and ^{1}H-NMR absorptions. On hydrogenolysis of the yellow oil in ethanol at atmospheric pressure over 5% palladium on charcoal, a yellow solid was obtained in 43% yield, which, on purification by recrystallization from ethyl acetate, gave N-(N-acetylprolyl)-N-nitrosoglycine: mp., 110 C (found: C, 44.5; H, 5.3; N, 17.1%; $C_9H_{13}N_3O_5$ requires C, 44.5; H, 5.4; N, 17.3%); λ_{max} (ethanol), 238, 389, 403, 426 nm (log ε, 3.76, 1.79, 1.97, 1.98); ν_{max} (nujol), 3 200–2 300, 1 740, 1 720, 1 590, 1 510 cm^{-1}; δ_H (acetone-d$_6$) 2.10 (3H,s), 1.7-2.4(4H,m), 3.5-3.9(2H,m), 4.6(2H,s), 5.5-5.9(1H,br m).

Rates of decomposition of (IV)

These reactions were monitored spectrophotometrically at λ_{max} 238 nm (and occasionally at 405 nm) in the temperature-controlled cuvette of a Unicam SP1800 instrument. The initial concentration of (IV) was usually about 5×10^{-5} mol/L. All the reported reactions showed excellent first-order behaviour over 3–4 half-lives, and pseudo-first-order rate coefficients (rate $= k_0$[IV]) were calculated graphically from the integrated rate expression. Errors in k_0 are about $\pm 8\%$.

Rates of formation and decomposition of N-nitrosopeptide in aqueous acid

These measurements were also carried out by monitoring the concentration of N-nitrosopeptide spectrophotometrically at λ_{max} 405 nm in the temperature-controlled cuvette of the SP1800 instrument. An aliquot of the peptide substrate (0.1 mol/L) in aqueous acid was equilibrated at 25°C in the cuvette. To this, 50 μL aqueous sodium nitrite were added to give the required concentrations of nitrous acid (usually 0.01 mol/L) in the cuvette. The absorbance usually increased, passed through a maximum, then decreased (Fig. 2). These changes correspond to the formation and decomposition (hydrolysis) of the N-nitrosopeptide.

Rates of the decomposition reaction (rate $= k_0$[III]) were calculated from the integrated rate expression for a pseudo-first-order process (the plots were linear over at least four half-lives). From the decomposition data, a theoretical maximum absorption for the N-nitrosopeptide was estimated by extrapolation. This extrapolated absorption was used as the 'infinity' to calculate the rate of N-nitrosopeptide formation. These reactions also followed a pseudo-first-order rate expression (rate $= k_0$[peptide]). Errors in both the rates of formation and decomposition of the N-nitrosopeptide were about $\pm$ 10%.

RESULTS

N-(N-Acetylprolyl)-N-nitrosoglycine (IV)

Compound (IV) was readily synthesized as the racemate by aprotic nitrosation of the benzyl ester of the parent peptide, followed by removal of the benzyl group by catalytic hydrogenolysis. It was obtained as an analytically pure, yellow solid, after recrystallisation from warm ethyl acetate.

Compound (IV) was found to be very soluble in water, acetone and low molecular weight alcohols, sparingly soluble in ether and ethyl acetate and insoluble in petrol and methylene chloride. It decomposed on melting, but was unexpectedly stable on heating in ethyl acetate (half-life, about 2 h at 60°C). This may explain why (IV), unlike N-nitrosoamides, gives a strong response in the Thermal Energy Analyzer.

The stability of (IV) was also examined in several aqueous media. In aqueous buffers at pH 1–7.4 and 25°C, decomposition occurred at an almost constant rate (Table 1), corresponding to a half-life of about 10 h. The lack of a well-defined pH-dependency implies that these reactions are largely thermal. Faster acid- and base-catalysed decomposition is apparent in strong acid and alkali, respectively. In acid, denitrosation (k_0^{NO}) and hydrolytic deamination ($k_0 N^2$) occur concurrently (Fig. 4), as observed previously for N-butyl-N-nitrosoacetamide (Berry & Challis, 1974). Denitrosation is the more strongly acid-catalysed pathway, which becomes predominant at high acidity (Fig. 5). Deamination of (IV) is also rapid in dilute aqueous sodium hydroxide at 25°C, but strong UV absorptions attributed to the diazoacetate product have hindered the acquisition of quantitative data.

Table 1. Rates of decomposition of N-(N-acetylprolyl)-N-nitroso-glycine (IV) in aqueous buffers at 25°C

Buffer	pH	$10^5 k_0{}^a$ (s^{-1})
0.10 mol/L HCl	1.00	2.46
0.01 mol/L HCl	1.98	2.38
0.1 mol/L HCO$_2$H/0.056 mol/L HCO$_2$Na	3.98	2.13
0.1 mol/L CH$_3$CO$_2$H/0.1 mol/L CH$_3$CO$_2$Na	4.78	1.62
0.25 mol/L KH$_2$PO$_4$/0.25 mol/L Na$_2$HPO$_4$	6.75	1.92
0.09 mol/L KH$_2$PO$_4$/0.03 mol/L Na$_2$HPO$_4$	7.40	2.53
0.1 mol/L Na$_2$B$_4$O$_7$	9.20	10.7

^{a} Rate $= k_0$[IV]

Fig. 4. Scheme of the denitrosation and hydrolytic deamination of *N*-(*N*-acetylprolyl)-*N*-nitrosoglycine

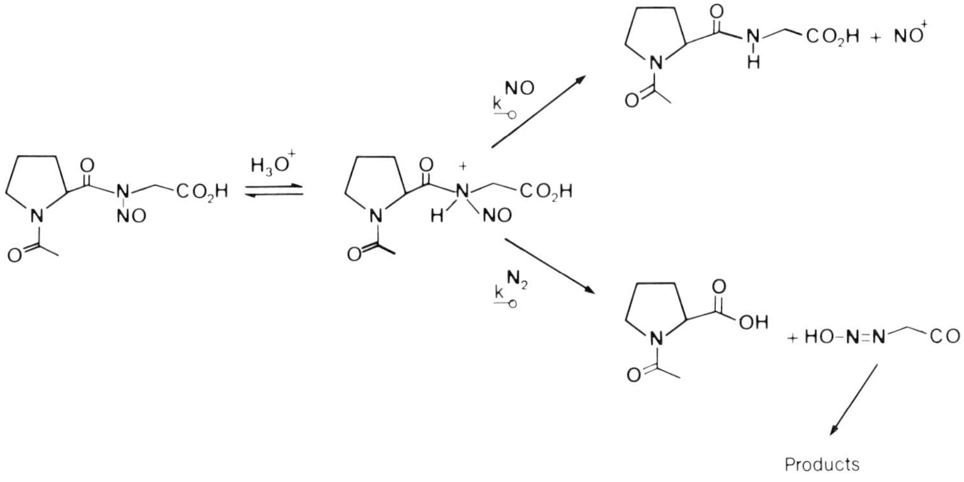

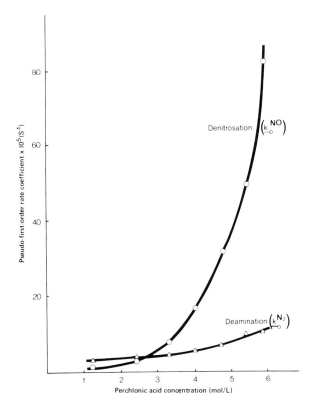

Fig. 5. Denitrosation and deamination (hydrolysis) of *N*-(*N*-acetylprolyl)-*N*-nitrosoglycine in aqueous perchloric acid at 25°C

The decomposition of (IV) in aqueous solution at 25°C was also measured in the presence of nucleophilic entities, and second-order rate coefficients (rate, k_2[IV][nucleophile]) are summarized in Table 2. These show that only powerful nucleophiles (e.g., cysteine) exert a significant effect. Added amino acids are relatively ineffectual; thus, it seems unlikely that the terminal carboxylate ion of (IV) is involved in any intramolecular reaction analogous to that claimed earlier for acylated *N*-nitroso-α-amino acids (Chow & Polo, 1980).

Formation and decomposition of N-*nitrosopeptide in strong acid*

Thus far, the unequivocal synthesis and isolation of *N*-nitrosopeptides with a terminal NH_3^+ group has proven difficult. Such compounds, however, form readily in strongly acidic media, then decompose by an acid-catalysed hydrolysis pathway (see Fig. 6). Above about 2 mol/L perchloric acid, for example, both formation and decomposition reactions can be studied kinetically.

Table 2. Nucleophilic catalysed decomposition of *N*-(*N*-acetylprolyl)-*N*-nitrosoglycine

Nucleophile	pH	$k_2{}^a$ (mol^{-1}Ls^{-1})
Sulfamic acid	2.0	$\leq 10^{-5}$
Hydrazine	4.0	4.0×10^{-4}
Glycine	9.2	3.3×10^{-3}
L-Prolylglycine	9.2	$\leq 10^{-5}$
L-Cysteine	9.2	0.27

^{a} Rate $= k_2$[IV][Nucleophile]

Fig. 6. Formation and hydrolysis of *N*-nitrosoglycylglycine in 8 mol/L perchloric acid at 25°C

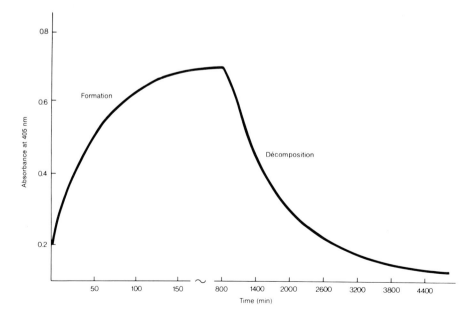

Typical results for glycylglycine, summarized in Table 3, show that the formation of the N-nitrosopeptide obeys the following equation.

$$\text{Rate} = k_2[\text{GlyGly}][\text{HNO}_2]$$

Similar findings apply to other peptides. Above 2 mol/L perchloric acid values of k_2 increase rapidly with acidity and reach a maximum at about 8 mol/L (Table 4). These findings are consistent with nitrosation of the conjugate acid of the peptide by the nitrosonium ion (NO^+), as shown in Figure 7. One other interesting feature of the results given in Table 4 is the small variation in the rate of nitrosation of different peptides when allowance is made (as in the case of pentaglycine) for the number of peptide N-atoms.

Table 3. Kinetic orders for the nitrosation of glycylglycine in perchloric acid at 25 °C

[HClO$_4$] (mol/L)	[GlyGly] (mol/L)	[HNO$_2$] (mol/L)	$10^2 k_2{}^a$ (mol^{-1}Ls^{-1})
6.75	0.1	0.005	5.52
6.75	0.1	0.01	5.57
6.75	0.1	0.02	5.06
5.70	0.049	0.005	1.69
5.70	0.10	0.005	1.56
5.70	0.192	0.005	1.63

^{a} Rate $= k_2[\text{GlyGly}][\text{HNO}_2]$

Table 4. Effect of acidity on the nitrosation of peptides in perchloric acid at 25 °C. Initial [Peptide] = 0.1 mol/L [HNO$_2$] = 0.01 mol/L

[HClO$_4$] (mol/L)	$10^3 k_2{}^a$ (mol^{-1}Ls^{-1})			
	GlyGly	ProGly	AcProGly	Pentagly^b
8.9	102	–	–	–
8.6	–	15.7	–	–
8.0	120	–	–	–
7.92	–	–	–	52.0
7.1	–	–	–	31.0
6.75	53.8	–	–	–
6.6	–	6.5	–	–
5.95	26.3	5.4	–	–
5.7	16.3	–	–	11.9
5.0	8.3	–	–	3.8
4.43	–	1.3	–	–
4.0	–	–	2.6	–
3.9	1.28	1.12	–	0.76
3.1	0.55	0.66	–	0.53
2.8	–	–	0.44	–

^{a} Rate $= k_2[\text{Peptide}][\text{HNO}_2]$
^{b} To allow for the statistical factor, observed k_2 values have been divided by 4

Fig. 7. Scheme of the nitrosation of the conjugate acid of glycylglycine by nitrosonium ion

$$HNO_2 \; + \; H_3O^+ \; \rightleftharpoons \; NO^+ \; + \; 2H_2O$$

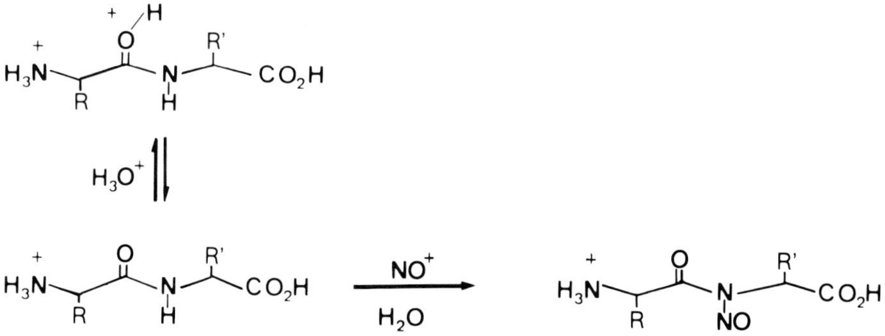

Table 5. Effect of acidity on the hydrolysis of *N*-nitrosopeptides in perchloric acid at 25 °C

[HClO$_4$] (mol/L)	$10^4 k_0{}^a$ (s^{-1})			
	GlyGly	ProGly	AcProGly	PentaGly
8.9	11.8	–	–	–
8.6	–	0.28	–	–
8.0	9.6	–	–	3.1
7.1	5.5	–	–	6.0
6.6	–	3.07	–	2.7
6.05	1.5	–	–	–
5.95	–	0.74	–	0.99
5.0	0.81	–	–	0.88
4.43	–	0.42	–	–
4.0	0.41	0.23	1.34	0.39
2.8	–	0.10	–	0.27
2.5	–	–	0.62	–

^{a} Rate = k_0[*N*-Nitrosopeptide]

The corresponding rates of hydrolysis of the *N*-nitrosopeptide (rate = k_0[*N*-nitrosopeptide]) in perchloric acid at 25°C are summarized in Table 5. These reactions are also acid-catalysed, but to a lesser extent than the formation of the *N*-nitrosopeptides. One consequence of this difference is that formation of the *N*-nitrosopeptides is more easily observed in concentrated perchloric acid than in dilute. Further, as with the formation of *N*-nitrosopeptides, their acid-catalysed hydrolysis is not strongly structure-dependent (Table 5).

DISCUSSION

Compound (IV) appears to be the first authentic *N*-nitrosopeptide isolated as an analytically pure compound. Its spectroscopic properties strongly support the postulated structure. The low intensity triplet in the electronic spectrum at 380–430 nm is very characteristic of the

–C(=O)NNO– group (Brundrett *et al.*, 1979) as are the (relatively high) C=O and N=O stretching vibrations in the infra-red spectrum at v_{max} 1 740 and 1 510 cm^{-1}, respectively (Djerassi *et al.*, 1961). Further, the ^{1}H-NMR absorption of the glycyl-CH$_2$ group is significantly deshielded (0.5 ppm) in the nitrosated product.

Not surprisingly, compound (IV) has similar chemical properties to *N*-nitrosoamides (Berry *et al.*, 1981). Thus, it decomposes themally and by acid-, base- and nucleophilic catalysed pathways. The acid-catalysed decomposition has a denitrosation component (Fig. 4) which implies that formation of *N*-nitrosopeptides from nitrous acid is reversible. The acid-base and nucleophilic-catalysed deaminations (e.g., Fig. 4) all generate a diazohydroxide intermediate, which is an alkylating agent relevant to the probable biological activity. Further, these reactions occur under mild conditions, similar to those obtaining *in vivo*. Compound (IV), however, is more stable than expected, and all the above decompositions proceed four to ten times more slowly than those for *N*-nitroso-*N*-methyl acetamide. The reason for this difference is not fully understood. At pH 1–7.4 and 25 C (but in the absence of strong nucleophiles), compound (IV) has a half-life of about 10 h, and in formate buffer (pH 3.98) at 37 C this decreases to 2 h. Thus, it is sufficiently stable for absorption from the digestive tract and interaction with cellular material.

There is clear evidence that peptide *N*-atoms undergo nitrosation in aqueous acidic solutions, and the kinetic behaviour of these reactions is consistent with a rate-limiting interaction of NO$^+$ with the conjugate acid of the peptide (Scheme 3). An interesting question is whether these reactions can occur under gastric conditions (pH 1–5, and about 20 µmol/L nitrous acid). A direct answer is probably precluded by the occurrence of subsequent acid-catalysed hydrolysis of the *N*-nitrosopeptides, but, thus far, human gastric aspirates have not been examined for the presence of *N*-nitrosopeptides.

ACKNOWLEDGEMENTS

We thank Smith, Kline & French Research Ltd, the Ministry of Agriculture, Fisheries and Food, the Science and Engineering Research Council and the Cancer Research Campaign for their support of our work.

REFERENCES

Berry, C.N. & Challis, B.C. (1974) Denitrosation and deamination of *N*-n-butyl-*N*-nitroso acetamide in aqueous acids. *J. chem. Soc., Perkin Trans. II,* 1638–1644

Berry, C.N., Challis, B.C., Gribble, A.D. & Jones, S.P. (1981) *Chemistry of some N-nitrosoamides.* In: Scanlan, R.A. & Tannenbaum, S.R., eds, N-*Nitroso Compounds (Am. Chem. Soc. Symp. Ser., No. 174),* Washington D.C., American Chemical Society, pp. 102–113

Bonnett, R. & Nicolaidou, P. (1979) Nitrosation and nitrosylation of haemoproteins and related compounds. Part 3. The reaction of nitrous acid with the side chains of α-acylamino acid esters. *J. chem. Soc., Perkin Trans. I,* 1969–1974

Bonnett, R., Holleyhead, R., Johnson, B.L. & Randall, E.W. (1975) Reaction of acidified nitrite solutions with peptide derivatives: Evidence for nitrosamine and thionitrite from ^{15}N-nmr studies. *J. chem. Soc., Perkin Trans. I,* 2261–2264

Brundett, R.B., Colvin, M., White, E.H., McKee, J., Hartman, P.E. & Brown, D.L. (1979) Comparison of mutagenicity, antitumour activity, and chemical properties of selected nitrosoureas and nitrosoamides. *Cancer Res., 39,* 1328–1333

Chow, Y.L. & Polo, J. (1980) *Nitrosamides derived from peptide models: their preparation and chemical behaviour.* In: Walker, E.A., Griciute, L., Castegnaro, M. & Börszönyi, M., eds, N-*Nitroso Compounds: Analysis, Formation and Occurrence (IARC Scientific Publications No. 31)*, Lyon, International Agency for Research on Cancer, pp. 3–14

Curtius, T. & Thompson, J. (1906) Einwirkung von Ammoniak auf Diazoacetyl-glycinester. *Chem. Ber.*, **39**, 3398–3409

Curtius, T. & Callan, T. (1910) Uber Diazoacetylglycyl-glycinhydrazid. *Chem. Ber.*, **43**, 2447–2457, and references cited therein

Djerassi, C., Lund, E., Bunnenberg, E. & Sjoburg, B. (1961) Optical rotary dispersion studies. XLVIII. The nitroso chromophore. *J. Am. chem. Soc.*, **82**, 2307–2312

Knowles, M.E., McWeeny, D.J., Couchman, L. & Thorogood, M. (1974) Interaction of nitrite with proteins at gastric pH. *Nature*, **247**, 288–289

Kurosky, A. & Hofmann, T. (1972) Kinetics of the reaction of nitrous acid with model compounds and proteins, and the conformational state of N-terminal groups in the chymotrypsin family. *Can. J. Biochem.*, **50**, 1282–1296

Magee, P.N., Montesano, R. & Preussmann, R. (1976) *N-Nitroso compounds and related carcinogens.* In: Searle, C.E., ed., *Chemical Carcinogens (Am. Chem. Soc. Monogr. No. 173)*, Washington DC, American Chemical Society, pp 491–625

Philpot, J.S.L. & Small, P.A. (1938) The action of nitrous acid on pepsin. *Biochem. J.*, **32**, 542–551

Pollock, J.R.A. (1982) *Nitrosation products of peptides.* In: Bartsch, H., O'Neill, I.K., Castegnaro, M. & Okada, M., eds, N-*Nitroso Compounds:Occurrence and Biological Effects (IARC Scientific Publications No. 41)*, Lyon, International Agency for Research on Cancer, pp. 81–85

White, E.H. (1955) The chemistry of the N-alkyl-N-nitrosoamides. I. Methods of preparation. *J. Am. chem. Soc.*, **77**, 6008–6010

PRODUCTION OF *N*-NITROSOIMINODIALKANOIC ACIDS BY NITRITE IN GASTRIC JUICE

J.R. OUTRAM & J.R.A. POLLOCK

Pollock and Pool Ltd, Ladbroke Close, Woodley, Reading RG5 4DX, UK

INTRODUCTION

The contribution of ingested nitrite to the formation of nitrosamines *in vivo* has been a question of interest for some time, and Walters *et al.* (1982) and Bavin *et al.* (1982) have made extensive quantitative studies of the formation of *N*-nitroso compounds, considered as a group, in gastric juice. The data of Walters *et al.* show interesting correlations with various pathological conditions. Pollock (1982), in connection with the work of Walters *et al.* (1982), reported that the substances being nitrosated in gastric juice might well be simple peptides, since a range of dipeptides yielded *N*-nitroso compounds upon nitrosation; and he suggested that these might be the *N*-nitrosamides in which the amide nitrogen had been nitrosated. It was later shown (Pollock, 1984) that the *N*-nitroso compounds formed during the nitrosation of dipeptides are not *N*-nitrosamides, but *N*-nitrosamines arising from a deaminative rearrangement of the form:

$$R_1 \cdot CH \cdot CO \cdot N \cdot CH(R_2)COOH \rightarrow \begin{array}{c} R_1 \cdot CH \cdot COOH \\ | \\ N \cdot NO \\ | \\ R_2 \cdot CH \cdot COOH \end{array}$$
$$\underset{NH_2}{|}$$

These compounds and the substances formed during the nitrosation of gastric juice do not undergo reactions characteristic of *N*-nitrosamides; thus, they remain as *N*-nitroso compounds after treatment with alkali and are much more thermally stable than would be expected of *N*-nitrosamides. The dipeptides, $H_2NCH(R_1) \cdot CONHCH(R_2) \cdot COOH$ and $H_2NCH(R_2) \cdot CONHCH(R_1) \cdot COOH$, give the same *N*-nitrosamine as a result of nitrosation.

As mentioned by Walters *et al.* (1982), at least 40% of the total *N*-nitroso compounds of nitrosated gastric juice can be accounted for by substances such as those discussed by Pollock (1982). We have therefore carried out controlled nitrosations of gastric juice in order to ascertain whether this type of reaction leading to the formation of nitrosamines may take place under conditions likely to occur *in vivo*.

EXPERIMENTAL

The gastric juice used in this work was a single sample of pooled material and was kindly supplied by Dr C. L. Walters.

Gastric juice (1–5 g) was placed in a conical flask (150-mL), adjusted in pH (as required) with dilute hydrochloric acid, and aqueous sodium nitrite was added in predetermined amounts. The flask was kept at 37 $\pm$ 2 °C for 16 h. The reaction was terminated by adding sulfamic acid (2 g). The mixtures were then treated successively with N-nitrosoazetidine-2-carboxylic acid (308 ng), to serve as internal standard, and dichloromethane (40 mL). Anhydrous sodium sulfate (40 g) was added to the constantly agitated mixture. After cooling to −5 °C for 30 min, the dichloromethane phase was decanted, treated with excess ethereal diazomethane and evaporated to about 0.1 mL. An aliquot of the concentrate (5 μL) was analysed by gas chromatography (GC), using a glass column (640 cm × 4 mm), packed with OV225 on Chromosorb B, at an initial temperature of 170 °C, which was increased at 2 °C/min to 230 °C. The detector was a Thermal Energy Analyzer (TEA) (Thermo Electron Corporation), with the pyrolyser temperature set at 475 °C. Yields of products were determined by comparison of their peak areas with that due to the internal standard, and were calculated as N-nitrosoproline (NPRO) (MW, 144).

RESULTS

The incubation of gastric juice (5 mL, pH 3.6) with sodium nitrite (0.5 g), followed by working-up as described above, gave a chromatogram with a large number of peaks (Fig. 1). If the methylation step were omitted, no such peak was observed. The N-nitroso compounds present ranged in volatility from the methyl ester of NPRO to the substances produced from phe.gly, phe.ala, pro.gly and pro.ala. (the last two are, respectively, N-nitrosopro.gly and N-nitrosopro.ala; the first two are N-nitrosoiminoacetic acid-3-phenylpropionic acid and its 1-methyl homologue, respectively). Between NPRO and these substances, many other TEA-responsive peaks were observed, 11 of which are present in varying amounts in the chromatogram of Figure 1.

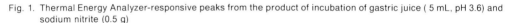

Fig. 1. Thermal Energy Analyzer-responsive peaks from the product of incubation of gastric juice (5 mL, pH 3.6) and sodium nitrite (0.5 g)

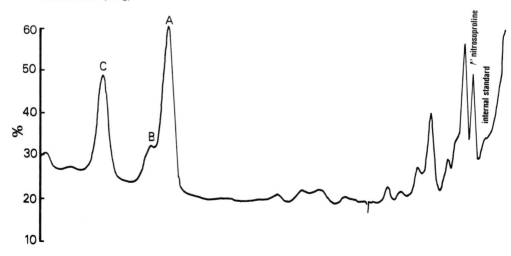

Fig. 2. Thermal Energy Analyzer-responsive peaks from the product of incubation of gastric juice (5 mL, pH 3.6) and sodium nitrite (2 mg)

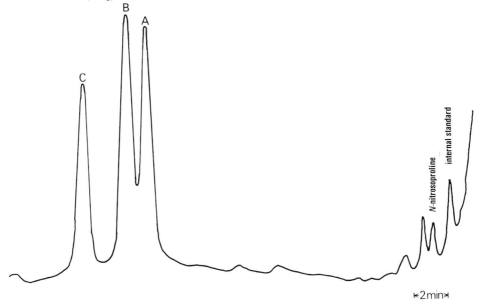

Fig. 3. Dependence of product yield on concentration of sodium nitrite added to gastric juice (1 mL, pH 3.6); X, *N*-nitrosoproline; ▲, compound C; ●, compound B; ■, compound A

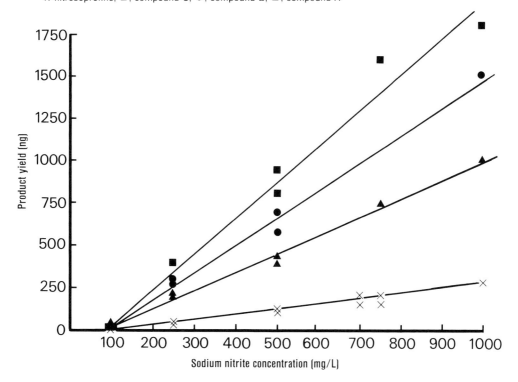

Such reactions, using high concentrations of nitrite, are generally informative, but have little direct bearing on in-vivo situations. The effects of reducing the concentration of nitrite were therefore studied. Smaller amounts of nitrosamines were produced in this case (Fig.2); the proportion of the added nitrite which was found as N-nitroso compounds that were volatile after derivatization was 1.1%. As the formation of compounds giving GC peaks required the methylation step, the parent substances of all the peaks observed contained acid functions.

The dependence of the observed concentrations of nitrosamines in the initial concentration of nitrite is illustrated in Figure 3. The concentrations of all the products decreased linearly with decreasing concentration of nitrite in the range 1 mg to 0.1 mg nitrite/mL gastric juice. Below this range, the yield of products was beneath our limit of detection (but see below). The yields of products were also dependent on pH, as might be expected: reaction was not evident at pH 6.5, but was substantial at pH 2.5, where, in addition, three new products were formed. The effects of pH on the formation of NPRO and three of the major nitrosamines are illustrated in Table 1.

An interesting and, for the present, unexplained feature of the pH-dependence of the nitrosation of the gastric juice was that when nitrosation was carried out for 2 h at pH 3.6, then completed at pH 2.5, the yield was increased by 30% compared with that obtained at a constant pH of 2.5.

Table 1.   Effect of pH on the formation of N-nitrosamine in gastric juice

pH	NPRO[a]	Substance A[a]	Substance B[a]	Substance C[a]
6.5	–	–	–	–
3.6[b]	0.6	0.38	0.27	0.2
2.5	1.25	1.25	0.6	0.3

[a] µg/mL gastric juice
[b] see also Fig. 2

Fig. 4. Thermal Energy Analyzer profile after treatment of gastric juice nitrosation product concentrate with alkali

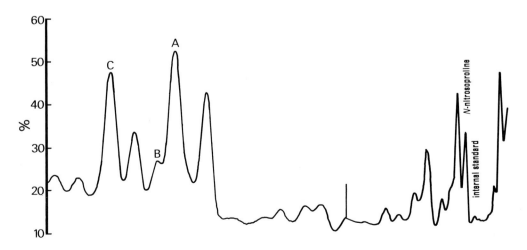

From Figure 3 it can be seen that the curves of nitrosamine concentration *versus* nitrite content might be extrapolated to zero response for nitrite concentrations of about 55 mg/L (1.2 µmol/L). At pH 3.6/2.5, the zero responses would occur with concentrations of about 0.8 µmol/L.

It was thought that it would be interesting to eliminate from the chromatograms any substances formed by the nitrosation of prolyl peptides, so as to be able to study only the nitrosoiminodialkanoic acids. Treatment of the nitrosation product of the gastric juice (nitrosated using a high concentration of nitrite) with aqueous sodium hydroxide led, as expected, to an increase of the peak due to NPRO (see Fig. 4), as well as of another substance of volatility similar to that of NPRO. In addition, three new peaks appeared in the region of the chromatograms at long retention time and there was a general enhancement of the peak size, so that the total observed *N*-nitrosamine content was approximately doubled by the treatment with alkali. This indicates that the original nitrosated solution contained many nitrosamines which are not volatile after methylation, but which can be hydrolysed to nitrosoiminodialkanoic acids. This is the behaviour that would be expected of amides of the nitrosoiminodialkanoic acids, such as would be formed on nitrosation of higher peptides and would give the simpler acids on alkaline hydrolysis:

$$
\begin{array}{ccc}
& R_1\text{--CH--COOH} & R_1\text{--CH--COOH} \\
& | & | \\
\text{Peptide} \rightarrow & N\cdot NO & \rightarrow \quad N\cdot NO \\
& | & | \\
& R_2\text{--CH--CONHCH}(R_3)\,\text{CONH}\ldots & R_2\text{--CH--COOH}
\end{array}
$$

CONCLUSIONS

The addition of nitrite to a gastric juice produced nitrosamines which were acids and which, apart from NPRO, NPRO.gly and NPRO.ala, were *N*-nitrosoiminodialkanoic acids. A further quantity of these nitrosamines was set free when the nitrosated mixture was treated with alkali, so that the total observed *N*-nitrosamine content was approximately doubled. Since about 40% of the total *N*-nitroso groups of nitrosated gastric juice could be accounted for as these nitrosoiminoacids without treatment with alkali, it is likely that about 80% of the total *N*-nitroso groups can be ascribed to free or bound compounds of this type.

The formation of these nitrosamines decreased linearly with concentration of added nitrite. In the particular gastric juice studied, the minimum concentration of nitrite that would give rise to the formation of these nitrosamines, allowing for those that would be liberated by treatment with alkali, was between 35 and 70 mg/L (0.75 and 1.5 µmol/L). Thus, there are substances in the gastric juice which react with nitrite before it can lead to production of the nitrosamines, and, when these are consumed, the formation of nitrosamines occurs by a process which is first order with respect to the remaining nitrite. It would be interesting to know how the competitive inhibitors, the presence of which is implied by the foregoing observations, vary in concentration in different gastric juices. The degree of formation of the nitrosamines, and their chemical natures, also depend on the concentrations and structures, respectively, of the peptides available to be nitrosated. As these nitrosamines seem to constitute the majority of the *N*-nitroso substances formed by the interaction of nitrite with gastric juice, and as they were formed with amounts of added nitrite that are not much greater than those which may be ingested naturally, it would be of great interest to know if they are physiologically active.

REFERENCES

Bavin, P.M.G., Darkin, D.W. & Viney, N.J. (1982) *Total nitroso compounds in gastric juice*. In: Bartsch, H., O'Neill, I.K., Castegnaro, M. & Okada, M., eds, N-*Nitroso Compounds: Occurrence and Biological Effects (IARC Scientific Publications No. 41)*, Lyon, International Agency for Research on Cancer, pp. 337–344

Pollock, J.R.A. (1982) *Nitrosation products from peptides*. In: Bartsch, H., O'Neill, I.K., Castegnaro, M. & Okada, M., eds, N-*Nitroso Compounds: Occurrence and Biological Effects (IARC Scientific Publications N. 41)*, Lyon, International Agency for Research on Cancer, pp. 81–85

Pollock, J.R.A. (1984) Formation of nitrosoiminodialkanoic acids during the nitrosation of peptides. *Food Cosmet. Toxicol.* (in press)

Walters, C.L., Smith, P.L.R., Reed, P.I., Haines, K. & House, F.R. (1982) N-*Nitroso compounds in gastric juice and their relationship to gastrointestinal disease*. In: Bartsch, H., O'Neill, I.K., Castegnaro, M. & Okada, M., eds, N-*Nitroso Compounds: Occurrence and Biological Effects (IARC Scientific Publications No. 41)*, Lyon, International Agency for Research on Cancer, pp. 345–356

PRESENCE IN HUMAN URINE OF NEW SULFUR-CONTAINING *N*-NITROSAMINO ACIDS: *N*-NITROSOTHIAZOLIDINE 4-CARBOXYLIC ACID AND *N*-NITROSO 2-METHYLTHIAZOLIDINE 4-CARBOXYLIC ACID

H. OHSHIMA, I.K. O'NEILL, M. FRIESEN, B. PIGNATELLI & H. BARTSCH

International Agency for Research on Cancer, 150, cours Albert Thomas, Lyon, France

SUMMARY

A new type of sulfur-containing *N*-nitrosamino acid, *N*-nitrosothiazolidine 4-carboxylic acid (NTCA) and *N*-nitroso 2-methylthiazolidine 4-carboxylic acid (NMTCA), was isolated and identified in the urine of human subjects. Identification was based on identical chromatographic and mass spectral data for the purified urine sample and the synthesized authentic compounds.

The amounts of NTCA and NMTCA excreted in 24-h urines of 15 volunteers varied from 0.9 to 35.9 µg/day and from 0.4 to 19.8 µg/day, respectively. These amounts were 2.4 and 1.6 times greater than that of *N*-nitrosoproline (NPRO) detected in the same urine samples.

Thiazolidine 4-carboxylic acid and its 2-methyl derivative were found to be nitrosated *in vitro* about 250–500 and 60–300 times more rapidly than proline, respectively. In addition, NTCA and NMTCA were also readily formed by reaction of a mixture of nitrite and L-cysteine, with formaldehyde and acetaldehyde, respectively.

Although their origin in human urine is unknown, preliminary results in one human volunteer have shown that some of these compounds are formed endogenously. Thus, measurement of these new sulfur-containing *N*-nitrosamino acids in the urine may (i) provide another index for endogenous nitrosation reactions in the human body and (ii) allow monitoring of exposure of humans to precursors such as aldehydes and nitrate/nitrite.

INTRODUCTION

We reported previously that *N*-nitrosamino acids such as N-nitrosoproline (NPRO) and N-nitrosarcosine (NSAR) can be measured in human urine as an indicator of endogenous *N*-nitrosation (Ohshima & Bartsch, 1981, 1982; Bartsch *et al.*, 1983). During analysis of human urine for these compounds by gas chromatography (GC) coupled with a Thermal Energy Analyzer (TEA) (Thermo Electron Inc., model 502), several unidentified substances (Figure 1 peaks 3–5) have frequently been detected.

These peaks appeared only after derivatization with diazomethane, suggesting that the unknown compounds may be *N*-nitrosamino acids carrying a carboxyl group(s). In view of the established carcinogenicity of most *N*-nitroso compounds in experimental animals, detection of hitherto unknown *N*-nitroso compounds in human urine may reveal a new source of

Fig. 1. Typical gas chromatographic-Thermal Energy Analyzer chromatogram of human urine extract after esterification with diazomethane. Peak 1, *N*-nitrososarcosine; peak 2, *N*-nitrosoproline; peaks 3, 4 and 5, unknown

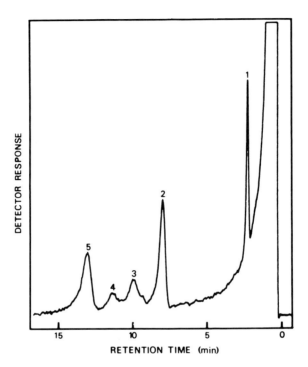

carcinogen exposure. Furthermore it is known that many *N*-nitrosamines are metabolized *in vivo* to *N*-nitrosamino acids which are subsequently excreted in the urine (Blattmann & Preussmann, 1973; Okada & Ishidate, 1977). We now report the isolation and identification of some previously unknown *N*-nitroso compounds in human urine.

EXPERIMENTAL

Reagents

N-Nitrosothiazolidine 4-carboxylic acid (NTCA) was synthesized by nitrosation of thiazolidine 4-carboxylic acid (TCA, Sigma Chemical Co.), as reported previously (Ohshima *et al.*, 1983). 2-Methylthiazolidine 4-carboxylic acid (MTCA; m.p. 162 °C) was prepared according to the method of Riemschneider and Hoyer (1962). The nitrosated product(s) of MTCA (NMTCA) was synthesized in a similar manner. NPRO and *N*-nitrosopipecolic acid (NPIC) were synthesized according to the method of Lijinsky *et al.*, (1970). The purity and identity of these compounds were verified by thin-layer chromatography, GC, mass spectrometry (MS) and Fourier transform nuclear magnetic resonance (^{1}H-FTNMR) spectroscopy. All other chemicals were commercially available products and were used without further purification.

Isolation and identification

In order to obtain enough of the compounds for anaysis by MS, 40 L of human urine were extracted. The method for isolation and purification of the unknown substance involved: (i) ethyl acetate extraction of urine in the presence of sodium chloride and ammonium sulfamate at pH 1; (ii) derivatization of the extract with excess diazomethane; (iii) washing of the derivatized extract with aqueous alkali and then acid solution (saturated aqueous sodium chloride adjusted to pH 10 with sodium hydroxide or to pH 1 with sulfuric acid); (iv) chromatographic clean-up on a Sephadex LH-20 column (dichloromethane elution) and then (v) on a silicic acid column by successive elution with mixtures (v/v) of dichloromethane : *n*-pentane (33 : 67), (50 : 50) and (25 : 75); (vi) preparative high-performance liquid chromatography (HPLC) using a Whatman Partisil M9 silica gel column (dichloromethane : pentane gradient from (25 : 75) to (50 : 50) in 50 min; flow rate, 4 mL/min) and (vii) reversed-phase HPLC using a Whatman Partisil PXS ODS-3 column (gradient from acetonile: water (50 : 50) to acetonitrile (100) in 25 min; flow rate, 1 mL/min). During these purification procedures, the presence of TEA responsive compounds of interest was monitored by GC-TEA. The final fractions (A & B) thus obtained were subjected to GC-MS analysis.

MS was performed using a Perkin Elmer, Sigma 3B, gas chromatograph coupled to a VG Micro Mass 70-70 F mass spectrometer, operated in the electron impact mode at 70 eV. A 0.25 mm i.d. × 50 m capillary column of OV-101 was used. ^{1}H-FTNMR spectra were obtained with a CAMECA 350 spectrometer at 350 MHz at 20 °C.

Stability of N-*nitrosamino acids*

Three *N*-nitrosamino acids (NPRO, NMTCA and NTCA) were dissolved at concentrations of 30 mg/L either in distilled water, basic solution (0.1 and 1 mol/L sodium hydroxide) or acidic solutions (0.1 and 1 mol/L hydrochloric acid and sulfuric acid). These solutions were incubated at 50 °C for 24 h and analysed for *N*-nitrosamino acids as described below.

Nitrosation in vitro

Experiments were carried out at 37 °C in 50 mmol/L aqueous citrate-citric acid buffer at a pH-range of 1.0 to 6.0. Nitrosation was initiated by adding a nitrite solution to the buffer solution containing an amino acid (L-proline, TCA or MTCA). The final volume was 6 mL, and the final concentration of nitrite and an amino acid was 2 mmol/L. The reaction was stopped after 30 min by adding an excess of ammonium sulfamate. Similarly, the reaction mixture containing a 2 mmol/L concentration of each L-cysteine, sodium nitrite and either formaldehyde or acetaldehyde in 50 mmol/L aqueous citrate buffer was incubated at 37 °C for 30 min. NPIC was added as internal standard to the reaction mixtures, from which aliquots were taken and extracted with ethyl acetate. The solvent extracts were dried over anhydrous sodium sulfate, and 0.5-mL aliquots were used for derivatization with diazomethane and subsequent GC-TEA analysis of *N*-nitrosamino acids formed.

Analysis of N-*nitrosamino acid in human urine*

Urine samples were collected for 24 h in plastic bottles containing 10 g sodium hydroxide. Aliquots were stored at −20 °C prior to analysis. A 15 mL sample of urine, to which 150 ng NPIC had been added as an internal standard, was extracted three times with 25 mL of 10% (v/v) methanol in dichloromethane in the presence of 5 g sodium chloride and 2 mL of 20% ammonium sulfamate in 1.8 mol/L sulfuric acid. The combined extracts were dried over anhydrous sodium sulfate and concentrated to dryness in a rotary evaporator at 30 °C. The residue was dissolved in 3 mL diethyl ether, derivatized with diazomethane and analysed by GC-TEA, as reported previously (Ohshima & Bartsch, 1981; Ohshima *et al.*, 1983). The average recoveries of NTCA, NMTCA, NPRO and NSAR added to the urine samples at a concentration of 20 µg/L were 92, 98, 85 and 81%, with minimum detectable levels of 0.5, 0.5, 0.5 and 0.1 µg/L, respectively.

RESULTS AND DISCUSSION

Identification of unknown N-*nitroso compounds in human urine*

A typical GC-TEA chromatogram of a human urine extract (after esterification) is shown in Figure 1; each substance detected is assumed to be an *N*-nitroso compound because (i) of the TEA specificity and (ii) these peaks disappeared after treatment either with UV-irradiation at 365 nm or hydrogen bromide/acetic acid (Krull *et al.*, 1979). In addition to peaks 1 and 2, corresponding to NSAR and NPRO, respectively, at least three unknown peaks (peaks 3–5) were frequently observed.

In order to identify their structures by GC-MS, the unknown substances were isolated from 40 L of human urine and purified as described above. Identification of the unknown *N*-nitroso compounds by initial GC-MS analysis of these purified samples (fractions A & B), however, was not successful, because they still contained many other substances. Therefore, approximately 40 different *N*-nitroso derivatives of amino acids were synthesized, including those of *N*-alkylamino acids and cyclic amino acids; their chromatographic data were then compared with those of the unknowns, using two different GC columns (5% FFAP and 3% OV-17).

Subsequently, the methyl ester of NTCA (NTCA-Me) was found to elute with the same GC-retention times as the unknown peak 5 on these two GC columns. The mass spectra of authentic NTCA-Me and that of the GC-peak eluting at the retention time of NTCA-Me in the chromatogram of the purified urine extract (fraction B) were compared (Figure 2A and B).

The peak found in the urine extract contained other interfering compounds, and the molecular ion at m/z 176 ($< 1\%$ relative intensity in authentic NTCA-Me) could not be detected. However, the relative intensities of the base peak at m/z 146 $(M–NO)^+$ and fragment ion peaks at m/z 117 $(M–CO_2CH_3)^+$, 87 $(M–NO–CO_2CH_3)^+$, 59 $(CO_2CH_3)^+$ and 30 $(NO)^+$ differed from those of authentic NTCA-Me by less than 15%. Thus, the unknown *N*-nitroso compound (peak 5) in human urine is identical to synthetic NTCA.

Two other hitherto unknown *N*-nitroso compounds (Figure 1, peaks 3 and 4) have been identified as epimeric isomers of NMTCA in a manner similar to that used for NTCA. The respective precursor amino acid, MTCA, was prepared by reaction of L-cysteine with acetaldehyde (Riemschneider & Hoyer, 1962). The isomeric nitrosation products of MTCA following diazomethane treatment gave two peaks with a peak area ratio of 4 : 1; their retention times were identical with those of the unknown peaks 3 and 4 on the two GC columns. GC-MS analysis of the synthesized material revealed that both the major and the minor peak produced essentially the same pattern of fragment ion peaks at 190 M^+, 175 $(M–CH_3)^+$, 160 $(M–NO)^+$, 131 $(M–CO_2–CH_3)^+$, 101 $(M–NO–CO_2–CH_3)^+$ and 86 $(M–NO–CH_3–CO_2CH_3)^+$, suggesting that they are epimeric isomers. It is known that L-cysteine reacts with aldehydes to produce epimeric mixtures of 2,4-*cis* and 2,4-*trans* 2-alkyl-1,3-thiazolidine-4-carboxylic acid (Szilagyi & Gyorgydeak, 1979). The two isomers formed from nitrosation of MTCA could be separated by silica gel column chromatography, eluting with a mixture of *n*-hexane and acetone, and finally two fractions (C and D) were obtained. Fractions C and D, following diazomethane treatment, were both found to contain two substances, the ratios being 9 : 1 and 4 : 6,

Fig. 2. Mass spectra of authentic N-nitrosothiazolidine-4-carboxylic acid methyl ester (A) and of unknown compound (peak 5) after purification steps i – vii (B)

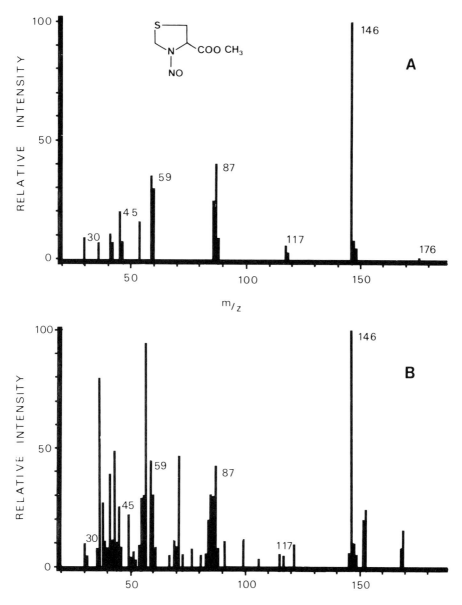

respectively. By ¹H-FTNMR examination of these fractions, the major peak of the original mixture was tentatively assigned to the *trans*-epimer and the minor peak to the *cis*-epimer (detailed data will be published elsewhere). From these results, we conclude that peaks 3 and 4 found in human urine are probably the *trans*- and *cis*-isomers, respectively, of NMTCA.

Stability of NTCA and NMTCA

Although NPRO was stable under all the conditions tested, NTCA and NMTCA were found to be much less stable than NPRO. When NTCA and NMTCA were dissolved in strong alkaline (1 mol/L sodium hydroxide) or acidic solutions (0.1 and 1.0 mol/L hydrochloric acid or sulfuric acid), more than 90% was decomposed after 24-h incubation at 50 °C, whereas the same compounds dissolved in distilled water or in 0.1 mol/L sodium hydroxide showed no apparent decomposition. Because NTCA and NMTCA are particularly acid labile and were found to be decomposed in considerable amounts during evaporation of the ethyl acetate extracts of urine prepared according to the previous method (Ohshima & Bartsch, 1981), we modified the analytical procedures as described above.

Formation in vitro of NTCA and NMTCA

The formation of NTCA and NMTCA by nitrosation of their respective precursors was compared with that of NPRO. As shown in Figure 3A, the yield of NTCA formed by nitrosation of TCA increased linearly with decreasing pH, and no optimum pH was observed in the pH range 1 to 6. On the other hand, the nitrosation of MTCA was optimal at pH about 3.5 (Figure 3B). TCA and MTCA were nitrosated about 250–500 and 60–300 times more rapidly than proline, respectively.

Fig. 3. pH dependence of *N*-nitrosothiazolidine-4-carboxylic acid (NTCA) (A) and *N*-nitroso-2-methylthiazolidine-4-carboxylic acid (NMTCA) (B) formation. □, nitrosation of thiazolidine-4-carboxylic acid; △, nitrosation of 2-methylthiazolidine-4-carboxylic acid; ○, nitrosation of L-proline; ■, nitrosation of L-cysteine and formaldehyde; ▲, nitrosation of L-cysteine and acetaldehyde

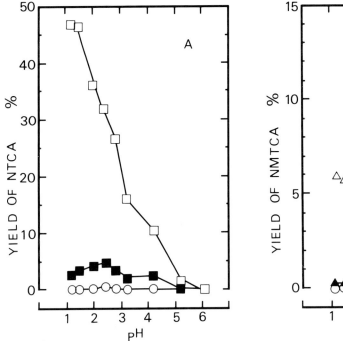
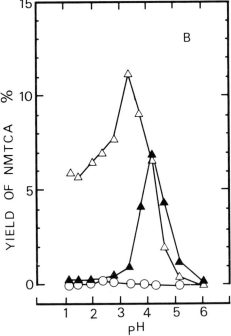

Because TCA and MTCA are easily formed by reaction of L-cysteine with formaldehyde and acetaldehyde, respectively, the yields of NTCA and NMTCA from the reaction mixture containing all these precursors (L-cysteine, aldehyde and nitrite) were determined. Both NTCA and NMTCA were found to be formed readily under such conditions; the pH optimum was 2.5 for the formation of NTCA and 4.5 for NMTCA. More detailed kinetic studies of the formation of these compounds are in progress in our laboratory.

Possible origin of NTCA and NMTCA in urine

The amounts of NTCA and NMTCA detected in 21 samples of the 24-h urine collected from 15 human volunteers varied from 0.9 to 35.9 and from 0.4 to 19.8 µg/day, respectively (Table 1). In comparison with the amount of NPRO in the same urine samples, NTCA and NMTCA occured at 2.4 (range: 0.4–5.2) and 1.6 (range: 0.06–4.73) times greater concentrations. Subjects who smoked cigarettes appeared to produce more *N*-nitrosamino acids (mean, 24.6 µg/day) than non-smokers (mean, 13.6 µg/day). These newly identified sulfur-containing *N*-nitrosamino acids have been detected in many of the human urine samples so far collected in the People's Republic of China, Finland, France and Italy (Bartsch *et al.*, 1983); individual levels will be reported elsewhere.

Table 1. Amounts of *N*-nitrosamino acids[a] detected in urine samples of human volunteers

Subject	NTCA	NMTCA[b]	NPRO	NSAR	Total[c]
			µg/24-h urine		
Nonsmoker					
A	11.4	0.6	10.5	0.9	23.4
	8.0	10.5	4.5	0.5	23.5
B	3.0	0.8	0.9	0.2	4.9
	2.8	1.0	1.7	0.3	5.8
C	21.4	2.2	10.3	–[c]	33.9
	1.7	1.1	1.1	–	3.9
D	11.6	0.8	2.4	–	14.8
E	6.0	5.2	14.3	–	25.5
F	4.6	10.4	2.2	0.5	17.7
G	2.7	3.8	1.4	0.4	8.3
H	2.0	0.4	1.5	–	3.9
I	1.0	2.7	1.1	0.7	5.5
J	0.9	0.6	1.6	–	3.7
Smoker					
A	35.0	5.0	12.4	0.6	53.9
	11.4	1.0	2.2	1.1	15.7
B	34.0	9.3	6.7	–	50.0
	3.1	2.5	1.6	–	7.2
C	4.3	9.7	3.7	0.6	18.3
	4.6	9.4	2.7	1.6	18.3
D	18.4	19.8	4.5	0.4	43.1
E	5.1	2.6	1.1	–	8.8

[a]NTCA, *N*-nitrosothiazolidine-4-carboxylic acid; NMTCA, *N*-nitroso-2-methylthiazolidine-4-carboxylic acid; NPRO, *N*-nitrosoproline; NSAR, *N*-nitrososarcosine
[b]Sum of *trans*- and *cis*- isomers of NMTCA
[c]Sum of four nitrosamino acids
[d]Not detectable (<0.1 µg/L)

Fig. 4. Possible origin of N-nitrosothiazolidine-4-carboxylic acid (NTCA) and N-nitroso-2-methylthiazolidine-4-
       carboxylic acid (NMTCA) found in human urine. cys, ʟ-cysteine; TCA, thiazolidine-4-carboxylic acid; MTCA,
       2-methylthiazolidine-4-carboxylic acid

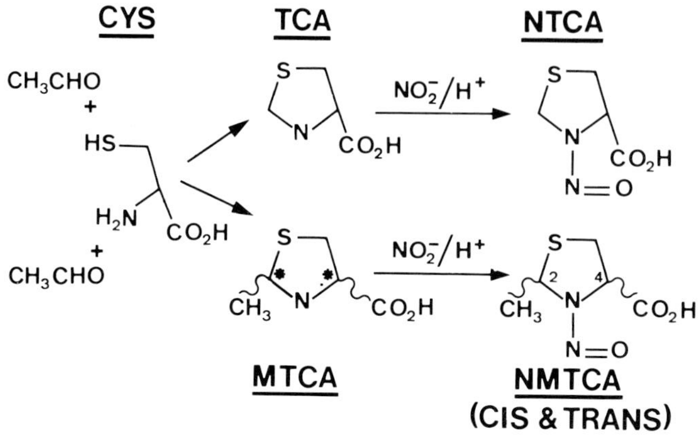

To our knowledge, no published report has appeared on the occurrence of NTCA and NMTCA in food products or biological materials. Similarly, no data are available to explain the origin of these compounds in human urine. Three possible sources, however, may be considered: (i) intake of preformed N-nitroso compound from foods and subsequent excretion in urine (NTCA was recently detected in smoked food products[1]; (ii) intake of (methyl) thiazolidine 4-carboxylic acid and subsequent nitrosation in vivo; and (iii) endogenous two-step synthesis by reaction of L-cysteine, an aldehyde and a nitrosating agent (Figure 4).

In our initial experiments (data not shown), intake of a diet supplemented with ascorbic acid appeared to reduce urinary excretion of NTCA and NMTCA. As ascorbic acid is a well-known inhibitor of nitrosation, this suggests that some of the NTCA and NMTCA may be formed endogenously. A similar inhibitory effect of ascorbic acid on urinary NTCA in human subjects was recently observed by S.R. Tannenbaum et al.[2]

CONCLUSION

We have shown the presence in human urine of a new type of sulfur-containing N-nitrosamino acids, NTCA and NMTCA. Their toxic and other adverse biological effects have not been reported. In view of the apparent wide exposure of the general human population (our studies) and the possibility that these N-nitrosothiazolidine 4-carboxylic acids may undergo decarboxylation in vivo to yield N-nitrosothiazolidine derivatives, both reported to be mutagenic (Sekizawa & Shibamoto, 1980), further studies on the biological significance of these compounds are especially desirable, and some are in progress in our laboratory. In addition, measurement of these newly-identified sulfur-containing N-nitrosamino acids in the urine may provide a further index for endogenous nitrosation in humans and may allow monitoring exposure of human subjects to precursors such as aldehydes and nitrate/nitrite.

---

[1] J.R.A. Pollock, personal communication
[2] Personal communication

The identification of these unknown *N*-nitroso compounds has also been reported by S.R. Tannenbaum[1] and Tsuda *et al.* (1983).

ACKNOWLEDGEMENTS

We wish to acknowledge our appreciation to Drs J.R.A. Pollock and S.R. Tannenbaum, for access to unpublished data; to Drs D. Fraisse, M. Bigois and Q.T. Pham, CNRS, Lyon, France, for collaboration in obtaining the MS, elemental analysis and FTNMR data. We also wish to thank Mrs E. Heseltine and Mrs M.B. D'Arcy for editorial and secretarial assistance, and Miss J. Michelon and Miss M-C. Bourgade for technical help. The TEA detector was provided on loan by the National Cancer Institute, Bethesda, MD, USA, under contract No. NOI CP-55715.

REFERENCES

Bartsch, H., Ohshima, H., Muñoz, N., Crespi, M. & Lu, S.H. (1983) *Measurement of endogenous nitrosation in humans: potential applications of a new method and initial results.* In : Harris, C.C. & Autrup, H.N., eds, *Human Carcinogenesis,* New York, Academic Press , pp. 833–856

Blattmann, L. & Preussmann, R. (1973) Zur Struktur von Metaboliten carcinogener Dialkylnitrosamine im Rattenurin. *Z. Krebsforsch., 79,* 3–5

Krull, I.S., Goff, E.U., Hoffmann, G.G. & Fine, D.H. (1979) Confirmatory methods for the thermal energy determination of *N*-nitroso compounds at trace levels. *Anal. Chem., 51,* 1706–1709

Lijinsky, W., Keefer, L. & Loo, J. (1970) The preparation and properties of some nitrosamino acids. *Tetrahedron, 26,* 5137–5153

Ohshima, H. & Bartsch, H. (1981) Quantitative estimation of endogenous nitrosation in humans by monitoring *N*-nitrosoproline excreted in the urine. *Cancer Res., 41,* 3658–3662

Ohshima, H. & Bartsch, H. (1982) *Quantitative estimation of endogenous nitrosation in humans by measuring excretion of* N*-nitrosoproline in the urine.* In : Sugimura, T., Kondo, S. & Takebe, H., eds, *Environmental Mutagens and Carcinogens,* Tokyo, University of Tokyo Press, pp. 577–585

Ohshima, H., Friesen, M., O'Neill, I.K. & Bartsch, H. (1983) Presence in human urine of a new *N*-nitroso compound, *N*-nitrosothiazolidine-4-carboxylic acid. *Cancer Lett., 20,* 183–190

Okada, M., & Ishidate, M. (1977) Metabolic fate of *N,N*-butyl-*N*-4-hydroxybutyl nitrosamine and its analogs; selective induction of urinary bladder tumors in the rat. *Xenobiotica, 7,* 11–24

Riemschneider, V.R. & Hoyer, G.A. (1962) Synthese und Eigenschaften einiger 2-substituierter Thiazolidin-4-carbonsäuren. *Z. Naturforsch., 17b,* 765–768

Sekizawa, J. & Shibamoto, T. (1980) Mutagenicity of 2-alkyl-*N*-nitrosothiazolidines. *J. agric. Food Chem., 28,* 781–783

Szilagyi, L. & Gyorgydeak, Z. (1979) Comments on the putative stereoselectivity in cysteine-aldehyde reactions. Selectivity C (2) inversion and C (4) epimerization in thiazolidine-4-carboxylic acids *J. am. chem. Soc., 101,* 427–432

Tsuda, M. Hirayama, T. & Sugimura, T. (1983) Presence of *N*-nitroso-L-thioproline and *N*-nitoso-L-methylthioproline in human urine as major *N*-nitroso compounds. *Gann, 74,* 331–333

---

[1] Personal communication

A NEW TYPE OF *N*-NITROSAMINO ACID, *N*-NITROSO-L-THIOPROLINE AND *N*-NITROSO-L-METHYLTHIOPROLINES, FOUND IN HUMAN URINE AS MAJOR *N*-NITROSO COMPOUNDS

M. TSUDA[1], T. HIRAYAMA & T. SUGIMURA

Biochemistry Division, National Cancer Center Research Institute, 1-1, Tsukiji 5 chome, Chuo-ku, Tokyo 104, Japan

T. KAKIZOE

National Cancer Center Hospital, 1-1, Tsukiji 5 chome, Chuo-ku, Tokyo, 104, Japan

SUMMARY

In addition to *N*-nitrosoproline (NPRO), *N*-nitrosamino acids of a new type containing sulfur were found as major *N*-nitroso compounds in the urine of seven healthy subjects. These compounds were detected using a gas chromatograph connected with a Thermal Energy Analyzer (GC-TEA), and they were identified as *N*-nitroso-L-thiazolidine-4-carboxylic acid (*N*-nitroso-L-thioproline, NTPRO) and the *cis* and *trans* isomers of *N*-nitroso-L-methylthiazolidine-4-carboxylic acid (*N*-nitroso-L-methylthioproline, NMTPRO) by using gas chromatography-mass spectrometry (GC-MS).

The amounts of NPRO, NTPRO and NMTPRO found in 100 mL samples of human urine were 65–471 ng, 67–2 250 ng and 275–5 825 ng, respectively. L-Thioproline was nitrosated 20–60 times faster than L-proline by nitrite over the whole range of acidic pH.

The precursors of these new-*N*-nitrosamino acids containing sulfur may be formed by the reaction of L-cysteine with formaldehyde and acetaldehyde in the human body. These sulfur-containing *N*-nitroso compounds, NTPRO and NMTPRO, in addition to NPRO, could be useful as probes for investigating the dynamics of nitrosation in the human body.

INTRODUCTION

Most *N*-nitroso compounds have been found to be potent carcinogens in a wide variety of animals and organs (Druckrey *et al.*, 1967; IARC, 1978). Humans are exposed daily to *N*-nitroso compounds in foods, beverages, drugs, cosmetics and the air (Woo & Arcos, 1981). In addition to such exogenous *N*-nitroso compounds, endogenously formed *N*-nitroso

---

[1] Author to whom correspondence should be sent

compounds have also been found to be important potential human carcinogens (Tannenbaum, 1980; Ohshima & Bartsch, 1981; Ohshima et al., 1982; Bartsch et al., 1983). However, there is as yet not convincing epidemiological evidence linking N-nitroso compounds to the aetiology of any human cancer. Recently, Ohshima and Bartsch (1981) reported that the amount of N-nitroso-L-proline (NPRO) in human urine was markedly increased after ingestion of nitrate and L-proline. This finding provided important evidence for the formation of N-nitroso compounds in the human body, and opened up a new way of studying the relation of N-nitroso compounds to cancer.

In this paper, we report the occurrence and structural determination of sulfur-containing N-nitrosamino acids, a new type of N-nitroso compound, in the urine of seven healthy subjects. The compounds were analysed with a gas chromatograph connected with a Thermal Energy Analyzer (GC-TEA) and by gas chromatography-mass spectrometry (GC-MS), and identified as N-nitroso-L-thazolidine-4-carboxylic acid (N-nitroso-L-thioproline, NTPRO) and the cis and trans isomers of N-nitroso-L-2-methylthiazolidine-4-carboxylic acid (N-nitroso-L-methylthioproline, NMTPRO). These new N-nitrosamino acids, NTPRO and NMTPROs, in addition to NPRO, should be useful probes for evaluating human exposure to endogenously formed N-nitroso compounds.

MATERIALS AND METHODS

Chemicals

N-nitrosoproline (NPRO), N-nitrososarcosine (NSAR) and N-nitrosopipecolic acid (NPIC) were synthesized by the method of Lijinsky et al. (1970). Sarcosine, L-cysteine hydrochloride, L-thioproline and p-toluenesulfonyl-N-methyl-N-nitrosamide were obtained from Tokyo Kasei Co. (Tokyo, Japan). L-Proline, sodium nitrite, formalin, acetaldehyde, methylene chloride and ethyl acetate were purchased from Wako Pure Chemicals (Tokyo, Japan). Ammonium sulfamate was obtained from Kanto Chemical Co. (Tokyo, Japan). All chemicals were used without further purification.

Collection and storage of human urine samples

Human urine samples were collected from seven healthy subjects, six males and one female of 32–46 years old on unrestricted diets. Urine samples were collected in 300-mL capacity plastic urine cups containing 10 mL of ammonium sulfamate solution (20% ammonium sulfamate in 1 mol/L sulfuric acid) and stored at $-20\,^{\circ}$C until analysis.

Analytical conditions by GC-TEA and GC-MS

A Shimadzu GC-7AG gas chromatograph (Kyoto, Japan) was used with argon carrier gas and interfaced to a TEA (Model 502A, Thermo Electron Corp., Waltham, MA, USA). GC-TEA analysis of the N-nitrosamino acids was performed after treating the compounds with diazomethane, prepared from p-toluenesulfonyl-N-methyl-N-nitrosamide. For GC, a 2.6 m × 2.6 mm i.d. glass column, packed with 5% OV-1 on Gaschrom Q (80–100 mesh), was programmed from $80\,^{\circ}$–$200\,^{\circ}$C at $4\,^{\circ}$/min. The argon carrier flow rate was 40 mL/min. OV-17 (5%) and PEG 20M (10%) columns were also used for GC analysis.

GC-MS spectra were recorded in a Varian MAT 44S gas chromatograph-mass spectrometer, using a 7 m × 0.2 mm capillary column with SP2100. The ionizing electron energy was 70 eV.

Extraction and esterification of N-*nitrosamino acids in human urine*

A 40-mL sample of human urine was applied to an Extrelut-20 column (Merck, Darmstadt, FRG) and extracted with 200 mL ethyl acetate. After complete evaporation, the residual materials were treated with diazomethane in dichloromethane. Excess diazomethane was removed by evaporation *in vacuo*, and the residue was extracted three times with 5 mL dichloromethane. The combined extract was filtered, and the filtrate was condensed to 0.1–0.2 mL by evaporation and subjected to GC-TEA analysis for *N*-nitroso compounds.

Syntheses for NTPRO and NMTPROs

L-Cysteine hydrochloride (1 mmol) was treated with 2 mmol of formaldehyde or acetaldehyde in 5 mL distilled water at room temperature for 2 h. The reaction products were extracted twice with 30 mL ethyl acetate. The extract was dried over anhydrous sodium sulfate and evaporate to dryness *in vacuo*. The dried material was treated with 5 mmol of sodium nitrite in 5 mL of 0.01 mol/L hydrochloric acid for 2 h at room temperature and the nitrosated materials were extracted twice with 50 mL ethyl acetate. The combined extract was dried over anhydrous sodium sulfate and evaporated to dryness. The products obtained were determined by GC-TEA and GC-MS.

Nitrosation of L-proline and L-thioproline by nitrite at various pH values

L-Proline (1 mmol/L) or L-thioproline (1 mmol/L) was treated at 37 °C for 2 h with 2 mmol/L sodium nitrite at various acidic pHs obtained with a 0.1 mol/L sodium citrate-0.1 mol/L hydrochloric acid buffer system. Reactions were terminated by addition of ammonium sulfamate. Sodium chloride (200 mg) was added to 1-mL aliquots of the reaction mixtures, which were then extracted three times with 4 mL ethyl acetate by shaking in a mixer. The combined extracts were dried over anhydrous sodium sulfate and evaporated to dryness. The resulting *N*-nitroso products were esterified with diazomethane in ethyl acetate-methanol (1:1, v/v), and the resulting methyl esters of NPRO and NTPRO were dissolved in dichloromethane for quantitative analysis of NPRO and NTPRO by GC-TEA. The GC conditions for this purpose were as follows: OV-1 (5%) at 130 °C; flow rate of argon carrier gas, 40 mL/min.

RESULTS

Detection of unknown N-*nitrosamino acids in human urine samples by GC-TEA*

Ethyl acetate extracts of human urine samples commonly exhibited three major peaks of unknown TEA-sensitive compounds in addition to NPRO (Fig. 1). The relative retention times (RRT) of the three unidentified peaks to that of NPRO (RRT = 1.00, 16.5 min) were 1.14, 1.17 and 1.21. Diazomethane treatment of urine extracts was necessary for detection of these unknown *N*-nitroso compounds by GC-TEA. When UV (365 nm) irradiation, which is known to cleave N-NO bonds photochemically (Doerr & Fiddler, 1977), was carried out for 45 min on a urinary extract in a capillary tube, all the peaks, including that of NPRO, disappeared. These results suggested that the TEA-positive compounds were *N*-nitroso derivatives of some amino acids with secondary amine functions, such as proline. These unknown TEA-positive peaks could not have been NSAR, NPIC or *N*-nitrosohydroxyproline (NHPRO), judging from their peak positions (Ohshima *et al.*, 1982).

Fig. 1. A typical gas chromatograph-Thermal Energy Analyzer chromatogram of human urine extract after esterification with diazomethane. For gas chromatography, a 2.6 m × 2.6 mm i.d. glass column, packed with 5% OV-1 on Gaschrom Q (80–100 mesh), was programmed from 80 °C to 200 °C at 4 °C/min. The argon flow rate was 40 mL/min.

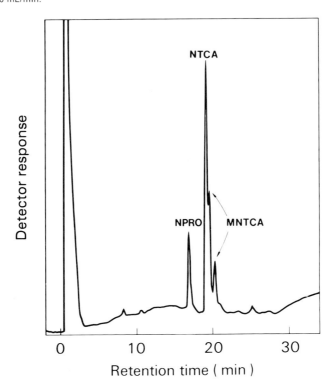

Characterization of NTPRO and NMTPROs

The nitrosated products formed by reaction of L-cysteine with formaldehyde, then with nitrite after esterification with diazomethane, gave a single TEA-positive peak with an RRT value of 1.14 in the OV-1 column system. This TEA-positive product was isolated by preparative thin-layer chromatography (TLC) (silica gel 60 F_{254}-CHCl$_3$, R_f 0.38). Its mass spectrum showed ion peaks at m/z 176 (M^+), 146 (M^+-NO) and 87 (M^+-NO-COOMe), and the compound was identified as the methyl ester of NTPRO. This compound was also synthesized directly from L-thioproline by treatment with nitrite. Nitrosated products formed by the reactions of L-cysteine with acetaldehyde followed by nitrite treatment gave two TEA-positive peaks with a peak height ratio of 8:2 and RRT values of 1.17 (major peak) and 1.21 (minor peak) in the OV-1 column system after esterification with diazomethane. Structural analysis of these synthetic N-nitrosamino acids was performed by GC-MS. The GC-MS spectra of the major (RRT = 1.17) and minor (RRT = 1.21) peaks both showed ion peaks at m/z 175 (M^+-Me), 160 (M^+-NO), 131 (M^+-COOMe), 101 (M^+-NO-COOMe) and 86 (M^+NO-Me-COOMe). From the mass spectral data, these TEA-positive compounds were identified as the *cis* and *trans* isomers of NMTPRO, with regard to the orientations of the 2-methyl and 4-carboxylic functions. The precise peak assignments of the *cis* and *trans* isomers of NMTPRO are now being studied.

Identification of unknown N-*nitrosamino acids found in human urine*

On the basis of preliminary results concerning the structures of the unidentified *N*-nitroso compound, available secondary amino acids were nitrosated and examined by GC-TEA. First, the possibility that the unknown materials were NSAR, NPIC and NHPRO were ruled out by their GC peak positions. Next, we examined the *N*-nitroso compounds derived from cyclic amino acids formed by the reactions of amino acids, such as cysteine, tryptophan, tyrosine and histidine with aldehydes (Riemschneider & Hoyer, 1962; Esterbauer, 1982; Nagasawa *et al.*, 1982; Wakabayashi *et al.*, 1983). Finally, we found that the unknown materials in human urine samples with an RRT value (OV-1) of 1.14 had the same retention time as authentic NTPRO in three GC column systems (OV-1, OV-17 and PEG 20M). Furthermore, the unknown materials with RRT values (OV-1) of 1.17 and 1.21 had the same mobilities as the major and minor isomers of NMTPRO, respectively, in the three GC column systems. From these chromatographic characteristics, we concluded that the unknown TEA-positive compounds found in human urine samples were the *N*-nitroso derivative of L-thiazolidine-4-carobxylic acid, and *cis*- and *trans*-*N*-nitroso-L-2-methylthiazolidine-4-carboxylic acids (Tsuda *et al.*, 1983).

Gas-chromatographic behaviour of NPRO, NTPRO and NMTPROs

In the OV-1 and OV-17 column systems, NPRO appeared first, followed by NTPRO, then the NMTPROs. However, when the PEG 20M column system (at 195°C; argon carrier; 50 mL/min) was used, the order of appearance of NTPRO and the NMTPROs was reversed, and the *cis* and *trans* isomers of NMTPRO were not separated. The relative retention times of NTPRO and the NMTPROs to NPRO (RRT = 1.00, 1.75 min) were 1.55 and 1.26, respectively.

Variation in the amounts of NPRO, NTPRO and NMTPROs in human urine

The amounts and ratios of NTPRO and NMTPROs to NPRO in human urine varied markedly from one healthy subjects to another. The amounts of NPRO, NTPRO and NMTPROs found in 100-mL samples of urine of the seven healthy subjects are summarized in Table 1.

pH-Dependency of nitrosations of L-proline and L-thioproline

The pH dependencies of NPRO and NTPRO formation are shown in Figure 2. The optimal pH was about 2.0 in both cases. An optimal pH of 2.25 was reported for the nitrosation of L-proline by Mirvish (1972). It is noteworthy that L-thioproline was nitrosated 20–60 times faster than L-proline.

DISCUSSION

In addition to NPRO, we found a new type of *N*-nitroso compound in the urine of healthy subjects; i.e., several *N*-nitrosamino acids containing sulfur. These compounds were found by GC-TEA after esterification with diazomethane and were identified as NTPRO and the *cis* and *trans* isomers of NMTPRO (Tsuda *et al.*, 1983). A possible pathway for the formation of these sulfur-containing *N*-nitrosamino acids in the human body is shown in Figure 3. It is noteworthy that the sum of the amounts of NTPRO and NMTPROs found in human urine in the present study were greater than that of NPRO, as indicated in Table 1. A high positive correlation

Fig. 2. pH-Dependence of nitrosation of L-proline and L-thioproline by nitrite: ●, *N*-nitrosoproline; o, *N*-nitroso-L-thioproline

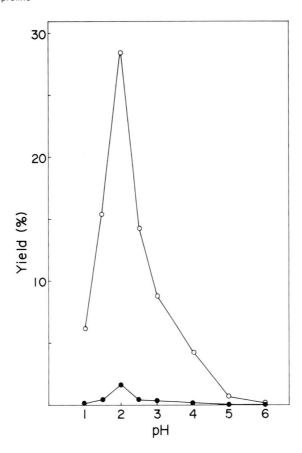

Table 1. Amounts of *N*-nitrosamino acids[a] found in 100-mL samples of urine of seven healthy subjects (ng per 100 mL of urine)

Subject	NPRO	NTPRO	NMTPROs[b]	Total amount[c]	R[d]
A [M.T.]	118	67	87	272	1.3
B [Y.N.]	65	275	385	725	10.2
C [H.K.]	471	278	264	1 013	1.2
D [T.K.]	200	796	362	1 358	5.8
E [K.W.]	379	299	929	1 607	3.2
F [M.T.]	418	1 438	920	2 776	5.6
G [M.T.]	250	2 250	3 325	5 825	22.3

[a] NPRO, *N*-nitrosoproline; TPRO, *N*-nitroso-L-thioproline; NMTPROs, *N*-nitroso-L-methylthioprolines
[b] Sum of *cis* and *trans* isomers
[c] Sum of NPRO, NTPRO and NMTPROs
[d] Ratio of NTPRO plus NMTPROs to NPRO

Fig. 3. Possible mechanism of formation of N-nitroso-L-thioproline (R = H) and N-nitroso-L-methylthioprolines (R = CH₃)

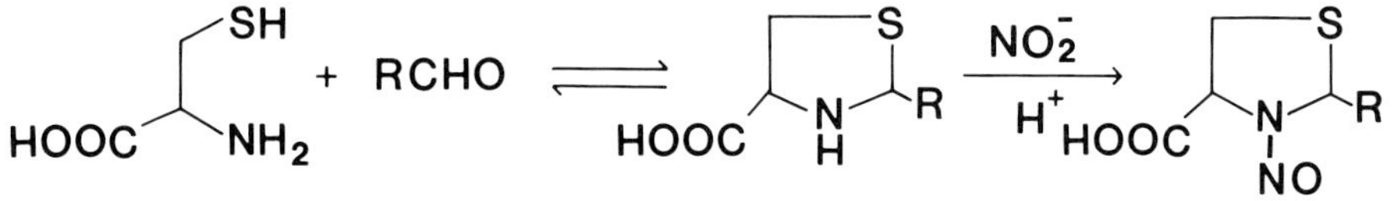

(r = 0.832) was observed between the amounts of NTPRO and NMTPROs, but not between the amounts of NPRO and NTPRO (r = 0.161) or between the amounts of NPRO and NMTPROs (r = 0.075).

The reaction of L-thioproline with nitrite was 20–60 times faster than that of proline over the whole range of acidic pH. From this result, and the ratios (R = 1.2–22.3) of NTPRO plus NMTPROs to NPRO (Table 1), thioproline and methylthioprolines seem to be more effective nitrite trapping agents than proline in the human body.

Formaldehyde has been shown to be a weak carcinogen (IARC, 1982). It seems likely that it is scavenged through NTPRO formation and excreted in the urine, as shown in Figure 3. However, the biological properties of these compounds, including their mutagenicity and carcinogenicity, are unknown and should be studied as soon as possible. In any event, these new sulfur-containing N-nitroso compounds should be useful, along with NPRO, as probes for studies of the dynamics of nitrosation in the human body.

ACKNOWLEDGEMENTS

This study was supported by Grants-in-Aid for Cancer Research from the Ministry of Education, Science and Culture and the Ministry of Health and Welfare of Japan. We wish to thank Dr Z. Yamaizumi for help with GC-MS analyses.

REFERENCES

Bartsch, H., Ohshima, H., Munoz, N., Crespi, M. & Lu, S.H. (1983) *Measurement of endogenous nitrosation in humans: potential applications of a new method and initial results*. In: Harris, C.C. & Autrup, H.N., eds, *Human Carcinogenesis*, New York, NY Academic Press, pp. 833–856

Doerr, R.C. & Fiddler, W. (1977) Photolysis of volatile nitrosamines at the picogram level as an aid to confirmation. *J. Chromatogr., 140*, 284–287

Druckrey, H., Preussmann, R., Ivankovic, S. & Schmähl, D. (1967) Organotrope carcinogene Wirkungen bei 65 verschiedenen N-nitroso-Verbindungen und BD-Ratten. *Z. Krebsforsch., 69*, 103–201

Esterbauer, H. (1982) *Aldehydic products of lipid peroxidation*. In: McBrien, D.C.H. & Slater, T.F., eds, *Free Radicals, Lipid Peroxidation and Cancer*, London, Academic press, pp. 101–128

IARC (1978) *IARC Monographs on the Evaluation of Carcinogenic Risks of Chemicals to Man*, Vol. 17, *Some N-nitroso Compounds*, Lyon, International Agency for Research on Cancer

IARC (1982) *IARC Monographs on the Evaluation of Carcinogenic Risks of the Chemicals to Man*, Vol. 29, *Some Industrial Chemicals and Dyestuffs*, Lyon, International Agency for Research on Cancer, pp. 345–389

Lijinsky, W., Keefer, L. & Loo, J. (1970) The preparation and properties of some nitrosamino acids. *Tetrahedron, 26*, 5137–5153

Mirvish, S.S. (1972) *Kinetics of* N-*nitrosation reaction in relation to tumorigenesis experiments with nitrite plus amines or ureas.* In: Bogovski, P., Preussmann, R. & Walker, E.A., eds, *N-Nitroso Compounds, Analysis and Formation, (IARC Scientific Publications No. 3)*, Lyon, International Agency for Research on Cancer, pp. 104–108

Nagasawa, H.T., Goon, D.J.W., Zera, R.T. & Yuzon, D.L. (1982) Prodrugs of L-cysteine as liver-protective agents. 2 (RS)-methylthiazolidine-4(R)-carboxylic acid, a latent cysteine. *J. med. Chem.*, **25**, 489–491

Ohshima, H. & Bartsch, H. (1981) Quantitative estimation of endogenous nitrosation in humans by monitoring *N*-nitrosoproline excreted in the urine. *Cancer Res.*, **41**, 3658–3662

Ohshima, H., Béréziat, J.-C. & Bartsch, H. (1982) Monitoring *N*-nitrosamino acids excreted in the urine and feces of rats as an index for endogenous nitrosation. *Carcinogenesis*, **3**, 115–120

Riemschneider, R. & Hoyer, G.-A. (1962) Synthese und Eigenschaften einiger 2-substituierter Thiazolidin-4-Carbonsäuren. *Z. Naturforsch.*, **17b**, 765–768

Tannenbaum, S.R. (1980) A model for estimation of human exposure to endogenous *N*-nitrosodimethylamine. *Oncology*, **37**, 232–235

Tsuda, M., Hirayama, T. & Sugimura, T. (1983) Presence of *N*-nitroso-L-thioproline and *N*-nitroso-L-methylthioprolines in human urine as major *N*-nitroso compounds. *Gann*, **74**, 331–333

Wakabayashi, K., Ochiai, M., Saito, H., Tsuda, M., Suwa, Y., Nagao, M. & Sugimura, T. (1983) The presence of 1-methyl-1,2,3,4-tetrahydro-β-carboline-3-carboxylic acid, a precursor of a mutagenic nitroso compound, in soy sauce. *Proc. natl Acad. Sci. USA*, **80**, 2912–2916

Woo, Y.-T. & Arcos, J.C. (1981) *Environmental chemicals.* In: Sontag, J.M., ed., *Carcinogens in Industry and the Environment*, New York, Marcel Dekker, pp. 200–225

INVESTIGATION ON THE MUTAGENICITY OF *N*-NITROSO-THIAZOLIDINE USING THE AMES *SALMONELLA* TEST

W. FIDDLER, A.J. MILLER, J.W. PENSABENE & R.C. DOERR

US Department of Agriculture, Agricultural Research Service, Eastern Regional Research Center, Philadelphia, PA, USA

INTRODUCTION

Two research groups, including our own, have recently identified *N*-nitrosothiazolidine (NTHZ) in bacon (Gray *et al.*, 1982; Kimoto *et al.*, 1982). Since the original identification of this compound, we have developed a dual-column chromatographic method for its simultaneous determination with *N*-nitrosodimethylamine and *N*-nitrosopyrrolidine (Pensabene & Fiddler, 1982) and conducted studies demonstrating that NTHZ is present in bacon as a result of smokehouse processing (Pensabene & Fiddler, 1983a).

Little is known about the toxicity of NTHZ, although this *N*-nitrosamine, formed from the Maillard-Browning reaction and nitrite, was found to be a direct-acting mutagen with *Salmonella typhimurium* TA100, the activity of which was suppressed by a $9\,000 \times g$ supernatant of rat liver homogenate (Mihara & Shibamoto, 1980; Sekizawa & Shibamoto, 1980).

As an initial toxicological evaluation, we carried out the Ames *Salmonella* test on NTHZ to verify the mutagenicity of this compound. Our findings are presented here.

MATERIALS AND METHODS

Materials

Cysteamine hydrochloride, thiazolidine, formaldehyde (37%), sodium nitrite and all other reagents were purchased from commercial suppliers and used without further purification.

N-Nitrosothiazolidine synthesis

Thiazolidine method: Sodium nitrite (0.30 mol) was added slowly to a cooled (0 °C), stirred, aqueous solution of thiazolidine (0.28 mol) and 4.5 mol/L sulfuric acid (0.28 mol). After addition, the cold mixture was stirred for an hour, then for another hour at room temperature. The reaction mixture was extracted with dichloromethane (DCM), the DCM was washed with 30% potassium hydroxide, dried over anhydrous sodium sulfate and concentrated on a rotary evaporator. The oily residue was vacuum distilled to obtain NTHZ (85 °C at 0.55 torr).

Cysteamine/formaldehyde method: An aqueous solution of cysteamine hydrochloride (0.18 mol) and formaldehyde (0.18 mol) was stirred at room temperature for 24 h. This solution was cooled to 0 °C and 4.5 mol/L sulfuric acid (0.18 mol) were added. Sodium nitrite (0.20 mol) was then added slowly and the mixture stirred at 0 °C for one hour, then at room temperature for another hour. NTHZ was isolated as described by Ray (1978), except that DCM was used instead of ether to extract the nitrosamine from the reaction mixture.

Caution: Nitrosamines are potential carcinogens. Exercise care in handling these materials.

N-*Nitrosothiazolidine confirmation*

N-Nitrosothiazolidine from both sources was confirmed by gas-liquid chromatography-mass spectrometry (GLC-MS) (Hewlett Packard, model 5992B), with no apparent difference in their spectra when these were obtained under conditions described previously (Kimoto *et al.*, 1982). No difference was observed in the spectra obtained from the NTHZs (10 µL/10 mL hexane) when scanned from 260 to 400 nm on a Hewlett-Packard Model 8450A UV/VIS spectrophotometer. Four major peaks were noted: λ_{max} 283, 360, 372, and 386. Both samples of NTHZ were more than 99% pure, as indicated by GLC, using a 1.8 m × 2 mm column containing 15% Carbowax 20M-TPA on 60/80 Gas Chrom P.

Mutagenicity assay

Mutagenicity assays were performed in accordance with the preincubation method described by Kitamura *et al.* (1981). *Salmonella typhimurium* TA100 (a gift of Dr B.N.Ames) was used as the indicator organism (Ames *et al.*, 1975). Approximately 2×10^8 cells were placed in sterile test tubes to which were added 100 µL dimethylsulfoxide, alone or with the dissolved test compound, and 500 µL phosphate buffer (0.1 mol/L, pH 7.4).The solutions were mixed and incubated for 20 min at 37 °C. At termination, 2 mL of 50 °C soft top agar (0.5%) were added to the incubating solutions. They were then mixed and poured onto minimal medium in petri dishes (Miller & Buchanan, 1983). Appropriate solvent and known mutagen (*N*-methyl-*N'*-nitro-*N*-nitrosoguanidine, 10µg/plate) controls were included each day with the experimental samples. Genetic markers were checked routinely according to the method of Ames *et al.* (1975). After an hour, the dried plates were inverted and incubated for 48 h at 37 °C. His^+ revertant colonies were counted using a Biotran automated colony counter (New Brunswick Scientific Co.). All experiments were performed at least twice, using triplicate plates per determination. A positive mutagenic response was defined as a minimum of twice the solvent-control reversion yield.

High-performance liquid chromatography (HPLC) analysis

Fifty µL of NTHZ distillate, obtained from cysteamine/formaldehyde/nitrite, were diluted with 50 µL hexane-DCM (1:1, v/v) and separated by HPLC (Milton Roy) using a 3.2 mm × 25 cm, 5 µ Spherisorb silica column and a variable-wavelength detector (Perkin-Elmer, Model 55) set at 365 nm, the maximum absorbance of NTHZ. A linear solvent gradient of 100% hexane to 100% DCM over a 15-min. interval was employed, with a flow rate of 1 mL/min. Sample fractions were collected after 2 min, for 4- or 6-min intervals, up to 30 min.

RESULTS AND DISCUSSION

N-Nitrosothiazolidine, synthesized by direct nitrosation of thiazolidine, was tested for mutagenicity by the Ames assay procedure. This compound was shown not to be mutagenic to TA100 over a 2 log dose range. However, when NTHZ was synthesized from cysteamine/

Fig. 1. Mutagenic activity of *N*-nitrosothiazolidine synthesized by two different procedures: □, cysteamine/formaldehyde/nitrite; o, thiazolidine/nitrite

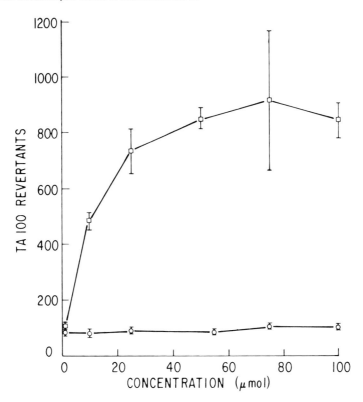

formaldehyde/nitrite according to the procedure of Mihara and Shibamoto (1980), the product was found to be mutagenic (maximum response was approximately nine times the spontaneous level). The mutagenic responses of NTHZ synthesized by the two different methods are shown in Figure 1. It is likely that the other investigators did not detect mutagenicity of NTHZ, but of some other compound. Our results suggest that the mutagenic species obtained by the cysteamine/formaldehyde/nitrite reaction, which we henceforth designate 'NTHZ', was either a trace contaminant, formed as a result of a side reaction, or a residual reaction precursor. For this reason, we tested formaldehyde, cysteamine, thiazolidine and nitrite individually for potential genotoxic activity, using the same conditions as for 'NTHZ'. The results for all compounds except nitrite are shown in Figure 2. Formaldehyde was strongly mutagenic at the 5-μmol level, but became cytotoxic at higher doses; Donovan *et al.* (1983) made a similar observation. However, it was thought that formaldehyde was not the mutagenic species observed in 'NTHZ', since its presence was unlikely, due to its volatility and high reactivity. Cysteamine was found not to be mutagenic over a 0-30-μmol dose range. This compound has, in fact, been shown to offer protection against genotoxic agents by what is thought to be radical scavenging activity (Bianchi *et al.*, 1982). Thiazolidine was tested because its mutagenic activity was reported by Mihara and Shibamoto (1980): we observed moderate mutagenicity at concentrations above 20 μmol/plate, which is not sufficient to account for the mutagenicity of 'NTHZ'. The results for nitrite, not shown on the figure, gave no evidence of mutagenic activity

Fig. 2. Mutagenic activity of '*N*-nitrosothiazolidine and its precursors: ○, *N*-nitrosothiazolidine; ★, thiazolidine; □, cysteamine; △ formaldehyde

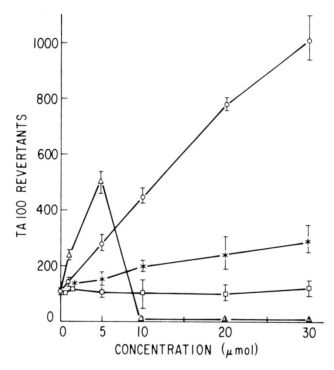

under the conditions employed, which involved the use of a buffer at pH 7.4. If the test had been run under acidic conditions, nitrite, or, more precisely, nitrous acid, would be expected to be mutagenic, since it is known to deaminate nucleotides such as adenine (Nicholson-Guthrie, 1970). Generally, these results and those shown in Figure 2 suggest that the genotoxic response observed with 'NTHZ' was not due to residual precursors.

Studies were then carried out to separate the 'NTHZ' by HPLC (using a silica column) to determine if a mutagenic contaminant was present. The chromatograph is shown in Figure 3. The fraction collected between 6 and 12 min, independently determined to contain NTHZ, exhibited no mutagenic activity, whereas, the fraction collected between 12 and 18 min (containing several small peaks) showed strong mutagenic potential, as indicated in the same figure. The other fractions were found to contain no mutagenic activity. These data suggest that the mutagenic activity observed with 'NTHZ' was due to one or more contaminants resulting from the cysteamine /formaldehyde/nitrite reaction. It should be noted that the contaminant(s) is probably present in a very low concentration and, given the relatively strong mutagenic response, would have to be considered a potent directly-acting mutagen. Most *N*-nitrosamines, but not nitroso-amides and ureas, require metabolic activation before they are mutagenic. The latter classes of compounds are potent directly acting mutagens and animal carcinogens and have been implicated epidemiologically in human gastric and oesophageal cancer (Mirvish, 1971; Correa *et al.*, 1975). Generally there is a good correlation between in-vitro mutagenicity and rodent carcinogenicity for promutagenic nitrosamines if the liquid preincubation technique is used, as described by Yahagi *et al.* (1977), yet some carcinogenic nitrosamines have been reported to be non-mutagenic and *vice versa* (Rao *et al.*, 1979).

Fig. 3. '*N*-nitrosothiazolidine': high-performance liquid chromatogram and mutagenic response of six sample fractions

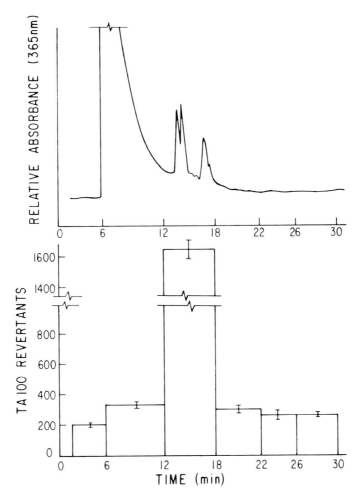

Investigators have sugggested that the discrepancies result from inappropriate in-vitro simulation of the in-vivo transformation that is necessary to form the active metabolite.

While the results of this study indicate that NTHZ is not mutagenic in our test system, the *N*-nitrosamine and the contaminant are still of toxicological concern. The fact that a mutagenic contaminant is formed during the synthesis of NTHZ by the cysteamine/formaldehyde/nitrite reaction and that NTHZ is present in bacon and other cured-meat products (Pensabene & Fiddler, 1983b), suggests the possibility that the mutagenic contaminant is also present in the latter. If the mutagen is found not to be a *N*-nitrosamine, it is possible that the Browning reaction, which forms thiazolidines from cysteamine and glucose (Kitamura *et al.*, 1981), can also form the mutagen or its precursor during the processing and/or cooking of cured meats. For this reason, it is important to identify the mutagen in 'NTHZ', determine how it is formed and develop means for its total or partial elimination. Research is currently in progress in these areas.

ACKNOWLEDGEMENTS

The authors thank Kathleen A. Fahy for her competent technical help in carrying out this study.

REFERENCES

Ames, B.N., McCann, J. & Yamasaki, E. (1975) Methods for detecting carcinogens and mutagens with the *Salmonella*/mammalian microsome mutagenicity test. *Mutat. Res., 31,* 347–364

Bianchi, M., Bianchi, N. Cortes, L. & Reigosa, M. (1982) Cysteamine protection of SCEs induced by UV and fluorescent light. *Mutat. Res., 104,* 281–286

Correa, P., Bolanos, O., Garcia, F.T., Gordillo, G., Duque, E. & Cuello, C. (1975) The cancer registry of Cali, Columbia – epidemiologic studies of gastric cancer. Recent results. *Cancer Res., 50* 155–169

Donovan, S.M., Krahn, D.F., Stewart, J.A. & Sarrif, A.M. (1983) *Mutagen activities of formaldehyde and hexamethylphosphoramide in reverse and forward* Salmonella typhimurium *mutagen assays.* In: *Proc. 14th Annu. Meet., Environmental Mutagen Society, San Antonio, Texas, March 3–6, 1983*

Gray, J.I., Reddy, S.K., Price, J.F., Mandagere, A. & Wilkins, W.F. (1982) Inhibition of *N*-nitrosamines in bacon. *Food technol., 36,* 39–45

Kimoto, W.I., Pensabene, J.W. & Fiddler, W. (1982) The isolation and identification of *N*-nitrosothiazolidine in fried bacon. *J. agric. Food Chem., 30,* 757–760

Kitamura, K., Wei, C.-I. & Shibamoto, T. (1981) Water-soluble thiazolidines formed in a cysteamine-D-glucose Browning model system. *J. agric. Food. Chem., 29,* 378–380

Mihara, S. & Shibamoto, T. (1980) Mutagenicity of products obtained from cysteamine-glucose Browning model systems. *J. agric. Food Chem., 28,* 62–66

Miller, A.J. & Buchanan, R.L. (1983) Detection of genotoxicity in fried bacon by the *Salmonella*/mammalian microsome mutagenicity assay. *Food Chem. toxicol., 21,* 319–323

Mirvish, S.S. (1971) Kinetics of nitrosamide formation from alkylureas, *N*-alkylurethans and alkylguanidines: Possible implication for the etiology of human gastric cancer. *J. natl Cancer Inst., 46,* 1183–1193

Nicholson-Guthrie, C.S. (1970) Nitrous acid effect on cleavage and development in fertilized frog legs. *Nature, 226,* 969–970

Pensabene J.W. & Fiddler, W. (1982) Dual column chromatographic method for determination of *N*-nitrosothiazolidine in fried bacon. *J. Assoc. off. anal. Chem., 65,* 1346–1349

Pensabene, J.W. & Fiddler, W. (1983a) Factors affecting the *N*-nitrosothiazolidine content of bacon. *J. Food Sci., 48,* 1452–1454

Pensabene, J.W. & Fiddler, W. (1983b) *N*-nitrosothiazolidine in cured meat products. *J. Food Sci., 48,* 1870–1871

Rao, T.K., Young, J.A., Lijinsky, W. & Epler, J.L. (1979) Mutagenicity of aliphatic nitrosamines in *Salmonella typhimurium. Mutat. Res., 66,* 1–7

Ray, S. (1978) Direct gas chromatograph analysis of cyclic *N*-nitrosamines. *J. Chromatogr., 153,* 173–179

Sekizawa, J. & Shibamoto, T. (1980) Mutagenicity of 2-alkyl-*N*-nitrosothiazolidines. *J. agric. Food Chem., 28,* 781–783

Yahagi, T., Nagao, M., Seino, Y., Matsushima, T., Sugimura, T. & Okada, M. (1977) Mutagenicities of *N*-nitrosamines on *Salmonella. Mutat. Res., 48,* 121–129

AMADORI- AND *N*-NITROSO-AMADORI COMPOUNDS AND THEIR PYROLYSIS PRODUCTS. CHEMICAL, ANALYTICAL AND BIOLOGICAL ASPECTS[1]

H. RÖPER[2] & S. RÖPER

Institute for Organic Chemistry and Biochemistry, University of Hamburg, Hamburg, FRG

B. MEYER

Department of Chemistry, University of Oldenburg, Oldenburg, FRG

SUMMARY

N-(1-Deoxy-D-fructos-1-yl)-L-amino acids (fructose amino acids), Amadori compounds, are formed by reaction of D-glucose and L-amino acids and Amadori rearrangement. They are detected in heat-processed natural products and various foodstuffs and are key products of the Maillard-Browning reaction. *N*-Nitroso-*N*-(1-deoxy-D-fructos-1-yl)-L-amino acids (*N*-NO-fructose amino acids), *N*-NO-Amadori compounds, are formed in high yields by reacting fructose amino acids with sodium nitrite in acidic aqueous solution. They constitute a new class of non-volatile, bis-β-oxidized nitrosamine derivatives with unknown biological (mutagenic and/or carcinogenic) activity.

N-NO-Fructose amino acids may be formed in nitrite-containing Maillard systems (e.g., cured-meat products, tobacco) or in the human stomach after ingestion of food containing fructose amino acids and nitrite in food or saliva.

Thirteen fructose amino acids and 13 *N*-NO-fructose amino acids (-gly, -ala, -val, -leu, -ileu, -ser, -thr, -met, -asp, -pheala, -tyr, -his, -trp) were prepared and investigated by high-resolution ¹H-nuclear magnetic resonance (NMR) and ¹³C-NMR spectroscopy. The percentage amounts of the sugar ring forms (β-pyranose, β-furanose, α-furanose and α-pyranose) of these compounds in D_2O mutarotation equilibrium were determined by ¹³C-NMR spectroscopy, together with the amounts (%) of E/Z isomers in the case of *N*-NO-compounds.

The nitrosation products of D-fru-L-tyr, D-fru-L-his and D-fru-L-trp were isolated and identified by spectroscopic methods (NMR, infra-red).

The *N*-NO-fructose amino acids can be separated by reversed-phase, ion-pairing, high-performance liquid chromatography. In some case the E/Z isomers are separated.

---

[1] Dedicated to Professor Dr Kurt Heyns on the occasion of his 75th birthday

[2] To whom correspondence should be addressed, at CPC Europe Industrial R & D Center, Havenstraat 84, B-1800 Vilvoorde, Belgium

The results of quantitative mutagenicity tests (Ames tests) of the N-NO-fructose amino acids in different strains of *Salmonella typhimurium* (with and without metabolic activation) are summarized. Ether extracts of N-NO-D-fru-L-val and N-NO-D-fru-L-leu pyrolysis products were mutagenic to TA100 (in the absence of metabolic activation). Dimethyl sulfoxide extracts of the pyrolysis products were non-mutagenic to TA100 (in the absence of metabolic activation).

INTRODUCTION

N-NO-N-(1-Deoxy-D-fructos-1-yl)-L-amino acids, N-nitroso fructose amino acids, are a new class of non-volatile, bis-β-oxidized nitrosamine derivatives (Heyns *et al.*, 1979; Röper *et al.*, 1982) of unknown biological activity. Their occurrence in environmental media, e.g., nitrite-containing Maillard systems (cured-meat products, tobacco etc.) is not yet proven, but likely. Formation in the human body also seems to be possible, because the precursor fructose amino acids (Röper *et al.*, 1983) were detected in a variety of natural products and foodstuffs.

The fructose amino acids are key products of the Maillard-Browning reaction, which takes place when aldoses react with amino acids and undergo subsequent Amadori rearrangement during the heating of natural products or food. They are readily nitrosated in the presence of nitrite in acidic aqueous medium to form the corresponding N-nitroso-fructose amino acids (Röper *et al.*,1982).

Coughlin (1979) has found D-glucose/L-tryptophan/$NaNO_2$ reaction mixtures to be non-mutagenic, whereas fructose-L-tryptophan/sodium nitrite reaction mixtures were mutagenic in *Salmonella typhimurium* TA98 and TA100.The mutagenic compound in the latter reaction, α-N-NO-D-fructose-L-tryptophan, was isolated and identified (Röper *et al.*, 1982). Since then, other representative N-NO-fructose amino acids have been prepared and studied by ^{1}HNMR and ^{13}C-NMR spectroscopy (Röper, 1983).

In view of the environmental significance of N-nitroso compounds in general, these compounds were tested by Pool *et al.*[1] and by Marquardt *et al.*[1] for mutagenicity in the *Salmonella typhimurium*/mammalian microsomal assay (Ames *et al.*, 1975). The results of these assays were used to set priorities in developing analytical procedures for screening foods containing potent mutagenic N-nitroso sugar amino acids.

MATERIALS AND METHODS

Fructose amino acids were prepared, purified and analysed by procedures described elsewhere (Röper *et al.*, 1983). N-Nitroso-fructose amino acids were prepared by reaction of the fructose amino acids (Amadori compounds) with sodium nitrite in acidic aqueous medium and characterized by [1]H-nuclear magnetic resonance (NMR) and ^{13}C-NMR spectroscopy (Heyns *et al.*, 1979; Röper *et al.*, 1982; Röper, 1983). Desalting of the N-NO-fructose amino acids was performed by ion-exchange chromatography on Dowex 50 WX8 (H^+) (100–200 mesh) and on Dowex 2X8 (OH^-) (20–50 mesh) and subsequent freeze drying (Röper,1983).

High-performance liquid chromatography (HPLC) was performed with a Waters ALC 100 instrument, with an ultra-violet detector (254 nm), differential refractometer (R.I.) and a U6K injection system. Column: 30 cm μ-Bondapak C_{18} (10 μm particles), 3.9 mm i.d. (Waters). Eluant, water: acetonitrile (9:1) with 0.05 mol/L tetrabutylammoniumphosphate (PIC A, Waters) as the ion-pairing reagent; flow-rate, 1mL/min[2].

---

[1] In preparation
[2] Röper, in preparation

The results of quantitative Ames assays with *N*-NO-fructose amino acids will be described in detail elsewhere[1]. In the present paper, the results are summarized.

Fig. 1. Prepared fructose amino acids (X = H) and *N*-NO-fructose amino acids (X = NO). Ring forms in D_2O mutarotation equilibrium as observed by nuclear magnetic resonance (NMR) spectroscopy. The probable conformations are depicted; only the $^2C_5$ chair of the β-pyranose form was established by ^1H-NMR spectroscopy

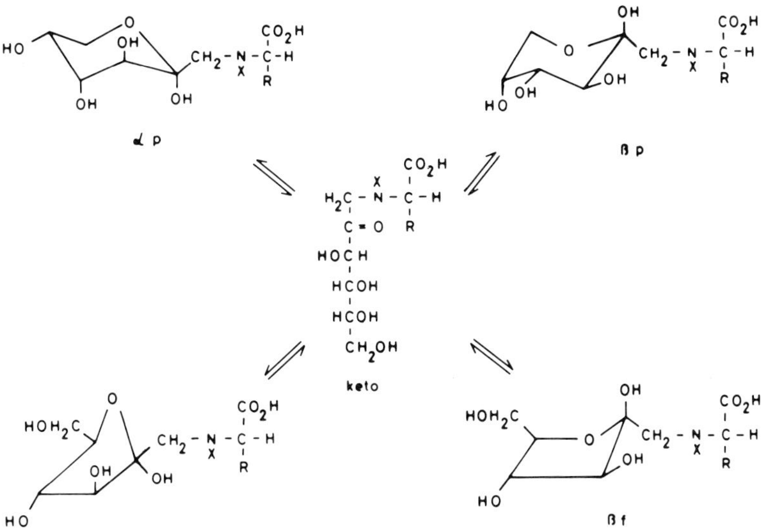

X = H	R	L-amino acid	X = NO
Frugly	– H	Glycine	N – NO – Frugly
Fruala	– Me	Alanine	N – NO – Fruala
Fruval	– CHMe$_2$	Valine	N – NO – Fruval
Fruleu	– CH$_2$CHMe$_2$	Leucine	N – NO – Fruleu
Fruile	– CH(Me)CH$_2$Me	Isoleucine	N – NO – Fruile
Fruser	– CH$_2$OH	Serine	N – NO – Fruser
Fruthr	– CH(OH)Me	Threonine	N – NO – Fruthr
Frumet	– CH$_2$CH$_2$SMe	Methionine	N – NO – Frumet
Fruasp	– CH$_2$CO$_2$H	Aspartic acid	N – NO – Fruasp
Frupheala	– Phenylmethyl	Phenylalanine	N – NO – Frupheala
Frutyr	– p-Hydroxyphenyl-methyl	Tyrosine	N – NO – Frutyr
Fruhis	– Imidazolylmethyl	Histidine	N – NO – Fruhis
Frutrp	– Indolylmethyl	Tryptophan	N – NO – Frutrp

[1] Pool *et al.*, in preparation; Marquardt *et al.*, in preparation

Table 1. ¹H-Nuclear magnetic resonance and ¹³C-Nuclear magnetic resonance studies

Fructose amino acids in D_2O mutarotation equilibrium

β-pyranose forms: 61–69%
β-furanose forms: 10–16%
α-furanose forms: 14–21%
α-pyranose forms: 0– 6%
keto forms: 0   %

N-NO-Fructose amino acids in D_2O mutarotation equilibrium

β-pyranose forms: 44–100%   (21–71% Z; 12–47% E)
β-furanose forms: 7– 32%   (3–16% Z; 6–22% E)
α-furanose forms: 4– 18%   (2–12% Z; 2– 6% E)
α-pyranose forms: 5– 8%
keto forms: 0   %

Fig. 2. Nitrosation products of F-fru-L-tyr, D-fru-L-his and D-fru-L-trp

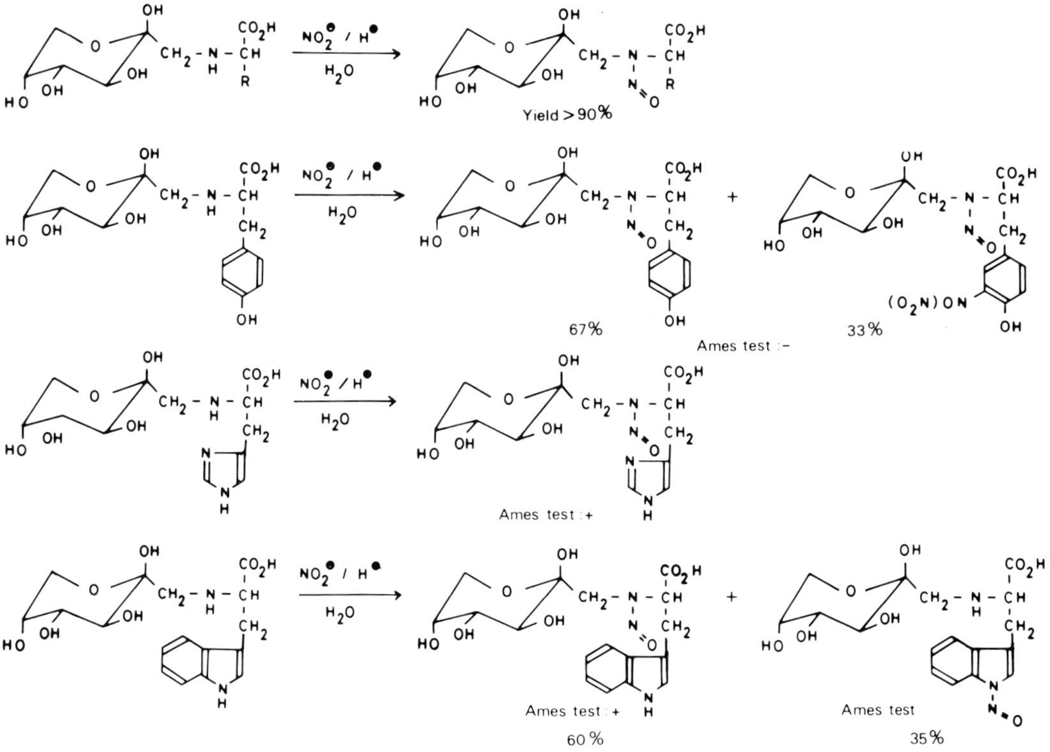

Table 2. High-performance liquid chromatographic analysis of N-NO-fructose amino acids by reversed-phase, ion-pairing chromatography[a]

N-NO-Fructose amino acid	Total retention time, t_R (min)
N-NO-D-Frugly	4.10
N-NO-D-Fru-L-ala	4.65
N-NO-D-Fru-L-val	7.55[b]
N-NO-D-Fru-L-leu	14.70[b]
N-NO-D-Fru-L-ileu	12.30 (20% Z)
	13.10 (80% E)
N-NO-D-Fru-L-ser[c]	4.00 (95% Z)
	4.65 (5% E)
N-NO-D-Fru-L-thr	3.85[b]
N-NO-D-Fru-L-met	10.40[b]
N-NO-D-Fru-L-asp	6.10
N-NO-D-Fru-L-phe	31.50
N-NO-D-Fru-L-tyr[d]	12.20 (40% Z)
	12.50 (60% E)
N-NO-D-Fru-L-his	9.90
α-N-NO-D-Fru-L-trp (F_1)	58.10 (70% Z)
	62.50 (30% E)
'Indolyl-NO'-D-fru-L-trp (F_2)	10.10
Sodium nitrite/water	4.60

[a] 30 cm μ-Bondapak C_{18} (10 μm) column (Waters); mobile phase: H_2O:H_3CCN (9:1, v/v) with 0.05 mol/L tetrabutylammoniumphosphate, pH 7.5 (PIC A, Waters) as the ion-pairing reagent; Ultra-violet detection (254 nm); flow rate 1 ml/min; detection limit, 5 ng
[b] Peak shoulders from E/Z isomers
[c] ^{13}C-NMR: 60% Z-, 40% E-isomer
[d] Additional peak with t_R = 22.0 min: aromatic substituted C-NO (C-NO$_2$) produkt

RESULTS

Figure 1 shows the prepared fructose- and N-NO-fructose amino acids, together with the sugar ring forms observed by high-resolution ^{1}H-NMR and ^{13}C-NMR spectroscopy. Table 1 shows the range of amounts of ring forms for the fructose amino acids in D_2O mutarotation equilibrium, as determined by ^{13}C-NMR spectroscopy, as well as those of the corresponding N-NO-fructose amino acids and the amounts of E/Z isomers. Figure 2 shows the nitrosation products of D-fru-L-tyr, D-fru-L-his and D-fru-L-trp.

Tables 3 and 4 show the results of quantitative Ames tests with N-NO-fructose amino acids with various strains of *Salmonella typhimurium* with and without metabolic activation (S9-Mix). The compounds were free from nitrite. The corresponding amino acids and D-fructose, tested under the same conditions, were not mutagenic.

Table 5 shows the preliminary results of mutagenicity tests (Ames tests) with dimethyl sulphoxide and ether extracts from pyrolysis of N-NO-D-fru-L-val and N-NO-D-fru-L-leu.

DISCUSSION

Fructose amino acids (Röper *et al.*, 1983) and N-NO-fructose amino acids (Heyns *et al.*, 1979; Röper *et al.*, 1982; Röper, 1983) (Fig. 1) were prepared as pure substances and were investigated by ^{1}H-NMR and ^{13}C-NMR spectroscopy. In the ^{13}C-NMR spectra of these

Table 3. Summary of quantitative mutagenicity test results with N-NO-D-fructose amino acids (Salmonella/microsome assays)[a] (B.L. Pool, German Cancer Research Center, Heidelberg, FRG)

	TA1535 −S9	TA1535 +S9	TA1537 −S9	TA1537 +S9	TA1538 −S9	TA1538 +S9	TA98 −S9	TA98 +S9	TA100 −S9	TA100 +S9
N-NO-D-fru-gly	−	−	−	−	−	−	−	−	−	−
N-NO-D-fru-L-ala	−	−	−	−	−	−	−	−	−	−
N-NO-D-fru-L-pheala	−	−	−	−	−	−	−	−	−	−
N-NO-D-fru-L-asp	−	−	−	−	−	−	−	−	−	−
N-NO-D-fru-L-tyr[b]	±[c]	−	−	−	−	−	−	−	−	−
N-NO-D-fru-L-ser	+	−	−	−	−	−	−	−	−	−
N-NO-D-fru-L-trp[d] (mixture)	+	+	+	+	+	+	+	+	+	+

N-NO-D-fru-L-ser

TA1535 (−S9)
dose (μg/plate)	0	0.5	5	50	500	2500	5000
rev./plate[e]	14	18	21	25	31	35	32
rev./μg	0	8	1.4	0.22	0.034	0.0084	0.0036

N-NO-D-fru-L-trp

TA1535 (−S9)
dose (μg/plate)	0	0.5	5	50	500	1000	2500	5000
rev./plate	25	27	36	61	84	94	ND	ND
rev./μg	0	4	2.2	0.72	0.118	0.069		

TA1535 (+S9)
dose (μg/plate)	0	0.5	5	50	500	1000	2500	5000
rev./plate	21	36	44	48	80	98	ND	ND
rev./μg	0	30	4.6	0.54	0.118	0.007		

TA1537 (−S9)
dose (μg/plate)	0	0.5	5	50	500	2500	5000
rev./plate	4	3	5	5	11	41	92
rev./μg	0	−2	0.2	0.02	0.014	0.0148	0.0176

TA1537 (+S9)
dose (μg/plate)	0	0.5	5	50	500	2500	5000
rev./plate	9	−2	12	8	11	34	51
rev./μg	0				0.004	0.01	0.0084

TA1538 (−S9)
dose (μg/plate)	0	0.5	5	50	500	2500	5000
rev./plate	6	17	10	4	12	ND	ND
rev./μg	0				0.004	0.018	

TA1538 (+S9)
dose (μg/plate)	0	0.5	5	50	500	2500	5000
rev./plate	22	24	27	22	23	37	42
rev./μg	0	4	1	0	0.002	0.006	0.004

TA98 (−S9)
dose (μg/plate)	0	0.5	5	50	500	2500	5000
rev./plate	28	26	26	28	39	105	165
rev./μg	0	−4	−0.4	0	0.022	0.0308	0.0274

TA98 (+ S9)	dose (µg/plate)	0	0.5	5	50	500	1 000	2 500	5 000
	rev./plate	32	37	33	34	36	ND	44	73
	rev./µg		10	0.2	0.04	0.008		0.0048	0.0082
TA100 (− S9)	dose (µg/plate)	0	0.5	5	50	500	1 000	2 500	5 000
	rev./plate	130	120	127	131	159	ND	281	395
	rev./µg		− 20	− 0.6	0.02	0.058		0.0604	0.053
TA100 (+ S9)	dose (µg/plate)	0	0.5	5	50	500	1 000	2 500	5 000
	rev./plate	171	164	164	168	181	ND	244	300
	rev./µg		− 14	− 1.4	− 0.06	0.02		0.0292	0.0258

[a] 0.5–5000 µg/plate in 6 concentrations, double determinations. Positive control (without metabolic activation S9) with NaN₃; for TA1535 (1410 rev./µg) and TA100 (860 rev./µg), positive control (+ S9) with 2-amino-anthracene for TA1535 (62 rev./µg), TA1537 (38 rev./µg), TA1538 (129 rev./µg), TA98 (113 rev./µg) and TA100 (114 rev./µg); positive control with 2-nitrofluorene (− S9) for TA1538 (69 rev./µg) and TA98 (68 rev./µg); positive control with 9-aminoacridine (− S9) for TA1537 (1 rev./µg)

[b] Mixture with 33% aromatic nitrosated (nitrated) product

[c] Borderline cases: doubling of spontaneous his⁺ revertants; L-amino acids and D-fructose, tested under identical conditions, were not mutagenic in any strain

[d] 'Indolyl-NO'-D-fru-L-trp was negative in qualitative spot tests in all strains (± S9); mixture containing 60% N-NO-D-fru-L-trp and 35% 'indolyl-NO'-D-fru-L-trp

[e] Mean value of his⁺ revertants calculated from a total of at least 18 plates of 6–9 individual experiments

Table 4.   Summary of quantitative mutagenicity tests[a] with N-NO-D-fructose amino acids (*Salmonella*/microsome assay with 30-min preincubation) (H. Marquardt et al., Dept. Toxicology, University of Hamburg Medical School, Hamburg, FRG)

	TA1535		TA1537		TA1538		TA98		TA100	
	−S9	+S9	−S9	+S9	−S9	+S9	−S9	+S9	−S9	+S9
N-NO-D-fru-L-met	−	−	−	−	−	−	−	−	−	−
N-NO-D-fru-L-leu	−	−	ND	ND	ND	ND	ND	ND	−	−
N-NO-D-fru-L-val	+	ND	−	−	−	−	−	−	+	+
N-NO-D-fru-L-thr	+	+	ND	ND	−	−	−	−	+	+
N-NO-D-fru-L-his	+	+	ND	ND	ND	ND	ND	ND	+	+

N-NO-D-fru-L-val

TA1535 (−S9)	dose (µg/plate)	0 (H₂O)	1 000	2 000	3 000	6 000	9 000
	rev./plate[b]	12	14		21		35
	rev./µg	0	0.002		0.003		0.0026
TA100 (−S9)	dose (µg/plate)	0 (H₂O)	1 000	2 000	3 000	6 000	9 000
	rev./plate	120	139	147	121	156	180
	rev./µg	0	0.019	0.0135	0.0003	0.006	0.0067
TA100 (+S9)	dose (µg/plate)	0 (H₂O)	1 000	2 000	3 000	6 000	9 000
	rev./plate	103	83	81	77	149	182
	rev./µg	0	−0.02	−0.011	−0.0087	0.0077	0.0088

N-NO-D-fru-L-thr

TA1535 (−S9)	dose (µg/plate)	0 (H₂O)	1 000	3 000	6 000	9 000
	rev./plate	6	4	7	11	69
	rev./µg	0	−0.002	0.0003	0.0008	0.007
TA1535 (+S9)	dose (µg/plate)	0 (H₂O)	1 000	3 000	6 000	9 000
	rev./plate	9	7	6	11	54
	rev./µg	0	−0.002	−0.001	0.0003	0.005
TA100 (−S9)	dose (µg/plate)	0 (H₂O)	1 000	3 000	6 000	9 000
	rev./plate	66	66	82	77	198
	rev./µg	0	0	0.0053	0.0018	0.0147
TA100 (+S9)	dose (µg/plate)	0 (H₂O)	1 000	3 000	6 000	9 000
	rev./plate	54	78	66	71	177
	rev./µg	0	0.024	0.004	0.0028	0.0137

N-NO-D-fru-L-his[c]

TA1535 (−S9)	dose (µg/plate)	0 (H₂O)	1 000	3 000	6 000
	rev./plate	6	56	101	138
	rev./µg	0	0.05	0.0317	0.022
TA1535 (+S9)	dose (µg/plate)	0 (H₂O)	1 000	3 000	6 000
	rev./plate	6	48	137	142
	rev./µg	0	0.042	0.0437	0.0227
TA100 (−S9)	dose (µg/plate)	0 (H₂O)	1 000	3 000	6 000
	rev./plate	88	154	265	360
	rev./µg	0	0.066	0.059	0.0453
TA100 (+S9)	dose (µg/plate)	0 (H₂O)	1 000	3 000	6 000
	rev./plate	96	163	244	333
	rev./µg	0	0.067	0.0493	0.0395

Sodium nitrite

TA1535 (−S9)	dose (µg/plate)	0 (H₂O)	10	100	500
	rev./plate	9	ND	18	62
	rev./µg	0	ND	0.09	0.106
TA100 (−S9)	dose (µg/plate)	0 (H₂O)	10	100	500
	rev./plate	53	73	75	97
	rev./µg	0	2.0	0.2	0.106

[a] Positive control (−S9) with NaN₃ for TA100 and TA1535; positive control (+S9) with 2-aminoanthracene for TA100 and TA1535
[b] Mean value of three plates per dose; compounds were NaNO₂-free as tested with Griess reagent
[c] D-fru-L-his is not mutagenic in *S. typhimurium* when tested at 6 000 µg/plate in TA1535 (±S9) or TA100 (±S9)

Table 5. Pyrolysis products of N-NO-fructose amino acids[a]. Results of qualitative mutagenicity tests (Ames tests) with dimethylsulfoxide and ether extracts (H. Marquardt, University of Hamburg, FRG)

	Dimethylsulfoxide extract TA100 −S9	Ether extract TA100 −S9
N-NO-D-fru-L-val (mutagenic)	−	+
N-NO-D-fru-L-leu (not mutagenic)	−	+

[a] N-NO-Fructose amino acids were heated in dry state in closed vessels up to 190 °C; after cooling, the pyrolysates were extracted with dimethylsulfoxide and ether. S9, metacyclic activation

compounds in D_2O mutarotation equilibrium, separated signals of the sugar ring forms (β-pyranose, β-furanose, α-furanose and α-pyranose) are observed. Their relative amounts can be calculated from the signal intensities (integrals) (Table 1). The β-pyranose forms are predominant, followed by the β-furanose-, α-furanose and α-pyranose forms. Signals from the keto forms are observed only in concentrated solutions ($> 2\%$). In the case of N-NO-fructose amino acids, signal doublings of ^{13}C resonances from E/Z isomers are observed. The relative amounts of these isomers can be determined as well for the different ring forms.

Nitrosation of D-fructose-L-tyrosine gives a mixture of 67% N-NO-fructose -L-tyrosine and 33% of N-NO-D-fructose-L-tyrosin, which is C-nitrosated or C-nitrated at the phenol ring system (Fig.2). The different nitrosation products can be separated by analytical HPLC (Table 2), but not yet on a preparative scale. The mixture of these nitroso compounds is not mutagenic (Table 3).

Nitrosation of D-fructose-L-histidine gives only one N-Nitroso product: N-NO-D-fructose-L-histidine, which was isolated in a pure state. The imidazolyl -NH is not nitrosated to give a stable dinitroso product. N-NO-D-fructose-L-histidine is mutagenic.

Two nitrosation products of D-fructose-L-tryptophan were isolated: N-NO-D-fructose-L-tryptophan (60%), which is mutagenic, and 'indolyl-N-NO'-D-fructose-L-tryptophan (35%), which is not mutagenic in the Ames test (Röper et al., 1982). A di-N-nitroso product of D-fructose-L-tryptophan is not formed.

For the analytical screening of foodstuffs which are suspected of containing N-NO-fructose amino acids, a method of separation and quantitative determination was developed. All prepared N-NO-D-fructose-L-amino acids can be separated by reversed-phase, ion-pairing HPLC (Table 2). In some cases, the E/Z isomer N-NO-compounds are separated or appear as peak shoulders. Their proportions calculated from the peak areas agree with those calculated from the ^{13}C-NMR spectra.

In Tables 3 and 4, the results of extensive quantitative mutagenicity tests (Ames tests) with different strains of *Salmonella typhimurium* ($\pm$ S9) are summarized. The results show that the N-NO-Amadori compounds fall into three categories with regard to their mutagenic action:

A. *Non-mutagenic N-NO-D-fructose-L-amino acids* (Tables 3 & 4)

N-NO-D-frugly, N-NO-D-fru-L-ala, N-NO-D-fru-L-pheala, N-NO-D-fru-L-leu, N-NO-D-fru-L-ser, N-NO-D-fru-L-met, N-NO-D-fru-asp and N-NO-D-fru-L-tyr were non-mutagenic in all tester strains – TA1535, TA1537, TA1538, TA100, TA98 – with and without metabolic activation over a dose range of 0.5–9 000 μg/plate. N-NO-D-fru-L-ser, however, seems to be weak mutagen (borderline case) in TA1535 (-S9), since the number of spontaneous *his*[+] revertants was more than doubled with 500, 2 500, and 500 μg/plate.

B. *Borderline cases (Table 4)*

N-NO-D-fru-L-val, shows clear dose-response relationships of the number of colonies formed in TA1535 (-S9) and TA100 ($\pm$ S9), with more than a doubling – TA1535 (-S9) – or nearly doubling of the number of *his* $^{+}$ revertants – TA100 ($\pm$ S9) – at the highest dosages (9 000 µg/plate). *N*-NO-D-fru-L-val is not mutagenic to TA1537 ($\pm$ S9), TA1538 ($\pm$ S9), TA1538 ($\pm$ S9) or TA98 ($\pm$ S9).

C. *Mutagenic N-NO-D-fructose-L-amino acids (Tables 3 & 4)*

N-NO-D-fru-L-thr (Table 4) is mutagenic in TA1535 ($\pm$ S9) and TA100 ($\pm$ S9) at dosages around 9 000 µg/plate, whereas it is not mutagenic in TA1538 ($\pm$ S9) or TA98 ($\pm$ S9). The compound was not tested in TA1537 ($\pm$ S9).

The mutagenicity of *N*-NO-D-fru-L-his in TA1535 ($\pm$ S9) and TA100 ($\pm$ S9) is clearly indicated by the results in Table 4 within the dosage range 1 000–6 000 µg/plate. The compound was not tested in TA 1537 ($\pm$ S9), TA1538 ($\pm$ S9) or TA98 ($\pm$ S9). The precursor D-fru-L-his was not mutagenic in TA1535 ($\pm$ S9) or TA100 ($\pm$ S9) at a dose of 6 000 µg/plate.

N-NO-D-fru-L-trp, tested in the dose range 0.5–5 000 µg/plate, showed strong mutagenic effects in all strains with and without S9 metabolic activation (Table 3). Doublings of the number of spontaneous *his* $^{+}$ revertants were observed with doses of only 50–500 µg/plate in TA1535 ($\pm$ S9) and TA1537 (-S9). In the other strains, the mutagenic effect appeared with higher dosages: > 1 000 µg/plate with TA1537 (+S9), TA1538 ($\pm$ S9), TA98 ($\pm$ S9) and TA100 ($\pm$ S9).

Table 4 shows also the results in the quantitative Ames assay with sodium nitrite in TA1535 and TA100 (-S9): 100 µg/plate and 500 µg/plate were mutagenic in TA1535 (-S9) and TA100 (-S9), respectively.

Whereas *N*-NO-D-fru-L-val, *N*-NO-D-Fru-L-thr and *N*-NO-D-fru-L-his seem to act as mutagens only by alkylation and base-pair substitution (in TA 1535, TA100), *N*-NO-D-fru-L-trp can act both by alkylation and base-pair substitution (in TA 1535, TA100), and as a frame-shift mutagen, by intercalation of the heterocyclic indole ring system between DNA double-strands of the bacteria.

The preliminary results of pyrolysis experiments with *N*-NO-D-fru-L-val (weak mutagen) and *N*-NO-D-fru-L-leu (non-mutagenic) show that mutagenic extracts of pyrolysis products are obtained with ether and non-mutagenic extracts with dimethyl sulfoxide. In the case of *N*-NO-D-fru-L-leu from a non-mutagenic *N*-NO-Amadori compound, mutagenic products of unknown structures can be formed by dry heating (Table 5).

The results of such mutagenicity tests could be used, therefore to screen nitrate- and/or nitrite-containing Maillard systems, e.g., cured meat products, tobacco, for the presence of mutagenic *N*-NO-Amadori compounds: *N*-NO-D-fru-L-met, *N*-NO-D-fru-L-his and *N*-NO-D-fru-L-trp. Even the corresponding precursor fructose amino acids should be taken into consideration because of their possible in-vivo formation in the human body.

ACKNOWLEDGEMENTS

We thank the Deutsche Forschungsgemeinschaft (DFG) for financial support and Mrs Renate Poehls for skillful assistance.

REFERENCES

Ames, B.N., McCann, J. & Yamasaki, E. (1975) Methods for detecting carcinogens and mutagens with the *Salmonella* /mammalian-microsome mutagenicity test. *Mutat. Res., 31,* 347

Coughlin, J.R. (1979) *Formation of* N-*nitrosamines from Maillard-Browning Reaction Products in the Presence of Nitrite,* Thesis, University of California

Heyns, K. Röper, S., Röper H. & Meyer, B. (1979) *N*-nitroso sugar amino acids. *Angew. Chem.,* **91,** 940–941; *Angew. Chem. Int. Ed. Engl.,* **18,** 878–880

Röper, H. (1983) *Organische Umweltkarzinogen. Spurenanalyse und Entstehung von* N-*nitroso-Verbindungen.* Habilitationsschrift, Fachbereich Chemie, Universität Hamburg

Röper, H., Röper, S., Heyns, K. & Meyer, B. (1982) N-*Nitroso sugar amino acids* (*N*-NO-D-fructose-L-amino-acids). In: Bartsch, H., O´Neill, I.K., Castegnaro, M. & Okada, M., eds, N-*Nitroso Compounds: Occurrence and Biological Effects (IARC Scientific Publications No. 41),* Lyon, International Agency for Research on Cancer, pp. 87–98

Röper, H., Röper, S., Heyns, K. & Meyer, B. (1983) NMR spectroscopy of *N*-(1-deoxy-d-fructos-1-yl)-L-amino acids ('fructose-amino acids'). *Carbohydr. Res.,* **116,** 183–195

PITFALLS TO AVOID IN DETERMINING *N*-NITROSO COMPOUNDS AS A GROUP

C.L. WALTERS & P.L.R. SMITH

Leatherhead Food Research Association, Leatherhead, Surrey, UK

P.I. REED

Gastrointestinal Unit, Wexham Park Hospital, Slough, Berkshire, UK

INTRODUCTION

While sensitive and selective methods are available for the determination of volatile *N*-nitrosamines, the great majority of precursors in a biological matrix would give rise to nonvolatile *N*-nitroso derivatives of amines, amides, guanidines, etc. Prime examples of such precursors are proline, hydroxyproline and sarcosine. Only a few of the non-volatile *N*-nitroso derivatives of such components have been evaluated for carcinogenicity, but the vast majority of *N*-nitrosamines, -amides, -ureas, -guanidines and -urethanes have induced tumours in a range of organs in experimental animals and sometimes in many different species.

Because of the considerable numbers of nitrosatable precursors in biological matrices, it would be impracticable to monitor large numbers of samples for each *N*-nitroso compound individually. It is therefore necessary to be able to screen samples for such compounds as a goup and to do so as selectively as possible to pinpoint those deserving more detailed examination. Any such method should be applicable to as many types of compounds as possible and should be capable of differentiating *N*-nitroso compounds from nitrite, nitrate and other compounds derived from them. A number of methods have been devised for the above purpose and this communication is intended to review them.

REVIEW OF METHODS

Stabilization of samples

Two prime objectives need to be considered in the selection of methods for the stabilization of samples to be analysed for *N*-nitroso compounds, namely (1) prevention of artefacts formed after sampling; and (2) retention of as many as possible of the compounds to be determined.

One of the first procedures to be adopted for the stabilization of *N*-nitroso compounds in biological systems was the addition of alkali to raise the pH to values at which the availability of undissociated nitrous acid and the possibility of bacterial intervention are extremely small. However, Challis *et al.* (1978) have demonstrated the case with which nitrosation can proceed at alkaline pH values, using dinitrogen trioxide and dinitrogen tetroxide. While the simple dialkyl and heterocyclic *N*-nitrosamines are considered to be stable in alkali, this is certainly not true of *N*-nitrosamides.

Sulfamic acid has two roles as a stabilizing agent, namely that of reducing the pH and thereby removing any nitrite present very rapidly and of preventing the bacterial reduction of nitrate. No excess formation of *N*-nitrosomorpholine has been observed from morpholine in aqueous solution containing nitrite concentrations of 1.0 mmol/L or 10 mmol/L at pH 3.0 or 7.0, following the addition of solid sulfamic acid to a concentration of 0.5 g in 100 mL (Smith & Walters, unpublished data). While no material destruction of *N*-nitrosamines occurs during storage in an aqueous solution of sulfamic acid, its pH is below that considered to be optimal (pH 4) for the stability of *N*-nitrosamides. Nevertheless, sulfamic acid is considered by Challis (1981) to be one of the two stabilizing agents that have the least effect on *N*-nitrosamides.

A system has been devised by Bavin *et al.* (1982) for the removal of nitrite at the pH value (4.0) anticipated to retain *N*-nitrosamides as effectively as possible. No details have been given concerning nitrosamide stability in the hydrazine solution employed, but this reagent, according to Challis (1981), promotes the breakdown of *N*-nitrosamides.

Ascorbic acid, an inhibitor of nitrosation, can also be used for the removal of nitrite, but its use can lead to the formation of oxides of nitrogen, which are themselves active nitrosating agents.

Determination of N-*nitroso compounds as a group*

All attempts to determine *N*-nitroso compounds as a group have been based on the common feature of the *N*-nitroso function which allows it to be cleaved to form either nitrite, a nitrosyl halide or nitric oxide. In 1964, for instance, Daiber and Preussmann reported that *N*-nitrosamines can be photolysed under alkaline conditions using ultra-violet irradiation, a major product being nitrite. In simple solution, the yield of nitrite can approach the theoretical; it can be markedly reduced, however, in the presence of co-extracted substances present in a biological sample (Walters *et al.*, 1970). Furthermore, a number of other types of nitrogenous compounds, including ammonia, can give rise to nitrite on photolysis with broad-wavelength ultra-violet light. Fan & Tannenbaum (1971) adopted the suggestion of Sander (1967) to employ a longer wavelength (360 nm) in order to increase the selectivity of the procedure. This eliminated interference by nitrate, but no information was given concerning the responses of other types of compounds containing oxygenated nitrogen atoms, such as *S*-nitrosothiols. Nevertheless, the method is potentially useful in that it is directly applicable to aqueous solutions.

The process of formation of *N*-nitroso compounds from nitrous acid and secondary amines is considered to be reversible, and it is difficult to ensure complete denitrosation of an *N*-nitrosamine in an aqueous environment. However, Eisenbrand and Preussmann (1970) succeeded in obtaining complete breakdown in acetic acid using hydrogen bromide. The nitrosyl bromide formed reacts as nitrite in the presence of added water and can therefore be determined spectrophotometrically as a red dye, using, for instance, sulfanilamide followed by *N*-(1-naphthyl)ethylenediamine. The denitrosation process with hydrogen bromide will tolerate water to an extent of about 10%, above which the process is almost completely suppressed. It is generally complete within a maximum of 15 min at room temperature, except for *N*-nitrosopyrrolidine, for which at least one hour is required (Castegnaro *et al.*, 1982). Denitrosation can also be accomplished in a water-immiscible solvent, such as hexane. At the end of the reaction, the product can be shaken with an aqueous solution of sulfanilamide to trap any nitrosyl bromide formed, the diazonium compound produced being converted to a red dye following the addition of *N*-(1-naphthyl)-ethylenediamine. While this procedure is very useful for monitoring *N*-nitrosamines in simple solution, the product of denitrosation, nitrosyl bromide, is very reactive and can interact with co-extracted phenols, amines, thiols, etc.

Nevertheless, the selectivity of the method of Eisenbrand and Preussmann for *N*-nitrosamines is high, and Walters *et al.* (1978) therefore set out to improve its sensitivity to approach that required for environmental studies. This improvement has been achieved by means of a number of modifications:

(1) a choice of conditions for denitrosation leading to rapid breakdown of nitrosyl bromide to nitric oxide, which is far less reactive, and to its immediate removal from the site of reaction in a stream of nitrogen, and

(2) the use of a chemiluminescence analyser for the sensitive and selective determination of nitric oxide.

The chemiluminescence analyser used is akin to that incorporated in the Thermal Energy Analyzer and relies upon the oxidation of nitric oxide by ozone to electronically activated NO_2^*, which emits light in the far-visible and near-infra-red regions as it decays to its ground state.

In order to ensure that the nitric oxide detected does not include a contribution from nitrite and other compounds derived from it, a sequential procedure is employed. Initially, thermally-labile compounds in an extract or solid matrix, such as *S*-nitroso derivatives of thiols, are cleaved in refluxing ethyl acetate. When any associated evolution of nitric oxide has ceased, acetic acid is introduced to decompose inorganic and organic nitrites. The amount of nitric oxide formed provides a measure of their concentration. The subsequent introduction of hydrogen bromide results in the evolution of nitric oxide from *N*-nitroso compound. Finally, nitric oxide can be derived from nitrate, *C*- and *N*-nitro compounds, etc., through the introduction of titanous chloride in the presence of hydrogen bromide. The application of the sequential procedure to an animal diet has been reported by Walters *et al.* (1980).

Subsequently, a similar method that it is claimed can estimate extractable *N*-nitroso compounds at the μg/kg level, was proposed by Drescher and Frank (1978). Again, denitrosation of *N*-nitroso compounds was accomplished using hydrogen bromide in glacial acetic acid, the amount of the latter being chosen so as to maintain a one-phase system in the presence of the dichloromethane extract under examination. The reaction is carried out at room temperature in a test tube attached to a degassing system by means of which nitric oxide is removed for determination by flushing with helium. All reactants are placed in the test tube, which is then immediately attached to the degassing system; thus, this method does not allow the differentiation of *N*-nitrosamines from nitrite and other compounds derived from it. Nitrite is therefore removed initially from extracts in dichloromethane by back-extraction into water, but this process was recognized to lead to losses of polar *N*-nitrosamines, such as *N*-nitrosoproline.

A third method that makes use of hydrogen bromide as denitrosating agent is that of Bavin *et al.* (1982). In this procedure, gastric juices are stabilized by treating them with a solution of hydrazine, buffered at pH 4, to remove nitrite. The treated gastric juice is then injected directly, without extraction, into refluxing ethyl acetate containing hydrogen bromide. The nitric oxide released at this stage is considered to represent the *N*-nitroso compounds present. The principal advantage of this method is speed, it being possible to carry out a determination within five minutes of sample collection.

A great advantage is claimed for a method due to Cox *et al.* (1982), in as much as the denitrosation process takes place in an aqueous environment, the active agent being 10% sodium iodide added to the sample and acidified with acetic acid and sulfuric acids. Both nitrate and nitrite interfere, the former only at concentrations above 4 mg nitrate nitrogen/L (0.29 mmol/L) and the latter at all levels. It is therefore necessary to remove these compounds initially by ion exchange, using the anion exchanger, Dowex IX-8. This process is capable of reducing the concentration of nitrate to an insignificant level, but a further treatment with sulfanilamide is necessary to eliminate completely the involvement of nitrite. The recoveries of N-nitrosodiethanolamine added to urine in amounts of 0.34 and 5.6 nmol/10 mL were 100% and 95%, respectively. Those of N-nitrosoatrazine ranged from 33% for an addition of 0.44 nmol to 50% for 7.5 nmol.

COMPARISONS BETWEEN METHODS

Direct use of samples

The methods to be compared are summarized in Table 1. Two of them (C and D) are capable of accepting solid samples directly, so that non-extractable N-nitroso compounds on a matrix can be determined. In addition, method C permits the preliminary dissipation of nitric oxide from nitrite and related compounds before the injection of hydrogen bromide to denitrosate N-nitroso compounds. However, nitrite is often present at concentrations greatly in excess of those of N-nitrosamines; in order, therefore, to remove the possibility of the nitrosation of co-extracted amines, it is preferable to stabilize samples with hydrazine or sulfamic acid.

Methods A, E and F can accept any amounts of water. For B, however, the volume of water should be less than 10% of that of the hydrogen bromide reagent in acetic acid, although this proportion can be increased through the use of acetic anhydride. Water has a deleterious action in method C when the amount exceeds about 2% (v/v) of the amount of ethyl acetate; even a single drop of water (0.04 mL) resulted in a 50% reduction in the detector response in method D, compared with that for a similar solution in pure dichloromethane. The detector signal was eliminated completely after the addition of 0.2 mL of water.

Table 1.   Summary of methods used for the determination of N-nitroso compounds as a group

Method	Originator(s)	Procedure	Effect of water[a]	Limit of detection (nmol)		Interference from[b]		
				in simple solution	in extract	heat-labile compounds	nitrite	nitrate
A	Sander (1967)	Photolysis	none	5	?	?	+	−
B	Eisenbrand & Preussmann (1970)	HBr	10%	5	700	?	+	−
C	Walters et al. (1978)	HBr	2%	0.2–0.5	0.2–0.5	−	−	+
D	Drescher & Frank (1978)	HBr	trace	0.02–0.5	?	?	+	?
E	Cox et al. (1982)	HI	none	?	0.3	?	+	+
F	Bavin et al. (1982)	HBr	none	?	?	+	−	?

[a] Upper limit tolerated
[b] When using method as described by authors; interference can be avoided in some instances; +, interference; −, no interference

Limits of detection

Both methods A and B require the determination of nitrite, of which the limit of detection by spectrophotometry is approximately 5 nmol. In both cases, however, the limit of detection is made worse by the presence of co-extracted compounds. In determining *N*-nitrososarcosine on powdered cornflakes, for instance, no response at all was obtained by method B when less than 720 nmol (equivalent to a concentration of 5 mg/kg) were added.

A limit of detection for *N*-nitrosodiethylamine of 0.02 nmol was claimed for method D. Apart from that value, the minimum amounts of *N*-nitroso compounds required for a significant response were, where quoted, similar to those obtained by methods employing a chemiluminescence analyser to determine liberated nitric oxide. In general, the limit of detection using method C is not influenced adversely by the presence of co-extracted biological components except for large quantities of lipids. The sensitivity obtainable when using a chemiluminescence analyser is generally adequate for the determination of *N*-nitroso compounds in biological systems.

Interfering compounds

A number of compounds potentially derived from nitrite, other than *N*-nitrosamines and *N*-nitrosamides, yield nitric oxide in a refluxing solvent. Methods A, B, D and E are carried out at room temperature, and the extent of interferences from such compounds has not been reported. In method C, the evolution of nitric oxide from heat-labile compounds is allowed to cease before the *N*-nitroso compounds are denitrosated. In method F, no similar opportunity is provided to segregate evolution of the gas from this source from that derived from *N*-nitrosamines, *N*-nitrosamides, etc. In fact, amounts of nitric oxide ranging from 2–108% of the theoretical have been found to arise from compounds derived from nitrite, such as pseudonitrosites, when using this method (Barnard *et al.*, 1982).

Allowance must be made for nitrite itself in methods A and B. Fan and Tannenbaum (1971) have introduced a procedure whereby the loss of nitrite during irradiation (method A) can be accounted for in a control run, omitting the extract under examination but using the same concentration of nitrite. Method C ensures the evolution of nitric oxide from nitrite before the denitrosation of *N*-nitroso compounds. In general, however, all methods using a chemiluminescence analyser favour the prior removal of nitrite by decomposing it with sulfamic acid, hydrazine or sulfanilamide, or by back-extracting it from an extract into water; not unexpectedly, the last-mentioned procedure is recognized to lead to losses of polar *N*-nitrosamines.

According to Fan and Tannenbaum (1971), interference from nitrate when using method A can be eliminated by using longer wavelength ultra-violet irradiation. No interference results from the presence of nitrate when using method B. However, a very small evolution of nitric oxide results from the treatment of nitrate with hydrogen bromide in refluxing ethyl acetate, and this can lead to significant interference when a considerable excess is present; this can generally be avoided by extraction of the *N*-nitroso compounds into an immiscible solvent. Interference from nitrate was also recognized in method E at levels above 4 mg nitrate-nitrogen, and excess nitrate was therefore removed by ion exchange, prior to the denitrosation of *N*-nitroso compounds present. No precaution with regard to interference by nitrate was cited in methods D and F.

Reproducibility

By no means all of the methods reviewed provide information concerning the reproducibility of the procedure. The reproducibility of that of Eisenbrand and Preussmann (method B) was studied by Downes *et al.* (1976). The coefficients of variation obtained by two uninformed workers using nominal 16-μg aliquots of *N*-nitrososarcosine were 4.9% and 5.9%. The corresponding values for 2.5-μg aliquots of *N*-nitrososarcosine in simple solution by the same two workers using method C were 9.2% and 7.0%. When nominal 2.0 μg amounts of *N*-nitrososarcosine were distributed as evenly as possible on 10 g powdered corn flakes, the mean values obtained by direct determination without extraction by two inexperienced workers using method C were 1.75 μg and 2.07 μg, with coefficients of variation of 9.7% and 13.8, respectively. The reproducibility of method F in determining *N*-nitrosocimetidine in unknown amounts was quoted by Barnard *et al.* (1983) to be ± 8–10%.

Range of N-*nitroso compounds covered*

No *N*-nitroso compound tested to date has failed to respond to denitrosation with hydrogen bromide under the conditions of at least one of the methods involving detection as nitric oxide, using a chemiluminescence analyser (C, D, E and F). Compounds examined have included *N*-nitrosodialkylamines, -diarylamines, -alkarylamines, heterocyclic amines, N-nitrosamines, -ureas, -guanidines, -urethanes and -sulphonamides. Some variations have been reported in the molar response of individual compounds. For instance, that of *N*-nitrosocarbazole was reported to be 99% and 55% using methods D and F, respectively. In general, however, the molar responses have approached 100% of the theoretical.

Fig. 1. Evolution of nitric oxide from extract of human bile (A) in refluxing ethyl acetate and (B) following addition of hydrogen bromide in acetic acid

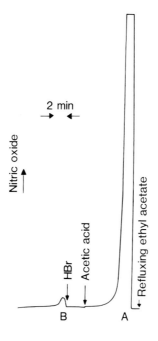

PRECAUTIONS RECOMMENDED IN DETERMINING *N*-NITROSAMINES AS A GROUP

Reagents

When determining low levels of *N*-nitrosamines by denitrosation, the hydrogen bromide reagent should be prepared by absorbing the gas in glacial acetic acid so as to reduce the blank response to a minimum. Massey and McWeeny (personal communication) have devised a procedure by means of which allowance can be made for the small blank response arising from heat-labile contaminants in the hydrogen bromide reagent. This involves the further addition of aliquots of hydrogen bromide to both the sample under examination and to the blank determination using the solvent alone. From the small responses obtained it is possible to calculate the contribution of the hydrogen bromide reagent itself to the nitric oxide released by the denitrosation of the *N*-nitroso compounds present.

Stabilization

In order to reduce to a minimum the potential formation of *N*-nitrosamines as artefacts from nitrite or oxides of nitrogen present, samples under examination should be stabilized. The method of choice will depend upon the information required, but consideration should be given to the following points:
(1) Hydrazine can be used effectively for stabilization at pH 4, at which *N*-nitrosamides are most stable, but is considered (Challis, 1981) to lead to their breakdown.
(2) Sulfamic acid requires a low pH to avoid artefact formation during stabilization, but is considered to have the least effect on *N*-nitrosamides (Challis, 1981).
(3) Ascorbic acid and nitrite lead to the formation of nitric oxide, which is oxidized in air to nitrogen dioxide, a very effective nitrosating agent.

Selective extraction

Extraction into an immiscible solvent should be undertaken whenever possible and particularly when large amounts of nitrate are present. When this is not feasible, nitrate can readily be removed by ion-exchange chromatography to levels excluding interference.

Determination stage

If the sample to be examined is aqueous, a method should be selected that will tolerate the amount of water involved. Nitric oxide from compounds other than *N*-nitrosamines, -amides, -ureas, -guanidines, -urethanes and -sulfonamides, which are labile under the conditions of the test procedure, should be dissipated before the denitrosation of *N*-nitroso compounds present. The necessity for this is illustrated by Figure 1, in which nitric oxide evolution from heat-labile compounds in an ethyl acetate extract of human bile was vastly greater than that produced following the subsequent denitrosation of putative *N*-nitroso compounds with hydrogen bromide. Thus, a grossly inaccurate value for *N*-nitroso compounds present would have been obtained had the sequential procedure not been employed.

ACKNOWLEDGEMENTS

C.L.W. and P.L.R.S. are grateful to the Cancer Research Campaign, London, for their financial support.

REFERENCES

Barnard, J., Bavin, P.M.G., Brimblecombe, R.W., Darkin, D.W., Durant, G.J. & Keighley, M.R.B. (1983) In: Magee, P.N., ed, *Nitrosamines and Human Cancer (Banbury Report No. 12)*, Cold Spring Harbor, N.Y., Cold Spring Harbor Laboratory, pp. 369–377

Bavin, P.M.G., Darkin, D.W. & Viney, N.J. (1982) *Total nitroso compounds in gastric juice.* In: Bartsch, H., O'Neill, I.K., Castegnaro, M. & Okada, M., eds, N-*Nitroso Compounds: Occurrence and Biological Effects (IARC Scientific Publications No. 41)*, Lyon, International Agency for Research on Cancer, pp. 337–343

Castegnaro, M., Michelon, J. & Walker, E.A. (1982) *Some detoxification methods for* N-*nitrosamine-contaminated wastes.* In: Bartsch, H., O'Neill, I.K., Castegnaro, M. & Okada, M., eds, N-*Nitroso Compounds: Occurrence and Biological Effects (IARC Scientific Publications No. 41)*, Lyon, International Agency for Research on Cancer, pp. 151–158

Challis, B.C. (1981) *The chemistry of formation of* N-*nitroso compounds.* In: Gibson, G.G. & Ioannides, C., eds, *Safety Evaluation of Nitrosatable Drugs and Chemicals*, London, Taylor & Francis Ltd., p. 16–55

Challis, B.C., Edwards, A., Hunma, R.R., Kyrtopoulos, S.A. & Outram, J.R. (1978) Rapid formation of N-nitrosamines from nitrogen oxides under neutral and alkaline conditions. In: Walker, E.A., Castegnaro, M., Griciute, L. & Lyle, R.E., eds, *Environmental Aspects of* N-*Nitroso Compounds (IARC Scientific Publications No. 19)*, Lyon, International Agency for Research on Cancer, pp. 127–142

Cox, R.D., Frank, C.W., Nikolalsen, L.D. & Caputo, R.E. (1982) Screening procedure for determination of total *N*-nitroso content in urine, *Anal. Chem., 54,* 253–256

Daiber, D. & Preussmann, R. (1964) Quantitative colorimetric determination of organic *N*-nitroso compounds by photochemical splitting of the nitroso amine bond, *Z. anal. Chem., 206,* 344–352

Downes, M.J., Edwards, M.W., Elsey, T.S. & Walters, C.L. (1976) Dermination of a non-volatile nitrosamine by using denitrosation and a chemiluminescence analyser, *Analyst, 101,* 742–748

Drescher, G.S. & Frank, C.W. (1978) Estimation of extractable *N*-nitroso compounds at the parts-per-billion level. *Anal. Chem., 50,* 2118–2121

Eisenbrand, G. & Preussmann, R. (1970) Eine neue Methode zur Kolorimetrischen Bestimmung von Nitrosaminen nach Spaltung der *N*-nitrosogruppe mit Bromwasserstoff in Eisessig. *Arzneimittel. Forsch., 20,* 1513–1517

Fan, T.Y. & Tannenbaum, S.R. (1971) Automatic colorimetric determination of *N*-nitroso compounds, *J. Agric. Food Chem., 19,* 1267–1269

Sander, J. (1967) Detection of nitrosamines. *Hoppe Seyler's Z. physiol. Chem., 348,* 852–854

Walters, C.L., Johnson, E.M. & Ray, N. (1970) Separation and detection of volatile and non-volatile *N*-nitrosamines, *Analyst, 95,* 485–489

Walters, C.L., Downes, M.J., Edwards, M.W. & Smith, P.L.R. (1987) Determination of a non-volatile *N*-nitrosamine on a food matrix, *Analyst, 103,* 1127–1133

Walters, C.L., Hart, R.J., Keefer, L.K. & Newberne, P.M. (1980) *The sequential determination of nitrite,* N-*nitroso compounds and nitrate and its application.* In: Walker, E.A., Griciute, L., Castegnaro, M. & Börzsönyi, M., eds, N-*Nitroso Compounds: Analysis, Formation and Occurrence (IARC Scientific Publications No. 31)*, Lyon, International Agency for Research on Cancer, pp. 389–399

A NEW THERMAL ENERGY ANALYZER FOR DIRECT HIGH-PERFORMANCE LIQUID CHROMATOGRAHIC AND GAS CHROMATO-GRAPHIC ANALYSIS OF N-NITROSAMIDES

D.H. FINE & D.P. ROUNBEHLER

New England Institute for Life Sciences, Waltham, MA 02154, USA

W.C. YU & E.U. GOFF

Thermo Electron Corporation, Waltham, MA 02254, USA

SUMMARY

The Thermal Energy Analyzer (TEA) has been modified to make it capable of detecting compounds such as *N*-nitrosamides. This modified TEA(amide) can be used with both gas chromatography (GC) and high-performance liquid chromatography (HPLC). Analysis of underivatized *N*-nitroso amides by GC-TEA(amide) and HPLC-TEA(amide) are also described.

INTRODUCTION

Using improved analytical techniques based on gas chromatography (GC), high-resolution mass spectrometry (HRMS) and GC-thermal energy analysis (TEA) (Fine, 1982), 13 *N*-nitrosamines have been found in various environments to which humans are exposed. Not a single *N*-nitrosamide (including *N*-nitrosoureas and *N*-nitrosoguanidines) has yet been shown to be present in the environment. This trend of finding relatively low molecular weight *N*-nitrosamines and not the non-volatile *N*-nitrosamides may only reflect the relative ease with which the analysis of the *N*-nitrosamines can now be carried out.

The lack of environmental data on non-volatile *N*-nitroso compounds is disturbing for several reasons:

First, it has been suggested by numerous workers that human gastric cancer may be caused, at least in part, by certain alkylnitrosamides which could be formed by intragastric nitrosation of alkylamides present in foods and drugs (Endo *et al.*, 1977).

Second, of the 86 *N*-nitrosamides that have been tested, 79 have been shown to be carcinogenic in animal experiments (National Academy of Sciences, 1981). Furthermore, *N*-nitrosamides are known to be direct alkylating agents without metabolic activation.

Third, precursors of *N*-nitrosamides are known to be present in the environment (Mirvish *et al.*, 1982). Nitrosatable guanidino compounds, for example, have been shown to be present in foodstuffs (Fujinaka *et al.*, 1978). Urea derivatives are also used as drugs (Mirvish & Chu, 1973), cosmetics (Cosmetic, Toiletry and Fragrance Association, 1977) and as agricultural pesticides (Thompson, 1975).

Fourth, compounds such as ethylurea are known to nitrosate at a rate many orders of magnitude faster than amines such as dimethylamine or even morpholine (Mirvish, 1975).

Fifth, the rate of nitrosation of amides depends on the concentration of nitrite to the first power, whereas amine nitrosation has a second-order dependence. Thus, at low concentrations of nitrite, ureas and amides nitrosate faster than do amines (Mirvish, 1975).

Sixth, recent analytical data of Walters *et al.* (1978), Bavin *et al.* (1982) and others on the total *N*-nitroso compound content of human body fluids have suggested the presence of relatively large amounts of as yet unidentified nonvolatile *N*-nitroso compounds.

Current methods for the analysis of N-nitrosamides

The analysis of *N*-nitrosamides in complex environmental or biological samples is made difficult by the lack of detection techniques. *N*-nitrosamides are much less stable than *N*-nitrosamines; they are generally non-volatile and decompose both thermally and photolytically.

A method for detection *N*-nitrosamides, in which they are hydrolysed under acidic conditions to liberate nitrite, was described by Preussmann and Schaper-Druckery (1972). In its simplest form, the nitrite which is released is detected colorimetrically, using Griess or similar reagents. Singer *et al.* (1977) interfaced the technique to reversed-phase high-performance liquid chromatography (HPLC). Walters *et al.* (1978) improved upon the sensitivity of the detection step by rapid release of the nitrosyl radical from the solution and detection by means of its chemiluminescent reaction with ozone. Drescher and Frank (1978) and Bavin *et al.* (1982) also detected the nitrosyl radical by chemiluminescence. The drawback of the technique is that it is too slow to be used as the detector for HPLC. For this reason, these procedures are used as a group detector for total *N*-nitroso compound content. Saul *et al.* (1982) were able to collect fractions from the HPLC, which they then analysed in batches, allowing them to construct a crude chromatogram.

Photolytic hydrolysis of *N*-nitroso compounds to release the nitrosyl radical was proposed by Daiber and Preussmann (1965). Tannenbaum[1] interfaced the photolytic hydrolysis technique to HPLC and used it for the analysis of *N*-nitrosamides. Other methods that have been used include HPLC with ultra-violet detection (Krull & Strauss, 1981) and derivation of the amide to a volatile product followed by GC-mass spectroscopy (MS) (Weinkam *et al.*, 1978; Smith *et al.*, 1981). Mirvish *et al.* (1979) denitrosated the nitrosoureas and then detected the parent urea by means of the Hunninglake and Grisolia spectrophotometric method.

None of the methods that has been used to date is adequately simple, rapid, sensitive or selective to be really useful in assessing the extent of man's exposure to *N*-nitrosamides. The goal of our research, therefore, was to find a way around the technological impasse, and to make the *N*-nitrosamides as easy to analyse as are the volatile *N*-nitrosamines.

Thermal denitrosation

Although the original work on the prototype TEA (Fine *et al.*, 1974) indicated that it exhibited a response to *N*-nitrosamides such as *N*-ethyl-*N*-nitrosourea (ENU), *N*-methyl-*N*-nitrosourethane (MNUT) and *N*-methyl-*N'*-nitro-*N*-nitrosoguanidine (MNNG), Hansen *et al.* (1979) and Mirvish *et al.* (1979) subsequently showed the response to be erratic, with poor yields. They advanced the theory that the nitrosoureas fragment during pyrolysis by a pathway

---

[1] Personal communication

Fig. 1. Thermal rearrangement of *N*-nitrosamides to diazo esters

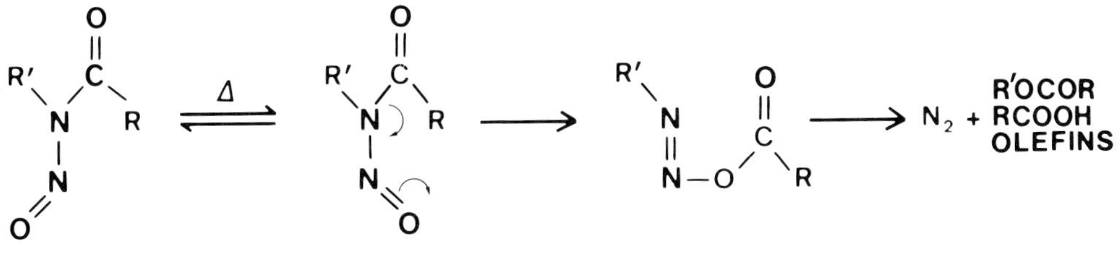

similar to their breakdown in electron-impact mass spectrometry. By analogy, mass spectrometric fragmentation of *N*-nitrosamines gives NO, whereas nitrosoureas cleave at the N-CO bond, followed by cleavage of the N-O bond of the resulting monoalkylnitrosamine ion, yielding the diazonium ion.

Another explanation comes from the work of Chow (1979). He showed that *N*-nitrosamides undergo irreversible thermal rearrangements at temperatures ranging from ambient to 100 °C to give diazo esters (Fig. 1). The diazo esters (III) themselves undergo rapid decomposition to give nitrogen gas, the carboxylic esters or acids and an olefin. The stability of the *N*-nitrosamides and the nature of the final products were shown to depend upon the nature of R′, the group attached to the N atom. The primary rearrangement step consists of the rotation of the N-NO bond to II and the intramolecular reorganization of the *N*-nitrosamide moiety, involving scission of the N-CO bond. The subsequent fragmentation of the diazo ester III is extremely sensitive to the nature of the R and R′ groups and also to the reaction conditions.

For the *N*-nitrosamides, therefore, the key to releasing the nitrosyl radical instead of nitrogen or nitrous oxide gas, would seem to be to prevent the thermal rearrangement of I to II. In principle, this can be achieved catalytically, by absorbing the *N*-nitrosamide on a suitable surface, thereby blocking its thermal rearrangement until it has stored enough energy to fragment at the N-NO bond. Also, vacuum produces a driving force which tends to eliminate highly volatile N_2. An increase in the pressure will tend to allow more time for the compound to release NO instead of N_2. These tentative concepts, although still unproven, provide a pictorial understanding on which the new detection approach to the analysis of *N*-nitrosamides is based.

EXPERIMENTAL

Materials

Authentic *N*-nitroso compounds, supplied by IIT Research Institute (Chicago, IL, USA), were made up in dichloromethane or methanol. All solvents were of glass-distilled grade (Burdick & Jackson, Muskedon, MI, USA). The solutions were stored in amber glass ampoules at −20 °C. At no stage of the sample handling were the *N*-nitroso compounds exposed to sun or fluorescent light.

HPLC-TEA

The HPLC system consisted of a solvent pump (Altex, Model 110) with an injector (Walters, Model U6K), connected to a modified TEA (Thermo Electron, 502LC). The gas plumbing of the TEA was modified by inserting a capillary flow restrictor between the catalytic pyrolyser and the vacuum chamber. The pressure drop thus occurred not within the pyrolyser, but after the furnace at the flow restrictor. Thus, the pyrolyser was forced to function at above atmospheric pressure, instead of under vacuum.

The catalyst supplied with the TEA was replaced by a new material that we have developed recently: a nickel-manganese-chromium alloy which was surface-oxidized and then passivated at 850 °C in an organo-fluoride atmosphere.

For most of the testing reported here, no HPLC column was inserted between the injector and the detector, allowing data to be taken more rapidly. A HPLC column was used, periodically, to check the performance of the system. A variable-wavelength ultra-violet detector (Schoeffel), connected in series between the injector and the TEA, was used for comparison purposes. The ultra-violet detector also ensured that the compounds had not decomposed prior to analysis.

GC-TEA

A gas chromatograph (Hewlett Packard, Model 5840A) was used, with a fused silica capillary column (SE54) 30 m long, 0.32 mm i.d.; carrier gas (helium) at a head pressure of 18 psi (124×10^3 Pa); temperature of injection port, 90–140 °C; column temperature programmed from the injector temperature to 200 °C at 8 °C/min. The detector was a TEA (Thermo Electron, Model 610) modified to the amide mode, as described above. The reaction chamber was held at 1.8 mm Hg (240 Pa), with an O_3 flow of 5 mL/min. A CTR (Thermo Electron) was used *in lieu* of a cold trap. The volume injected onto the column was 1.0 µL.

RESULTS AND DISCUSSION

HPLC-TEA(amide)

The improvement in performance of the modified HPLC-TEA(amide), compared with the conventional TEA supplied by Thermo Electron, is shown in Table 1). Both tests were carried out using 1 mL/min dichloromethane as the solvent. For the modified instrument, the

Table 1. Comparison of response and minimum detection limit for the high-performance liquid chromatograph-Thermal Energy Analyzer (HPLC-TEA) (amide)

Compound	Improvement over conventional TEA (fold)	Minimum detectable amount at S/N of 3/1 (ng)
N-Methyl-N-nitrosourea	+ 58	0.6
N-Ethyl-N-nitrosourea	+ 18	2.6
N-Trimethyl-N-nitrosourea	+ 5	0.2
N-Methyl-N'-nitro-N-nitrosoguanidine	+ 8	0.2
N-Nitroso-N-methylacetamide	+ 140	0.2
N-Methyl-N-nitrosourethane	+ 4.3	0.2
N-Nitrosocarbaryl	+ 9	0.5
N-Nitroso-p-toluenesulfomethylamide	+ 5.5	0.3
N-Nitrosodimethylamine	− 0.5	0.6

temperature of the pyrolyser was held at 400 °C; the conventional TEA was operated at a pyrolyser temperature of 500 °C.

From the table, it is seen that the response for *N*-nitroso-*N*-methylactamide showed the largest improvement, namely 140-fold; the improvement in response for the other *N*-nitrosamides was between 4- and 60-fold. Because the pyrolysis conditions are so mild, the response of *N*-nitrosodimethylamine was reduced to half its normal value.

The table also shows the minimal amount of *N*-nitrosamide that must be injected into the HPLC-TEA (amide) to give a response at a signal:noise ratio of greater than 3:1. For ENU, the minimum detectable amount was 2.6 ng. For the other *N*-nitrosamides, the detection limit was between 0.2 and 0.6 ng.

GC-TEA (amide)

Because of their thermal instability, *N*-nitrosamides have not previously been analysed directly by GC. However, recent work in our laboratory (Fine *et al.*, 1983) has shown that it is possible to analyse directly, without derivatization, thermally labile high explosives (nitrate

Fig. 2. Analysis of 84 ng *N*-methyl-*N*-nitrosourea in methanol on a fused silica capillary column (SE54) interfaced to a Thermal Energy Analyzer (TEA). A, conventional TEA; B, TEA (amide)

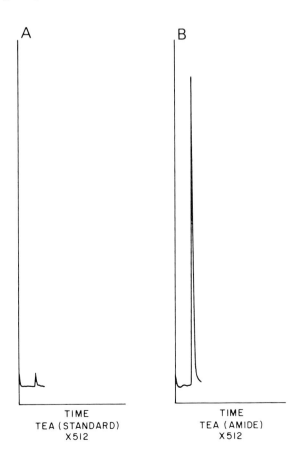

A

B

TIME
TEA (STANDARD)
X512

TIME
TEA (AMIDE)
X512

Fig. 3. Chromatograms of a mixture of *N*-methyl-*N*-nitrosourea (MNU), *N*-ethyl-*N*-nitrosourea (ENU) and *N*-nitrosomorpholine (NMOR) in methanol on capillary column gas chromatograph-Thermal Energy Analyzer (GC-TEA) (amide) with 1 µL injected in each case. The concentration of the test solution was diluted five-fold in B and 25-fold in C

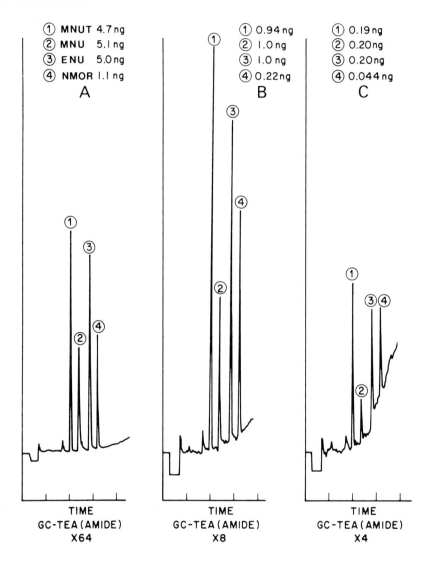

esters and nitramines), such as pentaerythritol tetranitrate and cyclo-1,3,5-trimethylene-2,4,6-trinitramine, by GC-TEA, using special capillary column procedures. In the case of the latter compound, the vapour pressure is also extraordinarily low (less than 10^{-8} mm Hg). We now applied the same chromatographic principles to highly unstable *N*-nitrosamides, such as *N*-methyl-*N*-nitrosourea and ENU.

Figure 2A is the chromatogram of 84 ng of MNU on the capillary column GC attached to a conventional TEA. As expected, only a small response was observed. However, when the

Fig. 4. Calibration plot of peak height *versus* number of mol injected on column, for the data in Figure 3; ●, *N*-nitrosomorpholine; △, *N*-methyl-*N*-nitrosourethane; ○, *N*-ethyl-*N*-nitrosourea; □, *N*-methyl-*N*-nitrosourea

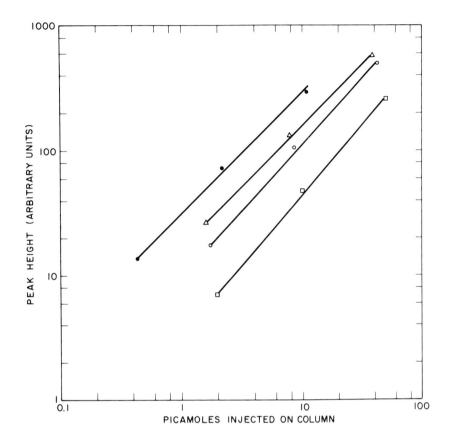

same column was interfaced to the TEA(amide) detector, 84 ng MNU now gave a 100-fold increase in detector response (Fig. 2B). Figure 3A is the resulting chromatogram of 1 μL of a mixture containing 4.7 ng/μL MNUT, 5.1 ng/μL MNU, 5.0 ng/μL ENU and 1.1 ng/μL *N*-nitrosomorpholine (NMOR). Figure 3B is a chromatogram of the same mixture diluted five-fold (approximately 1 ng injected on column); and Figure 3C is a chromatogram of a 25-fold dilution (approximately 0.2 ng injected on column).

Figure 4 is a plot of peak height *versus* the number of mol injected on column, corresponding to the data in Figure 3. The calibration is seen to be linear. However, unlike the situation with the conventional TEA, the response is sub-molar (a molar response would have given a single line, identical to that of NMOR). The fractional molar response, as compared to NMOR, is 0.16 for MNU, 0.37 for ENU and 0.53 for MNUT. The sub-molar response is probably due to two factors: first, less than quantitative breakdown of the compound to release NO in the TEA (amide) detector and, second, partial decomposition on the column. The peak for MNU, for example, is seen to have a broader base than these for the other compounds. The sensitivity, however, is still better than 0.1 ng injected on column, at a S:N ration of 3:1.

The descriptions 'thermally unstable' and 'nonvolatile' become meaningless when applied to the suitability of a compound for analysis by GC. The same chromatographic procedures as those described here will also, presumably, work for capillary column GC-MS.

Further work will be carried out shortly to minimize dead volumes and to optimize the catalytic parameters, temperature, flow rates, etc., so as to further improve the sensitivity of the method. The applicability of the GC approach to other *N*-nitrosamides, especially those with higher molecular weights, has still to be evaluated. Analytical extraction techniques that can incorporate this simple GC approach, still have to be developed.

CONCLUSION

Using a new type of TEA detector with a capillary GC column, a series of unstable, nonvolatile *N*-nitrosamides have been analysed by GC without prior derivatization. The technique is sensitive at the picogram level (33 pg at a S:N of 3:1 for MNUT, for example). A HPLC technique using the modified TEA has also been developed. While both techniques still need simplification and refinement, taken together they offer promise of making the *N*-nitrosamides amenable to routine analysis.

ACKNOWLEDGEMENTS

We gratefully acknowledge technical discussions with Brian Challis concerning the TEA (amide) instrument and with James Buckley concerning the capillary column GC. This investigation was supported, in part, by PHS Grant Number 1 RO1 CA 34837-01 awarded by the US National Cancer Institute, DHHS.

REFERENCES

Bavin, P.M.G., Darkin, D.W. & Viney, N.J. (1982) *Total nitroso compounds in gastric juice.* In: Bartsch, H., O'Neill, I.K., Castegnaro, M. & Okada, M., eds, N-*Nitroso Compounds: Occurrence and Biological Effects (IARC Scientific Publications No. 41)*, Lyon, International Agency for Research on Cancer, pp. 337–344

Chow, Y.L. (1979) *Chemistry of* N-*nitrosamides and related* N-*nitrosamino acids.* In: Anselme, F.P. ed. N-*nitrosamines, (ACS Symposium Series 101)*. Washington DC, American Chemical Society, pp. 13–38

Cosmetic, Toiletry and Fragrance Association (1977) *CTFA Cosmetic Ingredient Dictionary*, 2nd ed., Washington DC, Toiletry and Fragrance Association

Daiber, D. & Preussmann, R. (1965) Quantitative colimetrische Bestimmung organischer *N*-nitroso-Verbindungen durch photochemische Spaltung der Nitrosaminbindung. *Z. anal. chem., 206,* 344–352

Drescher, G.S. & Frank, C.W. (1978) *Anal. Chem., 50,* 2118–2121

Endo, H., Ishizawa, M., Endo, T., Takahashi, K., Utsunomiya, T., Kinoshita, N., Hidaka, K. & Baba, T. (1977) *A possible process of conversion of food components to gastric carcinogens.,* In: Hiatt, H.H., Watson, J.D. & Winston, J.A. eds, *Origins of human Cancer,* Cold Spring Harbor, NY, Cold Spring Harbor Laboratory, pp. 1591–1595

Fine, D.H. (1982) *Analytical methods for nitrosamines – an overview.* In: Magee, P., ed., *Nitrosamines and Human Cancer (Banbury Report No. 12)*, Cold Spring Harbor, NY, Cold Spring Harbor Laboratory, pp. 165–177

Fine, D.H., Rufeh, F. & Lieb, D. (1974) Group analysis of volatile and non-volatile N-nitroso compounds at the µg/kg level. *Nature, 247,* 309

Fine, D.H., Yu, W.C., Goff, E.U., Bender, E.C. & Reutter, D.J. (1983) Piogram analyses of explosive residues using the Thermal Energy Analyzer (TEA)[R]. *J. Forensic Sci., 29*, 732–746

Fujinaka, N., Masuda, Y. & Kurotsune, M. (1978) Methylguanidine content in food. *Gann, 67*, 679–683

Hansen, T.J., Archer, M.C. & Tannenbaum, S.R. (1979) Characterization of pyrolysis conditions and interference by other compounds in the chemiluminescence detection of nitrosamines. *Anal. Chem., 51*, 1526–1528

Krull, I.S. & Strauss, J. (1981) An improved trace analysis for *N*-nitrosourea from biological media. *J. anal. Toxicol., 5*, 42–46

Mirvish, S.S. (1975) Formation of *N*-nitroso compounds: chemistry kinetics and in-vivo occurrence. *Toxicol. appl. Pharmacol., 31*, 325–351

Mirvish, S.S. & Chu, C. (1973) Chemical determination of methylnitrosourea and ethylnitrosourea in stomach contents of rats after intubation with alkylureas plus sodium nitrite. *J. natl Cancer Inst., 50*, 745–750

Mirvish, S.S., Cairnes, D.A., Hermes, N.H. & Raha, C.R. (1982) Creatinine: A food component that is nitrosated-denitrosated to yield methylurea. *J. agric. Food Chem., 30*, 824–828

Mirvish, S.S., Sams, J.P. & Arnold, S.D. (1979) Spectrophotometric method for determining ureas applied to nitrosoureas, nitrosocyanamides and a cyanide. *Fresenius' Z. anal. Chem., 298*, 408–410

National Academy of Sciences (1981) *The Health Effects of Nitrate, Nitrite and N-Nitroso compounds*, Washington DC, pp. 9–27

Preussmann, R. & Schaper-Druckrey, F. (1972) Investigation of a colorimetric procedure for determination of *N*-nitrosamides and comparison with other methods. *Z. anal. Chem., 206*, 344–352

Saul, R.L., Bruce, W.R. & Archer, M.C. (1982) *An analytical method for simple N-nitrosamides*. In: Bartsch, H., O'Neill, I.K., Castegnaro, M. & Okada, M., eds, N-*Nitroso Compounds: Occurrence and Biological Effects (IARC Scientific Publications No. 41)*, Lyon, International Agency for Research on Cancer, pp. 175–184

Singer, G.M., Singer, S.S. & Schmidt, D.G. (1977) A nitrosamide specific detector for use with high-pressure liquid chromatography, *J. Chromatogr., 133*, 59–66

Smith, R.G., Blackstock, S.C., Cheung, L.K. & Loo, T.L. (1981) Analysis for nitrosourea antitumor agents by GC-MS. *Anal. Chem., 53*, 1205–1208

Thompson, W.T. (1975) *Agricultural Chemicals*, Indianapolis, IN, Thompson Publications

Walters, C.L., Downes, M.J., Edwards, M.N. & Smith, P.L.R. (1978) Determination of a non-volatile nitrosamine in a food matrix. *Analyst, 103*, 1127–1133

Weinkam, R.J., Wen, J.H.C., Furst, D.E. & Levin, V.A. (1978) Analysis for 1,3-bis(2-chloroethyl)-1-nitrosourea by chemical ionization mass spectroscopy. *Clin. Chem., 24*, 45–49

N-NITROSAMINE ANALYSIS IN FOODS: N-NITROSOAMINO ACIDS BY HIGH-PERFORMANCE LIQUID CHROMATOGRAPHY/THERMAL ENERGY ANALYSIS AND TOTAL N-NITROSO COMPOUNDS BY CHEMICAL DENITROSATION/THERMAL ENERGY ANALYSIS

R.C. MASSEY, P.E. KEY, D.J. McWEENY & M.E. KNOWLES

Ministry of Agriculture, Fisheries and Food, Food Science Laboratory, Queen Street, Norwich, NR2 4SX, UK

SUMMARY

The total N-nitroso content of foods can be measured by chemical denitrosation and chemiluminescent detection of the eliminated nitric oxide. Appropriate procedures substantially reduce the 'system response' to the denitrosating agent, so that total N-nitroso group contents down to 10 µg/kg can be measured on a one-gram sample. Using N-nitrosamine standards added to beer, the coefficients of variation are approximately 10% and 5% at N-nitroso contents of 19 and 94 µg/kg, respectively. In cured meats, the coefficient of variation for unidentified N-nitroso compounds is 26% for a 0.3-g sample containing 600 µg/kg. Some interference from non-nitroso compounds is possible, but, in some commodities at least, these interfering compounds are not detectable.

Conditions have been established that allow measurement of N-nitrosoamino acids in foods using a high-pressure liquid chromatograph interfaced to a Thermal Energy Analyzer, without the need for prior derivatization. After extraction of lipids with hexane, nitrosoamino acids are extracted with ethyl acetate and subjected to appropriate clean-up stages prior to high pressure liquid chromatography on Microbondapak CN with a hexane:ethanol:acetic acid mobile phase and Thermal Energy Analyzer detection. Recoveries from cured meat are in the 55–75% range for N-nitrososarcosine, N-nitrosoproline and N-nitrosohydroxyproline; elution is complete within seven minutes.

INTRODUCTION

Analysis of volatile nitrosamines in foods is now routinely carried out by gas chromatography-Thermal Energy Analyzer (GC-TEA) techniques; limits of detection of about 0.2 µg/kg are usual, and collaborative trials have established coefficients of variation (CV) of about 15% at the 2 µg/kg level (Marinelli *et al.*, 1982; Long, 1982).

The methods are not suitable for the determination of nonvolatile nitrosamines (unless they can be converted to volatile derivatives), but it must be assumed that these are formed along with volatile nitrosamines when nitrosating conditions are encountered. The present paper describes methods for the determination of total *N*-nitroso compounds by a modified chemical denitrosation procedure (limit, $\sim$ 10 µg/kg), and certain nitrosoamino acids.

MEASUREMENT OF TOTAL *N*-NITROSO COMPOUNDS

Principle of method

The sample is treated sequentially with acetic acid and hydrogen bromide:acetic acid; the nitric oxide evolved in these stages is measured (Walters *et al.*, 1978). Compounds containing acid-labile NO groups (e.g., inorganic nitrite and nitrosothiols) evolve nitric oxide on treatment with acetic acid. *N*-Nitroso compounds are stable to acetic acid, but release NO on treatment with hydrogen bromide:acetic acid; the amount of NO is directly proportional to the *N*-nitroso content of the sample. The method is sensitive to water and can give extremely high apparatus/reagent blanks ('system response') unless appropriate steps are taken.

Experimental procedure

Solid samples are weighed accurately on aluminium foil (about 2 × 2 cm) and the sample plus foil added to 50 ml of redistilled-in-glass ethyl acetate, containing 1% α-tocopherol, in a 250-mL three-necked flask. The flask is shaken vigorously for 30 sec and subjected to sonic-bath agitation for a further 30 sec to produce a fine suspension of the analyte. Liquid samples are added directly to the organic solvent and analysed without pretreatment. The flask is fitted with an injection port, an argon carrier-gas bubbler and an efficient reflux condenser, connected in series *via* three 6 mol/L potassium hydroxide traps, a solid carbon dioxide-isopropanol trap, a needle valve and a liquid nitrogen trap, to the reaction chamber of a Thermal Energy Analyzer operating at a pressure of 3 torr. The reaction mixture is brought to reflux and the system allowed to stabilize for 5 min. Glacial acetic acid (2 mL) is then injected into the reaction vessel and, when nitric oxide evolution ceases, another 2 mL acetic acid are added to ensure that the decomposition of acid-labile NO groups is complete. Two mL of 15% hydrogen bromide in acetic acid are then added to release nitric oxide from the *N*-nitroso groups in the sample. The 'system response' (see below) is estimated by a second injection of the hydrogen bromide reagent. Finally, the response of the system to the *N*-nitroso group is calibrated by injection of a standard solution of *N*-nitrosodimethylamine into the reaction mixture.

A typical total *N*-nitroso determination performed in the *absence* of sample is shown in Figure 1. A positive response is obtained for the first injection of the hydrogen bromide reagent and a smaller response for the second injection; further injections of hydrogen bromide (not shown in Fig. 1) produce the same response as the second injection.

The response to the first hydrogen bromide injection may be due, in part, to trace levels of *N*-nitroso impurities in the reagents. Another contribution arises from interaction of the denitrosation reagent with the glassware or connecting tubing of the apparatus itself; the response to the second hydrogen bromide injection arises solely from this source. The nature of the interaction is not known, but it may be considerably reduced by (i) treating the apparatus with an excess of hydrogen bromide reagent prior to analysis (i.e., each morning) and (ii) not cleaning the apparatus between analyses. With aqueous samples, it is necessary to rinse the condenser between analyses with acetone, followed by ethyl acetate, to remove hydrogen bromide dissolved in the droplets in the reflux condenser. The sample response is corrected for the 'system response', as follows:

corrected sample response = $c - (dc^1/d^1)$

where c = first response (sample assay)

d = second response (sample assay)

c^1 = first response ('system response' blank assay)

d^1 = second response ('system response' blank assay)

Fig. 1. Determination of total N-nitrosamine – blank assay; a, b, 2 mL acetic acid injected; c, d, 2 mL hydrogen bromide/acetic acid injected; e, N-nitrosodimethylamine standard injected.

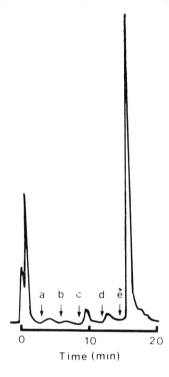

Fig. 2. Determination of total N-nitrosamine in beer (1 mL) fortified with NDMA; a, b, 2 mL acetic acid injected; c, d, 2 mL hydrogen bromide/acetic acid injected; e, N-nitrosodimethylamine standard injected.

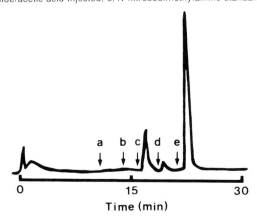

Fig. 3. Determination of total *N*-nitrosamine in cured meat (0.1 g); a, b, 2 mL acetic acid injected; c, d, 2 mL hydrogen bromide/acetic acid injected; e, *N*-nitrosodimethylamine standard injected.

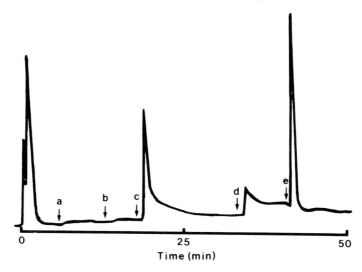

Time (min)

Analytical performance

Using the procedure described above, typical traces for 1 mL of beer fortified with *N*-nitrosodimethylamine or 0.1 g of cured meat are shown in Figures 2 and 3. The signal from beer shows a CV of 11.7% for peak height and 9.7% for peak area at 19 μg/kg *N*-nitroso compound; at this level, the signal is only two to three times greater than the system response. The corresponding CVs at 94 μg/kg are 9.4% and 5.1%, respectively. The signal from cured meat shows some peak broadening, probably related to the time required for the reagent to penetrate the meat particles and for the liberated NO to escape. The CVs are 36% and 26% for peak height and area, respectively, for 0.3 g meat at around 600 μg/kg *N*-nitroso compound.

Increasing amounts of water in the sample reduce the rate of NO evolution and lead to shallower, broader peaks which are less easily quantified; there is some signal suppression at high water levels. Peak areas from 0.25 mL, 0.5 mL, 1.0 mL and 2.0 mL of a standard solution in water were in the ratio 0.25, 0.54, 1.09 and 1.38; results for peak heights were substantially poorer.

Some chemical species other than *N*-nitroso compounds, e.g., nitrothiols, nitrolic acids and some aliphatic *C*-nitroso compounds, can give a response under the conditions employed (Walters *et al.*, 1979; Krull *et al.*, 1978). In practice, the contribution of these compounds to the total *N*-nitroso content in foods may be minimal, but it should be assumed *a priori* that they can be formed under the nitrosating conditions which lead to *N*-nitrosamine formation. The data obtained with the method described above may thus be regarded as indicating the maximum content of *N*-nitroso compounds. However, biscuits give a 'non-detectable' response, although they are often exposed to nitrogen oxides while being cooked in gas-fired travelling ovens; the occurence of 'false positives' is therefore by no means universal.

MEASUREMENT OF NITROSOAMINO ACIDS

Principles

After removal of most of the lipids, the nitrosoamino acids are extracted into ethyl acetate. After solvent exchange and a column adsorption/elution clean-up, the nitrosoamino acids are separated chromatographically, using a solvent system which allows long-term operation of cold traps and which gives low 'noise' with the Thermal Energy Analyzer (Massey *et al.*, 1982).

Experimental procedure

Solid samples are ground to a fine powder under liquid nitrogen with a pre-chilled mortar and pestle; a 5.0-g portion is then blended for 2 min with 50 mL 3mol/L phosphoric acid containing ammonium sulfamate (1 g) and sodium sulfate (15 g), pre-heated to 45°C. Lipids are extracted with hexane (2 × 130 mL), then the nitrosoamino acids are extracted from the aqueous suspension into ethyl acetate (4 × 100 mL); emulsions are broken by centrifugation. The organic extract is concentrated to dryness on a rotary evaporator at 45°C, and residual traces of water and acetic acid are removed by azeotropic distillation with acetone (100 mL) and cyclohexane (50 mL) on a rotary evaporator. The residue is extracted with acetone (2 × 10 mL), using sonic bath agitation. The extract is concentrated to dryness, re-dissolved in acetone (10 mL), cooled to 0–5°C for 10 min, and centrifuged. The supernatant is concentrated to dryness, taken up in 3 mL acetone:hexane (2:1) and applied to a Bond-Elut Aminopropyl column (Analytichem International, Harbor City, CA, USA).

After washing the column with 5-mL portions of acetone and 0.5% acetic acid in acetone, the nitrosoamino acids are eluted with 5 mL acetic acid:acetone (1:1) and the solvent removed by azeotropic distillation with cyclohexane (50 mL) on a rotary evaporator. The residue is extracted with acetone (1 mL), filtered and stored at 5°C in ambered vials pending analysis. The extract (20 µL) is analysed by HPLC-TEA using a Microbondapak CN column (25 cm × 4.5 mm id) and a 2 mL/min flow rate of hexane:ethanol:acetic acid (87:12:1). The eluate is fed into a TEA pyrolysis unit at 550°C, and the vapourized mobile phase condensed in two cold traps maintained at −78°C and −196°C; after reaction of NO with ozone, NO_2 is detected by the TEA/photomultiplier. Under these conditions, *N*-nitrosopipecolic acid (internal standard) is eluted after 3.6 min, *N*-nitrososarcosine at 4.4 min, *N*-nitrosoproline at 4.8 min and *N*-nitrosohydroxyproline at 6.6 min.

Analytical performance

Recoveries (five determinations) of nitrosoamino acids added to cured meat at a level of 200 µg/kg averaged 79.8% (standard deviation 8.1%) for *N*-nitrosopipecolic acid, 74.0% (SD 8.8%) for *N*-nitrososarcosine, 72.4% (SD 7.4%) for *N*-nitrosoproline and 55.0% (SD 3.9%) for *N*-nitrosohydroxyproline. The use of sodium chloride instead of sodium sulfate in the initial extraction from the phosphoric acid suspension leads to a low recovery of *N*-nitrosohydroxyproline. Recent work shows that *N*-nitrosothiazolidine-4-carboxylic acid reacts with co-extracted material during the concentration stage, and recoveries are poor.

However, if the ethyl acetate extract is applied directly to two Bond-Elut columns and eluted as described under *Experimental procedure*, above, good recoveries can be achieved, although there may be disadvantages with this much simplified clean-up, e.g., accelerated deterioration in column performance.

The chromatographic conditions avoid polar solvents (e.g., water, methanol), which induce severe instability in the TEA detector and reduce sensitivity by at least 100-fold; they avoid butanol, which in our experience causes baseline shift after a short time. The solvent has also been chosen so that it remains liquid at $-78°C$; this allows long HPLC runs through the use of high-capacity, low-dead-space traps.

CONCLUSIONS

Conditions have been established that allow routine measurement of certain N-nitrosoamino acids and of total N-nitroso compounds in a range of foods and beverages.

REFERENCES

Krull, I.S., Goff, E.U., Hoffmann, G.G. & Fine, D.H. (1978) Confirmatory methods for the thermal energy determination of N-nitroso compounds at trace levels. *Anal. Chem., 51,* 1706

Long, D.E. (1982) Analysis of N-nitrosodiethylamine in malted barley. *J. Inst. Brew., 88,* 266–271

Marinelli, N., Anderson, R., Fazio, T., Feit, M., Fiddler, W., Griffith, A., Hackbarth, J., Herwig, W., Issenberg, P., Kuroiwa, Y., O'Brien, T., Scanlan, R., Sen, N., Stebbins, P., Tebeau, C., Thomas, G. & McDougall, J. (1982) Report of ASBC sub-committee on N-nitrosamines in malt and beer for 1979–1980. Part II. *Am Soc. Brew. Chem., 39,* 35–40

Massey, R.C., Crews, C. & McWeeny, D.J. (1982) Method for HPLC measurement of N-nitrosamines in food. *J. Chromatogr., 241,* 423

Walters, C.L., Downes, M.J., Edwards, M.W. & Smith, P.L.R. (1978) Determination of a non-volatile N-nitrosamine in a food matrix. *Analyst, 103,* 1127

Walters, C.L., Hart, R.J., & Perse, S. (1979) The breakdown into nitric oxide of compounds potentially derived from nitrite in biological matrix. *Z. Lebensm. Untersuch. Forsch., 169,* 177

ON-LINE COMBINATION OF HIGH-PERFORMANCE LIQUID CHROMATOGRAPHY AND TOTAL N-NITROSO DETERMINATION APPARATUS FOR THE DETERMINATION OF N-NITROSAMIDES AND OTHER N-NITROSO COMPOUNDS, AND SOME RECENT DATA ON THE LEVELS OF N-NITROSOPROLINE IN FOODS AND BEVERAGES

N.P. SEN & S. SEAMAN

Food Research Division, Health Protection Branch, Ottawa, K1A OL2, Canada

SUMMARY

A simple high-performance liquid chromatographic chemiluminescence detection method has been developed for the quantitative determination of N-nitrosamides and is based on post-column denitrosation of the compounds with hydrogen bromide-acetic acid or hydrogen iodide-acetic acid, followed by detection of the liberated NO by a chemiluminescence detector (TEA™). The method was used for the simultaneous analysis of Diazald^R, N-nitroso-N-methylurea, N-methyl-N'-nitro-N-nitrosoguandine and streptozotocin standards, and for N-methyl-N-nitrosourea extracted from model-system reaction mixtures and spiked, cured meats. The minimum detection limit of N-methyl-N-nitrosourea was about 0.5 ng. The method for the determination of N-nitrosarcosine and N-nitrosoproline in foods and beverages has been improved by replacing diazomethane with a mixture of BF$_3$-methanol as the esterifying reagent and by simplifying the clean-up technique for purifying the prepared methyl esters. The average levels of N-nitrosoproline detected in 11 malts, 37 beers, 11 samples of fried bacon and 18 cured-meat products were found to be 24.1 µg/kg (5–113), 1.7 µg/kg (undetectable-6.0), 19.0 µg/kg (0.9–67.5), and 3.2 µg/kg (undetectable-21.6), respectively.

INTRODUCTION

Since the introduction and commercial availability of the Thermal Energy Analyzer (TEA™) detector, which is highly sensitive and specific for N-nitroso compounds, the analysis of foods and other complex matrices for N-nitrosamines has become much simpler and more precise. Once a difficult task, the trace analysis of foods and beverages for volatile nitrosamines has now become a routine process. The same statement cannot be made, however, for the analysis of the nonvolatile N-nitroso compounds. Although considerable progress has been made in developing sensitive methods for some of these compounds, e.g. N-nitrososarcosine (NSAR), N-nitrosoproline (NPRO), and N-nitrosodiethanolamine (NDELA), adequate methods for many others are still unavailable. For example, the nitrosamides, which are highly unstable, are not amenable to direct analysis by TEA. Under normal TEA pyrolysis conditions, most nitrosamides do not yield sufficient amounts of nitrosyl radical to be useful for detection by the TEA (Hansen *et al.*, 1979). For this reason, one has to resort to conventional methods of detection, such as colorimetric or ultra-violet spectrophotometry, which are not sufficiently specific for the analysis of complex matrices. There is thus a need to improve the method for these compounds.

From a review of the recent literature, two methods appeared to be promising enough for further improvement or investigation. One of them was a high-performance liquid chromatographic (HPLC)-photohydrolysis technique (Piacek-Llanes *et al.*, 1982), which was based on photochemical generation of nitrite and subsequent detection of the nitrite with Griess reagent; the other was the N-N = O determinatation (TND) method of Walters *et al.* (1980). The TND method involves denitrosation of *N*-nitroso compounds with hydrogen bromide-acetic acid and detection of the liberated NO by TEA, or any other chemiluminescence detector. We chose the TND procedure because of its higher specificity towards N – N = O compounds. This paper describes some recent results obtained by combining the TND apparatus with a HPLC system. Some improvements of our previous method (Sen *et al.*, 1982) for nitrosamino acids and our recent data on the occurrence of NSAR and NPRO in foods and beverages are also reported.

MATERIALS AND METHODS

HPLC-TND apparatus

The TND apparatus used was very similar to that described by Walters *et al.* (1980) and is shown in Figure 1. Ethyl acetate (30 mL) was added to the 250 mL three necked reaction flask and heated under reflux. Argon gas was bubbled through the solvent during the entire

Fig. 1. Schematic diagram of the high-performance liquid chromatography-total N-N = O determination (HPLC-TND) arrangement. Any part of the apparatus in contact with hydrogen bromide should be made of glass or Teflon[R] (e.g., Teflon-lined septum).

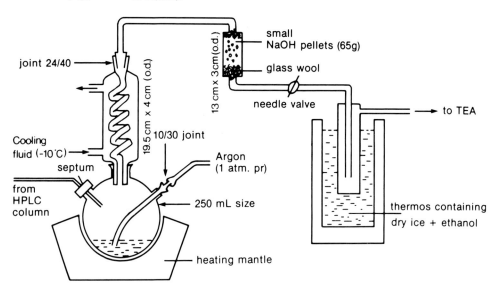

Fig. 2. High-performance liquid chromatography-total N-N=O determination (HPLC-TND) chromatogram obtained after injection of Diazald (550 ng), N-methyl-N'-nitro-N-nitrosoguanidine (MNNG) (575 ng), N-methyl-N-nitrosourea (MNU) (500 ng) and streptozotocin (850 ng). The programming was carried out using curve 10 setting of the programmer and was completed in 14 min. The dotted line gives the rate of increase in input from pump B, which contained methanol. At the end of each run, the system was switched to the original condition and pump A was switched to a column-conditioning solvent, 10% glacial acetic acid in n-hexane. After 5-10 min it was switched back to 15% acetone in n-hexane. Solvent flow rate was 2 mL/min troughout.

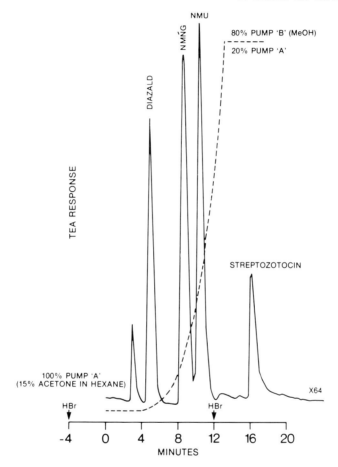

operation. The TEA (gas chromatographic or HPLC mode) chamber vacuum was maintained at 4-5 mm HG pressure (controlled using the needle valve). After the solvent had started to reflux for 3-5 min, a tube from the HPLC column was gently inserted through the septum and, at the same time, about 2 mL hydrogen bromide reagent (15%, in glacial acetic acid) was injected into the reaction flask. Immediately, a 25-μL aliquot of the nitrosamide(s) standard solution (in acetone or ethyl acetate) was injected into the HPLC column, and the response of the TEA detector was monitored continuously using a 1 mV recorder. After 10-12 min another 2-ml aliquot of hydrogen bromide reagent was injected to replenish that lost in the vacuum. The HPLC conditions used were as follows:

Column: 25 cm 4.6 mm (id) Lichrosorb-Si60 (5 μ). For analysing food extracts, a 3 cm × 4.6 mm (id) silica guard column should be used.

Mobile phase and programming conditions: See Figure 2.

Two Waters Associates Pumps (model 600A) and a Waters Associates solvent Programmer (model 660) were used.

At the end of the run, the TEA was switched to the vented position and the reaction flask dismantled and rinsed with acetone. The cold trap was also emptied occasionally, and sodium hydroxide pellets in the following trap were replaced every day. The fluid used to cool the condenser should preferably be kept at $-10\,°C$, but the TEA can be operated with the coolant at a higher temperature ($\simeq 5\,°C$).

Improvement in the method for N-*nitrosamino acids*

Two major changes were introduced: (1) replacement of the Preptubes™ with Clin Elut Extubes™ (Analytichem International, Harbor City, CA, USA), and (2) replacement of diazomethane with a mixture of BF_3-methanol as the esterifying agent. Briefly, the procedure is as follows:

A 15-20-g sample (malt, skim milk powder, fried bacon, etc) was mixed with 5-10 mL 0.5 mol/L sulfuric acid containing 1 % sulfamic acid and the mixture extracted with methanol, filtered and concentrated to 5-10 mL, as described previously (Sen *et al.,* 1982). The concentrated extract was mixed with 2 mL of 1.5 mol/L sulfuric acid and the mixture poured onto a 20-mL-capacity Clin Elut Extube. After 5 min, the tube was washed with 60-mL aliquot of *n*-hexane:dichloromethane (3:1, v/v) and the washing discarded (this washing, to remove pigments, was done only for malts). The tube was then eluted with 4×20-mL aliquots of ethyl acetate and the eluate dried over anhydrous sodium sulfate for 30 min, with occasional swirling. The ethyl acetate solution was filtered and concentrated to $\simeq 2$ mL, using a flash evaporator. The resulting solution was transferred (with adequate rinsing) to a 15-mL graduated test tube and carefully concentrated to 0.1-0.2 mL (avoiding evaporation to dryness) in a stream of nitrogen.

Finally, 1.0 mL BF_3-methanol reagent (Applied Science Laboratories, Rexdale, Ontario) was pipetted into the concentrated extract, the test tube stoppered and the mixture heated in a sand bath (60-70 °C) in the dark for 30 min. After cooling the sample to room temperature, about 4 mL water and exactly 1.0 mL dichloromethane were added, and the mixture was mixed vigorously for 2 min, using a Vortex mixer. A 6-μL aliquot of the dichloromethane layer was analysed by gas-liquid chromatography (GLC)-TEA. A 2.75 m × 3.2 mm (od) Ni column packed with 10% Carbowax 20M on 60-80 mesh Chromosorb W, HMDS treated, was used for GLC-TEA analysis. The GLC Oven was heated from 160-200 °C/min. Injection port and transfer line (from column to TEA) temperatures were 225 °C and 290 °C, respectively. Carrier gas (Ar) flow rate was 30-40 mL/min. The details of the method will be published elsewhere (Sen *et al.,* 1983).

For liquid samples (e.g., beer, urine), the initial extraction step with methanol was omitted. A 15-18-mL aliquot of the sample was mixed with 3 mL 1.5 mol/L sulfuric acid and 1 mL of 1% sulfamic acid, and the mixture was poured directly into the extraction tube. The rest of the procedure was the same as described above.

RESULTS AND DISCUSSION

The TND apparatus-HPLC combination worked fairly well. As a first step, four nitrosamides, namely, N-nitroso-N-methyl-*p*-toluenesulfonamide (Diazald^R), N-methyl-N'-nitro-N-nitrosoguanidine (MNNG), N-methyl-N-nitrosourea (MNU) and N-nitroso-N-D-glucosyl-(2)-methylurea (streptozotocin), were injected and were found to separate well from each other (Fig. 2). For MNU, a plot of peak height versus ng injected showed a linear relationship, at least in the range of 50-250 ng. The minimum detection limit for MNU was 0.5 ng (at attenuation 4). A comparison of peak areas obtained after injections of 2.5 µg MNU indicated that the TND-HPLC procedure produced an approximately 100-fold higher yield of nitrosyl radical than that obtained by the conventional HPLC-TEA technique. Therefore, an approximately one hundred-fold improvement in sensitivity was achieved. Since various components present in a sample extract are first separated on the HPLC column, a nitrosamide (if present) might be separated from many interfering materials (including other *N*-nitroso compounds), thereby increasing the specificity of the overall technique compared to that involving no preliminary HPLC separation. This will be particularly useful for the analysis of extracts of food-nitrite incubation mixture (if studying formation of nitrosamides), or of gastric juice, if studying (for example) in-vivo formation of *N*-nitrosocimetidine in patients undergoing treatment with cimetidine.

As reported by Cox *et al.* (1982) and Kawabata *et al.* (this volume), we have also investigated the possibility of using hydrogen iodide as a denitrosating agent in our system. Hydrogen iodide was generated *in situ* from 200 mg sodium iodide and 2 mL each of concentrated sulfuric acid and glacial acetic acid in a flask containing 30 mL ethyl acetate. This system seemed to be highly effective for detecting MNU but not for *N*-nitrosodimethylamine - a *N*-nitrosamine, the relative response for the two compounds being approximately 10. Therefore, the hydrogen iodide-HPLC system might be useful for the specific detection of MNU and possible other *N*-nitrosamides.

Furthermore, our technique has the following additional advantages: (1) it is simple to set up and does not require any additional investment; (2) it is not susceptible to interference from closely related chemicals, such as *C*-nitro (e.g., nitrohexane), *N*-nitro and *O*-nitro compounds (Krull *et al.*, 1979); and (3) it should be usable with both TEA models (502 and 543), as well as with other chemiluminescence analysers (e.g., Luminox 101A, British Oxygen).

A major disadvantage of the technique is that it results in broad peaks and is therefore incapable of separating peaks with closer retention times. Considering the fact that there is a large dead volume in the system and that the desorption of liberated NO from the reaction mixture is somewhat slow, both the peak-shape and peak-width obtained are highly satisfactory. If one is interested in the analysis of a large number of *N*-nitrosamides, the modified TEA technique for nitrosamides, reported by Fine *et al.* (See p. 121) should be chosen.

The HPLC solvent systems described here are given only as a guideline. Simpler systems can be worked out to suit specific needs. For example, if one is interested only in streptozotocin analysis, an isocratic run with 60% or 80% methanol in acetone would give a much sharper peak. The use of a solvent with a high methanol content, however, seemed to destroy (partly or completely) MNNG. An isocratic run with 15% of 20% acetone in hexane would be ideal for the analysis of Diazald, MNNG and MNU, singly or in a mixture. The above-mentioned destructive effect of methanol towards MNNG can be overcome by pumping 10% glacial acetic acid in *n*-hexane through the column for 10 min at the end of each run.

Thus far, the HPLC-TND technique has been applied to the determination of a few nitrosamide standards and to MNU extracted from model reaction media (e.g. reaction of methylguanidine or methylurea with nitrite) and from fried bacon spiked with MNU (100 µg/kg). The overall method gave nearly quantitative recovery ($\simeq 100\%$). The details of the clean-up method will be reported elsewhere. The method is currently being used to study the formation of nitrosamides in various foods after incubation with nitrite under simulated gastric conditions.

Changes to the method were necessary for measuring NSAR and NPRO for two reasons - the unavailability of the Preptubes and for safety (hazards of diazomethane). The Clin Elut Extubes worked extremely well if the sample was acidified with a minimum of 3 mL of 1.5 mol/L sulfuric acid. Otherwise, recoveries were low and irreproducible. A comparison of the

Table 1.   Levels of *N*-nitrosoproline (NPRO) in various foods and beverages

Commodity	No. of positive results/ total no. of samples	NPRO content	
		mean (μg/kg)	range
Malts (Canadian)[a]	11/11	24.1[b]	5–113[c]
Beer and ale (both domestic and imported)	28/37	1.7	trace–6.0
Fried bacon[a]	11/11	19	0.9–67.5
Other cured meats[a]	9/18	3.2	trace–21.6
Skim milk powder	0/6		

[a] Two samples of malt, 6 of fried bacon and 1 of cured meat contained, in addition to NPRO, traces (up to 4 μg/kg) of *N*-nitrososarcosine (not confirmed by mass spectrometry)
[b] Excluding a high (113 μg/kg) value obtained for an old sample
[c] In six samples of malt, the identity of NPRO (as methyl ester) was confirmed by gas-liquid chromatography-high-resolution mass spectrometry (monitoring for the molecular ion at a resolution of 10 000)

two methods of esterification (diazomethane versus BF_3-methanol) with standards, as well as with spiked food samples, gave comparable results. Recoveries of NSAR and NPRO added to malt, beer, skim milk powder, etc at spiking levels of 1-100 μg/kg were found to be over 80%. The simple clean-up technique of shaking the reaction mixture with water and 1 mL dichloromethane (to remove interfering BF_3-methanol reagent) resulted in a cleaner chromatogram and also gave a better separation of the NSAR peak from that of the solvent.

Our recent data (Table 1) indicate that only very low levels of NPRO are present in malt, beer, fried bacon and cured meats. Since NPRO is noncarcinogenic, these findings may have little health hazard significance to man. However, the presence of high levels (> 100 μg/kg) of NPRO in foods (e.g., bacon) that are cooked at a high temperature may be undesirable because of the possible conversion to *N*-nitrosopyrrolidine (NPYR), which is a potent carcinogen. Since the percentage conversion of NPRO to NPYR is very low (Sen *et al.*, 1980), only a small portion of the NPYR in fried bacon is formed by this process. The presence of NPRO, however, can be taken as an indicator of the presence of other nonvolatile *N*-nitroso compounds for which analytical methods are not yet available. Additional research along the present lines is necessary in order to develop new procedures which will be useful for both monitoring and research purposes.

REFERENCES

Cox, R.D., Frank, C.W., Nikolalsen, L.D. & Caputo, R.E. (1982) Screening procedure for determination of total *N*-nitroso content in urine. *Anal. Chem.*, *54*, 253-256

Hansen, T.J., Archer, M.C. & Tannenbaum, S.R. (1979) Characterization of pyrolysis conditions and interference by other compounds in the chemiluminescence detection of nitrosamides. *Anal. Chem.*, *51*, 1526-1528

Krull, I.S., Goff, E.U., Hoffman, G.G. & Fine, D.H. (1979). Confirmatory methods for the thermal energy determination of *N*-nitroso compounds at trace levels. *Anal. Chem.*, *51*, 1706-1709

Piacek-Llanes, B.G., Shuker, D.E.G. & Tannenbaum, S.R. (1982). N-*Nitrosamides of natural origin.* In: Bartsch, H., O'Neill, I.K., Castegnaro, M. & Okada, M., eds, N-*Nitroso Compounds: Occurrence and Biological Effects (IARC Scientific Publication No.41)*, Lyon, International Agency for Research on Cancer, pp. 123-130

Sen, N.P., Seaman, S. & McPherson, M. (1980) *Further studies on the occurrence of volatile and nonvolatile nitrosamines in foods.* In: Walker, E.A., Griciute, L., Castegnaro, M. & Börzsönyi, M., eds, N-*Nitroso Compounds: Analysis, Formation and Occurrence (IARC Scientific Publications No.31)*, Lyon, International Agency for Research on Cancer, pp. 457-465

Sen, N.P., Seaman, S. & Tessier, L. (1982) *A rapid and sensitive method for the determination of nonvolatile N-nitroso compounds in foods and human urine: Recent data concerning volatile* N-*nitrosamines in dried foods and malt-based beverages.* In: Bartsch, H., O'Neill, I.K., Castegnaro, M. & Okada, M., eds, N-*Nitroso Compounds: Occurrence and Biological Effects (IARC Scientific Publications No.41)*, Lyon, International Agency for Research on Cancer, pp. 185-197

Sen, N.P., Tessier, L. & Seaman, S. (1983) Determination of *N*-nitrosoproline and *N*-nitrososarcosine in malt and beer. *J. Agric. Food Chem., 31,* 1033–1036

Walters, C.L., Hart, R.J., Keefer, L.K. & Newberne, P.M. (1980) *The sequential determination of nitrite,* N-*nitroso compounds and nitrate and its application.* In: Walker, E.A., Griciute, L., Castegnaro, M. & Börzsönyi, M., eds, N-*Nitroso Compounds: Analysis, Formation and Occurrence (IARC Scientific Publications No.31)*, Lyon, International Agency for Research on Cancer, pp. 389-399

NONVOLATILE *N*-NITROSAMINE INVESTIGATIONS: METHODS FOR THE DETERMINATION OF *N*-NITROSOAMINO ACIDS AND PRELIMINARY RESULTS OF THE DEVELOPMENT OF A METHOD FOR THE DETERMINATION OF *N*-NITROSODIPEPTIDES *N*-TERMINAL IN PROLINE

S.J. KUBACKI

Institute of the Fermentation Industry, Department of Food Analysis, Warsaw, Poland, Visiting Scientist at the Food and Drug Administration, Bureau of Foods

D.C. HAVERY & T. FAZIO

Department of Health and Human Services, Food and Drug Administration, Washington DC 20204, USA

SUMMARY

The development of a rapid method for the determination of *N*-nitrosoamino acids is reported. Preliminary recoveries of *N*-nitrosoamino acids in ham fortified with 20 µg/kg generally ranged from 70 to 100%. The synthesis and instrumental characterization of four *N*-nitrosodipeptides *N*-terminal in proline from nitrite in aqueous acid solution are reported. Electron ionization-mass spectroscopy and infra-red spectroscopy strongly support the conclusion that only the amine nitrogen, and not the amide nitrogen at the peptide bond, is nitrosated. High-performance liquid chromatographic conditions are described for the separation of the synthesized *N*-nitrosodipeptides.

INTRODUCTION

It is well known that free amino acids occur in various kinds of foods primarily as the product of decomposition of proteins and peptides. For example, Lakritz *et al.* (1976) found that the concentration of proline and other free amino acids in pork bellies increased during storage at 2°C. Amino acids are also likely to form during food processing, cooking and digestion (Spinelli-Gugger *et al.*, 1980). Amino acids with secondary amine groups such as proline, hydroxyproline and sarcosine can be readily nitrosated to *N*-nitrosoamino acids at rates similar to that of morpholine (Mirvish *et al.*, 1973). Biological studies have demonstrated that *N*-nitrososarcosine (NSAR) is a weak carcinogen in rats (Druckrey *et al.*, 1967), but *N*-nitrosoproline (NPRO) and *N*-nitrosohydroxyproline (NHPRO) have failed to induce tumours (Garcia & Lijinsky, 1973). N-Nitrosoamino acids are thermolabile and may contribute to the formation of N-nitrosopyrrolidine, N-nitroso-3-hydroxypyrrolidine and N-nitrosodimethylamine. Lijinsky and Reuber (1982) have shown that although NPRO and NHPRO do not appear to be carcinogenic in themselves, they could lead to the formation of other carcinogenic N-nitroso compounds via transnitrosation in the presence of nitrosatable amines.

Data on the occurrence of N-nitrosoamino acids in meat products are inconsistent. Some authors have found up to a few hundred µg/kg (Kushnir et al., 1975; Dhont & van Ingen, 1976; Janzowski et al., 1978; Sen et al., 1978; Eisenbrand et al., 1978; Pensabene et al., 1979), while others report traces or no detectable amounts (Hansen et al., 1977; Baker & Ma, 1978; Sen et al., 1980). NPRO has been reported most frequently, while NHPRO and NSAR, if found, occur at lower levels. Concentrations of N-nitrosoamino acids reported in meat products have ranged from 2–1 138 µg/kg NPRO, 2–56 µg/kg NSAR and 5–161 µg/kg NHPRO. Bacon, dried cured meat products and malt are most likely to contain N-nitrosoamino acids (Sen et al., 1982, 1983); they have not been reported in fish.

Although several methods have been developed for the determination of N-nitrosoamino acids in environmental samples, including food, most of them are based on gas chromatography-thermal energy analysis (GC-TEA). Only a few procedures have been described using high-performance liquid chromatography (HPLC)-TEA for food analysis. Sen et al. (1980) analysed food samples by a procedure with a detection limit of 10-20 µg/kg, employing a silica column with a mobile phase consisting of dichloromethane/acetone/absolute ethanol/diethylamine-acetic acid buffer/water, Baker and Ma (1978) used a reversed-phase column with 5% acetic acid in water as the mobile phase; however, they found that reproducibility was poor when the TEA detector was operating in the liquid chromatographic mode. The detection limit of the method was approximately 5 µg/kg. Massey et al. (1982) used a silica column for HPLC-TEA analysis of N-nitrosoamino acids, eluting with a mixture of n-hexane/ethanol/acetic acid in a gradient mode. The limit of detection of the method was 5 µg/kg for meat products.

In the first section of this paper we describe a simple, rapid method for the determination of N-nitrosoamino acids in meat products by means of HPLC-TEA. Our aim was to develop a procedure for analysing N-nitrosoamino acids in foods and then to extend the method to include other groups of N-nitroso compounds such as N-nitrosopeptides and N-nitrosamides. Since some of these compounds are thermolabile, we selected HPLC-TEA instead of GC-TEA. The method is very rapid and could be used by food processors to check routinely the quality of their products.

Not only free amino acids, but also peptides are present in foods. Like amino acids, they can be formed by decomposition of protein during food processing or cooking. Digestion of protein in the alimentary tract leads to the formation of simple di- and tripeptides, which are further metabolized during passage through the intestine (Konturek, 1976). Those peptides that are N-terminal in proline or hydroxyproline can be nitrosated as amino acids themselves. Collagen, a very common protein, occurs in meats at levels up to 25% and is comprised roughly of 12% proline, 10% hydroxyproline and 33% glycine. Spinelli-Gugger et al. (1980) reported significant increases in the concentrations of free proline (52%) and glycine (41%) during processing of bacon bellies as a result of the decomposition of collagen. This suggests that simple peptides may be formed in addition to free amino acids. For these reasons we initiated investigations on the occurrence of N-nitrosopeptide in foods, especially cured products and those processed in the presence of nitrosating agents.

Although reports have been published on the synthesis (Stewart, 1969) and kinetics of nitrosation (Mirvish et al., 1973) of dipeptides, few attempts have been made to characterize the reaction products of dipeptides with nitrite in dilute aqueous acid. Pollock (1982) synthesized several N-nitrosodipeptides and concluded that nitrosation had occurred at the peptide bond. However, Kubacka et al. (1983), in a study of the same reaction, found that only the amine nitrogen was nitrosated and that the reaction proceeded faster than the nitrosation of free amino acids (Kubacka & Scanlan, 1983). Mirvish et al. (1973) also concluded that no nitrosation occurs at the peptide bond, and Bonnet and Holleyhead (1974a, b) saw no nitrosation on interaction of sodium nitrite with α-amino acids and peptide derivatives.

In the second section of this paper we report on the synthesis, characterization and preliminary chromatographic separation of four N-nitrosodipeptides N-terminal in proline.

MATERIALS AND METHODS

Apparatus and reagents

All reagents were analytical grade. Solvents were glass-distilled ultra-violet grade. NPRO NHPRO and NSAR were synthesized as described by Hansen et al. (1977), except that acetone instead of dichloromethane was used to extract the N-nitrosoamino acids from the reaction products. Proline and hydroxyproline were obtained from Kodak Chemical Co., Rochester, NY; sarcosine hydrochloride was obtained from Aldrich Chemical Co., Milwaukee, WI. Boron trifluoride-methanol reagent was obtained from Applied Science Laboratories Inc., Deerfield, IL. Anion exchange resin (Dowex 2 -X8) was purchased from Bio-Rad Laboratories. HPLC cyano and amide columns (25 cm, 5u) were purchased from Alltech Associates Inc., Richmond, CA. Prolyglycine, prolylisoleucine and prolylphenylalanine were purchased from Sigma Chemical Co., St Louis, MO and prolylglutamic acid from Bachem Inc., Torrence, CA.

Instrumentation

A gas chromatograph (Hewlett-Packard model 5710A), liquid chromatograph (Altex model 332), Thermal Energy Analyzer (TEA) (Thermo Electron Corporation model 502L), Elemental Analyzer (Perkin Elmer model 240B), electron microscope (ICI Super III), ultra-violet spectrophotometer (Beckman DU-7), mass spectrometer (MS) (Finnigan MAT CH5 DF), MS Data System (Varian V76) and infrared spectrometer (Digilab FTS 10) were used.

Instrumentation conditions

Liquid chromatograph: N-Nitrosoamino acids: cyano column; temperature, 90°C; mobile phase, hexane : dichloromethane : isopropanol (70 : 29.75 : 0.25); flow rate, 1.00 mL/min. N-Nitrosodipeptides: cyano and amide colums; temperature, ambient; mobile phase, hexane : dichloromethane : acetic acid (50 : 49 : 1); flow rate, 1.00 mL/min.

Thermal Energy Analyzer: furnace, 500°C; cold trap, ethanol-dry ice; operated at a pressure of approximately 1 torr (133.3 Pa).

Mass spectrometer: electron ionization spectra obtained from methanol solutions of N-nitrosodipeptides *via* solid probe; ionization energy, 70 eV; emission current, 300 μA; ion source temperature, 250°C; resolution, 800.

Infra-red spectrometer: potassium bromide discs; resolution 4 cm^{-1}.

Procedure

N-*Nitrosoamino acids:* The method described by Ohshima et al. (1982) for the determination of N-nitrosoamino acids in urine and faeces was modified for the analysis of food matrices. A 50 g aliquot of the ground samples was homogenized in a Waring blender for 3 min with 200 mL of a solution of 1 mol/L sodium chloride and 1% ammonium sulfamate adjusted to pH 1 with hydrochloric acid. The extract was filtered through glass wool. A 100-mL aliquot was adjusted to pH 1 with 6 mol/L hydrochloric acid, transferred to a 250-mL separatory funnel and gently extracted twice with 50-mL portions of *n*-hexane. The *n*-hexane layers were discarded. The aqueous phase was extracted four times with 100-mL portions of ethyl acetate. The ethyl acetate extracts were dried by passage through 75 g anhydrous sodium sulfate, held in a coarse sintered-glass funnel, into a 1-L round-bottomed flask. The extracts were concentrated to dryness with a rotary evaporator at 55 °C. The residue was transferred quantitatively with four 20-mL portions of dichloromethane to a 250-mL Kuderna-Danish evaporator concentrator. A Snyder column was attached and the extract rapidly concentrated as far as possible in an 80 °C water-bath and then to 0.1 mL under a stream of nitrogen. The sample was esterified by adding 2 mL boron trifluoride-methanol solution to the concentrator tube, and the mixture was heated in a 80 °C water-bath for 15 min. The sample was allowed to cool and mixed with 6 mL water. One mL dichloromethane was added and the mixture shaken vigorously for 30 sec. An aliquot of the dichloromethane layer was used for HPLC-TEA analysis.

Some samples require additional clean-up prior to HPLC-TEA. For these samples, the ethyl acetate extract obtained as described above was concentrated to dryness on a rotary evaporator at 55 °C. The residue was transferred quantitatively with four 20-mL portions of deionized water onto a column containing 5 g of anion-exchange resin. The column was drained and the walls of the column rinsed with three 5 mL portions of deionized water. The *N*-nitrosoamino acids were eluted, with 80 mL 1 mol/L sodium chloride adjusted to pH 1 with hydrochloric acid, into a 250-mL separatory funnel. The eluate was extracted with four 80-mL portions of ethyl acetate. The ethyl acetate was dried as described above and collected in a 1-L round-bottomed flask. The extract was evaporated under vacuum to dryness in a rotary evaporator at 55 °C. The residue was transferred quantatively to a 250-mL Kuderna-Danish concentrator with four 20-mL portions of dichloromethane, concentrated and esterified as described above.

A measured amount of an *N*-nitrosoamino acid standard solution in methanol containing known amounts of each *N*-nitrosoamino acid was esterified simultaneously with the samples. In order to avoid hydrolysis of the methylated derivatives, HPLC-TEA analysis was carried out on the same day in which the samples were prepared. Sample extracts and standards were introduced into the HPLC with a 20-μL loop.

N-*Nitrosodipeptides:* *N*-Nitrosodipeptides were synthesized by a modification of the procedure described by Kubacka *et al.* (1983) The dipeptides were nitrosated with sodium nitrite in dilute aqueous hydrochloric acid. The mixture was adjusted to pH 1 and dried by rotary evaporation. Traces of hydrochloric acid were removed by adding water to the residue and evaporating to dryness by rotary evaporation. This process was performed three times. The *N*-nitrosodipeptides were extracted with anhydrous acetone which was then removed by rotary evaporation. The residue was dried under vacuum [(0.05 torr (6.7 Pa)] at 55 °C for 3 h, over phosphorus pentoxide, followed by drying at ambient temperature for 12 h. The *N*-nitrosodipeptides were stored in a vaccum desiccator over phosphorus pentoxide.

RESULTS AND DISCUSSION

N-*Nitrosoamino acids*

Because of the ionic nature of *N*-nitrosoamino acids, the best systems for attaining HPLC separations are ion exchange or reversed-phase chromatography. However HPLC-TEA does not perform well with these systems. Attempts were made to separate the underivatized *N*-nitrosoamino acids by using a mobile phase containing an organic buffer

Fig. 1. High-performance liquid chromatography-Thermal Energy Analyzer chromatograms of *N*-nitrosoamino acids; A, 20 ng each of *N*-nitrososarcosine (NSAR) and *N*-nitrosoproline (NPRO); B, ham extract fortified with 20 µg/kg NSAR and NPRO; C, ham extract, unfortified

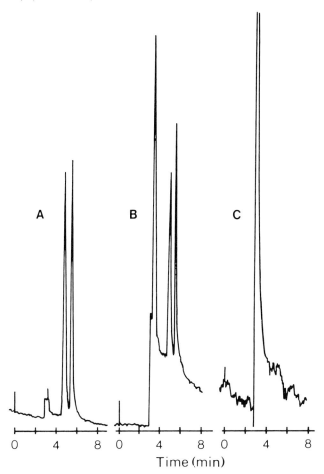

(diethylamine-acetic acid), as described by Sen *et al.*, (1980). Work with this system was discontinued because of very high TEA background noise. Methylation of the *N*-nitrosoamino acids allowed chromatographic separation with nonpolar solvents, such as *n*-hexane and dichloromethane, which did not affect the background noise level. The methylated derivatives of NSAR and NPRO were separated by HPLC-TEA using a cyano column. Initial chromatographic separation of the methylated derivatives resulted in the separation of *syn* and *anti* isomers of each N-nitrosamine. When the column temperature was increased to 90°C, the isomers merged, giving one peak for each *N*-nitrosoamino acid.

The method for the determination of *N*-nitrosoamino acids described here has been applied to ham. Samples were fortified with 20 µg/kg and analysed the same day by HPLC-TEA; recoveries ranged from 70–100%. Typical chromatograms of a ham extract (without additional clean-up), both blank and fortified with NSAR and NPRO, and the accompanying

N-nitrosoamino acid standards are shown in Figure 1. The procedure has shown to be amenable to GC-TEA analysis also.

Future research in this area will include market surveys of various foods, including cured meats and fish products.

Fig. 2. Structures of *N*-nitrosodipeptides

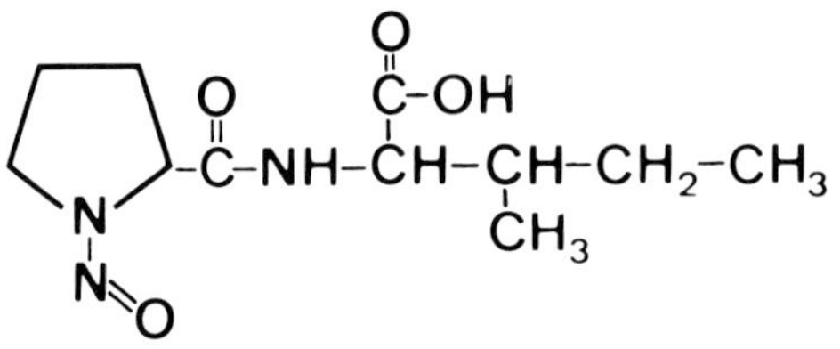

N-Nitrosoprolylisoleucine

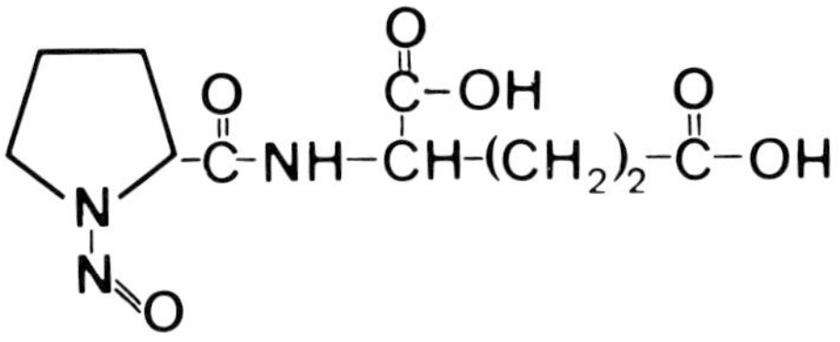

N-Nitrosoprolylglutamic acide

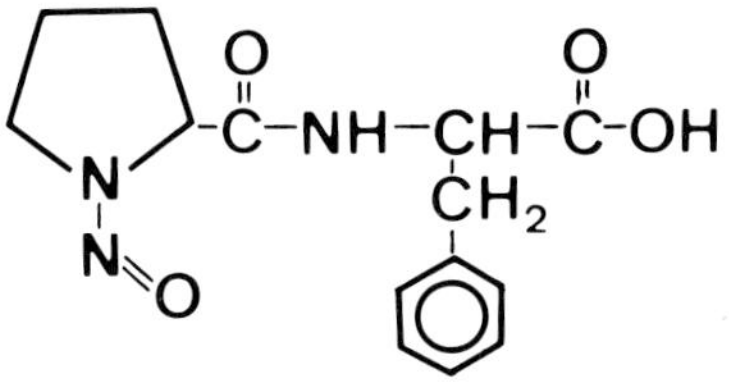

N-Nitrosoprolylphenylalanine

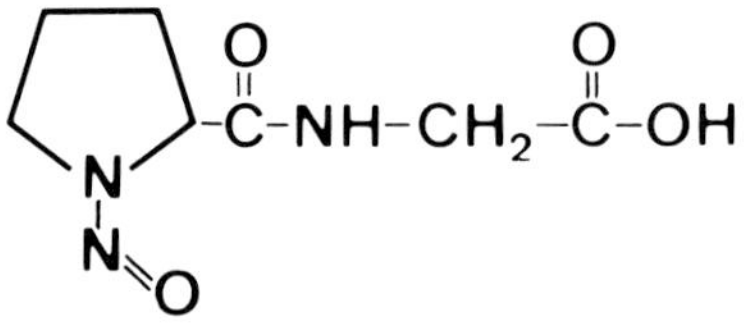

N-Nitrosoprolylglycine

N-*Nitrosodipeptides*

Four *N*-nitrosodipeptides *N*-terminal in proline were synthesized: *N*-nitrosoprolylglycine (NPRO-GLY), *N*-nitrosoprolylisoleucine (NPRO-ILE), *N*-nitrosoprolylphenylalanine (NPRO-PHE) and *N*-nitrosoprolylglutamic acid (NPRO-GLU). Their structures are shown in Figure 2. Previous attempts to synthesize *N*-nitrosodipeptides (Kubacka & Scanlan, 1983) resulted in yellow oils. All four synthesized *N*-nitrosodipeptides were extremely hygroscopic; when they were dried thoroughly, solid crystals were obtained; as soon as the crystals were exposed to air, yellow oils formed.

All four *N*-nitrosodipeptides were characterized by elemental analysis, electron microscopy, ultra-violet (UV) spectrophotometry, mass spectrometry and infra-red (IR) spectrophotometry. Although the laboratory performing the elemental analysis did not have the facilities for handling such hygroscopic compounds, the results obtained were in good agreement with theoretical calculations (Table 1). Residues for electron microscopic analysis were prepared by evaporation of solvent from a solution containing a *N*-nitrosodipeptide. This procedure produced an amorphous noncrystalline structure.

When solutions of the *N*-nitrosodipeptides in methanol were analysed by UV spectrophotometry, each exhibited two absorption bands characteristic of N-nitroso compounds – the first near 236 nm for the $N = N$ (II→II*) transition, the second near 350 nm for the $N = O$ (n→II*) transition (Table 2). The absorptions at 230 nm were approximately 60 times those at 350 nm.

The *N*-nitrosodipeptides were further characterized by electron ionization-mass spectrometry (EI-MS). A typical fragmentation pattern is shown in Figure 3 for NPRO-GLY, and Figure 4 shows its EI-MS spectrum. Weak molecular ions were observed for NPRO-GLY and NPRO-ILE but not for NPRO-PHE and NPRO-GLU; however, ions corresponding to $(M-NO)^+$ were observed for all compounds. In each spectrum, ions were observed at m/z 99 and 69, corresponding to the proline moiety. The ion at m/z 99 resulted from cleavage of *n*-nitrosopyrrolidine; ions at m/z 69 and 70 correspond to the pyrrolidine ring less the nitroso groups. Each of these ions was observed in the EI spectra of NPRO itself, which indicates the

Table 1. Elemental analysis of *N*-nitrosodipeptides

N-Nitrosodipeptide	Calculated (%)			Found (%)		
	C	H	N	C	H	N
N-Nitrosoprolylglycine	41.79	5.51	20.89	41.36	5.61	19.00
N-Nitrosoprolylphenylalanine	57.44	5.88	14.43	57.14	5.66	14.21
N-Nitrosoprolylisoleucine	51.31	7.44	16.33	51.86	7.20	15.85
N-Nitrosoprolylglutamic acid	43.96	5.52	15.37	43.25	5.71	15.85

Table 2. Ultra-violet absorption maxima of *N*-nitrosodipeptides

N-Nitrosodipeptide	Ultra-violet absorbance (nm)	
N-Nitrosoprolylglycine	236.5	352.5
N-Nitrosoprolylisoleucine	236.0	353.0
N-Nitrosoprolylphenylalanine	238.0	353.0
N-Nitrosoprolylglutamic acid	234.5	353.0

Fig. 3. Postulated electron ionization-mass spectrometric fragmentation of *N*-nitrosoprolylglycine

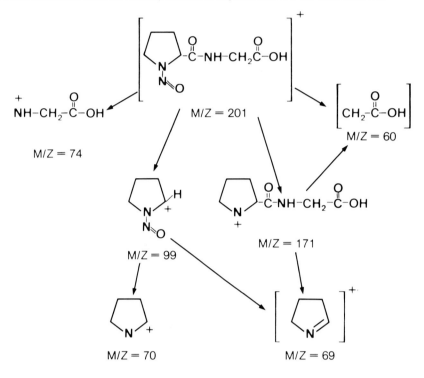

Fig. 4. Electron ionization-mass spectrum of *N*-nitrosoprolylglycine

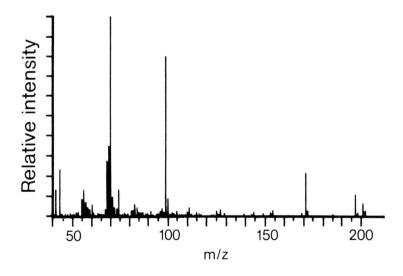

Table 3. Major characteristic infra-red absorption bands of dipeptides and the corresponding N-nitrosodipeptides (CM⁻¹)

Compound[a]	N–H[b]	⁺NH₂[c]	C=O[d]	C=O[b]	⁺NH₂[e]	N–H[f]	C=O[g]	N=O
PRO-ILE	3 242,3 065	2 800–2 000	–	1 680	1 612	1 462	1 584,1 382	–
NPRO-ILE	3 345,3 090	–	1 722	1 649	–	1 556	–	1 215
PRO-PHE	3 192,3 064	2 800–2 000	–	1 676	1 614	h	1 568,1 396	–
NPRO-PHE	3 341,3 065	–	1 738	1 662	–	1 541	–	1 202
PRO-GLU	3 264,3 047	2 800–2 000	1 719	1 672	1 612	1 568	1 585	–
NPRO-GLU	3 307,3 078	–	1 732	1 674	–	1 551	–	1 315
PRO-GLY	3 227,3 084	2 800–1 800	–	1 682	1 614	1 570	1 587,1 382	–
NPRO-GLY	3 300,3 079	–	1 739	1 664	–	1 549	–	1 312

[a] PRO-ILE, prolylisoleucine; NPRO-ILE, N-nitrosoprolylisoleucine; PRO-PHE, prolylphenylalanine; NPRO-PHE, N-nitrosoprolylphenylalanine; PRO-GLY, prolylglycine; NPRO-GLY, N-nitrosoprolylglycine; PRO-GLU, prolylglutamic acid; NPRO-GLU, N-nitrosoprolylglutamic acid
[b] in peptide bond
[c] in pyrrolidine ring
[d] in un-ionized COOH
[e] in pyrrolidine ring, in-plane deformation
[f] in peptide bond, in-plane deformation
[g] C- - - - - -O in ionized COOH
[h] overlapping by carboxylic band

presence of the nitroso group on the amine nitrogen of proline. Ions from the cleavage of the peptide bond were also observed, but no ion was present that would indicate a nitroso group on the amide nitrogen.

Fourier transform IR spectra were also obtained. The most important bands are shown in Table 3, and the spectra of prolylisoleucine and NPRO-ILE are shown in Figure 5. IR spectra of simple dipeptides are very complex due to ionic and nonionic configurations, and zwitterions are very characteristic of this group of compounds. IR spectra of simple dipeptides show a doublet at about 1500 cm^{-1} and about 1400 cm^{-1} due to the interaction of the carboxylic group with the amine of the pyrrolidine ring. However, when the amine nitrogen is nitrosated, the carboxylic group remains un-ionized, and a single C=O stretch is observed at about 1700 cm^{-1}. In simple dipeptides, the N–H stretches from the amine and amide groups generally overlap. Upon nitrosation, the N–H stretch of the amide can still be observed at about 1500 cm^{-1}. Due to hydrogen bonding between the carboxyl group and the nitroso group, the N=O stretch is observed at a lower frequency (about 1200 cm^{-1}) than expected (about 1300 cm^{-1}). Thus, the disappearance of the COO$^-$ bands, the presence of the C=O band of the amide group and the presence of the N–H band of the amide group after nitrosation provide strong evidence that the amine nitrogen was nitrosated while the amide nitrogen was not.

Fig. 5. infra-red spectra of (A) prolylisoleucine and (B0 *N*-nitrosoprolylisoleucine
(A) 1, C- - - - - -O symmetrical, in ionized COOH; 2, N–H in peptide bond, in-plane deformation; 3, C- - - - - -O asymmetrical, in ionized COOH; 4, $^+$NH$_2$ in pyrrolidine ring, in-plane deformation; 5, C=O in peptide bond; 6, N=H in peptide bond, *cis* and *trans*
(B) 1, N=O nitroso group; 2, N–H in peptide bond, in-plane deformation; 3, C=O in peptide bond; 4, C=O in unionized COOH; 5, N–H in peptide bond

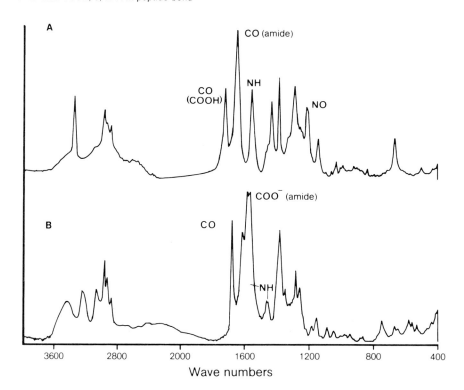

The physical and chemical characterization of *N*-nitrosodipeptides described here, especially by EI-MS and IR spectrophotometry, provide very strong evidence that the reaction of dipeptides with nitrite at acid pH results in the nitrosation of the amine group and not the amide nitrogen. Our work supports that of Kubacka *et al.* (1983), Bonnett *et al.* (1975) and Mirvish *et al.* (1973), but is in contrast to that described by Pollock (1982), who claimed that nitrosation occurs at both nitrogens under these conditions. On the basis of these findings, it appears that formation of *N*-nitrosodipeptides nitrosated at the amide nitrogen would be unlikely to occur in a food system. Nitrosation of the amide nitrogen of dipeptides may occur in other systems, however, such as in organic solvents with nitrogen tetroxide.

Establishing a HPLC separation of the *N*-nitrosodipeptides was the first step towards the development of a multi-detection method for the analysis of non-volatile *N*-nitrosamines in foods. HPLC separations of the *N*-nitrosodipeptides were obtained on cyano and amino columns, and both UV and TEA were used as detectors. The compounds were methylated by the same procedure described for *N*-nitrosoamino acids. Figures 6 and 7 show the chromatographic separations obtained. On the cyano column, NPRO-ILE and NPRO-PHE remained unresolved; the amine column appears to be more selective, since partial separation of the unresolved peaks was achieved.

Fig. 6. High-performance liquid chromatography (HPLC)-ultraviolet (UV) and HPLC-Thermal Energy Analyzer (TEA) chromatograms of methylated *N*-nitrosodipeptides on a cyano column: A, HPLC-UV of 5 µg each of 1, *N*-nitrosoproline; 2, *N*-nitrosoprolylisoleucine; 3, *N*-nitrosoprolylphenylalanine; 4, *N*-nitrosoprolylglutamic acid and 5, *N*-nitrosoprolylglycine. B, HPLC-TEA of 100 ng each of 1, *N*-nitrosoproline; 2, *N*-nitrosoprolylisoleucine; 3, *N*-nitrosoprolylphenylalanine; 4, *N*-nitrosoprolylglutamic acid and 5, *N*-nitrosoprolylglycine

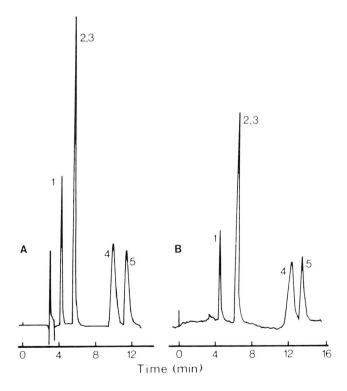

Fig. 7. High-performance liquid chromatography (HPLC-ultraviolet (UV) and HPLC-Thermal Energy Analyzer (TEA) chromatograms of methylated *N*-nitrosodipeptides on an amine column: A, HPLC-UV of 5 μg each of 1, *N*-nitrosoproline; 2, *N*-nitrosoprolylisoleucine; 3, *N*-nitrosoprolylphenylalanine; 4, *N*-nitrosoprolylglutamic acid and 5, *N*-nitrosoprolylglycine. B, HPLC-TEA of 100 ng each of 1, *N*-nitrosoproline; 2, *N*-nitrosoprolylisoleucine; 3, *N*-nitrosoprolylphenylalanine; 4, *N*-nitrosoprolylglutamic acid and 5, *N*-nitrosoprolylglycine

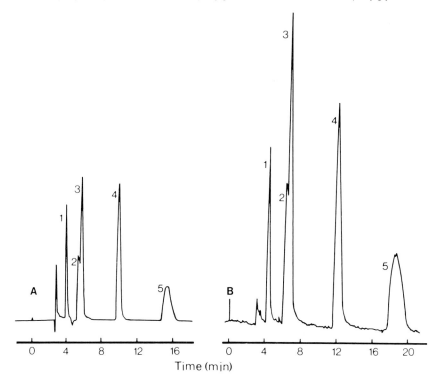

Fig. 8. High-performance liquid chromatography (HPLC)-ultraviolet (UV) chromatogram of *syn* and *anti* isomers of *N*-nitrosoprolylisoleucine on a silica column

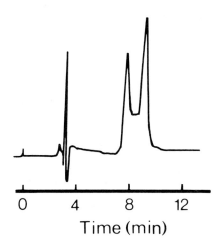

The efficiency of HPLC columns for analysing N-nitrosodipeptides is lower than that for other compounds, due apparently to the existence of *syn* and *anti* isomers and their tendency to separate under the chromatographic conditions used. Analysis of the N-nitrosodipeptides on a silica column with a mobile phase containing an organic buffer, as described by Sen *et al.* (1980), produced two peaks corresponding to the *syn* and *anti* isomers (Fig. 8). Although the tops of the peaks were well resolved, base separation was not achieved, probably because of the fast conversion between *syn* and *anti* isomers during chromatographic analysis.

Since the HPLC conditions for the separation of N-nitrosodipeptides and N-nitrosoamino acids are similar, application of a gradient elution system may facilitate separation of the two groups of compounds simultaneously. Work is continuing in this area.

It appears likely that N-nitrosodipeptides occur in foods together with N-nitrosoamino acids. It would be worthwhile, therefore, to investigate the in-vivo formation of N-nitrosodipeptides as well as their metabolism in live organisms. This is especially important since, in contrast to N-nitrosoamino acids, simple dipeptides are absorbed in the intestine, which suggests that N-nitrosodipeptides may also be absorbed.

ACKNOWLEGEMENTS

The authors are grateful to Dr William Brumley for carrying out the MS analysis and to Dr Jo-Yun Chen for carrying out the IR spectroscopy.

REFERENCES

Baker, JK. & Ma, C.Y. (1978) Determination of N-nitrosoproline in meat products. *J. Agric. Food Chem.,* **26,** 1253–1255

Bonnet, R. & Holleyhead, R. (1974a) *The interaction of nitrite with α-amino acid and peptide derivatives: the ^{15}N-nuclear magnetic resonance approach.* In: Bogovski, P. & Walker, E.A., eds, N-*Nitroso Compounds in the Environment (IARC Scientific Publications No. 9)* Lyon, International Agency for Research on Cancer, pp. 107–110

Bonnet, R. & Holleyhead, R. (1974b) Reaction of tryptophan derivatives with nitrite. *Perkin Trans. I, J. chem. Soc.,* **9,** 962–964

Bonnet, R., Holleyhead, R., Johnson, B.L. & Randall, E.W. (1975) Reaction of acidified nitrite solutions with peptide derivatives: evidence for nitrosamine and thionitrite formation from ^{15}N NMR studies. *Perkin Trans. 1, J. chem. Soc.,* **22,** 2261–2264

Dhont, J.H. & van Ingen, C. (1976) *Identification and quantitative determination of nitrosoproline and nitrososarcosine and preliminary investigations on nitrosohydroxyproline in cured meat products.* In: Walker, E.A., Bogovski, P. & Griciute, L., eds, *Environmental N-Nitroso Compounds: Analysis and Formation, (IARC Scientific Publications No. 14),* Lyon, International Agency for Research on Cancer, pp. 355–360

Druckrey, H., Preussmann, R., Ivankovic, S. & Schmähl, D. (1967) Oraganotrope carcinogene Wirkungen bei 65 verschiedenen N-Nitroso Verbindungen an BD Ratten. *Z. Krebsforsch,* **69,** 103–201

Eisenbrand, G., Spiegelhalder, B., Janzowski, C., Kann, J. & Preussmann, R. (1978) *Volatile and non-volatile N-Nitroso Compounds in foods and other environmental media.* In: Walker, E.A., Castegnaro, M., Griciute, L. & Lyle, R.E., eds, *Environmental Aspects of N-Nitroso Compounds, (IARC Scientific Publications No. 19),* Lyon, International Agency for Research on Cancer, pp. 311–324

Garcia, H. & Lijinsky, W. (1973) Studies of the tumorogenic effects of nitrosoamino acids and of low doses of nitrite to rats. *Z. Krebsforsch.,* **79,** 141–144

Hansen, T., Iwaoka, W., Green, L. & Tannenbaum, S.R. (1977) Analysis of N-nitrosoproline in raw bacon. Further evidence that nitrosoproline is not a major precursor of n-nitrosopyrrolidine. *J. Agric. Food. Chem.,* **25,** 1423–1426

Janzowski, C., Eisenbrand, G. & Preussmann, R. (1978) Occurrence of *N*-nitrosamino acids in cured meat products and their effect on formation of *N*-nitrosamines during heating. *Food Cosmet. Toxicol,* **16,** 343–348

Konturek, S. (1976) *The Physiology of Alimentary Tract,* Warsaw, Panstwowe Zuklady Wydawnictw Lekarskich, p. 99

Kubacka, W. & Scanlan, R.A. (1983) Kinetics of nitrosation of four dipeptides *N*-terminal in proline (in press)

Kubacka, W., Libbey, L.M. & Scanlan, R.A. (1983) Formation and chemical characterization of some nitrosodipeptides *N*-terminal in proline (in press)

Kushnir, I., Feinberg, J.I., Pensabene, J.W., Piotrowski, E.G., Fiddler, W. & Wasserman, A.E. (1975) Isolation and identification of nitrosoproline in uncooked bacon. *J. Food Sci.,* **40,** 427–428

Lakritz, L., Spinelli, A.M. & Wasserman, A.E. (1976) Effect of storage on the concentration of proline and other free amino acids in pork bellies. *J. Food Sci.,* **41,** 879–881

Lijinsky, W. & Reuber, M.D. (1982) *Transnitrosation by nitrosamines* in vivo. In: Bartsch, H., O'Neill, I.K., Castegnaro, M. & Okada, M., eds, N-*Nitroso Compounds: Occurrence and Biological Effects (IARC Scientific Publications No. 41),* Lyon, International Agency for Research on Cancer, pp. 625–631

Massey, R.C., Crews, C. & McWeeny, D.J. (1982) Method for high-performance liquid chromatographic measurement of *N*-nitrosamines in food and beverages. *J. Chromatogr.,* **241,** 423–427

Mirvish, S.S., Sams, J., Fan, T.Y. & Tannenbaum, S.R. (1973) Kinetics of nitrosation of the amino acids proline, hydroxyproline and sarcosine. *J. natl Cancer Inst.,* **51,** 1833–1839

Ohshima, H., Béréziat, J.C. & Bartsch, H. (1982) *Measurement of endogenous* N-*nitrosation in rats and humans by monitoring urinary and faecal excretion of* N-*nitrosamino acids.* In: Bartsch, H., O'Neill, I.K., Castegnaro, M. & Okada, M., eds, N-*Nitroso Compounds: Occurrence and Biological Effects (IARC Scientific Publications No. 41),* Lyon, International Agency for Research on Cancer, pp. 397–411

Pensabene, J.W., Feinberg, J.I., Piotrowski, E.G. & Fiddler, W. (1979) Occurrence and determination of *N*-nitrosoproline and *N*-nitrosopyrrolidine in cured meat products. *J. Food Sci.,* **44,** 1700–1702

Pollock, J.R.A. (1982) *Nitrosation products from peptides.* In: Bartsch, H., O'Neill, I.K., Castegnaro, M. & Okada, M., eds, N-*Nitroso Compounds: Occurrence and Biological Effects (IARC Scientific Publications No. 41),* Lyon, International Agency for Research on Cancer, pp. 81–85

Sen, N.P. Donaldson, B.A., Seaman, S., Iyengar, J.R. & Miles, W.F. (1978) *Recent studies in Canada on the analysis and occurrence of volatile and non-volatile* N-*nitroso compounds in foods.* In: Walker, E.A., Castegnaro, M., Griciute, L. & Lyle, R.E., eds, *Environmental Aspects of N-Nitroso Compounds, (IARC Scientific Publications No. 19),* Lyon, International Agency for Research on Cancer, pp. 373–393

Sen, N.P., Seaman, S. & McPherson, M. (1980) *Further studies on the occurrence of volatile and non-volatile nitrosamines in foods.* In: Walker, E.A., Griciute, L. Castegnaro, M. & Börzsönyi, M., eds, N-*Nitroso Compounds: Analysis, Formation and Occurrence (IARC Scientific Publications No. 31),* Lyon, International Agency for Research on Cancer, pp. 457–463

Sen, N.P., Seaman, S. & Tessier, L. (1982) *A rapid and sensitive method for the determination of non-volatile* N-*nitroso compounds in foods and human urine: recent data concerning volatile* N-*nitrosoamines in dried foods and malt-based beverages.* In: Bartsch, H., O'Neill, I.K., Castegnaro, M. & Okada, M., eds, N-*Nitroso Compounds: Occurrence and Biological Effects (IARC Scientific Publications No. 41),* Lyon, International Agency for Research on Cancer, pp. 185–197

Sen. N.P., Tessier, L. & Seaman, S. (1983) Determination of *N*-nitrosoproline and *N*-nitrososarcosine in malt and beer *J. Agric. Food Chem.,* **31,** 1033–1036

Spinelli-Gugger A.M., Lakritz, L. & Wasserman, A.E. (1980) Effect of processing on the amino acid composition and nitrosamine formation in pork belly adipose tissue. *J. Agric. Food. Chem.,* **28,** 424–427

Stewart, F.H.C. (1969) Peptide synthesis with the *N*-nitroso derivatives of sarcosine and proline. *Aust. J. Chem.,* **22,** 2451–2461

ENDOGENOUS FORMATION OF *N*-NITROSO COMPOUNDS

ANALYSIS FOR AND INTESTINAL METABOLISM OF PRECURSOR NITROSO COMPOUNDS IN NORMAL SUBJECTS AND IN PATIENTS WITH CHRONIC RENAL FAILURE

M.L. SIMENHOFF, S.R. DUNN & P.S. LELE

Department of Medicine, Division of Nephrology, Jefferson Medical College, Thomas Jefferson University, Philadelphia, PA 19107, USA

SUMMARY

We have demonstrated that patients with chronic renal failure generate increased amounts of both dimethylamine and *N*-nitrosodimethylamine in the small bowel in association with aerobic and anaerobic bacterial overgrowth. The significance of these findings in relation to the reported increased incidence of cancer in patients with chronic renal failure has not yet been defined.

INTRODUCTION

A human model exhibiting increased generation of dimethylamine (DMA), a precursor of *N*-nitrosodimethylamine (NDMA) was investigated in order to identify possible NDMA formation therefrom. Patients with chronic renal failure (CRF) fulfill the criteria for such a model (Simenhoff *et al.*, 1963, 1976); however, because of rapid degradation of NDMA in the liver, its formation in the gut would not be reflected accurately by blood NDMA levels (Simenhoff et al., 1982). Investigation of NDMA formation in uraemic patients is particularly desirable because of the reported increased incidence of cancer in patients with CRF. The presence of upper intestinal bacterial overgrowth adds further to the possibility that NDMA is produced *in situ* (Simenhoff *et al.*, 1978). The probable metabolic steps that occur in the intestine are illustrated in Figure 1.

MATERIALS AND METHODS

Fifteen patients with CRF (12 of whom were on thrice-weekly haemodialysis) and eight control subjects were studied by sampling blood and duodenal aspirates. The latter were obtained by intubation under sterile conditions (Simenhoff *et al.*, 1978). From a pool of 56 CRF patients, 39 were solicited randomly for the study, but only 21 consented. Of these, only 15 were successfully intubated.

Fig. 1. Proposed metabolic steps leading to the formation of *N*-nitrosodimethylamine (NDMA) in the intestine. *1, bacterial overgrowth in uraemia; *2, O = N–N⟨$^{CH_3}_{CH_3}$

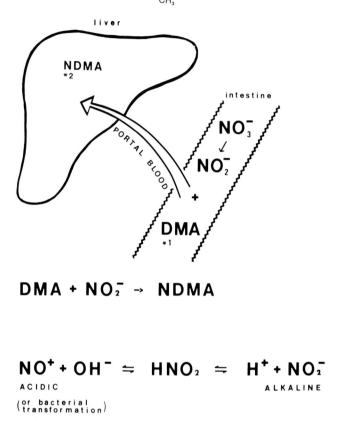

$$DMA + NO_2^- \rightarrow NDMA$$

$$NO^+ + OH^- \rightleftharpoons HNO_2 \rightleftharpoons H^+ + NO_2^-$$

ACIDIC   ALKALINE

(or bacterial transformation)

Methylamines and volatile nitrosamines were measured in blood. Bacterial culture, pH, methylamines and volatile nitrosamines were measured in the duodenal aspirate.

Collection and storage of specimens

Blood: Blood was drawn from the patient's arm vein into a standard 50-mL disposable syringe and was immediately transferred to two polypropylene centrifuge tubes (25-30 mL in one and 20-25 mL in the other). Fifty mg of ascorbic acid were added to one tube (#1), which was placed in a freezer (–15 °C). The blood in the other tube was allowed to clot and was then centrifuged at 2 500 rpm for 8–10 min. The serum was removed and placed in another tube (#2) and frozen at –15 °C. Tube #1 was assayed for volatile nitrosamines. Studies previously performed showed that two nitrosamines (NDMA and *N*-nitrosomethylethylamine) were stable for at least eight days under these conditions (Lakritz *et al.*, 1980). Tube #2 was assayed for volatile amines.

Duodenal aspirate: Duodenal aspirate was collected under sterile conditions. One portion was collected for both aerobic and anaerobic bacteria cultures and an additional portion collected into sterile polypropylene tubes (30–50 mL per tube). The pH was measured, and

30–50 mL were poured into a polypropylene centrifuge tube that contained about 50 mg ascorbic acid. This tube was frozen until the contents were assayed for volatile nitrosamines (usually the next day). The remaining aspirate was assayed for volatile amines.

All syringes, centrifuge tubes, rubber intubation tubing and sterilization fluids were checked for volatile nitrosamine contamination. Special care was taken to avoid exposure to direct sunlight and prolonged exposure to fluorescent light.

Analysis of blood and duodenal aspirate for volatile nitrosamines and volatile amines

Nitrosamines: Blood and duodenal aspirates were processed in the same manner. Weighed specimens (20.0 g minimum) were transferred to 1-L single-neck flasks, to which were added a few boiling chips, 50 mL of 'nitrosamine-free' deionized water, 30 mL 1N sodium hydroxide, 8 g hydrated barium hydroxide and 100 mg ascorbic acid. An internal standard of N-nitrosomethylethylamine (1.00 mL of 0.02 µg/mL) was added to follow recovery. The mixture was distilled at atmospheric pressure using grease-free, standard, tapered glassware. Aqueous distillate was collected until the distillation flask was dry.

The distillates were transferred to 250-mL separating funnels that contained 10 g sodium chloride. This solution was extracted three times with separate 80-mL volumes of dichloromethane (DCM). The extracts were combined and washed once with 50 mL 6N hydrochloric acid then once with 50 mL 5N sodium hydroxide. The DCM extract was then passed through 35 g granular anhydrous sodium sulfate held in a 60-mL coarse-fritted glass funnel and collected into a 500-mL Kuderna-Danish evaporator fitted with a 4-mL concentrator tube (Kontes Inc., Vineland, NJ, USA). The volume of the DCM extract was reduced to 4 mL using a steam bath. Reduction of the DCM extract to 1.0 mL was achieved using a micro Snyder column and a 65 °C water-bath. An aliquot (7–9 µL) of the DCM extract was injected into a gas chromatograph (GC) interfaced with a Thermal Energy Analyzer (TEA). The presence of NDMA in the samples was determined by comparing the retention time of the suspected NDMA in the sample to the retention time of a pure NDMA standard that was injected at various times during the day. The NDMA was quantified by peak height analysis using a calibrated external standard.

Patients' blood and duodenal specimens were always distilled at the same time. A water blank was run with every group of specimens and then 'subtracted' from the corresponding specimens. All glassware was rinsed with DCM prior to use. The DCM that was used was checked for TEA-positive peaks by evaporating 300 mL to 1.0 mL and assaying for TEA-positive peaks (Pensabene, J.W., 1980, personal communication). The 6N hydrochloric acid, 5N and 1N sodium hydroxide and water were also extracted with DCM to remove any TEA-positive peaks. Only polypropylene, glass and Teflon stoppers were used to close reagent bottles.

Aliphatic amines: The aliphatic amines, DMA and trimethylamine (TMA), were assayed for in serum and duodenal aspirate using gas-liquid chromatography. Frozen serum or duodenal aspirate was thawed, mixed and centrifuged. Amines were separated from biological fluids by adopting a modification of the procedure described by Conway (1950). A sealable porcelain micro-diffusion cell (Arthur H. Thomas, Philadelphia, PA, USA) was set up in duplicate (Fig. 2). The centre well (#1) contained 250 µL of 0.1N sulfuric acid. The intermediate well (#2) contained 'amine-free' deionized water and 1000 to 500 µL of either serum or duodenal aspirate. The outermost well (#3) contained 2.0 mL of a mixture of 50% v/v of saturated potassium carbonate and 12N potassium hydroxide (called the alkaline solution). This well acted as the sealing well. To the #2 well 1.00 mL of the alkaline solution was added carefully, and the cover was placed immediately on the dish. The dish was gently rocked for about 10–15 sec and allowed to set overnight (18 h). Each specimen was run in duplicate. Standards (usually four) were run with each set of specimens. After 18 h, the covers were carefully removed; the

Fig. 2. Conway micro-diffusion cell. Well #1 (collection well) contains 250 μL/0.1N H_2SO_4. Well #2 (reaction well) contains specimen (100-500 μL), water (500 μL) and KOH/K_2CO_3 (1000 μL). Well #3 (sealing well) contains 2000 μL KOH/K_2CO_3

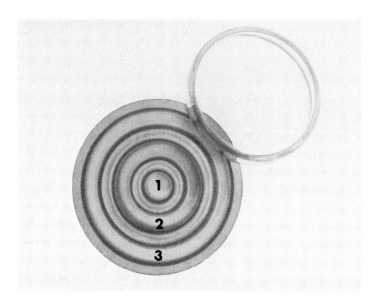

centre wells (#1) were transferred separately to tared polypropylene microcentrifuge tubes; the volume of each centre well was determined by weighing and tested to assure it was still acidic. This solution, containing the liberated volatile aliphatic amines from the specimens (now as acid salts of the amines), was then assayed for DMA and TMA. A portion (50 μL) of the acidic solution from the centre well was added to glass micro-test tubes, which contained the dry alkaline residue from 50 μL 1N potassium hydroxide that had been put into these tubes previously and allowed to evaporate in an oven at 90-100 °C. One μL of resulting alkaline solution was immediately injected into a gas chromatograph using conditions similar to those employed by Dunn *et al.* (1976), but with a slightly different column: 12% Amine 220 and 8% potassium hydroxide on 100/120 Chromosorb WAW. The column was run at 75 °C isothermal with nitrogen at 17 mL/min.

A second column, 6-ft (1.8-m) coiled glass packed with 4% Carbowax 20M and 0.8% potassium hydroxide on 60/80 Carbopack B (Supleco Inc. Bellefont, PA, USA) and operated at 75 °C isothermal, was used to confirm further the presence of DMA and TMA.

All specimens were corrected for recoveries of TMA and DMA, since the diffusion of each in the Conway cells is temperature dependent. Appropriate corrections were applied that accounted for the change in volume of the #1 well. To date, no satisfactory internal standard has been found.

Conditions for analysis by gas chromatography (GC)-Thermal Energy Analyzer (TEA)

The conditions used for GC-TEA analysis were the same as those reported by Fiddler *et al.* (1981).

Specimens that gave positive nitrosamine peaks were confirmed by the photolytic technique described by Doerr and Fiddler (1977), and, when enough nitrosamine was present, by mass spectrometry according to the technique described by Kimoto and Fiddler (1982).

Statistical analysis

Simple linear regression was performed for values of NDMA, DMA, TMA and pH in blood and duodenal fluids from CRF patients and controls. Mean levels of these same variables were tested for difference by an unpaired t test.

RESULTS

The only statistically different (at the $p = 0.05$ level) values for volatile nitrosamines and some of their specific biochemical precursors in blood and duodenal aspirate obtained from control subjects and CRF patients were those of DMA and NDMA.

Methylamine precursors

DMA: Differences between mean DMA levels in control and CRF patients' blood ($p < 0.05$) and duodenal aspirate ($p < 0.002$) were similar to those reported previously (Simenhoff *et al.*, 1976) and are illustrated in Figure 3.

TMA: Slight differences between controls and CRF were seen for the TMA content of blood but not of duodenal aspirate; again confirming previous reports (Simenhoff *et al.*, 1976) and are illustrated in Figure 4.

Fig. 3. Dimethylamine (DMA) in serum and duodenal aspirate from controls and from patients with chronic renal failure (CRF). Mean and SEM. For blood, control n = 8, CRF n = 15; for duodenal aspirate, control n = 7, CRF n = 14

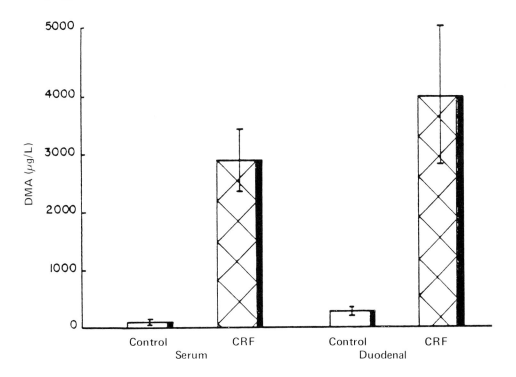

Fig. 4. Trimethylamine (TMA) in serum and duodenal aspirate from controls and from patients with chronic renal failure (CRF). Mean and SEM. For blood, control n = 8, CRF n = 15; for duodenal aspirate, control n = 7, CRF n = 14

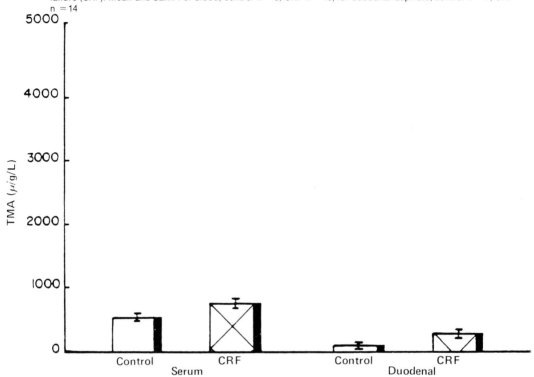

Fig. 5. *N*-Nitrosodimethylamine (NDMA) in blood and duodenal aspirate from controls and from patients with chronic renal failure (CRF). Mean and SEM. For blood, control n = 8, CRF n = 15; for duodenal aspirate, control n = 7, CRF n = 14

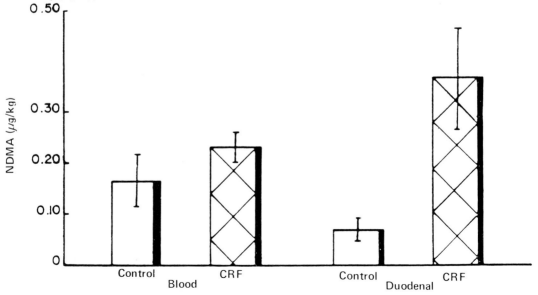

Monomethylamine was neither significantly nor consistently raised in either blood or duodenal aspirate.

Volatile nitrosamines

The only volatile nitrosamine found regularly in blood was NDMA (Fig. 5), at levels that were similar in both groups. However, in duodenal aspirate from CRF patients NDMA levels were significantly raised ($p < 0.05$) (Fig. 6).

No other volatile nitrosamine was seen in duodenal aspirates of control subjects, but four patients with CRF had N-nitrosopiperidine (NPIP) at levels of 12.0, 8.4, 1.2 and 2.1 µg/kg, respectively (Fig. 7).

The pH of the duodenal aspirates did not differ significantly (at the 0.05 level) between control and CRF subjects (means: control, 4.7 ± 2.4; CRF, 5.6 ± 2.2). Contamination of duodenal aspirate with gastric juice was often a problem and, therefore, the significance of the pH measurements is difficult to evaluate.

No linear correlation between NDMA, DMA, TMA and pH levels was noted for either blood or duodenal aspirate within each group.

Fig. 6. Individual levels of N-nitrosodimethylamine (NDMA) in blood and duodenal aspirates of controls and of patients with chronic renal failure (CRF). Mean and SEM.

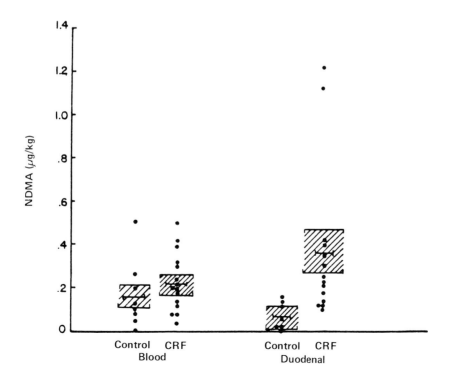

Fig. 7. Percentages of subjects with *N*-nitrosodimethylamine (NDMA) and *N*-nitrosopiperidine (NPIP) in blood and duodenal aspirate. Cont., controls; CRF, patients with chronic renal failure. Numerator shows the number of patients with the respective nitrosamine; denominator shows the total number surveyed

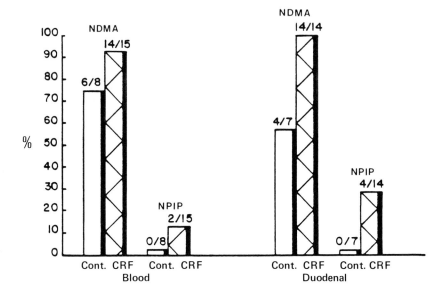

Fig. 8. Duodenal microflora in controls and in patients with chronic renal failure (CRF). Mean and SEM

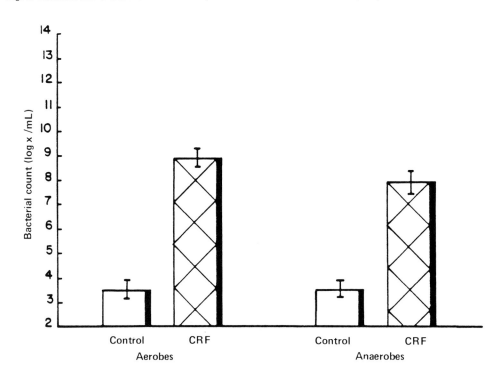

Bacterial overgrowth

The species characteristics of bacterial overgrowth in patients with chronic renal failure have been reported previously (Simenhoff *et al.*, 1978). The patients studied here exhibited similar abnormalities (Fig. 8).

DISCUSSION

These results show that patients with CRF have a significantly increased generation of NDMA high up in the small bowel (duodenum) when compared with control subjects (p = 0.043). This suggests an association with the presence of increased concentrations of the precursor compound DMA and bacterial overgrowth of both aerobic and anaerobic organisms.

Matas *et al.* (1975) described an increase in the incidence of cancer in patients with CRF; this was also reported subsequently by others (Lindner *et al.*, 1981). There is no direct evidence that their findings are related to an increased concentration of NDMA in the duodenum. It is clear, however, that there is a spectrum of NDMA duodenal levels, such that those patients who have concentrations within the normal range would probably be at less potential risk than patients with increased concentrations, if single measurements are representative of daily levels (Fig. 6). We have no information on diurnal or mensual variations.

Two CRF patients agreed to ingest 6 g vitamin C every day for two weeks and to be reintubated. Vitamin C should be capable of blocking nitrosation *via* interaction with available nitrite, thus decreasing NDMA formation. In one patient we were able to demonstrate a decrease in duodenal NDMA levels from 1.22 to 0.20 µg/kg; but, in the other, NDMA levels were not significantly different (0.23 to 0.25 µg/kg). A larger series of patients will be necessary to demonstrate if an antioxidant effect is present, and if it is sufficient to reduce NDMA formation in the duodenum.

NDMA formation might be anticipated in the presence of DMA and nitrite and at an appropriate pH – 3.4 is optimal for NDMA formation (Mirvish, 1970). In normal humans, these conditions are not usually met simultaneously. There is much discussion and disagreement concerning these optimal conditions.

Our results demonstrate significant increases in duodenal DMA in patients with CRF, the level always being higher than that in blood. This suggests that DMA reaches the lumen by ingestion or is produced *in situ;* in view of the fact that ours were fasting subjects, the latter is more likely. Quantitatively, salivary DMA could not account for this rise. Normally, nonabsorbed choline in the large gut is degraded in part to TMA by bacterial activity (Zeisel, 1981); TMA is then demethylated, probably in the liver, to DMA, which is an end metabolite. However, the potential enzymatic activities of the bacteria found in these patients could bring about sequential demethylation of TMA, and this has been shown *in vitro* (Colby & Zatmus, 1973).

Even in the presence of large increases in DMA in the duodenum, the conditions are not optimal for NDMA formation: measured nitrite levels have been variable and have not correlated with the measured NDMA levels; and the pH of the duodenal aspirate is usually alkaline (although contamination by the acid contents of the stomach has sometimes occurred). It has been speculated that metabolic bacterial activity is an essential condition for NDMA formation in this location (Klubes & Jondorf, 1971; Mills & Alexander, 1976). We have not yet had the opportunity of repeating the measurements following administration of non-absorbable antibiotics.

Although the suggestion from animal experiments (Asatoor & Simenhoff, 1965) is that DMA has both endogenous and exogenous sources, this paper has addressed only the exogenous formation of NDMA in the gut. We have no data on endogenous DMA formation.

ACKNOWLEDGEMENTS

This research was supported by grant No. CA 26 571 awarded by the National Cancer Institute, National Institutes of Health, DHHS.

We thank Steven Gorman of Jefferson Medical College, John Pensabene, Robert Gates, Walter Fiddler and Walter Kimoto from the US Department of Agriculture (ERRC) for technical assistance and advice.

All procedures that involved human subjects were carried out in accord with the Helsinki Declaration of 1975. Informed consent was obtained from all participants.

REFERENCES

Asatoor, A.M. & Simenhoff, M.L. (1965) The origin of urinary dimethylamine. *Biochem. biophys. Acta*, *111*, 384–392

Colby, J. & Zatman, L.J. (1973) Trimethylamine metabolism in obligate and facultative methylatrophs. *Biochem. J.*, *132*, 101–112

Conway, E.J. (1950) *Microdiffusion Analysis and Volumetric Error*. D. Van Nostrand Co.

Doerr, R. & Fiddler, W. (1977) Photolysis of volatile nitrosamines at the picogram level as an aid to confirmation. *J. Chromatogr.*, *140*, 284–287

Dunn, S.R., Simenhoff, M.L. & Wesson, L.G. (1976) Gas chromatographic determination of mono-, di- and trimethylamines in biological fluids. *Anal. Chem.*, *48*, 41–44

Fiddler, W., Pensabene, J.W. & Kimoto, W.I. (1981) Investigation of edible oils for volatile nitrosamines. *J. Food Sci.*, *46*, 603–605

Kimoto, W.I. & Fiddler, W. (1982) Confirmatory method for N-nitrosodimethylamine and N-nitro-soproline in food samples by multiple ion analysis with gas chromatography-low resolution mass spectrometry before and after U-V photolysis. *J. Assoc. off. anal. Chem.*, *65*, 1162–1167

Klubes, P. & Jondorf, W.R. (1971) Dimethylnitrosamine formation from sodium nitrite and dimethylamine by bacterial flora of rat intestines. *Res. Commun. Chem. Pathol. Pharmacol.*, *2*, 24–33

Lakritz, L., Simenhoff, M.L., Dunn, S.R. & Fiddler, W. (1980) N-Nitrosodimethylamine in human blood. *Food Cosmet. Toxicol.*, *18*, 77–79

Lindner, A.M., Farewell, V.T. & Sherrard, D.J. (1981) High incidence of neoplasia in uremic patients receiving long-term dialysis. *Nephron*, *27*, 292–295

Matas, A.J., Simmonds, R.L., Kjellstrand, C.M., Buselmeier, T.J. & Najarian, J.S. (1975) Increased incidence of malignancy during chronic renal failure. *Lancet*, *i*, 883–886

Mills, A.L. & Alexander, M. (1976) N-Nitrosamine formation of cultures of several microorganisms. *Appl. environ. Microbiol.*, *31*, 892–895

Mirvish, S.S. (1970) Kinetics of dimethyl nitrosation in relation to nitrosamine carcinogenesis. *J. natl Cancer Inst.*, *44*, 633–639

Simenhoff, M.L., Milne, M.D. & Asatoor, A.M. (1963) Retention of aliphatic amines in uremia. *Clin. Sci.*, *25*, 65–77

Simenhoff, M.L., Saukkonen, J.J., Burke, J.F., Wesson, L.G. & Schaedler, R.W. (1976) Amine metabolism and the small bowel in uremia. *Lancet*, *ii*, 818–821

Simenhoff, M.L., Saukkonen, J.J., Burke, J.F., Wesson, L.G., Schaedler, R.W. & Gordon, S. (1978) Bacterial populations of the small bowel in uremia. *Nephron*, *22*, 460–464

Simenhoff, M.L., Dunn, S.R., Fiddler, W. & Pensabene, J.W. (1982) *Presence of nitrosamines in blood of normal and diseased human subjects*. In: Magee, P.N., ed., *Nitrosamines and Human Cancer, Banbury Report 12*, Cold Spring Harbor, NY, Cold Spring Harbor Laboratory, pp. 283–293

Zeisel, S.H. (1981) Dietary choline: Biochemistry, physiology and pharmacology. *Ann. Rev. Nutr.*, *1*, 95–121

NITROSATION OF PIPERAZINE IN MAN

B.T.D. BELLANDER & L. HAGMAR

Department of Occupational Medicine, University Hospital, S-221 85 Lund, Sweden

B.-G. ÖSTERDAHL

National Food Administration, Uppsala, Sweden

SUMMARY

Piperazine, a secondary amine used as an anthelmintic drug, nitrosates rapidly *in vitro* to form two nitrosamines. Anhydrous piperazine and a drug formulation were found to have a content of 0.2–20 μg of the suspected carcinogen, *N*-mononitrosopiperazine, per gram of piperazine, but no detectable amount of the carcinogen, *N,N'*-dinitrosopiperazine.

The possible nitrosation of the drug piperazine in man was investigated, with the following results. Thirty min after oral administration of 480 mg piperazine to four, fasting, healthy, male volunteers, gastric juice contained 0.14–0.23 μg/mL *N*-mononitrosopiperazine, as determined by gas chromatography-thermal energy analysis. The total amount produced in the stomach is estimated to have been 30–66 μg. The nitrosamine was not detected in blood, but was excreted in the urine, mainly during the first 8 h (0.8–2.5 μg). Half had appeared within 3 h. Acidification of the urine did not affect the excretion. *N,N'*-Dinitrosopiperazine was never found in gastric juice, blood or urine.

Co-administration of 2 g ascorbic acid resulted in a significant, but incomplete and varying, inhibition of nitrosation in the stomach and of nitrosamine excretion in the urine.

INTRODUCTION

A great number of *N*-nitroso compounds are mutagenic and/or carcinogenic. Amines and nitrite may form *N*-nitroso compounds in the gastric content, as has been shown in a number of animal experiments and, in the case of proline, in healthy humans (Ohshima & Bartsch, 1981). The aim of the present study was to investigate the possible nitrosation of the drug piperazine in the human stomach and the excretion of nitrosation products in the urine.

Piperazine (PIP), a cyclic secondary amine, is used globally and extensively as an anthelmintic drug. In addition, occupational exposure to PIP occurs in the chemical and pharmaceutical industries. PIP nitrosates *in vitro* and in experimental animals to two *N*-nitrosopiperazines; *N*-mononitrosopiperazine (NPIP) and *N,N'*-dinitrosopiperazine (DNPIP) (Mirvish, 1975). DNPIP is mutagenic (Elespuru & Lijinsky, 1976) and carcinogenic

(Druckrey *et al.*,1967). NPIP has been reported to be both mutagenic (Braun *et al.*, 1977) and non-mutagenic (Elespuru & Lijinsky, 1976). Earlier reports concerning the carcinogenic properties of NPIP (Garcia *et al.*, 1970) were later questioned (Love *et al.*, 1977).

The present report deals with the nitrosation of PIP in man. Some of the first results of this study were presented as a letter to the editor of *The Lancet* (Bellander *et al.*, 1981).

MATERIALS AND METHODS

Chemicals

Piperazine syrup was obtained from ACO Läkemedel AB (Solna, Sweden). In this drug, PIP hexahydrate, corresponding to 48 mg PIP/mL, was formulated with saccharin (680 mg/mL), citric acid, citrus fruit tincture and methyl-*para*-hydroxybenzoate in water. Ascorbic acid L (+), dichloromethane, hydrochloric acid, sulfamic acid and kieselguhr (Extrelut®) were all of analytical grade (E. Merck A.G., Darmstadt, FRG) and were used without further purification. Sodium sulfamate solution was prepared from sulfamic acid and sodium hydroxide. Water was deionized or distilled. Sodium hydroxide (analytical grade) and PIP were purchased from a local supplier. Ammonium chloride was obtained from ACO Läkemedel AB. NPIP stock standard solution was obtained from Thermo Electron Corporation (Waltham, MA, USA). DNPIP stock standard solution was made from commercially available synthesized DNPIP.

Subjects

Four male, healthy (e.g., no symptom of urinary infection), non-smoking volunteers aged 31–45 of body weight 62 to 87 kg were studied. Routine biochemical liver and kidney tests gave normal results, and the urines were all negative to nitrite stick (Niturtest, Boehringer Mannheim; detection limit, approximately 0.5 mg/L or 10 µmol/L). One volunteer (No. 1) consumed a mainly vegetarian diet. The volunteers were fasted overnight (> 10 h). Two of the subjects (No. 3, 4) were given ammonium chloride before and during all experiments, so that the pH of their urine was adjusted to 5.

Administration and sampling

In all experiments, pre-exposure samples were taken in the morning for analysis of background levels and sample contamination and for recovery studies. Ten mL PIP syrup containing 480 mg PIP, the anthelmintic dose recommended to be taken twice daily for 2–7 days, was given with 50 mL tap water. In four experiments, 2 g ascorbic acid was added to the PIP syrup before intake.

Gastric juice was sampled repeatedly (*ca* 50 mL at a time) through a nasogastric tube. Ten-mL aliquots were promptly made alkaline with 10 mL 0.2 mol/L sodium hydroxide and put on a prepacked kieselguhr column. The column was extracted with 100 mL dichloromethane.

All *urine* was collected and, to 10- or 20-mL aliquots, 0.5 or 1 mL of 4% sodium sulfamate solution was added. In the first experiment (subjects nos 1, 2; gastric juice sampling; no ascorbic acid), sulfamic acid was used for sample preparation.

In four experiments, *blood* was collected for nitrosopiperazine analysis (after 45, 90, 135 min) in evacuated, heparinized tubes (Vacutainer®, Becton, Dickinson), without further treatment.

Table 1. Detection limits and recoveries at analysis of *N*-mononitrosopiperazine (NPIP) and *N,N'*-dinitrosopiperazine (DNPIP)

Compound	Medium[a]	Sample size (mL)	Detection limit (µg/mL)	Recovery		
				n	Amount added (µg/mL)	Recovery (%, mean ± SD)
NPIP	Gastric juice	10	0.0004	8	0.01–0.12	70 ± 14
				7	0.12–1.2	90 ± 10
	Urine	20	0.0002	14	0.002–0.02	85 ± 12
	Blood	5	0.002	10	0.002–0.02	24 ± 8
	PIP anhydrate	50 (mg)	0.03 (µg/g)	2	2 (µg/g)	74 and 90
	PIP syrup	1	0.004	2	0.2	86 and 65
DNPIP	Gastric juice	10	0.0005	4	0.002–0.02	89 ± 9
	Urine	20	0.0003	16	0.002–0.02	90 ± 12
	Blood	5	0.002	6	0.002–0.02	42 ± 9
	PIP anhydrate	50 (mg)	0.03 (µg/g)	–		
	PIP syrup	1	0.006	2	0.07	69 and 100

[a] PIP, Piperazine

Analysis of N-nitrosopiperazines

All extracts and samples for *N*-nitrosopiperazine determination were coded and mailed, reaching the laboratory within 24 h (at ambient temperature). They were stored at 5°C and analysed within a week. The sample code was unknown to the laboratory. Urine (2 × 10 or 20 mL) and blood (2 × 5 mL) were made alkaline and extracted in the same way as gastric juice. The extracts were concentrated and analysed using an isothermal gas-liquid chromatograph (GLC) interfaced to a Thermal Energy Analyzer (TEA), as described elsewhere (Bellander & Österdahl, 1983). The results were calculated using the external-standard calibration method and automatic peak-area integration. Detection limits and recoveries are summarized in Table 1. In most cases, duplicate samples were analysed and the result reported is the mean.

The identity of NPIP was confirmed tentatively by treating some extracts from samples of urine and gastric juice with ultra-violet light or hydrogen bromide in glacial acetic acid, followed by re-analysis in the GLC-TEA. Both procedures caused disappearance of the peak with the same retention time as the NPIP standard peak. Standard solutions and some samples contained traces of unidentified TEA-positive compounds with retention times about 5 s longer than those of NPIP and DNPIP. Unlike the last two, the unknown compounds were stable upon ultra-violet irradiation.

Artefactual formation of N-nitrosopiperazines

Low levels of NPIP were present in anhydrous PIP and in PIP hexahydrate (0.2–0.4 µg/g) as well as in the drug formulation tested (3–20 µg/g in three different batches). No DNPIP was found. A batch of the drug with a low content of NPIP was chosen for the experiments. The dose taken contained about 2 µg NPIP. Overnight storage of the drug with ascorbic acid did not affect its NPIP content.

The method of treatment of gastric juice samples was tested for artefactual nitrosamine formation by mixing gastric juice, sodium hydroxide, PIP (diluted syrup) and sodium nitrite (in that order) to final concentrations of: gastric juice, 77% (v/v); sodium hydroxide, 0.15 mol/L; PIP, 0.77 g/L (9.0 mmol/L) and sodium nitrite, 0.38 g/L (5.6 mmol/L). The mixture was promtly put on a kieselguhr column, extracted and sent for analysis. Only traces ($<$ 0.001 mg/L) of NPIP and NDPIP were present in the samples; the yield was thus of the order of 10^{-5} of the theoretical.

The treatment of urine samples was tested by mixing urine, PIP (from anhydrous PIP), sodium sulfamate and nitrite (in that order) to final concentrations of: urine, 94% (v/v); PIP, 0.28 g/L (3.3 mmol/L); sodium sulfamate, 1.9 g/L (15 mmol/L) and sodium nitrite, 2.1 mg/L (30 µmol/L). After 5 days' storage at room temperature, the NPIP concentration was less than 0.001 mg/L ($<$ 0.01 µmol/L). DNPIP could not be detected ($<$0.0003 mg/L). Sulfamic acid was less effective as a nitrite trap.

RESULTS

N-*Nitrosopiperazine in gastric juice*

No *N*-nitrosopiperazine could be detected in pre-exposure samples. NPIP, but never DNPIP, was found in gastric juice after intake of PIP (Fig. 1). The levels reached maximum values (0.14–0.23 µg/mL) in all subjects 30 min after the intake of the drug. In the two subjects

Fig. 1. *N*-Mononitrosopiperazine (NPIP) levels in gastric juice after intake of 480 mg piperazine in 4 subjects (data for subjects 1 and 2 in this challenge re-analysed from Bellander *et al.*, 1981)

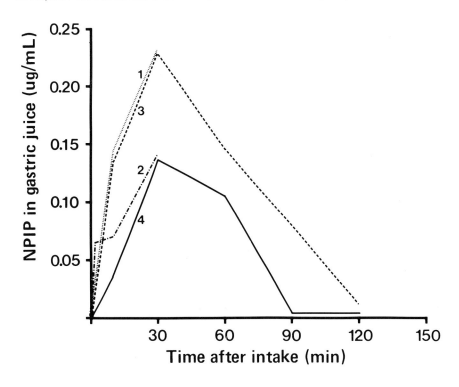

followed for 120 min, the level in the last sample was still above the detection limit. The total amount of NPIP sampled during the first 30 min is estimated to have been 21, 14, 14 and 5.2 μg (in subjects No. 1–4). The pH was 2–3 in the pre-exposure and last samples. Immediately after the intake of the drug, the pH rose by 2–3 units.

When the drug was mixed with 2 g ascorbic acid before intake, the NPIP concentration pattern in gastric juic was different (Fig. 2). The highest concentrations were lower (0.01–0.10 mg/L) and occurred earlier (at 10 min) than in the absence of ascorbic acid. In this experiment, the total amounts of NPIP sampled up to and including 30 min were 0.6, 1.0, 3.7 and 4.7 μg in the four subjects, respectively. In all four individuals, at least trace amounts were present in the last sample (at 150 min). The pH was 1.4–4.0 in the pre-exposure and last samples. Immediately after the intake of the drug, the pH rose by 0.2–2.0 units.

N-*Nitrosopiperazine in urine*

No *N*-nitrosopiperazine could be detected in pre-exposure samples. NPIP but not DNPIP, was excreted in the urine after intake. When no gastric juice was sampled, 0.8–2.5 μg was excreted during 8 h (Fig. 3). Two individuals (No. 3, 4), who were followed for an additional 29 and 32 h, excreted only 0.14 and 0.13 μg, respectively, in the latter period. Twenty-four hours from intake, the concentration in urine was below the detection limit. Half of the total amount excreted had appeared after about 3 h.

When the experiment was performed with gastric juice sampling, the four subjects excreted 0.12, 200, 1.8 and 0.96 μg, respectively, within 6 h. These values represent 18, 9 800, 240 and 51% of those in the experiment without gastric juice sampling. The highest amount excreted was more than 100 times greater than the next highest. This enormously high excretion is left out of the following comparisons.

When 2 g ascorbic acid were administered with the PIP dose (and gastric juice was sampled), 0.09, 0.36, 0.36 and 0.21 μg were excreted within 6 h, corresponding to 77, –, 20 and 21% of

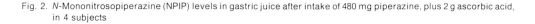

Fig. 2. *N*-Mononitrosopiperazine (NPIP) levels in gastric juice after intake of 480 mg piperazine, plus 2 g ascorbic acid, in 4 subjects

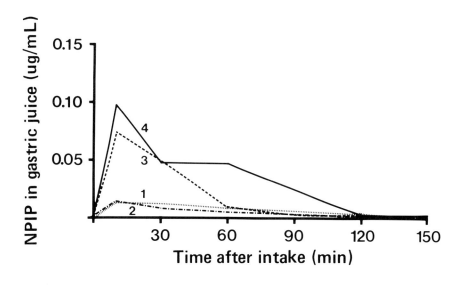

Fig. 3. Cumulated excretion of *N*-mononitrosopiperazine (NPIP) in urine after intake of 480 mg piperazine in 4 subjects (no gastric sampling)

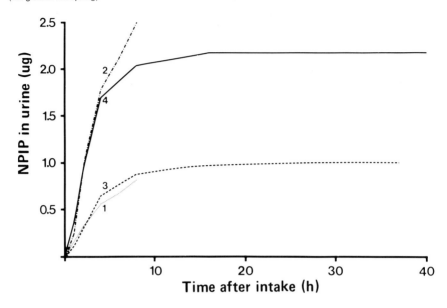

the amount excreted in the absence of ascorbic acid. In the two individuals followed until 16 h after intake (No. 1, 2), the level fell below the detection limit at 6 and 16 h, respectively.

In neither the experiments with nor without ascorbic acid was there a correlation between initial or peak pH of gastric juice and the peak NPIP level in gastric juice or the urinary NPIP excretion within 6 h.

In neither the experiments with nor without ascorbic acid was there a correlation between the peak concentration of NPIP in gastric juice and the excretion in the urine of the four individuals. Nor could the area under each gastric concentration curve be correlated with the urinary excretion. The two subjects (No. 3, 4) with urine adjusted to pH 5 did not have higher nitrosamine excretion then the other two.

DISCUSSION

The identity of NPIP was confirmed only tentatively; however, as the TEA detector exhibits extreme sensitivity and high specificity for *N*-nitrosamines (Fine & Rounbehler, 1975) and *N*-nitrosamines decompose upon ultra-violet irradiation or hydrobromic acid treatment, it is highly probable that the signal detected corresponded to NPIP. The fast work-up of the samples minimized the possibility of sampling artefacts, and the extracts were shown not to be sites of artefactual nitrosamine formation.

As the subjects were fasting, the nitrite level in saliva was probably low, even if some data indicate that a very high nitrate intake might cause elevated nitrite in saliva for as long as 21 h (Walters *et al.*, 1979). Furthermore, swallowed nitrite is rapidly consumed at the low pH obtaining at starvation. Thus, the amount of nitrite available for nitrosation in the stomach was probably small. In spite of this, considerable amounts of NPIP were formed in the stomach.

The gastric content is assumed to have been of the order of 200 mL. This crude estimate is supported by the fact that 60 mL liquid was given at the beginning of the experiments, that 110–220 mL gastric juice were sampled during the experiments (30–150 min) and that this removal did not greatly lower the excretion of PIP and NPIP. On the basis of this assumption, the maximum concentrations of NPIP correspond to total amounts of 27–47 μg (experiments without ascorbic acid). The total amount formed in the stomach may be 30–66 μg. This figure is arrived at by adding the approximate amounts already removed by sampling and subtracting the small amount (2 μg) present in the PIP syrup dose. This amount formed may be compared with the estimated daily intake of volatile N-nitrosamines from food in Sweden (0.1–1 μg; Slorach, 1981).

In urine, less than 10% of the NPIP estimated to have been formed in the stomach was excreted unchanged. The sampling of gastric juice lowered the urinary excretion only marginally. The finding that in one subject, one intake caused an enormously high excretion, is puzzling. As the value is the mean for two samples (divided after urination), artefact formation during the analytical procedure is unlikely. One possible explanation is that heavy contamination of the urine with nitrite or nitrite-forming bacteria occurred during urination. In favour of this interpretation is the fact that in this experiment (and in the similar experiment with subject No. 1), sulfamic acid was used as the nitrite trap. In all other cases, the more effective sodium sulfamate was used. Among other possible, but less likely, explanations are nitrosation in the stomach after the period studied or nitrosation elsewhere in the body during that experiment.

Acidification of the urine did not seem to affect the excretion of NPIP (pKa 6.8). This may indicate that the excretion mechanism is exclusively simple glomerular filtration.

Co-administration of ascorbic acid inhibited NPIP formation substantially. In gastric juice (calculated as above), the total amount formed was 3.0–24 μg. In urine, the excretion was 20–70% of that observed without ascorbic acid. Since nitrite reacts faster with PIP than with ascorbic acid (Mirvish, 1975), the incomplete inhibition observed with simultaneous administration is not surprising. In each experiment the results for different individuals differed considerably, but no subject had consistently lower or higher values in the different experiments. These observations clearly show that there are factors affecting the formation and excretion of NPIP which we did not control (e.g. amount of nitrite available) or of which we were unaware.

The reason that NPIP was not found in blood is most probably that the level never reached the detection limit. Assuming a blood volume of 5 L, the detection level would correspond to a momentary presence of 10 μg in the blood, which, in view of the limited excretion in urine, does not seem likely. Even if the level had reached the detection limit, masking could have withdrawn the NPIP from analysis (e.g., by conjugation).

The probable reason that no DNPIP was found in any medium is that the amount of NPIP was too low to compete successfully with the faster-reacting PIP (Mirvish, 1975) for the limited amount of nitrite. Our findings, therefore, do not rule out the possibility of DNPIP production under other circumstances; e.g., when nitrite is so high and PIP so low that most PIP is nitrosated.

The amounts of drug administered in this study were low compared with those usually employed in anthelmintic treatment. As nitrosation in the stomach seems to follow the theoretical kinetics (Ohshima & Bartsch, 1981), a preceding nitrate-rich meal should be expected to increase substantially the formation of NPIP and the risk of DNPIP formation. Although there is no conclusive evidence that NPIP is carcinogenic or that DNPIP may be formed, these possibilities are matters of concern. One way of reducing potential risk would be to formulate the drug with ascorbic acid. Exposure to preformed and/or endogenously formed NPIP (and perhaps DNPIP) due to industrial exposure to PIP should be investigated. Also, other readily-nitrosated drugs should be screened for preformed nitrosation products and endogenous formation of *N*-nitrosamines. Initial steps ought to be taken to evaluate the risk of prolonged occupational exposure to other nitrosatable amines.

ACKNOWLEDGEMENTS

We thank Åsa Amilon, Karin Annersten, Catarina Barkefors, Britt Englesson, Anita Hultberg, Christina Lilja, Ing-Marie Olsson and Bengt-Göran Svensson for valuable assistance and Professor Staffan Skerfving for critical discussion of the manuscript.

REFERENCES

Bellander, B.T.D., Hagmar, L.E. & Österdahl, B.-G. (1981) Nitrosation of piperazine in the stomach. *Lancet, ii,* 372

Bellander, B.T.D. & Österdahl, B.-G. (1983) Determination of *N*-mononitrosopiperazine and *N,N′*-dinitrosopiperazine in human urine, gastric juice and blood. *J. Chromatogr., 278,* 71–80

Braun, R., Schöneich, J. & Ziebarth, D. (1977) In-vivo formation of *N*-nitroso compounds and detection of their mutagenic acitivity in the host-mediated assay. *Cancer Res., 37,* 4572–4579

Druckrey, H., Preussmann, R., Ivankovic, S. & Schmähl, D. (1967) Organotrope carcinogene Wirkungen bei 65 verschiedenen *N*-Nitroso-Verbindungen an BD-Ratten. *Z. Krebsforsch., 69,* 103–201

Elespuru, R.K. & Lijinsky, W. (1976) Mutagenicity of cyclic nitrosamines in *Escherichia coli* following activation with rat liver microsomes. *Cancer Res., 36,* 4099–4101

Fine, D.H. & Rounbehler, D.P. (1975) Trace analysis of volatile *N*-nitroso compounds by combined gas chromatography and thermal energy analysis. *J. Chromatogr., 109,* 271–279

Garcia, H., Keefer, L., Lijinsky, W. & Wenyon, C.E.M. (1970). Carcinogenicity of nitrosothiomorpholine and l-nitrosopiperazine in rats. *Z. Krebsforsch., 74,* 179–184

Love, L.A., Lijinsky, W., Keefer, L.K. & Garcia, H. (1977) Chronic oral administration of l-nitrosopiperazine at high doses to MRC rats. *Z. Krebsforsch., 89,* 69–73

Mirvish, S.S. (1975) Formation of *N*-nitroso compounds: Chemistry, kinetics and in-vivo occurrence. *Toxicol. appl. Pharmacol., 31,* 325–351

Ohshima, H. & Bartsch, H. (1981) Quantitative estimation of endogenous nitrosation in humans by monitoring *N*-nitrosoproline excreted in urine. *Cancer Res., 41,* 3658–3662

Slorach, S.A. (1981) Dietary intake, in-vivo formation and toxicology of nitrates, nitrites and *N*-nitroso compounds. *Vår Föda, 33,* Suppl. 2, 171–184

Walters, C.L., Carr, F.P.A., Dyke, C.S., Saxby, M.J. & Smith, P.L.R. (1979) Nitrite sources and nitrosamine formation *in vitro* and *in vivo. Food cosmet. Toxicol., 17,* 473–479

IN-VIVO FORMATION OF *N*-NITROSODIMETHYLAMINE IN HUMANS AFTER AMIDOPYRINE INTAKE

B. SPIEGELHALDER & R. PREUSSMANN

*Institute of Toxicology and Chemotherapy, German Cancer Research Center,
Im Neuenheimer Feld 280, 6900 Heidelberg, FRG*

SUMMARY

Several authors have described the occurrence of *N*-nitrosodimethylamine (NDMA) in body fluids (e.g., blood and urine) and have interpreted this finding as an indication of endogenous formation of NDMA. Controlled excretion studies as well as careful control of artefacts showed, however, that, under normal conditions, NDMA formation *in vivo* cannot be monitored directly in urine due to a high metabolic conversion rate (more than 99.9%). Our own experiments showed an increased excretion rate (up to 2.4%) when ethanol was administrered simultaneously. This model was used in experiments to monitor in-vivo formation of NDMA. Amidopyrine, a compound that is easily nitrosated, was administered as a single oral dose of 500 mg to volunteers. With ingestion of 20–30 g ethanol NDMA could be detected in urine. Negative control experiments indicate that the appearance of NDMA in urine derives from in-vivo nitrosation of the drug. Between 0.5 and 10 μg NDMA were excreted within 8 h, and excretion was influenced by salivary nitrite concentrations, which ranged from 5–220 mg/L. By comparison with our earlier excretion studies in humans, it can be assumed that only 1–2% of endogenously formed *N*-nitrosamine was found in urine. To our knowledge, this is the first time that in-vivo formation of NDMA has been shown *directly* to occur in humans.

INTRODUCTION

Amidopyrine (AP) reacts with extreme ease with even low concentrations of nitrosating agent to form *N*-nitrosodimethylamine (NDMA) (Lijinsky *et al.*, 1972). It was demonstrated in animal experiments that simultaneous administration of AP and nitrite induced liver tumours in high yields, due to endogenous formation of NDMA (Lijinsky *et al.*, 1973) Since nitrite is a normal constituent of human saliva (Spiegelhalder *et al.*, 1976), in-vivo formation of NDMA in the acidic environment of stomach can be expected after oral administration of AP. In-vivo formation of NDMA from AP might be favoured by continuous excretion of AP *via* the salivary glands as long as appreciable amounts of the intact drug are present in the blood (Vesell *et al.*, 1975). Biological monitoring was proposed as a suitable tool to estimate the extent of in-vivo formation (Spiegelhalder *et al.*, 1982).

MATERIAL AND METHODS

Experimental design

Three volunteers (A,B,C) participated in this study. In all experiments a continental breakfast was taken about 1–2 h before beginning of the experiment. Urine and saliva samples were taken 1 h before, at the start of the experiment and every hour afterwards for up to 6 h. At the start (8:30 a.m.) volunteers received beverages and/or a nitrate-rich vegetable (radish, 250 g contained 200–300 mg nitrate), followed 1 h later by intake of 500 mg AP and then a beverage between 12:00 and 14:00 hours according to the following protocols:

(1) 500 mL beer; 500 mgAP; 500 mL beer
(2) 250 g radish + 500 mL beer; 500 mg AP; 500 mL beer
(3) 250 g radish + 500 mL mineral water; 500 mg AP; 500 mL mineral water
(4) 250 g radish + 500 mL beer; no AP; 500 mL beer

All volunteers followed protocols 1–4. They were allowed to take non-alcoholic drinks and a meal during the experiment but asked to avoid nitrate-rich items. Urine and saliva samples were made alkaline immediately after collection.

Nitrite-nitrate measurements

Nitrite and nitrate concentrations were determined in urine saliva and vegetable samples using a continuous flow analyser (Skalar Instruments), by standard methods (Gries colour reaction, cadmium reduction for nitrate analysis).

N-Nitrosamine measurements

NDMA concentrations in urine were determined by direct extraction with dichloromethane using Kieselguhr columns (Spiegelhalder et al., 1983) and measurement of the concentrated extracts by gas chromatography/chemoluminescence detection. The sensitivity of the method was greater than 0.1 μg/kg.

Amidopyrine measurements

Amidopyrine concentrations in saliva were determined by gas chromatography/mass spectrometry of dichloromethane extracts using the fragmentographic mode.

RESULTS AND DISCUSSION

Amidopyrine in saliva

AP was detected in the saliva of all volunteers after intake of 0.5 g; levels ranged from 3–5 μg/mL after 20 min and decreased to about 1–2 μg/mL after 6 h. The results of this study (Fig. 1) are comparable to those published previously. Vesell et al. (1975) determined its half-life in plasma to be 2.7 h and observed that plasma and saliva concentration of AP behave in a parallel fashion.

It would appear that in-vivo nitrosation occurs in two stages:
(1) Initially, a relatively large dose of AP enters the stomach. At this time, nitrosation is not favoured because the concentration of nitrite is low in relation to that of the drug and due to dilution by the stomach contents.

Fig. 1 Amidopyrine excretion in saliva of three volunteers after intake of 0.5 g

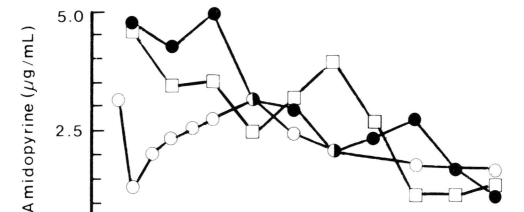

(2) After absorption and distribution in the blood of AP, it is excreted by the salvary glands over a long period (6–8 h) in µg/mL concentration. Together with nitrite, which is formed in the oral cavity from nitrate (Spiegelhalder *et al.*, 1976), the drug enters the acidic stomach in a continuous flow for several hours. The decreasing stomach content favours the nitrosation reaction. The total amount of AP secreted by salivary glands can be calculated to be 1–2 mg.

Nitrite and nitrate in saliva and urine

All urine and saliva samples were analysed for nitrite and nitrate. As expected, urine did not contain nitrite; nitrate concentrations showed wide variation, which seemed to be influenced partially by urine volume (Table 1). However, the absolute amount of nitrate excreted per hour in urine did not change greatly and could be related to the amount of nitrate ingested during the experiment.

Nitrite and nitrate levels in saliva showed individual differences and were strongly influenced by intake of dietary nitrate. In general, the results were comparable with those obtained in a more detailed study (Spiegelhalder *et al.*, 1976).

NDMA excretion in urine

All urines collected before intake of AP were free of detectable amounts of NDMA; 0.5–1 h after AP administration, NDMA appeared in urine in concentrations ranging from 0.4–1.3 µg/L after intake of ethanol. Peak concentrations were measured 1–4 h after AP intake; after intake of ethanol, the maximum NDMA concentrations were between 0.7 and 15 µg/L. Two volunteers (A and B) had higher maximum NDMA levels (see Table 1) after additional nitrate intake. With protocols resulting in high *N*-nitrosamine excretion (1 and 2) measurable levels of NDMA were still detectable 6 h after AP intake, so that some NDMA remained

Table 1.   Nitrite, nitrate and N-nitrosodimethylamine (NDMA) concentrations in urine and saliva

Volunteer	Protocol no.	max. NDMA concentration in urine (μg/L)	Concentration range of		
			Nitrite in saliva	Nitrate (mg/L)	Nitrate in urine (mg/L)
A	1	15	10–220	50–740	1–14
	2	0.7	20–32	70–210	30–110
	3	∼0.05	17–95	75–1 130	70–180
	4	ND	11–110	50–130	55–260
B	1	2.5	18–100	30–105	80–500
	2	1.6	5–7	6–20	8–17
	3	0.3	3–40	5–80	14–120
	4	Not determined			
C	1	1.8	7–30	11–50	50–470
	2	2.9	5–8	3–10	20–130
	3	0.2	3–11	13–23	15–60
	4	0.1	9–30	10–90	40–130

ND, not detected (<0.05)

undetected. The role of ethanol in increasing NDMA excretion can be seen clearly by comparing the results with protocols 1 and 3 (Table 1). This effect seems to be comparable to the increased excretion of NDMA after intake of preformed compound, as reported recently (Spiegelhalder et al., 1982). This phenomenon is probably due to a competitive inhibition of NDMA-metabolizing enzymes (Peng et al., 1982).

In the absence of AP intake, NDMA concentrations were either below or at the detection limit.

The extent of in-vivo formation of NDMA after AP intake was calculalted from the total amount of nitrosamine excreted (for the observed period) for each protocol for volunteers A, B and C: with protocol 1, the amounts were 9.3, 2.0 and 1.0 μg for each for the volunteers, respectively; with protocol 2, 0.6, 1.2 and 1.1 μg; with protocol 3, 0.2, 0.4 and 0.05 μg; and with protocol 4, none detected, not determined and 0.07 μg. These absolute amounts of NDMA excreted during the period of the experiment probably represent only a minor fraction of the total amount formed by in-vivo nitrosation. In excretion studies with preformed NDMA, an excretion rate of 0.5–2.4% was observed (Spiegelhalder et al., 1982). Thus, the total NDMA formed after AP intake might be 40 to 200 times higher than the fraction determined in urine, and the amount that might be formed in vivo after intake of 500 mg AP can be assumed to be in the order of 25–1 800 μg. These figures demonstrate the potential risk of the drug amidopyrine even under normal dietary conditions.

CONCLUSION

To our knowledge, this is the first time that in-vivo formation of NDMA had been shown to occur directly in humans. This observation could be made only by taking advantage of the fact that ethanol increases the excretion rate of NDMA. Using this ethanol method, it should be possible to monitor in-vivo formation of *N*-nitrosamines that are excreted at low rates. An increase in *N*-nitrosamine concentration after ethanol intake can therefore be interpreted as an indication of endogenous formation, as long as no exogenous factor has to be considered.

On the assumption that excretion rates of preformed NDMA and endogenously formed NDMA are comparable and are of the same order of magnitude, the total amount formed *in vivo* can be calculated. Exposure to NDMA after intake of 500 mg amidopyrine could be as high as 25–1 800 µg, which represents a considerable risk. Since amidopyrine is still available in some countries, the recommendation is made that its use be universally avoided.

ACKNOWLEDGEMENTS

We are grateful to Dr Scherf and Dipl.-Chem. Schreiber for their valuable contributions to this study.

REFERENCES

Linjinsky, W., Conrad, E. & van de Bogart, R. (1972) Carcinogenic nitroamines formed by drug nitrite interactions. *Nature, 239*, 165–167

Lijinsky, W., Taylor, H.W., Snyder, C. & Nettesheim, P. (1973) Malignant tumors of liver and lung in rats fed aminopyrine or heptamethyleneimine together with nitrite. *Nature, 244*, 176–178

Peng, R., Yong Tu, Y. & Yang, C.S. (1982) The induction and competitive inhibition of a high affinity microsomal nitrosodimethylamine demethylase by ethanol. *Carcinogenesis, 3*, 1457–1461

Spiegelhalder, B., Eisenbrand, G. & Preussmann, R. (1976) Influence of dietary nitrate on nitrite content of human saliva: Possible relevance to in-vivo formation of *N*-nitroso compounds. *Food Cosmet. Toxicol., 14*, 545–548

Spiegelhalder, B., Eisenbrand, G. & Preussmann, R. (1982) *Urinary excretion of N-nitrosamines in rats and humans.* In: Bartsch, H., O'Neill, I.K., Castegnaro, M. & Okada, M., eds, *N-Nitroso Compounds: Occurrence and Biological Effects (IARC Scientific Publications No. 41)*, Lyon, International Agency for Research on Cancer, pp. 443–449

Spiegelhalder B., Eisenbrand, G. & Preussmann, R. (1983) *Volatile N-nitrosamines in beer and other beverages by direct extraction using a kieselguhr column.* In: Preussmann, R., O'Neill, I.K., Eisenbrand, G., Spiegelhalder, B. & Bartsch, H., eds, *Environmental Carcinogens. Selected Methods of Analysis,* Vol, 6, *N-Nitroso Compounds. (IARC Scientific Publications No. 45)*, Lyon, International Agency for Research on Cancer, pp. 135–142

Vesell, E.S., Passananti, G.T., Glenwright, P.A. & Dvorchik, B.H. (1975) Studies on the disposition of antipyrine, aminopyrine, and phenacetin using plasma, saliva, and urine. *Clin. Pharmacol. Ther., 18*, 259

A SENSITIVE NEW METHOD FOR THE DETECTION OF
N-NITROSOMORPHOLINE FORMATION *IN VIVO*

J.B. MORRISON & S.S. HECHT

Naylor Dana Institute for Disease Prevention, American Health Foundation,
Valhalla, NY, USA

SUMMARY

A sensitive method was developed for quantitation of N-nitrosomorpholine (NMOR) formation *in vivo* in rats. A major metabolite of NMOR, N-nitroso(2-hydroxyethyl)glycine, was detected by gas chromatography-thermal energy analysis in the urine of rats treated with trace levels of NMOR or treated sequentially with morpholine and sodium nitrite. Since significant levels of 2-hydroxyethylglycine do not seem to occur in rat urine, even after treatment with morpholine, artefact formation was not a problem. Formation of 1 μg NMOR *in vivo* was readily detected. The formation of NMOR from morpholine and sodium nitrite *in vivo* in rats appeared to depend on the doses of morpholine and [sodium nitrite]^2 and occurred in higher yield than reported for formation of N-nitrosoproline, as expected. The formation of NMOR from morpholine and sodium nitrite under the conditions of the carcinogenicity study of Shank and Newberne was quantified. The daily levels of NMOR formation were highly variable, but the mean level was consistent with the tumorigenicity data in that dose-response study.

INTRODUCTION

Treatment of experimental animals with morpholine and sodium nitrite results in formation of N-nitrosomorpholine (NMOR) *in vivo* (Shank & Newberne, 1976). NMOR is also formed upon exposure of mice to morpholine and nitrogen oxides (Iqbal *et al.*, 1980; Mirvish *et al.*, 1983; Van Stee *et al.*, 1983). Humans are exposed to morpholine or its derivatives upon consumption of certain foods and drugs, through use of tobacco, and in the manufacture and use of rubber products. NMOR could therefore be formed *in vivo* in man. This paper describes a sensitive method for assessing in-vivo formation of NMOR based on quantitation of a major urinary metabolite of NMOR, N-nitroso(2-hydroxyethyl)glycine (NHEG; Fig. 1) (Hecht & Young, 1981).

Fig. 1. Metabolic formation of *N*-nitroso(2-hydroxyethyl)glycine from *N*-nitrosomorpholine

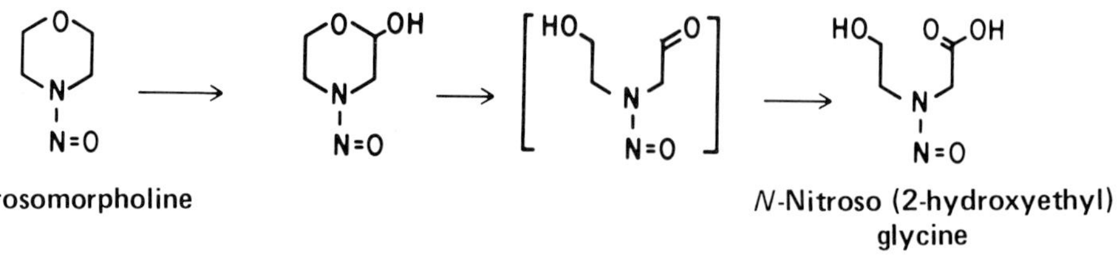

N-Nitrosomorpholine   *N*-Nitroso (2-hydroxyethyl)
                                                                      glycine

MATERIALS AND METHODS

Chemicals

NHEG was synthesized as follows: Iodoacetic acid (3 g, 16 mmol, Aldrich Chemical Co., Milwaukee, WI, USA) was added to an ice-cold, rapidly stirred solution of 2-aminoethanol (8.3 g, 136 mmol, MCB Manufacturing Chemists, Inc, Gibbstown, NJ, USA) in 8 mL distilled water. After the mixture had stood at room temperature for 20 h, water was removed by rotary evaporation. Absolute ethanol (8 mL) was added to the residue, and the resulting mixture was added slowly to 102 mL acetone : ethanol (94 : 8). A white precipitate was formed which was separated by filtration. A portion (0.5 g) of this precipitate was converted to the nitrosamine by the method used for *N*-nitroso-4-hydroxy-L-proline, as described by Lijinsky *et al.* (1970). NHEG was isolated as white crystals melting at 76–77 °C (m.p. 78.5–79.5 °C; Stewart, 1962).

[14]C-NHEG was synthesized as follows: A solution of [1-^{14}C]-iodoacetic acid (0.80 mg; 5.4 µmol; specific activity, 11.1 mCi/mmol; New England Nuclear, Boston, MA, USA) and 2-aminoethanol (2.8 mg, 46 µmol) in 100 µL distilled water in a 1-mL Reactivial (Pierce Chemical Co., Rockford, IL, USA) was allowed to stand at room temperature for 20 h. The solution was then basified to pH 11 by addition of 10 µL 1N sodium hydroxide and washed five times with 100-µL portions of ether. The remaining aqueous phase was acidified to pH 1 with 80 µL 1N hydrochloric acid and nitrosated by addition of sodium nitrite (795 µg, 11.5 µmol in 150 µL distilled water) and sonication for 2 h. After lyophilization to remove water, the residue was applied in acetone to a 5 × 20 cm silica gel thin-layer chromatography plate and developed with chloroform : methanol (1 : 1). The band at the R_f of standard NHEG was isolated by extraction with methanol to yield 10.6 µCi ^{14}C-NHEG (21% from iodoacetic acid) with a radiochemical purity greater than 99%, as demonstrated by radiochromatography (silica gel, chloroform : methanol, 2 : 3).

Analysis of NHEG in rat-urine

The 24-h rat urine was thawed, spiked with ^{14}C-NHEG (1.27×10^4 dpm, 170 ng), acidified by addition of 1 mL of a solution of 20% ammonium sulfamate in 3.6 N sulfuric acid, saturated with sodium chloride, and extracted six times with equal volumes of ethyl acetate. The combined ethyl acetate layers were dried (magnesium sulfate) and evaporated to dryness by rotary evaporation in a pear-shaped flask with a polished glass joint. Acetonitrile (1 mL, Sequanal grade, Pierce Chemical Co., Rockford, IL, USA) and 8 mL ether saturated with diazomethane were added. After the flask had been stoppered and allowed to stand at room temperature for 15 min, the solvent was removed under a stream of nitrogen. The residue was redissolved in 2 mL distilled water and passed through a Sep-Pak C_{18} cartridge (Waters Associates, Milford, MA, USA). The eluant was then extracted twice with 3 mL and thrice with

2 mL ethyl acetate. The pooled organic layers were dried (sodium sulfate) and evaporated to dryness by rotary evaporation. The residue was dissolved in 350 µL Regisil RC-2 (Regis Chemical Co., Morton Grove, IL, USA) and acetonitrile (silylation grade, Pierce), transferred to a 1-mL volumetric flask and immersed in a sonic cleaner for 10 min. Aliquots of this solution were analysed by gas chromatography with detection by a Thermal Energy Analyzer (GC-TEA), using a 3.7 m × 2 mm i.d. glass column packed with 3% OV-225 on Chromosorb W HP, 80/100 mesh (Analabs, Inc., New Haven, CT, USA), an oven temperature of 165 °C, an injection port temperature of 210 °C and argon as carrier gas with inlet pressure adjusted to 40 psi (276 kPa). Recoveries were determined with liquid scintillation counting by adding 1 mL distilled water and 10 mL Ready-Solv MP Cocktail (Beckman Instruments, Inc., Fullerton, CA, USA) to a 50-µL aliquot of this solution.

RESULTS

The methyl ester-trimethylsilyl ether derivative of NHEG was readily analysed by GC-TEA, the detection limit under the conditions used in this study being approximately 800 pg per injection. In order to test the reproducibility of the method for analysis of NHEG in rat urine, NHEG and ^{14}C-NHEG were added to four 10-mL samples of urine and analysed. The recovery of internal standard was 39 ± 5%, which was typical of all analyses carried out in this study. The average standard deviation of the analytical procedure for NHEG in rat urine was 9.1% of the mean. The detection limit was approximately 350 ng per 24-h urine sample.

Formation of NHEG from NMOR in Fischer 344 rats was then investigated. In preliminary experiments, we established that ≃ 95% of the NHEG was excreted within 24 h after treatment with NMOR. NMOR was administered in saline by intragastric gavage at various doses, as summarized in Table 1. The mean conversion of NMOR to urinary NHEG was 52% (range, 42–60%). Less than 10% of a dose of 3 µg N-nitrosodiethanolamine (NDELA) was converted to urinary NHEG by F344 rats.

The usefulness of the method as a monitor for in-vivo formation of NMOR was investigated by sequential administration by intragastric gavage to F344 rats of various levels of morpholine

Table 1. Formation of N-nitroso(2-hydroxyethyl)glycine (NHEG) from N-nitrosomorpholine (NMOR) in F344 rats[a]

Dose of NMOR		Number of rats	Urinary NHEG[b]		% Conversion of NMOR to NHEG
(µg)	(µmol)		(µg)	(µmol)	
50	0.43	3	26.1 ± 1.4	0.18 ± 0.01	42
10	0.086	3	7.2 ± 2.2	0.048 ± 0.014	56
5	0.043	3	3.1 ± 0.5	0.021 ± 0.003	49
1	0.0086	6	0.79 ± 0.12[c]	0.0052 ± 0.0008	60
0	0	2	<0.17	<0.0012	–
					mean ± SD, 52 ± 8

[a] NMOR in 0.8 mL saline was administered to F344 rats by intragastric gavage and the 24-h urine collected at −76 °C and analysed for NHEG
[b] Mean recovery of internal standard ^{14}C-NHEG, 34.7 ± 6.5%, n = 17
[c] A background peak corresponding to 0.17 µg was subtracted

Table 2. Detection of *N*-nitroso(2-hydroxyethyl)glycine (NHEG) in F344 rat urine after administration of morpholine and sodium nitrite[a]

Dose (µmol)		Urinary NHEG[b] (µmol)	Estimated percentage of morpho-line nitro-sated[c]
Morpholine	Sodium nitrite		
38.3	0	0.0016 ±0.0017	–
0	191	0.010 ±0.0024	–
38.3	191	1.01 ±0.91	5 ±5
19.2	95.7	1.20 ±0.34	12 ±3
3.83	19.1	0.072 ±0.025	4 ±1
1.92	9.6	0.0046[d]±0.003	0.5±0.3
0.92	4.8	0.0028[d]±0.0026	0.6±0.5

[a] Groups of F344 rats were treated by intragastric gavage with morpholine in 0.8 mL saline followed by sodium nitrite in 0.8 mL saline; 24-h urine collected at −76°C and analysed for NHEG
[b] Mean recovery of internal standard ^{14}C-NHEG, 33±6%, n=21
[c] µmol NMOR was estimated by dividing µmol NHEG by 0.52
[d] A background peak corresponding to 0.0012 µmol was subtracted

and a five-fold excess of sodium nitrite, as summarized in Table 2. When either 38.3 µmol morpholine or 191 µmol sodium nitrite were administered alone, a peak corresponding in retention time to that of NHEG was observed, but its magnitude was less than 1% of that obtained upon administration of the same amounts of both morpholine and nitrite. NHEG was detected each time that morpholine and nitrite were administered together. The lowest level tested, in which 0.0028 µmol (0.4 µg) NHEG was detected, is close to the detection limit of the method, as applied to rat urine. In each case, mol of NMOR formed was estimated by dividing mol of urinary NHEG by 0.52. A typical GC-TEA trace of NHEG in the urine of a rat treated with morpholine and sodium nitrite is illustrated in Figure 2.

It was possible that significant quantities of NHEG could have been formed in these experiments by nitrosation *in vivo* or during the analysis of 2-hydroxyethylglycine resulting from metabolic 2-hydroxylation of morpholine. In order to test this possibility, rats were treated with 38.3 µmol morpholine, and the 24-h urine was incubated with 14.5 mmol sodium nitrite at 37 °C for 0.5 h. The amount of NHEG detected (0.013 µmol) was less than 2% of the amount detected when 38.3 µmol morpholine and 191 µmol sodium nitrite were administered to rats. Thus, the artefactual formation under our conditions of significant amounts of NHEG can be excluded.

In-vivo formation of NMOR was further studied by intragastric intubation of various doses of morpholine and constant sodium nitrite or various doses of sodium nitrite and constant morpholine. A plot of NMOR formed as a function of dose of morpholine x [sodium nitrite]^2 is illustrated in Figure 3.

Daily formation of NMOR under the conditions of the carcinogenicity study reported by Shank and Newberne (1976) was estimated by adding 1000 mg/kg sodium nitrite and 50 mg/kg morpholine to the diet, as described. Excretion of NHEG was measured daily for each of five rats over a six-day period (Fig. 4). The mean level of NMOR formed per day was estimated to be 0.88 ± 0.59 µmol/rat.

Fig. 2. Typical gas chromatographic-Thermal Energy Analyzer (TEA) trace of N-nitroso(2-hydroxyethyl)glycine in the urine of a rat treated with morpholine and sodium nitrite. The peak corresponds to in-vivo formation of 8 μg N-nitrosomorpholine

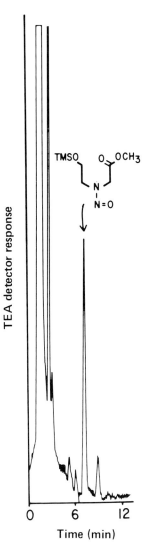

DISCUSSION

The method described in this paper involves use of NHEG, a stable metabolite of NMOR, as a monitor for in-vivo formation of NMOR. The use of NHEG is advantageous because it represents approximately 50% of the dose of NMOR, whereas, after low doses, less than 0.2% of NMOR is excreted unchanged in the urine (Spiegelhalder et al., 1982). NHEG can be

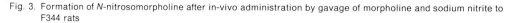

Fig. 3. Formation of N-nitrosomorpholine after in-vivo administration by gavage of morpholine and sodium nitrite to F344 rats

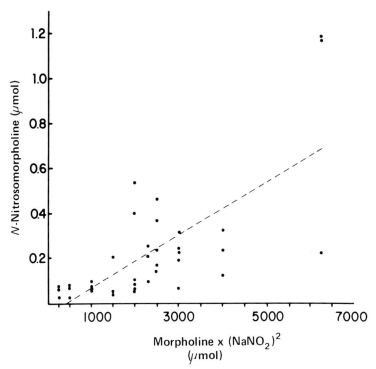

detected with excellent sensitivity by combined GC-TEA, and artefact formation seems to be minimal under our conditions. Thus, the detection of in-vivo formation of, or exposure to, as little as 0.6 µg NMOR is feasible in rats.

Only limited data are available on the levels of NMOR formed in the rat stomach after administration of morpholine and sodium nitrite. Mirvish *et al.* (1981) reported the formation of approximately 0.4 ± 0.05 µmol NMOR per gram of tissue in the rat stomach 2 h after administration of 116 µmol each of morpholine and sodium nitrite. These results seem similar to those reported here, although comparisons are difficult because the extent of metabolism of NMOR in the previous study is not known. In the present study, conversion of morpholine to NMOR ranged from 0.5–12%, depending on the dose of precursors administered by intragastric gavage. Although a large variability in NMOR formation from morpholine and nitrite was see, the levels of NMOR formed were generally in agreement with those expected on the basis of in-vitro studies in which dependence on [amine] x [nitrite]^2 has been established (Mirvish, 1975). The variability in NMOR formation greatly exceeded that observed in NMOR metabolism and was not markedly decreased by the use of buffered solutions and overnight fasting in the intragastric gavage experiments, as reported in studies on N-nitrosoproline formation (Ohshima *et al.*, 1982). Extensive variation in the in-vivo formation of N-nitrosamines has been observed in previous studies and is an indication of the complexity of the in-vivo situation (Sander *et al.*, 1974). Factors such as differing rates of decomposition of nitrous acid and stomach emptying, local variations in stomach pH and local catalysis in

Fig. 4. Daily formation of NMOR in rats fed a diet containing 50 mg/kg morpholine and 1 000 mg/kg sodium nitrite, as in the experiments of Shank and Newberne (1976); different symbols represent different animals

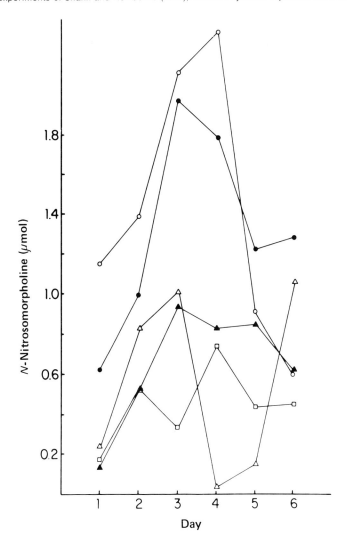

the stomach could contribute (Mirvish *et al.*, 1975). It will be important to identify those factors that can increase or decrease *N*-nitrosamine formation in individual rats.

The data illustrated in Figure 3 were obtained under conditions closely similar to those used in a study by Ohshima *et al.* (1982) on the in-vivo formation of *N*-nitrosoproline in rats. Comparison of the slope of the line in Figure 3 with that of the line obtained by plotting the data of Ohshima *et al.* indicates that the extent of nitrosation of morpholine *in vivo* is approximately 16 times as great as the extent of nitrosation of proline *in vivo*. The pH-dependent rate constant for nitrosation of morpholine *in vitro* has been reported to be 11 times as great as that for proline (Mirvish, 1975). The relatively good agreement between the data obtained *in vivo* and *in vitro* for nitrosation of morpholine and proline supports the use of *N*-nitrosoproline formation as a monitor for *N*-nitrosamine formation in man.

The results of the experiment in which we simulated the study of Shank and Newberne (1976) are consistent with their data. In their experiment, 58% of the rats treated with 5 mg/kg NMOR had liver-cell carcinomas, and 59% of rats treated with 1 000 mg/kg sodium nitrite and 50 mg/kg morpholine had liver-cell carcinomas. On the basis of a consumption of 41 g of diet per day, the daily dose of NMOR in the group treated with 5 mg/kg NMOR was 1.77 µmol. Our mean value for daily NMOR formation was 0.88 µmol/rat. Thus, the data on tumour induction and the daily doses of NMOR in the two groups agree quite closely. These data provide the first quantitative assessment of NMOR formation relating to tumour induction by morpholine and sodium nitrite.

ACKNOWLEDGEMENTS

This study was supported by US National Cancer Institute Grant CA 23 901.

REFERENCES

Hecht, S.S. & Young, R. (1981) Metabolic α-hydroxylation of *N*-nitrosomorpholine and 3,3,5,5-tetradeutero-*N*-nitrosomorpholine in the F344 rat. *Cancer Res., 41*, 5039–5043

Iqbal, Z.M., Dahl, K. & Epstein, S.S. (1980) Role of nitrogen dioxide in the biosynthesis of nitrosamines in mice. *Science, 207*, 1475–1477

Lijinsky, W., Keefer, L.K. & Loo, J. (1970) The preparation and properties of some nitrosamino acids. *Tetrahedron, 26*, 5137–5153

Mirvish, S.S. (1975) Formation of *N*-nitroso compounds: kinetics and *in vivo* occurrence. *Toxicol. appl. Pharmacol., 31*, 325–351

Mirvish, S.S., Patil, K., Ghadirian, P. & Kommineni, V.R.C. (1975) Disappearance of nitrite from the rat stomach: contribution of emptying and other factors. *J. natl Cancer Inst., 54*, 869–875

Mirvish, S.S., Issenberg, P. & Sams, J.P. (1981) N-*Nitrosomorpholine synthesis in rodents exposed to nitrogen dioxide and morpholine.* In: Scanlan, R.A. & Tannenbaum, S.R., eds, N-*Nitroso Compounds* (ACS Symposium Series 174), Washington DC, American Chemical Society, pp. 181–191

Mirvish, S.S., Sams, J.P. & Issenberg, P. (1983) The nitrosating agent in mice exposed to nitrogen dioxide: improved extraction method and localization in the skin. *Cancer Res., 43*, 2550–2554

Ohshima, H., Béréziat, J.-C. & Bartsch, H. (1982) Monitoring *N*-nitrosamino acids excreted in the urine and feces of rats as an index for endogenous nitrosation. *Carcinogenesis, 3*, 115–120

Sander, J., LaBar, J., Ladenstein, M. & Schweinsberg, F. (1974) *Quantitative measurement of* in vivo *nitrosamine formation.* In: Bogovski, P. & Walker, E.A., eds, N-*Nitroso Compounds in the Environment (IARC Scientific Publications No. 9)*, Lyon, International Agency for Research on Cancer, pp. 123–131

Shank, R.C. & Newberne, P.M. (1976) Dose-response study of the carcinogenicity of dietary sodium nitrite and morpholine in rats and hamsters. *Food Cosmet. Toxicol., 14*, 1–8

Spiegelhalder, B., Eisenbrand, G. & Preussmann, R. (1982) *Urinary excretion of* N-*nitrosamines in rats and humans.* In: Bartsch, H., O'Neill, I.K., Castegnaro, M. & Okada, M., eds, N-*Nitroso Compounds: Occurrence and Biological Effects (IARC Scientific Publications No. 41)*, Lyon, International Agency for Research on Cancer, pp. 443–449

Stewart, F.H.C. (1962) The preparation of some *N*-alkylsydnones containing a functional group in the side chain. *J. org. Chem., 27*, 687–689

Van Stee, E.W., Sloane, R.A., Simmons, J.E. & Brunnemann, K.D. (1983) *In vivo* formation of *N*-nitrosomorpholine in CD-1 mice exposed by inhalation to nitrogen dioxide and by gavage to morpholine. *J. natl Cancer Inst., 70*, 375–379

N-NITROSOPROLINE IN URINE FROM PATIENTS AND HEALTHY VOLUNTEERS AFTER ADMINISTRATION OF LARGE AMOUNTS OF NITRATE

G. ELLEN & P.L. SCHULLER

National Institute of Public Health, Bilthoven, The Netherlands

SUMMARY

Urines from 12 healthy volunteers, sampled from 0–24 h after the volunteers had been administered 9.5 g sodium nitrate intravenously or up to 10.5 g ammonium nitrate orally, were analysed for *N*-nitrosoproline (NPRO). The mean NPRO content in urines voided just before administration of nitrate was 4.1 µg/L. Mean NPRO levels remained low until 6 h after nitrate intake. Mean NPRO contents in urines voided 6–8 h, 8–10 h, 10–15 h and 15–24 h after nitrate administration were 10, 40, 74 and 53 µg/L. respectively. The highest NPRO content found was 320 µg/L. These findings demonstrate that intake of one large dose of nitrate leads to enhanced nitrosation in the body, which lasts at least one day. Surprisingly, in urine from 21 patients who had been ingesting 2.5–9 g ammonium nitrate daily for several months to prevent the redevelopment of calcium phosphate renal stones, only slightly enhanced NPRO levels were found: < 1–32 µg/L; mean value, 6.2 µg/L. In most of the urines, from the healthy volunteers as well as from the patients, *N*-nitrosothiazolidine-4-carboxylic acid was also detected. Results from the volunteers indicated that urinary excretion of this compound also increases several hours after intake of one large dose of nitrate.

INTRODUCTION

We reported recently our investigations on volatile *N*-nitrosamines in urine and saliva of healthy volunteers after administration of one large dose of nitrate (Ellen *et al.*, 1982a) and on volatile *N*-nitrosamines in blood and urine of patients who had ingested gram amounts of nitrate daily for longer periods of time (Ellen *et al.*, 1982b). It was found that if volatile *N*-nitrosamines are present in human urine and blood at all, it is only in trace amounts, mostly less than 0.1 µg/kg. No evidence was obtained that administration of large doses of nitrate had any influence on the levels of volatile *N*-nitrosamines in human blood and urine. It was realized, however, that those formed by nitrosation *in vivo*, for instance in the stomach, might be metabolized quickly at other sites in the body and thus escape detection on analysis of blood and urine. Ohshima and Bartsch (1981) and Ohshima *et al.* (1982) obtained evidence that monitoring of *N*-nitrosoproline (NPRO) in urine might give useful information about the extent of *in vivo* nitrosation. In order to obtain additional information about the influence of very high intakes of nitrate on in-vivo nitrosation, we determined NPRO contents in the urine samples that were still available from our two studies described above.

MATERIALS AND METHODS

Samples

From our study with healthy volunteers (Ellen *et al.*, 1982a), 53 urine samples from 12 volunteers were still available; from the study with patients (Ellen *et al.*, 1982b), 21 of the 23 urine samples were available for analysis. All urines had been stored at -10°C since the moment of sampling. Details of the identity of the samples are given in Tables 1 and 2.

Analytical method

Urine samples were analysed for NPRO by the method described by Ohshima and Bartsch (1981). Because our samples contained high levels of nitrate, some modification was necessary to overcome large interfering solvent peaks during analysis of the extracts by gas chromatography with a Thermal Energy Analyzer TM (GC-TEA) detector. In brief, the analytical procedure was as follows: to 15 mL urine 5 g sodium chloride and 1.5 mL of a 200g/L solution of ammonium sulfamate in 1.8 mol/L sulfuric acid were added, and this mixture was extracted three times with 25 mL ethyl acetate. The combined ethyl acetate extracts were dried on anhydrous sodium sulfate and evaporated to dryness under reduced pressure with a rotary evaporator. Two mL diethyl ether were added to the residue and, after swirling, the ether was transferred into a small glass tube; this operation was repeated twice with 1 mL ether. The combined ether extracts were purged by a stream of nitrogen, which had passed through an

Table 1. Contents of *N*-nitrosoproline (NPRO) in urine from 12 healthy volunteers after intravenous administration of 9.5 g sodium nitrate (Nos 1–12) or oral administration of 0.15 g/kg body weight of ammonium nitrate (Nos 13–24)

Volunteer No.[a]	Total amount of NH₄NO₃ taken (g)	NPRO content (µg/L) in urine collected during various periods after administration of nitrate							
		Blank[b]	0–2 h	2–4 h	4–6 h	6–8 h	8–10 h	10–15 h	15–24 h
1		–[c]	1.3	2.5	3.6	6.2	–	31	–
2		2.5	<1	–	<1	8.1	16	–	–
8		–	–	–	–	–	–	60	–
12		3.2	–	<1	3.9	12	20	28	36
13	9.5	–	1.0	1.8	3.8	–	22	–	–
14	8.0	6.1	1.2	1.9	<1	–	–	–	–
15	10.5	2.6	–	–	3.1	–	28	–	–
16	10.5	6.2	–	–	–	–	–	–	–
18	8.5	–	–	–	–	3.5	–	5.8	4.4
22	10.5	–	<1	2.8	2.0	3.7	18	19	8
23	7.0	–	<1	2.4	15	16	39	54	152
24	8.0	–	<1	5.0	3.0	24	140	320	–
Mean content		4.1	1.1	2.5	4.0	10	40	74	53

[a] Numbers of the volunteers are those given in Ellen *et al.* (1982a)
[b] Sample taken just before administration of nitrate
[c] –, sample no longer available for analysis

Table 2. N-Nitrosoproline (NPRO) in urine from patients ingesting large amounts of nitrate daily for long periods of time

Patient No.[a]	Amount of NH_4NO_3 taken daily (g)	Time (h) between intake of last portion of NH_4NO_3 and urine sampling	NPRO (µg/L)
1	2×3	2	2.0
2	2×1.5	4	3.4
3	2×3	14	5.8
4	3×2	2.5	7.8
5	3×2.25	5	2.8
6	3×3	22	3.6
7	2×1.5	17	1.8
8	2×2.25	19	6.7
10	3×1.5	5	2.9
11	2×1.5	13	2.1
12	2×3	4.5	6.3
13	2×4.5	4	32
14	2×3	19	12
15	2×2.25	24	2.3
16	1×6	16	<1
17	3×2.25	2.5	15
18	3×1.5	3	2.5
19	2×3	3	4.4
21	1×2.5	13	11
22	3×1.5	3	3.5
23	1×3	12	<1
		Mean	6.2

[a] Numbers of the patients are those given in Ellen *et al.* (1982b)

ethereal solution of diazomethane, until the extract became pale yellow. The solvent was evaporated with a stream of nitrogen and the residue was redissolved in 50 µL methanol; 5 µL of this methanolic extract were injected into the GC-TEA system. GC was performed on a 2.5 m × 3.2 mm o.d. nickel column, filled with 10% Carbowax 20M on Chromosorb WHP 80–100 mesh, at a temperature of 170°C and a nitrogen flow rate of 20 mL per minute.

Prior to analysis, all urine samples were spiked with N-nitrosopipecolic acid as an internal standard at a level of 10 µg/L. Contents of NPRO in urine were calculated by comparison of peak heights on the chromatograms of sample extracts with the peak height for an external standard. Results were corrected for recovery of the internal standard.

NPRO and N-nitrosopipecolic acid were synthesized according to the method of Lijinsky *et al.* (1970) and were converted to their methyl esters with diazomethane. The identity and purity of the two N-nitrosamino acids were checked by ^{1}H-nuclear magnetic resonance (NMR) and mass spectrometry (MS). The two methyl esters were analysed for identity and purity by ^{1}H-NMR, GC-MS, GC-TEA and GC with flame-ionization detection.

RESULTS AND DISCUSSION

NPRO in urine from healthy volunteers

The overall results for levels of NPRO in the 53 samples of urine from the volunteers are presented in Table 1. Twenty of these samples were also analysed by Mr H. Ohshima, IARC, Lyon, and the NPRO contents he found were in good agreement with our results. The data in Table 1 show clearly that up to six hours after administration of nitrate, the excretion of NPRO in urine remains low and fairly constant, but shows a sharp increase after that time. The highest NPRO contents were found in urine voided 10–15 h after administration of nitrate.

The relation between excretion of NPRO and time is even more clearly demonstrated in Figure 1, where mean NPRO contents in urine from the 12 volunteers are plotted against time after nitrate administration. Assuming that the NPRO in urine is due to endogenous formation from nitrite and other suitable precursors (e.g., proline), the path in Figure 1 can be well explained: nitrate administered orally or intravenously recirculates in part *via* the salivary glands, and part of the salivary nitrate is reduced to nitrite in the oral cavity; after swallowing, this leads to an increased nitrite burden in the stomach. In the stomach, nitrite may react with other substances to yield NPRO. After NPRO has been formed in the stomach, it is excreted *via* the urinary tract one to several hours later.

In our earlier study (Ellen *et al.*, 1982a), we found the highest nitrate and nitrite contents in saliva from 2–6 h after nitrate administration. This agrees well with the occurence of maximum NPRO contents in urine some hours later. The finding that the blank urine samples showed higher NPRO levels than urines voided up to 6 h after nitrate administration may be explained by the fact that, for most of the volunteers, the blank sample was the early morning urine, which is usually more concentrated than urine voided later in the day. Ohshima *et al.* (1982) found an average of 2.3 µg NPRO, corresponding to 1–1.5 µg/L in 24-h urines of a subject on a low-nitrate diet. Bearing in mind that the volunteers in our study ate diets of their own choice, the levels of NPRO we found after 0–6 h after nitrate administration conform well with those of Ohshima *et al.* (1982).

Fig. 1. Mean *N*-nitrosoproline (NPRO) content (µg/L) in urine from 12 volunteers collected during various periods after administration of nitrate

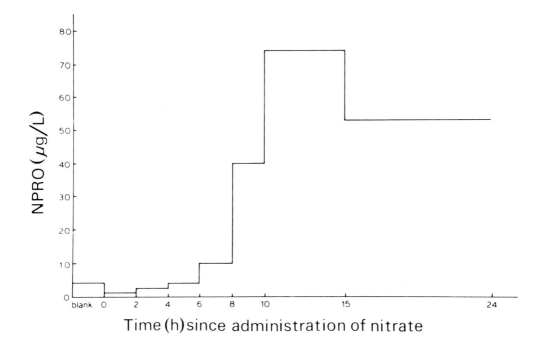

Our results lead us to conclude that administration of a single large dose of nitrate leads to an enhanced nitrosating potency in the body, which lasts longer than 24 h. As the subjects in our study consumed a free-choice diet, the results show that a normal western diet contains enough precursors of NPRO to elicit this nitrosating effect.

NPRO in urine from patients

In Table 2, the results are summarized for the 21 patients who were ingesting large amounts of ammonium nitrate daily for some months. Comparison of the data in Table 2 with those in Table 1 shows that 13 of the 21 patients had NPRO contents from < 1–5 µg/L, which is roughly the same range as found in samples from the volunteers up to 6 h after nitrate administration. Of the remaining eight patients, four had NPRO contents between 5 and 10 µg/L and the other four had 11–32 µg/L.

Apart from the value of 32 µg/L, these contents are much lower than might be expected in view of the results obtained with the volunteers (Table 1). For the moment we have no conclusive explanation for this difference. Since all the urine samples from the patients were voided between 10:00 and 14:00 hours, the NPRO contents might have been lowered, since NPRO formed from precursors in the supper had probably been excreted in the early morning urine. To obtain more information about whether regular high nitrate intakes lead to enhanced endogenous formation of NPRO, 24-h urines from patients maintained on ammonium nitrate will be analysed and the results compared with those obtained for 24-h urines from persons on a normal diet.

N-*Nitrosothiazolidine-4-carboxylic acid in urine*

In most of the chromatograms of the urine extracts, a peak other than NPRO was present, belonging to an unknown TEA-responsive compound. The retention time of this compound was 1.9 relative to N-nitrosopipecolic acid methyl ester. The unknown peak was not observed in urine extracts that had not been treated with diazomethane, and it disappeared after ultra-violet irradiation of extracts containing it. These observations suggested that the unknown was a N-nitrosamino acid. Ohshima *et al.* (1983) identified N-nitrosothiazolidine 4-carboxylic acid (NTCA) in urine, and comparison of their chromatograms with ours indicated that our unknown was probably also NTCA. Synthesis of NTCA from thiazolidine-4-carboxylic acid by the procedure of Lijinsky *et al.* (1970) and conversion of the product into its methyl ester gave a compound the ^{1}H-NMR, infra-red and MS spectra of which were in accordance with the expected structure of NTCA-methyl ester (NTCA-Me). The mass spectrum of NTCA-Me was identical with that published by Ohshima *et al.* (1983). The unknown compound in the urine extracts had the same retention time as NTCA-Me on GC-TEA analysis, and in two different urine extracts the presence of NTCA-Me was confirmed with GC-MS.

GC analysis of solutions and extracts containing NTCA-Me was sometimes problematical, due to decomposition of this compound: on a glass column filled with 10% Carbowax 20M on Chromosorb WHP 80–100 mesh, no decomposition was observed; on nickel and stainless-steel columns filled with 10% Carbowax 20M on Chromosorb WAW 80–100 mesh, severe decomposition of NTCA-Me occured; after we tried to inactivate the column by injecting 10–20 µL of a 10% solution of dimethyldichlorosilane in toluene, even more decomposition was observed, and sometimes no peak at all was seen on the chromatogram. When Chromosorb WHP was used instead of Chromosorb WAW in the nickel and stainless-steel columns, the decomposition of NTCA-Me was strongly reduced. Thus, the presence of NTCA in urine extracts might be missed using improper chromatographic conditions.

At the time we analysed the urine extracts for NPRO, the NTCA contents could not be established, since the identity of this compound was then still unknown. Scrutiny of the chromatograms later on revealed that the NTCA content of most of the urines containing it was probably less than 10 μg/L; however, it should be borne in mind that, under the chromatographic conditions used, partial decomposition of NTCA-Me may have taken place. In urines from two of the volunteers (Nos 2 and 13 in Table 1), who are identical twins, much higher levels of NTCA were present – up to more than 100 μg/L. These high levels were found only in urines voided more than 6 h after administration of nitrate, which suggests that NTCA may originate from endogenous formation enhanced by high nitrate intakes. The observation of Ohshima *et al.* (1983) that consumption of a diet supplemented with ascorbic acid – a known inhibitor of nitrosation – reduces urinary excretion of NTCA also indicates endogenous formation.

ACKNOWLEDGEMENTS

This work was carried out on behalf of the Chief Officer of Public Health (Foodstuffs) and the Chief Medical Officer, The Netherlands. We are indebted to Mr H. Ohshima for analysing 20 urine samples for NPRO and for information prior to publication about the identity of the unknown compound in urine. We wish to thank Miss E. Egmond for technical assistance with the experiments and Dr J. Freudenthal for carrying out the mass spectrometric measurements. The cooperation in this study of Dr E. Bruijns and Dr P.G.A.M. Froeling from the St Radboud University Hospital in Nijmegen is gratefully acknowledged.

REFERENCES

Ellen, G., Schuller, P.L., Bruijns, E., Froeling, P.G.A.M. & Baadenhuijsen, H. (1982a) *Volatile N-nitrosamines, nitrate and nitrite in urine and saliva of healthy volunteers after administration of large amounts of nitrate.* In: Bartsch, H., O'Neill, I.K., Castegnaro, M. & Okada, M., eds, N-*Nitroso Compounds: Occurence and Biological Effects (IARC Scientific Publications No. 41),* Lyon, International Agency for Research on Cancer, pp. 365–378

Ellen, G., Schuller, P.L., Froeling, P.G.A.M. & Bruijns, E. (1982b) No volatile *N*-nitrosamines detected in blood and urine from patients ingesting daily large amounts of ammonium nitrate. *Food Chem Toxicol., 20,* 879–882

Lijinsky, W., Keefer, L. & Loo, J. (1970) The preparation and properties of some nitrosamino acids. *Tetrahedron, 26,* 5137–5153

Ohshima, H. & Bartsch, H. (1981) Quantitative estimation of endogenous nitrosation in humans by monitoring *N*-nitrosoproline excreted in the urine. *Cancer Res., 41,* 3658–3662

Ohshima, H., Bereziat, J.C. & Bartsch, H. (1982) *Measurement of endogenous N-nitrosation in rats and humans by monitoring urinary and faecal excretion of* N-*nitrosamino acids.* In: Bartsch, H., O'Neill, I.K., Castegnaro, M. & Okada, M., eds, N-*Nitroso Compounds: Occurence and Biological Effects (IARC Scientific Publications No. 41),* Lyon, International Agency for Research on Cancer, pp.397–411

Ohshima, H., Friesen, M., O'Neill, I.K. & Bartsch, H. (1983) Presence in human urine of a new *N*-nitroso compound, *N*-nitrosothiazolidine 4-carboxylic acid. *Cancer Lett., 20,* 183–190

STUDIES ON THE EXCRETION OF ENDOGENOUSLY FORMED *N*-NITROSOPROLINE
I. PERCUTANEOUS EXCRETION OF *N*-NITROSOPROLINE IN HUMANS

P.A. BOGOVSKI & M.A. ROOMA

Institute of Experimental and Clinical Medicine, Tallinn, Estonia, USSR

J.M. KANN

Tallinn Polytechnical Institute, Estonia, USSR

SUMMARY

N-Nitrosoproline (NPRO) formed intragastrically after ingestion of 8 mg/kg body weight sodium nitrate and the same amount of proline was determined in the sweat of six volunteers during intensive sweating in a Finnish sauna (60–80 °C). The amounts of sweat and NPRO and the concentrations of this compound varied between individual volunteers and in the same subjects in consecutive experiments. Females excreted higher concentrations of NPRO in smaller amounts of sweat. During the second hour after the start of intragastric nitrosation of proline, the concentrations and amounts of NPRO in sweat decreased rapidly.

INTRODUCTION

Monitoring of *N*-nitrosoproline (NPRO) excreted by humans in urine after ingestion of sodium nitrate and proline has been proposed by Ohshima and Bartsch (1981) as a method for estimating the extent of nitrosation *in vivo* in epidemiological and clinical studies and for correlating nitrosation potential with cancer incidence. The absence of risk to human health of the NPRO method has been sufficiently established (Ohshima *et al.*, 1982).

Certain metabolic end products and xenobiotics are eliminated from the human organism not only in urine and in faeces, but also, in small amounts, in sweat. The chemical composition of sweat resembles that of urine; however, the concentrations of compounds in sweat are usually much lower than their levels in blood plasma, with the exception of lactic acid and some nitrogen compounds (Kuno, 1959). The amounts of sweat secreted vary with conditions, such as external temperature, from 500 to up to 10 000 mL and more over 24 h. In some pathological conditions, e.g., in uraemia, sweat can contain considerable amounts of urea and other nitrogen compounds.

We assumed that sweat contains NPRO after a subject has ingested its precursors, sodium nitrate and proline. Certain analytical aspects justify attempts to develop methods for measuring NPRO excreted in sweat as alternative techniques for determining the nitrosation potential of humans.

We investigated the excretion of endogenously formed NPRO in human sweat, individual variations of this process and some of its time trends.

MATERIALS AND METHODS

Intensive sweating was induced in six apparently healthy volunteers, aged from 44 to 68 years, two female and four male, one of whom (E, Table 1) was a smoker, by exposure to high ambient temperatures (60–80 °C) in a Finnish sauna, characterized by comparatively low humidity ($\sim 60\%$). Two hours before sweating started, 8 mg/kg body weight sodium nitrate were ingested as juice of red beetroots or as the same juice enriched with sodium nitrate or an aqueous solution of the compound. One hour before sweating, 8 mg/kg body weight proline were taken in aqueous solution. Sweat was collected into glass jars from the skin surface of the face, neck and pectoral, ventral and dorsal regions and limbs by means of adsorbing material (filter paper or hygroscopic cotton wool). The lids of the jars were opened as rarely as possible to minimize evaporation of the collected sweat. Individual jars and dry absorbent material were weighed before each experiment.

In the first four experiments, certain methodological aspects were not taken into account, e.g., the body surface was not thoroughly washed just before sweating.

Table 1. Excretion in sweat of intragastrically formed *N*-nitrosoproline (NPRO) in volunteers[a]

Volunteer				Experiment number				
Code	Age (years)	Weight (kg)	Sex	1	2	3	4	5
A	48	57	F	10/714 / 14	6.2/365 / 17	2.4/60 / 40	–	3.4/92 / 37
B	45	65	F	7.5/500 / 15	5.5/500 / 11	–	–	9.9/268 / 37
C	44	100	M	12.7/108 / 118	2.1/31 / 68	–	–	13.4/56 / 240
D	53	90	M	–	1.3/6 / 226	17.5/116 / 151	–	22.2/65 / 342
E	64	95	M	24.4/317 / 77	2.2/19 / 114	16.2/120 / 135	15.3/95 / 161	22.9/83 / 276
F	68	83	M	5.6/112 / 50	3.3/67 / 49	2.4/44 / 54	10.4/70 / 149	14.8/98 / 151

[a] Data presented as follows:

amount of NPRO in sweat (µg) / concentration of NPRO in sweat (µg/kg)
——————————————————————————————————————
amount of sweat (g)

In the first series of experiments (1–5), sweat was collected for 25 min. In the second series (6 and 7), sweat was collected from two volunteers starting 1 h after proline intake over three separate periods, each lasting 15 min, separated by two pauses of 10 min in a cooler room. Before and after each sweating period, a shower was taken, and the body surface was washed with soap. Sweat from each period was collected in separate jars.

The hermetically closed jars were stored for 12–15 h at 4 °C in a refrigerator, then weighed to determine the amount of sweat, which was then analysed for NPRO.

Analytical procedure

Sweat was extracted from adsorbing material by pouring boiling distilled water into the jar (up to 400 mL). Fat was removed from the filtrate by three extractions with 100 mL *n*-pentane in a separating funnel. The aqueous residue was acidified with 7 mol/L sulfuric acid to pH < 1. *N*-Nitrososarcosine as internal standard was added, and three extractions were carried out with 50 mL ethyl acetate. The ethyl acetate phase was dried over anhydrous sodium sulfate and concentrated in a rotary evaporator to 5 mL. After filtration through an absorbent to remove coloured admixtures, the residue was dried by evaporation and methylated with diazomethane in sulfuric ether. The mixture was concentrated to ~ 1 mL and sealed in vials before analysis by gas chromatography and thermal energy analysis (Thermal Energy Analyzer 502).

A glass column (1.5 m, 4 mm i.d.), packed with Chromaton N/AW HMDS, 80–100 mesh, was used for the analysis. The stationary phase was 20% 20M PEG; carrier gas (Ar) flow was 20 mL/min. The Thermal Energy Analyzer was operated at 475 °C pyrolyser temperature, –135–140 °C cold-trap temperature and residual pressure of ~ 3 torr (~ 400 Pa).

The rate of recovery of NPRO from sweat was 62 ± 5.5%. The limit of detection of the method was 1 µg/kg.

The Thermal Energy Analyzer responses coincided with the results of parallel colorimetric determinations at 520 nm of hydrogen bromide derivatives, using a calibration curve.

RESULTS

The first series of five experiments carried out at intervals of two to four weeks in six volunteers prove unequivocally that NPRO is excreted in sweat after ingestion of sodium nitrate and proline. The amounts of NPRO excreted are sufficient for analytical purposes.

Table 2. Excretion of intragastrically formed *N*-nitrosoproline (NPRO) in sweat from two volunteers after ingestion of sodium nitrate and proline

Volunteer	Sweating period (min after proline intake)	Experiment no. 6			Experiment no. 7		
		Amount of sweat (g)	Amount of NPRO in sweat (µg)	NPRO in sweat (µg/kg)	Amount of sweat (g)	Amount of NPRO in sweat (µg)	NPRO in sweat (µg/kg)
E	60– 75	146	9.2	63	125	9.6	77
	75–100	149	5.5	38	187	6.2	33
	110–125	82	1.9	23	150	2.3	15
F	60– 75	52	2.0	39	72	1.7	24
	75–100	52	1.1	22	92	1.4	15
	110–125	145	1.6	11	80	0.7	9

There were considerable differences between individual volunteers (Table 1); the amounts of sweat secreted varied, as did the amounts and concentrations of NPRO. Differences can also be seen in the same volunteers in subsequent experiments. Volunteer E was a smoker. Females tended to secrete less sweat with a higher concentration of NPRO than males.

The second series of experiments (6 and 7) in two of the volunteers, carried out with an interval of two days between the two series, provided more consistent data (Table 2; Fig. 1), since sweat collection techniques and washing of the body surface before sweating were standardized and improved in comparison with the first four experiments. The two volunteers differed distinctly with regard to the amounts and concentrations of NPRO excreted in their sweat during the second hour of intragastric nitrosation: much higher values were found in the sweat of volunteer E.

As can be seen in Figure 1, the amounts and concentrations of NPRO in sweat decreased rapidly in both volunteers, in spite of considerable differences in numerical values. The highest values were found at the beginning of the second hour after the start of intragastric nitrosation of proline.

DISCUSSION

The individual variations observed were due partly to slight differences in experimental conditions, such as different dietary regimens of the volunteers. In addition, some NPRO may have reached the skin surface by imperceptible perspiration during the hour between proline intake and start of intensive sweating; and the values in experiments 1–4 may have been higher as the body surface was not washed immediately before sweating.

Fig. 1. Excretion of *N*-nitrosoproline (NPRO) is sweat after ingestion of sodium nitrate and proline by two volunteers in two experiments, A and B (6 and 7, Table 2).
Volunteer E: ▲, amount of NPRO in sweat; ▼, concentration of NPRO in sweat
Volunteer F: ●, amount of NPRO in sweat; ■, concentration of NPRO in sweat

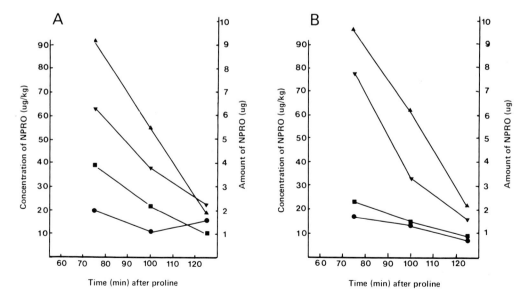

Nevertheless, some features of NPRO excretion in sweat seem to be individually determined. In females (volunteers A and B), the amounts of sweat tend to be smaller and the concentrations of NPRO higher than in males in comparable experiments. Smoking seems to increase the nitrosation potential and/or the excretion of NPRO in sweat.

Ohshima and Bartsch (1981) reported that one human volunteer excreted about 15 μg NPRO in daily urine after ingesting 375 mg nitrate and 250 mg proline. It is interesting to note that after forced sweating for 25–45 min, the amounts of NPRO eliminated from the organism were of the same order of magnitude or greater (by some subjects) after ingestion of about twice the quantities of precursors. The amounts of sweat secreted by our volunteers were usually less than half of the minimal value for daily sweat secretion (500 mL) under physiological conditions (Kuno, 1959).

Sweating over the entire body surface, with the exception of specific sites such as the axillary and pudendal regions, where apocrine sweat glands are situated, and the palms, is considered to be a necessary function for regulating body temperature, especially to prevent overheating. The excretory function has not been investigated extensively but seems to be of little importance: only about 1–1.5 g urea and nonproteinic nitrogen compounds are excreted daily, even when 5 L of sweat are secreted (Kuno, 1959).

Whether and to what extent sweating can serve to diminish the body burden of endogenously-formed nitroso compounds requires further investigation.

In view of the fact that the concentrations of chemical compounds in sweat are generally lower than those in blood plasma [since in sweat glands mainly diffusion of compounds takes place (Kuno, 1959) and not concentration, as in the kidneys], levels in blood plasma are probably reflected more closely by the values found in sweat than by those in urine.

The possibility of applying the measurement of NPRO excretion in sweat as an indicator of individual nitrosation potential will be investigated further, mainly by simplifying the techniques and correlating various environmental parameters as well as individual features with the amounts and concentrations of NPRO excreted in sweat.

CONCLUSIONS

(1) Endogenously formed NPRO is excreted by humans in sweat during forced sweating.

(2) The amounts and concentrations of NPRO in sweat vary between individuals under similar experimental conditions and in the same subjects in consecutive experiments.

(3) In females, the concentration of NPRO excreted in sweat tends to be higher and the amount of sweat lower than in males.

(4) During the second hour after the start of intragastric nitrosation of proline, the concentrations and amounts of NPRO in sweat decrease rapidly.

ACKNOWLEDGEMENTS

The authors wish to thank the National Cancer Institute, Bethesda, MD, USA, for the loan of the Terminal Energy Analyzer (Contract NO1 CP 75 975). We are grateful to Anu Hamburg and Lehti Kuldmäe for their skilful analytical work.

REFERENCES

Kuno, Y. (1959) *Human Perspiration,* Springfield, IL, Charles C. Thomas Publishers

Ohshima, H. & Bartsch, H. (1981) Quantitative estimation of endogenous nitrosation in humans by monitoring *N*-nitrosoproline excreted in the urine. *Cancer Res., 41,* 3658–3662

Ohshima, H., Béréziat, J.C. & Bartsch, H. (1982) *Measurement of endogenous N-nitrosation in rats and humans by monitoring urinary and faecal excretion of* N-*nitrosamino acids.* In: Bartsch, H., O'Neill, I.K., Castegnaro, M. & Okada, M., eds, N-*Nitroso Compounds: Occurrence and Biological Effects* (*IARC Scientific Publications No. 41*), Lyon, International Agency for Research on Cancer, pp. 397–411

N-NITROSOPROLINE EXCRETION IN URINE, FAECES AND MILK FROM COWS IN RELATION TO FEED COMPOSITION

L.W. VAN BROEKHOVEN, J.A.R. DAVIES & J.H. GEURINK

Centre for Agrobiological Research PO Box 14 6700 AA Wageningen, The Netherlands

SUMMARY

The technique of Ohshima and Bartsch for measuring the excretion of N-nitrosoproline (NPRO) was applied in a balance trial with cows to estimate the in-vivo formation of N-nitrosamines. In the first trial, a cow with a high milk production received rations of concentrates and hay with low or high contents of nitrate and free proline. Samples were taken from the urine, faeces and milk. In the second trial, two non-lactating cows were put on hay rations with different nitrate and free proline contents, and samples were taken from the rumenal fluid every 15 min to measure the formation of nitrite from the ingested nitrate. Samples of urine and faeces were also taken. It was found that dried roughage may contain considerable amounts of free proline, and the NPRO formed is related to the nitrate content. No NPRO was found in the urine and faeces when the NPRO content of the hay was low, not even when the ingested nitrate was reduced drastically to nitrite or when the concentration of free proline was high. When NPRO was present in the feed, it was recovered from the urine and faeces but was not transmitted to the milk.

INTRODUCTION

More intense use of grasslands over the last few decades has led to an increase in the use of nitrogen fertilizer and thus to the presence of nitrate in grass and grass products. Not only acute toxicity (nitrate poisoning) in cows, but also the possibility of formation of N-nitroso compounds must be considered. When N-nitroso compounds are present or are formed *in vivo* from precursors present in the feed, they may be transferred to meat or milk that is consumed by humans. In an earlier investigation, no formation of volatile N-nitrosamines was detected in the rumen fluid of cows fed nitrate-rich hay (van Broekhoven & Davies, 1981); this may have been due to a lack of appropriate secondary amines. Ohshima *et al.* (1982) have described a method in which excretion in the urine of N-nitrosoproline (NPRO) - a non-volatile nitrosamine, which is not metabolized in the body - is measured in order to estimate daily human exposure to endogenously formed N-nitroso compounds. This seemed a good method for investigating whether or not there is nitrosamine formation in cows in relation to the feed components and to look for a correlation between such formation and the nitrite content in the rumen.

This paper presents the results of two short balance trials with cows given different rations, some of which were supplemented with potassium nitrate and L-proline.

MATERIALS AND METHODS

Chemicals

L-Proline and DL-pipecolic acid were obtained from Sigma Chemical Co. (St Louis, MO, USA); *N*-methylnitrosourea for the preparation of diazomethane from ICN-K + K Laboratories, Inc. (Plainview, NY, USA); all other chemicals from Merck (Darmstadt, FRG). Preptube cartridges type 117 were purchased from Thermo Electron Corp. (Waltham, MA, USA). All chemicals were used without further purification. NPRO and *N*-nitrosopipecolic acid (NPIC) were synthesized according to the method of Lijinsky *et al.* (1970)

Feeding experiments

The balance trials were carried out with lactating and non-lactating Friesian cows in a digestion cowshed. One week before the start of the experiments, the animals were equipped with a device for the separate collection of faeces and urine (van Es & Vogt, 1959), including urinal and harness. Each experimental period consisted of a collection period of three days, after a preliminary adaptation period of three days. Each animal was fitted with a rumen fistula.

The composition of the feed used in the experiments is given in Table 1. Table 2 gives information about the daily intake of dry matter, nitrate, total nitrogen, proline and NPRO during the different collection periods. The daily ration was given in two portions (at 8:00 and 16:00 h). Only in the first experiment was the hay ration supplemented with a pelleted commercial dairy concentrate according to the requirements of a cow with an average daily milk production of 30 L. In the second collection period (Table 2; experiments I-2 and II-2), the daily ration was divided into a nitrate-rich portion in the morning (8:00 h) and a nitrate-poor portion in the afternoon (16:00 h). In the third and fourth periods, extra potassium nitrate and L-proline dissolved in 2.5 L water at about 35°C were given through the rumenal fistula.

Sampling

In order to sample the rumenal fluid, a perforated tube was pressed through the fistula almost to the bottom of the ventral sack, as described by Kemp *et al.* (1977). During the three-day collection period, milk, urine and faeces were collected, weighed, mixed and sampled every

Table 1. Composition of feed

Feed	Total nitrogen (g N/kg dry matter)	Nitrate (g N/kg dry matter)	Proline (g/kg fresh feed)	*N*-Nitrosoproline (μg/kg fresh feed)	Dry matter (g/kg fresh feed)
Concentrate	30.1	0.17	2.65	68.8	870
Hay A	20.5	0.05	0.98	41.9	809
Hay B	47.1	3.48	15.27	377.5	899
Hay C	18.6	0.68	0.89	13.0	882
Hay D	47.5	4.29	7.48	329.0	878

Table 2. Average daily intake of dry matter, nitrate, total nitrogen, proline and N-nitrosoproline (NPRO)

Expt no.	Cow (body weight in kg)	Collection no.	Concentrate (kg dry matter/day)	Hay (kg dry matter/day)	Composition[a]	Nitrate (g N/day)	Total nitrogen (g N/day)	Proline (g/day)	NPRO (µg/day)
I	Ada (527)	1	9.6	7.5	A	1.97	442.7	38.26	1 146.5
		2	9.6	4.1 + 4.0	A + B	16.06	564.0	104.19	2 698.6
		3	9.6	8.2	A	2.00 + 11.64[b]	468.7	39.05	1 180
		4	9.6	7.6	A	1.97 + 11.64[b]	456.4	38.36 + 10[c]	1 151
II	Agatha (451)	1	–	7.1	C	4.83	132.1	7.12	104
		2	–	2.6 + 4.4	C + D	14.15	205.3	26.14	1 016
		3	–	6.2	C	4.22 + 14.55[b]	115.3	5.52 + 19.1[c]	91
	Boukje (597)	1	–	8.8	C	5.98	163.7	8.9	130
		2	–	3.4 + 4.4	C + D	17.58	243.3	29.88	1 344
		3	–	7.1	C	4.83 + 16.22[b]	132.1	6.31 + 25.7[c]	104

[a] For composition, see Table 1.
[b] Extra dose of nitrate added as potassium nitrate
[c] Extra L-proline added

24 h. The bottles for collecting urine contained 250 mL 1 mol/L sodium hydroxide as a preservative and were cooled in ice-water; the bottles were changed twice a day. The faeces were caught in a stainless-steel tank and were collected several times a day in a barrel containing 500 mL 1 mol/L sodium hydroxide. All samples were stored at 4°C until analysis. The milk samples were worked up one hour after sampling. At the end of a collection period, representative samples of faeces and urine were mixed in appropriate proportions for the three-day period and worked up as soon as possible. Directly after collection, the rumen fluid samples were mixed with lead acetate to preserve them for analysis of nitrate and nitrite. These samples were also stored at 4°C until analysis (Vertregt, 1977).

Extraction of NPRO

A 20-g aliquot of the feed was mixed with 50 mL 1% sulfamic acid and 250 mL methanol and further extracted as described by Sen *et al.* (1982). For extraction of faeces, 75 g were mixed with 75 mL water. After centrifugation (30 min, 2000 rpm), 10 mL of the supernatant were mixed with 2 g sodium chloride, 2 mL 3.6 mol/L sulfuric acid and 1 mL 15% sulfamic acid in 1.8 mol/L sulfuric acid poured into a Preptube (prewetted with 10 mL ethyl acetate) and extracted with 4 × 20 mL ethyl acetate.

Urine samples were mixed before extraction with 2 g sodium chloride, 2 mL 3.6 mol/L sulfuric acid and 1.3 mL 15% sulfamic acid in 1.8 mol/L sulfuric acid per 10-mL sample; 50-mL samples were extracted with 3 × 50 mL ethyl acetate, and 10-mL samples were extracted, using a Preptube (prewetted with 10 mL ethyl acetate), with 4 × 20 mL ethyl acetate.

Milk samples were mixed with methanol (30 mL milk with 150 mL methanol) and further extracted as described by Sen *et al.* (1982).

Analysis of NPRO

To each sample, 520 ng NPIC were added as an internal standard. Blank runs (with water instead of sample) were performed throughout the experiments. The combined ethyl acetate layers were dried over sodium sulfate and concentrated in a rotary evaporator. The residue was treated with an excess of diazomethane in ether. Before concentrating to 0.5 mL in a stream of nitrogen, 0.5 mL methanol was added.

For the analysis, a gas chromatograph (GC)-Thermal Energy Analyzer (TEA) combination was used, with the following conditions: GC (Packard Becker 427; Packard Becker, Delft, The Netherlands): injection port, 220°C; column, stainless-steel (length, 3 m; o.d., 3.2 mm) containing 10% Carbowax 20M on Chromosorb WHP 80/100; oven, isotherm, 200°C; carrier gas, argon; inlet pressure, 0.3 MPa. TEA (model 502LC, Thermo Electron Co., Waltham, MA, USA): pyrolyser temperature, 450°C; reaction chamber pressure, 133-200 Pa; cold trap (liquid nitrogen-isopentane), -160 to -145°C. Typically, about 20 µL of the final solution were injected.

The percentage recoveries of 50 µg/kg aliquots of NPRO and NPIC added to the samples were found to be excellent (90-100%) using the extraction with Preptubes described by Sen *et al.* (1982); with extraction procedures not involving Preptube, recoveries of 50-70% have been found. Blank determinations were free of interference. No peak other than those of NPIC and NPRO was present in the chromatogram. The detection limit of the method is about 2-3 µg/kg for feed, urine and milk and about 6 µg/kg for faeces.

The rubber material used for the urinals and in the milking machine was investigated for release of *N*-nitrosamines under our experimental conditions. After extraction for 24 h with water at both pH 4 and 7 no *N*-nitrosamine was found.

Other analyses

Proline was determined as described by Richter *et al.* (1975); nitrate and nitrite according to Vertregt (1977). Total nitrogen and dry matter were determined by standard methods.

Table 3. Intake and excretion in faeces, urine and milk of N-nitrosproline (NPRO), and nitrite in rumenal fluid

Expt no.	Cow	Collection no.	NPRO intake (μg/day)	NPRO in faeces (μg/day) (% of intake)	NPRO in urine (μg/day) (% of intake)	NPRO in milk (μg/day)	Recovery (%)	Nitrite in rumenal fluid (mmol/L)[a]
I	Ada	1	1 146.5	934 (82)	232 (20)	<60[b]	102	<0.02
		2	2 698.6	983 (36)	1 306 (48)	<60	84	<0.02
		3	1 180	754 (64)	400 (34)	<60	98	<0.02
		4	1 151	1 011 (88)	286 (25)	<60	113	<0.02
II	Agatha	1	104	<120[c]	<20[d]	ND	ND	<0.02
		2	1 016	638 (63)	334 (33)	ND	96	0.98
		3	91	<120	<20	ND	ND	1.59
	Boukje	1	130	<120	<20	ND	ND	<0.02
		2	1 344	915 (68)	467 (35)	ND	103	1.23
		3	104	<120	<20	ND	ND	2.87

[a] Highest values only, measured at end of each three-day collection period
[b] Detection limit based on an average daily production of 30 L of milk
[c] Detection limit based on an average daily production of 20 kg faeces
[d] Detection limit based on an average daily production of 6 L urine
ND, not determined

RESULTS

It has been reported that under conditions of stress (e.g., high temperature), proline accumulates in plants (Aspinall & Paleg, 1981); thus, it was expected that free proline would be present in hay as a result of the drying process. The content found in the hay used in the experiments was more or less related to that of total nitrogen (Table 1). We also found NPRO in the feed samples (Table 1), in quantities somewhat dependent on the total nitrogen content, which was presumably formed during the drying of the hay. The origin of the proline and NPRO in the concentrate is unknown. Table 3 shows the intake and the excretion in faeces, urine and milk of NPRO and the nitrite concentrations in rumenal fluid found in the two experiments.

In experiment I, a cow was used which had an average daily milk production of 30 L. Data on this experiment are given in Tables 2 and 3. No detectable amount of nitrite was found in the rumenal fluid, even after feeding of nitrate-rich hay (collection period 2) or intrarumenal administration of extra potassium nitrate (collection periods 3 and 4). Intake of a ration rich in concentrates can cause lowering of rumenal pH, leading to less favourable conditions for nitrite accumulation. NPRO already present in the feed was excreted quantitatively by the cow, mostly in the faeces and a smaller amount in the urine; no NPRO was found in milk samples.

In experiment II (Tables 2 and 3), two non-lactating cows were fed hay only. Under these conditions, high levels of nitrite could be expected in the rumenal fluid in relation to the nitrate intake. Figure 1 shows the changes in the contents of nitrate and nitrite in the rumenal fluid

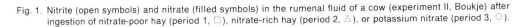

Fig. 1. Nitrite (open symbols) and nitrate (filled symbols) in the rumenal fluid of a cow (experiment II, Boukje) after ingestion of nitrate-poor hay (period 1, □), nitrate-rich hay (period 2, △), or potassium nitrate (period 3, ○).

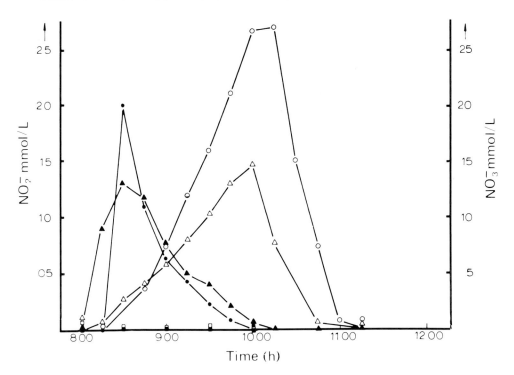

of one cow on the third day of each collection period, after administration of the different feeds. No formation of NPRO was found, even during collection period 2, when a relatively high amount of free proline was present in the hay and the nitrate available provided a high nitrite concentration in the rumenal fluid over a number of hours. In collection period 3, sufficient L-proline and potassium nitrate were administered to the rumen to provoke a situation similar to that in period 2. In both cows, the amounts of NPRO present were near the detection limit. Thus, it can be concluded that under these conditions no NPRO is formed endogenously. NPRO already present in the feed was recovered nearly quantitatively in the urine and faeces, in almost equal percentages.

After a period during which the animals adapted to the ration, the amounts of faeces and urine excreted during the collection periods were very regular, which may account for the good recoveries after three days.

In a preliminary assessment of grazing cows, urine samples were taken from three cows grazing on a pasture that had been treated with 1000 kg N/ha for one year. The nitrate content of the grass was 4.9 g N/kg dry matter. No NPRO was found in the urine samples.

DISCUSSION

One of the aims of this study was to look for a correlation between formation of nitrite in the rumenal fluid and endogenous formation of NPRO, which would make it possible to estimate the extent of endogenous nitrosation in cattle. However, the results show only that NPRO ingested with feed can be recovered. The feeding conditions used in the two experiments are comparable with those applied normally for lactating and non-lactating cows, respectively. No indication was found that the formation of NPRO was related to intake and output values. Most of the ingested NPRO was excreted in the faeces: thus, adsorption of NPRO from the intestinal tract was largely prevented. A similar effect, though to a lesser extent, was found by Ohshima *et al.* (1982) in their experiments with non-fasted rats.

It can be speculated that the reason that no formation of NPRO was found is that proteins and amino acids are readily degraded in the rumen, depending on the microbiological activity (Church, 1975), and thus the proline could have been degraded very rapidly. Moreover, due to a rather high pH ($\simeq 7$), conditions in the rumen may not have been suited to the formation of *N*-nitroso compounds, although the rennet-stomach, with a pH $\simeq 3$, seems to provide ideal conditions for their formation. Further experiments are needed to study the fate of proline and of NPRO in the rumen and the possible formation of NPRO in the rennet-stomach.

ACKNOWLEDGEMENTS

We wish to thank Mr E. Davelaar for performing the proline determinations, Mr B. de Bruin for his skillful assistance during the experiments and Mr D.J. den Boer (Research and Advisory Institute for Cattle Husbandry, Lelystad, The Netherlands) for the urine samples from grazing cows.

REFERENCES

Aspinall, D. & Paleg, L.G. (1981) *Proline accumulation: physiological aspects.* In: Paleg, L.G. & Aspinall, D., eds, *The Physiology and Biochemistry of Drought Resistance in Plants*, Sydney, Academic Press, pp. 206–241

Van Broekhoven, L.W. & Davies, J.A.R. (1981) The analysis of volatile *N*-nitrosamines in the rumen fluid of cows. *Neth. J. Agric. Sci., 29*, 173–177

Church, D.C. (1975) *Rumen metabolism of nitrogenous compounds.* In: Church, D.C., ed., *Digestive Physiology and Nutrition of Ruminants, Vol. 1, Digestive Physiology*, Corvallis, Oregon, pp. 227–252

Van Es, A.J.H. & Vogt, J.E. (1959) Separative collection of faeces and urine of cows. *J. Anim. Sci.,* **18,** 1220–1223

Kemp, A., Geurink, J.H., Haalstra, R.T. & Malestein, A. (1977) Nitrate poisoning in cattle. 2. Changes in nitrite in rumen fluid and methemoglobin formation in blood after high nitrate intake. *Neth. J. Agric. Sci.,* **25,** 51–62

Lijinsky, W., Keefer, L. & Loo, J. (1970) The preparation and properties of some nitrosamino acids. *Tetrahedron,* **26,** 5137–5153

Ohshima, H., Béréziat, J.C. & Bartsch, H. (1982) Monitoring *N*-nitrosamino acids excreted in the urine and faeces of rats as an index for endogenous nitrosation. *Carcinogenesis,* **3,** 115–120

Richter, R., Dijkshoorn, W & Vonk, D.R. (1975) Amino acids of barley plants in relation to nitrate, urea or ammonium nutrition. *Plant Soil,* **42,** 601–618

Sen, N.P., Seaman, S. & Tessier, L. (1982) *A rapid and sensitive method for the determination of non-volatile* N-*nitroso compounds in foods and human urine: Recent data concerning volatile* N-*nitrosamines in dried foods and malt-based beverages.* In: Bartsch, H., O'Neill, I.K., Castegnaro, M. & Okada, M, eds, *N-Nitroso Compounds: Occurrence and Biological Effects (IARC Scientific Publications No. 41)*, Lyon, International Agency for Research on Cancer, pp. 185–197

Vertregt, N. (1977) The formation of methemoglobin by the action of nitrite in bovine blood. *Neth. J. Agric. Sci.,* **25,** 243–254

DIETARY PHENOLICS AND BETEL NUT EXTRACTS AS MODIFIERS OF N-NITROSATION IN RAT AND MAN

H.F. STICH & B.P. DUNN

British Columbia Cancer Research Centre, Vancouver, Canada

B. PIGNATELLI, H. OHSHIMA & H. BARTSCH[1]

International Agency for Research on Cancer, Lyon, France

SUMMARY

Polyphenolic compounds (PPC) isolated from betel nuts and some dietary PPC were examined for their modifying effects on N-nitrosation *in vitro* and *in vivo*. The formation of N-nitrosodiethylamine (NDEA) and N-nitrosoproline (NPRO) was either enhanced or inhibited by PPC from betel nuts, depending on (1) the structure of the PPC, (2) the pH of the reaction medium, (3) the relative concentrations of nitrite and PPC, and (4) the nature of the nitrosatable amino compounds. Both catalysis and inhibition of endogenous nitrosation of proline were observed in rats, although to a lesser extent than *in vitro*. Caffeic and ferulic acids, as well as the PPC-containing beverages tea and coffee, exerted inhibitory effects on endogenous formation of NPRO in two human subjects. These results demonstrate that PPC can modify the yield of endogenously formed N-nitroso compounds, and may thus effect the carcinogen burden in man.

INTRODUCTION

Polyphenolic compounds (PPC) are commonly consumed in foodstuffs and beverages. The formation of N-nitroso compounds can be catalysed or suppressed by PPC, depending on their structure, on the pH and on the relative concentrations of nitrite and PPC in the reaction medium (Gray & Dugan, 1975; Davies *et al.*, 1978; Pignatelli *et al.*, 1980). Both catalysis and inhibition of N-nitrosation have been shown to occur *in vitro* and *in vivo* in rats (Bogovski *et al.*, 1972; Kawabata *et al.*, 1979; Pignatelli *et al.*, 1982, 1983; Stich *et al.*, 1982a, b) An increased risk of cancer of the upper digestive tract in man has been associated with the chewing of betel quids (Muir & Kirk, 1960; Hirayama, 1966; Jussawalla, 1976); betel nut contains large amounts of PPC, and N-nitrosation of betel nut alkaloids has been hypothesized to be involved in the aetiology of this disease (Wenke & Hoffmann, 1983).

The objectives of our studies are to examine those combinations of nitrate/nitrite, nitrosatable compounds and PPC mixtures that may inhibit or enhance N-nitrosation. We

---

[1] To whom correspondence should be addressed

focus on the modifying effect of PPC on the endogenous formation of *N*-nitrosoproline (NPRO) (Ohshima & Bartsch, 1981; Ohshima *et al.,* 1982) in rats and man and on the in-vitro nitrosation of diethylamine. The ultimate goal is to collect data on the rate of formation of *N*-nitroso compounds in man after ingestion of commonly consumed precursors and to explore possibilities for inhibiting their endogenous synthesis by dietary factors.

MATERIALS AND METHODS

Preparation of betel nut extracts

Total aqueous extract I: Ten g of ground betel nut were extracted four times each with 50 mL water (1 h, 21 °C, shaking), then filtered through a Millipore filter. Solid material on the filter was rinsed with 5 mL water. The combined filtrates (total volume, 220 mL) were used in the experiments and are referred to as 'aqueous betel nut extract I' (equivalent to 45.45 mg betel nut/mL of aqueous extract).

Total aqueous extract II: Whole, dry areca nuts were powdered in a blender and extracted twice with 500 mL *n*-hexane (30 min, 21 °C, shaking). After filtration, the *n*-hexane was evaporated. The dry residue was extracted five times with water (containing 0.1% sodium metabisulfite) with heating in a boiling water-bath for 10 min. The combined filtrates were centrifuged at 4 000 × *g* for 10 min and the supernatant freeze-dried. This extract is referred to as 'aqueous betel nut extract II'.

An amount of extract II (expressed as weight of freeze-dried extract) was equal to 1/10 the amount of extract I (the latter expressed as equivalent weight of betel nut).

Other extracts: Other phenolic extracts, enriched in tannins, flavonoids or catechins, were prepared as described previously (Stich *et al.,* 1983).

Assays for nitrosation of proline and diethylamine in vitro

A sodium nitrite solution was added to a solution of either proline or diethylamine (hydrochloride) (final volume, 1 mL), with or without addition of a betel nut extract. Precursor solutions were prepared gravimetrically prepared in 0.2 mol/L sodium citrate-citric acid buffer of defined pH. After 15 min incubation at 37 °C, residual nitrite was destroyed, and the amounts of NPRO or *N*-nitrosodiethylamine (NDEA) were measured.

Analysis of NPRO: Ten to 20 mL of the diluted reaction medium (or rat urine) were spiked with *N*-nitrosopipecolic acid (NPIC) as internal standard. NPRO was analysed by gas chromatography (GC) coupled with a Thermal Energy Analyzer (TEA) after conversion of the *N*-nitrosamino acids to their methyl esters (Ohshima & Bartsch, 1981; Ohshima *et al.,* 1982; Pignatelli *et al.,* 1982).

Analysis of NDEA: Ten to 20 mL of the reaction medium were diluted and spiked with *N*-nitrosodipropylamine (NDPA) as internal standard. The volatile nitrosamines were extracted (3 × 20 ml dichloromethane) in the presence of 5 g sodium chloride and 1.5 mL 20% ammonium sulfamate in 3.6N sulfuric acid. The organic phase was dried over anhydrous sodium sulfate and concentrated to 0.5–1 mL in a Kuderna-Danish apparatus. NPRO and NDPA were determined by GC-TEA, the chromatographic conditions being the same as those used for NPRO analysis, except that the temperature of the column was 120 °C.

Assays for nitrosation of proline in rats in vivo

Groups of 5 to 10 BD rats (300 g body weight, fasted for 20 h before starting the experiments) received 0.5 mL of an aqueous proline solution with or without the addition of a betel nut extract, followed immediately by 0.5 mL of a freshly prepared aqueous sodium nitrite solution.

The two precursor solutions were prepared gravimetrically in 0.2 mol/L sodium citrate-citric acid buffer (pH 4) or 0.2 mol/L citric acid (pH 1.9) and were given by stomach tube. NPRO excreted in the 24-h urine of rats (means $\pm$ SD) was measured as described above. The Wilcoxon test was applied for statistical evaluation of the amounts of NPRO excreted by rats who had ingested betel nut extracts *versus* that of control animals.

Measurement of NPRO in human urine

Samples of urine were preserved by the addition of 300 mg solid sodium hydroxide per 100 mL and were stored frozen prior to analysis; 15-mL samples of urine were acidified with 3 mL 20% ammonium sulfamate in 1.8 mol/L sulfuric acid, and spiked with NPIC. Urine samples were loaded onto 20-mL capacity extraction columns (unbuffered, style TE 3020, Fisher Scientific) and allowed to absorb. Columns were then eluted with 4×20 mL ethyl acetate which had been dried over 20 g anhydrous sodium sulfate. The organic extracts were decanted and evaporated to dryness. Residues were dissolved in a total of 4 mL methanol, and the methanol was evaporated to a volume of approximately 0.1 mL at 50 °C under a stream of nitrogen. Then, 0.5 mL boron trifluoride reagent (14% in methanol) was added and the samples capped and incubated for either 4 h at 50 °C, or overnight at room temperature. Then, 0.5 mL dichloromethane and 2 mL water were added, and the samples were shaken vigorously to extract the esterified *N*-nitrosamines into the chlorinated solvent. Daily calibration samples were prepared by esterifying 150 ng NPIC and NPRO in 0.5 mL boron trifluoride-methanol in a similar manner. Analysis of the *N*-nitrosamino acid esters was performed by GC-TEA (Ohshima & Bartsch, 1981; Ohshima *et al.*, 1982).

RESULTS

Modifying effects of aqueous betel nut extracts on the nitrosation of diethylamine and proline in vitro

In the presence of nitrite ([amine]/[nitrite] = 0.5), total aqueous betel nut extract I catalysed the formation of NDEA (Fig. 1A) and NPRO (Fig. 1B) at pH 4. The formation of both *N*-nitroso compounds formed increased as a function of the concentration of extract I and rose to a maximum with about 1.4 mg of freeze-dried aqueous extract/mL. The magnitude of catalysis depended on that of the amine substrate; the maximum yields of NDEA and NPRO were 25- and 7-fold greater, respectively, than those in control assays.

Figure 1C shows the effect of betel nut extract II on the nitrosation of proline ([amine]/[nitrite] = 2.5). At pH 4, it was catalysed at lower concentrations of betel nut extract II. At a 1-mg/mL concentration of betel nut extract II, the yield of NPRO increased by 6.5-fold; at 10-fold and 30-fold higher concentrations, betel nut extract II inhibited nitrosation by 50% and 96%, respectively. At pH 1.9, an inhibitory effect on NPRO formation was observed over the whole range of concentrations of betel nut extract II (Fig. 1D). The presence of 1 mg betel nut extract II/mL inhibited NPRO formation by 50%.

Modifying effects of phenolic subfractions from betel nut extracts on N-nitrosation of diethylamine and proline in vitro

The effect of tannin, flavonoid and catechin fractions prepared from betel nut on the nitrosation of diethylamine at pH 4 was investigated *in vitro*. NDEA formation was enhanced up to 20 times in the presence of a high concentration of nitrite and low amounts (1/10 of a

Fig. 1. Influence of total aqueous betel nut extracts I and II on nitrosation of diethylamine and proline *in vitro*
The assays contained 10 mmol/L diethylamine (hydrochloride salt) (A) or proline (B,C,D) and 20 mmol/L (A,B) or 4 mmol/L (C,D) sodium nitrite dissolved in citric acid-citrate buffer at pH 4 (A,B,C) or in citric acid at pH 1.9 (D). *N*-nitrosodiethylamine (NDEA) (A) and *N*-nitrosoproline (NPRO) (B,C,D) were measured (μmol/L) after 15 min incubation at 37 °C. Experiments were carried out either in the absence (○ in A), (△ in B), (◇ in C), (□ in D) or in the presence (● in A), (▲ in B), (◆ in C), (■ in D) of variable amounts (mg/mL) of total aqueous betel nut extract I (A,B) or II (C,D). The relative yields of NDEA (A) and NPRO (B,C,D) were calculated by taking the yield of the uncatalysed reaction (betel nut extract omitted) as 1 (- - - - - -).

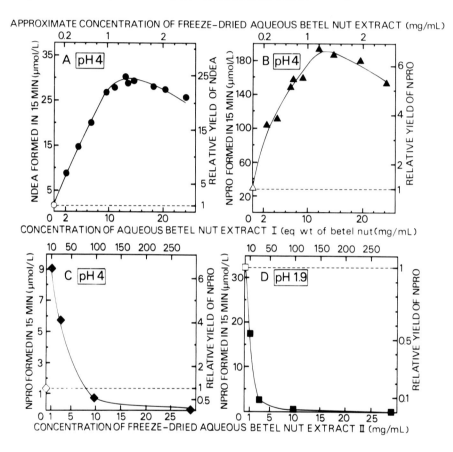

betel nut/mL) of phenolic extracts (data not shown). Tannin-catalysed nitrosation was concentration-dependent, and a maximal yield of NDEA was observed, as in the case of aqueous betel nut extract I (Fig. 1B).

Table 1 shows the effect of tannins, flavonoids, catechins and betel nut and of their mixtures (M_1, M_2) on the in-vitro nitrosation of proline at pH 4 and pH 1.9. The range of concentrations of betel nut extracts was chosen in order to simulate in-vivo conditions prevailing in humans chewing betel nuts or ingesting phenolic fractions (Stich *et al.*, 1983). Except for the lowest concentration of the catechin extract, all other samples exerted inhibitory effects on NPRO formation at pH 1.9. With increasing concentrations of the extracts, inhibition was also augmented. Flavonoids, catechins and mixture M_2 of betel nut extracts catalysed nitrosation

Table 1. Influence of tannins, flavonoids, catechins and mixtures (M₁, M₂) of extracts of betel nut on the nitrosation of proline *in vitro* at pH 4 and 1.9

Expt no.	Betel nut extract added to the precursors[a]	mg/mL	Ratio[b] (sodium nitrite)/(betel nut extract)	NPRO formed[c] at pH 4 μmol/L in 15 min	Relative[d] yield	at pH 1.9 μmol/L in 15 min	Relative[d] yield
1	O, Control (betel nut extract omitted)		—	1.4	1	32.2	1
2	Tannin extract	11.59	0.02	0.08	0.06	ND	ND
3	Tannin extract	3.86	0.07	0.94	0.7	ND	ND
4	Flavonoid extract	9.39	0.03	1.27	0.9	0.4	0.01
5	Flavonoid extract	3.13	0.09	10.5	7.5	6.3	0.2
6	Catechin extract	1.77	0.15	5.0	3.6	2.2	0.07
7	Catechin extract	0.59	0.46	ND	ND	30.4	0.94
8	Catechin extract	0.13	2.12	10.5	7.5	53.7	1.67
9	Mixture M₁ { Tannin extract / Flavonoid extract / Catechin extract }	5.68 / 2.90 / 2.34 / 0.44	0.05 / 0.09 / 0.12 / 0.63	1.0	0.7	ND	ND
10	Mixture, { Tannin extract / Flavonoid extract / Catechin extract }	1.89 / 0.96 / 0.78 / 0.15	0.15 / 0.29 / 0.35 / 1.84	4.8	3.4	5.6	0.17

[a] The assays contained 10 mmol/L of proline and 4 mmol/L of sodium nitrite
[b] Calculated by taking concentrations of nitrite and betel nut extracts expressed in mg/mL
[c] N-nitrosoproline formed (μmol/L) was measured after 15 min of incubation at 37°C.
[d] Calculated by taking the amount of NPRO in the control experiment (betel nut extract omitted) No. 1 as 1
ND, not determined

Table 2.   Effect ot total aqueous (I, II) and tannins extracts of betel nut on the formation of *N*-nitrosoproline (NPRO) *in vitro* and *in vivo* (in rats)

Expt no.	Ingredients[a]			pH[b]	NPRO formed		In vitro[d]	
	Proline (μmol)	Sodium nitrite (μmol)	Betel nut extract (mg in parentheses)		In vivo			
					nmol/24 h per rat (mean ± SD) (no. rats)	Relative[c] yield	nmol/ 15 min	Relative[c] yield
1	–	20	none (background)	4	3.0 ± 1.9 (5)	–	0	–
2	10	20	none (control)	4	12.9 ± 6.4 (10)	1	28.9	1
3	–	20	aqueous ext. I (24.27)	4	2.8 ± 1.0 (10)	–	ND	–
4	10	20	aqueous ext. I (24.27)	4	30.1 ± 6.0 (10)[s**]	2.3[s**]	152.2	5.2
5	10	20	tannins ext. (2.4)	4	36.8 ± 16.5 (10)[s**]	2.8[s**]	195.2	6.7
6	100	4	none (control)	4	8.4 ± 2.6 (5)	1	20.9	1
7	100	4	aqueous ext. II (0.96)	4	10.7 ± 5.4 (5)[ns]	1.3[ns]	73.2	3.5
8	100	4	aqueous ext. II (2.90)	4	14.6 ± 3.4 (5)[s***]	1.7[s***]	42.6	2.0
9	100	4	none (control)	1.9	48.9 ± 38.7 (5)	1	174.7	1
10	100	4	aqueous ext. II (2.90)	1.9	30.2 ± 10.6 (5)[ns]	0.6[ns]	19.4	0.1
11	100	4	aqueous ext. II (9.65)	1.9	7.6 ± 3.5 (5)[s*]	0.1[s*]	4.0	0.02

[a] Each rat received precursors (proline and nitrite) at the doses (μmol) indicated in parenthesis in buffered solutions (each precursor in 0.5 mL). Groups of rats received either no betel nut extracts (control exp. no. 2, 6 and 9) or a betel nut extract (added to the proline solution) at the dose (mg) indicated in parentheses and expressed either in equivalent weight of betel nut (expt nos 3–4) or in weight of freeze-dried extract (expt nos 5, 7, 8, 10, 11).

[b] Precursor solutions (proline and nitrite) prepared in either 0.2 mol/L citric acid – citrate buffer pH 4 (expt 1–8) or 0.2 mol/L citric acid pH 1.9 (expt 9–11) – pHs of both precursor solutions and reaction medium in *in vitro* experiments.

[c] Calculated by taking the amount of NPRO in control experiments no. 2, 3 and 9 as 1; s, Wilcoxon Test applied for statistical evaluation between amounts of NPRO excreted in rats who had ingested betel nut extracts *versus* control animals; *, p < 0.02; **, p < 0.01; *ns*, not significant

[d] Precursor solutions (proline without or with betel nut extract and nitrite) at the dose indicated were incubated at 37 °C for 15 min in 1 mL of solution either at pH 4 (expt no. 1–8) or at pH 1.9; mean of two or three experiments.

ND, not detected

Table 3. Effect of phenolic compounds and phenolic-containing beverages on urinary levels of N-nitrosoproline (NPRO) in two human subjects

Expt no.	Nitrite + proline + modifying agent[a]	NPRO excreted in urine over 10 h			
		Subject A		Subject B	
		μg/10 h	% control	μg/10 h	% control
1	None	8.3	100	6.4	100
2	Caffeic acid (subject A, 2 × 300 mg; subject B, 3 × 300 mg)	2.4	29	0.9	14
3	Ferulic acid, (2 × 300 mg)	1.9	23	1.8	28
4	Decaffeinated instant coffee, 2 cups[b]	3.8	45	1.3	20
5	Regular instant coffee, 1 cup	ND	ND	0.9	14
6	Indian tea, 1 cup	4.4	48	2.6	41
7	Chinese tea, 1 cup	2.3	27	1.6	25

[a] Individuals ingested 300 mg sodium nitrate at the start of the experiment, followed by 300 mg proline 0.5 h later. Inhibitor was consumed at the same time as proline; where two doses of inhibitor are indicated, one was taken with the proline and one after an additional 10 min.
[b] Equivalents of 1 or 2 cups were consumed in 20 mL water to avoid dilution effects in the stomach.
ND, not determined

of proline at pH 4 (expt nos. 5, 6, 8, 10); catalysis was increased when concentrations of the extracts were lowered. Tannins inhibited NPRO formation over the entire concentration range tested.

Effect of betel nut extracts on the nitrosation of proline in rats in vivo

Total aqueous extracts I and II and tannin betel nut extracts were co-administered to rats dosed with proline and nitrite (Table 2). In comparison with control animals given no PPC (expt nos. 2, 6, 9), all three extracts either catalysed (expt nos. 4, 5, 7, 8) or inhibited (expt nos. 10, 11) the nitrosation of proline when precursors were administered in buffered solutions either at pH 4 or at pH 1.9. The effects observed *in vivo* were qualitatively similar to those found *in vitro* (experiments carried out with the same precursor solutions used for the in-vivo experiments), although their magnitude was in general only 42 to 85% of that found *in vitro*.

Effect of phenolics and phenolic-containing beverages on the endogenous formation of NPRO in human subjects in vivo

Some phenolic compounds can react with nitrite and thus reduce the amount of nitrosating agents available for synthesis of N-nitrosamines in the stomach. In order to estimate endogenous nitrosation capacity in man and its modulation by phenolics, two volunteers ingested nitrate, then proline together with the modulating agent (Table 3). The effect of consuming certain phenolic compounds and PPC-containing beverages after nitrate and proline on the amount of NPRO excreted in 10 h is shown in Table 3. Both ferulic acid and caffeic acid sharply reduced (by 70–86%) the amount of NPRO excreted in the urine. Coffee, which contains large amounts of caffeic acid as well as chlorogenic acid, was also a strong

Fig. 2. Effects of phenolic compounds and phenolic-containing beverages on levels of *N*-nitrosoproline (NPRO) excreted in the urine

In each experiment, two human subjects ingested 300 mg nitrate and 300 mg proline. Immediately thereafter, they ingested phenolics or a beverage, followed 10 min later by a second intake of phenolics or beverage and, occasionally, a third intake (caffeic acid). The first urine sample was collected 180 min after the nitrate intake, and further collection of urine was pursued at 3-h intervals up to 24 h.

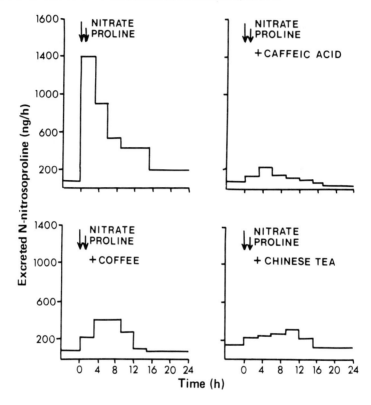

inhibitor of NPRO formation *in vivo* (Table 3; Fig. 2 B, C). Similar inhibition was brought about by Indian and Chinese teas (Table 3; Fig. 2D). Taken together, our results indicate that after ingestion of phenolic compounds or PPC-containing beverages, the amount of NPRO excreted is reduced by 50–80% of that excreted in control experiments. Since part of the NPRO excreted is derived from preformed dietary NPRO (which was not determined), the actual inhibition of NPRO formation in our experiments may be somewhat greater than that indicated in Table 3.

DISCUSSION

Our results indicate that the modifying effects (catalysis or inhibition) of phenolic constitutents depend not only on their structure but also on the pH, the relative concentration of nitrite *versus* phenolic compounds and on the nature of the nitrosatable amino compounds present. We found that PPC cause both catalysis and inhibition *in vivo*, although the effects were smaller than those observed *in vitro*. Because extrapolation of in-vitro kinetic data on nitrosation reactions to the situation occurring in the intact organism remains difficult, we gathered information by examining humans directly. Measurements of urinary NPRO following ingestion of nitrate and proline revealed that caffeic acid and ferulic acid exert a relatively strong inhibitory effect on nitrosation. Similarly, phenolic-containing beverages, like instant coffee, decaffeinated coffee and teas, reduce the levels of excreted NPRO. These inhibitory effects are most probably due to scavenging of nitrite by phenolics, which, at pH 2, dominated the nitrosation of proline. In our experiments (Table 3, Fig. 2), the amount of ingested phenolics probably exceeded that of nitrite present in the gastric juice, which may explain the absence of an enhancing effect; catalysis seems to occur only when the ratio of [nitrite]:[phenolics] was high enough (*in vitro*, Fig. 1C and Table 1, expt nos. 5, 6, 8, 10; and in rats *in vivo*, Table 2, expt nos. 4, 5, 7, 8). Similarly, a large excess of phenolic betel nut extract over that of nitrite led to an inhibition of NPRO formation both *in vitro* at pH 4 and pH 1.9 (Fig. 1 C, D), in rats *in vivo* (Table 2, expt no. 11) and in human subjects (Stich *et al.*, 1983).

Phenolics appear to exert their antimutagenic and anticarcinogenic effects in experimental animals, and possibly in man, by different mechanisms: (1) their nitrite-trapping capacity should protect against the induction of tumours that are induced by endogenously formed *N*-nitroso compounds; (2) they may interact with and inactivate electrophilic carcinogen-derived metabolites: it has been shown that ellagic, caffeic and ferulic acids block the mutagenicity of diol epoxides derived from polycyclic aromatic hydrocarbons (Wood *et al.*, 1982), (3) they may interfere with the metabolic activation reaction of carcinogens, i.e., 3-*tert*-butyl-4-hydroxyanisole inhibited the induction of stomach cancer by benzo[*a*]pyrene (BP) in mice probably by inhibiting its activation.

The observed inverse relationship between the amount of green-yellow vegetables consumed and incidences of cancer at several sites (Hirayama, 1966; Miller, 1982) is generally believed to be due to their contents of vitamins A and C. However, phenolic compounds could conceivably be partially responsible for this protective effect of vegetables: more than 60 mg caffeic acid and approximately 1 g flavonoids (Kühnau, 1976) are consumed daily in a 'regular' western diet; these quantities by far exceed the salivary nitrite swallowed normally by a healthy human subject during the course of one day. The effects of PPC on nitrosation in man can now be assessed using the NPRO method. Studies are currently under way in our laboratories to understand better the role of PPC as possible protective agents against certain types of cancers in man.

REFERENCES

Bogovski, P., Castegnaro, M., Pignatelli, B. & Walker, E.A. (1972) *The inhibiting effect of tannins on the formation of nitroso-amines.* In: Bogovski, P., Preussmann, R. & Walker, E.A., eds, N-*nitroso Compounds, Analysis and Formation (IARC Scientific Publications No. 3)*, Lyon, International Agency for Research on Cancer, pp. 127–129

Davies, R., Dennis, M.J., Massey, R.C. & McWeeney, D.J. (1978) *Some effects of phenol and thiol-nitrosation on N-nitrosamine formation.* In: Walker, E.A., Castegnaro, M., Griciute, L. & Lyle, R.E., eds, *Environmental Aspects of* N-*nitroso Compounds (IARC Scientific Publications No. 19)*, Lyon, International Agency for Research on Cancer, France, pp. 183–197

Gray, J.I. & Dugan, L.R. (1975) Inhibition of *N*-nitrosamine formation in model food system. *J. Food Sci., 40*, 981–984

Hirayama, T. (1966) An epidemiological study of oral and pharyngeal cancer in Central and South-East Asia. *Bull. World Health Org., 34*, 41–69

Jussawalla, D.J. (1976) The problem of cancer in India: an epidemiological assessment, *Gann, 18*, 265–273

Kawabata, T., Ohshima, H., Uibu, J., Nakamura, M., Matsui, M. & Hamano, M. (1979) *Occurrence, formation and precursors of N-nitroso compounds in Japanese diet.* In: Miller, E.C., Miller, J.A., Hirona,

J., Sugimura, T. & Takayama, S., eds, *Naturally Occuring Carcinogens-Mutagens and Modulators of Carcinogenesis,* Japanese Scientific Society Press, Tokyo/Baltimore, University Park Press, pp. 195–209

Kühnau, J. (1976) The flavonoids. A class of semi-essential food components: their role in human nutrition. *World Rev. Nutrit. Diet, 24,* 117–191

Miller, A.B. (1982) *Nutritional aspects of human carcinogenesis.* In: Bartsch, H. & Armstrong, B., eds, *Host Factors in Human Carcinogenesis (IARC Scientific Publications No. 39),* Lyon, International Agency for Research on Cancer, pp. 177–192

Muir, C.S. & Kirk, R. (1960) Betel, tobacco, and cancer of the mouth. *Br J. Cancer, 14,* 597–608

Ohshima, H. & Bartsch, H. (1981) Quantitative estimation of endogenous nitrosation in man by monitoring *N*-nitrosoproline excreted in the urine. *Cancer Res., 41,* 3658–3662

Ohshima, H., Béréziat, J.C. & Bartsch, H. (1982) Monitoring *N*-nitrosamino acids excreted in the urine and feces of rats as an index of endogenous nitrosation. *Carcinogenesis, 3,* 115–122

Pignatelli, B., Friesen, M.D. & Walker, E.A. (1980) *The role of phenols in catalysis of nitrosamine formation.* In: Walker, E.A., Griciute, L., Castegnaro, M. & Börzsönyi, M., eds, N-*Nitroso Compounds: Analysis, Formation and Occurrence (IARC Scientific Publications No. 31),* Lyon, International Agency for Research on Cancer, pp. 95–109

Pignatelli, B., Béréziat, J.C., Descotes, G. & Bartsch, H. (1982) Catalysis of nitrosation *in vitro* and *in vivo* in rats by catechin and resorcinol and inhibition by chlorogenic acid. *Carcinogenesis, 3,* 1045–1049

Pignatelli, B., Scriban, R., Descotes, G. & Bartsch, H. (1983) Inhibition of endogenous nitrosation of proline in rats by lyophilized beer constituents. *Carcinogenesis, 4,* 491–494

Stich, H.F., Rosin, M.P. & Bryson, L. (1982a) Inhibition of mutagenicity of a model nitrosation reaction by naturally occurring phenolics, coffee and tea. *Mutat. Res., 95,* 119–128

Stich, H.F., Chan, K.L. & Rosin, P. (1982b) Inhibitory effects of phenolics, teas and saliva on the formation of mutagenic nitrosation products of salted fish. *Int. J. Cancer, 30,* 719–724

Stich, H.F., Ohshima, H., Pignatelli, B. & Bartsch, H. (1983) Inhibitory effect of betel nut extracts on endogenous nitrosation in man. *J. natl Cancer Inst., 70,* 1047–1050

Wenke, G. & Hoffmann, D. (1983) A study of betel quid carcinogenesis. 1. On the *in vitro N*-nitrosation of arecoline. *Carcinogenesis, 4,* 169–172

Wood, A.W., Huang, T.-T., Chang, R.L., Newmark, H.L., Lehr, R.E., Yagi, H., Sayer, J.M., Jerina, D.M. & Conney, A.H. (1982) Inhibition of the mutagenicity of bay-region diol epoxides of polycyclic aromatic hydrocarbons by naturally occuring plant phenols: exceptional activity of ellagic acid. *Proc. natl Acad. Sci. USA, 79,* 5513–5517

MODULATION OF ENDOGENOUS SYNTHESIS OF *N*-NITROSAMINO ACIDS IN HUMANS

D.A. WAGNER, D.E.G. SHUKER, C. BILMAZES, M. OBIEDZINSKI, V.R. YOUNG & S.R. TANNENBAUM

Department of Nutrition and Food Science, Massachusetts Institute of Technology, Cambridge, MA, USA

SUMMARY

Endogenous production of *N*-nitrosoproline (NPRO) was demonstrated in human subjects ingesting a diet low in nitrate and NPRO. The daily endogenous synthesis of NPRO was 26 ± 10 nmol/day (mean $\pm$ SD). Upon administration of nitrate and proline, the NPRO excreted in urine ranged from 50–318 nmol/24 h. It was found that ascorbic acid and α-tocopherol did not lower the background endogenous synthesis of NPRO; however, ascorbic acid was very effective in preventing the nitrate-induced synthesis of NPRO in all subjects, while α-tocopherol was less effective in some subjects. Furthermore, it was demonstrated that administered ^{15}N-nitrate could be incorporated into NPRO, suggesting clearly that nitrosation reactions indeed occur in humans. Ascorbic acid significantly inhibited the incorporation of ^{15}N-nitrate into NPRO. The presence of another *N*-nitrosamino acid, *N*-nitrosothiazolidine-4-carboxylic acid (NTCA), was detected in the urine of many subjects even without nitrate intake. However, upon ingestion of nitrate, there was a six-fold increase in mean NTCA synthesis (25 ± 16 nmol/24 h), and all subjects had detectable levels of NTCA in the urine. Ascorbic acid completely blocked the nitrate-induced synthesis of NTCA, while α-tocopherol was not as effective.

INTRODUCTION

In recent years, growing attention has been focused on *N*-nitrosamines as causative agents in the induction of human cancer. Various attempts have been made to demonstrate in-vivo production of *N*-nitrosamines in humans. Following a meal of cooked bacon, spinach, tomatoes, bread and beer, volatile nitrosamines were reported in the blood of a human volunteer (Fine *et al.*, 1977). Wang *et al.* (1978) detected volatile *N*-nitroso compounds in human faecal material and suggested that they are produced in the lower gastrointestinal tract. Other workers have reported the presence of volatile nitrosamines in urine and blood of healthy volunteers (Kakizoe *et al.*, 1979; Lakritz *et al.*, 1980). However, all of these in-vivo determinations of *N*-nitrosamines have been shown to be potentially susceptible to analytical artefacts (Eisenbrand *et al.*, 1981; Lee *et al.*, 1981; Garland *et al.*, 1982).

The best technique used to date for determining in-vivo nitrosamine formation in humans is measurement of the nonvolatile nitrosamine, N-nitrosoproline (NPRO), in urine. Ohshima and Bartsch (1981) and Ohshima et al. (1982) and, more recently, Wagner et al., (1982) administered nitrate, followed by proline, to human volunteers and measured significant levels of NPRO in urine. This approach has been successful because NPRO is not metabolized to any extent (Chu & Magee, 1981), is stable and nonvolatile during analytical clean-up, is found in relatively high levels in urine, and is not a carcinogen (Mirvish et al., 1980). Therefore, NPRO excretion in urine can be used as a quantitative indicator of the amount of N-nitrosation in vivo.

We now report on additional experiments with human subjects which have been conducted to extend our original observations and to observe the effect of N-nitrosation blocking agents such as ascorbic acid and α-tocopherol. Experiments have been conducted to determine the extent of incorporation of $^{15}NO_3$ into NPRO in these subjects, using low-resolution mass fragmentography in conjunction with capillary gas chromatography. The use of ^{15}N as a tracer allows a clear-cut distinction between intragastric synthesis of NPRO and other contributions to urinary excretion. Results are also presented on the occurrence and modulation of another urinary compound, N-nitrosothiazolidine-4-carboxylic acid (NTCA).

METHODS

Subjects and diets

The subjects participating on these studies were students at the Massachusetts Institute of Technology, ranging in age from 19 to 27 years old. All subjects were judged to be healthy on the basis of a thorough physical examination and routine blood and urine analyses. Throughout the study, subjects were fed a controlled, low-nitrate diet, consisting of an egg omelette and liquid soya and milk formula. In initial studies, dried eggs were used, but they were replaced by fresh eggs, since analysis of the dried eggs showed a high concentration of NPRO. The liquid formula and egg omelette supplied 2 000 calories per day for a 70-kg man; the remaining calories were derived from protein-free cookies, cornstarch dessert and sucrose beverages. Each subject consumed a diet to meet all vitamin and trace mineral requirements on the basis of National Academy of Sciences/National Research Council recommendations.

NPRO analysis in urine

Twenty-four-hour urine collections were preserved with absolute ethanol (100 mL), dibasic sodium phosphate (10 g) and sodium bisulfite (1.5 g) and stored frozen ($-20\,°C$) to prevent bacterial growth and artefactual N-nitrosamine formation. NPRO was extracted from urine samples by methods described previously in detail (Wagner et al., 1982).

N-nitrosopipecolic acid (NPIC) was added as an internal standard to an aliquot of urine before analysis. The urine extract was derivatized with diazomethane to form the methyl ester of NPRO and NPIC and analysed by gas chromatography coupled with a Thermal Energy Analyzer (TEA). The retention times of NPRO methyl ester and NPIC methyl ester were 5 min and 4 min, respectively, on a 2-m column packed with 3% OV-225 on 100/120 Supelcoport (Supelco, Bellefonte, PA, USA) operating at 135 °C isothermally with a helium flow rate of 25 mL/min.

NTCA analysis in urine

We had found that while analysing urine samples for NPRO, an additional peak was detected on the TEA chromatogram. Since learning that Ohshima et al. (1983) and Tsuda et al. (1983)

had identified NTCA in human urine, we have confirmed the presence of this unknown peak on the TEA chromatogram as NTCA. The NTCA methyl ester had a retention time of 6 min on the column used for NPRO analysis.

^{15}N-NPRO analysis

In addition to the steps used to extract NPRO from urine for total NPRO analysis, urine samples underwent additional clean-up steps for mass fragmentographic analysis. This included passing samples through an anion exchange column (10 cm x 1 cm, Dowex 1, 200–400 mesh, formate form) and eluting NPRO with 60 mL 1N hydrochloric acid. Then, two high-performance liquid chromatographic steps were used to further separate NPRO from other organic acids in urine. Samples were first chromatographed on an amino column (250 mm × 5 mm), mobile phase, 2 mmol/L ammonium formate with 5% acetonitrile (pH 5), and then through a C18 column (150 mm × 5 mm), mobile phase 5 mmol/L ammonium formate with 1% acetonitrile (pH 3). NPRO was detected at a wavelength of 245 nm. Samples were methylated with diazomethane and then analysed by selected ion monitoring of m/z = 99 and m/z = 100 using a Hewlett Packard GC/MS (HP 5992) with a 35-m glass capillary column (Carbowax 20M). A complete mass spectrum of the urine sample was used to identify the peak of NPRO.

Experimental protocol

Two studies were carried out to observe the effect of nitrosation blocking agents on NPRO synthesis. In the first study, six subjects were placed on the low-nitrate diet described above and urine collected for five consecutive days. The dietary intake of ascorbic acid during this part of the study was 60 mg. On the sixth day of the study, on a fasted stomach, subjects were administered orally 3.5 mmol sodium ^{15}N-nitrate (99% ^{15}N) in 10 mL distilled water, followed by 200 mL water. One hour later, 4.3 mmol L-proline was administered in 10 mL water. Urine was collected for the following 48 h. A break period of one week from the low-nitrate diet followed, but subjects were administered 2 g ascorbic acid (500 mg tablets, four times per day). Following the break period, subjects were again placed on the low-nitrate diet but continued to consume 2 g ascorbic acid for one week. After five days, nitrate and proline were administered as described above; one 500-mg ascorbic acid tablet was administered with the nitrate, and three additional tablets were taken throughout the remainder of the day. A second study was conducted exactly as the first, except that four subjects were used and 400 mg α-tocopherol were included in the diet during the second phase of the study. When nitrate and proline was administered, α-tocopherol was administered one-half hour before administration of proline. The results obtained in the control periods of the two studies are combined in the results to increase the number of data points.

RESULTS

The first, surprising result was that with a low-nitrate diet (< 150 μmol/day), basal excretion of NPRO ranged from 5–49 nmol/day, with a mean excretion of 26 ± 10 nmol/day (Fig. 1). This basal excretion represents endogenous synthesis of NPRO, since the amount of NPRO in the diet had been subtracted from the total amount of NPRO found in the urine. In general, each subject excreted a relatively constant amount of NPRO per day. Upon administration of nitrate and proline, a significant rise in the excretion of NPRO was observed, ranging from 50–318 nmol/24 h, with a mean of 100 ± 81 nmol/24 h.

Fig. 1 Endogenous synthesis of N-nitrosoproline (NPRO) (Total urinary excretion – dietary NPRO) during three
     different dietary regime (mean ± SD)

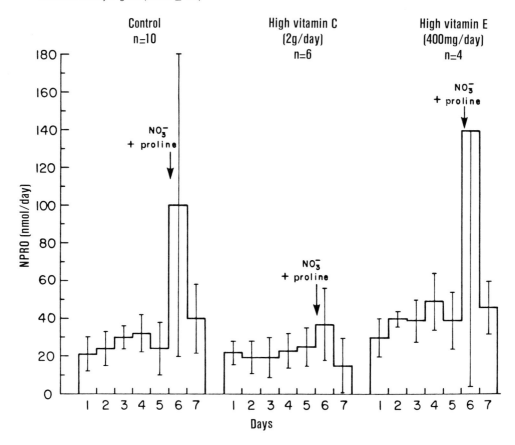

Administration of 2 g ascorbic acid or 400 mg α-tocopherol in the diet had no effect on the
background endogenous synthesis of NPRO (Fig. 1). However, when ascorbic acid was
administered with nitrate and proline, there was a significant decline in NPRO production, with
essentially complete inhibition of nitrate-induced NPRO synthesis. The mean excretion of
NPRO after nitrate and proline administration with ascorbic acid was 37 ± 19 nmol/24 h; but
α-trocopherol was not as effective in blocking nitrate-induced NPRO synthesis: complete
inhibition was seen in two subjects and none in the other two. This explains the large standard
deviation shown in Figure 1 during the α-tocopherol phase with administration of nitrate and
proline.

    Incorporation of ^{15}N-nitrate into NPRO was demonstrated by gas chromatograph-mass
sprectroscopy (Table 1). During the control period (low ascorbic acid in the diet), the amount
of ^{15}N-NPRO synthesis after nitrate and proline intake ranged from 3.86–43.7 nmol/24 h. In
contrast, after inclusion of ascorbic acid in the diet and following nitrate and proline
administration, the amount of ^{15}N-NPRO was significantly less, ranging from 0–8.67
nmol/24 h, and every subject showed inhibition of incorporation of ^{15}N-nitrate into NPRO.
Background endogenous synthesis of ^{14}N-NPRO was not effected by ascorbic acid treatment.

Table 1. Incorporation of ¹⁵N-nitrate into *N*-nitrosoproline (NPRO): Effect of ascorbic acid on NPRO synthesis induced by nitrate and proline

Subject no.	nmol/24 h			
	Total NPRO		¹⁵N-NPRO	
	low C [a]	high C [a]	low C	high C
1	29.0	27.0	3.86	1.84
2	49.1	17.9	9.94	0.57
3	84.2	13.2	43.7	0.00
4	50.5	61.3	14.9	8.67
5	55.6	43.2	13.4	0.57
6	77.9	36.5	36.5	0.19

[a] Low C diet consisted of 60 mg/day ascorbic acid, and high C diet consisted of 2 g/day

Fig. 2 Excretion of *N*-nitrosothiazolidine-4-carboxylic acid (NTCA) in urine during three different dietary regimes (mean ± SD)

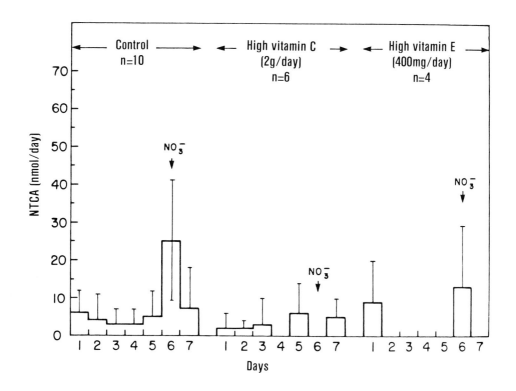

Analysis of the urine samples for NTCA showed a background level of this nitrosoamino acid (Fig. 2), which could not be accounted for by dietary intake. The mean excretion of NTCA was 4.2 ± 5.2 nmol/day. Not every subject on a low-nitrate diet excreted a detectable level of NTCA in urine, but, upon ingestion of nitrate, every subject excreted NTCA. Overall, there was a six-fold increase in NTCA synthesis with nitrate administration (25 ± 16 nmol/24 h).

Administration of ascorbic acid in the diet did not change the endogenous background level of NTCA in urine; however, ascorbic acid completely blocked nitrate-induced synthesis of NTCA (Fig. 2). The high-vitamin E diet appeared to be able to block the endogenous background production of NTCA, since NTCA was detected only on the first day in subjects on this diet. α-Tocopherol was not as effective in some subjects as ascorbic acid in blocking nitrate-induced synthesis of NTCA; in fact, the same two subjects in which α-tocopherol was ineffective in inhibiting NPRO synthesis also continued to synthesize high levels of NTCA following administration of nitrate.

DISCUSSION

Significant levels of NPRO were excreted in the urine of subjects ingesting a low-nitrate diet. Therefore, endogenous biosynthesis of NPRO occurs in humans, and this may be linked to endogenous production of nitrate in humans, previously reported by our group (Green et al., 1981). It is unclear where the endogenous synthesis of NPRO takes place. Although nitrate produced in the body is recirculated to the salivary glands and reduced to nitrite by bacteria in the oral cavity, exposing the stomach to nitrite and thus making it capable of participating in nitrosation reaction, it might be expected that ascorbic acid and/or α-tocopherol would inhibit the production of NPRO by this route. However, we found that inclusion of high amounts of either ascorbic acid or α-tocopherol in the diet did not lower the amount of endogenous NPRO appearing in urine (no nitrate and proline taken). Therefore, either endogenous NPRO synthesis occurs in the stomach at times when ascorbate or tocopherol is not present or there is nongastric synthesis of NPRO. The use of labelled proline, administered intravenously, may answer this question.

The demonstration of incorporation of ^{15}N-nitrate into NPRO shows clearly that a precursor-product relationship is conducted via N-nitrosation reactions. Furthermore, we found that ascorbic acid could block the incorporation of ^{15}N-nitrate into NPRO. There was a mean inhibition of ^{15}N-NPRO synthesis of 81% and four of six subjects had greater than 95% inhibition. The finding that α-tocopherol was not as effective a nitrosation inhibitor as ascorbic acid under the protocol used in these experiments may be explained by the different dosing regiments, which permitted ten times as much ascorbic acid as tocopherol to be administered. These doses were determined on the basis of known tolerance and clinical experience with these two vitamins. Similar results have been reported by Ohshima and Bartsch (1981). Additional studies on more subjects with different doses will be necessary to reach a firm conclusion.

The finding of an additional N-nitrosamino acid in human urine, NTCA, presents another analytical tool for assessing in-vivo nitrosation reactions. We have found that, upon ingestion of nitrate, the level of NTCA in urine is significantly increased. Ascorbic acid blocks this nitrate-induced increase, while α-tocopherol is not as effective.

We believe that this methodology is suitable for estimating in-vivo formation of N-nitrosamines in humans. It also allows the study of other possible nitrosation inhibitors that occur naturally in the diet (Pignatelli et al., 1982). Furthermore, the methodology may give valuable insight when constructing dietary intervention programmes in areas of high cancer risk.

ACKNOWLEDGEMENT

This investigation was supported by PHS Grant Number NCI-1-PO1-CA26731-04, awarded by the US National Cancer Institute, DHHS.

REFERENCES

Chu, C. & Magee, P.N. (1981) The metabolic fate of nitrosoproline in the rat. *Cancer Res.,* **41,** 3653–3657

Eisenbrand, G., Speigelhalder, B. & Preussmann, R. (1981) *Analysis of human biological specimens for nitrosamine contents.* In: Bruce, W.R., Correa, P., Lipkin, M., Tannenbaum, S.R. & Wilkin, T.D., eds, *Gastrointestinal cancer: Endogenous Factors (Banbury Report No. 7),* Cold Spring Harbor, NY, Cold Spring Harbor Laboratory, pp. 275–283

Fine, D.H., Ross, R., Rounbehler, D.P., Silvergleid, A. & Song, L. (1977) Formation *in vivo* of volatile *N*-nitrosamines in man after ingestion of cooked bacon and spinach. *Nature,* **265,** 753–755

Garland, W.A., Holowarchenko, H., Kunezig, W., Norkus, E.P. & Conney, A.H. (1982) *A high resolution mass spectrometry assay for N-nitrosodimethylamine in human plasma.* In: Magee, P.N., ed., *Nitrosamines and Human Cancer (Banbury Report No. 12),* Cold Spring Harbor, NY, Cold Spring Harbor Laboratory, pp. 183–196

Green, L.C., Ruiz de Luzuriaga, K., Wagner, D.A., Rand, W., Istfan, N., Young, V.R. & Tannenbaum, S.R. (1981) Nitrate biosynthesis in man. *Proc. natl Acad. Sci. USA,* **78,** 7764–7768

Kakizoe, T., Wang, T.T., Eng. W.S., Furrer, R., Dion, P. & Bruce, W.R. (1979) Volatile N-nitrosamines in the urine of normal donors and of bladder cancer patients. *Cancer Res.,* **39,** 829–832

Lakritz, L., Simenhoff, M.L., Dunn, S.R. & Fiddler, W. (1980) N-Nitrosodimethylamine in human blood. *Food Cosmet. Toxicol.,* **18,** 77–79

Lee, L., Archer, M.C. & Bruce, W.R. (1981) Absence of volatile nitrosamines in human faeces. *Cancer Res.,* **41,** 3992–3994

Mirvish, S.S., Bulay, O., Runge, R.G. & Patil, K. (1980) Study of the carcinogenicity of large doses of dimethylnitramine, *N*-nitroso-L-proline, and sodium nitrite administered in drinking water to rats. *J. natl Cancer Inst.,* **64,** 1435–1442

Ohshima, H. & Bartsch, H. (1981) Quantitative estimation of endogenous nitrosation in humans by monitoring *N*-nitrosoproline excreted in the urine. *Cancer Res.,* **41,** 3658–3662

Ohshima, H., Pignatelli, B. & Bartsch, H. (1982) *Monitoring of excreted N-nitrosamino acids as a new method to quantitate endogenous nitrosation in humans.* In: Magee, P.N., ed., *Nitrosamines and Human Cancer (Banbury Report No. 12),* Cold Spring Harbor, NY, Cold Spring Harbor Laboratory, pp. 287–318

Ohshima, H., Friesen, M., O'Neill, I.K. & Bartsch, H. (1982) Presence in human urine of a new *N*-nitroso compound, *N*-nitrosothiazolidine-4-carboxylic acid. *Cancer Lett.,* **20,** 183–190

Pignatelli, B., Béréziat, J.C., Descotes, G. & Bartsch, H. (1982) Catalysis of nitrosation *in vitro* and *in vivo* in rats by catechin and resorcinol and inhibition by chlorogenic acid. *Carcinogenesis,* **3,** 1045–1049

Tsuda, M., Hirayama, T. & Sugimura, T. (1983) Presence of *N*-nitroso-L-thioproline and *N*-nitroso-L-methylthioprolines in human urine as major *N*-nitroso compounds. *Gann,* **74,** 331–333

Wagner, D.A., Shuker, D.E.G., Hasic, G. & Tannenbaum, S.R. (1982) *Endogenous nitrosoproline synthesis in humans.* In: Magee, P.N., ed. *Nitrosamines and Human Cancer (Banbury Report No. 12),* Cold Spring Harbor, NY, Cold Spring Harbor Laboratory, pp. 319–333

Wang, T., Kakizoe, T., Dion, P., Furrer, R., Varghese, A.J. & Bruce, W.R. (1978) Volatile nitrosamines in normal human faeces. *Nature,* **276,** 280–281

THE BLOCKING EFFECTS OF CHINESE *ACTINIDIA SINENSIS* JUICE ON *N*-NITROSAMINE FORMATION *IN VITRO* AND *IN VIVO*

SONG PUJU, ZHANG LIN, LI YINZENG & DING LAN

*Department of Nutrition and Food Hygiene, Beijing Medical College, Beijing,
People's Republic of China*

S.R. TANNENBAUM[1] & J.S. WISHNOK

*Department of Nutrition and Food Science, Massachusetts Institute of Technology, Cambridge,
MA 02139, USA*

SUMMARY

Chinese gooseberry juice has been found to be an efficient inhibitor of nitrosation both *in vitro* and *in vivo*. This activity appears to be due partly to high concentrations of ascorbic acid and partly to an unidentified nitrite scavenger.

INTRODUCTION

Several authors have reported on the inhibitory effects of ascorbic acid and α-tocopherol on nitrosation reactions. Mirvish *et al.* (1972), Mirvish (1975) and Kamm *et al.* (1974) have shown that ascorbic acid blocks nitrosamine formation both *in vivo* and *in vitro*. Mergens *et al.* (1978, 1980) demonstrated similar effects with α-tocopherol. *Actinidia sinensis* Planch (Chinese gooseberry or kiwi fruit), a wild fruit originally found in China, is rich in ascorbic acid and other nutrients (Selman, 1983). The work reported here was undertaken to evaluate the possible role of the juice of this fruit as an inhibitor of nitrosamine formation.

MATERIALS AND METHODS

Sample preparation: Chinese gooseberry juice was produced by a factory in the People's Republic of China. Lemon juice was purchased in a supermarket in Boston, MA, USA. The juices were centrifuged at $10\,000 \times g$ for 10 min to remove pulp and other particulate matter. Solutions of L-ascorbic acid were prepared in citrate-phosphate buffer at concentrations

---

[1] To whom correspondence should be addressed

equivalent to those found in the Chinese juice. The pH of the Chinese juice was typically between 3.16–3.40, so the lemon juice (initial pH, 2.26–2.68), ascorbic acid solutions and buffer solutions were adjusted to pHs within that range prior to reaction. High-performance liquid chromatography or titrimetry (Sichuan Medical College, 1980) was employed for the determination of ascorbic acid concentrations. The ascorbic acid in some samples (see below) was destroyed by treatment with ascorbic acid oxidase in the presence of air.

Nitrosation of morpholine: Morpholine (stock solutions) was added to 5 mL of juice, ascorbic acid solution or buffer solution in a stoppered vial to give a final morpholine concentration of 2.0 mmol/L. The reactions were started by the addition of sufficient sodium nitrate to yield a concentration of 2.0 mmol/L and reaction mixtures were incubated at 37 °C for 1 or 2 h. The reactions were stopped by the addition of a large excess of ammonium sulfamate along with sufficient sulfuric acid to lower the pH to below 3. The reaction mixtures were allowed to stand for 15 min. Sodium hydroxide was used to bring the pH up to 5 for the extraction of *N*-nitrosomorpholine with methylene chloride (3 × 3 mL). The combined extracts were dried over anhydrous sodium sulfate and then concentrated to 2–3 mL with a stream of nitrogen. Analysis was carried out by gas chromatography, (Carbowax 20M/TPA/KOH at 175 °C) with a nitrosamine-specific Thermal Energy Analyzer as the detector (Fine & Rounbehler, 1975).

Nitrosation of aminopyrine: A model system simulating the conditions known to exist in the stomach (pH 3.3, 37 °C) was used in these experiments. Various concentrations of sodium nitrite and aminopyrine were incubated with Chinese juice, ascorbic acid solution or buffer solution for 1 h. Aliquots (0.1 mL) were then assayed for mutagenicity by standard methods (Ames *et al.*, 1975). *Salmonella typhimurium* strain TA100 was used for the detection of mutagenic activity due presumably to the formation of an *N*-nitroso mutagen from the reaction of sodium nitrite with aminopyrine (Lijinsky, 1979). Test samples and bacteria, with or without a metabolic activation system, were mixed with molten top agar and poured onto minimal agar plates. At least a two-fold increase in the number of induced revertants over the historical background of spontaneous revertants was required in order for a sample to be considered mutagenic (Skopek *et al.*, 1978).

Reaction of nitrite with juice: Sodium nitrite (1 mol/L stock solution) was added to Chinese juice, lemon juice, ascorbic acid solution or buffer solution to give a nitrite concentration of 2.0 mmol/L. Samples were taken at 0, 15, 30, 60, 120 and 180 min, and the nitrite concentrations were determined using Griess reagent.

Male Wistar rats, weighing 160–180 g, were distributed randomly into six groups of eight animals and dosed as shown in Table 1.

Table 1.   Dosing protocol[a]

Group	Sodium nitrite (mg/kg)	Aminopyrine (mg/kg)	Chinese juice (mL)	Ascorbic acid (mL)
1	19	19	–	–
2	19	19	3	–
3	19	19	–	3
4	19	–	–	–
5	–	19	–	–
6	–	–	–	–

[a] Animals were given the chemicals and juice by gavage twice a day over a period of 60 h and killed 7 h after the last dose. Serum glutamic-pyruvic transaminase was determined using standard procedures (Shanghai Medical Analytical Institute, 1979), and the livers were examined microscopically

RESULTS

The mean ascorbic acid content in Chinese juice was 254 (range, 215–384) mg/mL, and that of commercial lemon juice was 37 (range, 21–68) mg/mL. The pH ranges were 3.16–3.40 and 2.26–2.68 for Chinese juice and lemon juice, respectively.

The results suggest that the Chinese juice in the most effective of these compounds as a nitrosation inhibitor. The ascorbic acid present in the juice may contribute to this effect during the first hour, but – as can be seen in Table 2 – ascorbic acid is not effective during the second hour of reaction, while the effects of the Chinese juice do not change significantly during that period. In addition, the inhibitory properties of the Chinese juice are less strongly diminished by oxidation of the ascorbic acid than are those of the other compounds.

Nitrosation of morpholine

The results of these experiments are summarized in Table 2.

Reaction of nitrite with juice

Changes in the concentration of nitrite added to Chinese gooseberry juice, lemon juice and ascorbic acid solution were followed for 3 h: approximately 40% of the nitrite disappeared during the first 60 min in all three systems, i.e., the rates were indistinguishable during this period. After 180 min, however, somewhat more nitrite remained in the lemon juice and ascorbic acid solution (approximately 20%) than in the Chinese gooseberry juice (approximately 5%), but the difference was not dramatic. These results suggest that destruction of nitrite during the first hour or so is due largely to the presence of ascorbic acid in the juices. This conclusion would be consistent with the data shown in Table 2.

Nitrosation of aminopyrine

The results of these experiments are detailed in Table 3.

Table 2. Effect of fruit juice on the nitrosation of morpholine[a]

	N-Nitrosomorpholine (ppb)			% Inhibition		
	0.5 h	1.0 h	2.0 h	0.5 h	1.0 h	2.0 h
Chinese juice	19	62	78	99	96	98
Lemon juice	200	1 120	2 430	85	35	37
Ascorbic acid	32	182	1 336	98	89	66
Chinese juice (oxidized)	126	200	783	90	88	80
Lemon juice (oxidized)	453	1 556	1 920	65	10	51
Ascorbic acid (oxidized)	–	–	3 027	–	–	22
Buffer solution	1 300	1 732	3 885	–	–	–

[a] pH 3.13–3.28; 37 °C; ascorbic acid concentration of Chinese juice and ascorbic acid solution, 88.5 mg/mL; that of lemon juice, 21.2 mg/mL

Table 3. Nitrosation of aminopyrine-nitrite reaction mixtures

Test chemicals	Mutant ratio[a]				
	Concentration of aminopyrine-nitrite (mg/mL)				
	1.0	2.0	4.0	5.0	8.0
Aminopyrine-nitrite	1.14	1.21	1.85	2.44	2.43
Aminopyrine-nitrite (+ Chinese juice)	1.00	1.21	1.15	1.35	1.65
Aminopyrine-nitrite (+ ascorbic acid)	1.11	1.51	1.44	2.38	–

[a]Ratio of induced: spontaneous revertants; mean number of spontaneous revertants/plate was 187.2

Fig. 1. Reaction of juices with 30 mL of 1 mol/L sodium nitrite at 37 °C; pH, 3.13–3.24. ▲, ascorbic acid solution (15 mL); △, lemon juice (15 mL); ●, dilute Chinese juice (15 mL); ○, 0.3% citric acid solution (15 mL)

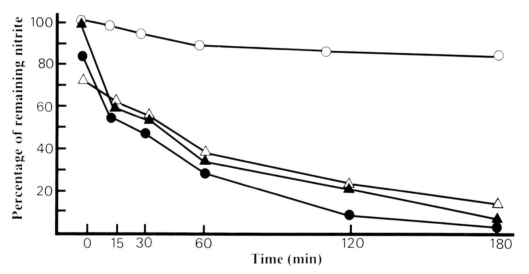

In-vivo inhibition of nitrosation

Pathological examination of the livers and the activity of serum glutamic-pyruvic transaminase of treated rats indicated that the Chinese gooseberry juice prevented or regressed hepatic lesions due apparently to the formation of N-nitroso compounds from aminopyrine and nitrite; transaminase activity remained normal when the juice was co-administered with those compounds. In the group not given the juice, body weight was reduced, centrilobular hepatic necrosis developed and serum glutamic-pyruvic transaminase increased. There was no observable changes in these characteristics among rats administered aminopyrine or sodium nitrite alone. The ascorbic acid solutions were significantly less effective than was the Chinese gooseberry juice.

CONCLUSIONS

The results described above suggest that Chinese gooseberry juice can inhibit the formation of *N*-nitroso compounds from sodium nitrite and aminopyrine or morpholine, both *in vivo* and *in vitro*. This effect appears to be due at least partly to a rapid reaction with nitrite or with one of the nitrosating species arising from nitrite. Both the rate and extent of destruction of nitrite by the Chinese gooseberry juice are greater than can be accounted for by the amount of ascorbic acid present in the juice, indicating the existence of one or more active substances other than ascorbic acid.

ACKNOWLEDGEMENTS

This investigation was supported by the World Health Organization and by PHS Grant Number 1-PO1-CA26731-04 awarded by the National Cancer Institute, DHHS. We thank Beijing Medical College, People's Republic of China, for samples of Chinese gooseberry juice, and Dr Yen-Ping Chin-Hsieh and Mr Walter W. Bishop for experimental assistance.

REFERENCES

Ames, B.N., McCann, J. & Yamasaki, E. (1975) Methods for detecting carcinogens and mutagens with the *Salmonella*/mammalian-microsome mutagenicity test. *Mutat. Res., 31*, 347–364

Fine, D.H. & Rounbehler, D.P. (1975) Trace analysis of volatile *N*-nitroso compounds by combined gas chromatography and thermal energy analysis. *J. Chromatogr., 109*, 271–279

Kamm, J.J., Dashman, T., Conney, A.H. & Burns, J.J. (1974) *The effect of ascorbate on amine-nitrite hepatoxicity*. In: Bogovski, P. & Walker, E.A., eds, N-*Nitroso Compounds in the Environment, (IARC Scientific Publications No. 9)*, Lyon, International Agency for Research on Cancer, pp. 200–204

Lijinsky, W.J. (1979) N-*Nitrosamines as environmental carcinogens*. In: Anselme, J.-P., ed., N-*Nitrosamines (ACS Symposium Series No. 101)*, Washington DC, American Chemical Society, pp. 165–173

Mergens, W.J., Kamm, J.J. & Newmark, H.L. (1978) *Alpha-tocopherol: uses in preventing nitrosamine formation*. In: Walker, E.A., Castegnaro, M., Griciute, L. & Lyle, R.E., eds, *Environmental Aspects of* N-*Nitroso Compounds, (IARC Scientific Publications No. 19)*, Lyon, International Agency for Research on Cancer, pp. 199–212

Mergens, W.J., Chau, J. & Newmark, H.L. (1980) *The influence of ascorbic acid and DL-a-tocopherol on the formation of nitrosamines in vitro gastrointestinal model system*. In: Walker, E.A., Griciute, L., Castegnaro, M. & Börzsönyi, M., eds, N-*Nitroso Compounds: Analysis, Formation and Occurrence (IARC Scientific Publications No. 31)*, Lyon, International Agency for Research on Cancer, pp. 259–267

Mirvish, S.S. (1975) Blocking the formation of *N*-nitroso compounds with ascorbic acid *in vitro* and *in vivo*. *Ann. N.Y. Acad. Sci., 258*, 175–180

Mirvish, S.S., Walcave, L., Eagen, M. & Shubik, P. (1972) Ascorbate-nitrite reaction: possible means of blocking the formation of carcinogenic *N*-nitroso compounds. *Science, 177*, 65–68

Selman, J.D. (1983) The vitamin C content of some kiwi fruits (*Actinidia sinensis* Planch., var. Hayward). *Food Chem., 11*, 63–75

Shanghai Medical Analytical Institute (1979) *Analysis of serum glutamic pyruvic transminase*. In: *Clinic Biochemical Analysis,* Shanghai, Shanghai Scientific Publisher, p. 332

Sichuan Medical College (1980) *Analysis of ascorbic acid*. In: *The Instruction Manual of Nutrition and Food Hygiene Analysis*

Skopek, T.R., Liber, H.L., Krolewski, J.J. & Thilly, W.G. (1975) Quantitative forward mutation assay in *Salmonella typhimurium* using –azaguanine resistance as a genetic marker. *Proc. natl Acad. Sci. USA, 75*, 410–414

EXPERIMENTAL MODEL FOR EVALUATING ANIMAL EXPOSURE TO ENDOGENOUS N-NITROSODI-n-BUTYLAMINE BY MEASURING ITS URINARY METABOLITES N-BUTYL-N-(4-HYDROXYBUTYL)-NITROSAMINE AND N-BUTYL-N-(3-CARBOXYPROPYL)NITROSAMINE

L. AIROLDI, C. SPAGONE, A. MACRI & R. FANELLI

Laboratory of Environmental Pharmacology and Toxicology
Istituto di Ricerche Farmacologiche Mario Negri
Via Eritrea 62, 20157 Milano, Italy

SUMMARY

Endogenous formation of N-nitrosodi-n-butylamine (NDBA) was studied in rats after administration of sodium nitrite or sodium nitrate and N,N-dibutylamine (DBA) by monitoring the urinary excretion of NDBA and its metabolites, N-butyl-N-(4-hydroxybutyl)-nitrosamine (BBN) and N-butyl-N-(3-carboxypropyl)nitrosamine (BCPN).

Animals were given sodium nitrite (0.2%) or sodium nitrate (0.5%), dissolved in the drinking-water. This treatment was started 24 h before DBA administration and was continued throughout the experiment. Animals were fasted overnight before receiving DBA, which was administered by gavage as three doses of 50 mg/kg, 8 h apart; 24-h urine samples were collected on ammonium sulfamate. NDBA, BBN and BCPN were extracted and analysed by GC-TEA, according to a method previously described.

Under the experimental conditions reported, NDBA and BBN (free or glucuronic acid-conjugated) were not detected in the urine of animals given nitrite or nitrate and DBA, but the presence of BCPN indicated that N-nitrosation had occurred in both groups of animals.

These results suggest that, when studying nitrosamines that are extensively metabolized, quantitative analysis of urinary metabolites is a better indicator of nitrosamine exposure than measurement of nitrosamine itself.

INTRODUCTION

N-Nitroso compounds are known to be formed *in vivo* in animals and humans (Fine, 1977; Lijinsky & Taylor, 1977) and it is accepted that exposure to endogenous N-nitroso compounds represents as great a risk for human health as exposure to exogenous ones. In order to assess this risk, Ohshima and Bartsch (1981) and Ohshima *et al.* (1982) developed a method for studying in-vivo nitrosation in humans and rats by measuring the urinary excretion of N-nitrosoproline, after administration of proline and sodium nitrite or sodium nitrate.

However, it is not easy to assess endogenous exposure to *N*-nitroso compounds quantitatively when dealing with volatile nitrosamines which are rapidly and extensively metabolized.

We have previously shown (Airoldi *et al.*, 1983) that only 0.3% of *N*-nitrosodi-*n*-butylamine (NDBA) administered by gavage to rats was excreted unchanged in the 24-h urine, whereas the acidic metabolite *N*-butyl-*N*-(3-carboxypropyl)nitrosamine (BCPN) appeared to be a better indicator of the degree of exposure, since its excretion represented about 18% of the administered NDBA.

In view of these results, we have investigated endogenous NDBA formation from the precursors *N*,*N*-dibutylamine (DBA) and sodium nitrite or sodium nitrate by monitoring the urinary excretion of NDBA and its metabolites *N*-butyl-*N*-(4-hydroxybutyl)nitrosamine (BBN) and BCPN, the latter being the proximate metabolite of NDBA and BBN which is responsible for the induction of urinary bladder tumours in rats (Okada & Ishidate, 1977). NDBA, BBN and BCPN were extracted from urine and assayed by gas chromatography-thermal energy analysis (GC-TEA). BBN was measured as the trimethylsilyl ether and BCPN as the trimethylsilyl ester.

MATERIALS AND METHODS

Reagents

N,*O*-Bis(trimethylsilyl)trifluoroacetamide (BSTFA), trimethylchlorosilane (TMCS) and pyridine (Pierce Chemical Co., USA).

CLIN ELUT™1020 extraction columns (Analytichem International, 24201 Frampton Ave., Harbor City, CA 90710, USA).

β-Glucuronidase/arylsulfatase (Boehringer).

Standards

NDBA (Eastman Kodak Co., USA); BBN and BCPN were synthesized according to the method of Okada *et al.* (1978a, b).

Experimental

Male CD-COBS rats from Charles River, Italy (body weight, 180 ± 10 g), were housed individually in metabolic cages. Treatment with sodium nitrite (0.2%) or sodium nitrate (0.5%) in the drinking-water was started 24 h before DBA administration and was continued throughout the experiment. DBA was dissolved in dilute hydrochloric acid to give a solution of pH > 6-< 7. The animals were fasted overnight before being given DBA, which was administered by gavage in three doses of 50 mg/kg, 8 h apart. Urine samples were collected for 24 h (from the time of the first DBA dose) on 500 mg ammonium sulfamate. NDBA, BBN and BCPN were extracted and analysed by a method previously described (Airoldi *et al.*, 1983), before and after hydrolysis with β-glucuronidase/arylsulfatase. Trimethylsilyl derivatives of BBN and BCPN were obtained by adding a reagent mixture containing pyridine : BSTFA : TMCS (50 : 45 : 5) to the dry samples. A DANI 3800 gas chromatograph equipped with a TEA 543 detector (Thermal Energy Analyzer, Thermo Electron, USA) was used. The glass column (2 m × 2 mm id) was packed with 3% OV-1 on Gas Chrom Q, 100–120 mesh. NDBA was analysed at 140 °C.

For analysis of BBN and BCPN, the oven temperature was kept at 140 °C for 2 min, then programmed from 140 to 170 °C at a rate of 15 °C/min. The carrier gas (helium) flow was 30 ml/min. The GC-TEA interface temperature was 250 °C, and the pyrolyser temperature was 500 °C.

Table 1. Urinary excretion of *N*-nitrosodi-*n*-butylamine (NDBA), *N*-butyl-*N*-(4-hydroxybutyl)nitrosamine (BBN) and *N*-butyl-*N*-(3-carboxypropyl)nitrosamine (BCPN) after administration of *N*,*N*-dibutylamine (DBA) and nitrite or nitrate

Treatment	No. of animals	Compound excreted (ng/24 h)		
		NDBA	BBN[a]	BCPN[b] (Mean ± SE)
$NaNO_2$[c] + DBA[d]	4	< 10	< 10	360 ± 200
$NaNO_3$[e] + DBA[d]	13	< 10	< 10	25 ± 5
$NaNO_2$[c]	4	< 10	< 10	< 10
$NaNO_3$[e]	4	< 10	< 10	< 10
DBA[d]	4	< 10	< 10	< 10

[a] Free or glucuronic acid/arylsulfate-conjugated
[b] Free acid
[c] Given as 0.2% solution in drinking-water
[d] 3 × 50 mg/kg p.o.
[e] Given as 0.5% solution in drinking-water

RESULTS AND DISCUSSION

As shown in Table 1, the administration of nitrite or nitrate in the drinking-water and gavage with DBA did not lead to detectable urinary excretion of either NDBA or its metabolite BBN (free or glucuronic acid-conjugated); but the presence of BCPN indicated that DBA was nitrosated endogenously in both groups of animals. The amount of BCPN excreted in the 24-h urine by nitrite-DBA-treated animals was about 14 times the amount found in the urine of nitrate-DBA-treated animals.

Assuming that the BCPN excreted is about 18% of the amount of NDBA formed *in vivo*, it can be calculated that the amount of NDBA formed was 10.6 nmol and 0.72 nmol, respectively, in the nitrite- and nitrate-treated animals under our experimental conditions. According to these calculations, 0.005% and 0.0003% of the administered DBA was nitrosated *in vivo* when sodium nitrite or sodium nitrate was dissolved in the drinking-water. In both instances, the amount of urinary NDBA was below the limit of sensitivity of the method (< 10 ng/24 h). DBA, nitrite or nitrate taken alone did not result in detectable urinary excretion of NDBA, BBN or BCPN.

Thus, quantitative analysis of urinary volatile nitrosamines does not appear to be a worthwhile indicator of endogenous exposure to these compounds, since they are extensively metabolized. Measurement of urinary metabolites, however, seems to be a better indicator of in-vivo nitrosation. Moreover, this procedure is useful for studying factors which might influence the endogenous nitrosation rate or the formation of carcinogenic metabolites.

ACKNOWLEDGEMENTS

This work was supported by the Italian National Council for Research, Contract No. 81.01403.96 (Control of Neoplastic Growth).

REFERENCES

Airoldi, L., Spagone, C., Bonfanti, M., Pantarotto, C. & Fanelli, R. (1983) Rapid method for quantitative analysis of *N,N*-dibutylnitrosamine, *N*-butyl-N-(4-hydroxybutyl)nitrosamine and *N*-butyl-*N*-(3-carboxypropyl)nitrosamine in rat urine by gas chromatography/thermal energy analysis. *J. Chromatogr., 276,* 402–407

Fine, D.H., Ross, R., Rounbehler, D.P., Silvergleid, A. & Song, L. (1977) Formation *in vivo* of volatile *N*-nitrosamines in man after ingestion of cooked bacon and spinach. *Nature, 265,* 753–755

Lijinsky, W. & Taylor, H.W. (1977) Feeding tests in rats on mixtures of nitrite with secondary and tertiary amines of environmental importance. *Food Cosmet. Toxicol., 1,* 269–274

Ohshima, H. & Bartsch, H. (1981) Quantitative estimation of endogenous nitrosation in humans by monitoring *N*-nitrosoproline excreted in the urine. *Cancer Res., 41,* 3658–3662

Ohshima, H., Béréziat, J.C. & Bartsch, H. (1982) *Measurement of endogenous* N-*nitrosation in rats and humans by monitoring urinary and faecal excretion of* N-*nitrosamino acids.* In: Bartsch, H., O'Neill, I.K., Castegnaro, M. & Okada, M., eds, N-*Nitroso Compounds: Occurrence and Biological Effects (IARC Scientific Publications No. 41),* Lyon, International Agency for Research on Cancer, pp. 397–411

Okada, M. & Ishidate, M. (1977) Metabolic fate of *N-n*-butyl-*N*-(4-hydroxybutyl)nitrosamine and its analogues. Selective induction of urinary bladder tumors in the rat. *Xenobiotica, 7,* 11–24

Okada, M., Suzuki, E. & Iiyoshi, M. (1978a) Syntheses of *N*-alkyl-*N*-(hydroxy- or oxo-alkyl)nitrosamines related to *N*-butyl-*N*-(4-hydroxybutyl)nitrosamine, a potent bladder carcinogen. *Chem. Pharm. Bull., 26,* 3891–3896

Okada, M., Suzuki, E. & Iiyoshi, M. (1978b) Syntheses of *N*-alkyl-*N*-(ω-carboxyalkyl)nitrosamines related to *N*-butyl-*N*-(3-carboxypropyl)nitrosamine, principal urinary metabolite of a potent bladder carcinogen *N*-butyl-*N*-(4-hydroxybutyl)nitrosamine. *Chem. Pharm. Bull., 26,* 3909–3913

OXIDATION OF AMMONIA AND HYDROXYLAMINE TO NITRATE IN THE RAT

R.L. SAUL[1] & M.C. ARCHER[2]

Department of Medical Biophysics, University of Toronto,
Ontario Cancer Institute, 500 Sherbourne St,
Toronto M4X 1K9, Canada

SUMMARY

We have demonstrated that ammonia is oxidized to nitrate in the rat. Male Sprague-Dawley rats gavaged with 1 000 µmol ^{15}N-ammonium chloride each day for five days were found to excrete low, but significant, amounts of excess ^{15}N-nitrate in their urines on the five days of treatment and on the five subsequent days. We recovered a total of 0.28 ± 0.03 µmol excess ^{15}N-nitrate (mean $\pm$ SE) per rat, which indicates that ammonia is converted to nitrate with a yield of about 0.0080%. ^{15}N-Hydroxylamine was oxidized in the rat to ^{15}N-nitrate with a yield of 4.7%, but oxidation of ^{15}N-labeled glycine and L-glutamic acid to ^{15}N-nitrate could not be detected. These results suggest that hydroxylamine, but not glycine or L-glutamic acid, may be an intermediate in the ammonia oxidation process. The injection of rats with Arochlor 1254 failed to stimulate nitrate synthesis, which indicates that the cytochrome P-450 drug metabolizing system is probably not involved in ammonia oxidation. Carbon tetrachloride, which causes hepatic lipid peroxidation, produced a small, but significant, increase in nitrate synthesis. Our results are consistent with the hypothesis that ammonia is oxidized *in vivo* by a non-enzymatic process involving reactive oxygen species. We estimate that a 215 g rat produces 3.0 µmol of nitrate per day by this process. The significance of our results to the problem of endogenous *N*-nitroso compound formation in man is discussed.

INTRODUCTION

Humans on low nitrate diets excrete more nitrate in their urine than they ingest (Tannenbaum *et al.*, 1978; Green *et al.*, 1981a). It has been proposed that this excess nitrate is synthesized endogenously *via* the oxidation of ammonia or other nitrogen-containing compounds. Green *et al.* (1981b) and Witter *et al.* (1981) showed that urinary nitrate levels in excess of dietary levels could be observed for germ-free, as well as conventional-flora rats,

---

[1] Present address: University of California, Biochemistry Department, Berkeley, CA 94720, USA
[2] To whom correspondence should be addressed

indicating that this effect is not produced by endogenous microorganisms. The excess nitrate is not derived from atmospheric oxides of nitrogen, since Saul and Archer (1983) demonstrated excess urinary nitrate for rats maintained in a nitrogen oxide-free environment. It therefore appears likely that ammonia, or a related compound, is oxidized to nitrate by a process of mammalian origin. The existence of such an oxidation process in man may be important, since nitrate and nitrite formed in this way could act as precursors of carcinogenic N-nitroso compounds. In this paper, we demonstrate that ammonia is oxidized to nitrate in the rat, and we suggest a mechanism for this process.

MATERIALS AND METHODS

For all animal experiments, male Sprague-Dawley rats, initially 42–46 days old and weighing 194 ± 7 g (mean $\pm$ SD), were housed individually in metabolic cages (Nalgene Co., Rochester, NY, USA) for periods of up to 13 days. The rats were allowed unlimited amounts of deionized drinking water and a casein- and corn starch-based diet which contained 3.8% nitrogen (Product No. 0902L, Bioserve Inc., Frenchtown, NJ, USA). Using the method of Sen and Donaldson (1978), we found the nitrate content in this diet to be 0.17 μmol/g, and detected no nitrite (detection limit, 0.01 μmol/g). Water bottles and food containers were changed daily and food consumption was measured. All ^{15}N-labeled chemicals had a minimum isotopic enrichment of 99% and were obtained from Stohler Isotope Chemicals (Waltham, MA, USA). Since ^{15}N-labeled ammonium chloride and hydroxylamine hydrochloride contained small amounts of ^{15}N-nitrate as an impurity, these chemicals were eluted with water through a 6×1 cm anion-exchange column (AG1-X8, 100–200 mesh, chloride form, Bio-Rad Laboratories, Richmond, CA, USA) to remove the contaminating nitrate prior to use.

In order to test ammonia as a precursor of nitrate, rats were gavaged with 1 000 μmol of ^{15}N-ammonium chloride at the beginning of each of days 4 to 8 (inclusive) of a 13-day experimental period. Urines were collected daily. Ten mL of 0.6 mol/L sodium hydroxide solution were added to each urine collection container before use, to prevent nitrate destruction or synthesis due to contaminating faecal microorganisms (Saul et al., 1981). In order to minimize the accumulation of faeces on the collection funnel, separating cone and urine ring, the metabolic cages were disassembled, washed in deionized water, and reassembled each day. The preserved urine samples were stored and analysed for total nitrate content (both ^{14}N- and ^{15}N-nitrate) by cadmium reduction of nitrate to nitrite and the Griess reaction for nitrite detection (Saul & Archer, 1983).

In order to determine the atom-percent excess ^{15}N of the urinary nitrate, the nitrate was derivatized to the volatile product, nitrobenzene, which was analysed by gas chromatography-mass spectroscopy (Green et al., 1982). In our method, chloride ion was precipitated from the urine samples with silver sulfate, prior to derivatization, since chloride inhibits nitration reactions. For the derivatization step, we used the method of Wu and Saschenbrecker (1977). The excess ^{15}N-nitrate in a given urine sample was calculated by multiplying the total urinary nitrate level by the atom-percent excess ^{15}N for the nitrobenzene derived from that sample.

Several possible intermediates in the ammonia oxidation process were administered to rats. ^{15}N-Glycine was given by gavage at a dose of 1 000 μmol per day, following the protocol described for ^{15}N-ammonium chloride. The other compounds were given by gavage as a single dose on day 4 of the experimental period, at doses of 500 μmol for ^{15}N-L-glutamic acid and 20 μmol for ^{15}N-hydroxylamine hydrochloride. The levels of excess ^{15}N-nitrate in the urines of these rats were determined as described above.

Carbon tetrachloride was administered intraperitoneally to rats on day 4 of the experimental period at a dose of 1 580 mg/kg. Aroclor 1254 was tested using the same protocol at a dose of 500 mg/kg. Corn oil, which was used as the vehicle for these compounds, was given alone to rats as a negative control. Urinary nitrate (unlabelled) was determined for these rats using the Griess reaction, as described above.

RESULTS

For rats administered ^{15}N-ammonium chloride, the average daily food consumption for days 1 through 13 was 19.2 ± 1.9 g (mean ± SD), which represents an average nitrate intake of 3.3 ± 0.3 µmol/day. The average urinary nitrate output (^{14}N plus ^{15}N) for these rats was 4.4 ± 0.7 µmol/day, which was consistently greater than dietary nitrate intake on all days by an average of 1.1 ± 0.7 µmol/day. No significant difference of dietary nitrate intake or urinary nitrate output is observed when treatment days (4 to 8) and non-treatment days are compared. The average weight gain over the entire experimental period was 7.0 ± 1.2 g/day.

The average excess ^{15}N-nitrate levels in the urines of the three rats given ^{15}N-ammonium chloride are shown in Figure 1. The average level measured for the urines collected during the control period (days 1 to 3) was 0.002 ± 0.002 µmol/day (mean ± SE). The levels for all five days on which the labelled compound was administered were significantly above the level of the control period (by t test, $p < 0.05$) and the levels remained this way for five days after the last gavage. The total amount of labelled nitrate recovered in the urine was 0.28 ± 0.03 µmol (mean ± SE), which is 0.0056% of the total administered label.

Hawksworth and Hill (1971) administered nitrate to 200-g Sprague-Dawley rats by gavage and found that 71 ± 11% (mean ± SE) of the nitrate was recovered in the urine. This recovery value is almost identical to that found by Saul and Archer (1983), who injected rats intravenously with nitrite, which was recovered as urinary nitrate with a yield of 70 ± 10% (mean ± 95% confidence limits). Assuming that nitrate that is formed *via* ammonia oxidation

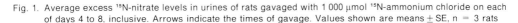

Fig. 1. Average excess ^{15}N-nitrate levels in urines of rats gavaged with 1 000 µmol ^{15}N-ammonium chloride on each of days 4 to 8, inclusive. Arrows indicate the times of gavage. Values shown are means ± SE, n = 3 rats

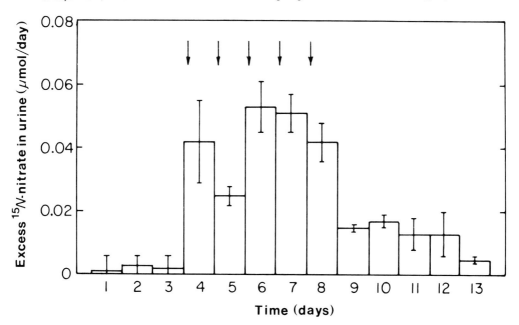

is also recovered with a yield of about 70%, we estimate that about 0.0080% of the administered ^{15}N-ammonia was converted to ^{15}N-nitrate in our rats.

Several control experiments were performed to determine whether our experimental protocol might lead to false-positive artefacts caused by in-vitro oxidation of ammonia during urine collection, storage or analysis. To test for artefacts formed during collection, some urine samples from ^{15}N-ammonium chloride-treated animals were divided into two. One half was stored immediately after collection as described above; the other half remained in the collection container at room temperature, exposed to the atmosphere, for an additional 120 h. There was no significant difference between the levels of ^{15}N-nitrate found in the samples exposed for 24 h and in those exposed for 144 h. In order to test for artefacts formed during storage and analysis, urine samples from untreated rats were spiked with 8 500 µmol ^{15}N-ammonium chloride and were stored and analysed as described in the Materials and Methods section. No excess ^{15}N-nitrate could be detected in these samples.

For the rats given 20 µmol ^{15}N-hydroxylamine hydrochloride, the total amount of labelled nitrate recovered was 0.66 ± 0.04 µmol (mean ± SE), or 3.3% of the administered label. After correcting this value for nitrate recovery, we estimate that about 4.7% of the administered ^{15}N-hydroxylamine was converted to nitrate. Most of the excess ^{15}N-nitrate for rats given this compound was observed in the urines on day 4.

No excess ^{15}N-nitrate was found in the urines of rats given either ^{15}N-glycine or ^{15}N-L-glutamic acid. The sensitivity and accuracy of our method was sufficient to detect a total excess ^{15}N-nitrate level of 0.020 µmol per experiment. After correcting this value for nitrate recovery, we estimate that the minimum amount of excess ^{15}N-nitrate that we could detect reliably would be 0.030 µmol per experiment. Therefore, during the period of our experiment, these amino acids were converted to nitrate in yields of less than 0.006% for L-glutamic acid and less than 0.0006% for glycine.

Carbon tetrachloride caused a greater than two-fold increase in excess nitrate excretion for days 4 and 5 (both levels significantly greater than control period levels; t test, p < 0.02). No corresponding increase was observed for the vehicle controls. No effect was observed for animals treated with Arochlor 1254 within seven days of treatment.

DISCUSSION

The recovery of ^{15}N-nitrate from ^{15}N-ammonium chloride-treated rats is direct proof that ammonia is oxidized to nitrate in the rat. One possible mechanism is that ammonia is first incorporated into an amino acid; the amino acid, or a metabolic product of the amino acid, is then oxidized to yield nitrate. We chose to test glycine and L-glutamic acid, since these are important intermediates in the biosynthesis of a number of nitrogenous compounds. However, when ^{15}N-labeled glycine and L-glutamic acid were administered to rats, no excess ^{15}N-nitrate could be detected. Alternatively, the first step of the ammonia oxidation process may be the direct oxidation of ammonia to hydroxylamine. This mechanism is supported by our finding that ^{15}N-hydroxylamine is oxidized to nitrate with a yield more than 500 times greater than that from ammonia.

The administration of Arochlor 1254 to rats did not stimulate nitrate synthesis, indicating that the cytochrome P-450 drug metabolizing system is probably not involved in ammonia oxidation. Carbon tetrachloride, however, caused a small, but significant, increase in the rate of endogenous nitrate synthesis. At the dose used in this study, carbon tetrachloride, is known to cause hepatic lipid peroxidation (Klaassen & Plaa, 1969). It is believed that the mechanism involves the formation of free radicals which initiate autocatalytic peroxidative breakdown of lipid membranes. Recently, Wagner and Tannenbaum (1982) showed that treatment of rats with a bacterial endotoxin stimulates nitrate synthesis. These authors suggested that the endotoxin causes the rats' reticuloendothelial system to produce reactive oxygen species which might oxidize ammonia or related compounds. Such species would include the superoxide anion, as well as the hydroxyl free radical which can be derived from superoxide *via* the Haber-Weiss reaction. The common factor in our carbon tetrachloride experiment and in the endotoxin experiment of Wagner and Tannenbaum (1982) may be the formation of free radicals which can act as oxidizing agents.

We have used our results from ^{15}N-ammonium chloride-treated rats to make a rough estimate of the total amount of nitrate formed by ammonia oxidation. Our rats consumed an average of 19.2 g/day of a diet which contained 3.8% nitrogen. These animals therefore ingested an average of 730 mg nitrogen per day, mainly as protein-nitrogen. Since the animals were increasing in weight at the rate of 7.0 g/day, and since tissue is about 3.0% nitrogen, the net amount of nitrogen incorporated into the animals would be about 210 mg per day, so that the remaining 520 mg of nitrogen per day would be excreted mainly as urea. Since urea and ammonia are interconverted within the body (Regoeczi *et al.*, 1965), we have made the assumption that the administered ^{15}N-ammonia was incorporated rapidly into the urea-ammonia pool of the rat. If the nitrogen in this pool is oxidized to nitrate with the same yield as the administered ^{15}N-ammonia (0.0080%), then the total amount of nitrate formed from ammonia oxidation would be approximately 41.6 µg nitrate nitrogen per day or 3.0 µmol/day. Our rats were therefore exposed to about 3.0 µmol/day of ammonia-derived nitrate and 3.3 µmol/day of dietary nitrate, for a total nitrate exposure of 6.3 µmol/day. Assuming that 70% of this total nitrate exposure is recovered in the urine, we would predict an average urinary output of 4.4 µmol/day. This rough estimate of urinary nitrate output is in surprisingly good agreement with the observed urinary nitrate output of 4.4 $\pm$ 0.7 µmol/day (mean $\pm$ SD). The amount of nitrate formed *via* ammonia oxidation may therefore be sufficient to account for most, if not all, of the observed excess urinary nitrate in our rats.

It is not known at this time whether ammonia oxidation occurs in man. It is known, however, that nitrate is synthesized endogenously in man, and we believe that ammonia oxidation is a likely mechanism. Green *et al.* (1981a) used an isotope-dilution technique to demonstrate that endogenous synthesis contributes about 650 µmol nitrate per day to urinary nitrate in humans. Since these authors recovered in urine about 60% of the nitrate administered to humans, their observations suggest that endogenous synthesis produces about 1 083 µmol or 64 mg nitrate per day in man.

The average North American consumes about 68 mg dietary nitrate per day (Hartman, 1982). A fraction of this nitrate is absorbed into the blood, secreted into the oral cavity by the salivary glands, reduced to nitrite by oral cavity microorganisms and passed into the stomach, where it may participate in acid-catalysed nitrosation reactions (reviewed by Archer, 1982). If man produces 64 mg nitrate per day through ammonia oxidation, then this process would contribute significantly to man's total nitrate exposure and would consequently contribute significantly to the amount of nitrite formed in the body from nitrate reduction. Nitrite might also be formed as an intermediate in the oxidation of ammonia to nitrate. In these two ways, ammonia oxidation may contribute to man's exposure to nitrite and therefore increase the amount of *N*-nitroso compounds that may be formed *in vivo*.

ACKNOWLEDGMENTS

The authors thank Louis Marai, Kwan Leung and Peter Zucker for their assistance. This research was supported by the Ontario Cancer Treatment and Research Foundation and the National Cancer Institute of Canada. Studentships from the Province of Ontario are gratefully acknowleged by R.L.S.

REFERENCES

Archer, M.C. (1982) *Hazards of nitrate, nitrite, and nitrosamines in human nutrition.* In: J.N. Hathcock, ed., *Nutritional Toxicology,* Vol. 1, New York, Academic Press, pp. 327–381

Green, L.C., Ruiz de Luzuriaga, K., Wagner, D.A., Rand, W., Istfan, N., Yang, V.R. & Tannenbaum, S.R. (1981a) Nitrate biosynthesis in man. *Proc. natl acad. Sci. USA, 78,* 7764–7768

Green, L.C., Tannenbaum, S.R. & Goldman, P. (1981b) Nitrate synthesis in the germfree and conventional rat. *Science, 212,* 56–58

Green, L.C., Wagner, D.A., Glogowski, J., Skipper, P.L., Wishnok, J.S. & Tannenbaum, S.R. (1982) Analysis of nitrate, nitrite, and $^{15}NO_3^-$ in biological fluids. *Anal. Biochem., 126,* 131–138

Hartman, P.E. (1982) *Nitrates and nitrites: Ingestion, pharmacodynamics, and toxicology.* In: F.J. deSerres & A. Hollaender, eds, *Chemical Mutagens,* Vol. 7, New York, Plenum, pp. 211–294

Hawksworth, G.M. & Hill, M.J. (1971) Bacteria and the *N*-nitrosation of secondary amines. *Br. J. Cancer, 25,* 520–526

Klaassen, C.D. & Plaa, G.L. (1969) Comparison of the biochemical alterations elicited in livers from rats treated with carbon tetrachloride, chloroform, 1,1,2-trichloroethane and 1,1,1-trichloroethane. *Biochem. Pharmacol., 18,* 2019–2027

Regoeczi, E., Irons, L., Koj, A., & McFarlane, A.S. (1965) Isotopic studies of urea metabolism in rabbits. *Biochem. J., 95,* 521–532

Saul, R.L. & Archer, M.C. (1983) Nitrate formation in rats exposed to nitrogen dioxide. *Toxicol appl. Pharmacol., 67,* 284–291

Saul, R.L., Kabir, S.H., Cohen, Z., Bruce, W.R. & Archer, M.C. (1981) Reevaluation of nitrate and nitrite levels in the human intestine. *Cancer Res., 41,* 2280–2283

Sen, N.P. & Donaldson, B. (1978) Improved colorimetric method from determining nitrate and nitrite in foods. *J. Assoc. off. anal. Chem., 61,* 1389–1394

Tannenbaum, S.R., Fett, D., Young, V.R., Land, P.C. & Bruce, W.R. (1978) Nitrite and nitrate are formed by endogenous synthesis in the human intestine. *Science, 200,* 1487–1489

Wagner, D. & Tannenbaum, S.R. (1982) *Enhancement of nitrate synthesis by* Escherichia coli *lipopolysaccharide.,* In: Magee, P.N., ed., *Nitrosamines and Human Cancer (Banbury Report No. 12),* Cold Spring Harbor, NY, Cold Spring Harbor Laboratory, pp. 437–441

Witter, J.P., Gatley, S.J. & Balish, E. (1981) Evaluation of nitrate synthesis by intestinal microorganisms *in vivo. Science, 213,* 449–450

Wu, W.S. & Saschenbrecker, P.W. (1977) Nitration of benzene as a method for determining nitrites and nitrates in meat and meat products. *J. Assoc. off. anal. Chem., 60,* 1137–1141

MAMMALIAN NITRATE BIOCHEMISTRY: METABOLISM AND ENDOGENOUS SYNTHESIS

D.A. WAGNER, V.R. YOUNG & S.R. TANNENBAUM

Departments of Nutrition and Food Science

D.S. SCHULTZ & W.M. DEEN

Department of Chemical Engineering, Massachusetts Institute of Technology, Cambridge, MA 02139, USA

SUMMARY

The metabolic fate of an oral dose of 3.5 mmol ^{15}N-labelled nitrate was investigated in young adults. An average of 60% of the ^{15}N-nitrate dose appeared in the urine within 48 h; less than 0.1 % appeared in the faeces. Some of the ^{15}N label of nitrate was found in the urine (3%) and faeces (0.2%) in the form of ammonia and urea; the remainder of the dose was attributed to nitrate loss *via* metabolism to other reduced nitrogen compounds. Studies with germ-free rats indicated that half of the nitrate metabolism is due to mammalian processes. These and previous studies show that not all of the nitrate excreted in the urine is of dietary origin but evolves from endogenous synthesis. An oral dose of ^{15}N-ammonium acetate was incorporated into urinary ^{15}N-nitrate in rats, suggesting that ammonia is a precursor of nitrate. Furthermore, *Escherichia coli* lipopolysaccharide was found to be a potent stimulus of nitrate excretion (nine-fold increase), due to an increased rate of synthesis. Two other types of experimentally induced inflammatory states – injection of carrageenan and of turpentine – enhanced nitrate synthesis. It is proposed that the pathway of nitrate biosynthesis may be the result of oxidation of reduced nitrogen compounds by oxygen radicals generated by an activated reticuloendothelial system.

INTRODUCTION

Several reports have suggested a causal relationship between high nitrate exposure and stomach cancer incidence (Hill *et al.*, 1973; Cuello *et al.*, 1976). It is believed that excess nitrate exposure can lead to increased formation of carcinogenic *N*-nitroso compounds. The potential harm of over-exposure to nitrate stems from its conversion to nitrite by bacterial reduction in the oral cavity and other parts of the body containing high concentrations of bacteria. Salivary nitrite concentration has been reported to be directly proportional to the amount of nitrate ingested (Spiegelhalder *et al.*, 1976). The swallowing of saliva exposes the stomach to nitrite, and the acidic environment found in the stomach favours formation of *N*-nitroso compounds. Recent evidence has demonstrated that administration of nitrate and an amine, such as proline, to humans results in production of an *N*-nitroso compound, in this case *N*-nitrosoproline (Ohshima & Bartsch, 1981; Wagner *et al.*, 1982). Therefore, to assess the role that nitrate may play in human carcinogenesis, we need to examine all the potential sources of nitrate exposure as well as the processes that remove this ion from the body.

SOURCES OF NITRATE EXPOSURE

A major source of nitrate exposure in man is food and water. It is not surprising to find nitrate widely distributed in water supplies and in almost all vegetable material, since nitrate is produced by heterotrophic organisms in rivers and lakes and in the soil. Some 85–90% of all ingested nitrate comes from vegetables (White, 1975): a typical diet contains between 1–1.5 mmol/day of nitrate. Additionally, nitrate levels in drinking-water can be a major source of nitrate exposure in some localities (National Academy of Sciences, 1981).Recent studies (Tannenbaum *et al.*, 1978); Green, *et al.*, 1981a) have confirmed an earlier report (Mitchell *et al.*, 1916) that the diet is not the only source of nitrate but that nitrate is synthesized endogenously from reduced nitrogen compounds. This conclusion was based on results of nitrate balance studies in human subjects ingesting a low-nitrate diet. The total amount of nitrate appearing in the urine exceeded dietary input by factors of two to 30. Hence, not all of the nitrate excreted in the urine is of dietary origin.

ENDOGENOUS NITRATE BIOSYNTHESIS

Although it was first thought that the origin of the excess urinary nitrate was microbial synthesis in the intestinal tract (Tannenbaum *et al.*, 1978), it has now been shown conclusively that intestinal microorganisms are not responsible for excess urinary nitrate, on the basis of nitrate-balance studies in conventional and germ-free rats (Green *et al.*, 1981b; Witter *et al.*, 1981). Additional evidence for nitrate biosynthesis in man comes from long-term (84 days) nitrate-balance studies of healthy young men, which showed that the amount of nitrate excreted in urine was an average of four-fold greater than the amount ingested over the entire 84-day experimental period (Green *et al.*, 1981a). This observation ruled out the hypothesis that the origin of excess urinary nitrate is the result of a slow wash-out of nitrate stored in the body. Furthermore, the use of ^{15}N-labelled nitrate showed that the source of the excess nitrate in urine was the endogenous biosynthesis of nitrate rather than the emptying of a body pool (Green *et al.*, 1981a; Wagner *et al.*, 1983a). Daily endogenous biosynthesis of nitrate in man is estimated to be about 1 mmol/day (Wagner *et al.*, 1983a).

Therefore, with the clear evidence that endogenous nitrate biosynthesis is a mammalian process, we recently investigated the mechanism of this synthesis using stable isotopes (Wagner *et al.*, 1983b). It is well known that the oxidation of ammonia to nitrate by microorganisms is a continuous process of nitrogen cycle. Thus, in order to determine whether ammonia could be converted to nitrate in mammals, we investigated whether isotopically labelled ammonia, when administered to rats, appears as labelled nitrate in urine.

Orally administered ^{15}N-ammonia was found to be incorporated into nitrate-nitrogen. The ^{15}N enrichment of nitrate (atom % excess ^{15}N) appearing in the urine of six rats was 2.2 ± 0.57% (mean ± SD). The amount of ^{15}N-nitrate in urine was 73 ± 32 nmol, corresponding to 0.004% of the administered dose of labelled ammonia. This finding shows that a pathway exists for the formation of nitrate from ammonia and suggests that ammonia is either a precursor or is in rapid equilibrium with a precursor to form nitrate endogenously. The low conversion of ammonia to nitrate is not surprising since ammonia is rapidly cleared from plasma and incorporated into the body pools of urea and glutamine (Freed & Gelbard, 1982). Nitrate biosynthesis thus appears to be a minor component of ammonia metabolism.

METABOLIC FATE OF NITRATE

The reported recovery of nitrate in urine following high nitrate intakes in humans has ranged from 50 to 90% (Radomski et al., 1978; Ellen et al., 1982). The recovery of large oral doses of nitrate in laboratory animals has been found to be between 35 and 92% (Green & Hiatt, 1954; Kilgore, et al., 1959). Since urinary recovery is incomplete and faecal excretion of nitrate has been found to be negligible (Saul et al., 1981), it is clear that nitrate is metabolized to a significant extent in the body.

The metabolic fate of nitrate can be studied more directly using ^{15}N-labelled nitrate. We recently investigated the metabolic fate of an oral dose of 3.5 mmol ^{15}N-labelled nitrate in 12 healthy young adults (Wagner et al., 1983a). Samples of urine, plasma and faeces were collected over a period of 48 h following administration of the dose. An average of 60% of the dose appeared in the urine as ^{15}N-nitrate within 48 h, less than 0.1% was excreted in the faeces. The 15N label of nitrate was also found in the urine (3%) and faeces (0.2%) in the form of ammonia and urea. The remaining 35% of the ^{15}N-nitrate has not been accounted for. One possible fate of this nitrate is metabolism to gaseous products which are exhaled in the breath or appear in flatus. Nitrate retention in the body carcass could not account for the missing nitrate recovery, since Wang et al. (1981) showed this to be negligible. Either bacterial or mammalian metabolism of nitrate could be responsible for the unaccounted nitrate.

Recently, we investigated the contribution of bacterial metabolism of nitrate to total nitrate clearance in rats. A dose of ^{15}N-nitrate was administered to germ-free rats (kept in laminar flow cubicles to maintain their germ-free status). Following two doses of 10 µmol/rat of nitrate, the germ-free rats were allowed to acquire an intestinal flora. This was accomplished by placing the faeces of conventional rats in the cages. A dose of labelled nitrate was administered two weeks later. The urinary recovery of ^{15}N-nitrate in germ-free rats was significantly higher (p < 0.05), 70.6 ± 3.80%), than the recovery after these rats acquired a flora, 57.7 ± 8.7%. Although there was a significant increase in nitrate recovery in these rats after they had acquired a bacterial flora, there still was not complete recovery of nitrate in the urine. This observation suggests that there are mammalian processes for metabolizing nitrate.

A one-compartment pharmacokinetic model was used to analyse the data on plasma and urine in the study of Wagner et al. (1983a). It was found that the removal of nitrate from the human body is primarily first-order in plasma nitrate concentration. The half-life of nitrate in the body was found to be approximately 5 h, and its volume of distribution was about 30% of body weight. The total clearance of nitrate from the body was calculated to be 2.9 L/h, while renal clearance was 1.6 L/h. This ratio of renal to total clearance (1.6 : 2.9), determined from the data for total nitrate ([14+15]N), provides an independent prediction of the fraction of nitrate presented to the body that will appear unmetabolized in urine. The urinary clearance was calculated to be 55% of total clearance, which was in good agreement with the recovery of 60% of the administered ^{15}N-nitrate in urine as nitrate.

In summary, clearance of nitrate from the body can result from three processes: urinary excretion accounts for 60%, bacterial metabolism for about 15%, and 25% through unknown mammalian processes.

Fig. 1. Induction of nitrate excretion in rats during an endotoxin-induced fever. On day 8, rats were injected intraperitoneally with *Escherichia coli* lipopolysaccharide; mean urinary nitrate excretion for six rats ± 95% confidence interval

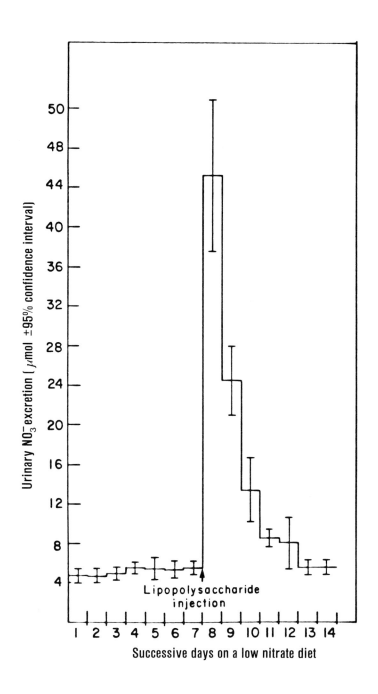

EFFECT OF INFLAMMATION ON NITRATE BIOSYNTHESIS

During the course of nitrate-balance studies in adult humans (Wagner & Tannenbaum, 1982), we observed an unexpected stimulation of nitrate biosynthesis in one subject who developed a fever and nonspecific intestinal diarrhoea. Urinary nitrate excretion increased nine-fold during this illness compared with that before the symptoms appeared. A similar elevation of urinary nitrate excretion was noted by Hegesh and Shiloah (1982) in infants suffering from diarrhoea. Therefore, we explored the possibility that rats exposed to *Escherichia coli* lipopolysaccharide (LPS), which can induce fever and diarrhoea, have enhanced nitrate biosynthesis (Wagner *et al.*, 1983b).

E. coli LPS endotoxin-induced fever had a striking effect on urinary nitrate excretion (Fig. 1), which increased nine-fold (45 $\pm$ 6.3 µmol/day) during the first day of the fever compared with an average nitrate excretion of 5.2 $\pm$ 0.13 µmol/day during the week preceeding LPS administration. As the fever subsided, nitrate excretion decreased, and nitrate levels returned to initial levels five days after injection. Control rats injected with 0.9% saline solution showed no increase in nitrate excretion.

The enhanced urinary excretion of nitrate during LPS administration was shown to be the result of an increased rate of nitrate synthesis, using ^{15}N-ammonium acetate as a N donor (Wagner *et al.*, 1983b). The increased excretion of nitrate after LPS administration was accompanied by increased incorporation of ^{15}N-ammonia into nitrate-nitrogen (Table 1). The fact that significantly more ^{15}N-nitrate was produced from labelled ammonia with LPS treatment suggests that more ammonia nitrogen is shunted into nitrate biosynthesis during LPS treatment.

Two other types of inflammatory states produced changes in nitrate biosynthesis. A carrageenan-induced inflammation produced a greater than two-fold increase in nitrate synthesis (Fig. 2); nitrate levels returned to baseline values after three days. Turpentine-induced inflammation produced a delayed pattern of enhancement of nitrate biosynthesis (Fig. 2): nitrate levels were not increased significantly for the first 24 h after turpentine administration, but thereafter were increased approximately three-fold. This finding is further evidence for induction of nitrate synthesis by an activated reticuloendothelial system.

These results support the hypothesis that activation of the reticuloendothelial system significantly increases nitrate biosynthesis. One possible mechanism for the increased nitrate

Table 1. Effect of lipopolysaccharide (LPS) administration on incorporation of [^{15}N]-ammonium acetate into [^{15}N]-nitrate [a]

Control			LPS administered		
Total urinary nitrate (µmol/24 h)	^{15}N in nitrate (nmol)	% of dose incorporated	Total urinary nitrate (µmol/24 h)	^{15}N in nitrate (nmol)	% of dose incorporated
2.68	40.5	0.002	17.0	602	0.030
3.41	87.0	0.004	71.6	3 000	0.150
2.60	39.0	0.002	21.7	710	0.036
2.56	56.6	0.003	25.3	660	0.033
3.62	80.4	0.004	7.52	266	0.013
1.58	18.6	0.001	27.0	1 345	0.067

[a] Rats were administered 2 mmol [^{15}N]-ammonium acetate intragastrically during the control period, and urinary nitrate was measured 24 h after dosing. After a break of one week, rats were given LPS (1 mg/kg) intraperitoneally and 2 mmol [^{15}N]-ammonium acetate.

Fig. 2. Effect of carrageenan and turpentine administration on nitrate excretion. On day 5, rats were injected with either 0.15 g carrageenan (intraperioneal) or 0.5 mL turpentine (subcutaneous); mean urinary nitrate excretion for six rats in each group ± SD

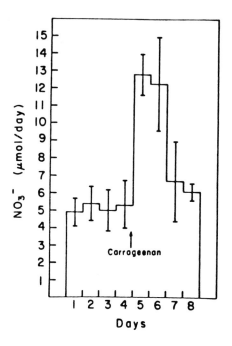 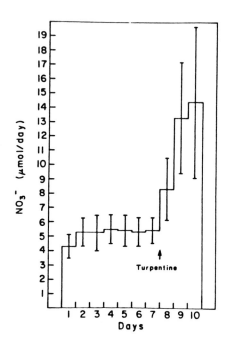

synthesis is the increased generation of reactive oxygen species capable of oxidizing reduced nitrogen compounds to nitrate. Potential oxidizing species, derived from an activated immune system, that could oxidize reduced nitrogen compounds to nitrate include superoxide, hydrogen peroxide, hydroxyl radical and singlet oxygen. Further experiments designed to block increased synthesis of reactive oxygen species after LPS administration will be necessary to test this hypothesis.

ACKNOWLEDGEMENTS

This investigation was supported by PHS Grant Number 1-PO1-CA26731-04, awarded by the US National Cancer Institute, DHHS

REFERENCES

Cuello, C., Correa, P., Haenszel, W., Gordillo, G., Brown, C., Archer, M. & Tannenbaum, S.R. (1976) Gastric cancer in Colombia. I. Cancer risk and suspect environmental agents. *J. natl Cancer Inst.,* **57,** 1015–1020

Ellen, G., Schuller, P.L., Bruijns, E., Froeling, P.G.A.M. & Baadenhuijsen, H.(1982) *Volatile N-nitrosamine, nitrate and nitrite in urine and saliva of healthy volunteers after administration of large amounts of nitrate.* In: Bartsch, H., O'Neill, I.K., Castegnaro, M. & Okada, M., eds, N-*Nitroso Compounds: Occurrence and Biological Effects (IARC Scientific Publications No. 41),* Lyon, International Agency for Research on Cancer, pp. 365–378

Freed, B.R. & Gelbard, A.S. (1982) Distribution of ^{15}N following intravenous injection of ^{15}N-ammonia in the rat. *Can. J. Physiol Pharmacol., 60,* 60–67

Green, L.C., Ruiz De Luzuriaga, K., Wagner, D.A., Rand, W., Isfan, N., Young, V.R. & Tannenbaum, S.R. (1981a) Nitrate biosynthesis in man. *Proc. natl. Acad. Sci. USA, 78,* 7764–7768

Green, L.C., Tannenbaum, S.R. & Goldman, P. (1981b) Nitrate synthesis in the germfree and conventional rat. *Science, 212,* 56–58

Greene, I. & Hiatt, E.P. (1954) Behavior of the nitrate ion in the dog. *Am. J. Physiol., 176,* 463–467

Hegesh, E. & Shiloah, J. (1982) Blood nitrates and infantile methemoglobinemia. *Clin. chim. Acta, 125,* 107–115

Hill, M.J., Hawksworth, G. & Tattersall, G. (1973) Bacteria, nitrosamines and cancer of the stomach. *Br. J. Cancer, 28,* 562–567

Kilgore, L., Almon, L. & Gieger, M. (1959) The effects of dietary nitrate on rabbits and rats. *J. Nutrit., 69,* 39–44

Mitchell, H.H., Shonle, H.A. & Gringley, H.S. (1916) The origin of the nitrates in the urine. *J. biol. Chem., 24,* 461–490

National Academy of Sciences (1981) *The Health Effects of Nitrate, Nitrite, and N-Nitroso Compounds.* Washington DC, National Academy Press, pp. 5–3–5–78

Ohshima, H & Bartsch, H. (1981) Quantitative estimation of endogenous nitrosation in humans by monitoring N-nitrosoproline excreted in the urine. *Cancer Res., 41,* 3658–3662

Radomski, J.L., Palmiri, C. & Hearn, W.L. (1978) Concentrations of nitrate in normal urine and the effect of nitrate ingestion. *Toxicol. appl. Pharmacol., 45,* 63–68

Saul, R.L., Kabir, S.H., Cohen, Z., Bruce, W.R. & Archer, M.C. (1981) Reevaluation of nitrate and nitrite levels in the human intestine. *Cancer Res., 41,* 2280–2283

Spiegelhalder, B., Eisenbrand, G. & Preussmann, R. (1976) Influence of dietary nitrate on nitrite content of human saliva: possible relevance to *in vivo* formation of N-nitroso compounds. *Food Cosmet. Toxicol., 14,* 545–548

Tannenbaum, S.R., Fett, D., Young, V.R., Land, P.D., & Bruce, W.R. (1978) Nitrite and nitrate are formed by endogenous synthesis in the human intestine. *Science, 200,* 1487–1489

Wagner, D.A. & Tannenbaum, S.R. (1982) *Enhancement of nitrate biosynthesis by Escherichia coli lipopolysaccharide.* In: Magee, P.N., ed., Nitrosamines in Human Cancer (Banbury Report No. 12), Cold Spring Harbor, NY, Cold Spring Harbor Laboratory, pp. 437–443

Wagner, D.A., Shuker, D.E.G., Hasic, G. & Tannenbaum, S.R. (1982) *Endogenous nitrosoproline synthesis in humans.* In Magee, P.N., ed. *Nitrosamines in Human Cancer (Banbury Report No. 12),* Cold Spring Harbor, NY, Cold Spring Harbor Laboratory, pp. 319–333

Wagner, D.A., Schultz, D.S. Deen, W.M., Young,V.R. & Tannenbaum, S.R. (1983a) Metabolic fate of an oral dose of ^{15}N-labeled nitrate in humans: Effect of diet supplementation with ascorbic acid. *Cancer Res., 43,* 1921–1925

Wagner, D.A. Young, V.R. & Tannenbaum, S.R. (1983b) Mammalian nitrate synthesis: Incorporation of ^{15}NH$_3$ into nitrate is enhanced by endotoxin treatment. *Proc. natl Acad. Sci. USA, 80,* 4518–4521

Wang, C.F., Cassens, R.G. & Hoekstra, W.G. (1981) Fate of ingested ^{15}N-labeled nitrate and nitrite in the rat. *J Food Sci., 46,* 745–748

White, J.W., Jr (1975) Relative significance of dietary sources of nitrate and nitrite. *J. Agric. Food Chem., 23,* 866–891

Witter, J.P. Gatley, S.J. & Balish, E. (1981) Evaluation of nitrate synthesis by intestinal microorganisms *in vivo. Science, 213,* 449–450

ABSORPTION, SECRETION AND EXCRETION OF DIMETHYLAMINE IN RATS

H. ISHIWATA, R. IWATA & A. TANIMURA

National Institute of Hygienic Sciences, 18-1, Kamiyoga 1-chome, Setagaya-ku, Tokyo 158, Japan

SUMMARY

The dimethylamine (DMA) concentration in the gastrointestinal tract of Wistar male rats fed a commercial diet containing 23.6 mg/kg DMA was highest (11.2 ± 2.1 mg/kg) in the stomach and decreased from the upper region to the lower region. In contrast, the highest DMA concentration (6.6 ± 2.5 mg/kg) in the upper small intestine was observed in rats fed a low-DMA diet containing 1.0 mg/kg DMA. DMA absorption was observed in the intestines and the absorbtion curves were monoexponential. The biological half-lives ($t\frac{1}{2}$) of DMA in the ligated stomach, upper and lower small intestine, caecum and large intestine were 198, 8.3, 11.6, 31.5 and 11.0 min, respectively. The DMA concentration in blood increased from 0.3 ± 0.1 mg/kg to 3.0 ± 1.0 mg/kg 5 min after injection of 250 μg DMA into the ligated upper small intestine.

The disappearance curve of DMA in blood was monoexponential and the half-life for the initial 15 min was 12.5 min when 250 μg DMA were injected through a femoral vein. Intestinal secretion of DMA (15.6 ± 12.6 mg/kg) was observed 15 min after the injection. Urinary DMA increased from 17.3 ± 9.4 to 139 ± 23 mg/kg within 30 min of intravenous injection of DMA. These results show that the behaviour of DMA in rats is as follows:

$$\text{ingestion} \rightarrow \underset{\text{absorption}}{\text{intestinal}} \rightarrow \text{blood} \rightarrow \underset{\text{excretion}}{\text{urinary}}$$
$$\uparrow \qquad \downarrow$$
$$\underset{\text{secretion}}{\text{intestinal}}$$

INTRODUCTION

Quantitative examinations of urinary excretion of dimetylamine (DMA) show that it is formed *in vivo* in man (Asatoor & Simenhoff, 1965; Asatoor *et al.*, 1967; Ishiwata *et al.*, 1978) and in rats (Ishiwata *et al.*, 1982). DMA is produced by two pathways, (1) from methylamine, to which methionine donates the methyl group, and (2) from lecithin, choline or trimethylamine oxide *via* trimethylamine. Lecithin is converted to choline in the intestines by bacterial lecithinase and choline is further metabolized to trimethylamine, then demethylated to DMA with intestinal bacterial *N*-dealkylating enzymes (Asatoor & Simenhoff, 1965).

Biochemical studies of secondary amines have been stagnant for 10 years, while many studies on the metabolism, formation and behaviour of nitrate and nitrite in the body have been reported. The present work examines the gastrointestinal absorption, intestinal secretion and urinary excretion of DMA in rats.

MATERIALS AND METHODS

Rats and diet

Male 15- to 20-week-old Wistar rats were fed a commercial diet containing 23.6 mg/kg DMA or a low-DMA diet containing 1.0 mg/kg DMA. The breeding room was maintained at 25 C and 60% humidity. The components of the low-DMA diet were 68% corn starch, 20% soy casein, 5% soya bean oil, 2% cellulose, 4% minerals and 1% vitamin mixture, according to Harper (1959).

Excision of the gastrointestinal tract

The low-DMA diet or the commercial diet and tap water were given freely to rats for one week prior to sacrifice. Rats were anaesthetized by intraperitoneal injection of sodium pentobarbital, and the stomach, the small intestine, the caecum and the large intestine were separated. The small intestine was cut into four equal lengths. The intestinal contents were washed out with 10 mL 0.05 mol/L hydrochloric acid. Blood was obtained by cardiac puncture. Killing was carried out in the morning.

Absorption, secretion and excretion tests

Rats fed the commercial diet were fasted overnight and anaesthetized. The abdomen was opened and the stomach and the caecum were ligated at both ends without closing the blood vessels. The upper and lower small intestine and the large intestine were separated into sections of about 5 cm in length by ligation. The site of the ligated section in the upper small intestine was 10 cm from the pylorus and that in the lower small intestine 10 cm from the ileo-caecal valve; 250 μg DMA were injected into each ligated section for the absorption tests. After a given time, the ligated sections were removed and the intestinal contents were washed out with 10 mL 0.05 mol/L hydrochloric acid. For the secretion test, an equal dose of DMA was injected through a femoral vein, and the ligated upper small intestine was removed at a given time. Urine in the bladder was collected through a syringe.

Determination of DMA

Biological materials and diets were steam-distilled under alkaline conditions with magnesium oxide, and the distillate was trapped in 1 mol/L hydrochloric acid. The distillate was treated with benzenesulfonyl chloride under alkaline conditions, using 5 mol/L sodium hydroxide solution. The derivative of DMA was extracted with *n*-hexane and determined by gas chromatography, using a Shimadzu (Kyoto, Japan) GC-4CM FP instrument, with a flame-photometric detector (Hamano *et al.*, 1979, 1980). Gas chromatographic conditions were as follows: detector temperature, 265 C; column, 3 mm i.d. × 1 m glass column, packed with 5% Silicon OV-101 on Gas Chrom Q (80–100 mesh); column temperature, 180 C; injection-port temperature, 230 C; carrier gas, nitrogen (flow rate 40 mL/min).

RESULTS

Distribution of DMA in the digestive tract

DMA in the contents of the gastrointestinal tract and in blood was determined after the rats had been fed the commercial or the low-DMA diet for a week (Fig. 1). The concentration of DMA in the gastrointestinal tract of the rats fed the commercial diet was high in the upper intestine and low in the lower intestine. When rats were fed the low-DMA diet, the DMA concentration was lowest (1.3 ± 0.5 mg/kg) in the stomach and highest (6.6 ± 2.5 mg/kg) in the upper small intestine and decreased in the lower small intestine and the caecum. The DMA concentration in the large intestine was higher than that in the caecum in both groups. The concentration of DMA in the contents of each ligated section in the rats fed the low-DMA diet was lower than that of the corresponding section in rats fed the commercial diet. Less than 1 mg/kg DMA was found in blood in both groups (Fig. 1). The DMA concentration in the intestinal contents of rats fed the low-DMA diet was higher than that in the diet, but that in the intestinal contents of the rats fed the commercial diet was lower than that in the diet.

Gastrointestinal absorption

The rates of disappearance of DMA from the stomach and the intestines after injection of 250 μg DMA are shown in Figure 2A. All rates were monoexponential over 30 min. The biological half-lives were 8.3, 11.6, 31.5 and 11.0 min for the upper small intestine, the lower small intestine, the caecum and the large intestine, respectively. Absorption of DMA from the stomach was barely observable (t½ = 198 min).

Fig. 1. Concentrations of dimethylamine (DMA) in the gastrointestinal contents of rats fed a commercial diet or a low-DMA diet. —, commercial diet containing 23.6 mg/kg DMA; . . . , low-DMA diet containing 1.0 mg/kg DMA; mean ± SD for 5 rats.

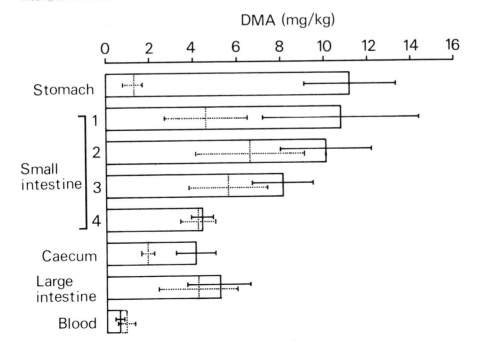

Fig. 2. Disappearance of dimethylamine (DMA) from the ligated digestive tract (A) and appearance of DMA in blood (B) (mean ± SD for 5 rats). ●, stomach; ○, upper small intestine; △, lower small intestine; □, caecum; ▲, large intestine. DMA in blood was determined after 250 μg DMA had been injected into the ligated upper small intestine.

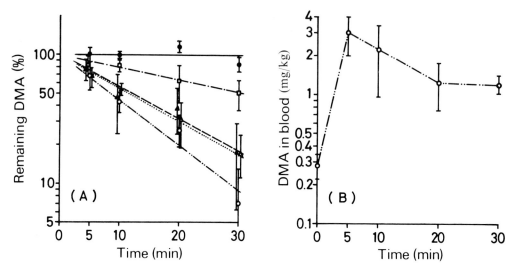

Fig. 3. Intestinal and urinary excretion of dimethylamine (DMA) in blood (mean ± SD for 5 rats). DMA was given in a dose of 250 μg through a femoral vein. △, urine; ○, upper small intestine; ●, blood.

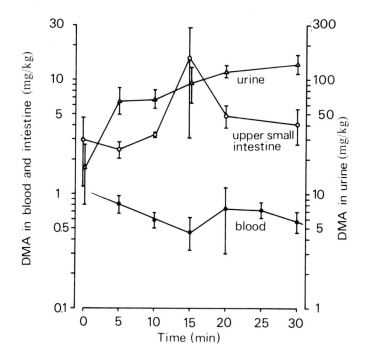

Decrease of DMA levels in blood and intestinal secretion

The initial half-life of DMA in blood was 12.5 min, and the disappearance curve was monoexponential. Urinary DMA concentration increased from 17.3 $\pm$ 9.4 mg/kg to 139 $\pm$ 23 mg/kg in 30 min. DMA was excreted not only in urine but also in the small intestine. The highest concentration of intestinal DMA (15.6 $\pm$ 12.6 mg/kg) was observed 15 min after intravenous injection of DMA (Fig. 3). When the intestinal DMA level decreased to the basic concentration, the blood DMA increased a little. The half-life for secondary disappearance of DMA in blood was 15.2 min.

DISCUSSION

DMA was not absorbed from the stomach, but was absorbed from the small intestine, the caecum and the large intestine. Absorbed DMA appeared in the blood, then disappeared rapidly. Most of the DMA in blood was excreted in the urine in a relatively short time and a small portion was secreted in the intestine. When rats were fed a commercial diet containing 23.6 mg/kg DMA, the concentration in the gastrointestinal tract was highest in the stomach and decreased from the upper intestine to the lower region. Since the DMA concentration in the lower intestines (about 4 mg/kg) was not affected by ingestion of DMA, most of the DMA ingested with the diet may be absorbed in the small intestine. The highest rate of absorption of DMA was observed in the upper small intestine, and was almost the same as that observed in guinea-pigs (Ishiwata *et al.*, 1977) The DMA found in the caecum and the large intestine may include an endogenous contribution, as reported by Asatoor and Simenhoff (1965) and by Johnson (1977). These authors concluded that intestinal bacteria form DMA from lecithin.

The gastrointestinal distribution of DMA in rats fed the low-DMA diet differed considerably from that in rats fed the commercial diet. The highest concentration of DMA (6.6 mg/kg), observed in the upper small intestine of rats fed the low-DMA diet, may be due to intestinal secretion of DMA from the blood. DMA secreted into the small intestine from blood (Fig. 3) can be re-absorbed. This is a probable explanation for the second maximum concentration of DMA observed in blood 25 min after intravenous injection of DMA. The disappearance rate between 25 and 30 min (t½ = 15.2) was almost the same as that between 5 and 15 min.

The higher concentration of DMA in the large intestine than in the caecum is considered to be due to the absorption of intestinal moisture. The site of DMA formation can be considered to be the lower digestive tract, although it may not always be the site of the highest DMA concentration.

ACKNOWLEDGEMENTS

This work was supported in part by a Grant-in-Aid for Cancer Research (56-39) from the Ministry of Health and Welfare, Japan.

REFERENCES

Asatoor, A.M. & Simenhoff M.L. (1965) The origin of urinary dimethylamine. *Biochem. biophys. Acta,* *111*, 384–392

Asatoor A.M., Chamberlain, M.J., Emmerson, B.T., Johnson, J.R., Levi, A.J. & Milne, M.D. (1967) Metabolic effects of oral neomycin. *Clin. Sci., 33*, 111–124

Hamano, T., Hasegawa, A., Tanaka, K. & Matsuki, Y. (1979) Quantitative analysis of aliphatic secondary amines as their derivatives with benzene sulphonyl chloride by means of a gas chromatograph equipped with flame photometric detector. *J. Chromatogr., 179*, 346–350

Hamano, T., Mitsuhashi, Y. & Matsuki, Y. (1980) Improved gas chromatographic method for the quantitative determination of secondary amines as sulphonamides formed by reaction with benzenesulfonyl chloride. *J. Chromatogr., **190,** 462–465*

Harper, A.E. (1959) Amino acid balance and imbalance. I. Dietary level of protein and amino acid imbalance. *J. Nutr., **68,** 405–417*

Ishiwata, H., Mizushiro, H., Tanimura, A., Takahashi, A., Omori, Y. & Murata, T. (1977) Metabolic fate of the precursors of *N*-nitroso compounds (I) Gastro-intestinal absorption of *N*-nitrosodimethylamine and its precursors in guinea-pigs. *J. Food Hyg. Soc. Jpn, **18,** 524–528*

Ishiwata, H., Mizushiro, H., Tanimura, A. & Murata, T. (1978) Metabolic fate of the precursors of *N*-nitroso compounds (II) Salivary secretion and urinary excretion of nitrosatable compounds in man. *J. Food Hyg. Soc. Jpn, **19,** 91–97*

Ishiwata, H., Iwata, R. & Tanimura, A. (1982) Urinary excretion of dimethylamine in rats. *J. Food Hyg. Soc. Jpn, **23,** 360–364*

Johnson, K.A. (1977) The production of secondary amines by the human gut bacteria and its possible relevance to carcinogenesis. *Med. Lab. Sci., **34,** 131–143*

FORMATION OF *N*-NITROSO COMPOUNDS. CATALYSIS, INHIBITION AND MECHANISMS

CATALYSIS AND INHIBITION OF *N*-NITROSATION REACTIONS

M.C. ARCHER

Department of Medical Biophysics, University of Toronto, Ontario Cancer Institute,
500 Sherbourne St., Toronto M4X 1K9, Canada

SUMMARY

A number of factors that can lead to an acceleration or inhibition of *N*-nitrosation reactions may play an important role in the formation of *N*-nitroso compounds in foods and other environmental samples and in the body. The anion thiocyanate is a particularly effective catalyst for nitrosamine formation. It occurs in normal human saliva, but at higher concentrations in the saliva of smokers. Although nitrosation reactions are accelerated in the normal manner with increasing temperature, rate enhancements are also observed in frozen systems, a phenomenon that may be important in frozen foods. Surfactants that form micellar aggregates can accelerate the nitrosation of hydrophobic amines. This may be important in foods in view of the presence of components such as lecithin, or in the body in view of the occurrence of bile acid micelles. Nitrosation reactions may also be accelerated in the presence of certain carbonyl compounds, thiols and nitrosophenols. A number of compounds readily convert nitrosating agents into innocuous products and hence inhibit nitrosation reactions. If reductones such as ascorbic acid are present, they may react much faster with nitrous acid than amines and therefore effectively scavenge the nitrosating agent. Rapid reaction of polyhydroxyphenols with nitrous acid is another example of how endogenous or exogenous nitrosation reactions may be inhibited. Many microorganisms can influence nitrosation reactions by converting nitrate to nitrite, a reaction that can take place in foods, but which is particularly important in the body.

INTRODUCTION

This short review is not an exhaustive survey of the literature but rather highlights a number of the more important findings concerning catalysis and inhibition of *N*-nitrosation reactions. The review does not cover nitrosation by gaseous nitrogen oxides.

Nitrosamines are usually prepared by the action of sodium nitrite on a secondary amine at pH < 5. The nitrosating agent is the nitrosonium ion, NO^+, which exists in free form in solutions of strong acid; but in dilute aqueous acids, it exists as NOX, where X is a nuclophilic anion (Ridd, 1961). NOX forms from the nitrous acidium ion (H_2ONO^+) in a rapid prequilibration step:

$$NO_2^- + H_3O^+ \rightleftharpoons HNO_2 + H_2O$$
$$HNO_2 + H_3O^+ \rightleftharpoons H_2ONO^+ + H_2O$$
$$H_2ONO^+ + X^- \rightleftharpoons NOX + H_2O$$
$$R_2NH_2^+ + H_2O \rightleftharpoons R_2NH + H_3O^+$$
$$R_2NH + NOX \rightarrow R_2NNO + HX$$

In the absence of other nucleophilic anions, nitrite itself acts as X^- to form N_2O_3, the anhydride of nitrous acid. For most secondary amines, the rate of their reaction with N_2O_3 is much slower than the rate of formation of N_2O_3. Since two mol of nitrous acid are required to produce a mol of N_2O_3, the reaction rate shows a second-order dependency on the nitrous acid concentration:

$$Rate = k_1[R_2NH][HNO_2]^2$$

Furthermore, only the free base form of the amine can be nitrosated. Since at low pH values the concentration of unprotonated amine is low, while at high pH values the concentration of undissociated nitrous acid is low, a bell-shaped pH-rate profile is observed (Mirvish, 1970; Fan & Tannenbaum, 1937a). The maximum rate occurs at about pH 3.4, which is the pKa for nitrous acid. In general, weak bases are more rapidly nitrosated than strong bases. Thus, dimethylamine, with a pKa of 10.7, has a rate constant of 5.4 M^{-2}/h, at pH 3.0, while morpholine with a pKa of 8.5, has a rate constant of 1 400 M^{-2}/h at the same pH (Mirvish, 1970; Fan & Tannenbaum, 1973a). For some amines, for example N-methylaniline (pKa 4.85), the nitrosation step is more rapid than N_2O_3 formation, which therefore becomes rate limiting (Kalatzis & Ridd, 1966). At pH 1, however, the concentration of nonionized N-methylaniline is so low that it becomes rate limiting.

Nitrosation of secondary amides (including ureas, guanidines and carbamates) is, in general, less facile than amine nitrosation. Thus Mirvish (1975) has shown that the major nitrosating agent for amides is not N_2O_3, but the more reactive nitrous acidium ion:

$$HNO_2 + H_3O^+ \rightleftharpoons H_2ONO^+ + H_2O$$
$$RNHCOR + H_2ONO^+ \rightarrow RN(NO)COR + H_2O$$
$$Rate = k_2[RNHCOR][HNO_2][H_3O^+]$$

In contrast to the nitrosation of secondary amines, this rate expression is first-order in nitrous acid concentration, and becomes progressively faster with increasing acidity.

CATALYSIS

The nitrosation of secondary amines is accelerated by nucleophilic anions, since the concentration of available nitrosating agent is increased. Furthermore, some of these reagents are more reactive than N_2O_3. The rate of nitrosation by NOX, shows a first-order dependency on the nitrous acid concentration:

$$Rate = k_3[R_2NH][HNO_2][H^+][X]^-$$

The effectiveness of the anion is related approximately to its nucleophilic strength. Thus, the ratios of the rate constants for nitrosation or morpholine in the presence of thiocyanate, bromide and chloride are 15 000 : 30 : 1 (Fan & Tannenbaum, 1973a). Buffer anions, such as acetate, may also take part in nitrosation reactions (Masui *et al.*, 1974). The rate enhancements produced by nucleophilic anions are greater for weakly basic than for more strongly basic amines (Boyland *et al.*, 1971; Fan & Tannenbaum, 1973a; Boyland & Walker, 1974); no catalysis is observed for amides, ureas or carbamates (Berry & Challis, 1974; Hallett *et al.*, 1980).

Since thiocyanate is present in considerable amounts in normal human saliva (10–30 mg/100 mL), while saliva of smokers contains three to four times the normal level, the catalytic effect of thiocyanate on nitrosamine formation may have important practical consequences, particularly for in-vivo nitrosation (Boyland *et al.*, 1971; Boyland & Walker, 1974).

Masui *et al.* (1979) demonstrated catalysis of dimethylamine nitrosation by thiourea at pH 4. In an investigation of the mechanism of this effect, Meyer and Williams (1981) showed that catalysis is caused by equilibrium formation of the *S*-nitroso adduct, which is a very potent nitrosating agent:

$$\underset{H_2N-\overset{\overset{\textstyle S}{\|}}{C}-NH_2}{} + N_2O_3 \rightleftharpoons [\underset{H_2N-\overset{\overset{\textstyle SNO}{\|}}{C}-NH_2}{}]^+ \; NO_2^- \rightarrow \underset{R_2NH}{R_2NNO} + \underset{H_2N-\overset{\overset{\textstyle S}{\|}}{C}-NH_2}{} + HNO_2$$

Catalysis occurs, then, in a similar manner to that with halide ions, but the formation constant for the *S*-nitroso derivatives is larger than for the nitrosylhalides, so that the order of efficiency for catalysis for morpholine, for example, is thiourea $> SCN^- > Br^-$ in the ratio 4 200 : 240 : 1.

In addition to specific anion effects, there are also the more general primary and secondary salt effects, which, for example, lead to inhibition of nitrosation resactions at pH > 3 with high levels of sodium chloride (Hildrum *et al.*, 1975; Cachaza *et al.*, 1978).

The nitrosation of morpholine at temperatures above 0 C follows the Arrhenius law in a classical manner (Fan & Tannenbaum, 1973b). When the reaction solution is frozen, however, the rate is considerably enhanced compared to that expected for a supercooled solution at the same temperature. This rate enhancement is explained by the exclusion of reactants from the ice lattice and hence their concentration in the unfrozen liquid phase. This phenomenon may be relevant to reactions taking place in frozen foods. At high temperatures (up to 180 C), nitrosamines have been shown to be formed from sodium nitrite and secondary amines even in low-moisture or dry systems (Gray & Dugan, 1974).

In a model food system in which dibutylamine and sodium nitrite were added to a matrix of carboxymethylcellulose and then freeze-dried, maximum nitrosamine formation occurred at 100–125 C, above which production decreased rapidly (Ender & Ceh, 1971). This decrease is most likely caused by expulsion of the amine from the system, since Fan and Tannenbaum (1972) have shown that nitrosamines are generally quite stable at 110 C. Other factors of importance for nitrosamine formation in these low-moisture systems are the nitrite: amine ratio and pH.

The rates of nitrosation of long-chain dialkylamines, such as dihexylamine, may be accelerated many fold in the presence of both synthetic and naturally occurring surfactants that form micellar aggregates (Okun & Archer, 1977a; Kim *et al.*, 1980). The magnitude of the catalytic effect depends on the chain length of the amine, since the amine becomes more soluble in the hydrophobic micellar phase as the chain length increases. The rate enchancements are explained in part by electrostatic interactions on the surface of the micelle, which destabilize the protonated amine relative to the free base form, and, in part, by the preferential dissolution of N_2O_3 in the micellar phase. An autocatalytic effect has also been observed during the nitrosation of dihexylamine (Okun & Archer, 1977b). The effect is caused by spontaneous emulsification of the product, nitrosodihexylamine, when its concentration exceeds its solubility in aqueous solution. Catalysis then takes place in the microdroplets in a manner analogous to that observed in the presence of added surfactant.

Catalytic effects on the nitrosation of long-chain dialkylamines have also been observed in heterogeneous model systems containing a 20% decane phase (Massey *et al.*, 1979). The mechanism for these rate enhancements is again probably similar to that for micellar catalysis. Since inhibiting effects have been observed in the nitrosation of dimethylamine in the presence of unsaturated lipids due to reaction of nitrous acid with the lipid itself (Kurechi & Kikugawa, 1979), prediction of the effect of lipophilic material on nitrosation, either in foods or in the digestive tract, will be difficult.

Very recently, Kim (1983) reported that the nitrosation rates of *N*-methylurea, *N*-butylurea, and *N*-octylurea decreased in the presence of taurocholate micelles. An explanation for this observation is that the nitrosating agent, H_2ONO^+, is excluded in this case from the micellar phase into which the ureas partition. The nitrosation reaction therefore takes place primarily in the bulk phase.

Another effect that may be important in the digestive tract or in foods, is the almost four-fold increase in the rate of nitrosation of dipropylamine in the presence of wheat bran (Wishnok & Richardson, 1979). Nitrosation of pyrrolidine and morpholine was not affected by bran, and the mechanism of the effect on dipropylamine nitrosation is unclear.

In 1973, Keefer and Roller showed that nitrosamine formation can occur under neutral or even basic conditions in the presence of certain carbonyl compounds such as formaldehyde. They found that acetaldehyde produced no catalysis, while chloral had a similar effect to formaldehyde. We showed subsequently (Archer *et al.*, 1976) that several benzaldehyde derivatives and also pyridoxal catalysed the nitrosation of morpholine. The likely mechanism for these reactions, proposed by Keefer and Roller (1973), and studied in detail by Casado *et al.*, (1981), involves reaction of the aldehyde and secondary amine to form an iminium ion (Fig. 1). Nucleophilic attack by nitrite ion on this intermediate forms the dialkylamino nitrite ester, which then collapses to form the nitrosamine. A similar mechanism has been proposed to explain the formation of nitrosamines from secondary amines and solid sodium nitrite in halogenated solvents such as dichloromethane (Roller *et al.*, 1980). In that case, the dichloromethane undergoes an SN2-type nucleophilic displacement reaction with the amine, producing the formaldiminium ion and an equivalent of acid (Fig. 1).

Kurechi *et al.* (1980a) have shown that malondialdehyde, which can be derived from lipids by peroxidation, decreased nitrosamine formation at pH 3, but increased it at pH 6–7. No mechanism for this effect was proposed, but the authors concluded that the promoting effect of malondialdehyde was different from that of formaldehyde.

Fig. 1. Nitrosamine formation in the presence of aldehydes or dichloromethane

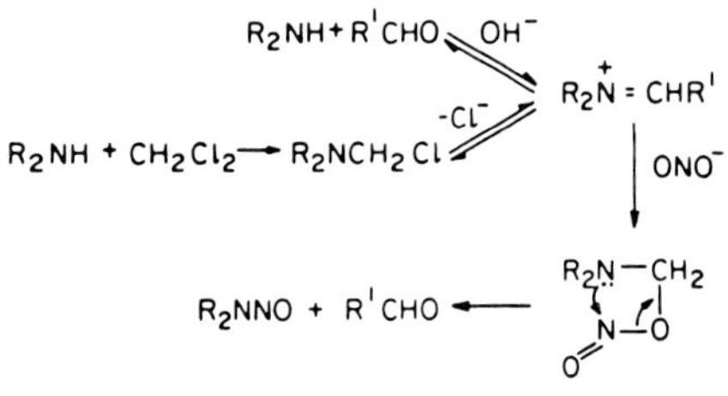

Fig. 2. Catalysis of nitrosamine formation by *p*-nitrosophenols

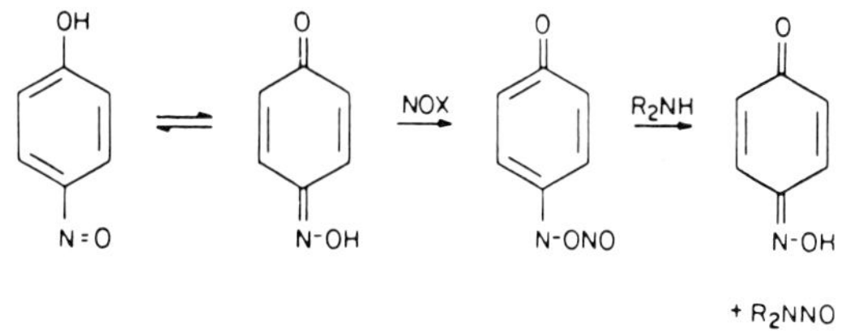

Nitrite ion in the presence of certain metal complexes can also generate nitrosamines from secondary amines. For example, nitrite in the presence of ferrocyanide at pH 11 and in 2,2'-dipyridine in the presence of cupric nitrate produces the nitrosating agents $[Fe^{III}(CN)_5NO]^{2-}$ and $[Cu^{II}(bipyr)ONO_2]$, respectively (Maltz *et al.*, 1971; Croisy *et al.*, 1980).

p-Nitrosophenols, which are known to occur in smoked meats, have been shown to catalyse the nitrosation of pyrrolidine and morpholine (Davies & . McWeeny, 1977; Davies *et al.*, 1980) and diethylamine (Walker *et al.*, 1979). The catalytic species is probably the quinone monoxime tautomer of the nitrosophenol which reacts rapidly with NOX to form the O-nitroso derivative (Fig. 2). This is followed by the slower attack on the O-nitroso derivative by the amine, resulting in nitrosamine formation and regeneration of the nitrosophenol (Walker *et al.*, 1979; Davies *et al.*, 1980). *p*-Nitroso-*N*-dialkylanilines catalyse nitrosamine formation by a similar mechanism (Davies *et al.*, 1980).

Phenols themselves react very rapidly with nitrous acid to produce nitrosophenols (Challis, 1973), and so an excess of phenol would inhibit nitrosation reactions. At high nitrite : phenol ratios, however, nitrosophenol formation will lead to catalysis. Pignatelli *et al.* (1980, 1982) showed that 1,3-dihydroxyphenols, but not 1,2- and 1,4-dihydroxyphenols, are potent catalysts of amine nitrosation. The mechanism involves initial formation of the dinitrosoresorcinols which react to form an *O*-nitroso derivative of the quinone oxime tautomer as before.

INHIBITION

A number of compounds are known to inhibit nitrosation reactions by rapidly converting nitrosating agents into products such as nitric oxide, nitrous oxide or nitrogen.

Of the compounds that reduce nitrous acid to nitric oxide, ascorbic acid is perhaps the best studied. This reductant is particularly valuable since it is obviously acceptable for human consumption and can be used to inhibit endogenous nitrosation reactions. Nitrosating agents, NOX, are rapidly reduced to nitric oxide by both ascorbic acid and ascorbate anion (pKa 4.3) (Bunton *et al.*, 1959). Oxidation proceeds *via* formation of the nitrite ester, which decomposes to the semiquinone (Fig. 3). Reaction of a further mol of nitrosating agent yields dehydroascorbate. Mirvish *et al.* (1972) first showed that ascorbic acid could effectively block nitrosamine formation from pH 1 to pH 4 by competing with secondary amines for nitrosating agent. In the presence of air, substantially more ascorbic acid is required for complete blocking of amine nitrosation than is necessary under anaerobic conditions (Archer *et al.*, 1975; Kim *et al.*, 1982), because reaction of nitric oxide with oxygen leads to formtion of additional oxidizing equivalents (nitrogen dioxide). Presence of oxygen could also lead to direct oxidation of ascorbate, again leading to oxidation of more than half a mol of ascorbic acid by one mol of nitrous acid. In addition to blocking nitrosation reactions in chemical and food systems,

Fig. 3. Oxidation of ascorbic acid by nitrosating agents in the absence of air

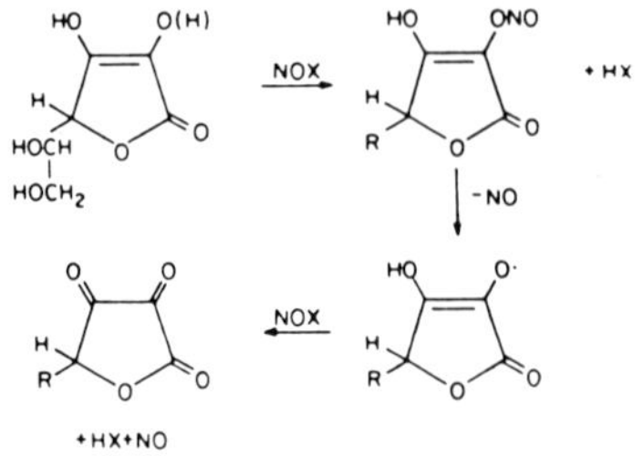

Fig. 4. Oxidation of α-tocopherol by nitrosating agents

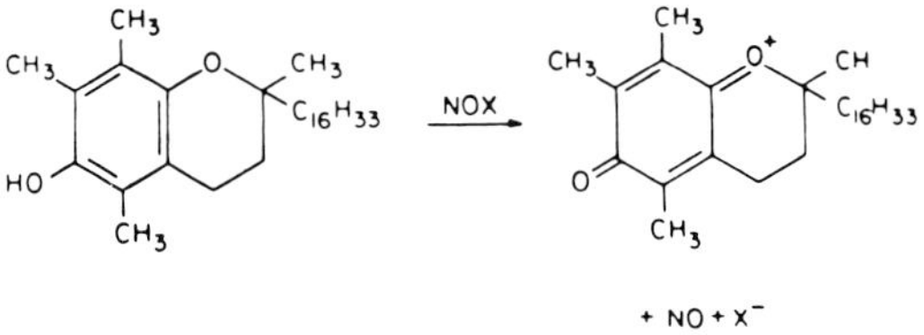

ascorbic acid has also been shown to block nitrosation *in vivo* (Mirvish, 1981; Ohshima & Bartsch, 1981).

It should be noted that in one report (Chang *et al.*, 1979) ascorbic acid was shown to accelerate nitrosation at pH 1–2 of the weakly basic amines *N*-methylaniline and diphenylamine, but not a series of more strongly basic secondary amines. The mechanism for this catalysis was attributed to interaction of ascorbic acid and nitrite to produce the nitrosating agent, oxyhyponitrous acid ($H_2N_2O_3$).

Since ascorbic acid is water soluble, it is most effective as a nitrite scavenger in aqueous environments. Various ascorbyl and erythorbyl esters and α-tocopherol have been shown to be more effective inhibitors in lipophilic environments, such as the fat phase of foods (Sen *et al.*, 1976; Pensabene *et al.*, 1976; Fiddler *et al.*, 1978; Mergens *et al.*, 1978). α-Tocopherol is oxidized to a quinonoid product by NOX with formation of NO (Fig. 4).

Phenolic compounds can effectively block *N*-nitrosation by rapid formation of *C*-nitrosophenols (Challis, 1973; Massey *et al.*, 1978; Kurechi *et al.*, 1979, 1980b). For example, the rate of nitrosation of phenol itself is 10^4 times that of dimethylamine nitrosation. It was noted above, however, that phenolic compounds can, under certain circumstances, catalyse nitrosamine formation *via* formation of nitrosophenols. Since nitrosophenols are oxidized in air to the stable nitrophenols, the effect of a phenol in a particular system in either catalysing or inhibiting nitrosation will depend on whether the steady-state concentration of nitrosophenol is sufficiently large to overcome the inhibitory effect of the phenol (Davies & McWeeny, 1977).

Pignatelli *et al.* (1980, 1982) have shown that, in contrast to 1,3-dihydroxyphenols (see above), 1,2- and 1,4-dihydroxyphenols, including naturally occurring derivatives, inhibit nitrosamine formation by their oxidation by N_2O_3 to the corresponding quinones, with formation of nitric oxide [earlier reports of catalysis by 4-methylcatechol (Challis & Bartlett, 1975) and gallic acid (Walker *et al.*, 1975) are incorrect due to artefactual nitrosamine formation during analysis]. Pignatelli *et al.* (1982) demonstrated inhibition of in-vivo nitrosation of proline by the 1,2-dihydroxyphenol chlorogenic acid.

There is a brief report on the activity of pyrrole as an inhibitor of nitrosation (Groenen, 1976), in which it was found to be a more effective inhibitor of morpholine nitrosation than ascorbic acid. It appears to act by reacting with nitrous acid to form the polymeric nitrosopyrrole black. Since pyrrole and its derivatives occur in food materials, the reaction may be important.

A number of inorganic compounds react rapidly and irreversibly with nitrous acid to produce a variety of products that are not nitrosating agents:

$$N_3^- + NOX \rightarrow N_2 + N_2O + X^-$$

$$NH_2NH_3^+ + \quad NOX \begin{array}{c} \text{High H}^+ \nearrow \quad HN_3 + H_3O^+ + HX \\ \\ \text{Low H}^+ \searrow \quad NH_4^+ + N_2O + HX \end{array}$$

$$NH_2SO_3H + NOX \rightarrow N_2 + H_2SO_4 + HX$$
$$NH_2OH + NOX \rightarrow N_2O + H_2O + HX$$
$$CO(NH_2)_2 + 2NOX \rightarrow 2N_2 + CO_2 + H_2O + 2HX$$

Such compounds can hence be used as nitrite scavengers in the study of nitrosation reactions. Since it is protonated at low pH, ammonia is a poor inhibitor. Ellisson and Williams (1981) have studied the relative efficiencies of a range of nitrite traps towards a number of nitrosating agents, with the following result: azide > hydrazine > sulfuric acid > hydroxylamine > urea. Ascorbic acid is also often used as a nitrite trap in chemical experiments; it has approximately the same reactivity as sulfamic acid towards NOBr but is considerably more reactive, particularly at lower acidities, towards NOSCN (Williams, 1978).

A number of simple alcohols and carbohydrates have been shown to inhibit N-nitrosation reactions through rapid equilibrium formation of the corresponding alkyl nitrite, which is virtually inactive as a direct nitrosating agent (Kurechi et al., 1980c; Aldred et al., 1982; Williams & Aldred, 1982):

$$ROH + NOX \rightleftharpoons RONO + HX.$$

Alkyl nitrites can act as nitrosating agents, however, in the presence of halide ion or thiourea catalysts due to the formation of the corresponding nitrosyl halide or nitrosothiourea adduct (Aldred & Williams, 1981). Challis and Shuker (1979) also demonstrated that alkyl nitrites with β-electron withdrawing substituents rapidly nitrosate secondary amines in 0.1 mol/L sodium hydroxide.

In a similar manner, thiols inhibit N-nitrosation by rapid formation of thionitrite esters (Gray & Dugan, 1975; Davies et al., 1978a; Aldred et al., 1982; Williams & Aldred, 1982). Thiols are more effective inhibitors than alcohols because of the virtual irreversibility of S-nitrosation at acidic pH compared to O-nitrosation under these conditions:

$$RSH + NOX \rightarrow RSNO + HX.$$

Under some conditions, particulary at pH > 5, thionitrites can act as nitrosating agents (Davies et al., 1978b; Dennis et al., 1979; Kunisaki & Hayashi, 1980). Evidence has been presented that thionitrites present in a polypeptide or protein can also effect nitrosation, though at a reduced rate (Massey *et al.*, 1978; Dennis -et, 1980). This reaction may be important however, in nitrite-treated foods.

THE ROLE OF MICROORGANISMS IN NITROSATION REACTIONS

It is now well established that microorganisms can facilitate nitrosation reactions. As pointed out by Scanlan (1975), various microorganisms may influence nitrosation by (a) reducing nitrate or nitrite (or, under certain conditions, oxidizing ammonia to nitrite); (b) lowering pH; and (c) producing substances or enzymes that directly catalyse nitrosation reactions.

Some microorganisms convert nitrate to ammonia or amino acids for ultimate synthesis of proteins, nucleic acids, etc. The enzyme involved in the first step of this process reduces nitrate to nitrite and is called 'assimilatory nitrate reductase'. Other organisms use nitrate as a terminal electron acceptor in place of oxygen, usually under anaerobic or partially anaerobic conditions. The enzyme involved in this process is called 'dissimilatory nitrate reductase'. Numerous organisms contain one or other type of nitrate reductase, which are generally flavomolybdoproteins (Nason, 1963; Payne, 1973). In many yeasts and bacteria, nitrite is reduced to ammonia by iron-containing enzymes that usually require NADPH and flavin cofactors (Prabhakararao & Nicholas, 1970). Nitrite can be made by certain aerobic microorganisms by oxidation of ammonia in a process known as 'nitrosification'; nitrite may also be oxidized to nitrate in a process known as 'nitrification' (both nitrosification and nitrification are often spoken of together as 'nitrification'). These processes have been reviewed by Schmidt (1978).

Formation of nitrite from nitrate by the nitrate reductase activity of microorganisms is an important process in the human body that can lead to endogenous nitrosamine formation. Sites of nitrite formation include the oral cavity, the abnormally hypochlorhydric or achlorhydric stomach and the infected urinary tract or bladder (reviewed by Archer, 1982).

There have been numerous reports of the catalysis of nitrosation reactions by microorganisms. Nonenzymatic, pH-dependent catalysis by one or more unidentified metabolic products has been proposed in suspensions of *Streptococcus* species (Collins-Thompson *et al.*, 1972), bacterial flora of the rat intestine (Klubes & Jondorf, 1971) and *Pseudomonas stutzeri* (Mills & Alexander, 1976). The nitrosation of several secondary amines is catalysed in the presence of microorganisms at pH 3.5 (Yang *et al.*, 1977). The magnitude of the rate enhancement depends on the alkyl chain length of the amine, as was found for surfactant catalysis. A nonenzymatic mechanism of nitrosamine formation was proposed, involving hydrophobic interactions of the precursor amine and cellular constituents.

In a number of viable microbial cultures, enzymatic catalysis of *N*-nitrosodimethylamine and *N*-nitrosodiethylamine formation has been proposed, but the enzyme(s) involved in such a reaction has never been isolated or characterized (reviewed by Archer, 1982). Recent work by Ralt and Tannenbaum (1981), however, has shown that the major role of a number of bacterial strains in the nitrosation of dimethylamine is reduction of nitrate to nitrite and/or the lowering of the pH of the medium. Furthermore, the complex media in which the microorganisms are cultured can catalyse nitrosation. It is likely that most, if not all, of the earlier reports on the involvement of enzymes in nitrosation reactions, were inadequately controlled, and a number may have been subject to artefactual synthesis or inadequate detection and quantification of nitrosamines. Clearly the utmost care is required in carrying out the microbiological and chemical techniques required in such studies, and all the appropriate controls must be performed before the result can be considered credible. There is, however, one case in which an enzyme is almost certainly involved in forming an $-N-N=O$ bond, and that is the biosynthesis of the antibiotic streptozotocin [2-deoxy-2-(3-methylnitrosoureido)-1)-glucopyranose] by *Streptoyces adromogenes* var. streptozoticus. Nothing is currently known about the synthesis of the nitrogen-nitrogen bond in this secondary metabolite (Singaram *et al.*, 1979).

ACKNOWLEDGEMENTS

The author is grateful for support from the Ontario Cancer Treatment and Research Foundation and the National Cancer Institute of Canada.

REFERENCES

Aldred, S. E. & Williams, D. L. H. (1981) Alkylnitrites as nitrosating agents. Kinetics and mechanism of the reactions of propyl nitrite in propal-1-ol. *J. chem. Soc. (Perkin II)*, 1021–1024

Aldred, S. E., Williams, D. L. H. & Garley, M. (1982) Kinetics and mechanism of the nitrosation of alcohols, carbohydrates and a thiol. *J. chem. Soc. (Perkin II)*, 777–782

Archer, M. C. (1982) *Hazards of nitrate, nitrite, and* N-*nitroso compounds in human nutrition*. In: Hathcoock, J. N., ed., *Nutritional Toxicology*, Vol. 1, New York, Academic Press, pp. 327–381

Archer, M. C., Tannenbaum, S. R., Fan, T. Y. & Weisman, M. (1975) Reaction of nitrite with ascorbate and its relation to nitrosamine formation. *J. natl Cancer Inst.*, **54**, 1203–1205

Archer, M. C., Tannenbaum, S. R. & Wishnok, J. S. (1976) *Nitrosamine formation in the presence of carbonyl compounds*. In: Walker, E. A., Bogovski, P. & Griciute, L., eds, *Environmental* N-*Nitroso Compounds: Analysis and Formation (IARC Scientific Publications No. 14)*, Lyon, International Agency for Research on Cancer, pp. 141–145

Berry, C. N. & Challis, B. C. (1974) The chemistry of nitroso compounds. Part VIII. Denitrosation and deamination of N-n-butyl-N-nitroso-acetamide in aqueous acids. *J. chem. Soc. (Perkin II)*, 1638–1644

Boyland, E. & Walker, S. A. (1974) Effect of thiocyanate on nitrosation of amines. *Nature*, **248**, 601–602

Boyland, E., Nice, E. & Williams, K. (1971) The catalysis of nitrosation by thiocyanate from saliva. *Food Cosmet. Toxicol.*, **9**, 639–643

Bunton, C. A., Dahn, H. & Loewe, L. (1959) Oxidation of ascorbic acid and similar reductones by nitrous acid. *Nature*, **183**, 163–165

Cachaza, J. M., Casado, J., Castro, A. & Lopez Quintela, M. A. (1978) Kinetic studies on the formation of nitrosamines. I. Formation of dimethylnitrosamine in aqueous solution of perchloric acid. *Z. Krebsforsch.*, **91**, 279–290

Casado, J., Castro, A., Lopez Quintela, M. A. & Vasquez Tato, J. (1981) Kinetic studies on the formation of *N*-nitroso compounds. V. Formation of dimethylnitrosamine in aqueous solution: effect of formaldehyde. *Z. Phys. Chem. neue Folge.*, **127**, 179–192

Challis, B. C. (1973) Rapid nitrosation of phenols and its implications for health hazards form dietary nitrites. *Nature*, **244**, 466

Challis, B. C. & Bartlett, C. D. (1975) Possible carcinogenic effects of coffee constituents. *Nature*, **254**, 532–533

Challis, B. C. & Shuker, D. E. G. (1979) Rapid nitrosation of amines in aqueous alkaline solutions by β-substituted alkyl nitrites. *J. chem. Soc. chem. Commun.*, 315–316

Chang, S. K., Harrington, G. W., Rothstein, M., Shergalis, W. A., Swern, D. & Vohra, S. K. (1979) Accelerating effect of ascorbic acid on *N*-nitrosamine formation and nitrosation by oxyhyponitrite. *Cancer Res.*, **39**, 3871–3874

Collins-Thompson, D. L., Sen, N. P., Avis, B. & Schwinghamer, L. (1972) Non-enzymic in-vitro formation of nitrosamines by bacteria isolated from meat products. *Can. J. Microbiol.*, **18**, 1968–1971

Croisy, A. F., Fanning, J. C., Keefer, L. K., Slavin, B. W. & Uhm, S.-J. (1980) *Metal complexes as promoters of N-nitrosation reactions: A progress report*. In: Walker, E. A., Griciute, L. Castegnaro, M. & Borzonyi, M., eds, N-*Nitroso Compounds: Analysis, Formation and Occurrence (IARC Scientific Publications No. 31)*, Lyon, International Agency for Research on Cancer, pp. 83–93

Davies, R. & McWeeny, D.J. (1977) Catalytic effect of nitrosophenols on N-nitrosamine formation. *Nature, 266,* 657–658

Davies, R. Massey, R.C. & McWeeny, D.J.: (1978a) A study of the rate of competitive nitrosations of pyrrolidine, p-cresol and L-cysteine hydrochloride. *J. Sci. Food Agric., 29,* 62–70

Davies, R., Dennis, M.J., Massey, R.C. & McWeeny, D.J. (1978b) *Some effects of phenol- and thiol-nitrosation reactions on N-nitrosamine formation.* In: Walker, E.A., Castegnaro, M., Griciute, L. & Lyle, R.E., eds, *Environmental Aspects of* N-*nitroso compounds (IARC Scientific Publications No. 19),* Lyon, International Agency for Research on Cancer, pp. 183–197

Davies, R., Massey, R.C. & McWeeny, D.J. (1980) The catalysis of the N-nitrosation of secondary amines by nitrosophenols. *Food Chem., 6,* 115–122

Dennis, J.M., Davies, R. & McWeeny, D.J. (1979) The transnitrosation of secondary amines S-nitrosocysteine in relation to N-nitrosamine formation in cured meats. *J. Sci. Food Agric., 30,* 639–645

Dennis, M.J., Massey, R.C. & McWeeny, D.J. (1980) The transnitrosation of N-methylaniline by a protein-bound nitrite model system in relation to N-nitrosamine formation in cured meats. *J. Sci. Food. Agric., 31,* 1195–1200

Ellison, G. & Williams, D.L.H. (1981) The relative effeciencies of a number of nitrite traps at different acidities and bromide ion concentrations. *J. chem. Soc. (Perkin II),* 699–702

Ender, F. & Ceh, L. (1971) Conditions and chemical reaction mechanisms by which nitrosamines may be formed in biological products with reference to their possible occurrence in food products. *Z. Lebensm.-Untersuch. Forsch., 145,* 133–142

Fan, T.Y. & Tannenbaum, S.R. (1972) Stability of N-nitroso compounds. *J. Food Sci., 37,* 274–276

Fan, T.Y. & Tannenbaum, S.R. (1973a) Factories influencing the rate of formation of nitrosomorpholine from morpholine and nitrite: Acceleration by thiocyanate and other anions. *J. Agric. Food Chem., 21,* 237–240

Fan, T.Y. & Tannenbaum, S.R. (1973b) Factors influencing the rate of formation of nitrosomorpholine from morpholine and nitrite. II. Rate enhancement in frozen solution. *J. Agric. Food Chem., 21,* 967–969

Fiddler, W., Pensabene, J.W., Piotrowski, E.G., Phillips, J.G., Keating, J., Mergens, W.J. & Newmark, H.L. (1978) Inhibition of formation of volatile nitrosamines in fried bacon by the use of cure-solubilized α-tocopherol. *J. Agric. Food Chem., 26,* 653–656

Gray, J.I. & Dugan, L.R. (1974) Formation of N-nitrosamines in low moisture systems. *J. Food Sci., 39,* 474–478

Gray, J.I. & Dugan, L.R. (1975) Inhibition of N-nitrosamine formation in model food systems. *J. Food Sci., 40,* 981–984

Groenen, P.J. (1976) *A new type of* N-*nitrosation inhibitor.* In: Tinbergen, B.J. & Krol, B., eds, *Proceedings of the 2nd International Symposium on Meat Products,* Wageningen, The Netherlands. Centre for Agricultural Publishing Documentation. pp. 171–173

Hallett, G., Johal, S.S., Meyer, T.A. & Williams, D.L.H. (1980) *Reactions of nitrosamines with nucleophiles in acid solution.* In: Walker, E.A., Griciute, L. Castegnaro, M. & Borzonyi, M., eds, N-*Nitroso Compounds: Analysis, Formation and Occurrence (IARC Scientific Publications No. 31),* Lyon, International Agency for Research on Cancer, pp. 31–41

Hildrum, K.I. Williams, J.L. & Scanlan, R.A. (1975) Effect of sodium chloride concentration on the nitrosation of proline at different pH levels. *J. Agric. Food Chem., 23,* 439–442

Kalatzis, E. & Ridd, J.H. (1966) Nitrosation, diazotisation and deamination. Part XII. The kinetics of N-nitrosation of N-methylaniline. *J. chem. Soc.,* 529–533

Keefer, L.K. & Roller, P.P. (1973) N-Nitrosation by nitrite ion in neutral and basic medium, *Science, 181,* 1245–1247

Kim, Y.L. (1983) N-*Nitrosation Reactions and their Inhibition in Aqueous and Micellar Solutions,* PhD Thesis, Massachusetts Institute of Technology

Kim, Y.K., Tannenbaum, S.R. & Wishnok, J.C. (1980) *Nitrosation of dialkylamines in the presence of bile acid conjugates.,* In: Walker, E.A., Griciute, L. Castegnaro, M. & Borzonyi, M., eds, N-*Nitroso Compounds: Analysis, Formation and Occurrence (IARC Scientific Publications No. 31),* Lyon, International Agency for Research on Cancer, pp. 207–214

Kim, Y.K., Tannenbaum, S.R. & Wishnok, J.C. (1982) *Effects of ascorbic acid on the nitrosation of dialkylamines.* In: Steib, P.A. & Tolbert, B.M., eds, *Ascorbic Acid: Chemistry, Metabolism and Uses (Advances in Chemistry Series 200),* Washington DC, American Chemical Society, pp. 571–585

Klubes, P. & Jondorf, W.R. (1971) Dimethylnitrosamine formation from sodium nitrite and dimethylamine by bacterial flora of rat intestine. *Res. Commun. Chem. pathol. Pharmacol., 2*, 24

Kunisaki, N. & Hayashi, M. (1980) Effects of ergothioneine, cysteine and gluthathione on nitrosation of secondary amines under physiological conditions. *J. natl Cancer Inst., 65*, 791–794

Kurechi, T. & Kikugawa, K. (1979) Nitrite-lipid reaction in aqueous system: Inhibitory effects on nitrosamine formation. *J. Food Sci., 44*, 1263–1266

Kurechi, T. Kikugawa, K. & Kato (1979) C-Nitrosation of sesamol and its effects on N-nitrosamine formation *in vitro. Chem. Pharm. Bull., 27*, 2442–2449

Kurechi, T., Kikugawa, K. & Ozawa, M. (1980a) Effect of malondialdehyde on nitrosamine formation. *Food cosmet. Toxicol., 18*, 119–122

Kurechi, T., Kikugawa, K. & Kato, T. (1980b) The butylated hydroxyanisole-nitrite reaction: Effects on N-nitrosodimethylamine formation in model systems. *Chem. Pharm. Bull., 28*, 1314–1317

Kurechi, T., Kikugawa, K. & Kato, T. (1980c) Effect of alcohols on nitrosamine formation. *Food Cosmet. Toxicol., 18*, 591–595

Maltz, H., Grant, M.A. & Navaroli, M.C. (1971) Reaction of nitroprusside with amines. *J. org. Chem., 36*, 363–364

Massey, R.C., Crews, C., Davies, R. & McWeeny, D.J. (1978) A study of the competitive nitrosations of pyrrolidine, ascorbic acid, cysteine and p-cresol in a protein-based model system. *J. Sci. Food Agric., 29*, 815–821

Massey, R.C., Crews, C. Davies, R. & McWeeny, D.J. (1979) The enhanced N-nitrosation of lipid soluble amines in a heterogeneous model system. *J. Sci. Food agric., 30*, 211–214

Masui, M., Nakahara, H., Ohmori, H. & Sayo, H. (1974) Kinetic studies on the formation of dimethylnitrosamine. *Chem. Pharm. Bull., 22*, 1846–1849

Masui, M., Ueda, T., Yasuoka, T. & Ohmori, H. (1979) Thioureas as effective catalysts for N-nitrosodimethylamine formation. *Chem. pharm. Bull., 27*, 1274–1275

Mergens, W.J., Kamm, J.J., Newmark, H.L., Fiddler, W., & Pensabene, J. (1978) *Alpha-tocopherol: Uses in preventing nitrosamine formation.* In. Walker, E.A., Castegnaro, M., Griciute, L. & Lyle, R.E., eds, *Environmental Aspects of* N-*nitroso compounds. (IARC Scientific Publications No. 19*), Lyon, International Agency for Research on Cancer, pp. 199–212

Meyer, T.A. & Williams, D.L.H. (1981) Catalysis of N-nitrosation and diazotisation by thiourea dn thiocyanate ion. *J. chem. Soc. (Perkin II)*. 361–365

Mills, A.L. & Alexander, M. (1976) N-Nitrosamine formation by cultures of several microorganisms. *Appl. environ. Microbiol., 31*, 892–895

Mirvish, S.S. (1970) Kinetics of dimethylnitrosamine nitrosation in relation to nitrosamines carcinogenesis. *J. natl Cancer Inst., 44*, 633–639

Mirvish, S.S. (1975) Formation of N-nitroso compounds: Chemistry, kinetics and in vivo occurrence. *Toxicol. appl. Pharmacol., 31*, 325–351

Mirvish, S.S. (1981) *Ascorbic acid inhibition of N-nitroso compound formation in chemical, food, and biological systems.* In: Zedeck, M.S. & Lipkin, M., eds, *Inhibition of Tumor Induction and Development,* New York, Plenum, pp. 101–126

Mirvish, S.S., Wallcave, L., Eagen, M. & Shubik, P. (1972) Ascorbate-nitrite reaction: Possible means of blocking the formation of carcinogenic N-nitroso compounds. *Science, 177*, 65–68

Nason, A. (1963) *Nitrate reductases.* In. Boyer, P.D., Lardy, H. & Myrback, K., eds, *The Enzymes,* Vol. 7, New York, NY, Academic Press, Inc. pp. 587–607

Ohshima, H. & Bartsch, H. (1981) Quantitative estimation of endogenous nitrosation in humans by monitoring N-nitrosoproline excreted in the urine. *Cancer Res., 41*, 3658–3662

Okun, J.D. & Archer, M.C. (1977a) Kinetics of nitrosamine formation in the presence of micelle-forming surfactants. *J. natl Cancer Inst., 58*, 409–411

Okun, J.D. & Archer, M.C. (1977b) Autocatalysis in the nitrosation of dihexylamine. *J. org. Chem., 42*, 391–392

Payne, W.J. (1973) Reduction of nitrogenous oxides by microorganisms. *Bacteriol. Rev., 37*, 409–452

Pensabene, J.W., Fiddler, W., Feinberg, J. & Wasserman, A.E. (1976) Evaluation of ascorbyl monoesters for the inhibition of nitrosopyrrolidine in a model system. *J. Food Sci., 41*, 199–200

Pignatelli, B., Friesen, M. & Walker, E.A. (1980) *The role of phenols in catalysis of nitrosamine formation.* In: Walker, E.A., Griciute, L. Castegnaro, M. & Borzonyi, M., eds, N-*Nitroso Compounds. Analysis, Formation and Occurrence (IARC Scientific Publications No. 31*), Lyon, International Agency for Research on Cancer, pp. 95–109

Pignatelli, B., Béréziat, J.C., Descotes, C. & Bartsch, H. (1982) Catalysis of nitrosation in vitro and in vivo in rats by catechin and resorcinol and inhibition by chlorogenic acid. *Carcinogenesis, 3,* 1045–1049

Prabhakararao, K. & Nicholas, D.J.D. (1970) The reduction of sulphite, nitrite and hydroxylamine by an enzyme from baker's yeast. *Biochim. biophys. Acta, 216,* 122–129

Ralt, D. & Tannenbaum, S.R. (1981) *The role of bacteria in nitrosamine formation.* In: Scanlan, R.A. & Tannenbaum, S.R., eds, *Nitroso Compounds (ACS Symposium Series No. 174),* Washington DC, American Chemical Society, pp. 157–164

Ridd, J.H. (1961) Nitrosation, diazotisation and deamination. *Q. Rev. chem. Soc., 15,* 418–441

Roller, P.P., Keefer, L.K. & Slavin, B.W. (1980) *Inhibitory agents and chemical mechanisms in the dihalomethane-mediated nitrosation of amines with solid nitrite.* In: Walker, E.A., Griciute, L. Castegnaro, M. & Borzonyi, M., eds, N-*Nitroso Compounds: Analysis, Formation and Occurrence (IARC Scientific Publications No. 31),* Lyon, International Agency for Research on Cancer, pp. 119–128

Scanlan, R.A. (1975) N-Nitrosamines in foods. *Crit. Rev. Food Technol., 5,* 357–402

Schmidt, E.L. (1978) *Nitrifying microorganisms and their methodology.,* In: Schlessinger, D., ed., *Microbiology-1978,* Washington DC, American Society for Microbiology, pp. 288–291

Sen, N.P., Donaldson, B., Seaman, S., Iyengar, J. & Miles, W.F. (1976) Inhibition of nitrosamine formation in fried bacon by propyl gallate and L-ascorbyl palmitate. *J. Agric. Food Chem., 24,* 397–401

Singaram, S., Lawrence, R.S. & Hornemann, U. (1979) Studies on the biosynthesis of the antibiotic streptozotocin (streptozocin) by *Streptomyces achromogenes* va. streptozoticus. *J. Antibiot., 32,* 379–385

Walker, E.A., Pignatelli, B. & Castegnaro, M. (1975) Effects of gallic acid on nitrosamine formation. *Nature, 258,* 176

Walker, E.A., Pignatelli, B. & Castegnaro, M. (1979) Catalytic effect of p-nitrosophenol on the nitrosation of diethylamine. *J. Agric. Food Chem., 27,* 393–396

Williams, D.L.H. (1978) Comparison of the efficiencies of ascorbic acid and sulphamic acid as nitrite traps. *Food Cosmet. Toxicol., 16,* 365–367

Williams, D.L.H. & Aldred, S.E. (1982) Inhibition of nitrosation of amines by thiols, alcohols and carbohydrates. *Food Chem. Toxicol., 27,* 1132–1134

Wishnok, J.S. & Richardson, D.P. (1979) Interaction of wheat bran with nitrosamines and with amines during nitrosation. *J. Agric. Food Chem., 27,* 1132–1134

Yang, H.S., Okun, J.D. & Archer, M.C. (1977) Nonenzymatic microbial acceleration of nitrosamine formation. *J. Agric. Food Chem., 25,* 1181–1183

N-NITROSAMINE FORMATION BY INTESTINAL BACTERIA

K. SUZUKI

Animal Physiology Laboratory, The Institute of Physical and Chemical Research,
Wako-shi, Saitama 351, Japan

T. MITSUOKA

Department of Biomedical Science, Faculty of Agriculture, University of Tokyo,
Bunkyo-ku, Tokyo 113 and Animal Physiology Laboratory, The Institute of Physical
and Chemical Research, Wako-shi, Saitama 351, Japan

SUMMARY

N-Nitrosamine formation by various intestinal bacteria was investigated. *N*-Nitroso-dimethylamine (NDMA) formation by viable resting cells of *Escherichia coli* A10 was proportional to the incubation time and the enzyme concentration, while boiled cells were incapable of nitrosation. The enzyme was optimal at pH 7.5 and showed about the same specificities for dimethylamine, diethylamine, dibutylamine, di-isobutylamine, piperidine and pyrrolidine, but high specificity for morpholine. The intestinal bacteria harbouring nitrosating enzyme were mainly aerobic, i.e., *Escherichia coli, Proteus morganii, Klebsiella pneumonia* and *Pseudomonas aeruginosa*. Only one of the 32 anaerobic intestinal bacterial species, i.e., *Peptococcus asaccharolyticus*, was positive. The enzyme activities of these nitrosating bacteria covered a range of 0.06–0.90 nmol NDMA formed per hour per mg protein.

These results support the theory of enzymatic catalysis of *N*-nitrosamine formation by microorganisms and suggest the possibility of endogenous nitrosation in the digestive tract.

INTRODUCTION

Nitrosation by intestinal bacteria is an important factor in the endogenous formation of *N*-nitrosamines in the gastrointestinal tract. There are, however, sharp differences of opinion concerning the microbial formation of *N*-nitrosamines: on the one hand, the enzymatic catalysis theory (Hawksworth & Hill, 1971; Klubes & Jondorf, 1971; Brooks *et al.,* 1972; Sherbet & Lakshmi, 1973; Hashimoto *et al.,* 1975; Coloe & Hayward, 1976; Mills & Alexander, 1976; Kunisaki & Hayashi, 1979; Hayashi *et al.,* 1982) and, on the other, the non-enzymatic catalysis theory (Klubes & Jondorf, 1971; Collins-Thompson *et al.,* 1972; Archer *et al.,* 1975; Mills & Alexander, 1976; Ralt & Tannenbaum, 1981). Since the foregoing reports were published, our understanding of this field has been considerably clarified, and it is not impossible that the differences reported in the earlier results were a consequence of differences in the experimental methods employed. The artefactual formation of N-nitrosamines seems to occur with relative ease during the assaying of N-nitrosamines because nitrosation occurs even under neutral or alkaline conditions (Tozawa, 1982) and is promoted by many chemicals (Boyland et al., 1971; Kunisaki & Hayashi, 1980; Tozawa, 1982). In fact, with regard to microbial nitrosation, many reports show that the background level of N-nitrosamines in the medium was higher than the amount formed by bacteria. In addition, earlier methods for detecting N-nitrosamines, without a Thermal Energy Analyzer (TEA) or mass spectrometer (MS), were less than perfect with regard to specificity.

In order to resolve these conflicting results, we have studied the properties of microbial nitrosation using resting cells of intestinal bacteria as the enzyme preparation and the TEA as the detector of N-nitrosamines.

EXPERIMENTAL

Preparation of enzyme

Fifty-four bacterial strains were used in this study. Forty-four were obtained from the culture collection of the Animal Physiology Laboratory, the Institute of Physical and Chemical Research, Wako-shi; one of Escherichia coli from Dr Kunisaki, Kagawa Nutrition College, Tokyo; and four of E. coli and one each of Proteus mirabilis, P. morganii, P. vulgaris, Klebsiella pneumonia and Pseudomonas aeruginosa from Dr Hashimoto, Yakult Institute for Microbiological Research, Tokyo.

Resting cell suspensions were prepared by culturing facultative and aerobic bacteria aerobically in a Trypticase soya broth (BBL). Anaerobes were cultured in EGL broth (Mitsuoka, 1980) in an anaerobic, steel-wool jar filled with oxygen-free carbon dioxide (Parker, 1955). After 24-h cultivation, the bacteria were collected aseptically and washed three times in sterile physiological saline by refrigerated centrifugation. The washed cells were resuspended in cold saline at a final cell density corresponding to about 15 mg protein per mL. This cell suspension was used as a crude enzyme solution.

Nitrosation reaction

The nitrosation reaction was carried out according to the method of Kunisaki and Hayashi (1979). Twenty mL of a reaction mixture containing 7.5 mmol/L dimethylamine (DMA), 25 mmol/L nitrite, 0.1 mol/L potassium phosphate buffer (pH 7.0) and a suitable amount of enzyme preparation were incubated at 37 C for 30 min.

The effect of pH on nitrosation in suspensions of resting cells of E. coli A10 was investigated. The procedure was similar to that used previously, except that the phosphate buffer was adjusted to various pH values.

Substrate specificity of secondary amines on nitrosation by E. coli A10 was also measured using a similar method. The amines used were dimethylamine (DMA), diethylamine (DEA), dibutylamine (DBA), di-isobutylamine (Di-BA), piperidine (PIP), pyrrolidine (PYR) and morpholine (MOR). Protein was measured by the method of Lowry et al. (1951), using bovine albumin as a standard.

Detection of N-nitrosamines

N-Nitrosamines produced in the reaction mixture were extracted with 10 mL dichloromethane for 3 min, using a shaker. The extracts were dehydrated with anhydrous potassium carbonate and the *N*-nitrosamines quantified by means of a gas-liquid chromatograph connected to a TEA (TEA 502, Thermo Electron) (Fine & Rounbehler, 1975). In all experiments, the values obtained with boiled cells (100 °C, 30 min) were used to correct the values for intact cells.

RESULTS

Kinetics of N-nitrosodimethylamine (NDMA) formation by E. coli *A10*

As shown in Figure 1, the formation of NDMA by *E. coli* A10 was proportional to the incubation time and the enzyme concentration. When the cells were boiled for 30 min at 100 °C before incubation, NDMA could not be detected, even with a high concentration of the enzyme. The blank value at the nitrosation reaction was 0.12 μmol/L NDMA.

Optimal pH for NDMA formation by E. coli *A10*

The amount of NDMA formed by *E. coli* A10 was observed over a limited pH range (6.5 to 8.5) and was optimal at pH 7.5 (Fig. 2). At pH 6.0, a large amount of NDMA was observed with the boiled cells, which could have been formed by a non-enzymatic process. No NDMA was observed at pH 9.0.

Substrate specificity of E. coli *A10*

Substrate specificity of the nitrosating enzyme of *E. coli* A10 for secondary amines is shown in Table 1. Only MOR showed marked specificity.

Fig. 1. Kinetics of *N*-nitrosodimethylamine (NDMA) formation by *Escherichia coli* A10.
Reactions were carried out in a medium containing 0.1 mol/L potassium phosphate buffer, 7.5 mmol/L dimethylamine, 25 mmol/L nitrite and 34.5 mg protein (1a) or 11.5 to 46 mg protein (1b) of intact cell suspension of *E. coli* A10 in a total volume of 20 mL. The temperature was 37 °C. (1b) shows NDMA formation in 10 min; ○, intact cells; △, boiled cells

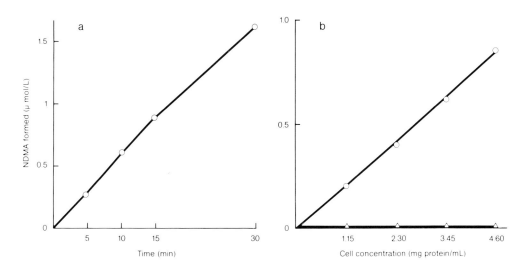

Fig. 2. Effect of pH on N-nitrosodimethylamine (NDMA) formation by *Escherichia coli* A10.
        Reactions were carried out in a medium containing 0.1 mol/L potassium phosphate buffer, 7.5 mmol/L
        dimethylamine, 25 mmol/L nitrite and 2 mL intact cell suspension (12 mg/mL as protein) of *E. coli* A10 in a total
        volume of 20 mL at 37 °C for 30 min

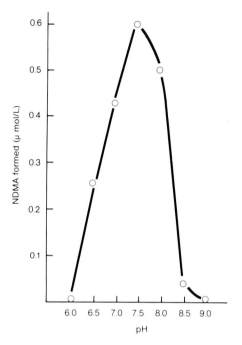

Table 1.   Substrate specificities of nitrosating enzyme
of *Escherichia coli* A10 for secondary amines[a]

Amine	Nitrosamine formed (μmol/L)
Dimethylamine	0.39
Diethylamine	0.51
Dibutylamine	1.66
Di-isobutylamine	0.94
Piperidine	0.79
Pyrrolidine	0.39
Morpholine	30.67

[a] Conditions: 7.5 mmol/L amine; 25 mmol/L nitrite;
1 mg/mL as protein of *E. coli*; 0.1 mol/L potassium
phosphate buffer, pH 7.5, at 37 °C for 30 min

Identification and activity of intestinal bacteria harbouring nitrosating enzymes

Of the 54 strains tested, 11 produced NDMA (Table 2). The following species include
NDMA-producing strains: *E. coli, P. morganii, K. pneumonia, P. aeruginosa* and *Peptococcus
asaccharolyticus. P. aeruginosa* showed the highest activity (0.9 nmol NDMA/h per mg
protein). Seven of nine *E. coli* produced NDMA at relatively high activities (0.28–0.75 nmol
NDMA/h per mg protein). Of the 34 anaerobes examined, only one, *P. asaccharolyticus,* was
positive for NDMA production.

Table 2. Nitrosating enzyme-producing species of intestinal bacteria and their activities

Species	No. of strains	No. of positive strains	Specific activity[a]
Facultative or aerobic bacteria			
Escherichia coli	9	7	0.28–0.75
Proteus mirabilis	1	0	0
Proteus morganii	1	1	0.06
Proteus vulgaris	1	0	0
Klebsiella pneumoniae	1	1	0.05
Pseudomonas aeruginosa	1	1	0.90
Streptococcus faecalis	1	0	0
Streptococcus faecium	1	0	0
Streptococcus spp.	4	0	0
Anaerobic bacteria			
Bacteroides fragilis	1	0	0
Bacteroides distasonis	1	0	0
Bacteroides ovatus	1	0	0
Bacteroides thetaiotaomicron	1	0	0
Bacteroides vulgatus	1	0	0
Bacteroides multiacidus	1	0	0
Bacteroides eggerthii	1	0	0
Fusobacterium necrogenes	1	0	0
Fusobacterium mortiferme	1	0	0
Bifidobacterium adolescentis	3	0	0
Bifidobacterium bifidus	1	0	0
Bifidobacterium breve	1	0	0
Bifidobacterium longum	1	0	0
Eubacterium aerofaciens	1	0	0
Eubacterium limosum	1	0	0
Eubacterium moniliforme	1	0	0
Eubacterium rectale	1	0	0
Eubacterium biforme	1	0	0
Peptococcus asaccharolyticus	1	1	0.17
Peptostreptococcus intermedius	1	0	0
Peptostreptococcus productus	1	0	0
Veillonella alcalescens	1	0	0
Veillonella parvula	1	0	0
Clostridium bifermentans	1	0	0
Clostridium indolis	1	0	0
Clostridium oroticum	1	0	0
Clostridium paraputrificum	1	0	0
Clostridium perfringens	1	0	0
Clostridium ramosum	1	0	0
Clostridium innocuum	1	0	0
Lactobacillus acidophilus	1	0	0
Lactobacillus salivarius	1	0	0

[a] nmol N-nitrosodimethylamine formed per hour per mg protein

DISCUSSION

By using resting cells as the enzyme preparation and the TEA as detector of N-nitrosamines, we have found that NDMA is produced in proportion to the incubation time and the cell concentration when $E.$ $coli$ cells are incubated with DMA and nitrite at neutral pH. In contrast, no NDMA is produced when boiled cells are used. This indicates that NDMA is produced from DMA and nitrite at neutral pH by the enzymic action of E. coli. Kunisaki and Hayashi (1979) have also reported that resting E. coli cells catalyse NDMA formation. However, the nitrosation activity reported by those authors was much higher than that observed here, perhaps because their method of N-nitrosamine detection (ultra-violet photolysis of the putative NDMA and measurement of the released nitrite) was less selective than ours.

Klubes and Jondorf (1971), Collins-Thompson et al. (1972), Mills and Alexander (1976) and Ralt and Tannenbaum (1981) concluded that nitrosation by some bacteria was non-enzymatic. In their experiments, however, the bacteria were incubated for a long time in a complex culture medium containing precursors of N-nitrosamines, so that the enzymatic nitrosation might occur simultaneously with an accelerating non-enzymatic mechanism, such as one involving a decrease of the pH of the medium and a catalytic effect of the bacterial or medium component. Archer et al. (1975) reported that longer-chain secondary amines are nitrosated catalytically at pH 3.5 in the presence of either intact or boiled cells. They proposed that the catalysis resulted from a non-enzymatic mechanism involving hydrophobic interactions of secondary amines and cellular constituents under acidic conditions.

The formation of NDMA in the presence of E. coli A10 was optimal at pH 7.5, whereas the non-enzymatic formation of NDMA is optimal at pH 3.4 (Mirvish, 1970).

Substrate specificity for secondary amines on nitrosation by E. coli was clarified by our experiment. The significance of the fact that MOR had marked specificity as a substrate of microbial nitrosation is not known, but even at acidic pH, the relative rate of nitrosation of MOR is higher than that of any other secondary amine we used (Mirvish, 1975).

Screening of intestinal bacteria for NDMA formation showed that nitrosating enzyme is widely distributed among facultative or aerobic bacteria. Since nitrosation is an oxidation reaction, it is possible that the anaerobic bacteria, except for P. asaccharolyticus, cannot catalyse the formation of nitrosamines. In contrast, seven of nine strains of the aerobic E. coli were positive for nitrosation.

With regard to nitrosation by E. coli, some conflicting eivdence exists; i.e., positive (Ayanaba & Alexander, 1973; Coloe & Hayward, 1976; Mills & Alexander, 1976), negative (Brooks et al., 1972; Collins-Thompson et al., 1972; Thacker & Brooks, 1974) and conditionally positive (Hawksworth & Hill, 1971; Hashimoto et al., 1975; Kunisaki & Hayashi, 1979; Hayashi et al., 1982). Hayashi et al. (1982) reported that E. coli formed considerable amounts of NDMA after 3 h incubation, but no NDMA was formed by E. coli at 22 h incubation. It seems possible that a catalytic effect of E. coli on nitrosation might be masked under certain conditions by high amounts of non-enzymatic nitrosation in the complex culture medium. Such non-enzymatic nitrosation could occur due to a lowering of the pH of the medium or the presence of catalysts such as cysteine, or perhaps other compounds that are known to catalyse nitrosation (Kunisaki & Hayashi, 1980). Earlier data obtained with complex culture media and with less specific detectors of N-nitrosamines may be open to question.

In conclusion, our results show that some intestinal bacteria are capable of forming N-nitrosamines from secondary amines and nitrite by enzymatic catalysis at neutral pH. These organisms may contribute to the endogenous production of N-nitrosamines in the gastrointestinal tract.

ACKNOWLEDGEMENTS

This research was supported by a Grant-in-Aid for scientific research from the Ministry of Education, Science and Culture of Japan.

REFERENCES

Archer, M.C., Yang, H.S. & Okun, J.D. (1975) *Acceleration of nitrosamine formation at pH 3.5 by microorganisms.* In: Walker, E.A., Castegnaro, M., Griciute, L. & Lyle, R.E., eds, *Environmental Aspects of N-Nitroso Compounds (IARC Scientific Publications No. 19)*, Lyon, International Agency for Research on Cancer, pp. 239–246

Ayanaba, A.K. & Alexander, M. (1973) Microbial formation of nitrosamines *in vitro. Appl. Microbiol., 25*, 862–868

Boyland, E., Nice, E.V. & Williams, K. (1971) The catalysis of nitrosation by thiocyanate from saliva. *Food Cosmet. Toxicol., 9*, 639–643

Brooks, J.B., Cherry, W.B., Thacker, L.V. & Alley, C.C. (1972) Analysis by gas chromatography of amines and nitrosamines produces *in vivo* and *in vitro* by *Proteus mirabilis. J. infect. Dis., 126*, 143–153

Collins-Thompson, D.L., Sen, N.P., Aris, B. & Schwinghamer, L. (1972) Non-enzymatic *in vitro* formation of nitrosamines by bacteria isolated from meat products. *Can. J. Microbiol., 18*, 1968–1971

Coloe, P.J. & Hayward, N.J. (1976) The importance of prolonged incubation for the synthesis of dimethylnitrosamine by enterobacteria. *J. med. Microbiol., 9*, 211–223

Fine, D.H. & Rounbehler, D.P. (1975) Trace analysis of volatile *N*-nitroso compounds by combined gas chromatography and thermal energy analysis. *J. Chromatogr., 109*, 271–279

Hashimoto, S., Kawai, Y. & Mutai, M. (1975) In vitro *N*-nitrosodimethylamine formation by some bacteria. *Infect. Immun., 11*, 1405–1406

Hawksworth, G. & Hill, M. (1971) Bacteria and the *N*-nitrosation of secondary amines. *Br. J. Cancer, 25*, 520–526

Hayashi, N., Ushijima, M., Kodaka, H., Teraoka, Y., Tanimura, A. & Kurata, H. (1982) Identification of nitrosodimethylamine-forming aerobic bacteria isolated from the gastric contents of the monkey, *Macara irus. Jpn. J. Bacteriol., 37*, 503–509

Klubes, P. & Jondorf, W.R. (1971) Dimethylnitrosamine formation from sodium nitrite and dimethylamine by bacterial flora of rat intestines. *Res. Commun. chem. Pathol. Pharmacol., 2*, 24–33

Kunisaki, N. & Hayashi, M. (1979) Formation of *N*-nitrosamines from secondary amines and nitrite by resting cells of *Escherichia coli* B. *Appl. environ. Microbiol., 37*, 279–282

Kunisaki, N. & Hayashi, M. (1980) Effects of ergothioneine, cysteine and glutathione on nitrosation of secondary amines under physiologic conditions. *J. natl Cancer Inst., 65*, 791–794

Lowry, O.H., Rosebrough, N.J., Farr, A.L. & Randall, R.J. (1951) Protein measurement with the Folin phenol reagent. *J. biol. Chem., 193*, 265–275

Mills, A.L. & Alexander, M. (1976) *N*-Nitrosamine formation by cultures of several microorganisms. *Appl. environ. Microbiol., 31*, 892–895

Mirvish, S.S. (1970) Kinetics of dimethylamine nitrosation in relation to nitrosamine carcinogenesis. *J. natl Cancer Inst., 44*, 633–639

Mirvish, S.S. (1975) Formation of *N*-nitroso compounds: chemistry, kinetics, and *in vivo* occurrence. *Toxicol. appl. Pharmacol., 31*, 325–351

Mitsuoka, T. (1980) *A Color Atlas of Anaerobic Bacteria*, Tokyo, Sobunsha

Parker, C.A. (1955) Anaerobiosis with iron wool. *Aust. J. exp. Biol. med. Sci., 33*, 33–38

Ralt, D. & Tannenbaum, S.R. (1981) *The role of bacteria in nitrosamine formation.* In: Scanlan, R.A. & Tannenbaum, S.R., eds, N-*Nitroso Compounds (ACS Symp. Ser. No. 174)*, Washington DC, American Chemical Society, pp. 159–164

Sherbet, G.V. & Lakshmi, M.S. (1973) Characterization of *Escherichia coli* surface by isoelectric equilibrium analysis. *Biochem. biophys. Acta, 298*, 50–58

Thacker, L. & Brooks, J.B. (1974) *In vitro* production of *N*-nitrosodimethylamine and other amines by *Proteus* species. *Infect. Immun., 9*, 648–653

Tozawa, H. (1982) *Effects of alkali and oxygen on nitrosation in dimethylamine-nitrite mixtures with and without reductants.* In: Bartsch, H., O'Neill, I.K., Castegnaro, M. & Okada, M., eds, N-*Nitroso Compounds: Occurrence and Biological Effects (IARC Scientific Publications No. 41)*, Lyon, International Agency for Research on Cancer, pp. 113–121

A NITROSATING AGENT FROM THE REACTION OF ATMOSPHERIC NITROGEN DIOXIDE (NO$_2$) WITH METHYL LINOLEATE: COMPARISON WITH A PRODUCT FROM THE SKINS OF NO$_2$-EXPOSED MICE

S.S. MIRVISH & J.P. SAMS

Eppley Institute for Research in Cancer, University of Nebraska Medical Center, Omaha, Nebraska, USA

SUMMARY

We showed previously that exposure of mice to atmospheric nitrogen dioxide (NO$_2$) leads to the formation of an ether-extractable nitrosating agent (NSA) in the skin, which produced *N*-nitrosomorpholine (NMOR) from morpholine *in vitro* but not *in vivo* (under our conditions). We now report that NO$_2$ bubbled into hexane solutions of methyl linoleate (MLIN) produced a similar NSA that reacted with morpholine in dichloromethane solution to produce NMOR. The NSA yield increased sharply as MLIN concentration was raised, with a maximum 0.1% yield of NSA from MLIN. The NSA yield from MLIN was four times that from methyl oleate and seven times that from methyl stearate. The NSA derived from MLIN travelled on thin-layer chromatography more slowly than the main weight fraction; whereas TLC of NSA in the skin lipids of NO$_2$-exposed mice and in untreated mouse skin lipids exposed *in vitro* to NO$_2$ produced NSA that travelled more rapidly than the main weight fraction.

INTRODUCTION

We have been studying the question of whether atmospheric NO$_2$ might nitrosate amines or amides *in vivo* to form *N*-nitroso derivatives. In our first report (Mirvish *et al.*, 1981), we showed that in mice exposed to about 50 ppm NO$_2$ for 4 h after they had been gavaged with morpholine no NMOR was formed, as detected by a system that prevented artefactual NMOR formation during the work-up. [Subsequently, Van Stee *et al.*, (1983) did detect a small extent of NMOR production under different conditions *in vivo*.] However, we observed NMOR formation when mice exposed to 50 ppm NO$_2$ for 4 h were homogenized with morpholine, confirming a report by Iqbal *et al.* (1980). This nitrosation was unlikely to be due to NO$_2$ itself and was attributed to the formation of NSA from NO$_2$ *in vivo*.

We decided to concentrate initially on identifying the NSA. We demonstrated that NSA occurred almost entirely in the skin, including the fur, of exposed mice, and was due to direct exposure of the skin to NO$_2$ and not to inhalation of NO$_2$ (Mirvish *et al.*, 1983). The NSA was extracted with ether from aqueous homogenates, i.e., was a lipid. Nitrite esters with electron-attracting (e.g., hydroxy) groups in the α position are known to act as NSA (Challis & Shuker, 1979), and Walters *et al.* (1979) showed that nitrosites (α-nitrosonitrite esters) can nitrosate amines. Hence, it seemed likely that the NSA produced by NO_2 consisted of nitrosates (α-nitronitrite esters), produced by the reaction of N_2O_4 (the dimer of NO_2) with ethylenic double bonds of unsaturated fatty acid moieties in lipids. Accordingly, we studied and here report on the chemical reaction of NO_2 with fatty acid esters to produce NSA, and on the chromatographic properties of the product and of NSA produced in mouse skin.

METHODS

In the 'standard' experiment, a freshly prepared solution of 50 mg methyl linoleate (MLIN) (Sigma Chemical Company, Milwaukee, WI, USA) in 100 mL *n*-hexane (MCB reagent grade, EM Science Industries Inc., Gibbstown, NJ, USA) and 6 g anhydrous sodium sulfate were placed in a 250-mL conical flask. An NO_2 sampler (catalog no. 7530-05, Ace Glass Inc., Vineland, NJ, USA) was inserted, the neck was closed with a plug of cotton, the flask was cooled in an ice bath, and NO_2 (50 ppm) in air was bubbled in at a rate of 1 L/min for 1 h. (The volume dropped to about 90 mL.) The solution was rotary-evaporated under vacuum to dryness; re-evaporated twice, each time after adding 30 mL hexane to remove unreacted NO_2; and brought up to 100 mL in hexane. Ten mL of this solution were added to a solution of 25 mg morpholine (Fisher Scientific Co., Pittsburgh, PA, USA) in 75 mL dichloromethane (DCM) (EM Science Industries), concentrated in a Kuderna-Danish apparatus and then with a stream of nitrogen to 1.5 mL, and left for 16 h in the dark at room temperature. Of this solution, 1–3 µL were analysed for *N*-nitrosomorpholine (NMOR) by gas chromatography-thermal energy analysis (GC-TEA) as described before (Mirvish *et al.*, 1983).

For the thin-layer chromatography (TLC) study, 426 mg MLIN in 100 mL hexane were reacted with NO_2 as described above. The solution was evaporated three times as described above and dissolved in 100 mL hexane. A 10-mL sample was reacted with morpholine and NMOR was determined. The remaining 90 mL were evaporated to a small volume and applied as an 18-cm strip to a fluorescent TLC plate (silica gel 60 F-254, 1 × 200 × 200 mm, EM Laboratories Inc.), which was developed with hexane : ethyl acetate (9 : 1). The plate was examined under long and short wavelength ultra-violet light. The TLC plate was divided on the basis of the ultra-violet absorption into five to six strips (fractions), each of which was scraped off and extracted with 100 mL DCM. Ten mL of each extract were evaporated to dryness and weighed; 80 mL were reacted with 25 mg morpholine in DCM, and NMOR was determined as described above.

In the in-vivo experiments, four adult male Swiss mice were exposed to 50 ppm NO_2 in air for 4 h as described before (Mirvish *et al.*, 1983). The mice were killed, and the skins were stripped off and homogenized in a Waring blender with 250 mL 0.9% sodiumchloride in water. The homogenate was extracted four times with 250 mL DCM [and not with ether as before (Mirvish *et al.*, 1983)]. The extract (1 120 mL) was stored at $-15\,°C$. Of a 100-mL sample containing 670 mg lipids, 10 mL were reacted with 25 mg morpholine in DCM, and NMOR was determined. The remaining 90 mL were concentrated and subjected to TLC. The TLC fractions were reacted with morpholine, and NMOR was determined.

In another experiment, the lipids of the skins of four unexposed mice were extracted with DCM as described above. A sample of the extract was evaporated to give 480 mg residue, and 50 ppm NO_2 were bubbled for 1 h into a solution of the residue in 100 mL hexane. The solution was evaporated three times and redissolved in 100 mL hexane. Of this solution, 10 mL were reacted with morpholine, and NMOR was determined; and 90 mL were concentrated and subjected to TLC, and the TLC fractions were reacted with morpholine.

RESULTS AND DISCUSSION

Since we suspected that the NSA was derived from polyunsaturated fatty acid moieties in lipids, we studied the reaction of atmospheric NO_2 with MLIN. In our standard procedure, NO_2 was bubbled into a solution of 50 mg MLIN in hexane, and the resulting NSA was reacted with morpholine in DCM. These conditions produced NSA in an amount equivalent to 15.1 μg NMOR/total sample (300 ng NMOR/mg MLIN), which was 10.8 times higher than the 'blank' value for NO_2 bubbled into hexane (Table 1). In preliminary experiments, various grades of ether were used, which produced high blank values and lower and more variable values for the standard conditions. Lower values were also obtained when sodium sulfate was omitted from the reaction mixture, indicating that anhydrous conditions were essential.

In experiments to check the standard conditions (Table 2), we showed that NMOR derived from the morpholine solution in DCM (probably present in the morpholine sample) was 5% of standard NMOR production and that relatively little NMOR was formed when the MLIN solution was worked up without NO_2 exposure, or when NO_2 was bubbled into hexane not containing MLIN. Air bubbled into MLIN solution produced 23% of the NMOR formed with NO_2, possibly due to NO_2 contamination of the bubbling apparatus and gas delivery tubes.

Table 1. Use of various solvents for steps 1 and 2[a] of the reaction of NO_2 with methyl lineolate (MLIN)

Solvent, step 1	Solvent, step 2	μg NMOR/sample, mean ± SD (no.)	
		Blank (− MLIN)	Exp. (+ MLIN)
Ether[b]	Ether[b]	6.3 ± 4.3 (3)	7.2 ± 3.9 (2)
Distilled ether[c]	Distilled ether[c]	1.3 ± 0.6 (5)	6.4 ± 2.2 (7)
Hexane	Distilled ether[c]	1.1 ± 0.7 (8)	5.4 ± 1.5 (7)
Hexane	Dichloromethane	1.4 ± 0.4 (5)	15.1 ± 2.6 (7)

[a] NO_2 (50 ppm, 1 L/min, 1 h) was bubbled into 50 mg MLIN/100 mL solvent (step 1). After NO_2 was removed, 1/10 was reacted with 25 mg morpholine/70 mL solvent (step 2)
[b] Mallinckrodt Nanograde
[c] Freshly distilled
NMOR, N-nitrosomorpholine

Table 2. Control experiments for standard conditions of the reaction of NO_2 with methyl lineolate (MLIN)

Experiment	μg NMOR/total sample, mean ± SD (no.)
Morpholine in DCM (step 2 only)	0.08 ± 0.03 (7)
MLIN soln. in hexane	1.0 ± 0 (2)
Air bubbled into MLIN soln.	3.5 ± 1.9 (3)
NO_2 bubbled into hexane, no MLIN	1.7 ± 0.7 (6)
NO_2 bubbled into MLIN soln. (standard conditions)	15.1 ± 2.6 (7)

NMOR, N-nitrosomorpholine; DCM, dichloromethane

Table 3. Variation of time during which NO_2 (50 ppm)
was bubbled into 50 mg methyl lineolate (MLIN)/
100 mL hexane

Time (h)	µg NMOR/total sample	
	Blank, no MLIN	With MLIN
0.5	1.3	7.7
1	2.8, 1.0	18.4, 14.9
2	1.5	26.9
4	2.7	20.7, 19.2
5	3.3	31.5

NMOR, N-nitrosomorpholine

Table 4. Thin-layer chromatography (TLC) of methyl lineolate (MLIN) after exposure
to NO_2 [a]

Fraction no.	Rf	Ultra-violet absorption	Weight (mg)	NMOR (µg)
1	0–0.06	+ +	0	6.1
2	0.06–0.24	+	13	7.3
3	0.24–0.41	+ + +	15	8.6
4	0.41–0.53	+	40	21.9
5	0.53–0.76	+	283	5.7
6	0.76–1.00	−	34	0.7
Total			385	50.4
Before TLC			397	36.0

[a] MLIN (482 mg) in 100 mL hexane was exposed to NO_2 (50 ppm, 1 h), evaporated, and
subjected to preparative TLC. Eluates of each band were reacted with morpholine.
NMOR, N-nitrosomorpholine

When the reaction was performed with different MLIN concentrations under otherwise standard conditions, the NMOR yield/total sample after subtracting the blank was 0.4 (for 6.25 mg MLIN), 0.8 (12.5 mg MLIN), 3.9 (25 mg MLIN), 13.9 (50 mg MLIN) and 40 (100 mg MLIN) µg, indicating that, at the higher MLIN levels, the formation of NSA increased more rapidly than did the MLIN concentration. The maximal amount of NSA, i.e., that producing 40 µg NMOR from 100 mg MLIN, corresponded to 0.10% yield from MLIN, assuming that 1 mol NSA produced 1 mol NMOR.

When the time during which NO_2 was bubbled into MLIN solution was varied under otherwise standard conditions (Table 3), the NSA yield increased up to 2 h and then remained more or less constant.

Use of various esters under otherwise standard conditions gave NMOR yields (after subtracting the blank of 1.6 µg NMOR) of 2.2 (for methyl stearate), 3.7 (methyl oleate) and 15.8 (MLIN) µg/total sample. (These are the results of single determinations, but similar results were obtained in earlier studies with ethereal solutions.) The difference between the results for methyl oleate, with one ethylenic group, and MLIN, with two ethylenes, indicated that NSA production increased more rapidly than the number of ethylene groups.

We then attempted to separate the NSA from MLIN reacted with NO_2, using TLC on silica gel with development by hexane : ethyl acetate (9 : 1). Each TLC fraction was reacted with morpholine, and NMOR was determined, i.e., each fraction was analysed for NSA. In an experiment using 482 mg MLIN (Table 4), most of the NSA was recovered from the TLC plate (compare last two rows of Table 4). The amount of NSA did not coincide with the unreacted MLIN, which was presumably the main fraction by weight, but travelled at lower Rf values of 0.06–0.41.

Mice were exposed to 50 ppm NO_2 for 4 h, as previously (Mirvish *et al.*, 1983), i.e., exposure to NO_2 took place *in vivo*. The skin lipids were then extracted and subjected to TLC, and each TLC fraction was reacted with morpholine as before. In contrast to the result with MLIN, the principal NSA fraction had an Rf of 0.68–1.00, ahead of the principal fraction by weight (Table 5). For comparison, the skin lipids of untreated mice were extracted, NO_2 was bubbled for 1 h into a hexane solution of these lipids, and the product was subjected to TLC and analysed as before (Table 6). As with the lipids reacted *in vivo*, the main NSA fraction had an Rf of 0.64–1.00, ahead of the main weight fraction.

Table 5.   Thin-layer chromatography (TLC) of skin lipids of five mice exposed to NO_2 (50 ppm, 4 h)[a]

Fraction no.	Rf	Ultra-violet absorption	Weight (mg)	NMOR (μg)
1	0–0.06	+ + +	0	0.11
2	0.06–0.31	–	22	0.17
3	0.31–0.56	+	239	0.16
4	0.56–0.68	+ +	55	0.45
5	0.68–1.00	+ +	84	3.53
Total			400	4.42
Before TLC			671	10.6

[a]Skins were homogenized in 0.9% sodium chloride and extracted with dichloromethane. The extract was subjected to TLC. Each TLC fraction was reacted with morpholine and *N*-nitrosomorpholine (NMOR) measured.

Table 6.   Thin-layer chromatography (TLC) of skin lipids of unexposed mice after lipids had been exposed to NO_2[a]

Fraction no.	Rf	Ultra-violet absorption	Weight (mg)	NMOR (μg)
1	0–0.06	+ + +	2	4.5
2	0.06–0.19	+	0	3.4
3	0.19–0.34	+	15	7.4
4	0.34–0.64	+	295	12.5
5	0.64–1.00	+ +	13	62.7
Total			325	90.5
Before TLC			421	150

[a]Skin lipids were extracted as usual, exposed to NO_2 in hexane, and subjected to TLC. Each fraction was reacted with morpholine to give *N*-nitrosomorpholine (NMOR).

Fig. 1. Possible nitrosating nitrite esters from reactions of methyl linoleate with nitrogen dioxide

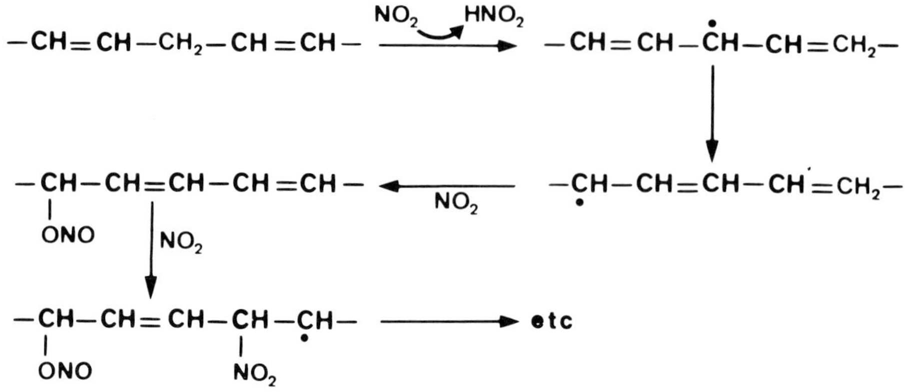

$$-CH=CH-CH_2-CH=CH- \xrightarrow{\;NO_2\;\;HNO_2\;} -CH=CH-\overset{\bullet}{C}H-CH=CH_2-$$

$$-CH-CH=CH-CH=CH- \xleftarrow{\;NO_2\;} -\overset{\bullet}{C}H-CH=CH-\overset{\bullet}{C}H=CH_2-$$
$$\;\;|$$
$$ONO \quad |NO_2$$

$$-CH-CH=CH-CH-\overset{\bullet}{C}H- \longrightarrow \; \bullet tc$$
$$\;\;|\qquad\qquad\qquad|$$
$$ONO\qquad\qquad\quad NO_2$$

The total NSA concentration of the crude lipids before TLC corresponded to 91 ng NMOR/mg lipid (36 µg/397 mg, see last two lines of Table 4) in the in-vitro experiment with MLIN, 16 ng NMOR/mg lipid (10.6 µg/671 mg) in the in-vivo experiment (Table 5), and a surprising 360 ng NMOR/mg lipid (150 µg/420 mg) for the in-vitro reaction of skin lipids with NO$_2$ (Table 6). It remains to (1) demonstrate whether the NSA obtained *in vivo* is derived from polyunsaturated fatty acids in the skin lipids and (2) discover the chemical identity of the in-vivo NSA and that derived from MLIN. For the last purpose, our results indicate that NSA yield would be increased by raising the MLIN concentration and NO$_2$ exposure time.

In conclusion, our previous results (Mirvish *et al.*, 1983) showed that production of the NSA from NO$_2$ *in vivo* occurred almost solely in the skin lipids. The present results show that NSA can be produced from the reaction of MLIN with NO$_2$ and that there was far less reaction with methyl stearate and methyl oleate. Despite the difference in TLC behaviour of NSA derived from mouse skin lipids and NSA derived from MLIN, the in-vivo NSA might be chemically similar to that obtained from MLIN. Active nitrite esters might arise by simple addition of N$_2$O$_4$ to an ethylene group to produce a nitrosate (see Introduction) or by a more complex series of free radical reactions, beginning with electron abstraction by NO$_2$ (Pryor & Lightsey, 1981) (Fig. 1). The latter type of reaction would occur mainly with polyunsaturated fatty acids and is hence favoured by our results.

It appears that we have discovered a lipid-soluble NSA in the skin of mice exposed to NO$_2$ and even in that of unexposed mice (Mirvish *et al.*, 1983), which might be derived from unsaturated lipids. This NSA reacts with amines *in vitro* to yield nitrosamines and might produce hazardous amounts of *N*-nitroso compounds *in vivo* under specific conditions. Similar compounds may also play a role in *N*-nitrosamine formation in foods such as beer and fried bacon, especially where there is exposure to NO$_2$ in the presence of lipids.

ACKNOWLEDGEMENTS

We thank Dr Phillip Issenberg of this Institute for valuable discussions. This work was supported by grant RO1 CA32192 from the National Institutes of Health and by a grant from the State of Nebraska.

REFERENCES

Challis, B.C. & Shuker, D.E.G. (1979) Rapid nitrosation of amines in aqueous alkaline solutions by beta-substituted alkyl nitrites. *J. chem. Soc., Chem. Comm.*, 315–316

Iqbal, Z.M., Dahl, K. & Epstein, S.S. (1980) Role of nitrogen dioxide in the biosynthesis of nitrosamines in mice. *Science, 207*, 1475–1477

Mirvish, S.S., Issenberg, P. & Sams, J.P. (1981) *A study of* N-*nitrosomorpholine synthesis in rodents exposed to nitrogen dioxide and morpholine.* In: Scanlan, R.A. & Tannenbaum, S., eds, N-*Nitroso Compounds (ACS Symposium Series No. 174)*, Washington DC, American Chemical Society, pp. 181–191

Mirvish, S.S., Sams, J.P. & Issenberg, P. (1983) The nitrosating agent in mice exposed to nitrogen dioxide: Improved extraction method and localization in the skin. *Cancer Res., 43*, 2550–2554

Pryor, W.A. & Lightsey, J.W. (1981) Mechanisms of nitrogen dioxide reactions: Initiation of lipid peroxidation and the production of nitrous acid. *Science, 214*, 435–437

Van Stee, E.W., Sloane, R.A., Simmons, J.E. & Brunnemann, K.D. (1983) *In vivo* formation of N-nitrosomorpholine in CD-1 mice exposed by inhalation to nitrogen dioxide and by gavage to morpholine. *J. natl Cancer Inst., 70*, 375–379

Walters, C.L., Hart, R.J. & Perse, S. (1979) The possible role of lipid pseudonitrosites in nitrosamine formation in fried bacon. *Z. Lebensmittel. Untersuch. Forsch., 168*, 177–180

IN-VIVO NITROSATION OF AMINES IN MICE BY INHALED NITROGEN DIOXIDE AND INHIBITION OF BIOSYNTHESIS OF N-NITROSAMINES[1]

Z.M. IQBAL

Department of Preventive Medicine, University of Illinois at Chicago, P.O.Box 6998, Chicago, IL, 60680, USA

SUMMARY

Inhalation of nitrogen dioxide (NO_2) by mice administered orally morpholine (MOR) or dimethylamine(DMA) resulted in the biosynthesis of N-nitrosomorpholine (NMOR) or N-nitrosodimethylamine (NDMA), respectively, as determined by the analysis of frozen whole-mouse powder, using gas chromatography with a Thermal Energy Analyzer detector.

Significant levels of NMOR were detected following exposure of mice to 0.38 mg/m³ NO_2 for 0.5 h (26 ng NMOR/mouse) and there was a two-fold increase when NO_2 exposure was extended to 4 h. NMOR levels also increased in a time-dependent manner at 28.4 and 47.3 mg/m³ NO_2 exposure levels, reaching a maximum of 450 and 725 ng NMOR/mouse, respectively, at 4 h. Oral administration of sodium ascorbate (50-250 mg), ammonium sulfamate (50-100mg) or DL-α-tocopherol (67-167 mg) immediately after MOR or DMA, but prior to NO_2 exposure, significantly inhibited both NMOR and NDMA biosynthesis, sulfamate being the most effective (>90% NMOR and NDMA inhibition), followed by ascorbate (83-90% NMOR and 58-90% NDMA inhibition) and α-tocopherol (22-42% NMOR and 46-69% NDMA inhibition). Low levels of NDMA were found in untreated control mice (<13 ng/mouse) and in most samples of commercially obtained animal feed (10-15 µg/kg); NMOR, however, was not detectable or was detected in negligible amounts in these cases. Various control experiments indicated that most of the recovered nitrosamine resulted from in-vivo nitrosation in mice, with only up to 1-2% of NMOR and approximately 10% of NDMA yields being attributed to artefact formation, possibly during work-up of the mouse-powder samples.

INTRODUCTION

Adverse biological effects and human health hazards posed by nitrogen oxides (NO_x) are well recognized and have been reviewed (National Academy of Sciences, 1977;Lee, 1980). Further concern arises from the accumulated evidence of NO_x-mediated nitrosation of amines, resulting

---

[1] This paper was originally scheduled for presentation at the previous meeting in this series in 1981.

in the formation of carcinogenic nitrosamines. These studies involved chemical and atmospheric model systems (e.g. Bretschneider & Matz, 1976; Challis & Kryptopoulous, 1977; Gehlert & Rolle, 1977; Challis *et al.*, 1978; Pitts *et al.*, 1978; Eisenbrand *et al.*, 1979; Janzowski *et al.*, 1980) and limited use of plasma and lung homogenates *in vitro* (Kaut, 1970; Challis *et al.*, 1980).

Recently, we demonstrated in-vivo nitrosation of two secondary amines, morpholine (MOR) and dimethylamine (DMA), after inhalation of NO_2 in mice, the biosynthesized *N*-nitrosamines (*N*-nitrosomorpholine, NMOR, and *N*-nitrosodimethylamine, NDMA) being recovered from powdered whole mice (Iqbal *et al.*, 1980, 1981).

Additional data available on in-vivo nitrosation appear to be confined to two preliminary and apparently conflicting reports: (1) NDMA was formed in different rat tissues after exposure to aminopyrine and NO_2 (Kusumoto *et al.*, 1980), which is consistent with the fact that NDMA is a known product of nitrite-aminopyrene reactions (Lijinsky *et al.*, 1972); (2) neither biosynthesis of NMOR in whole mouse and in rat blood and stomach content, nor in-vivo nitrosation of MOR by NO_2 was observed by Mirvish *et al.* (1981), leading those authors to conclude that the earlier demonstration of NMOR biosynthesis in whole mice (Iqbal *et al.*, 1980) could be due only to in-vitro nitrosation of MOR in homogenates of mice exposed to NO_2.

Further evidence of NMOR biosynthesis in mice is presented below, along with studies on the decay of biosynthesized NMOR and on the inhibition of biosynthesis of NMOR and NDMA in mice. Various control experiments confirm that observed yields of *N*-nitrosamine, with the possible exception of 1-10%, are due to their biosynthesis in mice.

MATERIALS

Sources of commercially obtained materials : Analytic grade(>99.8% pure)DMA-HCl, MOR and *N*-nitrosamine standards [NDMA, NMOR and *N*-nitrosodipropylamine (NDPA)] from Aldrich Chemical Co., Milwaukee, WI; pesticide-grade methanol from Fisher Scientific Co., Fair Lawn, N.J; glass-distilled dichloromethane (DCM) from Burdick & Jackson Laboratories, Inc., Muskegon, MI; sodium ascorbate, DL-α-tocopherol (Type V; mixed isomers from vegetable oil; ∼ 670 mg/g; sealed ampoules) and ammonium sulfamate from Sigma Chemical Co., St Louis, MO; liquid nitrogen from Liquified Industrial Gases, Inc., Hillside, IL; tanks of custom-grade, certified-standard NO_2 at specified concentrations from Matheson Co, Inc., Joliet, IL; Dynacal Permeation Devices (standard low-emission and wafer devices) from Metronics, Santa Clara, CA and unbuffered Ex-tubes (ToxElut, #3 020) from Analytichem International, Harbor City, CA; and male ICR mice (25-30 g; six weeks old) from Scientific Small Animal Farm, Arlington Heights, IL.

A Thermal Energy Analyzer (TEA) (Model 502; Thermo Electron Corp., Waltham, MA), interfaced to a Model 661 gas chromatograph (GC) (Thermo Electron Corp.) was used for *N*-nitrosamine determinations. A stainless-steel column (4.27m × 3.2 mm), packed with 10% Carbowax 20M plus 0.5% KOH on Chromosorb WHP 80/100, was used under isothermal conditions at 175 C. The argon carrier gas flow rate was 22 mL/minute at an inlet pressure of 4.08 atm (60 psi). Concentrated samples of DCM and methanol, DCM extracts of distilled water and all aqueous solutions were checked for contamination by NDMA and other *N*-nitrosamines; all solvents and solutions were *N*-nitrosamine-free (detection limit, 0.1 μg/L).

Mice were maintained on Purine Chow pellets for up to one week and starved in a wire-bottom cage for 18-20 h prior to test. Nalgene vacuum desiccators of approximately 7-L capacity (Nalge 5 310; Scientific Products, Inc., Mc Gaw Hill, IL), as modified by Iqbal *et al.*

(1980, 1981), were used as exposure chambers, with groups of three to four mice placed on a wire grid over a perforated desiccator plate (26.2 cm diam.) to prevent the ingestion of any urine or faeces excreted during exposure.

EXPERIMENTAL METHODS

NO$_2$ exposure

For exposures to concentrations of 70 to 84 mg/m^3, NO$_2$ gas from stock tanks was introduced directly into the exposure chambers[1].

NO$_2$ levels of 47.3 mg/m^3 were obtained by diluting stock NO$_2$ (78.4 or 84 mg/m^3) with air at appropriate flow rates. 'Dynacal' permeation devices were used to generate 0.38 and 28.4 mg/m^3 of NO$_2$ in the exposure chambers. For generating 0.38 mg/m^3 of NO$_2$, air (2.5 L/min) was introduced into a plastic tube (15 cm long, 1.5 cm i.d.) containing a metal wafer device (5.72 cm long, 1.43 cm in diameter) kept in a 35 C water bath. The other end of the plastic tube was connected to the exposure chamber. For generating 28.4 mg/m^3 of NO$_2$, a standard emission tube (10 cm long), kept at 42 C, was used. Both the wafer device and standard emission tubes were conditioned overnight prior to use. The accuracy of gas mixtures was checked by periodic monitoring of the chamber exhaust by the Greiss-Saltzman colorimetric assay, which was sensitive to 0.009 mg NO$_2$/m^3 (Katz, 1977).

NMOR biosynthesis and decay

Groups of three to four mice were gavaged with 2 mg MOR in 0.25 mL distilled water and exposed to 0.38, 28.4 and 47.3 mg/m^3 NO$_2$ (0.142 m^3/h; 20 volume changes/h) for 0.5, 1.2 and 4h at each NO$_2$ concentration. Concurrent controls consisted of groups of groups of three mice, exposed in separate chambers to the same NO$_2$ concentrations for the same periods. Additional controls consisted of groups of three to four mice gavaged with 2 mg MOR or 0.25 ml distilled water alone, followed by exposure to air for identical periods. After exposure, mice were frozen individually in liquid nitrogen and blended to a fine powder, 8 g aliquots of which were analysed for NMOR.

Experiments on the decay of biosynthesized NMOR involved two groups of mice gavaged with 2 mg MOR: sub-groups of three to four mice from one group were exposed to 3.8 mg/m^3 NO$_2$ for 0.5, 1, 1.5, 2, 4, 6 and 8 h, then frozen; the second group (15 mice) was exposed to 3.8 mg/m^3 NO$_2$ for 2 h, then to ambient room air, following which, five sub-groups of three mice were frozen after 0, 0.5, 1, 2 and 4 h in room air. Control groups received either MOR or NO$_2$ exposure alone, or were kept in room air for identical periods. Frozen mice were powdered for NMOR analysis.

Inhibition of N-nitrosamine biosynthesis

Groups of three to four mice were gavaged with 2 mg DMA in 0.25 mL distilled water. One of these groups was then gavaged with 50 mg sodium ascorbate, another with 50 mg ammonium sulfamate and a third with 67 mg DL-α-tocopherol. The same protocol was followed using 2 mg MOR in place of DMA, followed by 250 mg, 100 mg and 167 mg, respectively, of sodium ascorbate, ammonium sulfamate and DL-α-tocopherol. Mice gavaged with DMA were

---

[1] 1.89 mg NO$_2$/m^3 air $\simeq$ 1ppm at 25 °C

exposed to 78.4–84.1 mg/m^3 NO$_2$ for 2 h, while MOR-fed mice were exposed to 66–83.2 mg/m^3 NO$_2$ for 4 h; the exposure periods were selected for maximal NDMA and NMOR biosynthesis at the specified NO$_2$ levels. Positive control mice were fed DMA or MOR and equivalent volumes of distilled water (instead of inhibitors), then subjected to the specified NO$_2$ exposure. Additional controls underwent exposure to amine alone and to NO$_2$ alone.

Artefactual N-nitrosamines: control experiments

Groups of three to four mice were gavaged with an amine and exposed to NO$_2$ (2 mg MOR, 70 mg/m^3 NO$_2$ for 4 h; 2 mg DMA, 70 mg/m^3 NO$_2$ for 2 h). These concentrations and exposures are expected to yield maximal N-nitrosamine biosynthesis. Immediately after exposure, DMA-fed mice were gavaged with 2 mg MOR and quickly frozen and homogenized, while MOR-fed mice were gavaged with 2 mg DMA and frozen. Other groups of mice were fed DMA or MOR and exposed to NO$_2$ for 2 and 4 h, respectively, then frozen and powdered. To 8 g aliquots of powder, 2 mg MOR were added in the case of DMA-fed mice and 2 mg DMA in the case of MOR-fed mice, prior to homogenization and extraction. Control groups were exposed concurrently to DMA, MOR and NO$_2$ as described immediately above, then frozen, powdered and analysed without further treatment.

N-Nitrosamine analysis

NMOR, NDMA and other N-nitrosamines were determined quantitatively in frozen-mouse powder (Iqbal *et al.*, 1980, 1981). Approximately 8 g aliquots were taken from each powdered mouse and blended with 75 mL of ice-cold 35% aqueous methanol, with the addition of NDPA (240-260 ng) as an internal standard for recovery determinations. Homogenates were centrifuged, supernatants removed and the pellets extracted twice with 2 × 90 mL DCM. The organic layer was dried by passage through an 'Ex-tube' and concentrated to 2 mL in a Kuderna-Danish concentrator in a 65 C bath. Aliquots (20μL) of the concentrates from each of two or three powder samples were injected into the GC-TEA for N-nitrosamine analysis. Peaks were identified and quantified by comparing their retention times and heights with those of reference N-nitrosamines. Peak heights were corrected for N-nitrosamine contents of control mice and for NDPA recoveries from each powder sample.

RESULTS

No N-nitrosamine was found in distilled water solutions of the amines and inhibitors, or in the solvents, using TEA at a sensitivity of 0.1 μg/kg. However, low levels of NDMA (< 13 ng/mouse) and, rarely, NMOR (< 5 ng/mouse) were detected in occasional samples from untreated controls and from those treated with amine alone or NO$_2$ alone; no other N-nitrosamine was detected. The highest level of N-nitrosamine found in a control group was subtracted from all experimental values. The commercial animal feed used contained low levels of NDMA (10 μg/kg). Recovery of internal standard from mouse powder aliquots ranged from 82-96%. N-Nitrosamine levels generally varied by less than 5% from the average.

Figure 1 shows that exposure of MOR-exposed mice to 0.38 mg/m^3 NO$_2$ for 0.5 h resulted in significant NMOR yields (26 ng/mouse) with respect to controls, with a two-fold increase in NMOR level when exposure extended to 1 or 4 h; time-dependent increases of NMOR levels were also observed with 28.4 and 47.3 mg/m^3 NO$_2$, with maxima of 450 and 725 ng/mouse, respectively, at 4 h. Exposure of MOR-exposed mice to 3.8 mg/m^3 NO$_2$ also resulted in a

Fig. 1. Biosynthesis of *N*-nitrosomorpholine (NMOR) in mice exposed to 2 mg morpholine and NO₂; bars represent average ± SD (see text for details); ○, 47.3 mg/m³ NO₂; ●, 28.4 mg/m³ NO₂; △ , 0.38 mg/m³ NO₂

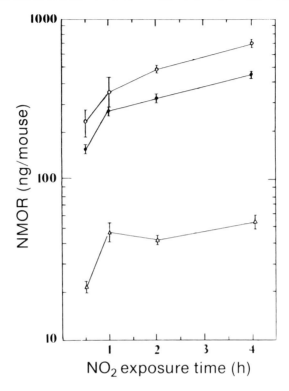

Fig. 2. Biosynthesis and decay of *N*-nitrosomorpholine (NMOR) in mice exposed to 2 mg morpholine and NO₂; solid line represents continuous exposure to 3.8 mg/m³ NO₂; dotted line indicates transfer of NO₂-exposed mice to ambient room air (see text for details)

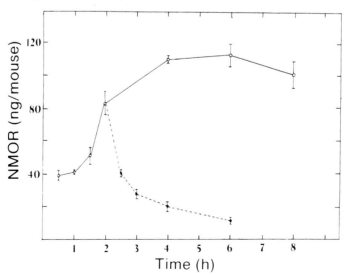

Table 1. Inhibition of N-nitrosamine biosynthesis in mice

Amine[a] (2 mg)	Inhibitor (mg)[b]			NO_2 (mg/m³)[c]	N-nitrosamine (ng/mouse)[a]		Inhibition (%)
	ASC	SULF	TOCO		NMOR	NDMA	
MOR	—	—	—	66 (4)	836.1 ± 21.1	—	0
MOR	50	—	—	66 (4)	147.8 ± 20.3	—	83
MOR	250	—	—	66 (4)	84.2 ± 10.3	—	90
MOR	—	—	—	72 (4)	908.6 ± 23.6	—	0
MOR	—	50	—	72 (4)	43.3 ± 3.2	—	95
MOR	—	100	—	72 (4)	29.1 ± 3.3	—	97
MOR	—	—	—	83 (4)	1 834.5 ± 36.8	—	0
MOR	—	—	67	83 (4)	1 436.5 ± 56.4	—	22
MOR	—	—	167	83 (4)	1 076.4 ± 30.6	—	42
DMA	—	—	—	84 (2)	—	67.4 ± 2.6	0
DMA	50	—	—	84 (2)	—	28.4 ± 2.5	58
DMA	250	—	—	84 (2)	—	6.9 ± 2.4	90
DMA	—	—	—	78 (2)	—	64.2 ± 3.1	0
DMA	—	50	—	78 (2)	—	4.7 ± 1.3	93
DMA	—	100	—	78 (2)	—	3.5 ± 0.7	95
DMA	—	—	—	83 (2)	—	69.3 ± 2.5	0
DMA	—	—	67	83 (2)	—	37.6 ± 2.1	46
DMA	—	—	167	83 (2)	—	21.6 ± 8.7	69

[a] MOR, morpholine; DMA, dimethylamine

[b] By gavage; ASC, sodium ascorbate; SULF, ammonium sulfamate; TOCO, DL-α-tocopherol

[c] Exposure time (h) in parentheses.

Table 2.   Control experiments for artefactual N-nitrosamine formation

Amine[a] (2 mg; gavaged)	NO$_2$ exposure time: 74 mg/m³ (h)	Post-exposure treatment[b]		N-nitrosamines formed[e] (ng/mouse)	
		Gavaged[c]	Homogenized[d] with	NDMA	NMOR
DMA	2	MOR	–	73.6 ± 4.9	7.9 ± 3.8
DMA	2	–	MOR	74.6 ± 5.5	49.3 ± 18.3[f, g]
DMA	2	–	–	76.2 ± 5.8[h]	2.6 ± 1.3[h]
MOR	4	DMA	–	15.4 ± 3.7	1 047.0 ± 123.0
MOR	4	–	DMA	18.8 ± 3.1[f]	1 032.0 ± 81.7
MOR	4	–	–	7.5 ± 4.6[h]	1 013.0 ± 84.0[h]

[a] DMA, dimethylamine; MOR, morpholine
[b] 2 mg of specified amine in 0.2 mL distilled-water
[c] Immediately after NO$_2$ exposure and quickly followed by freezing in liquid N$_2$
[d] 2 mg of specified amine, plus 240–260 ng NDPA (internal standard), were added to 8.01–8.09 g frozen mouse powder and the mixture homogenized with 75 mL ice-cold 35% aqueous methanol
[e] NDMA, N-nitrosodimethylamine; NMOR, N-nitrosomorpholine" corrected for recovery of internal stadard (82–96%). NDMA levels (<13 ng/mouse) generally observed in untreated control mice and negligible amounts of NMOR (<5 ng/mouse) in occasional samples were not subtracted
[f] Values calculated for total body weight of mice (22–34 g, MOR-addition group; 22–26 g, DMA-addition group). Actual amounts of NMOR or NDMA found in 8 g mouse powder homogenates, after addition of DMA or MOR (2 mg) were: 9.6 to 20.53 ng NMOR (0.00048 to 0.00103% of added MOR was nitrosated) and 4.2 to 5.5 ng NDMA (0.00021 to 0.00028% of added DMA was nitrosated; internal standard recovery 90–93%)
[g] Higher than average variation may be due to abnormal variations in internal standard recoveries (82, 89, 92% from three different aliquots)
[h] Control values

time-dependent increase of NMOR levels up to 4 h, with no significant further increase for times up to 8 h (Fig. 2); however, when MOR-fed mice were exposed to NO$_2$ for 2 h, then transferred to ambient room air, NMOR yields declined rapidly (from ~85 to 27 ng/mouse within 1 h), reaching 10 ng/mouse 4 h post-exposure. Our data also showed that, following oral administration of 2mg NMOR/mouse, recovery of NMOR from whole-mouse declined from 90% (zero-time) to 20 % (2 h), with a calculated half-life of 48-54 min[1]. Oral administration of ascorbate, sulfamate or α-tocopherol to MOR- or DMA-fed mice, prior to NO$_2$ exposure, significantly inhibited biosynthesis of the respective nitrosamines (Table 1); sulfamate (>100 mg toxic) was the most effective inhibitor (93-97%), followed by ascorbate and α-tocopherol.

Table 2 summarizes the results of control experiments carried out to quantify the extent of N-nitrosamine formation during the work-up of samples, as distinct from in-vivo formation. In mice exposed to DMA plus NO$_2$ and gavaged with 2 mg MOR immediately prior to freezing, very small quantities of NMOR were recovered (5.3 ng/mouse above control, amounting to 0.00023% of gavaged MOR or 0.5% of total NMOR recovered from MOR-fed mice after a 4-h exposure to the same NO$_2$ concentration), while NDMA yields (65-70 ng/mouse, or 0.003% of gavaged DMA) were comparable with positive DMA plus NO$_2$ controls and similar to those reported previously (Iqbal et al., 1981). Maximum possible artefactual formation of NMOR in similar experiments was estimated to be <200 ng/mouse (or <10%), of a maximum NMOR yield of 2300 ng/mouse (Iqbal et al., 1980). Addition of 2 mg MOR to 8 g powder aliquots from mice exposed to DMA and NO$_2$ resulted in slightly higher levels of NMOR (9.6–20.5 ng NMOR/8 g powder, amounting to 0.0005 to 0.001% of MOR added, or 1–2% of total NMOR recovered from MOR-fed mice after 4-h exposure to the same NO$_2$ concentration).

[1] Iqbal, unpublished results

Similarly, gavaging mice with 2 mg DMA immediately after MOR gavage and NO_2 exposure produced a small amount of NDMA ($\sim$ 8 ng/mouse above control, amounting to 0.0004% of DMA gavaged, or 10–11% of total NDMA recovered from DMA-fed mice after a 2-h exposure to the same NO_2 concentration) and high NMOR yields (average, $\sim$ 1050 ng/mouse, amounting to 0.05% of gavaged MOR), which were comparable to positive MOR + NO_2 control values. Addition of 2 mg DMA to powder from MOR-gavaged and NO_2-exposed mice produced lower NDMA yields (4.2–5.5 ng NDMA/8 g powder, amounting to 0.00021 to 0.00028% of added DMA, or 7% of total NDMA recovered from DMA-fed mice after a 2-h exposure to the same NO_2 concentration). In untreated and other controls, variable amounts of NDMA ($<$13 ng/mouse) were recovered.

DISCUSSION

These studies confirm the in-vivo nitrosation of exogenous and endogenous amines previously demonstrated in mice following NO_2 inhalation (Iqbal et al.,1980, 1981). It is also shown here that the biosynthesized NMOR in mice decays rapidly, which may be due to a variety of competing factors, including metabolism, binding and excretion; the rapid decay is consistent with the calculated half-life of 48–54 min. Biosynthesis of both NMOR and NDMA in mice was inhibited by administration of ascorbate and sulfamate prior to NO_2 exposure, which finding not only provides further evidence for formation of N-nitrosamines in vivo, but is also consistent with the well-recognized inhibitory effects of these agents on nitrite-induced nitrosation of amines, both in-vivo and in vitro (for review, see Mirvish, 1975). The control experiments (Table 2) also demonstrated that no more than 1–2% of NMOR and up to 10% of NDMA yields could be formed in vitro during work-up and that the rest represents in-vivo nitrosation of the respective amines by inhaled NO_2 in mice, a result consistent with our previous estimates of possible artefactual formation (Iqbal et al., 1980, 1981); higher estimates for NDMA may be due to its variable level in controls ($<$13 ng/mouse) and to lower yields (65–70 ng/mouse), compared to NMOR ($\sim$1 050 ng/mouse) at the same NO_2 concentration (Table 2). Additional support for in-vivo nitrosation is provided by the observation of NDMA formation in rats, following administration of aminopyrine and exposure to NO_2 (Kusumoto et al., 1980) and NMOR formation in whole carcasses and the gastrointestinal tract of mice, following chronic 30-week exposure to MOR and 1.9–3.8 mg/m^3 NO_2 (Van Stee et al., 1980).

Mirvish et al., (1981), however, have argued that our previous demonstration of NMOR biosynthesis in mice (Iqbal et al., 1980, 1981) was unsound, the NMOR being, in reality, synthesized during the extraction procedure. The arguments of Mirvish et al. do not appear to be adequately supported by their data. Some of the difficulties are as follows:

(1) Mirvish et al. confirmed NMOR formation when homogenates from mice exposed to MOR plus NO_2 were extracted as described by Iqbal et al. (1980). However, when another amine, 'cis-2,6-dimethylmorpholine' (DMM) was added to the homogenates and similarly extracted, significant levels of 'cis-2,6-dimethyl-N-nitrosomorpholine' (DMNM) and 'little' NMOR were detected. From this result, the authors concluded that the NMOR yields observed by Iqbal et al. (1980) were artefacts, produced during extraction rather than in vivo (different NMOR levels, however, were obtained in experiments with and without DMM (140 vs 4 ng/g) and no explanation of this finding was given). In addition, no significant formation of NMOR or DMNM was observed when homogenates from MOR + NO_2-treated mice were extracted with a 'stopping solution' (pH 1) containing large amounts of ascorbate and sulfamate (to prevent further nitrosation in vitro) and DMM (for monitoring in-vitro nitrosation).

A closer inspection of the foregoing results, however, does not entirely substantiate the conclusion that NO_2-induced NMOR biosynthesis in mice does not occur in vivo. The artefactual nitrosamine yields obtained by Mirvish et al. (e.g. 0.007% of the DMM or 0.007%

to 0.0085% of the MOR that was added to mouse powder homogenates, or tissues) were either comparable to those estimated previously ($< 0.001\%$ of MOR administered to mice, or added to powder homogenates; Iqbal *et al.*, 1980) or several-fold higher than those presented in Table 2 (0.00048% to 0.001% nitrosation of MOR added to homogenates).

(2) No internal *N*-nitrosamine standard (such as NDPA; Iqbal *et al.*, 1980, 1981) was used to estimate *N*-nitrosamine recoveries from homogenates. Reported recoveries of NMOR added to mouse homogenates and extracted with 'stopping solution' showed considerable variation ($101 \pm 57\%$).

(3) Experiments were not performed to demonstrate whether or not NMOR formation in mice exposed to MOR + NO$_2$ could be inhibited by oral administration of ascorbate or sulfamate (see Table 1 and Iqbal *et al.*, 1981). In view of the highly variable results and the fact that no internal *N*-nitrosamine standard was used to estimate recovery, the reported absence of any significant level of NMOR or DMNM in homogenates following extraction with 'stopping solution' does not appear to be conclusive.

(4) Rats administered MOR were exposed 30 min later to NO$_2$(22.7–39.7 mg/m^3 for 30 min), then transferred to room air for 30 min 'for nitrosation to proceed' prior to sacrifice. Detection of DMNM, combined with a lack of significant levels of NMOR, in the blood and stomach contents, led to the conclusion that nitrosation of MOR did not occur *in vivo*. However, the possible rapid decay of biosynthesized NMOR when rats were transferred to room air was not, apparently, considered (for comparable data from mice, see Fig. 2; NMOR half-life, 48–54 min). Other possible reasons for the apparent lack of NMOR are the expected low yields after such a brief exposure to low NO$_2$ concentrations (see data for mice, Fig. 1), the high variation in the DMNM recovery data (56 ± 23 and 118 ± 57 ng/g in rat stomach contents and blood) and the fact that only isolated tissues were analysed. Furthermore, estimates of artefactual nitrosamine formation from their data (0.003 to 0.006% of added DMM) are several-fold higher than those in Table 2.

The results presented here provide further evidence of the in-vivo nitrosating potential of NO$_2$, although the underlying mechanisms are as yet unknown. The public health implications of these results are clear, both with respect to the need for a short-term NO$_2$ standard and with respect to human exposure to NO$_x$ [up to 0.72 mg/m^3 in US urban air; $> 2\,880$ mg/m^3 in mainstream tobacco smoke (Neurath, 1972; National Academy of Sciences, 1977; Lee, 1980)], for which the current ambient and occupational NO$_2$ standards are 0.9 mg/m^3, annual average; 9 mg/m^3 for a 15-min ceiling concentration. Limited epidemiological studies have suggested the existence of some relationship between ambient NO$_2$ levels and an urban excess of cancer (Hickey *et al.*, 1970); Sprey *et al.*, 1973). Recent studies of carcinogenesis in mice exposed to MOR and NO$_2$ (1.9–3.8 mg/m^3) further heighten these concerns (Van Stee *et al.*, 1980).

ACKNOWLEDGEMENTS

The technical assistance of K. Dahl and R. Aslan is acknowledged. Work supported by US Environmental Protection Agency Co-operative Agreement # R-807293-10.

REFERENCES

Bretschneider, K. & Matz, J. (1976) *Occurrence and analysis of nitrosamines in air.* In: Walker, E.A., Bogovski, P. & Griciute, L., eds, *Environmental N-nitroso compounds. Analysis and Formation (IARC Scientific Publications No. 14)*, Lyon, International Agency for Research on Cancer, pp. 395–399

Challis, B.C. & Kyrptopoulous, S.A. (1977) Rapid formation of carcinogenic nitrosamines in aqueous alkaline solutions. *Br. J. Cancer, 35,* 693–696

Challis, B.C., Edwards, A., Hunma, R.R., Kyrptopoulous, S.A. & Outram, J.R. (1978) *Rapid formation of N-nitrosamines from nitrogen oxides under neutral and alkaline conditions.* In: Walker, E.A., Castegnaro M., Griciute, L. & Lyle, R.E., eds, *Environmental Aspects of N-Nitroso Compounds (IARC Scientific Publications No. 19)* Lyon, International Agency for Research on Cancer, pp. 127–142

Challis, B.C., Outram, J.R., & Shuker, E.G. (1980) *New pathways for the rapid formation of N-nitrosamines under neutral and alkaline conditions.* In: Walker, E.A., Griciute, L. Castegnaro, M. & Börszönyi, M., eds, *N-Nitroso compounds: Analysis, Formation and Occurrence (IARC Scientific Publications No. 31),* Lyon, International Agency for Research on Cancer, pp. 43–58

Eisenbrand, G., Spiegelhalder, B., Kann, J., Klein, R. & Preussmann, R. (1979) Carcinogenic *N*-nitrosodimethylamine as a contamination in drugs containing 4-demethyl-amino-2, 3-dimethyl-1-phenyl-3-pyrazolin-5-one (amidopyrine, aminophenazone) *Drug Res., 29,* 867–869

Gehlert, P. & Rolle, W. (1977) Formation of diethylnitrosamine by reaction of dimethylamine with nitrogen dioxide in gas phase. *Experientia, 33,* 579–581

Hickey, R.J., Boyce, D.E., Harner, E.B. & Clelland, R.C. (1970) *Ecological Statistical Studies on Environmental Pollution and Chronic Disease in Metropolitan areas of the US (RSRI Discussion Paper Series No. 35),* Philadelphia, Regional Science Research Institute

Iqbal, Z.M., Dahl, K. & Epstein, S.S. (1980) Role of nitrogen dioxide in the biosynthesis of nitrosamine in mice. *Science, 208,* 1475–1477

Iqbal, Z.M., Dahl, K. & Epstein, S.S. (1981) Biosynthesis of dimethylnitrosamine in dimethylamine-treated mice after exposure to nitrogen dioxide. *J. natl Cancer Inst., 67,* 137–141

Janzowski, C., Klein, R. & Preussmann, R. (1980) *Formation of N-nitroso compounds of the pesticides atrazine, simazine and carbaryl with nitrogen oxides,* In: Walker, E.A., Griciute, L. Castegnaro, M. & Börszönyi, M., eds, N-*Nitroso Compounds: Analysis, Formation and Occurrence (IARC Scientific Publications No. 31),* Lyon, International Agency for Research on Cancer, pp. 329–340

Katz, M., ed. (1977) *Methods of Air Sampling and Analysis,* 2nd ed., Washington DC, American Public Health Association, interdisciplinary Books and Periodicals, pp. 527–534

Kaut, U. (1970) Formation of nitrosamines in lung tissues after inhalation of nitrogen oxides. *Csesk. Hyg., 15,* 213–215

Kusumoto, S., Kimura, T., Nakajima, T. & Nakamura, A. (1980) *Formation of nitrosodimethylamine by NO₂ exposure in rats pretreated with aminopyrine.* In: *Eight International Conference on Occupational Health in the Chemical Industry, September 22–25, 1980,* Tokyo, Permanent Commission and International Association on Occupational Health, Nippon Press Center Hall

Lee, S.D., ed (1980) *Nitrogen Oxides and their Effects on Health,* Ann Arbor, Ann Arbor Science, p. 382

Lijinsky, W., Conrad, E. & Van de Bogart, R. (1972) Carcinogenic nitrosamines formed by drug/nitrite interaction *Nature, 239,* 165–167

Mirvish, S.S. (1975) Formation of *N*-nitroso compounds: Chemistry, kinetics and *in vivo* occurrence. *Toxicol. appl. Pharmacol., 31,* 325–351

Mirvish, S., Issenberg, P. & Sams, J.P. (1981) *A study on N-nitrosomorpholine synthesis in rodents exposed to nitrogen dioxide and morpholine,* In:Scanlan, R.A. & Tannenbaum, S.R., eds, N-*Nitroso Compounds (ACS Symposium Series 174),* Washington DC, American Chemical Society, pp. 181–191

National Academy of Sciences (1977) *Nitrogen Oxides,* Wahington DC, Committee on Medical and Biological Effects of Environmental Pollutants, Division of Medical Sciences, Assembly of Life Sciences, National Research Council, p. 333

Neurath, G. (1972) *Measurement of nitrogen oxides in tobacco smoke.* In: Bogovski, P., Preussmann, R. & Walker, E.A., eds, N-*Nitroso Compounds. Analysis and Formation (IARC Scientific Publications No. 3),* Lyon, International Agency for Research on Cancer, pp. 177–179

Pitts, J.N., Grosjean, D., Van Couwenberghe, K., Schmidt, J.P. & Fritz, D.R. (1978) Photoxidation of aliphatic amines under simulated atmospheric conditions; formation of nitrosamines, nitramines, amides and photochemical oxidant. *Environ. Sci. Technol., 12,* 946

Sprey, P.M., Takacs, I., Morson, J. & Allison, J.K. (1973) *A Study of Photochemical Pollutants and their Health Effects,* Rockville, MD, Environ. Control, Inc.

Van Stee, E.W., Boorman, G. & Haseman, J.K. (1980) Pulmonary adenomas in mice exposed to NO₂ by inhalation and morpholine by ingestion. *Pharmacologist, 22,* 158

FURTHER FACTORS INFLUENCING *N*-NITROSAMINE FORMATION IN BACON

J.I. GRAY, D.J. SKRYPEC, A.K. MANDAGERE, A.M. BOOREN & A.M. PEARSON

Department of Food Science and Human Nutrition, Michigan State University, East Lansing, MI 48824, USA

SUMMARY

The possible relationship of unsaturated fatty acids in adipose tissue to the formation of *N*-nitrosamines in bacon was evaluated by trials in which pigs were fed regular (control), tallow-, coconut fat- and corn oil-supplemented diets. Bacon prepared from pigs fed corn oil-supplemented diets contained significantly higher levels of *N*-nitrosopyrrolidine and *N*-nitrosodimethylamine than did control bacon samples; however, bacon produced from pigs fed a coconut fat-supplemented diet contained significantly lower levels of *N*-nitrosopyrrolidine. Fatty acid analyses of the adipose tissue of the bacon samples indicated that *N*-nitrosopyrrolidine levels in bacon correlated well with the degree of unsaturation of the adipose tissue. *N*-nitrosothiazolidine was detected in both brine-cured and dry-cured bacon at levels generally below 4 µg/kg. However, its formation was greatly reduced by the inclusion of α-tocopherol in the cure. The role of woodsmoke in *N*-nitrosothiazolidine formation in bacon is discussed.

INTRODUCTION

The presence of *N*-nitrosopyrrolidine (NPYR) and, to a lesser extent, *N*-nitrosodimethylamine (NDMA), in fried bacon, cook-out fat and the vapours produced during the frying process has resulted in many investigations into the mode of formation of these compounds. Coleman (1978) reported that the high temperature requirement, the inhibitory effects of water and antioxidants and the catalytic effect of lipid hydroperoxides are consistent with the involvement of a free radical in the formation of NPYR. Similarly, Bharucha *et al.* (1979) have suggested that, since *N*-nitrosamine formation occurs only after the bulk of the water has been expelled from the adipose tissue, the *N*-nitrosation reaction occurs mainly by a radical mechanism. Dennis *et al.* (1982) have shown that an oxygen-dependent mechanism is responsible for most of the *N*-nitrosamines produced during the frying of bacon. These authors proposed the oxidation of nitric oxide to be a key step in the reaction and implied that *N*-nitrosamine formation results from *N*-nitrosation reactions occuring during the frying process.

Recently, a new *N*-nitrosamine, *N*-nitrosothiazolidine (NTHZ), has been identified in fried bacon (Gray *et al.*, 1982; Kimoto *et al.*, 1982) and other cured meat products (Pensabene & Fiddler, 1983). Thiazolidine, the parent amine, has not been identified in foods (Sekizawa & Shibamoto, 1980); however, model system studies have shown that heterocyclic compounds, including thiazolidine, 2-methylthiazolidine and 2-ethylthiazolidine, are formed on heating a cysteamine/glucose model browning system (Sakaguchi & Shibamoto, 1978). Similarly, Russell (1983) reported the formation of NTHZ from the reaction of cysteamine/formaldehyde/nitrite. Further studies are necessary to quantify the levels of NTHZ in both brine-cured and dry-cured bacon and to establish its mode of formation in bacon, since some *N*-nitrosothiazolidines have shown positive mutagenic response in the Ames mutation assay (Sekizawa & Shibamoto, 1980). Recently, Pensabene and Fiddler (1983) reported that the formation of NTHZ in bacon appears to be associated with smokehouse processing.

The objective of the present study was two-fold: (1) to investigate the effect of diet and subsequently fatty acid composition of bacon adipose tissue on *N*-nitrosamine formation in bacon; and (2) to further investigate NTHZ formation and inhibition in bacon.

MATERIALS AND METHODS

Effect of diet on N-*nitrosamine formation in bacon*

Diets consisting of 15% added corn oil, coconut fat or tallow were prepared by adding the respective fat to a basic control ration. The basic ration was a commercial type corn-soy bean meal-based diet, supplemented with vitamins and minerals to meet nutritional requirements. Twenty pigs weighing 62–81 kg were separated at random into four groups of five and fed *ad libitum* for five weeks. The pigs were weighed initially and at the end of the feeding period. They consumed an average of 2.17 to 3.38 kg of feed/day and, depending on the group, average weight gains were 0.75 to 0.89 kg/day. Bellies from these pigs were stitched-pumped to 110% of their green weight with a brine containing 15% sodium chloride, 5.0% sucrose, 3.5% sodium tripolyphosphate, sodium nitrite (1 200 mg/kg) and sodium ascorbate (5 000 mg/kg). The bellies were equilibrated for 48 h and smoked, tempered, sliced and packaged as described previously (Gray *et al.*, 1982). After one week, the bacon was analysed for residual nitrite (Association of Official Analytical Chemists, 1975). The fried bacon and cook-out fat were analysed for *N*-nitrosamines by the gas chromatograph-Thermal Energy Analyzer procedure outlined by Reddy *et al.* (1982). The fatty acid composition of adipose tissue was determined by the method of Morrison and Smith (1964).

Formation and inhibition of N-*nitrosothiazolidine in fried bacon*

Dry-cured bacon was manufactured under carefully controlled processing conditions in the pilot plant at the Meat Laboratory, Michigan State University, USA, as described by Reddy *et al.* (1982). Target concentrations of the dry-curing ingredients were: salt, 2.5%; sugar, 0.83%; nitrite, 120 mg/kg; and sodium ascorbate, 550 mg/kg. Dry-cured bacon was also prepared with α-tocopherol-coated Alberger Fine Flake Salt (Diamond Crystal Salt Company, St Clair, MI, USA), the target concentration of α-tocopherol being 500 mg/kg. Brine-cured bacon samples were prepared as well, with the target α-tocopherol levels again being 0 and 500 mg/kg. The bellies in the control group (no tocopherol) were pumped with a brine containing regular Alberger Fine Flake Salt, while the α-tocopherol-coated bellies were prepared using salt coated with both α-tocopherol and lecithin (Gray *et al.*, 1982). All bellies were smoked, sliced and packaged as described by Gray *et al.* (1982).

The concentration of NTHZ in the bacon samples was determined using a Varian 3 700 gas chromatograph containing a 3 m × 2 mm i.d. glass column packed with Carbowax 20M on 80/100 mesh Chromosorb W (Supelco Inc. Bellefonte, PA, USA) and mounted in line with a Thermal Energy Analyzer. Gas chromatographic conditions included temperature programming from 100–160 °C at 20 °C/min and a carrier gas (nitrogen) flow rate of 30 mL/min.

Woodsmoke and its role in N-*nitrosothiazolidine formation*

Hickory woodsmoke condensate was obtained during a typical bacon smoking process, as described by Gray *et al.* (1982). The condensate was collected in a stainless-steel tray containing a 4-L Erlenmeyer flask filled with ice. Aliquots of the condensate (100 mL) were reacted with nitrite, cysteamine and nitrite, cystine and nitrite, and cysteine and nitrite. Another aliquot was treated overnight with sodium bisulfite to remove the aldehydes from the condensate, vacuum distilled, and the distillate reacted with cysteamine and nitrite. The pH of the reaction mixtures was adjusted to 5.0 and the reactions carried out for one hour at 30 °C. The reaction systems were extracted with dichloromethane and analysed for NTHZ.

To investigate further the possible role of smoking in NTHZ formation in bacon, pork bellies were analysed for NTHZ at various stages during processing and cooking. Experimental procedures were similar to those previously described.

RESULTS AND DISCUSSION

Diet and N-*nitrosamine formation in bacon*

The influence of diet on the formation of *N*-nitrosamines in fried bacon was investigated by feeding pigs regular (control), corn oil-, tallow- and coconut fat-enriched diets for five weeks. Results of the *N*-nitrosamine analyses (Table 1) indicate NPYR concentrations in the range of 4-9 µg/kg (average 5.7 µg/kg) for the control samples. These values are consistent with those recently reported in other studies, where NPYR levels are generally below 10 µg/kg (Mergens & Newmark, 1979). Bacon from the group of pigs fed coconut fat contained significantly ($p < 0.05$) lower levels of NPYR, an average concentration of 3.8 µg/kg being obtained. Bacon from the corn oil group averaged 10.6 µg/kg, indicating that corn oil supplementation has a significant ($p < 0.05$) effect on NPYR formation. Feeding tallow to the pigs for five weeks did not influence NPYR levels in the fried product. Similar trends were observed for NPYR levels in the cook-out fat.

Table 1.   *N*-Nitrosamine and residual nitrite concentrations in fried bacon and cook-out fat from pigs fed various oil-supplemented diets

Diet/Treatment	Fried bacon[a] (µg/kg)		Cook-out fat[b] (µg/kg)		Residual Nitrite (mg/kg)
	NPYR	NDMA	NPYR	NDMA	
Control	5.7 (4–9)	2.7 (1–4)	13.2	6.8	37 (32–45)
Tallow	5.6 (4–8)	2.7 (1–4)	8.9	2.5	43 (29–58)
Corn oil	10.6[c] (7–15)	4.0[c] (2–7)	18.6	8.3	43 (31–56)
Coconut fat	3.8[c] (2–5)	2.2 (1.7–3	tr	2.0	33 (28–39)

[a] Values in parentheses represent range of *N*-nitrosamine levels observed for five bellies per treatment
[b] Cook-out fat from five bellies per treatment was combined and analysed in triplicate
[c] Values are significantly different from the control at the $p < 0.05$ level

Table 2. Fatty acid composition of adipose tissue of bacon pigs fed various supplemented diets

Diet	Fatty acid composition (percent)[a]									Total un-saturated
	C12	C14	C16	C18	Total saturated	C16:1	C18:1	C18:2	C18:3	
Bacon adipose tissue										
Control	–	1.5	21.0	11.7	34.2	2.6	50.0	13.5	–	66.1
Tallow	–	1.2	17.2	14.0	32.4	2.7	51.9	12.9	–	67.5
Corn oil	–	1.1	21.1	7.9	30.1	1.4	38.1	29.8	0.6	69.9
Coconut fat	2.8	6.9	25.1	10.2	45.0	5.5	37.9	10.1	0.3	53.8

[a] Average from five pigs per treatment

The effect of diet on NDMA levels was not as pronounced, possibly due to the smaller quantities of this *N*-nitrosamine in cooked bacon. Significantly ($p < 0.05$) higher concentrations of NDMA were found in bacon produced from pigs fed the corn oil-enriched diet. Unlike the results obtained for NPYR, there was no significant difference between NDMA levels in the control bacon samples and bacon from the coconut fat-supplemented group.

The influence of dietary supplementation on the fatty acid composition of adipose tissue is summarized in Table 2. Supplementation of the diet with corn oil tended to increase the degree of unsaturation of the adipose tissue. Specifically, there was an approximately two-fold increase in linoleic acid content in bacon adipose tissue from the corn oil treatment. Coconut fat-supplementation decreased the unsaturation of the adipose tissue, particularly with respect to oleic acid. This decrease in total unsaturation of the lipids paralleled the formation of greatly reduced levels of NPYR in the bacon. Conversely, the fatty acid composition of the adipose tissue of bacon from the pigs fed the corn oil diet correlated well with the higher levels of NPYR observed in this study, an indication that increasing unsaturation of the lipid enhances *N*-nitrosamine formation in bacon. Tallow, when fed to pigs, did not alter appreciably the fatty acid composition of the adipose tissue of the bacon. *N*-Nitrosamine analyses also revealed no significant differences in NPYR and NDMA formation when pigs were fed the tallow-supplemented diet.

These results are interesting in terms of the possible relationship between *N*-nitrosamine formation and the relative unsaturation of bacon adipose tissue. Mottram *et al.* (1977) have shown that *N*-nitrosation occurs mainly in the adipose tissue and have postulated that the non-polar lipids provide and environment conducive to *N*-nitrosamine formation. Goutefongea *et al.* (1977) studied the interaction of nitrite with adipose tissue and suggested that nitrite reacts with unsaturated carbon-carbon bonds. Walters *et al.* (1979) also reported that unsaturated lipids can react with nitric oxide in a manner similar to that of simpler olefins, such as cyclohexenes. They demonstrated that pseudonitrosites of unsaturated triglycerides transnitrosate to secondary amines and suggested that similar derivatives of unsaturated lipids may be involved in *N*-nitrosamine formation in adipose tissue.

Frouin (1976) has hypothesized that much of the nitrite added to cured meat is rapidly converted to various forms of bound nitric oxide, i.e., by reaction with proteins, thiols, hydroxyls, carboxyls, reducing agents and haem pigments. *N*-Nitrosamine formation from bound nitric oxide may occur either by direct transnitrosation of the secondary amines or by an indirect process involving the initial release of the nitric oxide moiety (Dennis *et al.*, 1982). It is well recognized that nitric oxide is a poor *N*-nitrosating agent, but, in the presence of air, it is rapidly converted to higher oxides of nitrogen which are powerful nitrosating agents. Dennis *et al.* (1982) have shown that when bacon is fried in an inert atmosphere, *N*-nitrosamine formation is markedly reduced. The oxygen-dependent activity is consistent with a mechanism in which the oxidation of nitric oxide is a key step in *N*-nitrosamine formation in bacon.

In another related study, Pryor and Lightsey (1981) investigated the reactions of nitrogen dioxide with cyclohexene in methyl oleate and linoleate. Nitrogen dioxide reacts with cyclohexene almost exclusively by abstraction of allylic hydrogen. This reaction also initiates the autoxidation of the alkene in the presence of oxygen or air, but it leads to the production of nitrous acid, rather than of a product containing a nitro group attached to a carbon atom. The nitrous acid can react with secondary amines to produce *N*-nitrosamines. These authors also showed that the rate of *N*-nitrosation of the amine increases directly with the number of double bonds in the reaction medium, an indication that nitrous acid formed by the nitrite-unsaturated ester reactions is participating in the nitrosation of the amine. Formation of nitrous acid by nitrite-alkene reactions adds credence to the postulate that the unsaturated fatty acids are involved in *N*-nitrosamine formation in bacon.

It appears that adipose tissue serves as a reservoir for a number of potential *N*-nitrosating agents and that the extent of *N*-nitrosation is directly related to the amount of unsaturation of the component fatty acids. Further studies are necessary to elucidate the nature of the principal *N*-nitrosating agent in bacon adipose tissue.

Formation of N-nitrosothiazolidine in bacon

Recently, several reports have mentioned the presence of NTHZ in fried bacon (Gray *et al.*, 1982; Kimoto *et al.*, 1982). In the present study, both dry-cured and brine-cured bacon samples were analysed for NTHZ (Table 3). NTHZ levels in the brine-cured bacon to which no α-tocopherol was added (treatment 1) ranged from 3.4 to 4.9 µg/kg. Slightly lower NTHZ levels were obtained for the dry-cured bacon. Addition of α-tocopherol (treatment 2) to the bacon samples had a marked inhibitory effect on NTHZ formation in both brine-cured and dry-cured bacon. Average values of less than 2 µg/kg were recorded for both types of bacon.

Experiments were also carried out to investigate the possibility of artefactual formation of NTHZ during the mineral oil distillation procedure normally employed in the extraction of *N*-nitrosamines from cooked bacon. Kimoto *et al.* (1982), for example, reported preliminary data showing that most, but not all, of the NTHZ in fried bacon was produced as an artefact during the analytical procedure when residual nitrite was present prior to analyis. It was established in our studies that the addition of ammonium sulfamate (2 g) to the distillation flask immediately before distillation reduced such artefact formation. When morpholine was added to the distillation flask, no *N*-nitrosomorpholine was detected in the distillate.

The presence of NTHZ in selected bacon samples raises the question of its possible mode of formation. Although thiazolidine has not been reported in foods (Sekizawa & Shibamoto, 1980), Kimoto *et al.* (1982) reported that the expected precursors for thiazolidine formation, cysteamine and formaldehyde, should be present in bacon. Cysteamine can result from the decarboxylation of cysteine and formaldehyde by the fragmentation of sugar and, to a lesser extent, by the oxidation of pork lipids. Recently, Pensabene & Fiddler (1983) reported NTHZ data for bacon and other cured meat products which strongly suggest that NTHZ is formed as a result of wood-smoking. However, it was not determined whether NTHZ was formed during smoking and deposited on the bacon surface during processing, or whether one or more of the smoke components reacted with meat consitutents to form the *N*-nitrosamine.

In the present study, woodsmoke condensate was reacted with various compounds to determine the possible role of smoking in NTHZ formation in cured meats (Table 4). No NTHZ was detected in woodsmoke condensate, even after the addition of sodium nitrite. However, when cysteamine was added to the condensate, NTHZ was isolated and its identity confirmed by mass spectrometry. The presence of small amounts of NTHZ in the model system

Table 3.   *N*-Nitrosothiazolidine (NTHZ) levels and percent inhibition in brine-cured and dry-cured bacon samples

Bacon type	Treatment[a]	Fried bacon[b,c]		Cook-out fat	
		NTHZ (µg/kg)	Inhibition (%)	NTHZ	Inhibition (%)
Brine-cured	1	4.1 (3.4–4.9)	–	trace	–
	2	1.4 (0.6–3.2)	66	ND[d]	–
Dry-cured	1	2.8 (1.2–4.1)	–	trace	–
	2	1.9 (1.1–2.5)	32	ND	–

[a] Treatment 1, control samples; treatment 2, 500 mg/kg α-tocopherol added
[b] Each value represents the average of three analyses of five bellies per treatment
[c] Values in parentheses represent range of NTHZ levels obtained per treatment
[d] ND, not detected (limit of detection, 0.1 ng)

Table 4. *N*-Nitrosothiazolidine formation in woodsmoke condensate model systems.

Model System [a]	NTHZ [b] (µg)	NMTHZ (µg)	NMOR (µg)
Woodsmoke condensate	ND [c]	ND	ND
Woodsmoke condensate + nitrite	ND	ND	tr [d]
Woodsmoke condensate + cysteamine	0.4	ND	tr
Woodsmoke condensate + cysteamine + nitrite	1.550	14.4	tr
Woodsmoke condensate + cystine + nitrite	ND	ND	tr
Woodsmoke condensate + cysteine + nitrite	ND	ND	tr
Woodsmoke condensate treated with NaHSO₃ overnight, vacuum distilled, + cysteamine + nitrite	tr	ND	ND

[a] Consisted of 100 mL of woodsmoke condensate, to which were added cysteamine (25 mg), cystine (25 mg), cysteine (25 mg) or nitrite (25 mg), where appropriate. The pH of the stystems was adjusted to 5.0; reaction time 1 hour at 30 °C
[b] NTHZ, *N*-nitrosothiazolidine; NMTHZ, *N*-nitroso-2-methylthiazolidine; NMOR, *N*-nitrosomorpholine
[c] ND, not detectable
[d] tr, traces

Table 5. *N*-Nitrosothiazolidine levels in pork bellies at various stages of processing and cooking [a]

Sample	NTHZ (µg/kg) [a]
Pork belly	ND
Pork belly, smoked	tr
Pork belly, cured	ND
Pork belly, cured and smoked	2.5
Pork belly, fried	ND
Pork belly, smoked and fried	ND
Pork belly, cured and fried	ND
Pork belly, cured, smoked and fried	1.4

[a] Average value for two bellies per treatment, triplicate analyses per belly

containing only woodsmoke condensate and cysteamine suggests the probable presence of nitrogen oxides generated during the combustion process (NAS, 1982). These results indicate that woodsmoke does not contain NTHZ or thiazolidine *per se*, but that some component(s) of woodsmoke is capable of reacting with cysteamine to form thiazolidine. To further test this hypothesis, the aldehydes in the woodsmoke condensate were removed by forming the bisulfite addition complexes (Morrison & Boyd, 1976). After filtering and adjusting the pH to 10, the condensate was vacuum-distilled and the distillate was reacted with cysteamine and nitrite, as before. Only traces of NTHZ were detected, suggesting that a carbonyl compound, most probably formaldehyde, is involved in the formation of this *N*-nitrosamine. Formaldehyde is present in woodsmoke at concentrations of approximately 80 mg/100 g sawdust (Gorbatov *et al.*, 1971). Similarly, Ruiter (1979) reported a formaldehyde concentration of 710 mg/kg in a smoke solution obtained by exposing water-filled Petri dishes to smoke. Another *N*-nitrosamine, *N*-nitroso-2-methylthiazolidine (NMTHZ) was detected in the model system containing woodsmoke condensate, cysteamine and nitrite (Table 4). Acetaldehyde, which has been implicated in the formation of this *N*-nitrosamine (Sakaguchi & Shibamoto, 1978) has been identified in the low-boiling components of hickory smoke (Doerr *et al.*, 1966).

Pork bellies at various stages of processing and cooking were analysed for NTHZ (Table 5). Higher levels of NTHZ were found in raw pork belly which had been cured and smoked than in the fried counterpart. Although this study is rather limited, these preliminary data are in general agreement with those of Pensabene and Fiddler (1983), who reported that the NTHZ level in raw bacon was higher than that found in fried bacon and the cook-out fat combined.

While it is apparent that the primary mode of NTHZ formation in bacon is related to the smoking process, other possible sources of this *N*-nitrosamine cannot be discounted. Further studies are necessary to determine whether glucose in bacon can undergo fragmentation during frying to produce formaldehyde. Furthermore, although the concentrations of various amines in fresh and processed pork have been determined (Lakritz *et al.*, 1975), there is a paucity of data regarding the cysteamine content of meat products. It is possible that formaldehyde can react with cysteine to form thioproline (thiazolidine carboxylic acid), which could be converted to NTHZ during the cooking process. This mechanism, however, cannot account for the presence of NTHZ in raw smoked bacon, as the normal smoking temperature is approximately 135°F (58°C) and is not high enough to effect the decarboxylation reactions. Further studies are required to determine cysteamine levels in cured meats and also to ascertain whether NTHZ is formed during the frying process.

ACKNOWLEDGEMENT

This study was supported in part by grants from the American Meat Institute, United States Department of Agriculture, Grant No. 82-CRSR-2-2051, and National Cancer Institute, DHEW, Grant No. 1 RO1 CA 26576-03. Michigan Agricultural experiment Station Journal Article No. *10843.*

REFERENCES

Association of Official Analytical Chemists (1975) *Official Methods of Analysis,* 12th ed., Washington, DC

Bharucha, K.R. Cross, C.K. & Rubin, L.J. (1979) Mechanism of *N*-nitrosopyrrolidine formation in bacon. *J. Agric. Food Chem, 27,* 63–69

Celeman, M.H. (1978) A model system for the formation of *N*-nitrosopyrrolidine in grilled or fried bacon. *J. Food Technol., 13,* 55–69

Dennis, M.J., Massey, R.C. & McWeeny, D.J. (1982) The effect of oxygen on nitrosamine formation in bacon. *Z. Lebensm. Unters. Forsch., 174,* 114–116

Doerr, R.C., Wasserman, A.E. & Fiddler, W. (1966) Composition of Hickory sawdust smoke. Low-boiling constituents. *J. Agric. Food Chem., 14,* 662–665

Frouin, A. (1976) *Nitrates and nitrites; reinterpretation of analytical data by means of bound nitric oxide.* In: *Proc. 2nd Int. Symp. Nitrite in Meat Products,* Zeist, The Netherlands, Pudoc, pp. 115–120

Gorbatov, V.M., Krylova, N.N., Voloinskaya, V.P., Lyaskovskaya, Yu. N., Bazarova, K.I., Khlamova, R.I. & Yakovleva, G. Yu. (1971) Liquid smokes for use in cured meats. *Food Technol., 25*(1), 71–77

Goutefongea, R., Cassens, R.G. & Woolford, G. (1977) Distribution of sodium nitrite in adipose tissue during curing. *J. Food Sci., 42,* 1637–1641

Gray, J.I., Reddy, S.K., Price, J.F., Mandagere, A.K. & Wilkens, W.F. (1982) Inhibition of *N*-nitrosamines in bacon. *Food Technol., 36*(6), 39-45.

Kimoto, W.I., Pensabene, J.W., & Fiddler, W. (1982) Isolation and identification of *N*-nitrosothiazolidine in fried bacon. *J. Agric. Food Chem., 30,* 757–760

Lakritz, L., Spinell, A.M. & Wasserman, A.E. (1975) Determination of amines in fresh and processed pork. *J. Agric. Food Chem., 23,* 44

Mergens, W.J. & Newmark, H.L. (1979) *The use of alpha-tocopherol in bacon processing: an update.* In: *Proc. Meat Industry Research Conf.,* Chicago, Am. Meat Inst. Found., pp. 79–84

Morrison, R.T. & Boyd, R.N. (1976) *Organic Chemistry,* 3rd ed., Boston, Allyn and Bacon, Inc., pp. 638–639

Morrison, W.R. & Smith L.M. (1964) Preparation of fatty acid methyl esters and dimethylacetals from lipids with boron fluoride-methanol. *J. Lipid Res., 5,* 600–608

Mottram, D.S., Patterson, R.L.S., Edwards, R.A. & Gough, T.A. (1977) The preferential formation of volatile N-nitrosamines in the fat of fried bacon. *J. Sci. Food Agric., 28,* 1025–1029

NAS (1981) *The Health Effects of Nitrate, Nitrite and* N-*Nitroso Compounds.* Washington DC, Natl. Acad. Press

Pensabene, J.W. & Fiddler, W. (1983) N-Nitrosothiazolidine in bacon and other cured meat products. Paper presented at the 43rd. Annual Meeting of the Institute of Food Technologists, New Orleans, June 18–22

Pryor, W.A. & Lightsey, J.W. (1981) Mechanisms of nitrogen dioxide reactions: Initiation of lipid peroxidation and the production of nitrous acid. *Science, 214,* 435–437

Reddy, S.K., Gray, J.I., Price, W.F. & Wilkens, W.F. (1982) Inhibition of N-nitrosopyrrolidine in dry cured bacon by α-tocopherol-coated salt systems. *J. Food Sci., 47,* 1598–1602

Ruiter A. (1979) Color of smoked foods, *Food Technol. 33*(5), 54, 56, 58, 59–60, 63

Russel, G.F. (1983) *Nitrite interactions in model Maillard browning systems.* In: Waller, G.R. & Feather, M.S., eds., *The Maillard Reaction in Foods and Nutrition,* ACS Symposium Series 215, Washington, DC, Am. Chem. Soc., pp. 83–90

Sakaguchi, M. & Shibamoto, T. (1978) Formation of heterocyclic compounds from the reaction of cysteamine and D-glucose, acetaldehyde, or glyoxal. *J. Agric. Food Chem., 26,* 1179–1183

Sekizawa, J. & Shibamoto, T. (1980) Mutagenicity of 2-alkyl-N-nitrosothiazolidine. *J. Agric. Food Chem., 28,* 781–783

Walters, C.L., Hart, R.J. & Perse, S. (1979) The possible role of lipid pseudonitrosites in nitrosamine formation in fried bacon. *Z. Lebensm. Unters. Forsch., 168,* 177–180

NITROSATION BY ALKYL NITRITES. CATALYSIS BY INORGANIC SALTS

R. DABORA, M. MOLINA, V. NG, J.S. WISHNOK & S.R. TANNENBAUM

Department of Nutrition and Food Science, Massachusetts Institute of Technology, Cambridge, MA, USA

SUMMARY

Isobutyl nitrite is an effective nitrosating agent at acidic, neutral and basic pH in the presence of species arising from phosphate ion. The reaction is first-order in isobutyl nitrite and amine. In the reaction of isobutyl nitrite with sulfanilamide, the pH dependence reflects the change in concentration of the various protonated forms of phosphate, with H_3PO_4 and $H_2PO_4^-$ most strongly affecting the rate. In the reaction of isobutyl nitrite with dipropylamine, the pH dependence also reflects the change in the concentration of unprotonated amine.

INTRODUCTION

The formation of *N*-nitroso compounds *via* reaction of amines with various nitrosating agents, especially those arising from inorganic nitrite, has been investigated extensively during the past several years (Mirvish, 1975, 1977; Magee, 1982 and references). This attention has been due largely to concern over the general carcinogenicity of *N*-nitroso compounds and their consequent possible involvement in human cancer (Druckrey *et al.*, 1967; Magee *et al.*, 1976; Magee, 1982). Somewhat less attention has been devoted to nitrosation by gaseous nitrogen oxides or by alkyl nitrites, due partly to a focus on the stomach as the major in-vivo nitrosation compartment for possible endogenous formation of *N*-nitroso compounds, and partly to the fact that simple alkyl nitrites are generally poor nitrosating agents, except under non-polar conditions (Challis & Shuker, 1979; Aldred & Williams, 1981) i.e., in neither case would extensive formation of *N*-nitroso compounds be expected from participation of organic nitrites.

We have nonetheless been interested in the potential behaviour of some specific alkyl nitrites in physiological situations, e.g., intestinal micelles. Absorption of dietary cholesterol, for example, is accomplished largely *via* incorporation into mixed micelles along with bile acids and lecithin (Harper *et al.*, 1977). It is well known that deamination reactions are catalysed by micelles (Moss & Lane, 1967,; Hutchinson & Stedman, 1973) and that significant enhancement of the rate of formation of *N*-nitrosamines can be obtained when the reactions are carried out in the presence of micelles (Okun & Archer, 1977; Kim *et al.*, 1982). The cholesterol, of course, arrives in the intestine *via* the acidic conditions in the stomach, where, in the presence of nitrite, it could react to give the compound cholesteryl nitrite (Djerassi *et al.*, 1963).

The properties of cholesteryl nitrite are not well known, but it has been shown that - in contrast to simple alkyl nitrites - some activated alkyl nitrites are capable of N-nitrosation under neutral or alkaline conditions (Challis & Shuker, 1979; Oae *et al.*, 1978; Yamamoto *et al.*, 1979). It is thus conceivable that cholesteryl nitrite is an effective nitrosating agent under these conditions, i.e., incorporation into micelles may lead to enhanced reactivity.

Because of some early technical problems with cholesteryl nitrite and because of interest in the physiological behaviour of the more readily available simple alkyl nitrites, we studied the latter compounds. Our results to date are presented below.

MATERIALS AND METHODS

Sodium nitrate, sodium nitrite, sulfanilamide and naphthylethylenediamine dihydrochloride were of analytical reagent grade and were purchased from Malinkrodt (St Louis, MO, USA). Amines were purchased from Aldrich or Baker, and, except for morpholine, were shown to be free from nitrosamine impurities and were used as obtained. Morpholine was distilled prior to use. Commercial ('street') formulations of alkyl nitrites, labeled 'Rush' and 'Hardware', were obtained from shops in the Boston adult-entertainment district and were shown by nuclear magnetic resonance and gas-chromatograph-mass spectrometry to be virtually pure isobutyl nitrite (the nitrous acid ester of 2-methyl-1-propanol). Stock solutions of the alkyl nitrites (1:300 in acetonitrile) were used for kinetic runs.

Gas chromatography was carried out on a Varian Model 200 with glass columns packed with Carbowax 20M/TPA/KOH, SP-2100, or OV-17. The detector was a Thermal Energy Analyzer (Fine *et al.*, 1973). Mass spectral analyses were done on a Hewlett-Packard 5992A gas-chromatograph-mass spectrometer with glass or fused silica capillary columns coated with Carbowax 20M or SP-2100.

Kinetic runs with sulfanilamide were carried out using a Hewlett-Packard 8550 UV-Visible spectrophotometer interfaced with a Hewlett-Packard HP-85 desktop computer. For a typical kinetic run with sulfanilamide, a 1-mL solution containing buffer (borate or dimethyl glutarate), sulfanilamide (0.232 mol/L), 1-naphtylethylenediamine dihydrochloride (0.232 mol/L) and disodium orthophosphate (0.081 mol/L), at the desired pH, was brought to 25°C in a water-jacketed cuvette. Alkyl nitrite was added (4.8 µL of the stock solution) to start the reaction, and the absorbance at 500 nm was measured for 1 s every 2 s for 10 min. For experiments with carbonate, water was boiled to remove dissolved carbon dioxide prior to addition of sodium carbonate. Stock solutions of sodium carbonate were then prepared at a pH below that desired for the experiment in order to minimize changes in the concentration of carbonate due to loss of carbon dioxide. Experiments with dialkylamines were carried out in Reactivials, which were placed in shaker baths at 37°C. Aliquots were removed at desired time intervals, and the reactions were quenched by the addition of ammonium sulfamate. The quenched solutions were extracted with methylene chloride in Eppendorf tubes, which were then centrifuged to separate the layers.

RESULTS

Nitrosation by isobutyl nitrite

Preliminary experiments with isobutyl nitrite and dimethylamine in rat blood suggested that nitrosation in whole blood proceeds slightly faster than in buffered saline solution, and that the reaction is faster still in plasma. This has been confirmed in more carefully controlled experiments, but the difference in results between plasma and aqueous buffer is significant only when the concentration of isobutyl nitrite approaches saturation, i.e., it is probably not physiologically meaningful. Inconsistent behaviour in phosphate-buffered aqueous control systems indicated that the reaction was affected by phosphate, and this effect was then studied in more detail in dilute solutions *via* reactions of isobutyl nitrite with Griess reagent. This effect is reproduceable both with sulfanilamide (Griess reagent) and with di-*n*-propylamine. The rates were studied with various concentrations of amine, isobutyl nitrite and phosphate, and at various acidities, yielding the empirical rate equation for reaction with sulfanilamide shown below:

$$\text{Rate (mol L}^{-1}\text{s}^{-1}) = [\text{Alkyl Nitrite}][\text{Amine}][0.013[H_3PO_4] + 26.2[H_2PO_4^-]]$$

The results of these experiments are summarized in Tables 1 and 2 and Figure 1. Note that the logarithms of the reaction rates vary linearly with pH over the ranges 5.0-7.5 for reaction with sulfanilamide (r = 0.99 for reaction with and without phosphate) and 6.5-8.5 for the reaction with di-*n*-propylamine (r = 0.97). Sulfate appears to have had a slight effect on the reaction at pH 5.0 and 7.4 (approximately 70 % of the effect of phosphate at pH 5 and approximately 14% of the effect of phosphate at pH 7.4), while carbonate had no effect over

Table 1. Reaction of isobutyl nitrite with sulfanilamide in the presence of phosphate. Effect of pH

pH	Reaction rate × E9 (mol L^{-1}s^{-1})		
	Control[a]	Phosphate added[a]	Calculated[b]
5.0	4.5 (0.15;n=2)	13.3 (1.1;n=4)	13.8
5.5	2.7 (0.07;n=2)	8.0 (0.3;n=4)	6.5
6.0	0.7 (0.06;n=2)	4.6 (0.5;n=4)	4.1
6.5	0.3 (0.04;n=2)	3.1 (0.3;n=5)	3.0
7.0	0.1 (0.01;n=3)	2.1 (0.1;n=5)	2.1
7.5	0.05 (0.05;n=2)	1.0 (0.1;n=5)	1.1

[a] Mean rate (SD; number of observations)
[b] Calculated from equation 1

Table 2. Nitrosation of sulfanilamide by isobutyl nitrite and by sodium nitrite. Effect of pH and of phosphate

pH	Reaction rate × E9 (mol L^{-1}s^{-1})	
	Isobutyl nitrite	Sodium nitrite
5.0	23[a]	1
5.0	6	0.08
7.5	1[a]	0.01
0.05	7.5	0.01

[a] Phosphate added

DABORA *ET AL.*

Fig. 1. Effect of pH and phosphate on nitrosation of sulfanilamide by isobutyl nitrite; △, phosphate added; ○, no
phosphate

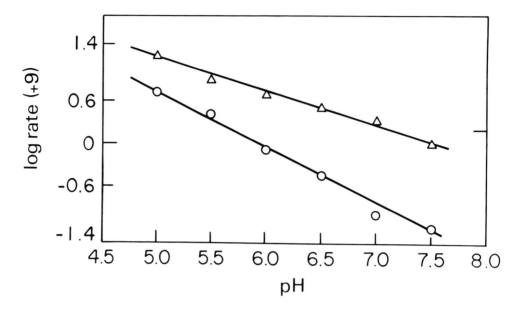

the pH range 5.0-7.0. The rate of nitrosation by equimolar concentrations of sodium nitrite
was, under all conditions studied, lower than the rate of nitrosation by isobutyl nitrite (Table
2). When isobutyl nitrite was added to Griess reagent in human plasma at the same
concentrations as in the experiments summarized in Table 1, there was essentially no reaction
with or without added phosphate. The phosphate-catalysed reaction did occur in plasma that
had been subjected to ultrafiltration to remove constituents with molecular weights greater than
25000, but the rate of reaction was not significantly greater than in phosphate-containing
aqueous saline solution or resuspended filtrate.

DISCUSSION

Exploratory experiments with dialkyl amines and isobutyl nitrite indicated that isobutyl
nitrite was a more effective nitrosating agent than sodium nitrite in the pH range of
physiological interest. Erratic behaviour in phosphate-buffered control systems suggested that
the reaction was catalysed by the buffer. This was borne out by subsequent kinetic experiments
on the pH-dependence of the rate of nitrosation of sulfanilamide by isobutyl nitrite. The
nitrosatable nitrogen on sulfanilamide remained unprotonated over the pH range of our
experiments, and it was consequently possible to demonstrate that the effect of pH on the rate
of this nitrosation could be attributed entirely to the changing relative concentrations of H_3PO_4
and $H_2PO_4^-$ as the pH was changed. The rate of the reaction of di-*n*-propylamine, which has
a pKa of about 11, depends additionally on the amount of unprotonated amine. For the pH
range 6.5 to 7.5, taking into account only the concentration of unprotonated amine, the rate
of nitrosation of di-*n*-propylamine would be expected to increase about 10-fold. The effect due
to phosphate, however, would be expected to lead to a three-fold decrease in rate. The observed
increase of about three-fold is in good agreement for these two effects combined.

Comparison of rates of nitrosation by isobutyl nitrite and by sodium nitrite (Table 2) indicates that—even at pH as low as 5 and in the absence of catalysts—isobutylnitrite is a more effective nitrosating agent than sodium nitrite, i.e., nitrosation *via* isobutyl nitrite does not necessarily involve prior hydrolysis to nitrite ion, as is apparently the case at pH 2.8-3.0 (Shenton & Johnson, 1972). Challis and Shuker (1980) demonstrated an accelerating effect on *N*-nitrosation by β-substituted alkyl nitrites. This presumably arose *via* anchimeric assistance from lone electron pairs on the substituents. In our experiments, we observed nitrosation by unsubstituted alkyl nitrites and accelerated nitrosation when the reaction was carried out in the presence of phosphate. Whether or not these observations are related or, instead, represent three separate mechanisms, is at present not understood.

ACKNOWLEDGEMENT

This work was supported by NIEHS Grant No. 2-PO1-ES00597-13. The nuclear magnetic resonance spectrum of 'Rush' (isobutyl nitrite) was obtained by Mr Mark St Lezin.

REFERENCES

Aldred, s.E. & Williams, D.L.H. (1981) Alkyl nitrites as nitrosating agents. Kinetics and mechanism of the reactions of propyl nitrite in propan-l-ol. *J. chem. Soc., Perkin Trans. II*, 1021–1024

Challis, B.C. & Shuker, D.E.G. (1979) Rapid nitrosation of amines in aqueous alkaline solution by beta-substituted alkyl nitrites. *J. chem. Soc., Chem. Commun.*, 315–316

Challis, B.C. & Shuker, D.E.G. (1980) Chemistry of nitroso compounds. Part 16. Formation of *N*-nitrosamines from dissolved NOC1 in the presence of alkanolamines and related compounds. *Food Cosmet. Toxicol.*, *18*, 283–288

Djerassi, C., Wolf, H. & Brunnenberg, E. (1963) Optical rotatory dispersion studies. LXXXV. Circular dichroism and optical rotatory dispersion of the nitrite and nitro chromophores. *J. Am. chem. Soc.*, *85*, 2842

Druckrey, H., Preussmann, R., Schmahl, D. & Ivankovic, S. (1967) Organotrope carcinogene Wirkung bei 65 verschiedenen *N*-nitroso-Verbindungen an BD-Ratten. *Z. Krebsforsch.*, *69*, 103–201

Fine, D.H., Rufeh, H. & Gunther, B. (1973) A group specific procedure for the analysis of both volatile and non-volatile *N*-nitroso compounds in picogram amounts. *Anal. Lett.*, *6*, 731–733

Harper, A.L., Rodwell, V.W. & Mayes, P.A. (1977) *Review of Physiological Chemistry*, 19th ed., Lange Los Altos, pp. 205–210

Hutchinson, M. & Stedman, G. (1973) Micellar catalysis of the deamination of *O*-hydroxylamines. *J. chem. Soc. Perkin Trans. II*, 93–95

Kim, Y.-K., Tannenbaum, S.R. & Wishnok. J.S. (1982) *Effects of ascorbic acid on the nitrosation of dialkylamines*. In: Seib, P.A. & Tolbert, B.M., eds, *Ascorbic Acid: Chemistry, Metabolism and Uses, (Advances in Chemistry 200)* Washington DC, American Chemical Society, pp. 571–585

Magee, P.N., ed. (1982) *Nitrosamines and Human Cancer (Banbury Report 12)*, Cold Spring Harbor, NY, Cold Spring Harbor Laboratory

Magee, P.N., Montesano, R. & Preussmann, R. (1976) N-*Nitroso compound and related carcinogens*. In: Searle, C.E., ed., *Chemical Carcinogens*, Washington, DC, American Chemical Society. pp. 491–625

Mirvish, S.S. (1975) *N*-Nitroso compounds: their chemical and *in vivo* formation and possible importance as environmental carcinogens. *J. Toxicol. environ. Health*, *2*, 1267–1277

Mirvish, S.S. (l977) Formation of *N*-nitroso compounds, nitrite, and nitrate: possible implications for the causation of human cancer. *Prog. Water Technol.*, *8*, 5655–5661

Moss, R.A. & Lane, S.M. (1967) Solvolysis of alkyl diazotates. II. Stereochemistry of internal return in the 2-octyl system. *J. Am. chem. Soc.*, *89*, 5655–5661

Oae, S., Asai, N. & Fujimori, K. (1978) Alkaline hydrolyses of alkyl nitrites and related carboxylic acids. *J. chem. Soc., Perkin Trans. II*, 1124

Okun, J.D. & Archer, M.C. (1977) Kinetics of nitrosamine formation in the presence of micelle-forming surfactants, *J. natl Cancer Inst., 58,* 409–411

Shenton, A.J. & Johnson, R.M. (1972) A comparative kinetic study of the *N*-nitrosation of sulfanilamide by cyclohexyl nitrite and nitrous acid. *Int. J. chem. Kinet., 4,* 235–242

Yamamoto, M., Yamada, T. & Tanimura, A. (1979) The effects of ethanol, glucose and sucrose on nitrosation of secondary amines following alkalization of reaction mixture. *J. Food Hyg. Soc. (Jpn), 20,* 15

NITROSAMIDE CARCINOGENESIS: NITROSATION OF AMIDE LINKAGES AND FACILE DECOMPOSITION OF RESULTING NITROSAMIDES

Y.L. CHOW[1], S.S. DHALIWAL & J. POLO

Department of Chemistry, Simon Fraser University, Burnaby, British Columbia, Canada

SUMMARY

Nitrite ions interact readily with N-methylacetamide and N-acetylglycine in aqueous buffer solution of pH < 4 to give the transient nitrosamides, N-nitroso-N-methylacetamide and N-nitroso-N-acetylglycine. These nitrosamides could not be isolated under these conditions because they decompose rapidly, as demonstrated by ultra-violet spectroscopic traces. The gas chromatographic identification of the products indicates that diazo esters and diazoalkanes are the intermediates in these decompositions. The kinetic analysis of the nitrosation in buffered solution shows that the rate constants are proportional to the hydrogen ion concentration in the pH < 4 range. Evidence in support of the participation of a carboxylate group in the nitrosation of N-acetylglycine is discussed. Possible implications of the presence of nitrite in carcinogenesis in digestive tracts are discussed on the basis of facile formation and decomposition of nitrosamides and the intermediacy of diazo compounds.

INTRODUCTION

In contrast to the enormous activity and concern aroused by N-nitrosamines, very little interest has been shown, until recent years, in the possible carcinogenic behaviour of nitrosamides. While N-nitroso derivatives of ureas, urethane and guanidines have been shown to be tumorigens (Druckrey *et al.*, 1967; Mirvish, 1971), it is only recently that N-nitroso-N-methylacetamide and N-nitroso-N-methylbenzamide have been shown to be proximate carcinogens, as opposed to the indirect, organotropic, nitrosamine carcinogens that require metabolic activation (Bulay *et al.*, 1979). Biological activation of nitrosamines has been attributed to the α-hydroxylation reaction converting nitrosamines to α-hydroxynitrosamines, which are proximate carcinogens (Joshi *et al.*, 1977). It is therefore not surprising that the chemically related nitrosamides are also proximate carcinogens.

A question we have asked for a long time concerns the possible participation of the peptide linkage of proteins in nitrosation reactions, to give nitrosamides (N-nitroso-peptides) with

---

[1] To whom requests for reprints should be addressed

nitrite from dietary sources and/or generated by microbial reduction *in vivo*. How do these nitrosopeptides behave under biological conditions? Is their chemical behaviour linked to carcinogenicity? It may be noted that simple nitrosamides are known to be unstable towards heat ($< 100°C$) (Bieren & Dinan, 1970) and light (Chow, 1979; Chow & Polo, 1981).

MATERIALS AND METHODS

Glycine was acetylated with acetic anhydride, and *N*-acetylglycine was recrystallized from ethanol: m.p., 205–208: ^{1}H-nuclear magnetic resonance spectra (NMR) in deuterated dimethyl sulfoxide, 1.88(s,3H) and 3.77(2,sH) ppm; ^{13}C-NMR (D_2O) 177.5(s), 176.3(s), 43.9(t), 24.3(q) ppm. *N*-methylacetamide (MA) and inorganic chemicals were of chemically-pure grade and were used as supplied from commercial sources. The ultra-violet (UV) visible spectra were recorded with a Cary 210 spectrophotometer. Gas chromatography (GC) was performed with a Hewlett-Packard 5792A, equipped with an OV-1 capillary column (12.5m × 0.20 mm i.d.). Kinetic measurements were carried out in 50-mL flasks, immersed in a controlled-temperature bath, and the nitrite absorptions at 300–450 mm were monitored. After nitrosation, the products were isolated by a combination of distillation and extraction and analysed by gas chromatography, using authentic samples for comparison.

RESULTS

Aqueous solutions of sodium nitrite at pH 5–9 showed a diffused peak at λ_{max} 355 nm with $\varepsilon = 23$. In view of the $pK_a = 3.37$ for nitrous acid, nitrite ions must exist mainly as NO_2^- above pH 4, showing the broad peak, and as HNO_2 below pH 3, showing the structured absorption spectrum (see Fig. 1). *N*-Acetyl-*N*-nitrosophenylalanine and other nitrosamides [λ_{max}, 420 nm (ε, $\simeq 45$), 405($\simeq 40$) and 390] derived from several α-amino acids were prepared by the N_2O_4 nitrosation procedure (Polo, 1980). Attempts to prepare and isolate *N*-nitroso-*N*-acetylglycine (NAG) by nitrosation of *N*-acetylglycine (AG) were not successful because of the solubility in water and the instability of the nitrosamides. *N*-nitroso-*N*-methylacetamide (NMA) was more stable and can be prepared by a similar method from MA. It exhibited typical absorptions, with $\lambda_{max} = 423$ nm ($\varepsilon = 95$), 404(100) and 390 in water.

The reaction of nitrite (5 mmol/L) and MA (50 mmol/L) in phosphate buffer at pH 1–5 was monitored by UV spectroscopy. The spectral traces, shown in Figures 1a and 1b, indicated that accumulation of NMA in the solution was rapid at the beginning and tapered off after 3–4 h. The intensity of NMA absorptions above 400 nm at the stationary state was relatively high at pH 1 (Fig. 1a) and decreased sharply as the pH increased to 2 (Fig. 1b). Above pH 2, the NMA absorptions could barely be detected. In several experiments, nitrosated solutions gave small amounts of methyl acetate, detected by GC analysis. Obviously, NMA decomposition occurred concurrently with formation to give azo ester **1**, then methyl acetate, by a mechanism outlined in Figure 2. At pH > 2, the rate of decomposition was much faster than the formation rate, resulting in failure to observe NMA absorption in the UV spectra above 400 nm.

The nitrosation of AG under similar conditions was followed by UV spectroscopy at pH 1–5. As shown in Figure 1c, even at pH 1, only weak absorptions typical of nitrosamides, plus monotonic decreases of the HNO_2 absorptions, could be observed. GC analysis of the nitrosated products showed the presence of acetic acid and glycolic acid. Again, both spectral and product analysis demonstrated that NAG was formed and decomposed rapidly under the conditions obtaining, *via* intramolecular reactions, as shown in Figure 3 (Chow & Polo, 1981).

Fig. 1. Ultra-violet (U V) spectrometric traces of the reaction of sodium nitrite (5 mmol/L) and *N*-methylacetamide (5 mmol/L) in phosphate buffer at pH 1.05 (a) and at pH 2.00 (b). Traces Nos 1 to 7 were recorded at about 0. 60, 120, 180, 240, 300, and 360 min, respectively. (c), UV traces of the reaction of sodium nitrite (5 mmol/L) and *N*-acetylglycine (5 mmol/L) in phosphate buffer at pH 1.00. traces Nos 1 to 7 were recorded at one-hour intervals, starting from zero time.

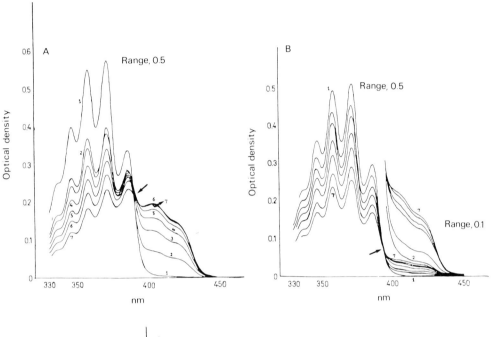

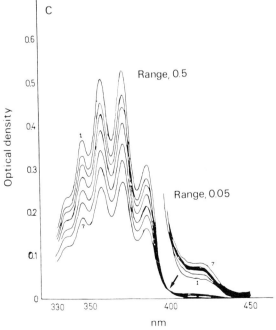

Fig. 2. Formation and decomposition of N-nitroso-N-methylacetamide (NMA); MA, N-methylacetamide

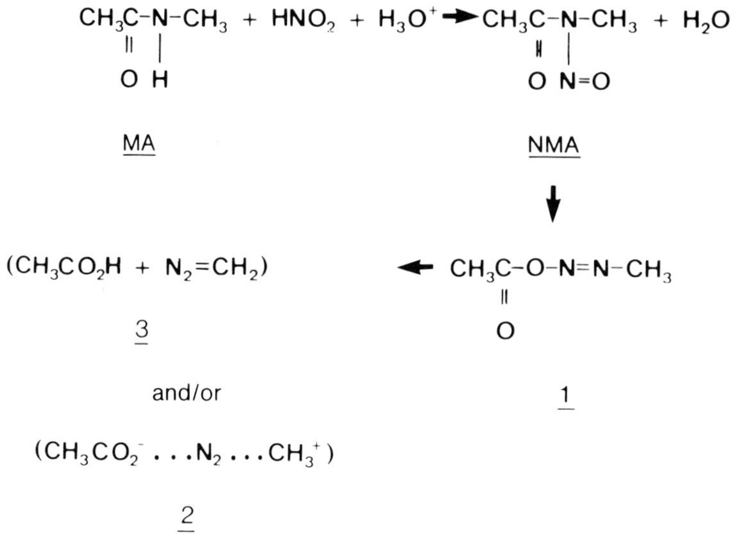

$$CH_3C-N-CH_3 + HNO_2 + H_3O^+ \rightarrow CH_3C-N-CH_3 + H_2O$$

with groups:

CH_3C (‖ O) $-N$ (| H) $-CH_3$ + HNO_2 + H_3O^+ → CH_3C (‖ O) $-N$ (| N=O) $-CH_3$ + H_2O

MA   NMA

$(CH_3CO_2H + N_2=CH_2)$ ← $CH_3C-O-N=N-CH_3$ (‖ O)

3   1

and/or

$(CH_3CO_2^- \ldots N_2 \ldots CH_3^+)$

2

Fig. 3. Formation and decomposition of N-nitroso-N-acetylglycine (NAG); AG, N-acetylglycine

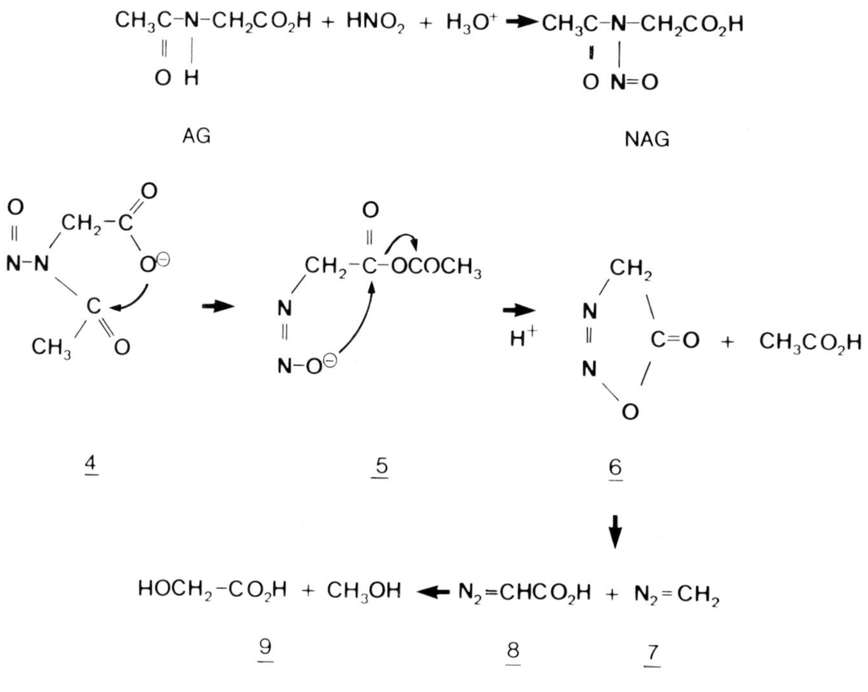

CH_3C (‖ O) $-N$ (| H) $-CH_2CO_2H$ + HNO_2 + H_3O^+ → CH_3C (‖ O) $-N$ (| N=O) $-CH_2CO_2H$

AG   NAG

4   5   6

$HOCH_2-CO_2H + CH_3OH \leftarrow N_2=CHCO_2H + N_2=CH_2$

9   8   7

In the nitrosation of alkylureas and amides, the rate was assumed to follow the expression given in equation 1. In these experiments, in order to simplify the kinetic analysis, the pH was kept constant with a buffer and a 10-fold excess of amides was used,

Rate $= k_3[\text{Amide}][\text{HNO}_2][\text{H}^+]$ equation 1
Rate $= k_2[\text{Amide}][\text{HNO}_2]$, where $k_2 = k_3[\text{H}^+]$ equation 2
Rate $= k_1[\text{HNO}_2]$, where $k_1 = k_2[\text{Amide}]$ equation 3

with respect to sodium nitrite. Under these conditions, the kinetic behaviour corresponded to the pseudo-first-order expression in equation 3. The value of k_1 in equation 3 was ascertained by plotting log $\Delta A/\Delta t$ against log$[\text{HNO}_2]$, where $\Delta A/\Delta t$ is the initial rate of HNO_2

Fig. 4. Nitrosation of *N*-methylacetamide (x) and *N*-acetylglycine (●) in phosphate buffers

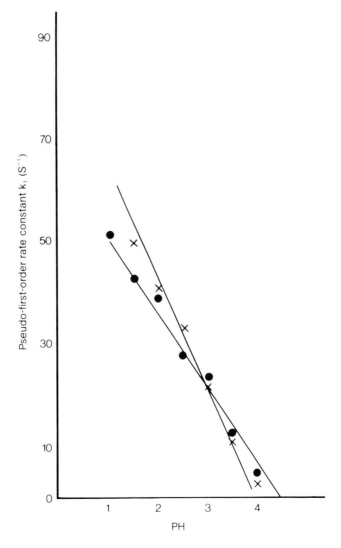

Fig. 5. Nitrosation of *N*-methylacetamide (x) and *N*-acetylglycine (●) in acetate buffers

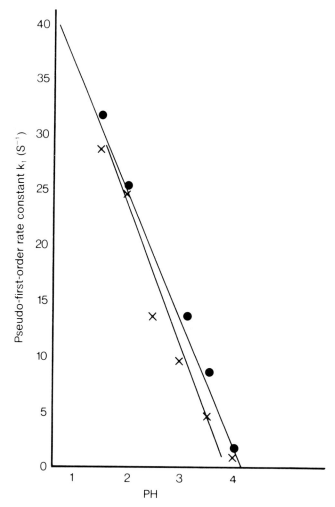

disappearance. The slope of 0.91 in this plot indicated that the order of HNO_2 in equation 3 is indeed unity, within experimental error.

The nitrosation of amides was carried out in the pH range 1 to $\simeq 4$, at $35°C$ in phosphate buffer solution. The initial concentrations were sodium nitrite, 5mmol/L, amides 50 mmol/L and buffer 50 mmol/L. The plots of the logarithm of HNO_2 concentration against time were analysed by a least-squares method to give the pseudo-first-order rate constants at various pH values, with correlation coefficients of 0.99 or better. In Figure 4, the pseudo-first-order rate constants for the nitrosation of AG and MA are plotted against pH. Similar experiments with acetate buffer are shown in Figure 5. These two plots show that the nitrosation rates were indeed proportional to the hydrogen ion concentrations in the pH range 1–4. In acetate buffers, furthermore, the rate constants are indistinguishable for the two nitrosations, and the two plots

Table 1.   Second order rate constants, k_2, of nitrosation

pH	Temperature (°C)	$k_2 \times 10^4$ (mol^{-1}Ls^{-1})	
		N-Acetylglycine	N-Methylacetamide
2.0	35	7.68	8.14
2.5	25	4.75	4.42
2.5	45	9.29	10.26
3.0[a]	30	3.91	2.40
3.0	35	4.75	4.29
3.0	45	6.30	5.77
3.5	25	2.45	1.57
3.5	35	2.57	2.19
3.5	45	3.21	2.14
4.0	25	0.57	0.34
4.0	35	0.99	0.44
4.0	45	1.06	0.89

[a] This experiment was carried out with 40 mmol/L of the reactant in 0.1 mol/L phosphate buffer, and the rate constant was calculated using the integrated second-order rate equation. The other reactions were carried out with sodium nitrite (5 mmol/L) and an amide (50 mmol/L) in 50 mmol/L phosphate buffer solution.

are nearly parallel. In phosphate buffers, however, the two plots for AG and MA cross at pH slightly < 3.

The second order rate constants, k_2, of the nitrosation of AG and MA in phosphate buffers, obtained from equation 2 at temperatures 25–45°C, are collected in Table 1. These rate constants were calculated from the pseudo-first-order plots, using the first-order rate constants and the known amide concentrations. The data indicate that at pH < 2.5, k_2 is larger for MA nitrosation than for AG nitrosation, but above pH 2.5 the situation is reversed. Above pH 4, the rates became too slow, and accurate measurements could not be obtained. The pseudo-first-order rate constants obtained in the presence and absence of thiocyanate ions were nearly identical, within experimental error.

DISCUSSION

The results described above allow us to draw the following conclusions. Firstly, both MA and AG can be nitrosated at the amide site with aqueous nitrous acid in solution of pH < 4 to give the corresponding NMG and NAG. Secondly, the presence of the isobestic points (see arrows in Fig. 1) indicate that the nitrosamides NAG and NMA are the only products obtained in both nitrosation reactions. Finally, both nitrosamides decompose faster than they are formed at pH < 4, according to the mechanism depicted in Figures 2 and 3. Nitrosation of AG rapidly yields glycolic acid, **9**, and acetic acid as the final products, owing to the facile intramolecular attacks of the carboxylate groups in NAG. In this scheme, oxadiazo intermediate **6** and/or diazo derivatives **7** and **8** are likely intermediates. Although NAG has not been isolated, its pKa is expected to be lower than that of AG itself, due to the electron-withdrawing nitrosoamido group, and can be assumed to be about 2. In the region of pH > 1, the rearrangement is facilitated by the presence of the carboxylate form, **4**, and much faster than that of NMA, as shown by the time-dependent UV profiles (Fig. 1).

Fig. 6. Mechanism of catalytic participation of a carboxylate group in nitrosation

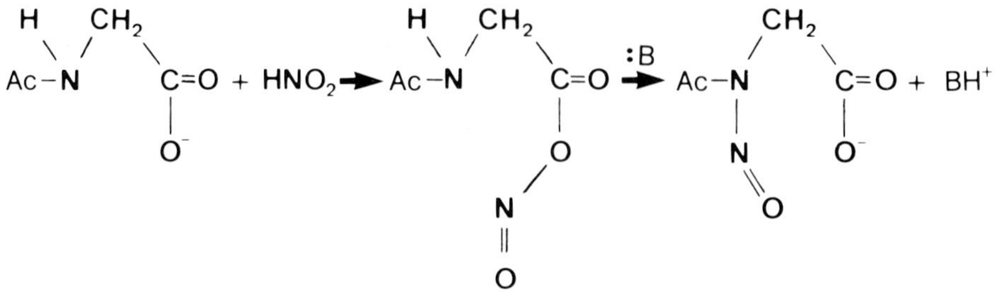

Close examination of Figures 4 and 5 indicates that the carboxylate group in AG may participate catalytically in nitrosation. The crossing of the rate constant-pH plots for MA and AG in phosphate buffers occurs at about pH 3 (Fig. 4), which coincides approximately with the onset of a significant concentration of N-acetylglycinate anions, since the pK_a of AG is known to be 3.6–3.7. As the HNO_2 (pK_a, 3.36) concentrations fall rapidly at pH above 4, more dramatic differences between the nitrosation of AG and MA could not be observed. A similar tendency can be observed from the bimolecular rate constants measured over 25–45°C in phosphate buffers (Table 1). It is more instructive to compare these results with the rate constant-pH profiles for both nitrosations in acetate buffers. In the latter nitrosations, the effects of the carboxylate group of AG are probably overshadowed by the common presence of a high concentration of acetate ions in the bulk solution. While the evidence obtained is not dramatic, a catalytic participation of the carboxylate group is established and may be interpreted by means of a mechanism shown in Figure 6.

Diazomethane derivatives and carbonium ions are known to be electrophilic alkylating agents (Bieren & Dinan, 1970) and have been proposed to be intermediate species in the decomposition of N-nitroso derivatives, directly from nitrosoureas and indirectly from nitrosamines after metabolic activation (Joshi *et al.*, 1977). They are also proposed as the precursors responsible for carcinogenesis at the molecular level. Thus, NAG, NMA and the allied nitrosamides, as well as any nitrosated peptide, must be regarded as potential proximate carcinogens. It follows that, under conditions in which the flux of peptide linkage and acidity are high, nitrite ions may act alone to generate a wide range of endogeneous nitrosamide carcinogens. Among the human organs that are most vulnerable to such conditions is, naturally, the digestive tract, which explains why stomach cancer can be induced readily in animals by nitrosoureas or nitrosourethanes. Furthermore, since microbial reduction of nitrate is significant in human saliva (Hill, 1979), it is also conceivable that the present nitrosation-decomposition pathway plays a role in the etiology of oesophageal and forestomach cancer (Li *et al.*, 1980).

ACKNOWLEDGEMENT

Y.L. Chow wishes to express his thanks to the Natural Sciences and Engineering Research Council of Canada for financial support.

REFERENCES

Bieren, J.F. & Dinan, F.J. (1970) *Rearrangement and elimination of the amido group.* In: Zabichi, J., ed., *The Chemistry of Amides,* New York, Interscience, pp. 245–288

Bulay, O., Mirvish, S.S., Garcia, H., Pelfrene, A.F., Gold, B. & Eagan, M. (1979) Carcinogenicity tests of six nitrosamides and nitrosocyanamide administered orally to rats. *J. natl Cancer Inst., 62,* 1523–1528

Chow, Y.L. (1979) *Chemistry of* N-*nitrosamides and related* N-*nitrosamino acids.* In: Anselme, J.P., ed., *Nitrosamines, (Am. chem. Soc. Symp. Ser.* No.101), Washington, DC, The American Chemical Society, pp. 13–37

Chow, Y.L. & Polo, J. (1981) Rearrangement of carboxylates derived from *N*-acetyl-*N*-nitroso-α-amino acids. *J. chem. Soc. chem. Commun.,* 297–299

Druckrey, H., Preussmann, R., Ivankovic, S. & Schmähl, D. (1967) Organotrophe Carcinogen Wirkungen bei 65 verschiedenen N-nitroso-Verbindungen an BD-Ratten. *Z. Krebsforsch., 69,* 103–201

Hill, M.J. (1979) *In-vivo bacterial* N-*nitrosation and its possible role in human cancer.* In: Miller, E.C., ed., *Naturally Occurring Carcinogens-Mutagens and Modulators of Carcinogenesis,* Tokyo, Japan Scientific Society Press, pp. 229–240

Joshi, S.R., Rice, J.M., Wenk, M.L., Roller, P.P. & Keefer, L.K. (1977) Selective induction of intestinal tumours in rats by methyl(acetoxymethyl)nitrosamine, an ester of the presumed reactive metabolite of dimethylnitrosamine. *J. natl Cancer Inst., 58,* 1531–1535

Li, M.X., Li, P. & Li, B.R. (1980) Recent progress in research on esophageal cancer in China. *Adv. Cancer Res., 33,* 173–249

Mirvish, S.S (1971) Kinetics of nitrosamide formation from alkylurea, N-alkylurethanes and alkylguanidines : possible implications for the etiology of gastric cancer. *J. natl Cancer Inst., 46,* 1183–1193

Polo, J. (1980) *Chemistry of N-Nitrosamines derived from a-Amino Acids,* Ph D thesis, Simon Fraser University, Burnaby, BC, Canada

Tannenbaum, S.R., Archer, M.C., Wishonok, J.S., Correa, P., Cuello, C. & Haenszel, W. (1977) *Nitrate and the etiology of gastric cancer.* In: Hatt, H.H., Watson, J.D. & Winster, J.A., eds, *Origins of Human Cancer, (Cold Spring Harbor Conferences on Cell Proliferation,* Vol. 4), Book C, *Human Risk Assessment,* Cold Spring Harbor, NY, Cold Spring Harbor Laboratory, pp. 1609–1625

NITROSATING PROPERTIES OF BIS-METHYLTHIO-DIIRON-TETRANITROSYL (ROUSSIN'S RED METHYL ESTER), A NITROSO COMPOUND ISOLATED FROM PICKLED VEGETABLES CONSUMED IN NORTHERN CHINA

A. CROISY

INSERM, U219- Institut Curie, Section de Biologie, 91405 Orsay, France

H. OHSHIMA & H. BARTSCH

International Agency for Research on Cancer, 150 cours Albert-Thomas, Lyon, France

SUMMARY

Bis-methylthio-diiron-tetranitrosyl (Roussin's red methyl ester, RRME), recently identified in pickled vegetables consumed in a high incidence area of oesophageal cancer in Northern China, was examined for its activity as a nitrosating agent *in vivo* and *in vitro*. Freshly synthesized RRME nitrosated secondary amines (morpholine and pyrrolidine) slowly in the presence of air; it failed to nitrosate these amines under strictly anaerobic conditions. In experiments in rats, a fresh sample of RRME was found to be a weak nitrosating agent, whereas partially decomposed RRME showed a strong nitrosating activity comparable to that of nitrite. Possible mechanisms for nitrosation by RRME are discussed.

INTRODUCTION

Oesophageal cancer is a common neoplasia in several areas of the People's Republic of China, and in Linxian County in Northern China there is a very high incidence. Environmental and dietary factors have been suspected to play a role; the etiology of the disease has been reviewed (Miller 1975, 1977; Li *et al.*, 1980; Yang, 1980, 1982; Lu & Lin, 1982). Epidemiological studies in Linxian County showed a positive correlation between consumption of pickled vegetables and incidence rates for oesophageal cancer (Li *et al.*, 1980; Yang, 1980; Lu & Lin, 1982). Pickled vegetables extracts were reported to be carcinogenic in rats (Department of Chemical Etiology, 1977), and showed mutagenic, transforming and promoting activity in cultured cells (Cheng *et al.*, 1980) as well as mutagenic effects in *Salmonella typhimurium* (Lu *et al.*, 1981).

Examination of contaminants occurring in these foods by sophisticated analytical techniques made possible the detection of a nitroso compound, Roussin's red methyl ester (RRME) or bis-methylthio-diiron-tetranitrosyl (Wang *et al.*, 1980) (Fig. 1). Its occurrence at mg/kg levels

CROISY *ET AL*

Fig. 1. Chemical structure of Roussin's red methyl ester

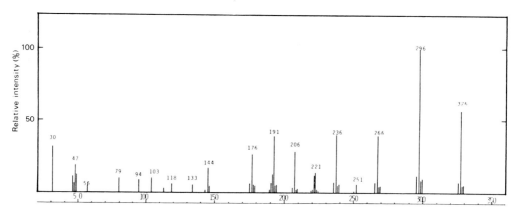

in samples of pickled vegetables collected in Linxian was reported recently (Zhang *et al.*, 1983). In view of reports mentioning the presence of nitrite, nitrate and traces of *N*-nitrosodimethylamine and *N*-nitrosodiethylamine in some pickled vegetables (Lu & Lin, 1982), the occurrence of this inorganic tetra-nitrosyl compound in the diet of inhabitants in a high-incidence area for oesophageal cancer merits attention. In this study we therefore investigated whether RRME can act as a nitrosating agent *in vivo* and *in vitro*.

EXPERIMENTAL

Chemicals

Roussin's red methyl ester (m.p., 93 °C) was synthesized as reported earlier (Wang *et al.*, 1980; Lu *et al.*, 1981), and purified by repeated crystallizations from ethanol. Purification and storage was done under an inert atmosphere, since this compound is air-sensitive, even in the solid state (Seyferth & Gallagher, 1981).

The mass spectrum of RRME (Fig. 2) confirmed the authenticity of the compound. In a previously published mass spectrum of synthetic RRME (Lu *et al.*, 1981), the peak at m/z 176

Fig. 2. Mass spectrum of Roussin's red methyl ester

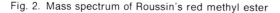

was erroneously labelled 186; and Wang *et al.* (1980) cited a mass spectrum of RRME from the published literature in which the ion m/z 176 was completely missing. Our spectrum was virtually identical to those for synthetic RRME published earlier by Wang *et al.* (1980).

Partially decomposed RRME was obtained from RRME stored for about one year at $-20\,^\circ$C in the presence of air. Nitrite contamination of freshly synthesized and partially decomposed RRME was determined as follows: about 500 mg of the material were well dispersed in 10 mL distilled water, then separated from the water by filtration through a No. 111 Durieux filter paper. Nitrite dissolved in the filtrate was determined colorimetrically with Griess reagents. Fresh and partially decomposed RRME contained 0.002% and 1.4% Griess reagent-positive substance(s) (calculated as sodium nitrite), respectively.

All other chemicals were of analytical grade, and all solutions were prepared freshly prior to experiments.

Apparatus

Infra-red spectra were recorded on a Nicolet 5MX FT/IR spectrometer. The mass spectrum of RRME was determined on an AEI MS50 spectrometer at 70 eV using the direct probe insertion technique (probe temperature, 150 °C).

N-Nitrosamines for in-vitro studies were analysed using an Aerograph 1800 gas chromatograph equipped with a flame-ionization detector. Analysis of *N*-nitrosoproline (NPRO) in in-vivo studies was performed using a Tracor 550 gas chromatograph, interfaced to a Thermal Energy Analyzer. In both cases, a 10% Carbowax 20M column was used at 170 °C.

In-vitro nitrosation

RRME was reacted with morpholine and pyrrolidine in anhydrous medium by keeping dichloromethane containing 0.245 mmol/L RRME and 0.96 mmol/L amine at reflux temperature or at room temperature either under argon or air. Reactions in aqueous medium were carried out at 37 °C, using 1.5 mL solutions of RRME (0.01 mol/L) in acetone, 20 µL amine and 1 mL of the appropriate buffer solutions (0.1 mol/L). The final pH was verified after mixing.

In-vivo nitrosation

Procedures similar to those used in previous studies on endogenous transnitrosation from *N*-nitrosodiphenylamine to proline in rats (Ohshima *et al.*, 1982a) were used to investigate in-vivo nitrosation by RRME. Six fasted rats were given 0.5 mL of an aqueous 0.1 mol/L proline solution by gavage, immediately followed by 0.5 mL of 0.02 mol/L RRME in acetone. Groups of three rats received either proline or RRME alone, or 1 mL of acetone:water (1:1, v/v). In order to compare the nitrosating activity of RRME with that of nitrite, the gavage sequence was: first, 0.25 mL of 0.2 mol/L proline solution, then 0.5 mL acetone, followed by 0.25 mL of 0.04 mol/L nitrite solution. When several compounds were tested for their catalytic of inhibitory effects, they were dissolved either in the proline solution (water-soluble substances) or in the RRME solution (water-insoluble substances).

The rats were placed in metabolic cages, and the urine was collected for 24 h in tubes containing 5 mL of 1 mol/L sodium hydroxide. Analysis of NPRO was carried out according to a published procedure (Ohshima *et al.*, 1982b) after conversion of NPRO to its methyl ester with diazomethane.

RESULTS

In-vitro nitrosation

Under strictly anaerobic conditions, freshly prepared RRME failed to nitrosate secondary amines (morpholine or pyrrolidine) in dichloromethane solution, even at reflux temperature. However, in the presence of air, a slow reaction was observed, and the final yield of *N*-nitrosomorpholine (NMOR) was 100% after three days at room temperature.

In buffered aqueous acetone solution, and in the presence of air, nitrosation of morpholine proceeded slowly and afforded a maximum yield of 20% NMOR after seven hours at pH 1, whereas at high pH (pH 13) the final yield was only 12.5% (Fig. 3). At intermediary pH, NMOR formation was very slow, and the yield never exceeded 3-5%, even after two days (Fig. 3).

Pyrrolidine, which is a much more basic amine than morpholine, was not nitrosated easily by RRME under acidic conditions (Fig. 4). Formation of *N*-nitrosopyrrolidine increased linearly with increasing pH, and the final yield at pH 13 was about 5% after two hours at 37 °C.

Fig. 3. Formation of *N*-nitrosomorpholine as a function of reaction time at different pH in a buffered aqueous acetone solution: ▲, pH 1; ○, pH 4; △, pH 7; □, pH 9; ●, pH 11.2; ■, pH 13

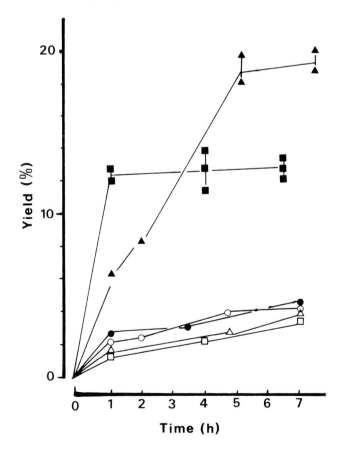

Fig. 4. Nitrosation by Roussin's red methyl ester in buffered aqueous acetone after 2 h reaction as a function of pH at 37°C (each point corresponds to the mean of four determinations): ●, pyrrolidine; ○, morpholine

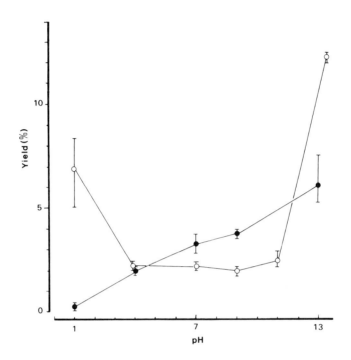

In-vivo nitrosation

The results obtained are summarized in Table 1. A dose of either RRME or proline alone did not significantly increase the urinary levels of NPRO above the background level. Co-administration of proline with RRME, however, resulted in excretion of 2.46 nmol NPRO, about 15 times more than in the controls (expt No. 6 *versus* 1, 2 and 3). The RRME (fresh) used in the experiments contained trace amount of Griess-reagent-positive substance (0.95 nmol/10 μmol RRME). However, the amount of NPRO excreted (2.46 nmol) was about 2.6 times more than the nitrite content, so that the increased amounts of NPRO cannot be accounted for by nitrite contamination alone but may result from nitrosation by RRME *in vivo*.

Thiocyanate has been reported to enhance endogenous nitrosation of proline in rats by nitrite or *N*-nitrosodiphenylamine (Ohshima *et al.*, 1982a,b). However, no catalytic effect of thiocyanate on nitrosation by RRME was observed (expt No. 7 *versus* 6).

The nitrosating capacity of RRME was compared with that of nitrite. When sodium nitrite and proline were given to rats under the same conditions as in the experiments with RRME, 531 nmol NPRO were found in the urine (expt No. 9). Thus, the yield of NPRO after nitrosation by RRME *in vivo* was about 216 times less than that after reaction with nitrite (expt No. 9 *versus* 6).

When a partially decomposed (old) sample of RRME was administered to rats together with proline, the levels of NPRO found in the urine were as high as 901 nmol, which was about 366

Table 1.   Endogenous nitrosation by Roussin's red methyl ester (RRME) of proline in rats

Expt no.	Dose of reagent (µmol/rat)				No. of rats	nmol NPRO formed per (mean ± SD)
	RRME	Nitrite	Proline	KSCN		
1	0	0	0	0	3	0.01 ± 0.06
2	10 [a]	0	0	0	3	0.05 ± 0.03
3	0	0	50	0	3	0.11 ± 0.05
4	10 [a]	0	0	50	3	0.27 ± 0.13
5	0	0	50	50	3	0.07 ± 0.02
6	10 [a]	0	50	0	6	2.46 ± 1.08 [c]
7	10 [a]	0	50	50	6	2.52 ± 0.96
8	0	10	0	0	3	0.58 ± 0.08
9	0	10	50	0	6	531 ± 593
10	10 [b]	0	0	0	3	5.63 ± 2.76
11	10 [b]	0	50	0	6	901 ± 584

[a] Freshly synthesized RRME
[b] Partially decomposed RRME
[c] Comparison of results of expt no. 6 *versus* 1, 2 and 3 (p < 0.003)

and 1.7 times more than that found after administration of fresh RRME and nitrite, respectively (expt No. 11 *versus* 6 and 9). This sample of RRME contained 0.66 µmol Griess-reagent-positive substance(s) per 10 µmol RRME (calculated as sodium nitrite). Endogenous formation of NPRO by the old RRME was strongly inhibited by co-administration of sodium ascorbate, ammonium sulfamate, cysteine and α-tocopherol. The reaction was enhanced by potassium thiocyanate and potassium iodide.

DISCUSSION

Freshly prepared RRME nitrosated secondary amines slowly in the presence of air, but not under strictly anaerobic conditions. In addition, RRME appeared to nitrosate morpholine efficiently only under extreme pH conditions at which it seems relatively unstable. Its decomposition thus appears to be a limiting factor for nitrosation, although the pK of the amino substrate also seems to play a role, as illustrated by the inefficiency of RRME in nitrosating pyrrolidine at acidic pH (Fig. 4). The latter would indicate a nucleophilic reaction of the amine either at the coordinated nitrosyl or at the nitrogen of a higher nitrogen oxide, formed during the oxidative decomposition of the complex. Such a substitution would be strongly affected by protonation of the NH group of a strong base, as observed with pyrrolidine.

In the in-vivo experiments in rats, a fresh sample of RRME was found to be a weak nitrosating agent, whereas partially decomposed (old) RRME had strong nitrosating activity comparable to that of nitrite. Nitrosation of proline with this 'old' sample was enhanced by thiocyanate or iodide, and was inhibited by ascorbic acid, α-tocopherol, L-cysteine and ammonium sulfamate. These compounds are well-known catalysts and inhibitors of nitrosation by nitrite. However, nitrosation of proline by fresh RRME in rats was not affected by thiocyanate, which is a known catalyst for nitrosation by nitrite or for transnitrosation by *N*-nitrosodiphenylamine (Ohshima *et al.*, 1982a,b).

A coordinated nitrosyl can be assumed to have an electrophilic character on the basis of the linear structure of the metal-N = O bond (Bottomley, 1978) and of the NO stretching frequency

Fig. 5. Fourier transform-infrared spectrum of Roussin's red methyl ester and its derivatives (nujol) with electronic subtraction of nujol bands. *A*, Roussin's red methyl ester (RRME); *B*, partially decomposed RRME ('old' sample)

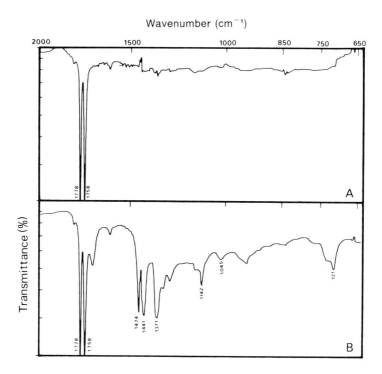

in infra-red spectra ($\nu NO > 1850$ cm^{-1}) (Eisenberg & Meyer, 1975; Bottomley, 1978). The Fe-N=O bond in RRME appears, on the basis of crystallographic studies, to be relatively linear (Thomas *et al.*, 1958); however, the stretching frequencies of the nitrosyls are less than 1850 cm^{-1} (Fig. 5a), and nucleophilic attack at the coordinated NO group would be surprising.

Although nitrosation by RRME at high pH values is consistent with the reaction of nitroprusside ion with amines (Maltz *et al.*, 1971; Keefer, 1976), the oxygen dependency of the reaction is more indicative that RRME acts only as a NO carrier, releasing higher nitrogen oxides(s) (NO$_2$ and/or N$_2$O$_3$) into the medium under the action of atmospheric oxygen.

Although freshly prepared RRME nitrosated proline very slowly *in vivo* (Table 1), partially decomposed RRME was much more efficient as a nitrosating agent under the same conditions. Therefore, in addition to the nitrosation process described above, a different reaction may be involved in the case of old RRME. The infra-red spectrum of the sample showed the appearance of absorption bands in the region 1350-1540 cm^{-1}, which might be explained by coordination of nitrogen oxide(s) of higher oxidation state than NO (Fig. 5b); however, the absence of absorption bands between 800 and 850 cm^{-1} completely excludes the possibility of a coordinated nitrite (Nakamoto, 1978). However, coordinated nitrates have also been reported as efficient nitrosating species (Croisy *et al.*, 1980), and RRME may easily be decomposed to such compounds. Therefore further attempts should be made to characterize the RRME derivatives which act as potential nitrosating species and which may be present or formed in pickled vegetables consumed in the high incidence area of oesophageal cancer in Northern China.

ACKNOWLEDGEMENTS

We wish to thank J.-C. Béréziat, M.C. Bourgade and J. Michelon for technical assistance and M.B. D'Arcy for secretarial work. The Thermal Energy Analyzer was provided on loan by the National Cancer Institute of the United States under contract No. 1 CP-55715.

We are grateful to Dr S.R. Tannenbaum, Cambridge MA, USA, for drawing our attention to an error in a previously published mass spectrum of Roussin's red methyl ester.

REFERENCES

Bottomley, F. (1978) Electrophilic behavior of coordinated nitric oxide, *Acc. Chem. Res., 11*, 158–163

Cheng, S.J., Sala, M. Li, M.H. Wang, M.Y. Pot-Deprun, J. & Chouroulinkov, I. (1980) Mutagenic, transforming and promoting effect of pickled vegetables from Linxian County, China. *Carcinogenesis, 1*, 685–692

Croisy, A., Fanning, J.C., Keefer, L.K. & Slavin, B.W. (1980) *Metal complexes as promoters of N-nitrosation reactions: A progress report.* In: Walker, E.A., Griciute, L., Castegnaro, M. & Börzsönyi, M., eds, N-*Nitroso Compounds: Analysis, Formation and Occurrence (IARC Scientific Publications No. 31)*, Lyon, International Agency for Research on Cancer, pp. 83–93

Department of Chemical Etiology of the Cancer Institute of the Chinese Academy of Medical Sciences and Linxian Research Team for Prevention and Treatment of Oesophageal Cancer (1977) Preliminary investigation on the carcinogenicity of extracts of pickles in Linxian. *Res. Cancer Prev. Treat., 2*, 46–49

Eisenberg, R. & Meyer, C.D. (1975) The coordination chemistry of nitric oxide. *Acc. chem. Res., 8*, 26–34

Keefer, L.K. (1976) *Promotion of N-nitrosation reactions by metal complexes.* In: Walker, E.A., Bogovski, P. & Griciute, L., eds, *Environmental N-Nitroso Compounds: Analysis and Formation (IARC Scientific Publications No. 14)*, Lyon, International Agency for Research on Cancer, pp. 153–159

Li, M.X., Li, P. & Li, B. (1980) Recent progress in research on esophageal cancer in China. *Adv. Cancer Res., 33*, 173–249

Lu, S.H. & Lin, P. (1982) Recent research on the etiology of oesophageal cancer in China. *Z. Gastroenterol., 20*, 361–367

Lu, S.H., Camus, A.M., Tomatis, L. & Bartsch, H. (1981) Mutagenicity of extracts of pickled vegetables collected in Linshien county, a high-incidence area for oesophageal cancer in Northern China. *J. natl Cancer Inst., 66*, 33–36

Maltz, H., Grant, M.A. & Navardi, M.C. (1971) Reaction of nitroprusside with amines. *J. org. Chem., 36*, 363–364

Miller, R.W. (1975) High esophageal cancer rates in human and chickens in North China. *J. natl Cancer Inst., 54*, 535

Miller, R.W. (1977) Partial report on cancer in the people's republic of China. *Child. Cancer Etiol. Newsl., 44*, 1–4

Nakamoto, K. (1978) *Infrared and Raman Spectra of Inorganic and Coordination Compounds,* 3rd ed., New York, Wiley-Interscience, pp. 220-226

Ohshima H., Béréziat J.-C. & Bartsch H. (1982a) *Measurement of endogenous N-nitrosation in rats and humans by monitoring urinary and faecal excretion of N-nitrosamino acids.* In: Bartsch, H., O'Neill, I.K., Castegnaro, M. & Okada, M., eds, N-*Nitroso Compounds: Occurrence and Biological Effects (IARC Scientific Publications No. 41)*, Lyon, International Agency for Research on Cancer, pp. 397–411

Ohshima H., Béréziat, J.-C. & Bartsch, H. (1982b) Monitoring *N*-nitrosamino acids excreted in the urine and feces of rats as an index for endogenous nitrosation. *Carcinogenesis, 3*, 115–120

Seyferth, D. & Gallagher, M.K. (1981) Roussin's red salt, $(\mu\text{-}S)_2Fe_2 (NO)4^{2-}$; some chemistry and an interesting comparison with $(\mu\text{-}S)_2Fe_2(CO)_6{}^{2-}$. *J. organomet. Chem., 218*, C5–C10

Thomas, J.T., Robertson, J.H. & Cox, E.G. (1958) The crystal structure of Roussin's red ethyl ester. *Acta Cryst., 11*, 599–604

Topping, G. (1965) Infrared assignments and force constants in metal-nitrato complexes. *Spectrochim. Acta, 21*, 1743–1751

Wang, G.H., Zhang, W.X. & Chai, W.G. (1980) The identification of Roussin's red methyl ester. A product isolated from pickled vegetables. *Adv. Mass Spectr., 8B*, 1369–1374

Yang, C.S. (1980) Research on oesophageal cancer in China: a review. *Cancer Res., 40*, 2633–2644

Yang, C.S. (1982) *Nitrosamines and other etiological factors in the oesophageal cancer in Northern China.* In: Magee, P.N., ed., *Nitrosamines and Human Cancer (Banbury Report* No. 12), Cold Spring Harbor, NY, Cold Spring Harbor Laboratory, pp. 487–501

Zhang, W.X., Xu, M.S., Wang, G.H. & Wang, M.Y. (1983) Quantitative analysis of Roussin's red methyl ester in pickled vegetables. *Cancer Res., 43*, 339–341

RAPID FORMATION OF *N*-NITROSODIMETHYLAMINE FROM GRAMINE, A NATURALLY OCCURRING PRECURSOR IN BARLEY MALT

M.M. MANGINO

Department of Pathology, Northwestern University Medical School,
303 E. Chicago Ave., Chicago, IL 60611, USA

R.A. SCANLAN

Department of Food Science and Technology, Oregon State University,
Corvallis, OR 97331, USA

SUMMARY

The two tertiary amine alkaloids, hordenine and gramine, which are biosynthesized in malt during germination, were subjected to nitrosation under conditions typical for the study of tertiary amine nitrosation. At 65°C in dilute aqueous acid (pH 4.4 or pH 6.4), nitrosation of both amines resulted in formation of *N*-nitrosodimethylamine (NDMA). At 24°C in dilute acid (pH 3.4), the initial rate of NDMA formation from gramine was nearly equal to the initial rate of NDMA formation from dimethylamine. At the same temperature, the ratio of initial rates of formation of NDMA from gramine and trimethylamine was 6250:1. At 23°C, the ratio of initial rates of formation of NDMA from gramine and hordenine was 5200:1. The rapid reaction of gramine with nitrous acid and the nature of the gramine nitrosation reaction products both indicated that gramine did not undergo nitrosation by the expected mechanism of nitrosative dealkylation. A new mechanism if proposed to explain the labile nature of the dimethylamino group of gramine and to account for the fact that NDMA is the only *N*-nitrosamine formed during the nitrosation of gramine.

INTRODUCTION

It is now well documented that the carcinogen, *N*-nitrosodimethylamine (NDMA), may be present at low levels in beer (Spiegelhalder *et al.*, 1979; Scanlan *et al.*, 1980). Extensive analytical studies have shown that the source of NDMA in beer is barley malt dried by direct-fired kilning, a process in which nitrogen oxides are formed and come into direct contact with malt during drying (Mangino *et al.*, 1981). Challis and Kyrtopoulos (1978) have shown that nitrous anhydride and nitrogen tetroxide are both extremely effective nitrosating agents when formed in neutral or alkaline solution from their component gases. Nitrous anhydride is also known to be the principal nitrosating agent present in dilute aqueous acid during the nitrosation of amines *in vitro*.

MANGINO & SCANLAN

Fig. 1. Structures of compounds studied: *1*, hordenine; *2*, gramine; *3*, aminopyrine; *4*, 5-methoxygramine; *5*, N,N-dimethyl-5-methoxytryptamine; *6*, N-nitroso-N-methyl-3-amino-methylindole; *7*, N'-nitroso-N-nitroso-N-3-aminomethylindole; *8*, indole-3-carboxaldehyde; *9*, indole-3-carbinol; *13*, 2-(N,N-dimethylaminomethyl)-pyrrole

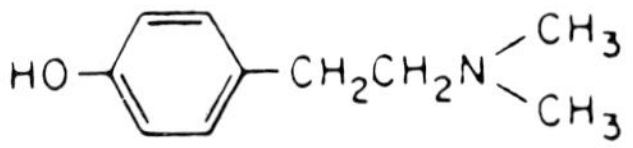

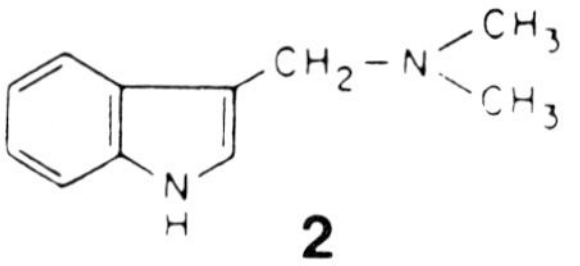

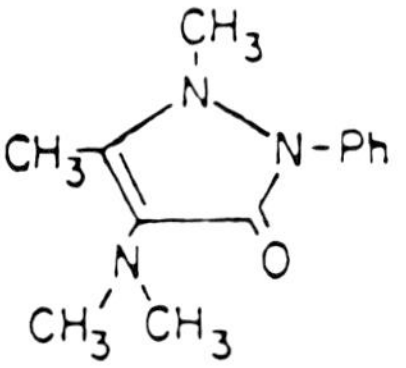

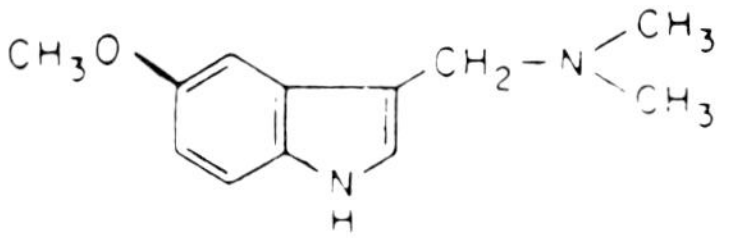

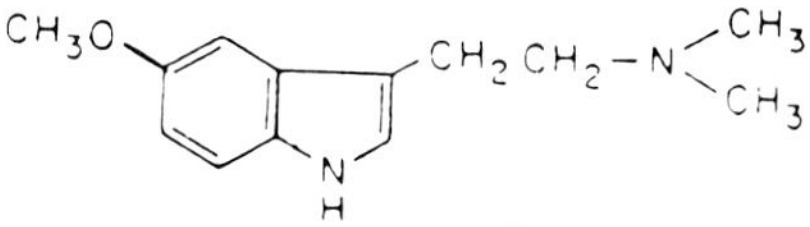

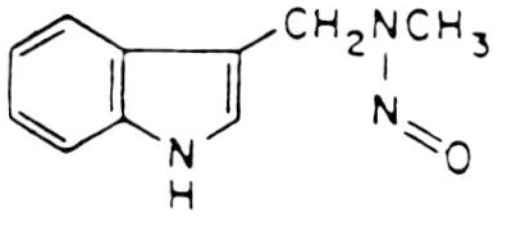

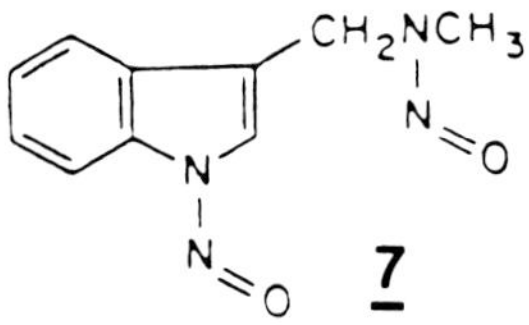

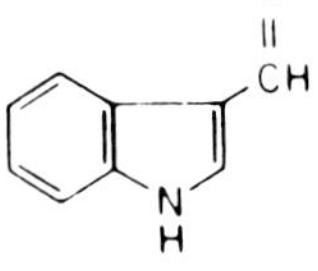

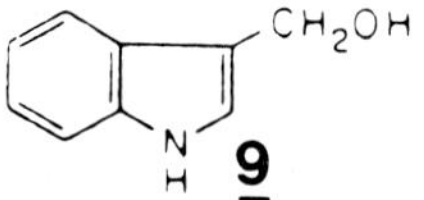

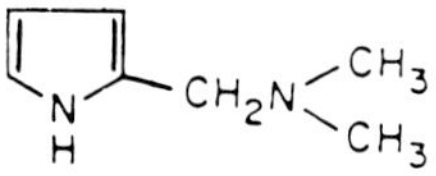

Information concerning the amine precursor of NDMA in green malt might be useful for devising a programme to inhibit NDMA formation. Any acceptable hypothesis concerning the precursor(s), however, must account for the fact that NDMA is by far the most abundant volatile *N*-nitrosamine in dried malt (Mangino *et al.*, 1981).

Amines that could be NDMA precursors in malt would include dimethylamine and the alkaloids, hordenine, *1*, and gramine, *2* (Fig. 1). Dimethylamine is reported to be present in beer (Drews *et al.*, 1957; Singer & Lijinsky, 1976), and malt is the most likely source of this volatile amine, since it was reported not to be formed during fermentation. Hordenine and gramine are tertiary amines formed by biosynthesis in malt during germination (Frank & Marion, 1956; Gower & Leete, 1963).

We have presented evidence showing that gramine is higly susceptible to nitrosation to liberate NDMA under conditions normally used to study the nitrosation of tertiary amines (Mangino *et al.*, 1981). We now present data confirming the unusual reactivity of gramine and offer a hypothesis to account for its facile nitrosation.

MATERIALS AND METHODS

The following compounds were obtained from the Aldrich Chemical Co. (Milwaukee, WI, USA): dimethylamine hydrochloride, trimethylamine hydrochloride, aminopyrine, *N*-*N*-dimethyl-5-methoxytryptamine, 5-methoxygramine and indole-3-carbinol. Gramine, hordenine hemisulfate and indole-3-carbox-aldehyde were obtained from the Sigma Chemical Co. (St Louis, MO, USA).

Nitrosation of amines and determination of NDMA yields

Nitrosation of amines for 16 h: The reactions were carried out in the following buffer solutions: (a) 60% acetic acid raised to pH 4.4 by addition of anhydrous sodium acetate; (b) (pH 6.4) 6.9 parts of dibasic sodium phosphate (0.2 mol/L) plus 3.1 parts of citric acid (0.1 mol/L). Sodium nitrite (0.35 g) was added to solutions of the amines (0.1 mol/L, 10 mL) in 25-mL KIMAX glass tubes. Each tube was sealed with a TEFLON-lined screw cap and placed in a water-bath at $65° \pm 1°$ for 16 h. The tubes were cooled to room temperature and the contents extracted with two 10-mL portions of dichloromethane (DCM). The combined DCM extracts were dried over sodium sulfate and the volume made up to 25 mL with DCM. The NDMA concentrations were determined by gas chromatography-thermal energy analysis (GC-TEA), using a Varian 3700 GC, interfaced to a Thermal Energy Analyser (Thermo Electron Corp., Waltham, MA, USA). The GC column was a 3.05 m × 3.2 mm i.d. stainless-steel column, packed with 20% Carbowax 20M plus 2% sodium hydroxide on Cromosorb W-AW (oven temp., 140° or 170°; helium flow rate, 25 mL/min). Quantification was carried out by comparing peak heights of NDMA in samples and external standards (NDMA solutions).

Since gramine was found to be highly reactive with nitrous acid, a third buffer solution was prepared from 15% acetic acid, raised to pH 3.4 with anhydrous sodium acetate and used for the nitrosation of gramine and dimethylamine at 23–25°C for 6 h.

Formation of NDMA from gramine and secondary and tertiary amines: Buffered solutions were made up as follows: 15% acetic acid solution was raised to pH 3.15 by addition of anhydrous sodium acetate and was used to make 0.1 mol/L solutions of gramine, 5-methoxygramine and *N*,*N*-dimethyl-5-methoxytryptamine, all with final pH 3.4. A second buffer was made with 15% acetic acid plus anhydrous sodium acetate (pH 3.45), and was used to make 0.1 mol/L solutions of dimethylamine hydrochloride, trimethylamine hydrochloride and hordenine hemisulfate (final pH 3.4).

Samples of amine solutions (10 mL) were nitrosated in 20-mL KIMAX glass tubes. Reactions at 23–24°C were initiated by addition of 0.69 g sodium nitrite and the tubes sealed with TEFLON-lined screw-caps. Reactions were quenched by pouring the mixtures into ice-cold solutions of 6.2 mol/L ammonium sulfamate (5 mL, pH 1.5). When foaming subsided, the mixtures were extracted with three 5-mL portions of chloroform and the extracts combined and made up to 25 mL. The NDMA concentration was determined by GC-TEA, as outlined above. For reactions at elevated temperature, each amine solution was preincubated in a water-bath to 37 ± 0.5°C or 65 ± 0.5°C, before addition of sodium nitrite. Heated tubes were cooled in ice-salt baths before opening and quenching.

NDMA recovery determinations were carried out using known solutions of NDMA dissolved in the pH 3.45 acetic acid-acetate buffer. After addition of 0.69 g sodium nitrite, the reaction tubes were capped and allowed to stand at ambient temperature for 30 min. Quenching, extraction and NDMA determination were carried out as described above. NDMA recoveries from six determinations were plotted as a function of the theoretical yields of NDMA. The resulting recovery curve was used to correct the NDMA yield from each nitrosation reaction.

Analysis of gramine nitrosation using high-performance liquid chromatography (HPLC)

Solutions of gramine (0.1 mol/L) in acetate buffer (pH 3.4) were nitrosated at 20°C by addition of 0.35 g sodium nitrite. After a specified time, acetonitrile was added to the reaction tube and the contents shaken to ensure complete solution. Aliquots were injected onto a Spectra-Physics 8700 HPLC (Spectra-Physics Corp.; San Jose, Cal.; USA) equipped with 10 μm Spherisorb C_{18} reversed-phase column (4.6 mm × 250 mm), using a gradient mobile phase (75% water: 25% methanol to 60% water: 40% methanol) at a flow rate of 2 mL/min, with detection at 254 nm. The peak corresponding to NDMA increased with time, as did peaks with retention times of 18.4 min and 19 min. These three peaks were the major reaction products after 60 min. A minor peak with retention time 16.4 min co-eluted with a standard of indole-3-carbinol. No peaks co-eluted with indole-3-carboxaldehyde, which would have been detected easily if present at a level of 0.5% in any reaction product.

RESULTS

The yields of NDMA from the nitrosation of dimethylamine, trimethylamine, hordenine and gramine were determined in dilute acid at 65° for 16 h at pH 4.4 and pH 6.4 (these conditions represent intermediate values of temperature and time and extreme values of pH encountered during kilning). Hordenine and gramine were both nitrosated to give NDMA (Table 1). Nitrosation of gramine to yield NDMA was also found to be facile at ambient temperature: for example, at 23°C in a three-fold excess of nitrite at pH 3.4, a 61% yield of NDMA was obtained in 6 h. Under the same conditions, nitrosation of dimethylamine produced a 60% yield of NDMA.

In order to confirm the conclusion that the nitrosation of gramine to liberate NDMA is an unusually facile reaction and to investigate the mechanism of the reaction, some 'comparative nitrosation' experiments were carried out. All nitrosation reactions were run at pH 3.4, with a ten-fold excess of nitrite to ensure that measureable yields of NDMA would be obtained.

Figure 2 shows the rates of NDMA formation from aminopyrine, gramine, dimethylamine and trimethylamine at 24°C. The initial reaction of aminopyrine with nitrite was so fast that accurate data could not be determined at times less than 2.5 min. Under the conditions used, no difference in the initial rates of nitrosation of gramine and dimethylamine could be observed,

Table 1. Yields (%) of N-nitrosodimethylamine after nitrosation of potential amine precursors[a]

Amine	pH 4.4[b]	pH 6.4[c]
Dimethylamine	78	65
Trimethylamine	8	0.8
Hordenine	11	2
Gramine	76	5

[a] Conditions: 0.1 mol/L amine in 0.5 mol/L $NaNO_2$ at 65°C for 16 h
[b] Acetate buffer
[c] Citrate-phosphate buffer

but the yield curves diverged after 5 min. After 2 h at 24°C, the yield of NDMA from trimethylamine was only 0.19%. The rates of NDMA formation from gramine and hordenine at 23°, 37° and 65° are compared in Figure 2B, 2C and 2D; the difference in reactivity is illustrated dramatically in Figure 2D: at 65°C, gramine was quantitatively converted to NDMA in 10 min, whereas the conversion of hordenine was only 7.2% complete after 30 min. From the initial rate data for nitrosation of gramine and hordenine at the three temperatures used, Arrhenius plots for the temperature range 23–65° indicated that the activation energies for NDMA formation were 14.2 Kcal/mol and 23.6 Kcal/mol, respectively.

The formation of NDMA from gramine, 5-methoxygramine and N,N-dimethyl-5-methoxytryptamine is shown in Figure 3. The same pattern of NDMA yield curves was observed at 23° and 37°C. These results strongly suggest that the N-substituted indole-3-methylene group is an essential element in the observed reactivity of gramine and 5-methoxygramine; elongation of the indole-3-methylene group by an additional methylene group caused complete loss of the enhanced reactivity (5-methoxygramine *versus* N,N-dimethyl-5-methoxy-tryptamine).

The fast reaction of gramine with nitrous acid to give high yields of NDMA indicated that gramine might not undergo nitrosation by the expected mechanism of nitrosative dealkylation (Smith & Loeppky, 1967). According to Figure 4, N,N-dimethyl substituted tertiary amines such as gramine should undergo extensive demethylation as a result of steric factors in the transition state for *syn* cyclic elimination of NOH from a preformed nitrosammonium ion. If demethylation were occurring during the nitrosation of gramine, the expected products would include N-nitroso-N-methyl-3-aminomethylindole, *6* (Fig. 1) and N'-nitroso-N-nitroso-N-methyl-3-aminomethylindole, *7* (Fig 1). Another product to be expected from nitrosative dealkylation of gramine is the carbonyl compound, indole-3-carboxaldehyde, *8* (Fig. 1).

Analysis of the nitrosation reaction of gramine by HPLC revealed the following:

(1) N-Nitrosamines *6* and *7* were not formed after 1 h of gramine nitrosation at 20°C in a five-fold excess of nitrite at pH 3.4. Under these conditions, compounds *6* and *7* are sufficiently stable (Mangino *et al.*, 1982) to be detectable, and either would have been observed if present at concentrations representing as little as 1% of the reaction product (based on the starting amine). The corresponding yield of NDMA under these conditions is approximately 40%.

(2) Indole-3-carboxaldehyde, *8,* was not formed from the nitrosation of gramine at ambient temperature or at 65°C in a large excess of nitrite. The aldehyde was stable under these conditions, as determined by heating authentic samples of *8* in aqueous acetic acid at 65°C (pH 3.4) in the presence of excess nitrite.

Fig. 2. Rates of formation of *N*-nitrosodimethylamine (NDMA) from gramine and secondary and tertiary amines at pH 3.4. A, NDMA formation from aminopyrine (△), dimethylamine (□), gramine (○) and trimethylamine (◇); B, NDMA formation from gramine (○) and hordenine (△) at 23°C; C, NDMA formation from gramine (○) and hordenine (△) at 37°C; D, NDMA formation from gramine (○) and hordenine (●) at 65°C

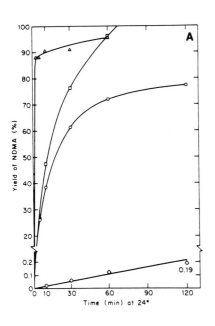

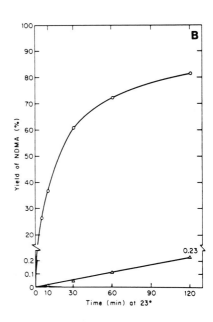

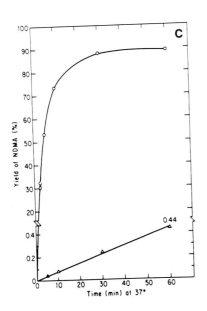

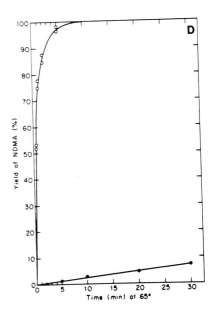

Fig. 3. A, Formation of *N*-nitrosodimethylamine (NDMA) from gramine (○), 5-methoxygramine (□) and *N*,*N*-dimethyl-5-methoxytryptamine (◇) at 23°C, pH 3.4; B, NDMA formation from gramine (○), 5-methoxygramine (□) and *N*, *N*-dimethyl-5-methoxytryptamine (◇) at 37°C, pH 3.4

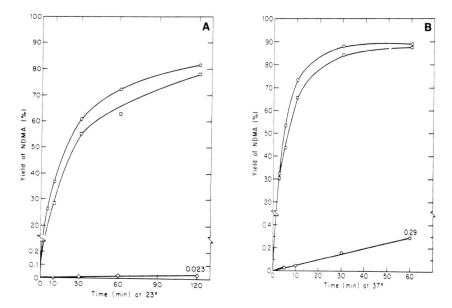

Fig. 4. Mechanism of nitrosative dealkylation

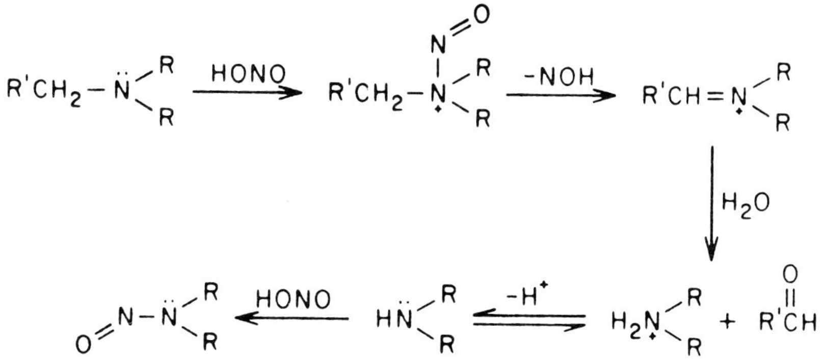

DISCUSSION

The results, which indicate that gramine does not undergo nitrosative dealkylation in nitrous acid, can be summarized as follows:

(1) The reaction with nitrous acid to yield NDMA is fast even at ambient temperature. The initial rate of nitrosation of gramine to yield NDMA appears to be nearly as fast as that of dimethylamine. The activation energy ($E_a = 14.2$ kcal/mol) for the transformation of gramine

Fig. 5. Mechanism to explain the facile nitrosation of gramine; *9*, indole-3-carbinol; *10*, attack of unprotonated nitrite ion on the imminium cation; *11*, nitrite ester; *12* nitro compound

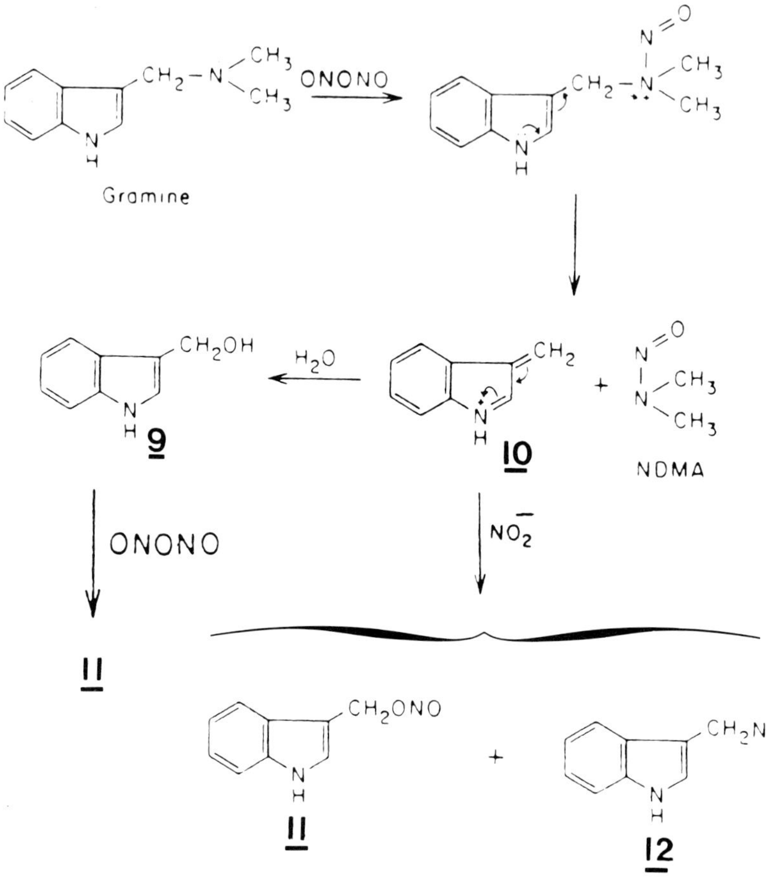

to NDMA at pH 3.4 was reasonably close to that expected for the nitrosation of a secondary amine (Fan & Tannenbaum, 1973; Mirvish *et al.*, 1973). In contrast, the activation energy observed for the nitrosative dealkylation of triethylamine at pH 3.8 was 20.3 kcal/mol (Gowenlock *et al.*, 1979).

(2) At elevated temperature, under conditions normally used to study tertiary amine nitrosation, the reaction of nitrous acid with gramine gave a quantitative yield of NDMA. Therefore, the expected loss of a methyl group from gramine by nitrosative cleavage could not have occurred.

(3) Investigation of the reaction products from nitrosation at ambient temperature showed that indole-3-carboxaldehyde was not formed after a time sufficient to obtain a 40% yield of NDMA. Indole-3-carboxaldehyde is the expected carbonyl by-product if NDMA were formed from gramine as a result of nitrosative dealkylation. A product was observed which co-eluted on HPLC with indole-3-carbinol, *9*, (Fig. 1).

(4) The two indolic *N*-nitrosamines, *6* and *7* (Fig. 1), were not formed during the nitrosation of gramine at ambient temperature. These two *N*-nitrosamines would be expected to form, in addition to NDMA, if gramine were subject to nitrosative demethylation.

In agreement with these experimental results, a mechanism is proposed (Fig. 5) to explain the facile nitrosation of gramine. This mechanism is a type of S_N1 reaction in which breakdown of an initial nitrosammonium ion results in direct elimination of NDMA. Attack of unprotonated nitrite ion on the imminium cation, *10*, could result in formation of the nitrite ester *11*, and the nitro compound, *12*. Nitrite ion is an ambident nucleophile which attacks electrohpilic species to give nitrite esters and nitro compounds (March, 1968). Alternatively, hydration of the imminium cation would lead to indole-3-carbinol, *9*, which could be nitrosated to give the nitrite ester, *11*.

We are now working on further characterization of reaction products from the nitrosation of gramine in dilute aqueous acid. Obviously, determination of the fate of the indole-3-methylene moiety is essential for verification of the mechanism proposed in Figure 5.

Following our initial report on the nitrosation of gramine, Loeppky *et al.* (1982) reported rapid nitrosation of 2-(*N,N*-dimethylaminomethyl)pyrrole, *13*. This amine was found to undergo nitrosation in acetic acid at 65°C to give NDMA in 80% yield in 5 min in a ten-fold excess of nitrite. At 25°C, the same compound gave a 75% yield of NDMA in 5 min; NDMA was the only *N*-nitrosamine detected under all reaction conditions employed. The results were consistent with a mechanism not involving nitrosative dealkylation. Because compound *13* is a Mannich base analogue of gramine, there may be a close relationship between the mechanism of nitrosation of the two compounds, a possibility which was also recognized by Loeppky *et al.* (1982).

Although care must be exercised in extrapolating from nitrosation in aqueous acid to nitrosation during the drying of green malt, it now seems reasonable to conclude that gramine could be an important precursor of NDMA in barley malt. Other workers have concluded that hordenine must be the principal precursor, since hordenine is present in green malt at higher concentration than gramine (Slack & Wainwright, 1981). These workers did not, however, take into account the large difference in rates of NDMA formation from the two compounds.

ACKNOWLEDGEMENTS

This investigation was supported in part by Grant Number CA25002 awarded by the National Cancer Institue, DHHS and in part by a grant from the United States Brewers Association, Inc. Appreciation is extended to the Great Western Malting Co. (Vancouver, WA, USA) for loan of a Thermal Energy Analyser and to Dr Richard Loeppky, University of Missouri, for valuable discussion. The technical assistance of Ms Carol Fish and Mr James Barbour was greatly appreciated. "Oregon Agricultural Experiment Station Technical Paper Number 6927".

REFERENCES

Challis, B.C. & Kyrtopoulos, S.A. (1978) The chemistry of nitroso compounds. Part 12. The mechanism of nitrosation and nitration of aqueous piperidine by gaseous dinitrogen tetraoxide and dinitrogen trioxide in aqueous alkaline solutions. Evidence for the existence of molecular isomers of dinitrogen tetraoxide and dinitrogen trioxide. *J. chem. Soc. Perkin Trans. II*, 1296–1302

Drews, B., Just, F. & Drews, H. (1957) Vorkommen und Bildung von Aminen in Malz, Würze, und Bier. *Proceedings of the European brewing Convention*, Copenhagen, Elsevier, pp. 167–172

Fan, T.-Y. & Tannenbaum, S.R. (1973) Factors influencing the rate of formation of nitrosomorpholine from morpholine and nitrite: acceleration by thiocyanate and other anions. *J. agric. Food Chem.*, **21**, 237–240

Frank, A.W. & Marion, L. (1956) The biogenesis of alkaloids. XVI. Hordenine metabolism in barley. *Can. J. Chem.*, **34**, 1641–1646

Gowenlock, B.G., Hutchison, R.J., Little, J. & Pfab, J. (1979) Nitrosative dealkylation of some symmetrical tertiary amines. *J. chem. Soc. Perkin Trans. II*, 1110–1114

Gower, B.G. & Leete, E. (1963) Biosynthesis of gramine; the immediate precursors of the alkaloid. *J. Am. chem. Soc.*, **85**, 3683–3685

Loeppky, R.N., Tomasik, W. Outram, J.R. & Feicht, A. (1982) Nitrosamine formation from ternary nitrogen compounds. In: Bartsch, H., O'Neill, I.K., Castegnaro, M. & Okada, M., eds, N-*Nitroso Compounds: Occurrence and Biological Effects (IARC Scientific Publications No. 41)*, Lyon, International Agency for Research on Cancer, pp. 41–56

Mangino, M.M., Scanlan, R.A. & O'Brien, T.J. (1981) N-*Nitrosamines in beer*. In: Scanlan, R.A. & Tannenbaum, S.R., eds, N-*Nitroso compounds (Am. chem. Soc. Symp. Ser. No. 174)*, Washington DC, American Chemical Society, pp. 229–246

Mangino, M.M., Libbey, L.M. & Scanlan, R.A. (1982) *Nitrosation of* N-*methyltyramine and* N-*methyl-3-amino methylindole, two barley malt alkaloids*. In: Bartsch, H., O'Neill, I.K., Castegnaro, M. & Okada, M., eds, N-*Nitroso Compounds: Occurrence and Biological Effects (IARC Scientific Publications No. 41)*, Lyon, International Agency for Research on Cancer, pp. 57–69

March, J. (1968) *Advanced Organic Chemistry: Reactions, Mechanism, and Structure*, New York, McGraw-Hill

Mirvish, S.S., Gold, B., Eagen, M. & Arnold, S. (1974) Kinetics of the nitrosation of aminopyrine to give dimethylnitrosamine. *Z. Krebsforsch.*, **82**, 259–268

Mirvish, S.S., Sams, J., Fan, T.-Y. & Tannenbaum, S.R. (1973) Kinetics of nitrosation of the amino acids proline, hydroxyproline, and sarcosine. *J. natl Cancer Inst.*, **51**, 1833–1839

Scanlan, R.A., Barbour, J.F., Hotchkiss, J.H. & Libbey, L.M. (1980) N-Nitrosodimethylamine in beer. *Food cosmet. Toxicol.*, **18**, 27–29

Singer, G.M. & Lijinsky, W. (1976) Naturally occurring nitrosatable compounds. I. Secondary amines in foodstuffs. *J. agric. Food Chem.*, **24**, 550–553

Slack, P.T. & Wainwright, T. (1981) Hordenine as the precursor of NDMA in malt. *J. Inst. Brew.*, **87**, 259–263

Smith, P.A.S. & Loeppky, R.N. (1967) Nitrosative cleavage of tertiary amines. *J. Am. chem. Soc.*, **89**, 1147–1157

Spiegelhalder, B., Eisenbrand, G. & Preussmann, R. (1979) Contamination of beer with trace quantities of N-nitrosodimethylamine. *Food cosmet. Toxicol.*, **17**, 29–30

FORMATION OF NITROSAMINES IN NON-IONIC AND ANIONIC EMULSIONS IN THE PRESENCE AND ABSENCE OF INHIBITORS

B.L. KABACOFF[1]

Revlon Research Center, Edison, NJ 08818, USA

M.L. DOUGLASS[1]

Colgate-Palmolive, Piscataway, NJ 08854, USA

I.E. ROSENBERG[1]

Clairol, Stamford, CT 06922, USA

L.W. LEVAN, J.K. PUNWAR, S.F. VIELHUBER[2] & R.J. LECHNER

Hazleton Raltech, Madison, WI 53704, USA

SUMMARY

Nitrosation of water-soluble (diethanolamine) and oil-soluble (dodecylmethylamine and dicyclohexylamine) amines in the absence and presence of inhibitors in model anionic and non-ionic emulsions was studied. Nitrosation of diethanolamine occurred at similar rates in non-ionic and anionic emulsions. Surprisingly, dodecylmethylamine and dicyclohexylamine were readily nitrosated in non-ionic emulsions, but not in anionic emulsions. Sodium bisulfite and ascorbyl palmitate were effective inhibitors, but the activity of ascorbic acid was lower. Considerably less effective were potassium sorbate, α-tocopherol and butylated hydroxyanisole. The results of this study will help formulators of emulsion products to minimize *N*-nitrosamine contamination.

INTRODUCTION

This study is a continuation of a project the purpose of which is to reduce the level of *N*-nitrosamine contamination in emulsions by the inclusion of nitrosation inhibitors of appropriate reactivity and solubility. The need to investigate the effect of an oil/water system

---

[1] These authors represent the Nitrosamine Task Force of the Cosmetic, Toiletry and Fragrance Association, Washington, DC 20005, USA
[2] Present address: D & S Associates, Madison, WI 53711, USA

on nitrosation was discussed in an earlier work which dealt with the nitrosation of water-soluble diethanolamine (DELA) in an anionic emulsion (Kabacoff *et al.*, 1981).

The present report describes the nitrosation of DELA in both a non-ionic emulsion and that of two oil-soluble amines, dodecylmethylamine (DOMA) and dicyclohexylamine (DCHA), since oil-soluble nitrosamines have recently been detected in cosmetic products (Morrison *et al.*, 1983). Three water-soluble and three oil-soluble nitrosation inhibitors have been examined and the results used to formulate guiding principles for minimizing *N*-nitrosamine production in emulsion products.

MATERIALS AND METHODS

Composition and preparation of model emulsions

The compositions of the emulsions are shown in Table 1. The method of preparation has been described elsewhere (Kabacoff *et al.*, 1981). The nitrite (10 mg/L as NO_2^-) and water-soluble inhibitors were added to the finished emulsions in aqueous solution. The oil-soluble inhibitors were added to the oil phase during emulsion preparation. Each inhibitor was added to provide an inhibitor/nitrite molar ratio of 10.

Nitrosation rate experiments

The finished emulsions were stored at 37 °C under a nitrogen atmosphere. At given times, aliquots were quenched with 10% ammonium sulfamate to destroy residual nitrite and refrigerated until analysis. Samples were then analysed for the appropriate *N*-nitrosamine, using the following methods.

Table 1. Composition of emulsions

Oil Phase	Water Phase
A. Components common to all emulsions	
1% mineral oil	0.1% benzoic acid
1% stearic acid	
2% cetyl alcohol	
B. Components specific to individual emulsions	
Anionic (DELA)	
	0.2% DELA
	1% SLS
	94.7% water
Nonionic (DELA)	
0.4% non-ionic emulsifier [b]	0.2% DELA
	95.3% water
Anionic (DCHA, DOMA)	
0.2% DCHA or DOMA	1% SLS
	94.7% water
Nonionic (DCHA, DOMA)	
0.2% DCHA or DOMA	94.86% water
0.84% non-ionic emulsifier [a]	

[a] 94 parts Polysorbate 60, 6 parts sorbitan monostearate
[b] DELA, diethanolamine; SLS, sodium Lauryl sulfate; DCHA, dicyclo-hexylamine; DOMA, dodecylmethylamine

Analytical method for N-*nitrosodiethanolamine (NDELA)*

The method used was that of Kabacoff *et al.* (1981), except that with non-ionic emulsions, 0.5 mL of 10 mol/L sodium hydroxide was added after addition of the calcium chloride. The samples were heated for 15 min at 50 °C, and the final extracts were neutralized with 50 μL glacial acetic acid before analysis by high-performance liquid chromatography.

Analytical method for N-*nitrosododecylmethylamine (NDOMA) and* N-*nitrosodicyclohexyl-amine (NDCHA)*

Non-ionic emulsions: Each 3-g emulsion sample was extracted with pentane. After concentration to 1–2 mL, the pentane solution was applied to an alumina column, and the *N*-nitrosamine was eluted with 20–25% ethyl ether in pentane. The solvent was removed, and the residue was dissolved in an internal standard solution containing 1 mg/L NDCHA in isooctane (for NDOMA analysis) or 1 mg/L NDOMA in isooctane (for NDCHA analysis).

A 5-μl aliquot was analysed by gas chromatography, using a nitrogen-phosphorus thermionic detector (4 mm i.d. × 175 cm glass column, packed with 3% OV-1 on 80–100 Gas Chrom Q, 180 °C, 60 mL/min helium flow rate).

Anionic emulsions: Analysis was carried out by the same method employed for non-ionic emulsions except that saturated sodium chloride was added to the emulsion sample before pentane extraction. The extract was washed with acetonitrile:water (2:1, v/v) before concentration.

RESULTS AND DISCUSSION

Nitrosation and inhibition

Table 2 shows the initial rates of nitrosation of DELA, DOMA and DCHA. Table 3 summarizes the results concerning the inhibition of NDELA formation in non-ionic and anionic oil/water (o/w) emulsions and of NDOMA formation in the non-ionic emulsions. The effect of inhibitors on NDOMA formation in the anionic emulsion was not studied because of the slow nitrosation rate.

Table 2. Nitrosation of water- and oil-soluble amines in various media

Nitrosamine precursor	Medium	Initial nitrosation rate (μmol/L per day)	SD	No. of expts
Diethanolamine	Aqueous solution	1.00	0.43	2
Diethanolamine	Aqueous solution containing SLS[a]	0.93	0.30	2
Diethanolamine	Non-ionic emulsion	2.46	0.34	3
Diethanolamine	Anionic emulsion	1.90	0.15	3
Dodecylmethylamine	Non-ionic emulsion	8.35	1.55	3
Dodecylmethylamine	Anionic emulsion	0.00	–	2
Dicyclohexylamine	Non-ionic emulsion	0.95	0.16	2
Dicyclohexylamine	Anionic emulsion	0.033	0.002	2

[a] Aqueous solution of sodium lauryl sulfate at the same pH and concentration used in the anionic emulsion

Table 3. Effect of nitrosation inhibitors on formation of *N*-nitrosodiethanolamine (NDELA) and *N*-nitrosododecyl-methylamine (NDOMA) in emulsions

Inhibitor	NDELA inhibition				NDOMA inhibition	
	Non-ionic emulsion		Anionic emulsion		Non-ionic emulsion	
	%	SD	%	SD	%	SD
Ascorbic acid	98	4	79	3	67	8
Potassium sorbate	65	3	32	16	22	6
Sodium bisulfite	98	2	100	0	96	1
Ascorbyl palmitate	91	0.4	90	10	96	1
Butylated hydroxyanisole	62	2	16	11	52	4
α-Tocopherol	21	12	4 [a]	–	72	5

[a] Calculated value of 8% was not statistically significant.

Effect of emulsions on the rate of nitrosation

The observed variations in rate are explained by the physical nature of o/w emulsions and of the species involved in the nitrosation reaction (Equation 1), the concentrations of which are governed by equilibria 2–4.

$$R_2NH + N_2O_3 \rightarrow R_2NNO + HONO \qquad (1)$$
$$H^+ + NO_2^- \rightleftharpoons HONO \qquad (2)$$
$$2HONO \rightleftharpoons N_2O_3 + H_2O \qquad (3)$$
$$R_2NH^+{}_2 \rightleftharpoons R_2NH + H^+ \qquad (4)$$

In o/w emulsions, molecules of surfactant species are concentrated at the interface between the oil droplet and the water phase. They are so oriented that the hydrophobic (hydrocarbon) tails lie largely within the oil globule and the polar ends lie largely within the aqueous phase. If the polar ends are ionic, this orientation leads to a charged electrical double layer at the interface, consisting of the charged group of the surfactant and the oppositely charged counter-ion. The concentration of the counter-ion is much greater at the interface than elsewhere in the aqueous phase.

Nitrosation of DELA was more rapid in both o/w emulsions than in water, possibly due to an increased effective concentration of N_2O_3 in oil (i.e., equilibria (2) and (3) were shifted to the right). Rate enhancement in lipophilic heterogeneous media has already been reported (Mirvish *et al.*, 1978). Catalysis by the micelles present in aqueous sodium lauryl sulfate (SLS) was not observed. The concentration of the micellar oil phase in aqueous SLS is less than 25% of the present in the anionic o/2 emulsion.

Nitrosation of DOMA would be expected to be slower than that of DELA, because it is more basic. In non-ionic o/w emulsions, DOMA was nitrosated much faster than DELA. The oil phase contains not only the reactive species, N_2O_3, but also the hydrophobic amine. The hydrocarbon chains of DOMA are dissolved in the hydrocarbon interior of the oil droplet, and the hydrophilic amino groups lie at the o/w interface. In the presence of neutral emulsifier, the positively charged surface of the oil drops attracts nitrite ions. Electrostatic interaction between the positive ammonium head-groups favour deprotonation, to form the reactive amine; i.e., equilibrium (4) is shifted to the right. Thus, the effective concentrations of the two N-nitrosamine precursors are greatly increased. Similar rate enhancements were observed by Okun and Archer (1977) for nitrosation of long-chain amines in the presence of micelles of cationic and non-ionic surfactants.

The lower rate of DCHA nitrosation in the non-ionic o/w emulsion was probably due to steric hindrance. The rate of DELA nitrosation in the non-ionic o/w emulsion was not further increased, because its polar groups disfavour migration of the amine into the oil phase.

The dramatic inhibition of DOMA and DCHA nitrosation in the o/w emulsion stabilized by the anionic emulsifier, SLS, is explained similarly. The effective concentration of nitrite at the o/w interface is reduced because it is replaced by the negative sulfate end-group of SLS. The negative charge at the interface further reduces the nitrosation rate by increasing the ratio of non-reactive protonated amine to free amine. The rate of nitrosation of DELA was again unaffected by the anionic emulsifier, as was the case in non-ionic emulsion, because little of the amines resides in the oil phase.

Inhibition of nitrosation

The most active inhibitor for both the water-soluble DELA and the oil-soluble DOMA was bisulfite. Ascorbic acid is much less reactive toward nitrite than is bisulfite[1] and thus was less effective than bisulfite in inhibiting both NDELA and NDOMA formation. In the non-ionic emulsions containing ascorbic acid, more NDOMA formed than NDELA, because DOMA was nitrosated faster than DELA in that medium.

Oil-soluble ascorbyl palmitate was much more effective than ascorbic acid in preventing nitrosation of DOMA. It is concentrated in the oil phase, with the palmitoyl groups dissolved in the oil and the polar ascorbyl groups aligned on the globule surface. The relatively high concentration of the ascorbyl group at the o/w interface lessened nitrosation of DOMA by nitrite present in the water phase.

As discussed above, the presence of an oil phase in emulsions doubled the rate of DELA nitrosation. Thus, the concentration of ascorbyl palmitate at the o/w interface made it more effective than ascorbic acid in inhibiting nitrosation of DELA in both types of emulsions.

The relatively weak inhibitors, sorbate, butylated hydroxyanisole and α-tocopherol, were much less active in preventing DELA nitrosation in anionic emulsion than in non-ionic emulsion. The negative lauryl sulfate emulsifier present in the oil globules, at the interface, displaced nitrite and prevented its reaction with the inhibitors dissolved in the oil phase.

The results of this study lead to several practical generalizations useful in minimizing N-nitrosamine contamination of emulsion products which contain organo-nitrogen compounds susceptible to N-nitrosamine formation.

Anionic emulsifiers are far superior to non-ionic or cationic emulsifiers in inhibiting nitrosation of hydrophobic amines.

A hydrophilic organo-nitrogen ingredient in an anionic emulsion requires a nitrosation inhibitor.

Non-ionic or cationic emulsions require larger amounts of inhibitors than do anionic emulsions, regardless of the solubility characteristics of the amine.

Inhibitors should be selected on the basis of their reactivity with nitrite and their oil- or water-solubility characteristics.

Inhibitors should be added to the formulation to destroy nitrite before any organo-nitrogen ingredients are added.

---

[1] Govil, A. & Stadnick, R., personal communication

REFERENCES

Kabacoff, B.L., Lechnir, R.J., Vielhuber, S.F. & Douglass, M.L. (1981) *Formation and inhibition of N-nitrosodiethanolamine in an anionic oil-water emulsion.* In: Scanlan, R.A. & Tannenbaum, S.R., eds, N-*Nitroso Compounds (Am. chem. Soc. Symp. Ser. No. 174),* Washington DC, American Chemical Society, pp. 149–156

Mirvish, S.S., Karlowski, K., Sams, J.P. & Arnold, S.D. (1978) *Studies related to nitrosamide formation: nitrosation in solvent: water and solvent systems, nitrosomethylurea formation in the rat stomach and analysis of a fish product for ureas.* In: Walker, E.A., Castegnaro, M., Griciute, L. & Lyle, R.E., eds, *Environmental Aspects of* N-*Nitroso compounds, (IARC Scientific Publications No. 19),* Lyon, International Agency for Research on Cancer, pp. 161–173

Morrison, J.B., Hecht, S.S. & Weinninger, J.A. (1983) *N*-nitroso-*N*-methyloctadecylamine in hair-care products. *Food Chem. Toxicol., 21,* 69–73

Okun, J.D. & Archer, M.C. (1977) Kinetics of nitrosamine formation in the presence of micelle-forming surfactants. *J. natl Cancer Inst., 58,* 409–411

ESTER-MEDIATED NITROSAMINE FORMATION FROM NITRITE AND SECONDARY OR TERTIARY AMINES

R.N. LOEPPKY, W. TOMASIK & T.G. MILLARD

Department of Chemistry, University of Missouri-Columbia, Columbia, MO 65211, USA

SUMMARY

N-Nitrosamines are formed from the heating of either a secondary or a tertiary amine with sodium nitrite in the presence of a high-boiling ester such as 2-acetoxyethanol in ethylene glycol. The four secondary and six tertiary amines examined were found to produce *N*-nitrosamines in yields ranging from 4% to 80% when equimolar amounts of amine and ester were heated at 120 °C with one- to ten-fold equivalents of sodium nitrite in ethylene glycol. Secondary amines competitively produced acetamides at a rate slightly greater than *N*-nitrosamine formation. Preincubation of a large excess of sodium nitrite and ester led to the rapid formation of *N*-nitrosamines in high yield. The reaction of tribenzylamine resulted in the formation of both benzaldehyde and dibenzylnitrosamine. *N,N*-Dimethylbenzylamine reacted to give nearly equimolar amounts of *N*-nitrosodimethylamine and *N*-nitroso-*N*-methylbenzylamine. It is proposed that the nitrosating agent is a nitrous ester, and it is shown that 2-benzoxyethyl nitrite rapidly nitrosates secondary and tertiary amines under these reaction conditions. It is also proposed that these transformations are good models for the environmental formation of *N*-nitrosamines in foods and commercial products.

INTRODUCTION

We reported previously that *N,N*-dialkylamides react with sodium nitrite upon heating to give variable yields of *N*-nitrosamines (0.3–27%), as indicated in equation (1) (Loeppky *et al.*, 1982).

$$\underset{R}{\overset{R'}{\diagdown}}N\!-\!\overset{\overset{\textstyle O}{\|}}{C}\!-\!R'' + NO_2^- \xrightarrow[120-180\,°C]{\triangle} R\!-\!\overset{\overset{\textstyle NO}{|}}{N}\!-\!R' + R''\!-\!COO^- \qquad (1)$$

We found that both the yield and rate of *N*-nitrosamine formation were markedly increased upon the introduction of ethylene glycol or glycerol. Additional experimentation in our laboratory has permitted us to postulate a mechanism for this reaction and the unusual role of the polyhydric solvents. The first step involves the transfer of an acyl group from the amide to the alcohol function of the solvent. The resulting ester is attacked by ionic nitrite to yield the nitrosating species, an alkyl nitrite. The nitrous ester then reacts with the amine produced in the first transformation, to give the *N*-nitrosamine. In the course of verifying this hypothesis we have investigated the reaction of secondary amines with the acetate esters of ethylene glycol and sodium nitrite in ethylene glycol. These experiments have been performed to answer the question: can esters and ionic nitrite lead to extensive nitrosation of secondary and tertiary amines? The results presented in this paper demonstrate that the answer is yes. Moreover, we believe that this general reaction scheme is mainly responsible for the production of *N*-nitrosamines in cosmetics, metal-working fluids, shampoos and other toiletry articles, as well as certain cooked and cured meats.

EXPERIMENTAL

Secondary amine nitrosation

The nitrosation reactions were conducted either in flasks connected to a reflux condenser, which was sealed at the top with a rubber septum, or in a septum-sealed vial. The flasks were heated in an oil bath at 120 °C and the vials were heated in a metal block at the same temperature. All experiments employed ethylene glycol as a solvent and sodium nitrite, ethylene glycol diacetate and the desired amine as reactants. Reactions were conducted in an atmosphere of argon. A typical procedure involved the heating of 0.306 g (4.43 mmol) sodium nitrite, 0.29 g (4.4 mmol) ethylene glycol diacetate and 30 mL ethylene glycol in a 50-mL flask for 2.7 h at 120 °C. Pyrrolidine (0.33 g, 4 mmol) was added by syringe below the surface of the hot liquid mixture. Samples were taken through the septum at specific intervals. When the reactions were conducted in vials, each point in the kinetic analysis was obtained from a separate vial, the contents of which were 'quenched' as described below.

Tertiary amine nitrosation

Tertiary amine nitrosations were conducted in a manner similar to the secondary amine nitrosation, except that the preincubation of the solvent, ester and sodium nitrite, was found to have little effect on the time-course of the transformation and was therefore eliminated. A typical procedure follows: two solutions were prepared. Solution 1 consisted of 0.9523 g (6.52 mmol) ethylene glycol diacetate and 0.4405 g (6.38 mmol) sodium nitrite, dissolved in enough ethylene glycol to bring the volume to 25.0 mL. Solution 2 consisted of a 5.37×10^{-2} mol/L solution of tribenzylamine in ethylene glycol (a saturated solution). Solutions 1 and 2 were brought to 120 °C in an oil bath. Reaction vials were charged with 1.50 mL of solution 1 and 0.50 mL of solution 2, sealed with Teflon-lined caps and heated at 120 °C, with occasional shaking. Sample vials were removed from the heating block at specific times, cooled rapidly, and 50-µL samples were taken and added to methanol in a 10-mL volumetric flask. After the samples had been diluted to a volume of 10.0 mL, analysis was performed by high-pressure liquid chromatography (HPLC), as indicated below.

Nitrosation of tribenzylamine with 2-benzoxyethyl nitrite

Tribenzylamine (0.013 g, 0.045 mmol) was weighed into each of 12 vials. The co-reactant was prepared by diluting 2.028 g of 55% 2-benzoxyethyl nitrite with 50.0 mL ethylene glycol in volumetric flask. Four mL of the solution was then placed in each vial. The vial headspace was purged with argon, and the vials were sealed. They were then heated at 120 °C, removed at specific times, cooled and diluted to 25.0 mL with methanol. Analyses were performed by HPLC, as described below.

Analyses

The majority of *N*-nitrosamine analyses were performed by reversed-phase HPLC, using a Waters instrument, equipped for gradient elution and employing an autosampler with a variable-volume injection system and an ultra-violet detector, operating at 254 nm. As an example, *N*-nitrosopyrrolidine (NPYR) was determined in the quenched sample, diluted to standard volume with methanol, by injection (10 μL) onto a duPont Zorbax-CN column (4.6 mm × 25 cm) which was eluted with methanol: water (2 mL/min at 20:40 to 40:60–4 min). The elution volume for NPYR was 6.4 mL and quantification was carried out using a standard curve obtained with external standards. Each point represents the repetition of three determinations. Benzaldehyde produced in the nitrosation of tribenzyl amine was also determined by HPLC, using a similar technique. Specific details of the chromatographic determination of various compounds can be obtained from the authors.

N-Acetylpyrrolidine and NPYR were analysed by gas chromatography (GC) as well. Samples from the nitrosation of pyrrolidine were prepared by passing a 0.5-mL sample through a small column containing 2 mL of AG 1-x8 anion-exchange resin with distilled water until 10.0 mL had been collected. The amide and nitrosamine were detected by a flame-ionization detector (FID) using a 2-m OV-225 column for separation (75 °C/min; 5 °C/min to 100 °C; 10 °C/min to 250 °C). Under these conditions, the retention time for NPYR was 6.24 min and that of *N*-acetylpyrrolidine 7.5 min. Nitrite ion consumption in this experiment was determined spectrophometrically, using Shin's reagent.

RESULTS

Secondary amine nitrosation

Typical nitrosation experiments were performed by heating the desired amine and sodium nitrite with an equilibrium mixture of monoacetyl and diacetyl ethylene glycol in ethylene glycol in a sealed container. The ester was added as diacetyl ethylene glycol and pre-equilibrated with ethylene glycol to give the mixture of esters, which was composed principally of monoacetyl ethylene glycol. Initial experiments were conducted at 180 °C but a reaction temperature of 120 °C was found to be much better for convenient study of the transformations, and all subsequent reactions were done at this temperature. Figure 1 demonstrates that the ester-mediated nitrosation of pyrrolidine is much faster and more extensive than the production of this nitrosamine from *N*-acetylpyrrolidine or the parent amine under the same conditions. The amine in these reactions is involved in two competitive transformations – nitrosation and reversible *N*-acylation. The equilibrium significantly favours amide formation (*N*-acylation) under the reaction conditions. The product ratio of *N*-nitrosamine to amide can be manipulated by adjusting the initial reaction conditions. The time course of a typical transformation involving pyrrolidine is shown in Figure 2. In this case, the ester and the sodium nitrite were preincubated at 120 °C for 2.5 h, prior to introduction of the amine. The results of a similar experiment employing a 25-fold excess of ester and sodium nitrite are shown in Figure 3. It can be seen that it led to very rapid and extensive formation of *N*-nitrosopyrrolidine.

A number of amines of varying basicity and structure have been nitrosated by the general procedure described above. The results are reported in Table 1. Generally, we made no attempt to maximize the yield of *N*-nitrosamine, since we have demonstrated that this can be done by manipulating the initial reactant concentrations and the reaction conditions. The

Fig. 1. Formation of *N*-nitrosopyrrolidine (NPYR) from the heating of 1.5 mol/L amine or amide and sodium nitrite at 180 °C in glycol; ◆, amine + ROAc + NO₂⁻; ●, amide + NO₂⁻; ▲, amine + NO₂⁻.

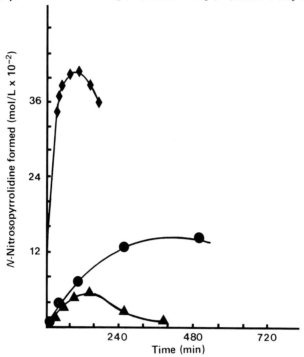

Fig. 2. % Formation of *N*-nitrosopyrrolidine (■) and *N*-acetylpyrrolidine (○) and % consumption of NO₂⁻ (●) as a function of time (Table 1, entry 2).

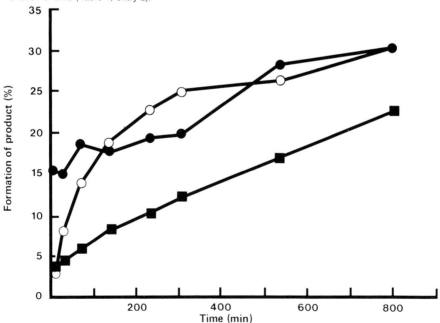

Fig. 3. % Formation of *N*-nitrosopyrrolidine as a function of time (Table 1, entry 1).

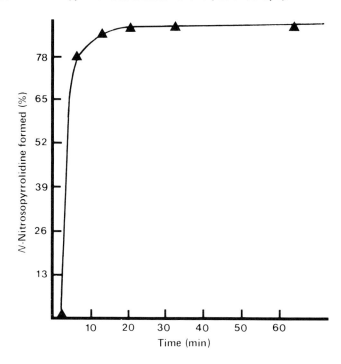

Time (min)

Table 1.   Ester-mediated nitrosation of secondary amines

Entry	Amine	Reactant ratio[a]			Yield[b] (%/h)	$10^2 \, k^c$ (min^{-1})
		Amine	Ester	Nitrite		
1	Pyrrolidine	1	25	25	67/12	139
2	Pyrrolidine	1	2.21	1.1	32/13.5	2.72
3	Diethyl	1	1.2	1	53/45	2.71
4	Diethanol	1	1.2	1	25/14.5	2.7
5	Dibenzyl	1	2.8	10	80/122	2.3

[a] [reactant]/[amine]
[b] % Yields based on amine at the time indicated
[c] Observed rate constants from plots of 1n(% reaction) versus time

ester-mediated transformations of the amine to amide and *N*-nitrosamine are kinetically complex because of the parallel and competitive steps involving both the ester and the amine. A better understanding of the reaction mechanism will require further kinetic experiments, but manipulation of the data given in Figure 2 reveals the interesting feature that a plot of time *versus* (log % reaction) is linear for this transformation and for the other transformations noted in Table 1. In several instances, points at longer times had to be dropped, but the reaction obeys this kinetic law up to the percent reaction given in Table 1. The slopes of these plots are reported as pseudo first-order rate constants in Table 1. An interesting feature of these rate constants is that, within experimental error, they are all equal (Table 1, entries 2–5), despite the differences in amine basicity and structure.

The nitrous ester, 2-acetoxyethyl nitrite, is a possible intermediate in this transformation and may be the active nitrosating agent (Loeppky *et al.*, 1982). Since the report by Challis and Shuker (1979), that secondary amines can be nitrosated by activated nitrous esters, we have synthesized 2-acetoxyethyl nitrite and 2-benzoxyethyl nitrite and shown that both compounds nitrosate secondary amines very rapidly at 120 °C. The latter ester is purified more easily than the former.

Tertiary amine nitrosation

The heating of tribenzylamine, sodium nitrite and diacetyl glycol in ethylene glycol at 120 °C in a sealed vial results in the slow production of equal molar quantities of *N*-nitrosodibenzylamine and benzaldehyde (equation 2).

$$(\varnothing CH_2)_3 N + NaNO_2 + AcOCH_2CH_2OAc \xrightarrow[120]{\triangle} \varnothing \overset{O}{\overset{\|}{C}}-H + (\varnothing CH_2)_2 N-NO \qquad (2)$$
$$\underset{OH \quad\quad OH}{}$$

The reaction must be protected from light in order to avoid the photodecomposition of *N*-nitrosodibenzylamine, which also gives benzaldehyde. Five other structurally-varied tertiary amines have been shown to produce *N*-nitrosamines when heated with sodium nitrite under these conditions. The data are given in Table 2. The time *versus* % reaction data were treated in a manner similar to those for the secondary amines, and the apparent rate constants, although considerably less precise, are reported. It can be seen that the apparent rate varies with the structure of the starting amine. *N,N*-Dimethylaniline was quite reactive, while *N*-butylpyrrolidine was relatively unreactive under the conditions of the transformation. Tribenzylamine represented the only case in which we attempted to identify the product cleaved from the amine nitrogen.

Table 2. Ester-mediated nitrosation of tertiary amines

Entry	Amine	Reactant ratio[a]			Yield[b] (%/h)	$10^5 \, k^c$ (min^{-1})
		Amine	Ester	Nitrite		
1	Tributyl	1	1.28	4.88	22/14	3.0
2	*N,N*-Dimethylaniline	1	1.1	4.59	45/14	7.0
3	*N*-Butylpyrrolidine	1	1.19	4.85	4.1/91	–
4	*N,N*-Dimethylbenzyl (NMBzA)	1	1.22	5.0	24/161	2.9
5	*N,N*-Dimethylbenzyl (NDMA)	1	1.22	5.0	17/161	1.8
6	Triethyl	1	1.2	1.0	17/26	1.0
7	Tribenzyl	1	2.83	10.2	7.5/33	4.1

[a] [reactant]/[amine]
[b] % Yields based on amine in the time indicated
[c] Approximate observed rate constants determined from plots of 1n (% reaction) versus time. These constants should be used only as a rough gauge of reactivity, since it is not clear that the reaction exhibits pseudo first-order kinetics.

Fig. 4. % Formation of *N*-nitrosodimethylamine (●) and *N*-nitroso-*N*-methylbenzylamine (■) from ester-mediated nitrosation of *N*,*N*-dimethylbenzylamine as a function of time. ▲, sum of % yields.

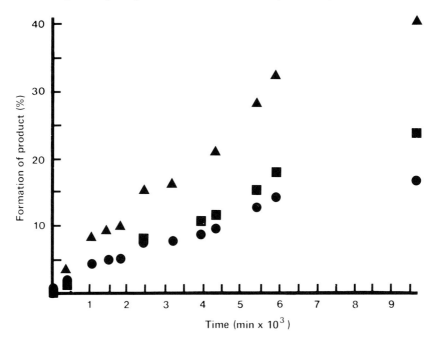

N,*N*-Dimethylbenzylamine reacted with sodium nitrite in the presence of the ester to produce both *N*-nitrosodimethylamine (NDMA) and *N*-nitroso-*N*-methylbenzylamine (equation 3).

$$\varnothing CH_2N(CH_3)_2 + NaNO_2 + AcOCH_2CH_2OAc \xrightarrow[\underset{OH\quad OH}{}]{\triangle \ 120} (CH_3)_2NNO + \varnothing CH_2\overset{NO}{\underset{|}{N}}CH_3 \qquad (3)$$

The time course of this transformation is shown in Figure 4. It can be seen that NDMA and *N*-nitroso-*N*-methylbenzylamine are formed in approximately equal molar amounts throughout the course of the reaction.

Since secondary amines are proposed intermediates in the acidic nitrosation of tertiary amines, we examined the reaction of tribenzylamine for the presence of dibenzylamine or its *N*-acetyl derivative. Neither of these substances was found. As was discussed in the case of secondary amine nitrosation, we have hypothesized that a nitrous ester might be the effective nitrosating agent in these transformations. Because of the difficulties we encountered in the preparation of 2-acetoxyethyl nitrite, we worked here with 2-benzyloxyethyl nitrite, which was much more easily prepared and purified. This nitrous ester reacted rapidly with tribenzylamine to form N-nitrosodibenzylamine, but no significant quantity of benzaldehyde (equation 4).

$$\emptyset\text{--}\overset{\displaystyle O}{\overset{\displaystyle \|}{\text{C}}}\text{--OCH}_2\text{CH}_2\text{--O--N}=\text{O} + (\emptyset\text{CH}_2)_3\text{N} \xrightarrow[120]{\triangle} (\emptyset\text{CH}_2)_2\text{NNO} + ? \qquad (4)$$

When a 10-fold molar excess of the ester was employed, the reaction exhibited pseudo first-order rate behaviour up to 89% production of N-nitrosodibenzylamine (reaction time 2.3 h). The observed rate constant under these conditions was $(1.3 \pm 0.2) \times 10^{-2}$ min^{-1}.

DISCUSSION

The results described above provide ample evidence that acetate esters of ethylene glycol promote the nitrosation of both secondary and tertiary amines by ionic nitrite. N-Nitrosamine formation has been shown to result from a wide range of structurally varied amines of different basicity. The nitrosation of secondary amines occurs with competitive formation of amides from the ester, but this reaction is reversible, and we have demonstrated that heating of amides with ionic nitrite in ethylene glycol or glycerine results in N-nitrosamine formation.

While the reaction has not been investigated from the perspective of the structure of the ester, our preliminary investigations suggest that esters of high-boiling alcohols will be effective in promoting the nitrosation of amines by the scheme discussed here. Methyl and ethyl esters of carboxylic acids are not anticipated to be effective in promoting nitrosation reactions, because the alkyl nitrites formed from them are so volatile. We observed this previously when examining the reaction between sodium nitrite and ethyl-N-acetylproline (Loeppky et al., 1982).

The data on secondary amine nitrosation reactions presented here strongly suggest that production of the nitrosating agent is the rate-limiting step in this transformation. The data of Table 1 support this hypothesis. Structurally different amines gave similar rate constants for nitrosation. Preincubation of nitrite with the acetate ester led to more rapid nitrosation of the amine. Preincubation of relatively large amounts of ester and nitrite (compared to amine) prior to introduction of the amine led to rapid and extensive N-nitrosamine formation. The precise nature of the nitrosating agent or agents under these conditions is not yet known. We have shown that a nitrous ester of ethylene glycol is capable of nitrosating both secondary and tertiary amines under the reaction conditions described and that the reaction takes place rapidly. It is also possible, however, that the reaction involves a species such as that shown in Figure 5.

The data on tertiary amine nitrosation display several interesting features. Tribenzylamine nitrosation follows the same course as it does in acidic media, producing both N-nitrosodibenzylamine and benzaldehyde (Smith & Leoppky, 1967). The reaction, however, must occur by a different mechanism than that involved in the acidic nitrosation of tertiary amines. Several lines of evidence point to this conclusion. First of all, the nitrosation of N-nitroso-N-methylbenzylamine and NDMA. We have demonstrated that the acidic nitrosation of this same amine results in the preferential formation of the former N-nitrosamine at a three-to-one ratio. This altered selectivity in the cleavage of the alkyl group from nitrogen is strongly suggestive of a new pathway for the nitrosation reaction. The acidic nitrosation of tribenzylamine and other tertiary amines investigated by Smith and Loeppky (1967) involves an intermediate N,N-dialkylimminium ion. This imminium ion is hydrolysed by the water in the acidic solution to produce a secondary amine and an aldehyde. The secondary amine is then

Fig. 5. Scheme for nitrosating reactions of a nitrous ester with secondary and tertiary amines.

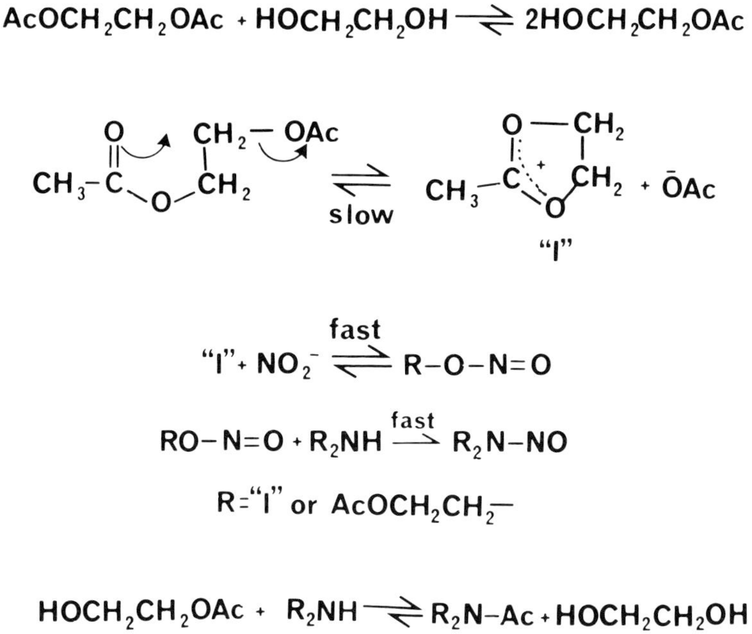

$$AcOCH_2CH_2OAc + HOCH_2CH_2OH \rightleftharpoons 2HOCH_2CH_2OAc$$

$$CH_3-\overset{O}{\overset{\|}{C}}\diagup_{O}\diagdown CH_2-OAc \underset{slow}{\rightleftharpoons} CH_3-\overset{O\;-\;CH_2}{\underset{O}{\overset{\cdot\cdot}{C}\diagdown}}\overset{+}{CH_2} + \bar{O}Ac$$

"I"

$$\text{"I"} + NO_2^- \overset{fast}{\rightleftharpoons} R-O-N=O$$

$$RO-N=O + R_2NH \overset{fast}{\longrightarrow} R_2N-NO$$

$$R = \text{"I" or } AcOCH_2CH_2-$$

$$HOCH_2CH_2OAc + R_2NH \rightleftharpoons R_2N-Ac + HOCH_2CH_2OH$$

presumed to be nitrosated to give the *N*-nitrosamine. We have not been able to detect secondary amines or their amides as intermediates in the nitrosation of tertiary amines by esters and ionic nitrite. Lijinsky *et al.* (1972) and Keefer and Roller (1973) have suggested an alternative mode of *N*-nitrosamine formation from an imminium ion, which could account for the formation of both *N*-nitrosodibenzylamine and benzaldehyde in this reaction. The imminium ion produced by the elimination of NOH from the nitrosated tertiary amine is envisioned to react with ionic nitrite to generate an α-aminonitrous ester. This species is presumed to decompose directly to the *N*-nitrosamine and the aldehyde. It is interesting that the nitrosation of tribenzylamine with 2-benzoxyethyl nitrite does not result in the production of benzaldehyde, although it does give *N*-nitrosodibenzylamine. This suggests yet another mode of tertiary amine nitrosation. Obviously, more work must be done before a detailed understanding of this reaction mechanism and the nature of the nitrosating agent become evident. In spite of this, the elaboration of these reactions provides a missing link in the environmental production of *N*-nitrosamines from ionic nitrite.

There have been numerous reports of environmental *N*-nitrosamine formation in which the reactants have not encountered an acidic environment. Previous work by Keefer and Roller (1973), Croisy *et al.* (1980), Challis and Shuker (1979), Challis and Outram (1979) and Challis and Kryptopoulos (1979) have demonstrated how *N*-nitrosamine formation can occur in an alkaline medium. Keefer's group has demonstrated how formaldehyde and metal ions can catalyse nitrosation, while Challis' group has demonstrated how oxides of nitrogen and nitrous esters can be effective nitrosating agents in alkaline media. Although it is difficult to be sure that *N*-nitrosamine formation is occuring in the absence of any oxides of nitrogen, there are many cases of environmental *N*-nitrosamine occurrence and formation which involve neither acidic nor alkaline aqueous mixtures.

Fig. 6. Scheme for *N*-nitrosamine formation in the cooking of nitrite-cured meats.

GLYCERIDE + H$_2$O   GLYCEROL + ACID

GLYCEROL + PEPTIDE   AMINE + ESTER

GLYCERIDE + NITRITE   GLYCERYL NITRITE + CARBOXYLATE

GLYCERYL NITRITE + AMINE   NITROSAMINE + GLYCEROL

Probably the best-known example involves the formation of NPYR in the cooking of nitrite-cured meats. These meats, of course, contain esters of glycerol (fat). We believe that *N*-nitrosamine formation occurs by the route we have discussed in this paper and which is sketched out in Figure 6. Cosmetic and metal-working fluid formulation often contain *N*-nitrosamines formed from alkanolamines and frequently contain either amides, esters or fatty acids. Temperatures as high as 100 °C are often reached during the formulation of these materials. One can understand how trace amounts of *N*-nitrosamines could be formed from adventitious nitrite or nitrite formed from the hydrolysis of oxides of nitrogen under the alkaline conditions present in metal-working fluids, for example. It is also possible that this general route could apply to the formation of *N*-nitrosamines during tobacco smoking. If the active nitrosating agent in these reactions is a nitrous ester, there is good reason to believe that this type of nitrosation reaction can be inhibited relatively easily. Nitrous esters are very reactive substances and may be chemically scavenged more easily than nitrous acid, and certainly more easily than ionic nitrite. Our research is proceeding on this subject.

RECOMMENDATION

We recommend that the IARC sponsor the development of a nitrosation test similar to the WHO acidic nitrosation test. This test would involve heating formulations at 100 °C for a fixed time, followed by analysis for *N*-nitrosamines.

ACKNOWLEDGEMENT

The support of this research by the National Cancer Institute under grant CA26914 is gratefully acknowledged.

REFERENCES

Challis, B.C. & Kryptopoulos, S.S. (1978) The mechanisms of nitrosation and nitration by gaseous dinitrogen tetraoxide and dinitrogen trioxide in aqueous solutions. *J. chem. Soc. Perkin*, *II*, 1296–1302
Challis, B.C. & Outram, J.R. (1979) The chemistry of nitroso-compounds. Part 15. Formation of *N*-nitrosamine in solution from gaseous nitric oxide in the presence of iodine. *J. chem. Soc. Perkin*, *I*, 2768–2775
Challis, B.C. & Shuker, D.E.G. (1979) Rapid nitrosation of amines in aqueous alkaline solutions by β-substituted alkyl nitrites. *J. chem. Soc. chem. Commun.*, 315–316

Croisy, A.F., Fanning, J.C., Keefer, L.K., Slavin, B.W. & Uhm, S.J. (1980) *Metal complexes as promoters of N-nitrosation reactions: a progress report.* In: Walker, E.A., Castegnaro, M., Griciute, L. & Börzsönyi, M., eds, N-*Nitroso Compounds: Analysis, Formation and Occurrence (IARC Scientific Publications No. 31)*, Lyon, International Agency for Research on Cancer, pp. 83–93

Keefer, L.K. & Roller, P.P. (1973) N-nitrosation by nitrite ion in neutral and basic medium. *Science, 181,* 1245–1247

Lijinsky, W., Keefer, L., Conrad, E. & Van De Bogart, R. (1972) Nitrosation of tertiary amines and some biological implications. *J. natl. Cancer Inst., 49,* 1239–1249

Loeppky, R.N., Tomasik, W., Outram, J.R. & Feicht, A. (1982) *Nitrosamine formation from ternary nitrogen compounds.* In: Bartsch, H., O'Neill, I.K., Castegnaro, M. & Okada, M., eds, N-*Nitroso Compounds: Occurrence and Biological Effects (IARC Scientific Publications No. 41)*, Lyon, International Agency for Research on Cancer, pp. 41–56

Smith, P.A.S. & Loeppky, R.N. (1967) Nitrosative cleavage of tertiary amines. *J. Am. chem. Soc., 89,* 1147–1157

PHOTOCHEMISTRY OF *N*-NITROSAMINES IN NEUTRAL MEDIA

C.J. MICHEJDA & T. RYDSTROM[1]

LBI-Basic Research Program, Chemical Carcinogenesis Program, NCI-Frederick Cancer Research Facility, Frederick, MD 21701, USA

SUMMARY

N-Nitrosamines have long been held to be photostable in solution in absence of acid, although a few reports to the contrary have been published. This paper reports a study of the photolysis of *N*-nitrosopiperidine and *N*-nitrosodiisopropylamine in aprotic and protic solvents. It is shown that the cleavage of the N-N bond is a very facile process. In the absence of radical scavengers, however, reformation of the nitrosamines is very rapid, giving little or no net photolysis. In the presence of scavengers, photolysis proceeds with high efficiency to give non-nitrosamine products. When the trapping agent is oxygen, the net reaction is photo-oxygenation to the corresponding nitramine. The nitramine, in turn, is photolabile and undergoes photolysis to give cleavage products. The formation of the nitramine proceeds through the initial photochemical cleavage of the nitrosamine to the aminyl radical and nitric oxide, followed by the oxidation of the nitric oxide to nitrogen dioxide and the recombination of the latter with the aminyl radical. These results have some important implications for the destruction of nitrosamine wastes.

INTRODUCTION

The photochemistry of nitrosamines has been the subject of numerous studies. Acid-catalysed photochemistry has been elucidated largely through the efforts of Chow and co-workers (1973, 1979). The salient feature of their work was the finding that the photochemical homolysis of the N-N bond is facilitated by coordination of the nucleophilic oxygen of the nitrosamines with a proton. These studies led Chow and co-workers, as well as other investigators, to utilize nitrosamine photolysis for many clever synthetic applications.

The photochemistry of nitrosamines in neutral media, however, has not been explored extensively because of the widespread assumption that, in the absence of acid, nitrosamines are photostable. Thus, for example, Michejda and co-workers (1976) found that photolysis of unsymmetrical nitrosamines in neutral media led to photo-catalysed E/Z isomerization, but no

---

[1] Present address: Department of Organic Chemistry, University of Umeå, 90187 Umeå, Sweden

net photolysis. There are reports in the literature, however, that contradict the notion of photostability of nitrosamines in non-acidic media. Daiber and Preussmann (1964) reported that dialkylnitrosamines could be cleaved quantitatively by photolysis in strongly alkaline solutions. These results were generally supported by the work of Sander (1967). Thus, there was a need to examine the photolysis of nitrosamines in the absence of acid. The present paper reports our initial findings in this area. These indicate that nitrosamines are indeed photolabile under certain conditions.

MATERIALS AND METHODS

Instruments and apparatus

The photochemical apparatus consisted of a 450W Hanovia, medium pressure, mercury vapour lamp, inserted into a water-jacketed quartz immersion well. The well was placed in the centre opening of a photochemical 'merry-go-round' device, which ensured that all samples received the same amount of light. The entire apparatus was immersed in a light-shielded water-bath which was maintained thermostatically at $25 \pm 0.2\,°C$. Product quantification was carried out on a Perkin-Elmer Sigma II gas chromatograph, using a 4 mm i.d. $\times$ 6 ft (1.83 m) glass column, packed with 10% Carbowax 20M and 2% potassium hydroxide on Chromasorb WHP. The peaks were visualized using a flame-ionization detector or a nitrogen-phosphorus detector. Quantification was carried out by comparison of experimental peak areas with those obtained using standard solutions. Identification of components was carried out by gas-chromatography-mass spectrometry, using a Finnigan mass spectrometer and comparison with spectra of authentic samples.

Chemicals

Nitrosamines were prepared by standard methods. N-Formylpiperidine and N-formyldiisopropylamine were prepared in high yield by refluxing a solution of the amine in ethylformate; N-formyldiisopropylamine was a commercial sample. Diisopropylnitramine was prepared in high yield (> 90%) by oxidation of the corresponding nitrosamine with trifluoroperacetic acid. Solvents were analytical quality reagents which were dried by distillation over appropriate drying agents.

Photochemical experiments

Samples were prepared by dissolving weighed amounts of reagents in appropriate solvents in volumetric flasks. Aliquots of these solutions were placed in tubes which were degassed under vacuum ($< 10^{-5}$ torr), using at least three freeze-pump-thaw cycles, and sealed. The tubes were then placed in the photochemical apparatus for appropriate periods of time. At least one tube was set aside as a dark control. Samples were withdrawn periodically and analysed. Experiments using oxygen were carried out in solutions which were attached to the immersion well. Oxygen was slowly bubbled into the solutions during photolysis.

RESULTS

Reactions in absence of oxygen

Photolysis of N-nitrosopiperidine (NPIP) and N-nitrosodiisopropylamine (NDiPA) in degassed benzene solutions was slow. For example, the photolysis of a 10 mmol/L solution of

NPIP required 30 h for half of the nitrosamine to be consumed. Addition of methanol to the photolysis sample, however, increased the rate of photolysis markedly. Thus, the half-life of a benzene solution of NPIP was 12 h in the presence of 10% methanol, less than 4 h in the presence of 50% methanol and about 2.5 h in pure methanol. Addition of two equivalents of the antioxidant, butylated hydroxytoluene (BHT), to a degassed benzene solution of the nitrosamine, resulted in rapid photolysis (half-life < 1 h). These data are presented in Table 1.

Reactions in presence of oxygen

The photolysis of NDiPA in the presence of air or oxygen was very rapid. The data in Table 1 show that, in the presence of oxygen, the nitrosamine decayed over 300 times faster than would have been predicted for photolysis in a neutral, degassed solvent, such as benzene. Photolysis of the nitrosamine in the presence of air was a little slower than in oxygen, presumably due to the dilution factor.

Products of photolysis

The photolysis of the nitrosamines under vacuum led to the formation of the corresponding amine if a hydrogen-atom donor was present, and also to the formation of the formamide when the photolysis was carried out in methanol. The formation of N,N-diisopropylformamide from NDiPA occurred in small amounts in benzene and methanol and required oxygen, but the formation of N-formylpiperidine from NPIP required only methanol. In fact, the photolysis of NPIP in pure methanol under vacuum resulted in the formation of a 46% yield of piperidine and a 39% yield of the N-formyl derivative. The photolysis of NDiPA in air or oxygen resulted in the initial formation of diisopropylnitramine, which was also photolabile. In one experiment

Table 1. Rates of photolysis[a] of nitrosamines[b] under various conditions

Nitrosamine	Solvent[c]	Atmosphere	Initial concentration (mmol/L)	Half-life (h)	k[d] 10^7 mol/sec^{-1}	Relative rate
NPIP	Bz	vacuum	9.88	29.84	0.46	1
	Bz:Me (9:1)	vacuum	9.88	11.96	1.15	2.5
	Bz:Me (1:1)	vacuum	9.88	3.74	3.67	8.0
	Me	vacuum	10.63	2.67	5.52	12.0
			9.53	2.46	5.39	11.7
			10.12	2.49	5.64	12.2
			100.22	29.68	4.69	10.2
	Bz + BHT[e]	vacuum	9.88	<1	>13.6	~30
NDiPA	Me	air	9.57	0.46	28.89	62.8
	Me	oxygen	95.68	0.64	213	351
	Me	vacuum	9.59	2.76	4.82	10.5
	Me	vacuum	10.43	2.73	5.29	11.5

[a] Samples were contained in Pyrex tubes which block light of wavelength >290 nm
[b] NPIP, N-nitrosopiperidine; NDiPA, N-nitrosodiisopropylamine
[c] Bz, benzene; Me, methanol
[d] k, rate constants were calculated from the initial zero-order part of the reaction curves. These were generally linear for at least 50% of the reaction. $-d(N)/dt = k$, then $kt = (N_o)-(N)$, but at $t_{1/2}$, $(N) = (N_o)/2$ then $k = (N_o)/2 \cdot t_{1/2}$ where N_o = initial nitrosamine concentration. The half-lives were calculated by linear regression analysis
[e] Butylated hydroxytoluene (20 mmol/L)

(NDiPA in methanol and air), it was shown that the nitramine concentration reached a maximum (9.6%) after 15 min and declined to zero after 1 h of photolysis. Photolysis of NDiPA in benzene gave the largest amount of the nitramine (13.4% after 1 h), but that also decayed rapidly on further photolysis. Photolysis of authentic diisopropylnitramine in methanol and air led to substantially the same products as the photolysis of NDiPA in methanol and air, namely the amine and the N-formyl derivative.

DISCUSSION

The principal conclusion of this work is that N-nitrosodialkylamines are not stable to photolysis. The key question concerns the apparent slowness of photolysis in degassed solvents, such as benzene. Gowenlock et al. (1978) reported that the photolysis of N-nitrosodiethylamine in cyclohexane proceeded with a quantum yield of 0.10, which rose to 0.72 in methanol. These results are in excellent agreement with those presented here. For example, the photolysis of NPIP in methanol was 12 times faster than in benzene under the same conditions. It is also interesting to note that the initial concentration of the nitrosamines does not affect the rate of photolysis appreciably. Our data are best accounted for by the following mechanism:

$$R_2NNO \overset{h\upsilon}{\rightleftarrows} R_2N\cdot + NO$$
$$R_2N\cdot + NO + R'H \rightarrow \text{non-radical products}$$
$$2NO + O_2 \rightarrow 2NO_2$$
$$R_2N\cdot + NO_2 \rightarrow R_2NNO_2$$

$$R_2NNO_2 + R'H \overset{h\upsilon}{\rightarrow} \text{non-radical products}$$

This mechanism accounts for all observations. Photolysis of nitrosamines in degassed solvents which are not good H-atom donors is very slow because the N-N bond fission is reversible. Although the rate constant for the reverse reaction is not known, the rate would be expected to be close to diffusion-controlled. The eventual decay of the nitrosamines in those solvents is probably due to disproportionation reactions between the two radical partners. Methanol is a good H-atom donor and is thus able to scavenge at least the aminyl radical. Evidence for this is provided by the presence of the formamides in the reactions containing methanol. Formation of N-formylpiperidine during the photolysis of N-nitropiperidine in methanol has been previously noted by Chow and co-workers (1979). The possibility that the enhanced rate of photolysis of the nitrosamines in methanol was due to the hydroxyl group was negated by the finding that photolysis of NPIP in degassed solutions in benzene containing 10% or 50% of t-butyl alcohol had virtually the same rates as in benzene alone.

Photolysis of NDiPA in the presence of air or oxygen resulted in the initial formation of the nitramine. The photooxidation reaction probably occurs by initial dissociation of the nitrosamine to the aminyl radical and nitric oxide, followed by the rapid oxidation of the latter to nitrogen dioxide ($k_{H_2O} = 8.8 \times 10^6$ Lmol^{-1}S^{-1}) (Pogrebnaya et al., 1972), then combination to the nitramine. The photochemistry of nitramines has been examined by Chow et al. (1979).

The photolysis of nitrosamines is greatly enhanced by the presence of a good H-atom donor. Thus, BHT was found to be very effective in this respect. Emmett et al. (1980) had noted that ascorbic acid or ascorbate seemed to catalyse the photolysis of N-nitrosodimethylamine. Those substances are also excellent radical scavengers. The observation of the photochemical E/Z isomerization of unsymmetrical nitrosamines (Michejda et al., 1976) can be rationalized in terms of the proposed mechanism. Initial breakage of the N-N bond, followed by recombination, will lead to a photo-stationary state in which a non-thermodynamic population of the E and Z rotamers may be achieved.

CONCLUSION

N-Nitrosodialkylamines can be photolysed to non-nitrosamine products, provided that conditions are such that re-synthesis of the nitrosamines can be prevented. This can be done by the inclusion of good free-radical scavengers, such as H-atom donors or oxygen, in the photolysis solution. The understanding of the chemistry of the process may make it feasible to dispose safely of dilute nitrosamine wastes by photochemical means (Polo & Chow, 1976), provided that other criteria are also kept in mind (Emmett *et al.*, 1980).

ACKNOWLEDGEMENTS

Research sponsored by the National Cancer Institute, DHHS, under contract No. NO1-CO-23909 with Litton Bionetics, Inc. The contents of this publication do not necessarily reflect the views or policies of the Department of Health and Human Services, nor does mention of trade names, commercial products, or organizations imply endorsement by the US Government.

Tomas Rydstrom was supported by a fellowship from Arbetarskyddsfonden, Stockholm, Sweden.

REFERENCES

Chow, Y.L. (1973) Nitrosamine photochemistry: Reactions of aminium radicals. *Acc. chem. Res.*, **6**, 354–360

Chow, Y.L., Richard, H., Williams Snyder, R. & Lockhart, R.W. (1979) Generation of aminyl and aminium radicals by photolysis of *N*-nitrodialkylamines in solution. *Can. J. Chem.*, **57**, 2936–2943

Daiber, D. & Preussmann, R. (1964) Quantitative Colorimetrische Bestimmung Organischer *N*-nitroso-Verbindungen durch photochemische Spaltung der Nitrosaminbindung. *Fresenius' Z. anal. Chem.*, **206**, 344–352

Emmett, G.C., Michejda, C.J., Sansone, E.B. & Keefer, L.K. (1980) *Limitations of photodegradation in the decontamination and disposal of chemical carcinogens*. In: Walters, D.B., ed., *Safe Handling of Chemical Carcinogens, Mutagens, Teratogens and Highly Toxic Substances*, Vol. 2, Ann Arbor, MI, Ann Arbor Science Publishers, Inc., pp. 535–553

Gowenlock, B.G., Pfab, J. & Williams, G.C. (1978) Quantum yields for the photolysis of some nitrosamines in solution. *J. chem. Res.*, **(S)**, 362–363

Michejda, C.J., Davidson, N.E. & Keefer, L.K. (1976) Photochemical perturbation of Z/E equilibria in nitrosamines. *J. Chem. Soc., Chem. Commun.*, 633–634

Pogrebnaya, V.L., Usov, A.P. & Varanov, A.V. (1972) Kinetics of the oxidation of nitric oxide by oxygen in aqueous solution. *Izv.Vyssh. Vcheb. Zaved. Khim. Tekhnol.*, **15**, 1697

Polo, J. & Chow, Y.L. (1976) Efficient photolytic degradation of nitrosamines. *J. natl Cancer Inst.*, **56**, 997–1001

Sander, J. (1967) Eine Methode zum Nachweis von Nitrosaminen. *Hoppe-Seyler's Z. physiol. Chem.*, **348**, 852–854

DECOMPOSITION N-NITROSOHYDROXYALKYLUREAS AND N-NITROSOOXAZOLIDONES IN AQUEOUS BUFFER

S.S. SINGER

LBI-Basic Research Program, Chemical Carcinogenesis Program, NCI-Frederick Cancer Research Facility, Frederick, MD 21701, USA

SUMMARY

The decomposition of N-nitroso-2-hydroxyethylurea, N-nitrosooxazolidone, N-nitroso-2-hydroxypropylurea and N-nitroso-5-methyloxazolidone in pH 7.4 phosphate buffer was studied. The aldehydes and ketones formed in the decompositions were monitored through the formation of dinitrophenylhydrazine derivatives, which were then analysed by high-performance liquid chromatography. N-Nitroso-2-hydroxyethylurea gave a 25% yield of acetaldehyde dinitrophenylhydrazone, while N-nitrosooxazolidone gave only 2%. The major product from the latter is 1,3-dioxolane-2-one (ethylene carbonate); ethylene glycol is a major product from both. The other two compounds studied gave similar products, but in much lower yields.

INTRODUCTION

The closely related compounds, N-nitroso-2-hydroxyethylurea (I, NHEU), N-nitroso-oxazolidone (II, NOX), N-nitroso-2-hydroxypropylurea (III, NHPU) and N-nitroso-5-methyl-oxazolidone (IV, NMOX) (Fig. 1) are all potent carcinogens, both when tested on mouse skin and when given intragastrically to rats (Lijinsky & Reuber, 1982). In the latter instance, there were marked differences in organ specificity, with both oxazolidones giving mainly forestomach tumours. In contrast, NHEU induced a broad spectrum of tumours at many sites and NHPU induced mainly thymic leukaemias and lymphomas. Since little is known about the decomposition of these compounds, we are studying their decomposition pathways to see if mechanistic differences are related to the carcinogenic organotropic effects.

The decomposition of N-nitrosoureas (Fig. 2) is generally believed to proceed *via* the mechanism of Hecht and Kozarich (1973), with the diazo compound produced being an alkylating species which could be responsible for carcinogenic activity through alkylation of DNA. Nitrosooxazolidones also decompose *via* a diazo species, but the product would be quite different from that produced from the related urea. Hassner and Ruess (1974) studied extensively the decomposition of substituted nitrosooxazolidones in methoxide/methanol and found that the nature of the substituents (aliphatic *versus* aromatic *versus* proton) determined the reaction pathway and product distribution (Fig. 3).

Fig. 1. Structures of compounds studied: I,NHEU, *N*-nitroso-2-hydroxy-ethylurea; II,NOX, *N*-nitrosooxazolidone; III,NHPU, *N*-nitroso-2-hydroxypropylurea; IV,NMOX, *N*-nitroso-5-methyloxazolidone

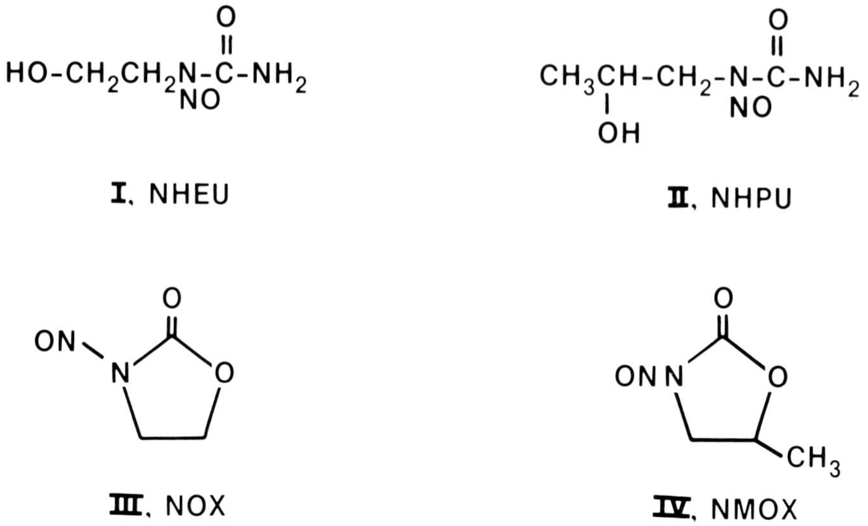

I, NHEU

II, NHPU

III, NOX

IV, NMOX

Fig. 2. Decomposition of *N*-nitrosoureas

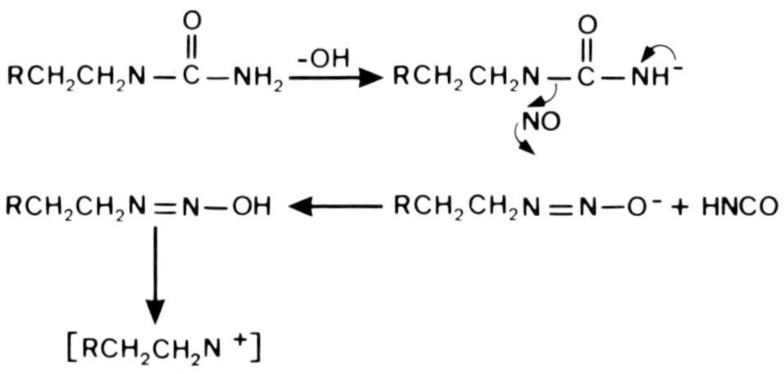

MATERIALS AND METHODS

Chemicals

Inorganic chemicals were of Fisher ACS reagent grade. Solvents for high-pressure liquid chromatography (HPLC) were from Burdick and Jackson (Muskegan, MI, USA) distilled-in-glass grade. The *N*-nitroso compounds were provided by Dr W. Lijinsky of the Frederick Cancer Research Facility (Frederick, MD, USA).

Fig. 3. Reaction pathways and product distribution of nitrosooxazolidones

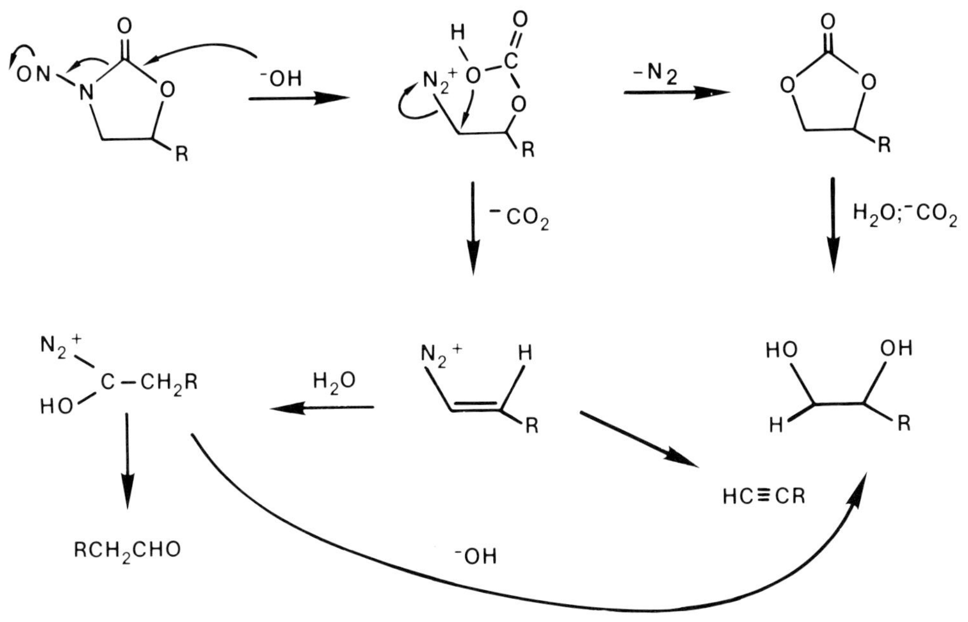

Table 1. Decomposition products from compounds tested

Compound[a]	Dinitrophenylhydrazine yield (%)			N_2[b]	Glycol	Car-bonate
	Acetal-dehyde	Acetone	Propional-dehyde			
I (NHEU)	25	$-$[c]	$-$	105	16	$-$
II (NOX)	2	$-$	$-$	92	15[d]	>60%
III (NHPU)	$-$	2.9	1.5	100	1.8	$-$
IV (NMOX)	$-$	0.2	0.1	100	22	20

[a] NHEU, N-nitroso-2-hydroxyethylurea; NOX, N-nitrosooxazolidone; NHPU, N-nitroso-2-hydroxypropylurea; NMOX, N-nitroso-5-methyloxazolidone
[b] Yield at 5 hours reaction time
[c] $-$, product not possible
[d] Under certain isolation conditions 90% yields of ethylene glycol and no carbonate will be obtained

Analyses

The dinitrophenylhydrazones (DNP) were analysed by HPLC on a Waters (Milford, MA, USA) Model 440, equipped with two 6000A pumps and a Model 660 solvent programmer. The column was an Altex (Palo Alto, CA, USA) Ultrasphere ODS, 15 cm x 4.1 mm, using 60% acetonitrile/water, 1 mL/min. Gas liquid chromatography (GLC) analyses were performed on a Tracor (Austin, TX, USA) MT220, using a 2.04 m $\times$ 2 mm glass column, packed with

Ultrabond PEGS (Ultra Scientific Corp., Hope, RI, USA), 60 mL/min He flow, programme 90° (5-min hold) to 140° at 5°/min. Decompositions: The nitrosoamide (0.3–0.4 mmol) was weighed into a 5-mL Reactivial (Wheaton Scientific) and 5 ml of pre-warmed, 1/15 mol/L, pH 7.4 phosphate buffer were added. When gas evolution was followed, the effluent gas was led into an inverted, water-filled burette. Otherwise, a condensing tube was placed on the Reactivial and the compound allowed to decompose overnight.

When decomposition was complete (the absence of starting material was shown by HPLC analysis), aldehyde and ketone formation was measured in the following manner: 200 µL reaction mixture were added to a mL DNP reagent. A yellow precipitate indicated DNP formation. The mixture was then extracted with isooctane, and the isooctane was extracted with acetonitrile, which was analysed directly by HPLC for acetaldehyde, propionaldehyde or acetone DNP, as appropriate (Table 1).

RESULTS AND DISCUSSION

Compounds I–IV were dissolved in 0.067 mol/L phosphate buffer at pH 7.4 at 37 °C. Gas evolution was rapid from the N-nitrosoureas (NHEU and NHPU) and somewhat slower for the N-nitrosooxazolidones, with NMOX decomposing at the slowest rate. In similar studies of bis-chloroethylnitrosourea by Montgomery et al. (1967), the gas evolved was found to be exclusively nitrogen, with any carbon dioxide produced remaining in the buffer. On this basis, yields of nitrogen produced by these four compounds ranged from 87–105%. In methoxide/methanol, NOX has been shown to give a 12% yield of acetylene (Newman & Kutner, 1951). We have not yet determined whether acetylenes are formed under the much milder conditions employed here, but that possibility cannot be discounted.

The decomposition products of compounds I to IV are shown in Table 1. It is clear that there are major differences in aldehyde formation among the four compounds. NHEU gave ten times as much acetaldehyde as did the corresponding oxazolidone (NOX). NHPU gave low yields of both propionaldehyde and acetone (1.5 and 2.9, respectively), but these were still slightly higher than the yields of these compounds obtained from NMOX (0.1–0.2%).

The reaction mixtures were also analysed by glc for the formation of other products. Ethylene glycol was anticipated to be the major product from both NHEU and NOX (see Fig. 3), and indeed, was formed from both. Yields of ethylene glycol from NHEU have been determined to be 16% of theoretical. The yield of glycols obtained from NOX and NMOX were in the range of 15–20%, while both compounds gave cyclic carbonates -1,3-dioxolane-2-one (ethylene carbonate) and 4-methyl-1,3-dioxolane-2-one (propylene carbonate) – as major products. Studies to quantify product formation and to improve the material balance are proceeding. Other low molecular weight products, such as acetylenes or cyclic alkane oxides or alcohols, may account for the 'missing' material, and the possible formation of polymeric compounds cannot be discounted.

At this point we do not have sufficient information to postulate a chemical mechanism to explain the differences in carcinogenic specificity of these four compounds. However, it is already clear that the nitrosoureas and the nitrosoxazolidones decompose by different mechanisms. It is of interest to note that the more chemically stable oxazolidones give rise to forestomach tumours, while the nitrosoureas, which decompose much more rapidly in buffered media, give rise to tumours at many sites in the rat. Studies are underway to determine the variation of mode and rate of decomposition with pH and other experimental conditions.

ACKNOWLEDGEMENTS

Research sponsored by the US National Cancer Institute, DHHS, under contract No. N01-CO-23909 with Litton Bionetis, Inc. The contents of this publication do not necessarily reflect the views or policies of the Department of Health and Human Services, nor does mention of trade names, commercial products, or organizations imply endorsement by the US Government.

REFERENCES

Hassner, A. & Reuss, R.H. (1974) Pathways in the base-catalyzed decomposition of cyclic *N*-nitroso carbamates. *J. org. Chem.*, **39**, 553–560

Hecht, S.M. & Kozarich, J.W. (1973) Mechanism of the base-induced decomposition of *N*-nitroso-*N*-methylurea. *J. org. chem.*, **38**, 1821–1824

Lijinsky, W. & Reuber, M.D. (1982) Carcinogenicity of the hydroxylated alkylnitrosoureas and of nitrosooxazolidones by mouse skin painting and by gavage in rats, *Cancer Res.*, **43**, 214-221

Montgomery, J.A., James, R., McCaleb, G.S. & Johnston, T.P. (1967) The modes of decomposition of 1,3-bis(2-chloroethyl)-1-nitrosourea and related compounds. *J. med. Chem.*, **10**, 668-674

Newman, M.S. & Kutner, A. (1951) New reactions involving alkaline treatment of 3-nitroso-2-oxazolidones. *J. Am. chem. Soc.*, **73**, 4199-4204

EFFECTS OF SACCHARIN AND URINE ON THE DECOMPOSITION OF N-NITROSOMETHYLUREA

C.T. MILLER[1]

Toxicology Research Division, Food Directorate, Health Protection Branch, Health and Welfare Canada, Tunney's Pasture, Ottawa, Ontario K1A OL2, Canada

SUMMARY

Addition of either saccharin or rat urine to aqueous N-methyl-N-nitrosourea (MNU) caused concentration-dependent loss of the ultraviolet absorption of MNU. The shapes of the absorption spectra of the residual MNU products were different and characteristic of either saccharin (flat-sided) or urine (symmetrical) as reaction matrix. In the presence of urine from rats fed 2.5% saccharin in the diet, the flat-sided curve characteristic of MNU-saccharin products was always observed. Further, the half-life of the MNU products in urine from saccharin-treated rats was shorter than the half-life observed in control urine, suggesting that saccharin ingestion might alter both the nature and rate of MNU decomposition *in vivo*. A molecular hypothesis for the mechanism of the MNU/saccharin interaction is proposed.

INTRODUCTION

The nitrosoureas have been found to decompose under physiological conditions, yielding methylating species and isocyanate (Magee *et al.,* 1976). The alkylating species bind to DNA, RNA and protein (Lawley & Thatcher, 1970), while the isocyanate moiety carbamoylates amino acid residues in proteins (Jump *et al.,* 1980). The possibility that carbamoylation of biological materials might contribute to the physiological effects of nitrosoureas was recognized during studies of these compounds used in cancer chemotherapy (Schmall *et al.,* 1973).

Both the alkylating and carbamoylating entities result from spontaneous decomposition of the nitrosoureas at physiological pH. Further, decomposition is susceptible to generalized base catalysis by certain buffer anions (Garrett *et al.,* 1965). For example, with N-methyl-N-nitrosonitroguanidine, the yield of nitrocyanamide was less in the presence of phosphate buffer than in the presence of Tris-HCl buffer at the same pH (Lawley & Thatcher, 1970). Thus, changes in the solute surrounding a nitrosamide could modify its biological effects with respect to either the alkylating (genetic?) or the carbamoylating (epigenetic?) potential of these 'complete' carcinogens.

---

[1] Present address: Priority Issues Directorate, Environment Canada, Hull, Québec K1A 1C4, Canada

Saccharin, although metabolically inert, has some nucleophilic character and might function as a generalized base catalyst. The present study was undertaken to determine whether saccharin could modify qualitatively or quantitatively the decomposition pathway of N-methyl-N-nitrosourea (MNU).

MATERIAL AND METHODS

Sodium saccharin (prepared by the Sherwin-Williams Co., batch 1777, drum no. 2, containing approximately 3 mg/kg organic solvent soluble impurities) was kindly supplied by Dr B. Stavric. MNU (lot 87730) was supplied by Koch and Koch Laboratories, Inc., Plainview, NY.

Spectrophotometry of saccharin/NMU reaction products

Solutions at the required concentration of saccharin were prepared in deionized water, and aliquots of 0.9 mL were pipetted into matched quartz cells in a Beckman DB-GT dual-beam spectrophotometer, with ultraviolet light source and automatic scanning and recorder. MNU was dissolved at 100 μg/mL in deionized water, and 0.1 mL was added to the test cell. The saccharin concentration in the reference cell was adjusted by addition of 0.1 mL deionized water. The ultraviolet absorption spectrum of the MNU was immediately scanned from 300 nm to 200 nm.

Spectrophotometry of urine/MNU reaction products

Fresh-voided urine samples were obtained after light ether anaesthesia from female, adult Sprague-Dawley rats maintained on standard rat chow or on rat chow supplemented with 2.5% (w/w) sodium saccharin. To determine the effect of urine solutes on MNU decomposition, the fresh urine was first diluted to provide 0.01 to 0.05 mL (as specified) per mL deionized water. Aliquots of 0.9 mL dilute urine were placed in the test and reference cells, and 0.1 mL deionized water (reference) or 0.1 mL MNU in deionized water (test) was added, and the spectrum was recorded as above.

To determine the half-life of the residual products, absorbance at a fixed wavelength was recorded over time. A plot of log absorbance *versus* time was approximately linear, indicating first-order exponential decay. The half-life was estimated from $\log A_t = A_o - kt$.

Mutagenicity testing

Salmonella typhimurium strain TA1535 was grown overnight in broth culture, as described by Ames *et al.* (1973). The bacteria from aliquots of 0.8 mL broth culture were sedimented by centrifugation at 2 000 g for 5 min, washed in phosphate-buffered saline (PBS, pH 7.4) and resuspended in 0.8 mL PBS, or in 0.8 mL filter-sterilized urine adjusted to pH 7.4 with mol/L potassium hydroxide, with and without added saccharin. The bacterial suspensions were treated with 0.2 mL of the appropriate dilution of MNU in sterile deionized water, and allowed to react for 10 min at 24 °C. The bacteria were then pelleted at 2 000 g and resuspended in 1.0 mL PBS. Treated bacteria (0.1 mL) were pipetted into top agar containing restrictive histidine and biotin, and plated. All assays were performed in triplicate. Colonies were counted after 48 h.

Samples of urine-treated and PBS-treated bacteria (without MNU) were diluted serially and were plated onto complete nutrient agar to estimate the effect of urine on survival.

RESULTS

The ultraviolet absorption spectra of MNU in deionized water (pH 5.5) and in saccharin solutions in deionized water were recorded. With each increase in saccharin concentration between 0.005% and 0.02%, there was progressive loss of absorption at wavelengths below 232 nm, giving rise to a flat-sided curve, without loss of absorption at the wavelength of maximum absorption ($\lambda_{max} = 232$ nm). Further increase in the concentration of saccharin was associated with decomposition of the residual absorbing moiety. The saccharin-dependent loss of absorption of MNU was identical when PBS at pH 7.4 was substituted for deionized water at pH 5.5 (Fig. 1). This interaction between saccharin and MNU took place within the 2 to 3 sec required to add MNU to the saccharin solution and activate the spectrophotometer.

Decomposition of MNU was also catalysed by diluted rat urine. With increasing amounts of rat urine added to the reaction mixture, the maximum absorption due to MNU (A_{max}) decreased steadily, and the position of λ_{max} shifted to higher wavelengths. The flat-sided curve characteristic of saccharin-MNU solutions did not occur.

Figure 2 shows a comparison of the absorption spectra of MNU in deionized water (dashed lines) and after addition of 0.02 volumes of urine from control rats (Fig. 2A) and rats fed 2.5% saccharin in the diet (Fig. 2B). The absolute amount of MNU decomposition induced by the urine varied somewhat between animals. However, all of the urine from saccharin-fed rats induced the flat-sided curve characteristic of a saccharin/MNU interaction, while all of the control urines gave symmetrical curves, with a shift in λ_{max} proportional to the loss of A_{max}.

Fig. 1. Effect of saccharin on decomposition of *N*-methyl-*N*-nitrosourea (MNU). The relative ultraviolet absorbance due to MNU (10 mg/L reaction mixture),

$$A_{rel} = \frac{A(+saccharin)}{A(-saccharin)}$$

is plotted against saccharin concentration. A_{rel} for MNU was measured for reactions in deionized water, at 240 nm (●); and for reactions in phosphate-buffered saline pH 7.4 at 240 nm (+)

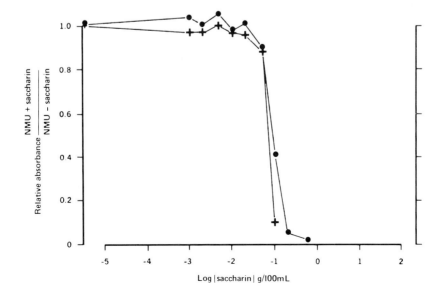

The interaction described above occurred essentially instantaneously. However, the residual absorbing products were themselves unstable. After the initial reaction, the residual absorption decayed with time, without further shift in the position of λ_{max}. The half-life of the residual MNU products for each concentration of urine from control of saccharin-fed rats, assuming exponential decay, is presented in Figure 3. The residual ultraviolet-absorbing MNU products in the presence of urine from saccharin-fed rats were less stable than those in urine from control animals. Dilution of urine was necessary because the rate of reaction without dilution was too fast to be measurable by this technique.

In order to provide initial characterization of the biological impact of MNU reaction in the presence of saccharin, the ability of reaction mixtures to revert *S. typhimurium* TA1535 was assessed. Human urine (without dilution) effectively reduced the mutagenicity of MNU relative to that of the PBS control (Table 1). The addition of saccharin caused a further concentration-dependent *decrease* in the mutagenicity (revertants per plate) of 100 μg/mL MNU.

The estimated survival was 7.5×10^7 colonies per plate after treatment with PBS alone, and 7.2×10^7 colonies per plate after treatment with human urine alone. Thus, the urine is not itself sufficiently toxic to reduce the number of viable bacteria exposed to the MNU.

Rat urine negated the mutagenicity even more effectively than human urine (Table 2). After dilution of the urine by one-half, the mutagenicity of MNU still could not be detected.

Fig. 2. Effect of saccharin exposure *in vivo* on the decomposition of *N*-methyl-*N*-nitrosourea (MNU) in rat urine. Reaction mixture contained MNU (10 mg/L) and 0 or 0.02 mL rat urine per ml mixture. Ultraviolet absorption spectra were recorded immediately after mixing; ———, MNU absorption spectrum in deionized water; A, MNU absorption spectra in dilute urine from 3 different control rats; B, MNU absorption spectra in dilute urine from 4 rats fed 2.5 L% saccharin in the diet

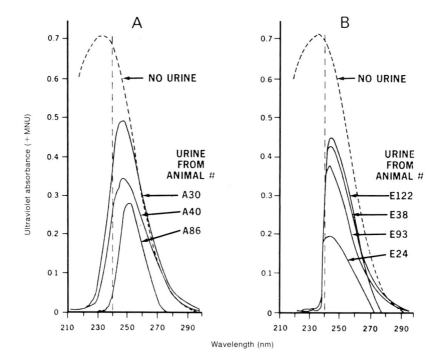

Fig. 3. Rate of decomposition of residual *N*-methyl-*N*-nitrosourea (MNU) products in dilute urine from control and saccharin-fed rats. The half-life $(t_{1/2})$ of MNU was estimated, assuming exponential decay of absorbance at λ_{max}, in the presence of the urine concentrations shown; ●, urine from control rats; +, urine from rats fed 2.5% saccharin in the diet

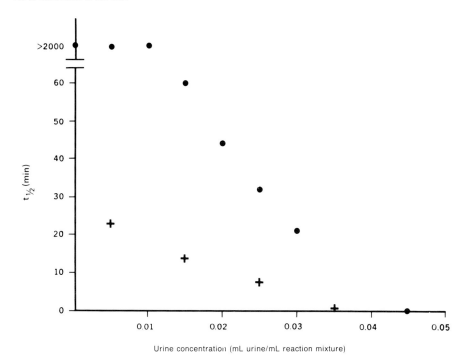

Urine concentration (mL urine/mL reaction mixture)

Table 1.   Solute effects on MNU mutagenicity: human urine ± saccharin

MNU (μg/mL)	MNU in buffer, pH 7.4	MNU in human urine, pH 7.4 ± saccharin		
	Saccharin added (g/100 mL)			
	0	0.01	0.1	1
	TA1535 revertants per plate (mean of triplicates)			
0	7	11	14	9	4
10	7	10	14	10	8
50	47	14	14	9	11
100	621	90	56	44	28

However, in the presence of 1% (10 g/L) saccharin added to urine, the number of revertant colonies tripled. After further dilution of the urine to one-quarter, the mutagenicity of MNU could be detected, and the number of revertants *increased* after addition of saccharin.

Table 2.   Solute effects on MNU mutagenicity: rat urine±saccharin[a]

Rat urine pH 7.4	Saccharin added (g/100 mL)				
	0	0.001	0.01	0.1	1
	TA1535 revertants[a] per plate (mean of triplicates)				
Undiluted	27	17	27	26	33
Diluted 1:2	30	44	41	55	90
Diluted 1:4	115	NT	NT	166	182

NT, not tested
[a] All reaction mixtures contained 100 µg/mL MNU

DISCUSSION

Assessment of the ultraviolet absorption spectra of MNU and its products indicated an effect on MNU decomposition by both saccharin and urine. The ultraviolet-absorbing products from MNU in the presence of saccharin were characterized by a peculiar flat-sided spectrum. Further, the saccharin/MNU products decomposed faster than urine/MNU products. Thus, the presence of saccharin in urine altered the pathway and the rate of MNU decomposition.

It was proposed (Cram & Hammond, 1964) that the base-catalysed hydrolysis of N-nitroso-N-alkylamides actually occurred *via* the diazoesters that are tautomers of the nitrosamides. More recent work has shown that N-nitroso-N-alkylamides undergo competitive reaction at the nitroso nitrogen and the carbonyl carbon, with production of either isocyanate or an ester. The competition is sensitive to the alkyl group, the group attached to the carbonyl carbon atom, the solvent and the nature of the base (Magee *et al.*, 1976). Either formation of the diazoalkane or formation of carbonium ion products may follow. The pathways for hydrolysis of N-nitrosoalkylureas are summarized below.

It is proposed that saccharin alters the nitrosamide/diazoester tautomerism. Such a tautomeric shift is consistent with the spectral changes observed. This 'solute' effect of saccharin could alter the proportions of isocyanate and ester produced and alter the extent of inactivation through denitrosation or the extent of carbamoylation. Although the present work demonstrates both qualitative and quantitative effects of saccharin on MNU decomposition, the chemical identity of the reaction products remains to be demonstrated.

The preliminary mutagenicity testing reported here is based on only one rat urine sample and one human urine sample, and it would be premature to assume a real species difference in the urine/MNU/saccharin interaction. However, the data do serve to emphasize the sensitivity of MNU-induced effects to changes in the surrounding solute. The potential effects of saccharin on naturally-occurring nitroso compounds might be worthy at least of consideration as a possible mechanism underlying the 'epigenetic' carcinogenicity of saccharin (Ashby *et al.*, 1978).

REFERENCES

Ames, B.N., Darston, W., Yamasaki, E. & Lee, F. (1973) Carcinogens are mutagens: a simple test system combining liver homogenates for activation and bacteria for detection. *Proc. natl. Acad. Sci.*, USA, **70**, 2281–2285

Ashby, J., Styles, J.A., Anderson, D. & Paton, D. (1978) Saccharin: an epigenetic carcinogen/mutagen? *Food Cosmet. Toxicol.*, **16**, 95–103

Cram, D.S. & Hammond, G.S. (1964) *Nucleophilic substitution at saturated carbon.* In: *Organic Chemistry,* McGraw-Hill, p. 252

Garrett, E.R., Goto, S. & Stubbins, J.F. (1965) Kinetics of solvolyses of various N-alkyl-N-nitrosoureas in neutral and alkaline solutions. *J. pharm. Sci., 54,* 119–123

Jump, D.B., Sudhakar, S., Tew, K.D. & Smulson, M. (1980) Probes to study the effect of methylnitrosourea on ADP-ribosylation and chromatin structure at the subunit level. *Chem.-biol. Interact., 30,* 35–51

Lawley, P.D. & Thatcher, C.J. (1970) Methylation or deoxyribonucleic acid in cultured mammalian cells by N-methyl-N'-nitro-N-nitrosoguanidine. *Biochem. J., 116,* 693–707

Magee, P.N., Montesano, R. & Preussmann, R. (1976) *N-Nitroso compounds and related carcinogens.* In: Searle, C.E., ed, *Chemical Carcinogens (Am. chem. Soc. Monogr. 173),* Washington DC, pp. 491–625

Schmall, B., Cheng, C.J., Fujimura, S. & Gersten, N. (1973) Modification of proteins by 1-(2-chloroethyl)-3-cyclo-hexyl-1-nitrosourea (NSC-79037) *in vitro. Cancer Res., 33,* 1921–1924

SAFE DESTRUCTION

DESTRUCTION OF CARCINOGENIC AND MUTAGENIC
N-NITROSAMIDES IN LABORATORY WASTES

G. LUNN & E.B. SANSONE[1]

Environmental Control and Research Program

A.W. ANDREWS

*Microbial Mutagenesis Laboratory, Program Resources, Inc.,
NCI-Frederick Cancer Research Facility, Frederick, MD 21701, USA*

M. CASTEGNARO, C. MALAVEILLE, J. MICHELON & I. BROUET

*Unit of Environmental Carcinogens and Host Factors, Division of Environmental Carcinogenesis,
International Agency for Research On Cancer, Lyon, France*

L.K. KEEFER

*Laboratory of Comparative Carcinogenesis, Division of Cancer Etiology,
National Cancer Institute, Frederick, MD 21701, USA*

SUMMARY

The chemical degradation of five N-nitrosamides used widely for the experimental induction of cancer has been studied with the goal of identifying, and experimentally validating, reliable methods that can be recommended for the destruction of carcinogenic N-nitrosoureas and related compounds in laboratory wastes. Although data are not yet complete, preliminary evidence indicates that none of the five methods studied thus far is ideal for hazard-control purposes. Decomposition with 1 mol/L potassium hydroxide solution destroyed the N-nitrosamides, but generated diazoalkanes, which are carcinogenic, toxic and potentially explosive. Treatment with strong acid in the presence of sulfamic acid or iron filings completely decomposed all N-nitrosamides without forming diazoalkanes, but failed in the presence of solvents which were immiscible with water. Cleavage with hydrogen bromide in glacial acetic acid proceeded to a point of maximum degradation, following which gradual reformation of the N-nitrosamide was observed; this resynthesis could be avoided by carefully bubbling nitrogen through the reaction mixture, but degradation was slow or failed completely in the presence of hydroxylic solvents. Permanganate oxidation was effective in sulfuric acid solution,

[1] To whom correspondence should be addressed

but was incomplete when an alcohol or dimethyl sulfoxide was present. *Salmonella typhimurium* tester strains TA1535, TA1530 and TA100, which detect base-pair substitutions in DNA, detected mutagenic degradation products in each of the destruction methods, with the exception of the hydrobromic acid/acetic acid procedure.

INTRODUCTION

N-Nitrosamides are widely used in research laboratories for the experimental induction of tumours (IARC, 1974a, 1978). In addition to hazards associated with their carcinogenicity and mutagenicity, some of these compounds can detonate on storage (Sparrow, 1973). Reliable methods for the safe destruction of these substances and their residues are therefore needed.

An experimental comparison of five methods for the destruction of *N*-nitrosamides has been carried out. The *N*-nitrosamides considered were *N*-methyl-*N*-nitrosourea (MNU), *N*-ethyl-*N*-nitrosourea (ENU), *N*-methyl-*N'*-nitro-*N*-nitrosoguanidine (MNNG), *N*-methyl-*N*-nitrosourethane (MNUT) and *N*-ethyl-*N*-nitrosourethane (ENUT). The results are reported here.

Preliminary considerations

One well-known method for the degradation of *N*-nitrosamides is the action of a strong base. Unfortunately, the concomitant generation of the toxic (Bachmann & Struve, 1942; Redemann *et al.*, 1955), explosive (de Boer & Backer, 1963) and carcinogenic (IARC, 1974b) diazoalkanes (Scheme 1) constitutes a disadvantage and can make this approach unacceptable for waste disposal. We found, however, that decomposition of *N*-nitrosamides with acid (Preussmann & Schaper-Druckrey, 1972) does not generate diazoalkanes. We first tried acid treatment alone. Initial experiments

$$
RCHN_2 \xleftarrow[-HOY]{OH^-} \overset{\overset{\textstyle NO}{|}}{Y-N-CH_2R} \xrightleftharpoons{H^+X^-} \overset{\overset{\textstyle H}{}}{Y-N-CH_2R} + XNO
$$

Scheme 1

using solutions that were 3 mol/L in hydrochloric acid showed that, although the *N*-nitrosamides were largely destroyed, traces were found in the reaction mixtures. This was consistent with the equilibrium process shown in Scheme 1 and suggested that destruction or removal of the *N*-nitrosating species would drive the reaction to the right and completely destroy the *N*-nitrosamide. Accordingly, we investigated three methods (A, B, C) using acid, and explored a fourth method, D, which used a strong oxidizing agent. For purposes of comparison, base decomposition (Method E) was also studied, verifying that the *N*-nitrosamide was destroyed and providing quantitative data on the concomitant production of diazoalkanes.

N-Nitrosamides are known to be mutagens in the Ames *Salmonella*/mammalian-microsome mutagenicity assay (Lijinsky & Andrews, 1979). This test was used to determine the presence of the test chemicals and/or mutagenic products of their decomposition after completion of each of the destruction methods.

Methods studied

A. Hydrochloric acid with sulfamic acid: Sulfamic acid is an effective nitrite trap (Carson, 1951).

B. Hydrochloric acid with iron filings: We postulated that the reducing action of an iron/acid mixture (Fieser & Fieser, 1967) would completely destroy any *N*-nitrosating intermediate.

C. Hydrobromic acid in acetic acid: This has been used for efficient cleavage of *N*-nitroso compounds (Eisenbrand & Preussmann, 1970). In this case, we planned to remove the *N*-nitrosating species by flushing the solution with nitrogen (Downes *et al.*, 1976) or by means of chemical scavengers.

D. Potassium permanganate/sulfuric acid: This reagent is known to oxidize many organic compounds (Mellor, 1932).

E. Potassium hydroxide: Many *N*-nitrosamides have been shown to decompose under alkaline conditions with generation of diazoalkanes (Fieser & Fieser, 1967).

MATERIAL AND METHODS

MNNG was obtained from the Aldrich Chemical Co. (Milwaukee, WI, USA), MNU and ENU were obtained from Sigma Chemical Co. (St Louis, MO, USA) and ENUT was obtained from Pfaltz and Bauer (Stamford, CT, USA). MNUT was supplied by Dr J. Saavedra.

Analysis for unreacted N-nitrosamides

Reaction mixtures were analysed for residual *N*-nitrosamides by high-pressure liquid chromatography (Milton Roy mini-pump, Riviera Beach, FL, USA) with the UV absorption detector set at 254 nm. The detector was a Gilford 240 UV/VIS spectrophotometer (Gilford Instruments, Oberlin, OH, USA) fitted with an 8 µL flow cell (Hellma Cells, Jamaica, NY, USA). A 25 cm Spherisorb ODS column of 4.6 mm i.d. (Supelco, Bellefonte, PA, USA) was used with 20:80 (v/v) methanol:water as eluant for MNU, ENU and MNNG, and with 60:40 methanol:water for MNUT and ENUT. The injector loop volume was 100 µL. The *N*-nitrosamides were quantified using a constant injection volume and integrating the area of the peaks obtained, using a Columbia Supergrator-3 computing integrator (Columbia Scientific Industries, Austin, TX, USA). Elution times at a flow rate of 0.84 mL/min in this system were 7.8 min for MNU, 7.3 min for MNUT, 11.3 min for MNNG, 15.8 min for ENU and 8.3 min for ENUT.

Analysis for diazoalkanes

The reaction mixture was swept continuously with nitrogen ($\simeq$ 50 mL/min) for 2 h into diethyl ether containing butyric acid. After neutralization by washing with saturated sodium bicarbonate solution, gas chromatography was used to measure the amount of methyl or ethyl butyrate present, as an index of the amount of diazomethane or diazoethane generated. A Hewlett-Packard 5830A gas chromatograph, fitted with a 1.8 m x 2 mm i.d. silanized glass column, flame-ionization detector and a computing integrator, was used with *n*-butanol or 2-ethoxyethanol as internal standards. The column was packed with 28% Penwalt 223 + 4% potassium hydroxide on 80/100 Gas Chrom R. Approximate retention times with a flow rate of 43 mL/min of nitrogen carrier gas were: methyl butyrate, 4 min; ethyl butyrate, 7 min.

Mutagenicity testing

The mutagenicity tests were conducted using tester strains TA1535, TA1530 and TA100 in the plate incorporation assay. The tests were performed for destruction methods A, B and E as recommended by Ames *et al.* (1975), with the modifications of Andrews *et al.* (1978).

Aliquots of 0.1 mL from the coded samples (approximately 1.5 mg of test compound) were tested with and without the addition of liver homogenate from Aroclor-1254-pretreated male Sprague-Dawley rats (S9), at a concentration of 3 mg of protein per plate. The tests for destruction methods C and D were also performed as recommended by Ames *et al.* (1975), with 60 min preincubation at 37 °C before the addition of soft agar. Aliquots of test compound (0.1 mL, see below) were assayed with and without liver S9 (100 µL/plate) from Aroclore-1254-treated female BD VI rats. For the hydrochloric acid/sulfamic acid method (A) and the hydrochloric acid/iron filings method (B), the test samples were neutralized with solid sodium bicarbonate before testing. For the hydrogen bromide method (C), test samples were basified with sodium hydroxide solution, extracted with dichloromethane, evaporated to dryness under reduced pressure and dissolved in dimethyl sulfoxide (DMSO). Tests were also performed directly using the reaction mixture flushed with nitrogen and neutralized with sodium hydroxide. With the potassium permanganate/sulfuric acid method (D), test samples were treated with ascorbic acid to destroy excess permanganate, basified with sodium hydroxide solution to pH 13-14, cooled, centrifuged and adjusted to pH 7 with hydrochloric acid. For the potassium hydroxide method (E), each test solution was neutralized by the addition of 5 mL glacial acetic acid per 100 mL test sample volume. Plates were incubated for 48 h at 37 °C, and revertant colonies were counted using a hand-held tally. The number of revertants above the spontaneous background considered to be significant was set at greater than twice the mean value of the "cells only" and "cells plus solvent" controls.

Warning

N-Nitrosamides are carcinogenic, may be explosive and should be handled with care. Appropriate protective equipment should be used and manipulations should be performed under a properly-functioning fume hood. Hydrochloric acid, sulfuric acid and hydrogen bromide in acetic acid are corrosive. Diluting hydrochloric and sulfuric acids with water and mixing 6 mol/L hydrochloric acid with other solvents are highly exothermic processes. Appropriate protective clothing should be worn at all times. Flushing with nitrogen generates toxic vapours and should be carried out only under an operating fume hood. Reactions involving diazoalkane generation should be performed only under a fume hood with smooth glass and plastic or rubber apparatus, behind a safety shield (de Boer & Backer, 1963).

RESULTS

Methods A and B. Hydrochloric acid/sulfamic acid; hydrochloric acid/iron filings

A solution of the *N*-nitrosamide in methanol, ethanol, acetone or DMSO (about 30 g/L) was mixed with an equal volume of 6 mol/L hydrochloric acid. To every litre of this solution, 35 g of sulfamic acid (A) or iron filings (B) were added, and the reaction mixture was stirred overnight. No *N*-nitrosamide (limit of detection, 0.5% of the starting material) and no diazoalkane was found (limit of detection, 0.3% of the theoretical yield); however, large quantities of unreacted *N*-nitrosamides were found when dichloromethane was used as solvent.

These two methods were studied collaboratively (Castegnaro *et al.*, 1983c) and, although traces of unreacted *N*-nitrosamides were detected occasionally, the methods were found to be at least 99% efficient in all cases.

Method C. Hydrobromic acid in acetic acid

While quick denitrosation was obtained using this reagent, there was a tendency for reformation of the *N*-nitrosamides on standing, as illustrated in Figure 1. The following

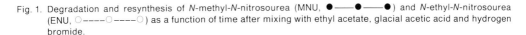

Fig. 1. Degradation and resynthesis of N-methyl-N-nitrosourea (MNU, ●——●——●) and N-ethyl-N-nitrosourea (ENU, ○----○----○) as a function of time after mixing with ethyl acetate, glacial acetic acid and hydrogen bromide.

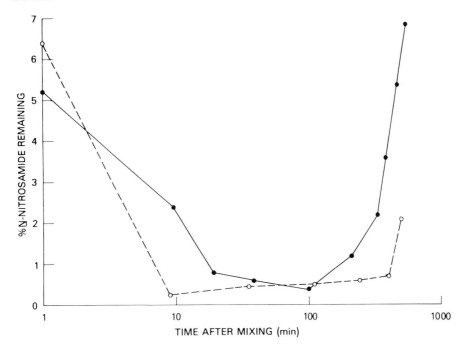

conditions were used: 100 mg MNU or ENU were taken up in 2 mL ethyl acetate, then 5 mL hydrogen bromide (30 g/L in glacial acetic acid) were added. Aliquots were removed and analysed at various times.

Ethanol and methanol, added to the ethyl acetate solution of the N-nitrosamide, were both found to reduce drastically the rate of denitrosation. Up to eight hours were necessary to degrade 99.5% of the N-nitrosamide in the presence of 20% ethanol or methanol.

It was also crucial to exclude water from the reaction mixture. When one volume of water was deliberately added to four volumes of reaction mixture 15 to 30 min after mixing the N-nitrosoureas with hydrogen bromide/acetic acid, up to 19% MNU and 13% ENU were detected. Since the reaction mixtures contained less than 1% residual N-nitrosamide (Fig. 1) immediately before adding the water, we conclude that addition of water caused extensive reformation of N-nitrosamide. It seems possible that gradual absorption of water from the air was responsible for the resynthesis, noted in Figure 1, following the time of maximum degradation of the N-nitrosoureas.

Various scavengers (e.g., ascorbic acid, potassium iodide, sulfamic acid) of the nitrosonium ion (NO^+) were tested, but their action was greatly limited by their insolubility in the medium; even addition of ascorbyl palmitate, which was soluble, did not improve the degradation.

We found, however, that flushing the reaction medium thoroughly with nitrogen permitted complete degradation, presumably by removing the nitrosyl bromide liberated, thus preventing the reformation of the N-nitrosamide. In one experiment, for example, when the reaction mixture was diluted with an equal volume of water 30 min after mixing the MNU with hydrogen bromide/acetic acid, it was found that 6% of the starting amount of MNU was present. In an otherwise identical experiment in which a 30-min flush with nitrogen (using a sintered-glass bubbling tube) was begun 30 min after mixing the N-nitrosamide with the hydrogen bromide/acetic acid, no MNU was seen (limit of detection, 0.05% in this case) after water addition.

The most complete inactivation was obtained when 100 mg of the N-nitrosamide in 2 mL ethyl acetate or dichloromethane were allowed to react with 10 mL hydrogen bromide (30 g/L in glacial acetic acid). After 30 min, the reaction was flushed with nitrogen for 30 min (about 180 mL/min), using a sintered-glass bubbling tube. For ethanol solutions, a modified procedure was used: 25 mg MNNG in 1.5 mL ethanol were allowed to react with 17 mL hydrogen bromide (30 g/L in glacial acetic acid) for 18 h before being flushed with nitrogen, as above. For all cases in which thorough nitrogen flushing was carried out, no N-nitrosamide was detected in the final mixture after quenching with water (detection limit, 0.5%). However, when flushing was conducted as above, but with a plain glass tube rather than a fritted-glass bubbler, unreacted N-nitrosamide was detected.

Method C was also tested during the collaborative study (Castegnaro et al., 1983c). Although traces of unreacted N-nitrosamide were detected occasionally, the method was found to be at least 99.5% efficient in all cases, provided that thorough nitrogen flushing was used.

Method D. Oxidation by potassium permanganate/sulfuric acid

To 100 mg N-nitrosamide, 10 mL of a 3 mol/L sulfuric acid solution were added, plus enough potassium permanganate to make the medium 0.3 mol/L in permanganate. The mixture was shaken vigorously. Aliquots taken at 5, 15 and 25 min after permanganate addition were treated with ascorbic acid to destroy the excess oxidizing agent and analysed directly by high-pressure liquid chromatography. No N-nitrosamide was found in any reaction mixture (detection limit, 0.01% of the starting material), except in the case of ENU, where 0.03% of the N-nitrosamide remained undegraded after 5 min of reaction.

Control experiments carried out in sulfuric acid solution (without permanganate) showed that degradation is not as effective in the absence of the oxidizer; after 2.5 h, 95.9% of the MNU, 97.9% of the MNNG and 99.9% of the ENU was destroyed, compared to >99.99% in the presence of permanganate.

The effect of methanol, ethanol and DMSO was tested by replacing the 10 mL of 3 mol/L aqueous sulfuric acid solution used above with 10 mL of 20% methanol, ethanol or DMSO, 3 mol/L in sulfuric acid. In some cases, detectable N-nitrosamide (up to 0.5%) remained undegraded after 25 min of reaction.

Method E. Destruction by potassium hydroxide

Each N-nitrosamide (30 mg per mL methanol) was treated with an equal volume of 1 mol/L potassium hydroxide solution. All N-nitrosamides were destroyed completely under these conditions (limit of detection, 0.5% of the starting material). However, diazoalkanes were detected as products in all reactions studied. The diazoalkane yields (percentage of the theoretical maximum) from the various N-nitrosamides were MNUT, 14%; ENUT, 0.06%; MNU, 19%; ENU, 1%; MNNG, 33%.

Mutagenicity testing

The data obtained with TA1535 and TA100 are shown in Tables 1-5. Those obtained with TA1530 agreed with those obtained with TA1535, except as noted below. When Method A was used, the destruction products of MNU and ENU were not mutagenic in TA1535 or TA100; however, the top layer of the reacted MNNG-acetone solution contained a direct-acting

Table 1. Number of revertants induced by products of destruction-method A (hydrochloric acid/sulfamic acid)

Test Compound	Solvent	TA1535		TA100	
		− S9	+ S9	− S9	+ S9
None	cells only	15	17	128	102
	methanol	15	15	104	107
	ethanol	15	18	117	92
	acetone T[a]	14	14	118	95
	B[b]	17	20	114	90
	DMSO	15	13	133	91
MNU	methanol	22	20	119	92
	ethanol	17	30	105	91
	acetone T	17	24	133	95
	B	23	22	132	107
	DMSO	14	28	136	92
ENU	methanol	10	27	120	107
	ethanol	12	16	125	113
	acetone T	12	11	136	88
	B	12	22	141	96
	DMSO	19	17	109	85
MNNG	methanol	14	14	141	81
	ethanol	19	26	124	94
	acetone T	<u>32</u>[c]	34	<u>536</u>	115
	B	11	15	<u>140</u>	109
	DMSO	20	12	137	113
MNUT	methanol	26	24	149	125
	ethanol	21	30	154	108
	acetone T	32	29	346	132
	B	<u>12</u>	18	<u>286</u>	145
	DMSO	18	19	<u>113</u>	101
ENUT	methanol	<u>120</u>	<u>175</u>	175	117
	ethanol	<u>70</u>	<u>139</u>	201	158
	acetone T	<u>110</u>	<u>41</u>	335	120
	B	<u>22</u>	<u>14</u>	<u>263</u>	122
	DMSO	<u>124</u>	26	<u>358</u>	93

[a] T = Top layer
[b] B = Bottom layer
[c] Underlining of numbers indicates that the number of revertants is significant

mutagen which was detected by both tester strains, and both the top and bottom layers of the MNUT acetone solution were mutagenic, without the addition of a metabolic activation system, in strain TA100, but only the top layer was mutagenic in TA1535. All test samples of ENUT contained mutagens. The methanol and ethanol test samples were not mutagenic in TA100, but were mutagenic, with and without metabolic activation in TA1535. The top layer from the acetone mixture was direct-acting in both strains, while the bottom layer was direct-acting only in TA100. Mutagenic activity was observed without activation in the presence of the DMSO solution.

With Method B, the acetone solution gave varied mutagenic response: with MNU, only the top layer was mutagenic and required metabolic activation; the ENU-acetone top layer

Table 2. Number of revertants induced by products of destruction-method B (hydrochloric acid/iron filings)

Test Compound	Solvent	TA1535		TA100	
		− S9	+ S9	− S9	+ S9
None	cells only	15	17	128	102
	methanol	19	14	192	107
	ethanol	14	17	166	140
	acetone T[a]	14	15	213	131
	B[b]	13	15	213	131
	DMSO	8	16	106	150
MNU	methanol	18	28	218	212
	ethanol	18	13	Tx	161
	acetone T	Tx[c]	10	149	<u>946</u>[d]
	B	9	18	202	<u>140</u>
	DMSO	2	18	157	135
ENU	methanol	16	26	191	110
	ethanol	5	14	Tx	110
	acetone T	Tx	450	Tx	2 306
	B	17	<u>10</u>	<u>493</u>	<u>136</u>
	DMSO	14	22	99	169
MNNG	methanol	<u>58</u>	<u>34</u>	61	152
	ethanol	<u>18</u>	20	140	157
	acetone T	68	377	1 233	3 712
	B	<u>14</u>	<u>12</u>	<u>137</u>	<u>135</u>
	DMSO	2	13	135	157
MNUT	methanol	15	28	180	213
	ethanol	2	26	137	142
	acetone T	160	<u>44</u>	178	100
	B	<u>18</u>	<u>15</u>	173	125
	DMSO	8	16	162	191
ENUT	methanol	16	29	158	274
	ethanol	20	14	149	143
	acetone T	<u>30</u>	16	165	124
	B	<u>10</u>	19	144	134
	DMSO	10	12	197	185

[a] T = Top layer
[b] B = Bottom layer
[c] Tx = Test sample is toxic to bacteria
[d] Underlining of numbers indicates that the number of revertants is significant

contained a potent mutagen, and the addition of a metabolic activation system detoxified the test sample; the bottom layer was direct-acting only in TA100. The MNNG-methanol product was mutagenic with and without metabolic activation only in strain TA1435. The top acetone layer, and not the bottom layer, was a potent direct-acting mutagen in both strains. The reaction product in the MNUT-acetone top layer gave the only mutagenic response of the test samples of MNUT: it was direct-acting only in strain TA1535 and was slightly inactivated by the addition of the metabolic activation system. The ENUT destruction mixtures were essentially not mutagenic; a direct result in TA1535 without activation was marginal.

When Method C was used, no mutagenicity was seen in either tester strain with any of the extracts. However, when reaction mixtures were tested directly, significant levels of

Table 3. Number of revertants induced by products of destruction-method C (hydrobromic acid in acetic acid)

Test Compound	TA1535		TA100	
	− S9	+ S9	− S9	+ S9
MNU (2.5)[a]	13	22	84	91
Control	13	22	82	91
ENU (1.2)	14	21	91	94
Control	14	21	91	94
MNNG (1.2)	5	10	75	101
Control	5	10	67	101
MNUT (2.5)	18	22	103	91
Control	13	22	82	91
ENUT (2.5)	14	21	91	94
Control	14	21	91	94

[a] The values in parentheses indicate the amount of the compound (in mg/plate) before decomposition

Table 4. Number of revertants induced by products of destruction-method D (potassium permanganate/sulfuric acid)

Test Compound	TA1535		TA100	
	− S9	+ S9	− S9	+ S9
MNU (1.2)[a]	Tx[b]	1 226[c]	Tx	119
Control	17	21	105	113
ENU (1.2)	Tx	1 200	Tx	113
Control	17	21	105	113
MNNG (1.1)	Tx	12	Tx	105
Control	9	12	68	105
MNUT (1.07)	Tx	2 466	100	109
Control	17	21	100	109
ENUT (0.7)	Tx	2 048	Tx	117
Control	17	21	100	109

[a] The values in parentheses indicate the amount of the compound, in mg/plate, before decomposition
[b] Test sample is toxic to bacteria
[c] Underlining of numbers indicates that the number of revertants is significant

mutagenicity were detected in strain TA1530 after degradation of MNU. None of the other residues was mutagenic in either strain.

With Method D, only strain TA1535 gave mutagenic responses. The MNU test sample was toxic without metabolic activation and was a potent mutagen with activation. ENU, MNUT and ENUT were all potent mutagens, with or without activation. None of the MNNG test

Table 5. Number of revertants induced by products of destruction-method E (potassium hydroxide)

Test Compound	TA1535		TA100	
	− S9	+ S9	− S9	+ S9
None	18	20	111	114
Blank	19	18	94	101
MNU	22	24	127	109
ENU	19	27	105	109
MNNG	> 10⁴	609 [a]	> 10⁴	769
MNUT	17	33	115	124
ENUT	26	28	125	133

[a] Underlining of numbers indicates that the number of revertants is significant

samples was mutagenic in either strain. However, when the oxidant: N-nitrosamide ratio was doubled and the reaction allowed to proceed overnight, no mutagenic effect was detected in either strain.

With Method E, only MNNG provoked a potent mutagenic response, with or without activation in both strains.

DISCUSSION

While the above results show that all five methods lead to extensive degradation of the N-nitrosamides studied, each procedure had identifiable limitations, and none appeared to be ideal for every application. Moreover, we have not tested any of these methods systematically under the wide variety of conditions (different concentrations, presence of possible inhibitors, etc.) that might be encountered in the laboratory, so that any general conclusion must be regarded as provisional at this point.

It should also be emphasized that comprehensive data concerning the identities and amounts of products generated in these procedures are not yet available. Such information is crucial for selecting a destruction method for hazard control purposes, because it could be dangerous to use a method which rapidly and quantitatively consumes the starting material but converts it to final products that are themselves carcinogenic or otherwise potentially hazardous. Thus, we cannot recommend treatment with strong base, despite its demonstrated efficiency for N-nitrosamide destruction, because it produces toxic, carcinogenic and explosive diazoalkanes.

The mutagenicity data, however, give useful information concerning the potential biological hazards associated with the decomposition products, allowing the following tentative conclusions to be drawn regarding the scope and limitations of the remaining four methods (A–D). Methods A and B were relatively insensitive to the type of hydrophilic solvent and could be used to degrade N-nitrosamides in ethanol, methanol or DMSO in one step. Possible disadvantages are that the methods did not completely destroy N-nitrosamides in solvents that are immiscible with water (e.g., dichloromethane) unless the solvent was first evaporated. They were also relatively slow, and the concentrated acid required is potentially hazardous.

Hydrobromic acid in acetic acid (Method C) was relatively fast, but it was not as effective without prior removal of hydroxylic solvents when they were present; the method was unreliable unless thorough nitrogen flushing was used. However, solutions in dichloromethane could easily be degraded without evaporation.

Potassium permanganate/sulfuric acid (Method D) was also rapid, but the presence of certain organic solvents left traces of the N-nitrosamides undegraded. This method does have the advantage that other hazardous compounds [e.g., aflatoxins, nitrosamines, polycyclic aromatic hydrocarbons and hydrazines (Castegnaro et al., 1980, 1982, 1983a, b, respectively)] are also degraded. Thus, the method can be used to treat mixtures of hazardous compounds when more specific methods might destroy only one class of compound.

Tester strains TA1535 and TA100 detect mutagens which cause base-pair substitutions in DNA. N-Nitrosamides are known to provoke mutation in these strains (Lijinsky & Andrews, 1979). TA100 is usually considered to be the more sensitive strain and should therefore be capable of detecting a wider range of mutagens. The results of these experiments show the value of simultaneously testing with both strains, since there were instances where TA1535 detected mutagens and TA100 did not.

ACKNOWLEDGEMENTS

We thank J. Saavedra for providing the MNUT and C. Brown and P. Johnson for technical assistance in carrying out the mutagenesis assays. Research was supported in part by the National Cancer Institute under Contract No. NO1-CO-23910 with Program Resources, Inc. and by the National Institutes of Health under contract NO1-DS-2-2130.

REFERENCES

Ames, B.N., McCann, J. & Yamasaki, E. (1975) Methods for detecting carcinogens and mutagens with the *Salmonella*/mammalian-microsome mutagenicity test. *Mutat. Res., 31,* 347–364

Andrews, A.W., Thibault, L.H. & Lijinsky, W. (1978) The relationship between carcinogenicity and mutagenicity of some polynuclear hydrocarbons. *Mutat. Res., 51,* 311–318

Bachmann, W.E. & Struve, W.S. (1942) *The Arndt-Eistert synthesis.* In: Adams, R., Bachmann, W.E., Fieser, L.F., Johnson, J.R. & Snyder, H.R., eds, *Organic Reactions,* Vol. 1, New York, John Wiley & Sons, pp. 38–62

de Boer, T.J. & Backer, H.J. (1963) *Diazomethane.* In: Rabjohn, N., ed., *Organic Syntheses, Coll.,* Vol. 4, New York, John Wiley & Sons, pp. 250–253

Carson, W.N. (1951) Gasometric determination of nitrite and sulfamate. *Anal. Chem., 23,* 1016–1019

Castegnaro, M., Hunt, D.C., Sansone, E.B., Schuller, P.L., Siriwardana, M.G., Telling, G.M., Van Egmond, H.P. & Walker, E.A., eds (1980). *Laboratory Decontamination and Destruction of Aflatoxins B_1, B_2, G_1, G_2 in Laboratory Wastes (IARC Scientific Publications No. 37).* Lyon, International Agency for Research on Cancer

Castegnaro, M., Eisenbrand, G., Ellen, G., Keefer, L., Klein, D., Sansone, E.B., Spincer, D., Telling, G. & Webb, K., eds (1982) *Laboratory Decontamination and Destruction of Carcinogens in Laboratory Wastes: Some N-Nitrosamines (IARC Scientific Publications No. 43),* Lyon, International Agency for Research on Cancer

Castegnaro, M., Grimmer, G., Hutzinger, O., Karcher,W., Kunte, H., Lafontaine, M., Sansone, E.B., Telling G. & Tucker, S.P., eds (1983a) *Laboratory Decontamination and Destruction of Carcinogens in Laboratory Wastes: Some Polycyclic Aromatic Hydrocarbons (IARC Scientific Publications No. 49),* Lyon, International Agency for Research on Cancer

Castegnaro, M., Ellen, G., Lafontaine, M., Van der Plas, H.C., Sansone, E.B. & Tucker, S.P. eds (1983b) *Laboratory Decontamination and Destruction of Carcinogens in Laboratory Wastes: Some Hydrazines (IARC Scientific Publications No. 54),* Lyon, International Agency for Research on Cancer

Castegnaro, M., Benard, J., Van Broekhoven, L.W., Fine, D., Massey, R., Sansone, E.B., Smith, P., Spiegelhalder, B., Stacchini, A., Telling, G. & Vallon, J.J., eds (1983c) *Laboratory Decontamination and*

Destruction of Carcinogens in Laboratory Wastes: Some N-*Nitrosamides (IARC Scientific Publications No. 55)*, Lyon, International Agency for Research on Cancer

Downes, M.J., Edwards, M.W., Elsey, T.S. & Walters, C.L. (1976) Determination of a non-volatile nitrosamine by using denitrosation and a chemiluminescence analyser. *Analyst, 101,* 742–748

Eisenbrand, G. & Preussmann, R. (1970) A new method for the colorimetric analysis of nitrosamines by cleaving the nitroso-group with hydrogen bromide in glacial acetic acid (in German). *Arzneim. Forsch., 20,* 1513–1517

Fieser, L.F. & Fieser, M. (1967) *Reagents for Organic Synthesis,* Vol. 1, New York, John Wiley & Sons, pp. 191–195, 519

IARC (1974a) *IARC Monographs on the Evaluation of Carcinogenic Risk of Chemicals to Man,* Vol. 4, *Some Aromatic Amines, Hydrazine and Related Substances,* N-*Nitroso Compounds and Miscellaneous Alkylating Agents,* Lyon, International Agency for Research on Cancer, pp. 183–195

IARC (1974b) *IARC Monographs on the Evaluation of Carcinogenic Risk of Chemicals to Man,* Vol. 7, *Some Anti-thyroid and Related Substances, Nitrofurans and Industrial Chemicals,* Lyon, International Agency for Research on Cancer, pp. 223–230

IARC (1978) *IARC Monographs on the Evaluation of the Carcinogenic Risk of Chemicals to Humans,* Vol. 17, *Some* N-*Nitroso Compounds,* Lyon, International Agency for Research on Cancer, pp. 191–215, 227–255

Lijinsky, W. & Andrews, A.W. (1979) The mutagenicity of nitrosamides in *Salmonella typhimurium. Mutat. Res., 68,* 1–8

Mellor, J.W. (1932) *A Comprehensive Treatise on Inorganic and Theoretical Chemistry,* Vol. 12, London, Longmans, Green & Co., pp. 323–325

Preussmann, R. & Schaper-Druckrey, F. (1972) *Investigation of a colorimetric procedure for determination of nitrosamides and comparison with other methods.* In: Bogovski, P., Preussmann, R., & Walker, E.A., eds, N-*Nitroso Compounds: Analysis and Formation (IARC Scientific Publications* No. 3), Lyon, International Agency for Research on Cancer, pp. 81–86

Redemann, C.E., Rice, F.O., Roberts, R. & Ward, H.P. (1955) *Diazomethane.* In: Horning E.C., ed., *Organic Syntheses, Coll.* Vol. 3., New York, John Wiley & Sons, pp. 244–248

Sparrow, A.H. (1973) Hazards of chemical carcinogens and mutagens. *Science, 181,* 700–701

METABOLISM OF *N*-NITROSAMINES AND *N*-NITRAMINES

COMPARATIVE METABOLISM OF *N*-NITROSAMINES IN RELATION TO THEIR ORGAN AND SPECIES SPECIFICITY

M. OKADA

Tokyo Biochemical Research Institute Tokyo, Japan

The principal target organ for tumour induction in rats by the homologous series of symmetrical *N*-nitrosodialkylamines is the liver (Druckrey *et al.*, 1967). Interest in the study of the structure-activity relationships of *N*-nitrosodi-*n*-butylamine (NDBA) and related compounds arose mainly because of the somewhat unusual ability of this symmetrical *N*-nitrosodialkylamine to induce urinary bladder tumours (Okada *et al.*, 1975; Okada, 1976; Okada & Ishidate, 1977). NDBA induces tumours of the liver, oesophagus and bladder in rats after oral administrations; a shift of organ specifity was observed after subcutaneous injections, when the bladder became the main target organ (Druckrey *et al.*, 1964). Druckrey *et al.* (1964) first noted that the bladder-specific carcinogenic effect of NDBA is related to terminal (ω) hydroxylation of one of the butyl groups, giving rise to a metabolite, *N*-nitrosobutyl-(4-hydroxybutyl)amine (NBHBA-4), which was found to be a selective and potent bladder carcinogen.

In order to elucidate a possible relationship between the metabolism and the organotropic effect on the urinary bladder of NDBA and NBHBA-4, the metabolic fate of these nitrosamines with the di-*n*-butyl structure was investigated in rats. After oral administration of NBHBA-4 or NDBA, urinary metabolites which retained the nitrosamino moiety were separated and characterized. On the basis of the urinary metabolites characterized, the metabolic pathways of NBHBA-4 (Okada & Suzuki, 1972; Suzuki & Okada, 1980a) and NDBA (Blattmann & Preussmann, 1973, 1974; Okada & Ishidate, 1977; Okada *et al.*, 1975; Suzuki & Okada, 1980b) in rats were determined. (Figure 1).

The major urinary metabolite of NBHBA-4, occurring as more than 40% of the dose, was *N*-nitrosobutyl(3-carboxypropyl)amine (NBCPA). Several other *N*-nitroso compounds were characterized as minor metabolites: glucuronic acid conjugates of NBHBA-4 and NBCPA; subsequent transformation products of NBCPA after β-oxidation according to the Knoop mechanisms, i.e., *N*-nitrosobutyl(2-hydroxy-3-carboxypropyl)amine, *N*-nitrosobutyl(carboxymethyl)amine (NBCMA) and *N*-nitrosobutyl(2-oxopropyl)amine (NBOPA).

NDBA underwent metabolic transformation *in vivo* in at last three ways. First, it was metabolized to NBHBA-4 by ω-oxidation of the one butyl chain, also giving NBCPA as a major urinary metabolite (about 10% of dose); secondly, it underwent (ω-1)-oxidation of one butyl group; and, thirdly, but to a lesser extent, (ω-2)-oxidation (β-oxidation) of one alkyl chain. The monohydroxylated metabolites, *N*-nitrosobutyl(3-hydroxybutyl)amine (NBHBA-3) and *N*-nitrosobutyl(2-hydroxybutyl)amine (NBHBA-2), were in turn conjugated with glucoronic acid to form the glucuronides, or they underwent further oxidative metabolic transformation *via* the corresponding oxo compounds, *N*-nitrosobutyl(3-oxobutyl)amine

Fig. 1. Metabolic fate of *N*-nitrosobutyl(4-hydroxybutyl)amine (NBHBA-4) and *N*-nitrosodibutylamine (NDBA). Compounds shown in parentheses have not been isolated and identified as urinary metabolites. NBCPA, *N*-nitrosobutyl(3-carboxypropyl)amine; NBHBA-3, *N*-nitrosobutyl(3-hydroxybutyl)amine; NBOBA-3, *N*-nitrosobutyl(3-oxobutyl)amine; NBHBA-2, *N*-nitrosobutyl(2-hydroxybutyl)amine; NBOBA-2, *N*-nitrosobutyl(2-oxobutyl)amine; NBCEA, *N*-nitrosobutyl(2-carboxyethyl)amine; NBCMA, *N*-nitrosobutyl(carboxymethyl)amine; NBOPA, *N*-nitrosobutyl(2-oxopropyl)amine.

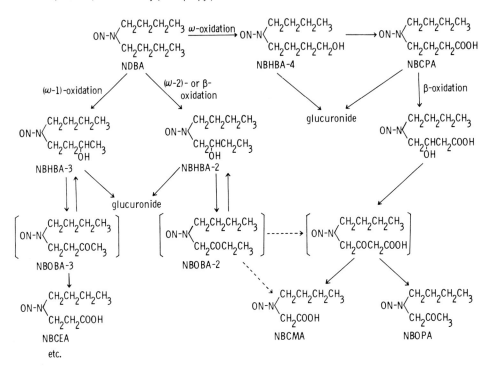

Fig. 2. Microsomal metabolism of *N*-nitrosodibutylamine (NDBA). Compounds and steps shown in parentheses have not yet been identified or demonstrated. NBHBA-1, *N*-nitrosobutyl(1-hydroxybutyl)amine; NBHBA-4, *N*-nitrosobutyl(4-hydroxybutyl)amine; NBHBA-3, *N*-nitrosobutyl(3-hydroxybutyl)amine; NBHBA-2, *N*-nitrosobutyl(2-hydroxybutyl)amine.

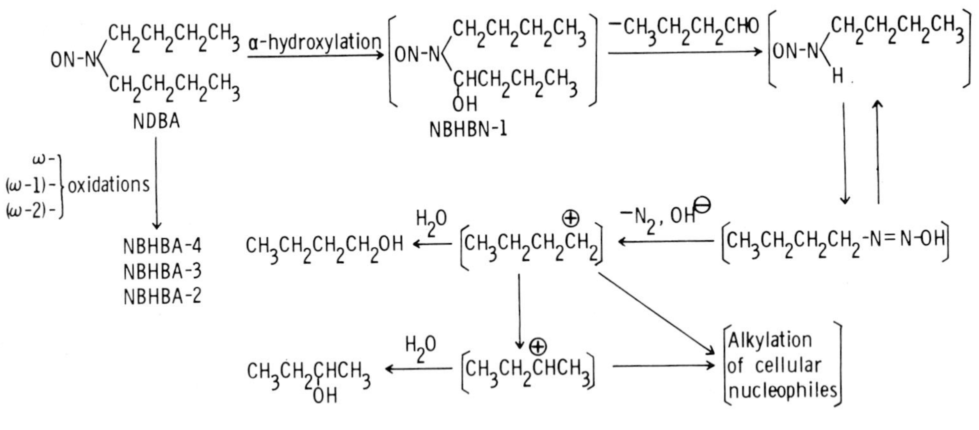

(NBOBA-3) - to *N*-nitrosobutyl(2-carboxyethyl)amine (NBCEA), NBCMA, etc - and *N*-nitrosobutyl(2-oxobutyl)amine (NBOBA-2) - to NBOPA, NBCMA, etc (Blattmann & Preussmann, 1975, Okada, 1976).

Because of the instability of α-hydroxy nitrosamines (Mochizuki *et al.*, 1980, 1982), the α-oxidation pathway of NDBA metabolism has not yet been demonstrated *in vivo*. In contrast to metabolism *in vivo*, α-hydroxylation is the predominant metabolic pathway of NDBA *in vitro*. Blattmann and Preussmann (1977) first demonstrated that butyraldehyde is produced as a major product after incubation of NDBA with liver microsomes prepared from rats (not treated with inducers). Metabolism of NDBA by liver microsomes prepared from rats treated with phenobarbital and polychlorinated biphenyls yielded butyraldehyde and/or two isomeric butyl alcohols (*n*- and *sec*-, the ratio of which was approximately 3:1), together with NBHBA-4, NBHBA-3 and NBHBA-2, of which NBHBA-3 occurred in an overwhelmingly greater quantity (Suzuki *et al.*, 1983a). Much less of these metabolites, especially butyraldehyde and butyl alcohols, was produced when liver microsomes prepared from untreated rats were used. In the presence of microsomes from treated animals, increased production of butyraldehyde, with a concomitant enhancement of the mutagenic effect of NDBA toward *Salmonella typhimurium* TA1535, was demonstrated.

On the basis of the reaction scheme for the generation of alkylating species from *N*-nitrosodialkylamines following microsomal α-hydroxylation, NDBA would be expected to produce butyraldehyde and isomeric butyl alcohols (*n*- and *sec-*), as shown in Figure 2.

Thus, α-hydroxylation may play a key role in the metabolic activation of NDBA. Support for this hypothesis comes from the finding that *N*-nitrosobutyl(1-acetoxybutyl)amine, yielding *N*-nitrosobutyl(1-hydroxybutyl)amine (NBHBA-1) on hydrolysis, has potent mutagenic activity toward bacterial strains of *Salmonella typhimurium* and *Escherichia coli* (Mochizuki *et al.*, 1979) in the absence of a 9000 × *g* supernatant preparation from rat liver. It was also mutagenic to V79 Chinese hamster cells (Huang *et al.*, 1981), and it was shown to have a primarily local carcinogenic effect (Takahashi *et al.*, 1982).

Incubation of NDBA with 9000 × *g* supernanant fractions prepared from livers of rats treated with inducers gave products oxidized at the ω, ω-1, and ω-2 positions, i.e., NBHBA-4, NBCPA, NBHBA-3, NBOBA-3 and NBHBA-2 (NBHBA-3 also being the major product under experimental conditions) and butyl alcohols in much larger quantities than with microsomes, but no butyraldehyde (Suzuki *et al.*, 1983b). Accordingly, higher mutagenic ability was observed with 9 000 × *g* supernatant fractions than with microsomes prepared from rats treated with inducers.

Incubation of NDBA with microsomes in the presence of SKF 525-A resulted in very small amounts of products derived by α-hydroxylation (butyraldehyde and butyl alcohols) but there was only a slight inhibitory effect on the formation of the (ω-1)-hydroxylation product (NBHBA-3). The enzyme involved in the α-hydroxylation of NDBA is considered to be cytochrome P-450, on the basis of the requirements of the reaction for NADPH and oxygen and the responses to SKF 525-A and 7,8-benzoflavone. The different effects of phenobarbital and polychlorinated biphenyls on α and ω-1 hydroxylation activities raise the possibility that a distinct cytochrome P-450 mediates each hydroxylation in hepatic microsomes (Suzuki *et al.*, 1983a).

The carcinogenic effects of NBHBA-4 and NDBA and their metabolites were examined in ACI rats (Okada & Hashimoto, 1974; Okada *et al.*, 1976b). Selective induction of bladder cancer in 100% of animals was observed with NBHBA-4 as reported earlier by other investigators, while NDBA produced no bladder cancer but only hepatomas under the experimental conditions used. NBCMA was considered not to be carcinogenic; more than 60% of the dose was recovered unchanged from the urine of rats. Hepatomas were induced by treatment with NBOPA. NBHBA-3 produced no tumours under these experimental conditions, although degenerative changes in the liver were noticed histologically in a few treated rats. NBOBA-2 and NBOBA-3 induced hepatomas, as did NBOPA. The carcinogenic effects of the other metabolites have not yet been examined.

NBCPA, the principal urinary metabolite of NBHBA-4 and of NDBA, was found to be an even more selective and potent bladder carcinogen in rats after oral administration (Hashimoto *et al.*, 1972), although more than 40% of the dose was recovered unchanged from the urine. Moreover, a direct carcinogenic action of NBCPA on bladder epithelium was demonstrated by intravesicular instillation in female rats (Hashimoto *et al.*, 1974a). In addition, neoplastic transformation by NBCPA of epithelial cells of rat bladder was demonstrated *in vitro* (Hashimoto & Kitagawa, 1974). It seems reasonable, therefore, to conclude that the induction of bladder cancer by NBHBA-4 and NDBA is due to the common major urinary metabolite, NBCPA.

In order to study the structural requirements for *N*-nitrosodialkylamines to act as bladder carcinogens, we carried out a series of studies on the synthesis (Okada *et al.*, 1978 a, b), metabolism (Suzuki & Okada, 1981 a, b; Suzuki *et al.*, 1981 a, b, c) and carcinogenicity (Okada & Hashimoto, 1974; Okada *et al.*, 1976b) of various compounds related to NBHBA-4, NDBA and their metabolites (Okada *et al.*, 1975; Okada, 1976; Okada & Ishidate, 1977).

The requirement that a 4-hydroxybutyl group be present for a compound to induce selective bladder carcinogenesis was confirmed by studies of the homologues and analogues of NBHBA-4. All the lower homologues of NBHBA-4 in which the butyl group is replaced by methyl (NMHBA-4), ethyl (NEHBA-4) and/or propyl (NPHBA-4) groups were found to be bladder carcinogens. However, possession of a 4-hydroxybutyl group alone is not sufficient for bladder carcinogenesis: the lack of carcinogenicity of *N*-nitroso-*tert*-butyl(4-hydroxybutyl)-amine (N*t*BHBA-4) is apparently associated with the absence of an α-hydrogen in the *tert*-butyl group. No induction of bladder cancer was observed with the amyl homologue of NBHBA-4 (NAHBA-4), although papillomas of the bladder were observed in a few treated rats. The carcinogenic activities of those NBHBA-4 homologues so far examined are the following: NEHBA-4 > NBHBA-4 = NMHBA-4 > NPHBA-4 > NAHBA-4 > N*t*BHBA-4, the last being inactive. On the basis of these observations, it is suggested that NEHBA-4 be used instead of NBHBA-4 as an effective and specific bladder carcinogen, at least in rats.

The principal metabolites of these homologues of NBHBA-4, except NAHBA-4, are the corresponding 3-carboxypropyl compounds; urinary excretion was estimated to be more than 40% of the dose, the highest (75%) being seen with N*t*BHBA-4. *N*-Nitrosoethyl(3-carboxypropyl)amine (NECPA), the principal metabolite of NEHBA-4, was found to be as selective and potent a bladder carcinogen as NEHBA-4 itself (Hashimoto *et al.*, 1974b), indicating that this metabolite is responsible for the organotropic carcinogenicity of NEHBA-4 to the bladder, as in the case with NBCPA and NBHBA-4. By the same logic, it is reasonable to predict that the 3-carboxypropyl compounds derived metabolically from NMHBA-4 and NPHBA-4 are also bladder carcinogens, whereas no bladder carcinogenicity should be expected from the 3-carboxypropyl compound produced from N*t*BHBA-4. The weak carcinogenicity of NAHBA-4 may be explained by the different metabolic transformation of the compound, which results in reduced availability of a metabolite with a 3-carboxypropyl group.

Decreasing the length of the alkyl chain of the 4-hydroxybutyl group changes the target specifity or abolishes the carcinogenicity of a compound. The main target organs of *N*-nitrosobutyl(2-hydroxyethyl)amine, like *N*-nitrosoethyl(2-hydroxyethyl)amine (Druckrey *et al.*, 1967), were the liver and oesophagus, while *N*-nitrosobutyl(3-hydroxypropyl)amine was noncarcinogenic 52 weeks after commencement of treatment (Okada *et al.*, 1976b). *N*-Nitrosoethyl(3-hydroxypropyl)amine, a lower homologue of *N*-nitrosobutyl(3-hydroxy-propyl)amine, was also inactive. The major urinary metabolites of these 3-hydroxypropyl and 2-hydroxyethyl analogues of NBHBA-4 were the corresponding 2-carboxyethyl and carboxymethyl compounds. Urinary excretion of the carboxylic acids amounted to 40 - 70%

- levels comparable to or higher than those of the 3-carboxypropyl metabolites observed with NBHBA-4 homologues. It can therefore be concluded that neither *N*-nitroso-alkyl(2-carboxyethyl)amine nor *N*-nitrosoalkyl(carboxymethyl)amine induces bladder tumours in rats.

Three *N*-nitrosobis(ω-hydroxyalkyl)amines - *N*-nitroso(2-hydroxyethyl)(4-hydroxybutyl)-amine, *N*-nitroso(3-hydroxypropyl)(4-hydroxybutyl)amine and *N*-nitrosobis(4-hydroxybutyl)-amine - all of which have a 4-hydroxybutyl group, induced neither bladder nor any other tumours in rats. The principal urinary metabolite of these dialkanolnitrosamines was the corresponding 3-carboxypropyl derivative, urinary excretion of which was estimated to be 30 - 60 %.

These results demonstrate that the presence of the di-*n*-butyl structure in *N*-nitroso-dialkylamines is not indispensable for them to induce bladder cancer in rats, as assumed previously (Druckrey *et al.*, 1964). An essential structural and metabolic requirement for *N*-nitrosodialkylamines to induce bladder cancer selectively is a 4-hydroxybutyl chain, which undergoes metabolic transformation to a 3-carboxypropyl group, resulting in considerable urinary excretion of a 3-carboxypropyl metabolite. That the presence of a 4-hydroxybutyl chain is not sufficient, however, is illustrated by the cases of N*t*BHBA-4, NAHBA-4 and *N*-nitroso-(ω-hydroxyalkyl)(4-hydroxybutyl)amines.

Metabolically, *N*-nitrosoalkylbutylamines such as *N*-nitrosomethylbutylamine, *N*-nitroso-ethylbutylamine, *N*-nitrosopropylbutylamine, and *N*-nitrosobutylamylamine could be expected to induce bladder tumours, since these asymmetric *N*-nitrosodialkylamines with a butyl chain would yield *N*-nitrosoalkyl(3-carboxypropyl)amines by metabolic ω-oxidation of the butyl group. However, they did not produce bladder tumours in rats but induced tumours in the oesophagus and liver under the experimental conditions used (Druckrey *et al.*, 1967; Okada *et al.*, 1976b). Urinary excretion of metabolites with a 3-carboxypropyl group was found to be considerably less than that observed with NDBA, which induced bladder tumours as well as hepatic and oesophageal tumours. Animals treated with these nitrosamines, however, died early of hepatic and oesophageal tumours, and it is possible that the short survival time precluded the development of bladder tumours.

Lijinsky and Taylor (1975) reported that oral treatment of rats with *N*-nitrosomethyl-*n*-dodecylamine (NMDA) gave rise to a 100% incidence of bladder tumours. We therefore investigated the metabolic fate of this long-alkyl chain nitrosamine. The principal urinary metabolite of NMDA in rats was not NMCPA, as expected, but *N*-nitrososarcosine, the urinary excretion of which was estimated to be about 3 and 15% of the dose (Okada *et al.*, 1976a, Suzuki *et al.*, 1981e), respectively. Administration of *N*-nitrososarcosine in relatively high doses was reported to induce oesophageal tumours in rats (Druckrey *et al.*, 1967). The butyl homologue of this nitrosamino acid, NBCMA, was found to be nontumorigenic to the bladder, although a large portion of the dose was excreted as such in the urine (Okada *et al.*, 1976b). In view of the fairly long-term (50 weeks) treatment with NMDA used by Lijinsky and Taylor, it seemed reasonable to suppose that NMCPA was responsible for the bladder carcinogenesis attributed to NMDA.

On the basis of the metabolic shortening of the alkyl chain by successive removal of two carbon fragments, according to the Knoop β-oxidation mechanism of fatty acid metabolism, and the finding that neither the *N*-nitrosoalkyl(2-carboxyethyl)amine nor the *N*-nitrosoalkyl-(carboxymethyl)amine could be involved in the bladder carcinogenicity of *N*-nitrosodialkyl-amines, it was predicted (Okada *et al.*, 1976a) that only even-numbered alkyl chain compounds would give rise to bladder tumours. This hypothesis was supported by the observation that all four *N*-nitrosomethyl-*n*-alkylamines tested (*N*-nitrosomethyl-*n*-octylamine, *N*-nitrosomethyl-*n*-decylamine, NMDA and *N*-nitrosomethyl-*n*-tetradecylamine) which have an even number of carbon atoms in the long chain induced a high incidence of bladder tumours in rats (Lijinsky *et al.*, 1981), but that liver and lung tumours were produced by the odd-numbered undecyl

(Lijinsky *et al.,* 1978) and nonyl (Lijinsky *et al.,* 1981) homologues. It was proposed recently (Singer *et al.,* 1981) that *N*-nitrosomethyl(2-oxopropyl)amine, a common, minor urinary metabolite of the even-numbered *N*-nitrosomethylalkylamines, might be a (more) proximate carcinogen in the bladder. This oxo compound could be formed by β-oxidation of NMCPA followed by decarboxylation, as in the case of NBOPA formation from NBCPA. In the light of previous findings on the carcinogenicity and target organs of *N*-nitrosoalkyl(2-oxoalkyl)amines (Okada & Hashimoto, 1974; Okada *et al.,* 1976b), however, it would hardly be expected that bladder tumours would be induced in rats by oral administration of *N*-nitrosomethyl(2-oxopropyl)amine.

Species differences in the susceptibility of animals to the bladder carcinogens NBHBA-4, NBCPA and NEHBA-4 were observed when the nitrosamines were administered in drinking-water (Hirose *et al.,* 1976). Thus NBHBA-4 selectively induced a high incidence of bladder cancer in rats (100%) and mice (63%), but not in Syrian golden hamsters or guinea-pigs being the least susceptible of the four species. Rats, mice and hamsters were susceptible to NEHBA-4, while no tumour was produced by this compound in guinea-pigs. It has also been suggested that different susceptibilities to NDBA exist among different animal species (Ivankovic & Bücheler, 1968; Okada & Ishidate, 1977; Suzuki *et al.,* 1981d). It is reasonable to assume that the differences in response are related to differences in metabolism and activation.

The metabolic fate of NBHBA-4, NDBA, NBCPA and NEHBA-4 was also investigated in other animal species, namely guinea-pigs, mice, hamsters and dogs (Suzuki *et al.,* 1981 e, 1983 c, d). All those urinary metabolites with a nitrosamino moiety were separated and characterized in the case of rats and guinea-pigs, but only acidic metabolites (expecially NBCPA and NECPA) were determined as their methyl esters colorimetrically after thin-layer chromatographic separation or by gas-liquid chromatography.

About 10% of a dose of NDBA was recovered as urinary NBCPA after oral administration to rats, while nearly 30% was recovered after subcutaneous injection. This finding may explain the earlier report (Druckrey *et al.,* 1964) that a much higher incidence of bladder cancer occurred after subcutaneous (more than 90%) than after oral ($\simeq$ 35%) administration of NDBA to rats. Urinary excretion of NBCPA in guinea-pigs after oral administration of NBHBA-4, NDBA or NBCPA was much less than that in rats, while excretion of NBCMA was greater in guinea-pigs than in rats. High excretion of the glucuronides of NBHBA-4 and NBHBA-3 observed in guinea-pigs given NBHBA-4 and NDBA, respectively, demonstrating greater glucuronylation activity in this animal species than in rats. As for the excretion of NBCPA and NBCMA, similar results were obtained with mice, hamsters and dogs. These findings have been confirmed recently (Suzuki *et al.,* 1983 d) in experiments involving a dose approximately equal to the daily doses used in chronic carcinogenicity assays. Accordingly, previous observations concerning species variations in response to NBHBA-4, NDBA and NBCPA may be explained on the basis of the different urinary excretion of NBCPA after administration of these compounds.

This explanation does not, however, appear to be applicable to mice, since both NBHBA-4 and NDBA induce bladder tumours relatively readily in this species. An acidic polar metabolite other than those described above was thought to be involved in inducing bladder tumours in mice, since it was found in fairly large amounts only in the urine of mice given NBHBA-4 or NDBA. This metabolite was isolated and identified (by direct comparison with an authentic synthetic sample) as the glycine conjugate of NBCPA (Suzuki *et al.,* 1983c). When given orally to mice, it was found to be partly hydrolysed to NBCPA, which was excreted in the urine (about 7% of the dose), while about 13% of the dose was recovered unchanged from the urine. Since 6% of a dose of NBHBA-4 was recovered as NBCPA from the urine of mice, we made no further attempt to test the carcinogenicity of this novel conjugate.

A relatively high urinary excretion of NECPA was observed after oral administration of NEHBA-4 to rats (59% of dose), mice (35%) and hamsters (49%), which were susceptible to NEHBA-4 while little excretion of the proximate carcinogen was found in guinea-pigs (4%), which were the least susceptible of the four species tested (no tumour was produced in this species). Thus, from the metabolic point of view, species variations in response to the urinary bladder carcinogens, NBHBA-4, NDBA, NBCPA and NEHBA-4, may be closely related to differences in the extent of urinary excretion of the active metabolites (proximate carcinogens) of these nitrosamines, NBCPA and NECPA.

Inter-strain differences in susceptibility to bladder carcinogenesis induced by NBHBA-4 were studies in rats by Ito *et al.* (1975). The incidence of bladder cancer was highest in ACI (100%) followed by Wistar (86%) and Sprague-Dawley (40%) strains. It was reported recently that analbuminaemic rats (established from Sprague-Dawley stock) are highly susceptible to NBHBA-4 (Kakizoe *et al.*, 1982): the incidences of bladder cancer in analbuminaemic rats and in Sprague-Dawley rats were 100 and 17%, respectively. No marked difference in the urinary excretion of NBCPA was demonstrated among these rat strains, however (Suzuki *et al.*, 1983d), and the inter-strain differences in susceptibility cannot therefore, be explained simply on the basis of the extent of urinary excretion.

ACKNOWLEDGEMENT

Work reported in this paper was supported in part by Grants-in-Aid for Cancer Research from the Ministry of Education, Science and Culture and the Ministry of Health and Welfare, Japan.

REFERENCES

Blattmann, L. & Preussmann, R. (1973) Struktur von Metaboliten Carcinogener Dialkylnitrosamine im Rattenurin. *Z. Krebsforsch.*, *79*, 3–5

Blattmann, L. & Preussmann, R. (1974) Biotransformation von carcinogenen Dialkylnitrosaminen. Weitere Urinmetaboliten von Di-*n*-butyl- und Di-*n*-pentylnitrosamin. *Z. Krebsforsch.*, *81*, 75–78

Blattmann, L. & Preussmann, R. (1975) Metaboliten von (2-Hydroxybutyl)-*n*-butylnitrosamin in Rattenurin. *Z. Krebsforsch.*, *83*, 125–127

Blattmann, L. & Preussmann, R. (1977) Oxidative biotransformation of di-*n*-butylnitrosamine. Formation *in vitro* of aldehydes in the presence of rat liver microsomes. *Z. Krebsforsch.*, *88*, 311–314

Druckrey, H. Preussmann, R., Ivankovic, S., Schmidt, C.H., Mennel, H.D. & Stahl, K.W. (1964) Selektive Erzeugung von Blasenkrebs an Ratten durch Dibutyl- und N-Butyl-N-butanol-(4)-nitrosamin. *Z. Krebsforsch.*, *66*, 280–290

Druckrey, H., Preussmann, R., Ivankovic, S. & Schmähl, D. (1967) Organotrope carcinogen Wirkungen bei 65 verschiedenen N-Nitroso-Verbindungen an BD-Ratten. *Z. Krebsforsch.*, *69*, 103–201

Hashimoto, Y. & Kitagawa, H.D. (1974) *In vitro* neoplastic transformation of epithelial cells of rat urinary bladder by nitrosamines. *Nature*, *252*, 497–499

Hashimoto, Y. Suzuki, E. & Okada, M. (1972) Induction of urinary bladder tumors in ACI/N rats by butyl(3-carboxypropyl)nitrosoamine, a major urinary metabolite of butyl(4-hydroxybutyl)-nitrosoamine. *Gann*, *63*, 637–638

Hashimoto, Y., Suzuki, K. & Okada, M. (1974a) Induction of urinary bladder tumors by intravesicular instillation of butyl(4-hydroxybutyl)nitrosoamine and its principal urinary metabolite, butyl(3-carboxypropyl)nitrosoamine in rats. *Gann*, *65*, 69–73

Hashimoto, Y., Iiyoshi, M. & Okada, M. (1974b) Rapid and selective induction of urinary bladder cancer in rats with N-ethyl-N-(4-hydroxybutyl)nitrosamine and by its principal urinary metabolite. *Gann*, *65*, 565–566

Hirose, M., Fukushima, S., Hamanouchi, M., Shirai, T., Ogiso, T., Takahashi, M. & Ito, N. (1976) Different susceptibilities of the urinary bladder epithelium of animal species to three nitroso compounds. *Gann, 67,* 175–189

Huang, G.-F., Mochizuki, M., Anjo, T. & Okada, M. (1981) Mutagenicity of N-alkyl-N-(α-acetoxyalkyl)nitrosamines in V79 Chinese hamster cells in relation to alkylating activity. *Gann, 72,* 531–538

Ito, N., Arai, M., Sugihara, S., Hirao, K. Makiura, S., Matayoshi, K. & Denda, A. (1975) Experimental urinary bladder tumours induced by N-butyl-N-(4-hydroxybutyl)nitrosamine. *Gann Monogr. Cancer Res, 17,* 367–381

Ivankovic, S. & Bücheler, J. (1968) Leber- und Blasen-Carcinoma beim Meerschweinchen nach Di-*n*-butylnitrosamin. *Z. Krebsforsch., 71,* 183–185

Kakizoe, T., Komatsu, H., Honma, Y., Niijima, T., Kawachi, T., Sugimura, T. & Nagase, S. (1982) High susceptibility of analbuminaemic rats to induced bladder cancer. *Br. J. Cancer, 45,* 474–476

Lijinsky, W. & Taylor, H.W. (1975) Induction of urinary bladder tumors in rats by administration of nitrosomethyldodecylamine. *Cancer Res., 35,* 958–961

Lijinsky, W. Taylor, H.W. Mangino, M. & Singer, G.M. (1978) Carcinogenesis of nitrosomethylundecylamine in Fischer rats. *Cancer Lett., 5,* 209–213

Lijinsky, W., Saavedra, J.E. & Reuber, M.D. (1981) Induction of carcinogenesis in Fischer rats by methylalkylnitrosamines. *Cancer Res., 41,* 1288–1292

Mochizuki, M., Suzuki, E., Anjo, T., Wakabayashi, Y & Okada, M. (1979) Mutagenic and DNA-damaging effect of N-alkyl-N-(α-acetoxyalkyl)nitrosamines, models for metabolically activated N′,N-dialkylnitrosamines. *Gann, 70,* 663–670

Mochizuki, M., Anjo, T. & Okada, M. (1980) Isolation and characterization of N-alkyl-N-(hydroxymethyl)nitrosamines from N-alkyl-N-(hydroperoxymethyl)nitrosamines by deoxygenation. *Tetrahedron Lett., 21,* 3693–3696

Mochizuki, M., Anjo, T., Takeda, K., Suzuki, E., Sekiguchi, N., Huang, G.-F. & Okada, M. (1982) *Chemistry and mutagenicity of α-hydroxy nitrosamines.* In: Bartsch, H., O′Neill, I.K., Castegnaro, M. & Okada, M., eds, N-*Nitroso Compounds: Occurrence and Biological Effects (IARC Scientific Publications No. 41),* Lyon, International Agency for Research on Cancer, pp. 553–559

Okada, M. (1976) *Metabolic aspects in organotropic carcinogenesis by dialkylnitrosamines.* In: Magee, P.M., Takayama, S., Sugimura, T. & Matsushima, T., eds, *Fundamentals in Cancer Prevention (Proceedings of the 6th international Symposium of the Princess Takamatsu Cancer Research Fund),* Tokyo, University of Tokyo Press, pp. 251–266

Okada, M. & Hashimoto, Y. (1974) Carcinogenic effect of N-nitrosoamines related to butyl(4-hydroxybutyl)nitrosamine in ACI/N rats, with special reference to induction of urinary bladder tumors. *Gann, 65,* 13–19

Okada, M. & Ishidate, M. (1977) Metabolic fate of N-*n*-butyl-N-(4-hydroxybutyl)nitrosamine and its analogues. Selective induction of urinary bladder tumours in the rat. *Xenobiotica, 7,* 11–24

Okada, M. & Suzuki E. (1972) Metabolism of butyl(4-hydroxybutyl)nitrosamine in rats. *Gann, 63,* 391–392

Okada, M., Suzuki, E., Aoki, J., Iiyoshi, M. & Hashimoti, H. (1975) Metabolism and carcinogenicity of N-butyl-N-(4-hydroxybutyl)nitrosamine and related compounds, with special reference to induction of urinary bladder tumors. *Gann Monogr. Cancer Res., 17,* 161–176

Okada, M., Suzuki, E. & Mochizuki, M. 1976a) Possible important role of urinary N-methyl-N-(3-carboxypropyl)nitrosamine in the induction of bladder tumors in rats by N-methyl-N-dodecyl-nitrosamine. *Gann, 67,* 771–772

Okada, M., Suzuki, E. & Hashimoto, Y. (1976b) Carcinogenicity of N-nitrosamines related to N-butyl-N-(4-hydroxybutyl)nitrosamine and N,N-dibutylnitrosamine in ACI/N rats. *Gann, 67,* 825–834

Okada, M., Suzuki, E. & Iiyoshi, M. (1978a) Syntheses of N-alkyl-N-(hydroxy- or oxo-alkyl)nitrosamines related to N-butyl-N-(4-hydroxybutyl)nitrosamine, a potent bladder carcinogen. *Chem. Pharm. Bull (Tokyo), 26,* 3891–3896

Okada, M., Suzuki, E., & Iiyoshi, M. (1978b) Syntheses of N-alkyl-N-(ω-carboxyalkyl)nitrosamines related to N-butyl-N-(3-carboxypropyl)nitrosamine, principal urinary metabolite of a potent bladder carcinogen N-butyl-N-(4-hydroxybutyl)nitrosamine. *Chem. Pharm. Bull. (Tokyo), 26,* 3909–3913

Singer, G.M., Lijinsky, W., Buettner, L. & McClusky, G.A. (1981) Relationship of rat urinary metabolites of N-nitrosomethyl-N-alkylamine to bladder carcinogenesis. *Cancer Res., 41,* 4942–4946

Suzuki, E. & Okada, M. (1980a) Metabolic fate of N-butyl-N-(4-hydroxybutyl)nitrosamine in the rat. *Gann, 71*, 856–862

Suzuki, E. & Okada, M. (1980b) Metabolic fate of N,N-dibutylnitrosamine in the rat. *Gann, 71*, 863–870

Suzuki, E. & Okada, M. (1981a) Metabolic fate of N,N-dipropylnitrosamine and N,N-diamylnitrosamine in the rat, in relation to their lack of carcinogenic effect on the urinary bladder. *Gann, 72*, 552–561

Suzuki, E. & Okada, M. (1981b) Metabolic fate of asymmetric N,N-dialkylnitrosamines having a butyl group in the rat. *Gann, 72*, 910–920

Suzuki, E., Iiyoshi, M. & Okada, M. (1981a) Metabolic fate of N-butyl-N-(4-hydroxybutyl)nitrosamine homologs in the rat, in relation to their organotropic carcinogenicity to the urinary bladder. *Gann, 72*, 113–122

Suzuki, E., Iiyoshi, M. & Okada, M. (1981b) Metabolic fate of N-alkyl-N-(4-hydroxypropyl and 2-hydroxyethyl)nitrosamines in the rat, in relation to the induction of bladder cancer by N-butyl-N-(4-hydroxybutyl)nitrosamine and its homologs. *Gann, 72*, 254–258

Suzuki, E., Takeda, Y. Mochizuki, M., Hashimoto, Y. & Okada, M. (1981c) Metabolic fate and carcinogenicity of N-(ω-hydroxyalkyl)-N-(4-hydroxybutyl)nitrosamines, analogs of N-butyl-N-(4-hydroxybutyl)nitrosamine, in the rat. *Gann, 72*, 539–546

Suzuki, E., Aoki, J. & Okada, M. (1981d) Metabolic fate of N-butyl-N-(4-hydroxybutyl)nitrosamine and N,N-dibutylnitrosamine in the guinea pig, with reference to their carcinogenic effects on the urinary bladder. *Gann, 72*, 547–551

Suzuki, E., Mochizuki, M. & Okada, M. (1981e) Metabolic fate of N-methyl-N-dodecylnitrosamine in the rat, in relation to its carcinogenicity to the urinary bladder. *Gann, 72*, 713–716

Suzuki, E., Mochizuki, M., Wakabayashi, Y. & Okada, M. (1983a) *In vitro* metabolic activation of N,N-dibutylnitrosamine in mutagenesis. *Gann, 74*, 51–59

Suzuki, E., Mochizuki, M., Shibuya, K. & Okada, M. (1983b) N,N-Dibutylnitrosamine metabolism by rat liver S9 fraction and oxidation by chemical model systems. *Gann, 74*, 41–50

Suzuki, E., Anjo, T., Aoki, J. & Okada, M. (1983c) Species variations in the metabolism of N-butyl-N-(4-hydroxybutyl)nitrosamine and related compounds in relation to urinary bladder carcinogenesis. *Gann, 74*, 60–68

Suzuki, E., Mochizuki, M. & Okada, M. (1983d) Relationship of urinary N-butyl-N-(3-carboxypropyl)nitrosamine to susceptibility of animals to bladder carcinogenesis by N-butyl-N-(4-hydroxybutyl)nitrosamine. *Gann, 74*, 360–364

Takahashi, M., Kurokawa, Y. Maekawa, A., Kokubo, T., Furukawa, F., Mochizuki, M., Anjo, T., & Okada, M. (1982) Comparative carcinogenicities of model compounds of metabolically activated N,N-dibutylnitrosamine in rats. *Gann, 73*, 687–694

DISTRIBUTION AND METABOLISM OF
N-NITROSOBIS(2-HYDROXYPROPYL)AMINE IN RATS

Y. MORI, H. TAKAHASHI, H. YAMAZAKI & K. TOYOSHI

Laboratory of Radiochemistry, Gifu Pharmaceutical University, Mitahora-higashi 5-6-1, Gifu 502, Japan

T. OBARA, T. MAKINO, D. NAKAE, S. TAKAHASHI & Y. KONISHI

Department of Oncological Pathology, Cancer Center, Nara Medical College, Kashihara, Nara 634, Japan

SUMMARY

The metabolic fate of the lung carcinogen N-nitrosobis(2-hydroxypropyl)amine (ND2HPA) in male Wistar rats was studied. The blood level after a single intraperitoneal (i.p.) injection of [1-^{14}C]-ND2HPA at a dose of 3 g/kg body weight reached a maximum within 1 h. Most of the administered ^{14}C was eliminated *via* the urine; 90.8% of the ^{14}C was excreted in urine within 24 h, 5.5% in faeces, and 3.2% in expired air. About 11% of the ^{14}C was detected in bile collected over 24 h. A relatively high concentration of ^{14}C was found in the blood and target organs, such as the lung, liver, thyroid gland and kidney 1 h after treatment. Analysis by high-pressure liquid chromatography showed that the ^{14}C in the blood and urine was mostly accounted for by unchanged ND2HPA, together with smaller amounts of N-nitroso-(2-hydroxypropyl)(2-oxopropyl)amine (N2HP2OPA). ND2HPA and N2HP2OPA were also detected in the lung and liver of rats 30 min to 12 h after the administration and were present in higher concentrations in the blood and lung than in the liver and pancreas. Besides ND2HPA and N2HP2OPA, N-nitrosomethyl(2-hydroxypropyl)amine (NM2HPA) was also found in urine collected over 6 h. ND2HPA, N2HP2OPA and NM2HPA showed mutagenicity in the *Salmonella* assay system with metabolic activation by a 9 000 × *g* supernatant of rat liver, and N2HP2OPA was also mutagenic in the presence of a rat lung preparation. These data suggest that N2HP2OPA and NM2HPA might be important intermediates in the metabolic activation of ND2HPA to its ultimate carcinogenic form in rats.

INTRODUCTION

Subcutaneous injection of N-nitrosobis(2-hydroxypropyl)amine (ND2HPA) induced a high incidence of pancreatic carcinomas in Syrian golden hamsters, whereas the pancreas is not a susceptible organ in other laboratory animal species (Pour & Wilson, 1980). We previously reported (Konishi *et al.*, 1976, 1978, 1979) that a high incidence of lung carcinomas was induced by oral or a single intraperitoneal (i.p.) administration of ND2HPA in rats and mice. In the present experiment we investigated the disposition and metabolism of ND2HPA using the radioactive tracer technique for the study of lung carcinogenesis by systemic administration of ND2HPA in rats. Some work on the *in vitro* metabolic activation of ND2HPA and its metabolites is also reported.

MATERIALS AND METHODS

Chemicals

ND2HPA, *N*-nitroso(2-hydroxypropyl)(2-oxopropyl)amine (N2HP2OPA), *N*-nitroso-methyl-(2-hydroxypropyl)amine (NM2HPA), *N*-nitrosobis(2-oxopropyl)amine (ND2OPA) and *N*-nitrosomethyl(2-oxopropyl)amine (NM2OPA) were synthesized in our laboratory (Mori *et al.*, 1983) and used for chromatographic comparison. [1-^{14}C]ND2HPA (58.3 µCi/mmol) was synthesized from DL-sodium lactate-1-^{14}C (Amersham Japan Ltd, Tokyo, Japan) according to the method described by Kupper *et al.* (1978). The compound was above 98% chemically and radiochemically pure, as determined by high-pressure liquid chromatography (HPLC).

Animals and treatments

Male Wistar rats (Shizuoka Laboratory Animal Center, Shizuoka, Japan), weighing from 180 to 200 g each, were used. Rats were housed in individual metabolic cages designed to enable the separate collection of urine, faeces and bile, and given food and water *ad libitum*. [1-^{14}C]ND2HPA or ND2HPA at a dose of 3 g/kg body weight was administered intra-peritoneally after overnight fasting. To prepare rats bearing a polyethylene biliary fistula, surgery was performed under light ether anaesthesia. The rats were killed by exsanguination from the abdominal aorta.

Tissue distribution and radioactive measurement

Blood samples were obtained from the tail vein at various intervals after administration of [1-^{14}C]ND2HPA. To study the tissue distribution of radioactive compound, main internal organs were taken 1 and 24 h after the injection and were rinced, blotted and weighed. A portion of the organs (0.1-0.2 g), or whole organs, and aliquots of faeces or blood were processed in an Aloka sample oxidizer (Aloka Instrument Co., Tokyo, Japan). Aliquots of urine and bile were dissolved directly in Oxifluor®-H$_2$O (New England Nuclear Corp., Boston, MA, USA). Expired ^{14}CO$_2$ was collected from rats maintained in a desiccator and was trapped by bubbling through a solution of ethanolamine:methanol (1:2, v/v) in three glass traps in series and measured in toluene phosphor. Radioactivity was determined in an Aloka model LSC-651 liquid scintillation spectrometer.

Isolation of metabolites from blood, tissue and urine

Blood samples were obtained from the abdominal aorta of rats and were heparinized. Livers and lungs were perfused *in situ* with 1.15% potassium chloride, and the tissues were homogenized in 1 volume of 1.15% potassium chloride. The homogenate, blood or urine was extracted with two volumes of ethyl acetate. The extract was clarified by centrifugation and passage through a Toyo membrane filter (0.45 µm pore size; type TM-2P) (Toyo Roshi Co. Ltd., Tokyo, Japan), then examined directly by HPLC. A portion of the urine *per se*, after treatment with a membrane filter, was also analysed by HPLC. HPLC was performed using a Jasco model Trirotor-II (Japan Spectroscopic Co. Ltd., Tokyo, Japan). Samples (6 μl) were injected into the HPLC directly and measured at 239 nm (0.02-1.28 absorbance unit full scale). ND2HPA and its metabolites were separated on a Jasco Finepak SIL C_{18} or Finepak SIL chromatographic column (25 cm × 4.6 mm i.d.). *N*-Nitrosamines were eluted with 40% (v/v) acetonitrile, acetonitrile or dichloromethane:isopropyl alcohol (99:1), and the solvent flow rate was 0.5 or 1.0 mL/min. Tissue, blood and urine (0.6-1.0 g or mL) were spiked with appropriate quantities of the nitrosamines, extracted and analysed as described above. The calculated recoveries include ND2HPA, 36%;N2HP2OPA, 64%; and ND2OPA, 89%. The limit of sensitivity (at 0.02 absorbance unit full scale) for detecting the *N*-nitrosamines was about 1 ng.

Mutagenesis assay

Salmonella typhimurium TA100 was used. The assay and tissue preparations have already been described (Mori *et al.*, 1983).

RESULTS

Excretion and tissue distribution

ND2HPA was rapidly absorbed in rats after i.p. administration. The blood level after a single i.p. dose of 3 g/kg of [1-^{14}C]ND2HPA reached a maximum at 1 h, and most of the ^{14}C was eliminated from blood within 24 h. The elimination half-life was 3.9 h, as calculated by linear regression analysis. Figure 1 shows the excretion of ^{14}C in urine, faeces, expired air and bile.

Fig. 1. Cumulative excretion of radioactivity (mean ± SE for 3 animals) after i.p. injection of [1-^{14}C]-*N*-nitrosobis(2-hydroxypropyl)amine (ND2HPA) to male Wistar rats at a dose of 3 g/kg b.w.; ▓ , urine; ⧮ , faeces; ■ , CO$_2$, □ , total; ▨ , bile

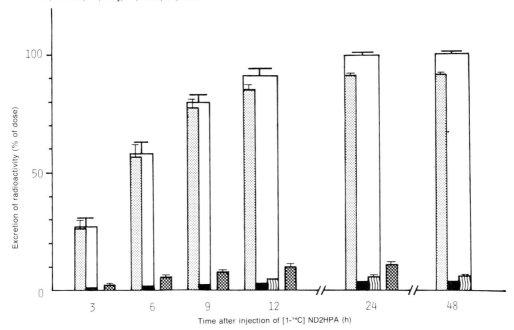

MORI *ET AL.*

Table 1. Tissue concentrations of total radioactivity in rats 1 and 24 h after a single i.p. injection of [1-^{14}C]-*N*-nitrosobis(2-hydroxypropyl)amine (ND2HPA)[a]

Tissue/Organ	1 h		24 h	
	(mg/g)	(% dose/organ)	(mg/g)	(% dose/organ)
Blood	3.47 ± 0.18		0.12 ± 0.07	
Kidney	3.72 ± 0.16	1.06 ± 0.00	0.08 ± 0.00	0.02 ± 0.00
Lung	3.42 ± 0.11	0.71 ± 0.05	0.06 ± 0.00	0.01 ± 0.00
Liver	3.28 ± 0.03	4.75 ± 0.26	0.13 ± 0.01	0.21 ± 0.02
Spleen	2.89 ± 0.08	0.39 ± 0.01	0.07 ± 0.01	0.01 ± 0.00
Thyroid gland	2.83 ± 0.57	0.01 ± 0.00	0.03 ± 0.02	< 0.005
Testis	2.76 ± 0.09	0.89 ± 0.17	0.01 ± 0.01	< 0.005
Submaxillary gland	2.66 ± 0.23	0.20 ± 0.02	0.03 ± 0.00	< 0.005
Brain	2.56 ± 0.37	0.62 ± 0.09	0.02 ± 0.01	< 0.005
Sublingual gland	2.44 ± 0.25	0.10 ± 0.01	0.05 ± 0.00	< 0.005
Muscle	2.36 ± 0.39		0.02 ± 0.01	
Stomach	2.35 ± 0.31	0.49 ± 0.04	0.04 ± 0.00	0.01 ± 0.00
Thymus	2.28 ± 0.32	0.22 ± 0.02	0.04 ± 0.00	< 0.005
Urinary bladder	2.21 ± 0.53	0.04 ± 0.01	0.03 ± 0.00	< 0.005
Adrenal gland	2.19 ± 0.47	0.02 ± 0.00	0.07 ± 0.02	< 0.005
Heart	2.05 ± 0.41	0.30 ± 0.07	0.03 ± 0.00	< 0.005
Sigmoid colon	2.00 ± 0.44		0.05 ± 0.01	
Pancreas	1.61 ± 0.14		0.04 ± 0.01	
Brown fat	1.44 ± 0.20		0.04 ± 0.01	
Trachea	1.42 ± 0.59		0.06 ± 0.00	
Oesophagus	1.29 ± 0.15		0.04 ± 0.01	
Fat	0.94 ± 0.43		0.02 ± 0.00	

[a] Values are means ± SE for three rats and are expressed as mg ND2HPA equivalent per wet weight of organ

The main excretion route of [1-^{14}C]ND2HPA appears to be the urine. Of the radioactive ND2HPA given, as much as 94% of the 48-h urinary excretion appeared in the first 12 h. About 11% of the administered ^{14}C was recovered in bile 24 h after the treatment, and 5.5% of that was excreted in faeces 24 h after the treatment. Respiratory elimination as ^{14}C-carbon dioxide was a minor factor (3.6% of the dose in 48 h).

The distribution of total radioactivity 1 and 24 h after administration of [1-^{14}C]ND2HPA to rats is summarized in Table 1. ^{14}C was found at high concentration in the blood and had reached all tissues examined 1 h after treatment. The highest concentrations of ^{14}C (mg ND2HPA equivalent/g tissue) were found in the kidney, lung and liver; the ^{14}C tissue:blood ratios were 1.07, 0.99 and 0.95, respectively. The thyroid gland showed the next highest concentration: relatively lower concentrations of ^{14}C were found in other tissues, such as the sigmoid colon and the pancreas. Within 24 h, 99.5% of the administered dose had been excreted, as shown in Figure 1, and less than 0.25% of the dose remained in the tissue (Table 1); there was no evidence of a specific affinity for these tissues 24 h after the treatment.

Identification of metabolites

ND2HPA metabolites in blood, tissues and urine were identified by HPLC profiles in three solvent systems, using authentic standards. The results are shown in Figure 2. Following the i.p. administration of ND2HPA to rats, ND2HPA was identified in the blood, pancreas, lung and liver. The levels of ND2HPA were highest from 30 min to 1 h, then decreased with time in all cases.

Fig. 2. Concentrations of ND2HPA and N2HP2OPA in blood and organs of rats given a single dose of ND2HPA (3 g/kg b.w.; i.p.). ND2HPA and N2HP2OPA were extracted from blood (O), lung (△), liver (□) and pancreas (X) and separated by HPLC, as described in Materials and Methods section

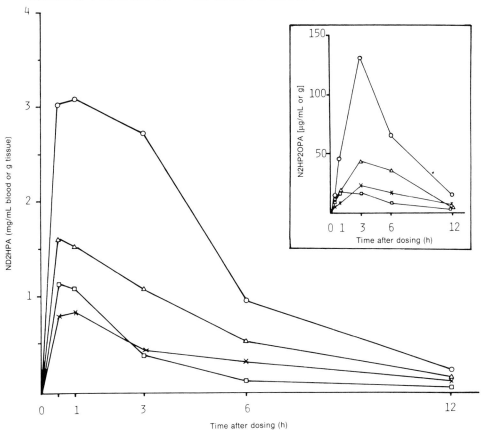

Smaller amounts of N2HP2OPA were also identified in the blood and the organs cited above. Levels of N2HP2OPA were highest 3 h after treatment. The concentrations of ND2HPA and N2HP2OPA in the lung were higher than those in the other organs examined, although lower than in the blood. The concentration of ND2HPA in the blood at 1 h was 3.1 ± 0.1 mg/g. This is consistent with the result for ^{14}C activity in the blood 1 h after i.p. administration of [1-^{14}C]ND2HPA (Table 1). NM2HPA was detected as a minor urinary metabolite, in addition to ND2HPA and N2HP2OPA. HPLC analysis of the urine *per se* revealed that, unlike the blood and tissue levels, urinary levels of ND2HPA increased with time, and 91.3% of the dose was recovered as ND2HPA in the 24-h urine. The levels of ND2OPA and NM2OPA in the blood, the organs and urine were below the limits of detection at the sensitivity range chosen (0.02 absorbance unit full scale, 0.2 µg/mL or g).

Mutagenicity of ND2HPA metabolites

ND2HPA showed mutagenicity in the presence of a 9 000 × *g* supernatant preparation (S9) from liver of rats pretreated with polychlorinated biphenyls (PCB), but not in the presence of S9 from kidney, lung, spleen or pancreas from treated rats or liver S9 from non-treated rats.

In contrast, N2HP2OPA and NM2HPA were mutagenic in the presence of liver S9 from non-treated rats; N2HP2OPA was also mutagenic in the presence of lung S9 from PCB-treated rats.

DISCUSSION

[1-^{14}C]ND2HPA was efficiently absorbed in rats, but only a trace of ^{14}C was left in the blood 24 h after the i.p. injection. [1-^{14}C]ND2HPA was highly concentrated in the kidney, lung and liver. The concentration of ^{14}C in the above organs was almost the same as that in the blood, and the rate of elimination of ^{14}C from the organs was similar to that from blood. Gingell *et al.* (1979) reported that when hamsters and rats were given i.p. injections of [1-^{14}C]ND2HPA, the rate of ND2HPA metabolism to carbon dioxide was less in rats than in hamsters. This finding is consistent with that of the present study. The greater part of the dose (more than 90%) was recovered in the urine, and low levels (less than 6%) were recovered in the faeces and expired ^{14}C-carbon dioxide. Accumulation of [1-^{14}C]ND2HPA in the kidney of rats may be due to its excretion, whereas that in the liver suggests metabolism. ND2HPA and N2HP2OPA were detected in the blood and in the liver, lung and pancreas soon after administration of ND2HPA; but ND2OPA, another oxidative metabolite of ND2HPA, was not detected by HPLC analysis. It has been reported (Pour *et al.*, 1980; Lawson *et al.*, 1981) that NM2HPA and NM2OPA, possible methylating metabolites, were found in the blood, urine and some organs of hamsters given NM2OPA or ND2OPA. This study reports for the first time that, in addition to ND2HPA and N2HP2OPA, NM2HPA was also found in the urine of rats given ND2HPA. However, most of the ^{14}C in the blood and urine of rats given i.p. injections of [1-^{14}C]ND2HPA was unchanged ND2HPA. ND2HPA was activated to a mutagen by rat liver, but not by rat lung; NM2HPA was more mutagenic than ND2HPA in the presence of rat liver S9. The present results suggest that N2HP2OPA could be a potent lung carcinogen in rats, and N2HP2OPA and NM2HPA might be important intermediates in the metabolic activation of ND2HPA to its ultimate carcinogenic form in rats.

REFERENCES

Gingell, R., Brunk, G., Nagel, D. & Pour, P. (1979) Metabolism of three radiolabeled pancreatic carcinogenic nitrosamines in hamsters and rats. *Cancer Res., 39,* 4579-4583

Konishi, Y., Denda, A., Kondo, H. & Takahashi, S. (1976) Lung carcinomas induced by oral administration of *N*-bis(2-hydroxypropyl)nitrosamine in rats. *Gann, 67,* 773-780

Konishi, Y., Kondo, H., Inui, S., Denda, A., Ikeda, T. & Kojima, K. (1978) Organotropic effect of *N*-bis(2-hydroxypropyl)nitrosamine (DHPN). Production of lung and liver tumors by oral administration of DHPN in mice. *Gann, 69,* 77-84

Konishi, Y., Ikeda, T. & Yoshimura, H. (1979) Carcinogenic effect of *N*-bis(2-hydroxypropyl)nitrosamine by a single administration in rats. *Cancer Lett., 6,* 115-119

Kupper, R., Nagel, D., Gingell, R. & Brunk, G. (1978) Synthesis of ^{14}C-labeled *N*-nitrosobis(2-hydroxypropyl)amine. *J. Labelled Comp. Radiopharm., 15,* 175-179

Lawson, T.A., Helgeson, A.S., Grandijean, C.J., Wallcave, L. & Nagel, D. (1981) The formation of *N*-nitrosomethyl(2-oxopropyl)amine from *N*-nitrosobis(2-oxopropyl)amine *in vivo. Carcinogenesis, 2,* 845-849

Mori, Y., Niwa, T., Takahashi, H., Toyoshi, K., Denda, A., Takahashi, S. & Konishi, y. (1983) Mutagenicity of *N*-nitrosobis(2-hydroxypropyl)amine and its related compounds in the presence of rat lung and liver S9. *Cancer Lett., 18,* 271-275

Pour, P.M. & Wilson, R.B. (1980) *Experimental tumors of the pancreas.* In: Moossa, A.R., ed., *Tumors of the Pancreas,* Baltimore/London, Williams & Wilkins, pp. 37-158

Pour, P., Gingell, R., Langenbach, R., Nagel, D., Grandijean, C., Lawson, T. & Salmasi, S. (1980) Carcinogenicity of *N*-nitrosomethyl(2-oxopropyl)amine in Syrian hamsters. *Cancer Res., 40,* 3585-3590

COMPARATIVE METABOLISM OF β-OXIDIZED NITROSAMINES

D. NAGEL[1], A.S. HELGESON, R. LEWIS & T. LAWSON

*Eppley Institute for Research in Cancer, University of Nebraska Medical Center,
Omaha, NE, USA*

SUMMARY

Several β-oxidized nitrosamines have been shown to induce pancreatic cancer in Syrian hamsters. *N*-Nitrosobis(2-oxopropyl)amine (ND2OPA) is the most specific, but it also induces either colonic or prostatic tumours in MRC-Wistar rats. In-vivo and in-vitro metabolic studies show that *N*-nitrosomethyl(2-oxopropyl)amine is a metabolite of ND2OPA in hamsters but not in rats. ND2OPA is also present in higher concentrations in hamster pancreas than in the liver. No similar effect occurs in rats. These factors may explain, in part, the organotropism and species specificity of this nitrosamine.

INTRODUCTION

Several β-oxidized nitrosamines induce pancreatic adenocarcinomas in Syrian golden hamsters, which resemble morphologically tumours found in man (Pour *et al.*, 1981). Within this series of nitrosamines, *N*-nitrosobis(2-oxopropyl)amine (ND2OPA) is the most specific for the hamster pancreas: a single dose of 20 mg/kg ND2OPA induces, almost solely, tumours of the pancreas (Pour *et al.*, 1978). In contrast, when ND2OPA is administered to MRC Wistar rats it produces colonic tumours (subcutaneous administration; Pour *et al.*, 1979) or tumours of the prostate (oral administration; Pour, 1983).

Our work over the past several years has centred on elucidating the mechanism of activation of ND2OPA in hamster pancreas and determinating the factors responsible for the unique organotropism and species specificity of this nitrosamine.

Studies utilizing [1-^{14}C]- and [2,3-^{14}C]-ND2OPA indicate that DNA of hamster pancreas is almost solely methylated, while DNA of hamster liver is both methylated and alkylated with a longer alkyl chain (Lawson *et al.*, 1981). Since *N*-nitrosamines are generally believed to be activated by α-hydroxylation *via* mixed-function oxidases, this observation prompted our searches for a nitrosamine metabolite of ND2OPA containing an *N*-methyl group. *N*-nitrosomethyl(2-oxopropyl)amine (NM2OPA) appeared to be a prime candidate, since it also

---

[1] To whom correspondence should be addressed.

induced a high incidence of pancreatic tumours at a lower single dose (2.5 mg/kg) than
ND2OPA (Pour *et al.*, 1980).

Examination of blood and urine samples from rats and hamsters following administration
of ND2OPA revealed no NM2OPA or its hydroxy analogue, *N*-nitrosomethyl(2-hydroxy-
propyl)amine (NM2HPA) (Pour *et al.*, 1980). The principal urinary metabolites of ND2OPA
were found to be *N*-nitroso(2-hydroxypropyl)(2-oxopropyl)amine (N2HP2OPA) and
N-nitrosobis(2-hydroxypropyl)amine (ND2HPA). There was no significant quantitative or
qualitative difference in ND2OPA metabolism between rats and hamsters (Gingell *et al.*, 1979).

We report here several experiments which have elucidated, in part, the mechanism of action
of ND2OPA and suggest factors which may be responsible for its tissue and species specificity.

EXPERIMENTAL

Male Syrian golden hamsters and male MRC-Wistar rats (both eight weeks old) were
obtained from the Eppley Institute colonies. ND2OPA, containing no detectabe amount of
ND2HPA, N2HP2OPA, NM2HPA or NM2OPA by gas chromatographic analysis, was
injected subcutaneously at a dose of 10 mg/kg body weight. Hamsters were killed in pairs by
exsanguination by cardiac puncture. Each pancreas and liver was rapidly excised and
immediately frozen in liquid nitrogen and stored therein until required.

The tissues were homogenized in a Polytron homogenizer for 5 sec at setting 5 in five volumes
of phosphate buffer (pH 7.4) saturated with sodium chloride. The homogenate was extracted
with two volumes of dichloromethane containing 5% (v/v) ethanol. The mixture was clarified
by centrifugation and the organic layer removed and concentrated to about 500 μL in a stream
of nitrogen. The extract was examined directly by gas chromatography.

Gas chromatography was performed on a Varian 3700 apparatus equipped with a thermionic
specific detector. Selected extracts were also determined using gas chromatography coupled
with Thermal Energy Analyzer. The all-glass column (2 m × 2 mm) contained 10% SP-2100
on 100/200 Supelcoport. The injection temperature was 190°C, and the flow rate of helium was
15 mL/min. The initial column temperature of 70°C was maintained for 2 min, raised 4°C/min
to 170°C and held for 2 min. The retention times found were ND2HPA, 22.7 min; ND2OPA,
17.0 min; N2HP2OPA, 19.3 min; NM2HPA, 11.6 min; and NM2OPA, 9.2 min.

Tissue samples (0.5–1.0 g) were spiked with appropriate quantities of the nitrosamines,
extracted and analysed as described above. The calculated recoveries were: ND2HPA, 30%;
N2HP2OPA, 70%; ND2OPA, 85%; NM2OPA, 85% and NM2HPA, 80%. The profiles of the
gas chromatograms obtained in the recovery study indicated that the individual compounds
were pure and that the ND2OPA metabolites observed *in vivo* were not formed during the
extraction procedure.

Cytochrome P-450 containing microsomal proteins was isolated from hamster tissues by
differential centrifugation. The reaction mixture contained microsomal protein (2 mg), NADP
(10 mmol/L), glucose-6-phosphate (10 mmol/L),glucose-6-phosphate dehydrogenase (5 units)
and ND2OPA (10–50 mmol/L) in 2 ml Tris-magnesium chloride-sucrose buffer (pH 7.4).

DISCUSSION

Table 1 gives the concentrations of ND2OPA and metabolites present in hamster liver and
pancreas tissues following ND2OPA administration. ND2OPA and the metabolites ND2HPA,
N2HP2OPA, and NM2OPA were present in higher concentrations in the pancreas than in the
liver. Similar determinations on other hamster tissues, including lung, kidney and salivary

gland (not shown), showed lower concentrations of the nitrosamine in those tissues than in the pancreas, suggesting that ND2OPA is taken up selectively by the hamster pancreas relative to the liver and other organs and that ND2OPA is metabolized in that tissue. This selective uptake of ND2OPA may explain, in part, the specificity of this nitrosamine for the hamster pancreas. Alternatively, since the metabolism of ND2OPA → N2HP2OPA → ND2HPA is known to be reversible (Gingell *et al.*, 1979), it can be argued that the selectivity is due to uptake of N2HP2OPA or ND2HPA with metabolism back to ND2OPA. This possibility seems less likely.

Table 1. Concentrations (μg/g tissue) of N-nitrosobis(2-oxopropyl)amine (ND2OPA) and its metabolites in tissues of Syrian hamsters given a single subcutaneous dose of 10 mg/kg body weight ND2OPA

Tissue	Time after dosing (min)	Concentration (μg/g tissue) [a]				
		ND2OPA	ND2HPA	N2HP2OPA	NM2OPA	NM2HPA
Liver [b]	10	0.1 ± 0.01	1.7 ± 0.6	0.2 ± 0.01	0.01 ± 0.01	ND
	15	0.6 ± 0.10	1.0 ± 0.5	0.2 ± 0.02	0.01 ± 0.01	ND
	20	0.4 ± 0.01	11.2 ± 0.9	1.7 ± 0.2	0.05 ± 0.01	ND
	30	ND	9.1 ± 0.5	ND	0.10 ± 0.4	ND
	45	ND	8.1 ± 0.4	ND	ND	ND
	60	ND	7.4 ± 0.4	ND	ND	ND
Pancreas [b]	10	0.2 ± 0.02	1.1 ± 0.1	1.2 ± 0.1	0.04 ± 0.02	0.06 ± 0.01
	15	0.4 ± 0.01	1.1 ± 0.1	1.2 ± 0.1	0.05 ± 0.01	ND
	20	0.4 ± 0.01	11.9 ± 0.1	1.3 ± 0.5	0.05 ± 0.1	ND
	30	3.7 ± 0.2	–	20.9 ± 0.3	0.20 ± 0.05	ND
	45	3.4 ± 0.5	14.8 ± 1.0	4.7 ± 0.8	0.40 ± 0.01	ND
	60	0.8 ± 0.1	18.9 ± 1.4	2.0 ± 0.2	0.02 ± 0.01	ND

[a] Mean ± SD; 3 animals/point; ND2HPA, N-nitrosobis(2-hydroxypropyl)amine; N2HP2OPA, N-nitroso(2-hydroxypropyl)-(2-oxopropyl)amine; NM2OPA, N-nitrosomethyl(2-oxopropyl)amine; NM2HPA, N-nitrosomethyl(2-hydroxypropyl)-amine
[b] Approximately 1 g of liver and 0.5 g of pancreas were extracted
ND, not detected (> 0.005 μg/g tissue)

Table 2. Concentrations (μg/g tissue) of N-nitrosobis(2-oxopropyl)amine (ND2OPA) and its metabolites in tissues of MRC-Wistar rats given a single subcutaneous dose of 10 mg/kg body weight ND2OPA

Tissue	Time after dosing (min)	Concentration (μg/g tissue) [a]				
		ND2OPA	ND2HPA	N2HP2OPA	NM2OPA	NM2HPA
Liver [b]	15	0.7 ± 0.1	ND	0.3 ± 0.1	ND	ND [c]
	30	1.9 ± 0.2	3.6 ± 0.4	0.5 ± 0.1	ND	ND
	45	13.1 ± 2.7	19.5 ± 1.8	1.7 ± 0.8	ND	ND
	60	25.4 ± 2.9	7.1 ± 0.7	0.8 ± 0.2	ND	ND
Pancreas [b]	15	ND	ND	2.9 ± 0.4	ND	ND
	30	2.9 ± 0.9	5.6 ± 1.2	3.3 ± 0.1	ND	ND
	45	1.8 ± 0.5	7.2 ± 0.7	22.2 ± 3.0	ND	ND
	60	1.3 ± 0.4	4.4 ± 0.3	7.1 ± 0.5	ND	ND

[a] Mean ± SD; 6 animals/point; ND2HPA, N-nitrosobis(2-hydroxypropyl)amine; N2HP2OPA, N-nitroso(2-hydroxypropyl)-(2-oxopropyl)amine; NM2OPA, N-nitrosomethyl(2-oxopropyl)amine; NM2HPA, N-nitrosomethyl(2-hydroxypropyl)-amine
[b] Approximately 1 g of liver and 0.5 g of pancreas were extracted
ND, not detected (> 0.005 μg/g tissue)

Table 2 shows the results of a similar study conducted with MRC-Wistar rats. Unlike the situation in hamster, the concentrations of ND2OPA and ND2HPA are lower in rat pancreas, but the levels of N2HP2OPA are higher. Neither NM2OPA nor NM2HPA was detected in the rat tissues examined.

Table 3 gives the results obtained from incubation of ND2OPA with hamster liver and pancreatic microsomes. NM2OPA, N2HP2OPA and ND2HPA are metabolites of both liver and pancreas. Slightly greater amounts of NM2OPA are produced in the pancreas than the liver. In similar studies conducted with microsomes obtained from pancreas and liver from MRC-Wistar rats (Table 4), ND2HPA and N2HP2OPA were metabolites of ND2OPA, but we could not detect NM2OPA. This result is in agreement with our earlier in-vivo results (Table 2).

These results suggest that NM2OPA is involved in the initiation by ND2OPA of pancreatic cancer in hamsters. NM2OPA is a more potent pancreatic carcinogen than ND2OPA, inducing tumours after a single dose of 2.5 mg/kg body weight. α-Hydroxylation of NM2OPA on the oxopropyl chain would certainly yield a methylating electrophile, which would account for the predominant methylation observed in pancreatic DNA following ND2OPA administration.

A second mechanism that may account for the observed methylation also appears likely. We reported recently that base-catalysed decomposition of ethyl *N*-nitroso-2-oxopropylcarbamate

Table 3. In-vitro metabolism of (ND2OPA) *N*-nitrosobis(2-oxopropyl)amine by Syrian hamster microsomal incubations[a]

Tissue	Amount of ND2OPA added (mmol)	Metabolites (nmol/mg microsomal protein)[b]			
		NM2OPA	ND2OPA	N2HP2OPA	ND2HPA
Pancreas	10	212 ± 10	6 400 ± 500	2 000 ± 600	600 ± 50
	50	425 ± 10	24 000 ± 4 000	300 ± 50	800 ± 100
Liver	10	50 ± 10	6 000 ± 900	1 100 ± 30	700 ± 100
	50	110 ± 10	22 500 ± 5 000	1 250 ± 100	800 ± 200

[a] 10-min incubations
[b] Values are averages of 8 determinations; NM2OPA, *N*-nitrosomethyl(2-oxopropyl)amine; ND2OPA, *N*-nitrosobis(2-oxopropyl)amine; N2HP2OPA, *N*-nitroso(2-hydroxypropyl)(2-oxopropyl)amine; ND2HPA, *N*-nitrosobis(2-hydroxypropyl)amine

Table 4. In-vitro metabolism of *N*-nitrosobis(2-oxopropyl)amine (ND2OPA) by Wistar rat microsomal incubations[a]

Tissue	Amount of ND2OPA added (mmol)	Metabolites (nmol/mg microsomal protein)[b]			
		NM2OPA	ND2OPA	N2HP2OPA	ND2HPA
Pancreas	10	ND	6 100 ± 200	500 ± 50	700 ± 40
	50	ND	23 900 ± 1 000	300 ± 40	500 ± 40
Liver	10	ND	7 200 ± 800	500 ± 200	640 ± 40
	50	ND	24 100 ± 2 050	400 ± 50	960 ± 250

[a] 10-min incubations
[b] Values are averages of 8 determinations; NM2OPA, *N*-nitrosomethyl(2-oxopropyl)amine; ND2OPA, *N*-nitrosobis(2-oxopropyl)amine; N2HP2OPA, *N*-nitroso(2-hydroxypropyl)(2-oxopropyl)amine; ND2HPA, *N*-nitrosobis(2-hydroxypropyl)amine

(pH 7.4) produces methanol in 40% yield (Lewis & Nagel, 1983). Diazoacetone is also produced in high yield, but this product is relatively stable at physiological pH. This suggests that, following α-hydroxylation, ND2OPA can yield a methylating electrophile. Recent studies by Leung and Archer (1983), utilizing N-nitrosoacetoxymethyl-2-oxopropylamine, also support this hypothesis. This compound methylated DNA. Hence it appears that the alkylation of hamster liver DNA following ND2OPA administration probably results from α-hydroxylation of ND2HPA or selective α-hydroxylation of N2HP2OPA on the oxopropyl chain.

ACKNOWLEDGEMENT

This work was supported by US National Cancer Institute Grants R01-CA31016 and R26-CA20198.

REFERENCES

Gingell, R., Brunk, G., Nagel, D. & Pour, P. (1979) Metabolism of three radiolabeled carcinogenic nitrosamines in hamsters and rats. *Cancer Res., 39*, 4579–4583

Lawson, T., Gingell, R. & Nagel, D. (1981) Methylation of hamster DNA by the carcinogen N-nitrosobis(2-oxopropyl)amine. *Cancer Lett., 11*, 251–254

Leung, K.-H. & Archer, M.C. (1983) Mechanism of DNA methylation by N-nitrosodipropylamine. *Proc. Am. Assoc. Cancer Res., 47*, 313

Lewis, R. & Nagel, D. (1983) Studies with a model of an activated form of beta-oxidized nitrosamines. *Proc. Am. Assoc. Cancer Res., 24*, 451

Pour, P. (1983) Prostatic cancer induced in MRC rats by N-nitrosobis-(2-oxopropyl)amine and N-nitrosobis(2-hydroxypropyl)amine. *Carcinogenesis, 4*, 49–55

Pour, P. Salmasi, S.Z. & Runge, R.G. (1978) Selective induction of pancreatic ductular tumors by single doses of N-nitrosobis(2-oxopropyl)amine in Syrian golden hamsters. *Cancer Lett., 4*, 317–323

Pour, P., Salmasi, S., Runge, R., Gingell, R., Wallcave, L., Nagel, D. & Stepan, K. (1979) Carcinogenicity of N-nitrosobis(2-hydroxypropyl)amine and N-nitrosobis(2-oxopropyl)amine in MRC rats. *J. natl Cancer Inst., 63*, 181–189

Pour, P., Gingell, R., Langenbach, R., Nagel, D., Grandjean, C., Lawson, T. & Salmasi, S. (1980) Carcinogenicity of N-nitrosomethyl(2-oxopropyl)amine, a potent pancreatic carcinogen in Syrian hamsters. *Cancer Res., 40*, 3585–3590

Pour, P.M., Runge, R.G., Birt, D., Gingell, R., Lawson, T., Nagel, D., Wallcave, L. & Salmasi, S.Z. (1981) Current knowledge of pancreatic carcinogenesis in the hamster and its relevance to the human disease. *Cancer, 47*, 1573–1587

METABOLISM OF NITROSAMINES BY CYTOCHROME P-450 ISOZYMES

C.S. YANG, Y.Y. TU, J. HONG & C. PATTEN

Department of Biochemistry, UMDNJ-New Jersey Medical School, Newark, NJ 07103, USA

SUMMARY

Results are presented to show that *N*-nitrosodimethylamine demethylase is P-450 mediated and *N*-nitrosodimethylamine is efficiently metabolized by specific P-450 isozymes inducible by a group of new inducers. The P-450-mediated *N*-nitrosodimethylamine demethylase also responds differently to inhibitors when activities are compared with those of classical monooxygenase systems.

INTRODUCTION

It is well recognized that metabolic activation of nitrosamines is required prior to the carcinogenic or cytotoxic actions of these compounds. However, the enzymes that catalyse such activation and the factors that affect the metabolism of nitrosamines are not clearly understood (Lai & Arcos, 1980). Although the involvement of cytochrome P-450 (P-450) in *N*-nitroso-dimethylamine (NDMA) metabolism has been demonstrated (Czygan *et al.*, 1973; Guengerich, 1977), the importance of P-450 in nitrosamine metabolism has been questioned, and alternative pathways have been suggested (Lake *et al.*, 1976a, b). Part of the controversy derives from the fact that microsomal NDMA demethylase (NDMAd) activity is not induced by classical P-450 inducers, such as phenobarbital and 3-methylcholanthrene (Lai & Arcos, 1980); nor is the NDMAd inhibited by commonly-used P-450 inhibitors such as SKF 525A (Lake *et al.*, 1976b). The presence of multiple K_m values for NDMAd has also puzzled many investigators (Lai & Arcos, 1980). Many problems, however, become understandable if we consider the multiplicity of P-450. It is known that there are different types of P-450 isozymes, each with different substrate specificities and inducibilities; the isozymes efficient in metabolizing nitrosamines may be different from the isozymes responsive to classical inducers and substrates. This report demonstrates that NDMA is indeed metabolized by P-450 and is most efficiently metabolized by a new type of P-450 isozyme inducible by a new class of inducers.

RECOVERY OF NDMAd IN MICROSOMES

It has been reported that only about 50% of the NDMAd activity in the postmitochondrial supernatant is recovered in the microsomal fraction and the activity is enhanced upon addition of the 100 000 × *g* supernatant (Lake *et al.*, 1976a).We have investigated this by following the recovery of not only NDMAd but also P-450. After centrifuging the postmitochondrial supernatant (derived from a 14% liver homogenate in 50 mmol/L Tris : 154 mmol/L potassium chloride, pH 7.4) at 100 000 × *g* for 90 min, 90% of the NDMAd was recovered in the microsomes. This was accompanied by a 83% recovery of P-450 and a 92% recovery of NADPH-cytochrome c reductase. About 10% NDMAd was present in the 100 000 × *g* supernatant; it is not known how much of this activity is attributable to unsedimented endoplasmic reticulum. Similar recoveries of NDMAd and P-450 in microsomes were also observed with postmitochondrial supernatant from rats pretreated with isopropanol, in which the total NDMAd activity was induced about four-fold by the treatment. Because mitochondria and nuclei have very low, if any, NDMAd activity, it is concluded that the NDMAd occurs predominantly in the endoplasmic reticulum, corresponding to the distribution of P-450 in hepatocytes.

INDUCTION OF NDMAd AND P-450 ISOZYMES

During the past two years, we have systematically investigated the induction of NDMAd and discovered a group of inducers. Rat liver microsomal NDMAd activity is induced two-to five-fold by fasting (Tu & Yang, 1983), diabetes (Peng *et al.*, 1983), acetone or isopropanol (Tu *et al.*, 1983), ethanol (Peng *et al.*, 1982) and pyrazole (Tu *et al.*, 1981). Kinetic analyses indicate that this is due mainly to the induction of a high-affinity form of NDMAd with K_m values of 50 to 70 μmol/L. The induction is accompanied by intensification of polypeptides with molecular weights of 50 000 to 52 000. Several lines of observation suggest that these polypeptides are P-450 isozymes, and this is confirmed by the purification-reconstitution approach described in the next section.

The above treatments also enhance the microsomal metabolism of NDMA. The metabolism of *N*-nitrosomethylbenzylamine and *N*-nitrosomethylaniline is enhanced by fasting, isopropanol and ethanol, but not by diabetes. The results suggest that, in addition to a common form of P-450, other P-450 isozymes are also induced by factors such as fasting, acetone or ethanol, and they may account for the enhanced activity with nitrosamines such as *N*-nitroso-methylaniline.

The mechanism of induction is still under investigation. The fact that both fasting and diabetes cause ketogenesis and that acetone is an inducer of NDMAd suggest that ketone bodies may be inducers for specific P-450 isozymes. These endogenous compounds may be an important class of P-450 inducers, which may also affect the metabolism of drugs and hormones. Ethanol consumption (for more than two days) would also result in ketogenesis. This factor may contribute to the induction of NDMAd. Ethanol itself has been shown to be an inducer; with a single intragastric dose of ethanol (4 g/kg), the induction is potentiated by aldoxime, an inhibitor of alcohol dehydrogenase (unpublished data). Pyrazole, a strong inducer of NDMAd, is also an inhibitor of alcohol dehydrogenase and can increase plasma levels of ethanol and acetone. The role of these two compounds in the induction of NDMAd by pyrazole, however, is not known.

METABOLISM OF NDMA BY P-450 ISOZYMES

P-450 isozymes were purified from control, acetone-, fasting- and pyrazole-induced rat liver microsomes by a procedure modified from Cheng and Schenkman (1982). It involved fractionation of the solubilized microsomes with a lauric acid-AH-Sepharose 4B column and removal of the solubilizing detergent, Emulgen 911, with a hydroxylapatite column. The preparation usually contained 6–9 nmol P-450/mg protein. In preparations that had been subjected to a carboxymethyl-Sepharose CL-6B column prior to hydroxylapatite, the P-450 contents were 12–14 nmol/mg. SDS-polyacrylamide gel electrophoresis indicated that the enzyme preparation contained a protein band with a molecular weight of 52 000 (Lanes B-E in Fig. 1), with minor impurity bands in the 49 000–50 000 region and around 35 000. The lower molecular weight impurity could be eliminated by carboxymethyl-Sepharose chromatography (Lane 1). The P-450 isozymes isolated from untreated rats appeared to have molecular weights slightly less than 52 000 (lanes F and G). P-450 was also purified from phenobarbital-induced

Fig. 1. SDS-polyacrylamide gel electrophoresis of monooxygenase enzymes. Conditions were similar to those of Tu and Yang (1983). P-450 preparations in the various Lanes were: phenobarbital-induced (A), fasting-induced (B), acetone-induced (C), pyrazole-induced (D, E), untreated (F,G) and acetone-induced with higher purity (I). Lanes H and J contained protein molecular weight standards and purified rat liver NADPH-cytochrome P-450 reductase, respectively.

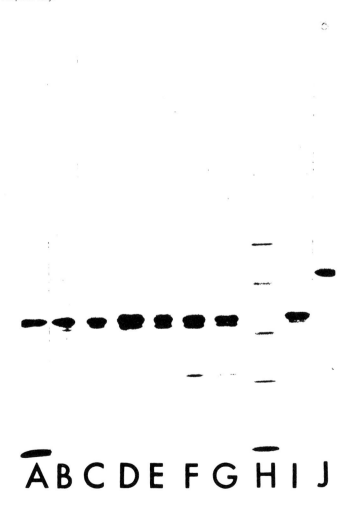

Table 1.   Activities of reconstituted monooxygenase system[a]

Type of P-450	N-Nitrosodimethylamine demethylase	Benzphetamine demethylase
Control	1.58	ND[b]
Pyrazole-induced	4.30	1.46
Acetone-induced	5.01	6.94
Phenobarbital-induced	0.41	12.16

[a] The reaction mixture contained 0.25 to 0.85 nmol P-450, 4.5 units of reductase (which reduced 4.5 µmol cytochrome c/min), 22 µg of dilauroylphosphatidyl-choline, 2 mg bovine serum albumin and 4 mmol/L N-nitrosodimethylamine (or 1 mmol/L benzphetamine) in 0.5 mL and was incubated for 20 min. Other conditions were similar to those of Tu and Yang (1983). Activity is expressed in nmol formaldehyde/min per nmol P-450.
[b] Not determined

Table 2.   Inhibition of P-450 mediated monooxygenase activities[a]

Inhibitor	Microsomes (% inhibition)		NDMAd by P-450 (% inhibition)	
	Benzphetamine demethylase	NDMAd	Acetone-induced	Pyrazole-induced
SKF 525A (0.01 mmol/L)	63	2	0	0
Pyrazole (1 mmol/L)	9	78	33	36
3-Amino-1,2,4-triazole (10 mmol/L)	17	87	96	ND[b]
2-Phenylethylamine (1 mmol/L)	24	100	81	84

[a] The incubation mixture contained acetone-induced microsomes (0.23 mg protein) or the reconstituted system (similar to that of Table 1) in 0.5 mL. The incubation period was 10 min with benzphetamine (1 mmol/L) and 20 min with N-nitrosodimethylamine (4 mmol/L). In the absence of inhibitors, the microsomal benzphetamine and N-nitrosodimethylamine demethylase (NDMAd) activities were 4.75 and 5.16 nmol/min per nmol, respectively, and the reconstituted NDMAd activities were 2.42 and 4.30 nmol/min per nmol, respectively, with acetone- and pyrazole-induced P-450.
[b] Not determined

microsomes by the method of West *et al.* (1979) to a purity of 14 nmol P-450/mg protein, showing a single band of molecular weight 52 000 (Lane A).

The purified P-450 isozymes exhibited NDMAd activity when reconstituted with purified NADPH-cytochrome P-450 reductase (Yang *et al.*, 1978) and dilauroylphosphatidylcholine. No activity was observed when either P-450 or the reductase was omitted from the incubation mixture. The phospholipid was required for maximal activity, although activity was also observed in its absence. Bovine serum albumin (or glutathione) was shown to prolong the linear portion of the time curve and therefore was included routinely in the incubation mixture.

The partially purified P-450 isozymes showed distinct substrate specificities (Table 1). When assayed with 4 mmol/L NDMAd, the pyrazole- or acetone-induced isozyme was about three times as active as the isozyme from untreated rats, whereas the phenobarbital-induced form was only 6% as active. With regard to benzphetamine demethylase, a classic monooxygenase, the phenobarbital-induced form had high activity; the acetone-induced form had lower activity;

and the pyrazole-induced form the lowest. It is possible that the P-450 preparation from acetone-induced rats contained more than one isozyme, some with high NDMAd activity and others with high benzphetamine demethylase activity.

With the reconstituted system, low K_m values of 50–70 µmol/L were observed with P-450 preparations from control, acetone-induced and pyrazole-induced rats; but high K_m values still existed in a manner similar to that observed with the corresponding microsomes (Tu *et al.*, 1979, 1983). Because the P-450 preparation may still contain more than one species of P-450 isozyme, it is not known whether the multiple K_m was due to one species of P-450 or to different P-450 isozymes. The question will be answered when pure P-450 becomes available (work in progress). At the present stage of purity, however, the P-450 preparations are useful with regard to several questions concerning the actions of inhibitors. The involvement of P-450 in NDMAd activity has been questioned, because the activity is not inhibited by SKF 525A, but by pyrazole and 3-amino-1,2,4-triazole. The possible involvement of monoamine oxidase has been suggested, because NDMA metabolism *in vivo* is inhibited by monoamine oxidase substrates or inhibitors such as 2-phenylethylamine (Phillips *et al.*, 1982). This pattern of inhibition was reproduced with acetone-induced microsomes (Table 2). With the exception of SKF 525A, all compounds are strong inhibitors of NDMAd but not of benzphetamine demethylase. When tested in a system reconstituted with acetone- and pyrazole-induced P-450 isozyme, SKF 525A was not an inhibitor, but 3-amino-1,2,4-triazole and 2-phenylethylamine were strong inhibitors of NDMAd. The results suggest that 2-phenylethylamine may affect NDMA metabolism by inhibiting P-450 and further strengthen the idea that NDMAd activity is that of a P-450-dependent monooxygenase system.

REFERENCES

Arcos, J.C., Bryant, G.M., Venkatesan, N. & Argus, M.F. (1975) Repression of dimethylnitrosamine-demethylase by typical inducers of microsomal mixed-function oxidase. *Biochem. Pharmacol., 24,* 1544–1547

Cheng, K.-C. & Schenkman, J.B. (1982) Purification and characterization of two constitutive forms of rat liver microsomal cytochrome P-450. *J. biol. Chem., 257,* 2378–2385

Czygan, P., Greim, H., Garro, A.J., Hutterer, F., Schaffner, F., Popper, H., Rosenthal, O. & Cooper, D.Y. (1973) Microsomal metabolism of dimethylnitrosamine and the cytochrome P-450 dependency of its activation to a mutagen. *Cancer Res., 33,* 2983–2986

Guengerich, F.P. (1977) Separation and purification of multiple forms of microsomal cytochrome P-450. *J. biol. Chem., 252,* 3970–3979

Lai, D.Y. & Arcos, J.S. (1980) Dialkylnitrosamine bioactivation and carcinogenesis. *Life Sci., 27,* 2149–2165

Lake, B.G., Phillips, J.C., Heading, C.E. & Gangolli, S.D. (1976a) Studies on the in vitro metabolism of dimethylnitrosamine by rat liver. *Toxicology, 5,* 297–309

Lake, B.G., Minski, M.J., Phillips, J.C., Gangolli, S.D. & Lloyd, A.G. (1976b) Investigation into the hepatic metabolism of dimethylnitrosamine in the rat. *Life Sci., 17,* 1599–1606

Peng, R., Tu, Y.Y. & Yang, C.S. (1982) The induction and competitive inhibition of a high affinity microsomal nitrosodimethylamine demethylase by ethanol. *Carcinogenesis, 3,* 1457–1461

Peng, R., Tennant, P., Lorr, N.A. & Yang, C.S. (1983) Alternation of microsomal monooxygenase system and carcinogen metabolism by streptozotocin-induced diabetes in rats. *Carcinogenesis, 4* (in press)

Phillips, J.C., Bex, C., Lake, B.G., Cettrell, R.C. & Gangolli, S.D. (1982) Inhibition of dimethylnitrosamine metabolism by some heterocyclic compounds and by substrates and inhibitors of monoamine oxidase in the rat. *Cancer Res., 42,* 3761–3765

Tu, Y.Y. & Yang, C.S. (1983) High affinity dealkylase system in rat liver microsomes and its induction by fasting. *Cancer Res., 43,* 623–629

Tu, Y.Y., Sonnenberg, J., Lewis, K.F. & Yang, C.S. (1981) Pyrazole-induced cytochrome P-450 in rat liver microsomes: an isozyme with high affinity for dimethylnitrosamine. *Biochem. biophys. Res. Commun.,* **103,** 905–912

Tu, Y.Y., Peng, R., Cheng, Z.-F. & Yang, C.S. (1983) Induction of a high affinity nitrosamine demethylase in rat liver microsomes by acetone and isopropanol. *Chem.-biol. Interact.,* **44,** 247–260

West, S.B., Hueng, M.-T., Miwa, G.T. & Lu, A.Y.H. (1979) A simple and rapid procedure for the purification of phenobarbital-inducible cytochrome P-450 from rat liver microsomes. *Arch. Biochem. Biophys.,* **193,** 42–50

Yang, C.S., Strickhart, F.S. & Kicha, L.P. (1978) Interaction between NADPH-cytochrome P-450 reductase and hepatic microsomes. *Biochem. biophys. Acta,* **509,** 326–337

ALTERNATIVE BIOACTIVATION ROUTES FOR β-HYDROXYNITROSAMINES. BIOCHEMICAL AND CHEMICAL MODEL STUDIES

R.N. LOEPPKY, W. TOMASIK, D.A. KOVACS, J.R. OUTRAM & K.H. BYINGTON

Departments of Chemistry and Pharmacology, University of Missouri-Columbia, Columbia, MO 65211, USA

SUMMARY

The biochemical retroaldol-like fragmentation of β-hydroxynitrosamines has been investigated further. The extent of fragmentation of 2-hydroxy-2-methylpropyl-methylnitrosamine (HMPMN) to *N*-nitrosodimethylamine and acetone induced by metabolic activation increases as the NADPH level is decreased. 2-Hydroxy-2-phenylethyl-methylnitrosamine (HPhEMN) undergoes competitive oxidation to 2-oxy-2-phenylethyl-methylnitrosamine (OPhEMN) and fragmentation to benzaldehyde and *N*-nitroso-dimethylamine in the presence of a metabolic activation system from rat liver. The extent of the oxidation was increased by preinduction of the rats with phenobarbital, or separate addition of NADPH and NAD, but was decreased by addition of dimethyl sulfoxide. The fragmentation was observed most readily when oxidation was inhibited or was not induced by cofactors. When HPhEMN was administered to a rat intraperitoneally, benzaldehyde (fragmentation) was found in the urine with OPhEMN and the substrate, but only the last two substances were found in liver and blood. These experiments provide evidence for retroaldol-like fragmentation of β-hydroxynitrosamines both *in vitro* and *in vivo*. In a related investigation, it was found that *N*-nitroso-*N*-4-chlorophenyl-2-aminoethanal (NCAE) is extremely reactive and induces spontaneous generation of 4-chlorobenzenediazonium ion in chloroform, as trapped by 2-naphthol. NCAE reacts with dimethylamine in chloroform, benzene or methanol to give *N*-nitrosodimethylamine and 4-chloroaniline, among other products. This suggests that β-nitrosaminoaldehydes produced by the biooxidation of their corresponding alcohols could produce cell alteration through alkylation, deamination or transnitrosation.

INTRODUCTION

The biochemical transformations of β-hydroxy and β-ketonitrosamines present challenges to the principal hypothesis linking the metabolic activation of *N*-nitrosamines with their carcinogenicity – the α-hydroxylation hypothesis. It was first shown by Krüger (1973), then

– 429 –

verified and extended by Archer and Leung (1981), that C-1 of N-nitrosodipropylamine (NDPA) or β-oxo- or β-hydroxypropylpropylnitrosamine is incorporated into rat liver nucleic acids as a methyl group. These latter two β-oxidized N-nitrosamines are metabolites of NDPA. Singer et al. (1981) have demonstrated that long-chain alkylmethylnitrosamines undergo bioconversion to β-oxo- and β-hydroxypropylpropylnitrosamines. Krüger (1973) proposed a mechanism of chain shortening, involving the β-ketonitrosamine, similar to that of fatty acid metabolism to account for the incorporation of C-1 into RNA as methyl group. We have shown that β-hydroxynitrosamines undergo both a chemical and a biochemical fragmentation reaction which could also account for nucleic acid methylation (Loeppky & Outram, 1982; Loeppky et al., 1982). β-Keto- and β-hydroxynitrosamines are in dynamic equilibrium in the mammalian organism. We have demonstrated that N-nitrosamino alcohols incapable of oxidation to ketones undergo the biochemical fragmentation. Nevertheless, both Krüger's and our hypotheses for chain shortening must be considered viable at this time. These hypotheses do not obviate the α-hydroxylation proposal. They foresee fragmentation of the β-oxidized N-nitrosamine to an alkylmethylnitrosamine prior to α-hydroxylation. Support for these hypotheses is provided by the finding that the in-vivo metabolism of bis-2-oxy-propylnitrosamine produces β-hydroxypropylmethylnitrosamine (Lawson et al., 1981). Other experiments and proposals relating to chain shortening and bioactivation modes for β-oxidized N-nitrosamines have been reviewed by us (Loeppky et al., 1981).

Long-term feeding and excretion studies by Preussmann et al. (1982) have shown recently that N-nitrosodiethanolamine (NDELA) has a carcinogenic potency similar to that of N-nitrosodimethylamine (NDMA), despite the unusually large percentage of this compound which is excreted unchanged. Extensive studies by Lethco et al. (1982) on the disposition of orally and topically administered ^{14}C-NDELA in rats have detected the production of a single, unidentified urinary metabolite and no incorporation of ^{14}C-labelled fragments in the nucleic acids. Preussmann has proposed that either our β-hydroxynitrosamine fragmentation or, an alternative hypothesis of Michejda's, alkylation (Koepke et al., 1979) may be involved in the bioactivation of NDELA. The α-hydroxylation of NDELA followed by decomposition is ultimately predicted to produce the 2-hydroxyethyl carbonium ion. A large body of chemical information relating to the properties of other 2-hydroxy alkyl carbonium ions suggests that this cation should either have a high propensity for rearrangement to protonated acetaldehyde (a comparatively poor electrophile) or it should produce a more stable electrophile such as ethylene oxide or 1,2,3-oxadiazoline. Another possible activation route for NDELA may involve its oxidation to an aldehyde. Okada's group (Suzuki & Okada, 1979) has reported that 2-(N-butylnitrosamino)ethanal is chemically unstable and upon standing at room temperature produces directly acting mutagens in the Ames assay. These considerations have caused us to broaden our enquiry into the mechanisms by which β-hydroxynitrosamines induce tumour formation in experimental animals.

RESULTS AND DISCUSSION

Biochemical fragmentation of β-hydroxynitrosamines

We reported previously that incubation of either 2-hydroxy-2-phenylethylmethylnitrosamine (HPhEMN) or 2-hydroxy-2-methylpropylmethylnitrosamine (HMPMN) results in the production of NDMA and benzaldehyde and acetone respectively (Loeppky & Outram, 1982). These transformations induced by rat liver 9 000 × g supernatant preparations (S9) have been investigated further and the stated products verified by gas chromatography-mass spectroscopy. In addition to benzaldehyde and NDMA, 2-oxo-2-phenylethyl-methylnitrosamine (OPhEMN) is produced during the incubation of HPhEMN (Fig. 1). Figure

2 shows that percent yield of NDMA and OPhEMN decreases at high concentration of S9. We previously observed decreases in product yields (after a maximum) with increasing incubation time and speculated that reductions in yields in these two types of experiment could result from further biotransformation of the reaction products. Such processes would be favoured, as the microsomal content of the incubation mixture increased, but would require the presence of an adequate supply of NADPH if oxidative metabolism were responsible.

Since our assay of the retroaldol-like cleavage of β-hydroxy nitrosamines has relied principally on the detection of NDMA, we initiated further experiments to test the hypothesis that it may be consumed oxidatively following its production in the cleavage reaction. Initial experiments involved HPMN, which is oxidized competitively to its ketone (OPMN), but we had difficulty in reproducing our earlier work with this substrate and chose to work with HMPMN, for which we had found the highest percent cleavage. Although the concentrations

Fig. 1. Reaction products of incubation of 2-hydroxy-2-phenylethylmethylnitrosamine (HPhEMN) with rat liver 9 000 × g supernatant preparation (S9); NDMA, N-nitrosodimethylamine; OPhEMN, 2-oxo-2-phenylethyl-methylnitrosamine.

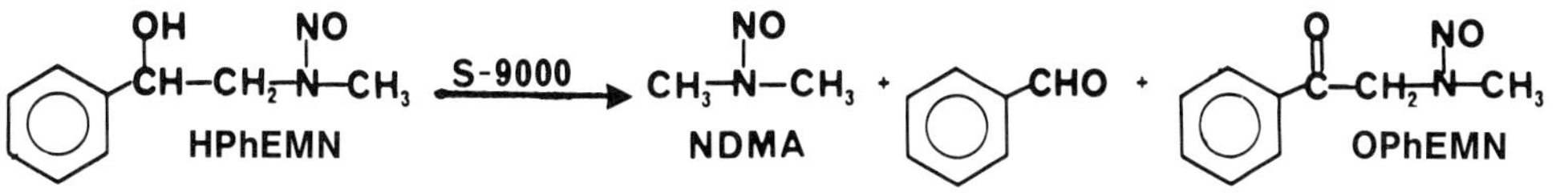

Fig. 2. % Yields of N-nitrosodimethylamine (●) and 2-oxo-2-phenylethylmethylnitrosamine (○) after incubation of 2-hydroxy-2-phenylethylmethylnitrosamine with rat liver 9 000 × g supernatant preparation (S9) as a function of protein concentration.

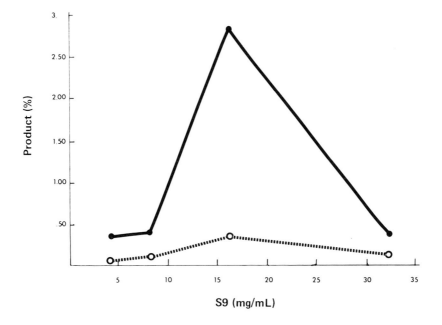

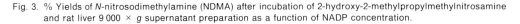

Fig. 3. % Yields of *N*-nitrosodimethylamine (NDMA) after incubation of 2-hydroxy-2-methylpropylmethylnitrosamine and rat liver 9 000 × *g* supernatant preparation as a function of NADP concentration.

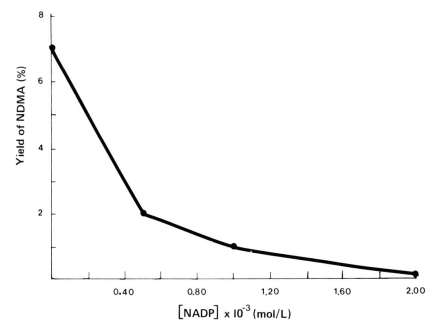

of substrate (0.023 mol/L) and S9 protein (8.25 mg/mL) were lower than in our previous experiments, cleavage of HMPMN to NDMA was again observed. The transformation was detected by high-performance liquid chromatographic separation and determination of DNMA after protein precipitation with trichloracetic acid, separation and clean-up using our ion-exchange method. The substrate was shown to be free of NDMA at a confidence level of 0.00012% (NDMA) by standard addition techniques, and this same procedure was used to quantitate the NDMA concentration (reversed-phase C-18 high-performance liquid chromatography with ultra-violet detection at 254 nm). Figure 3 shows that the percent yield of NDMA decreases as the concentration of NADP added to the NADPH generating system is increased in the incubation mixture. We conclude, therefore, that our ability to detect the retroaldol cleavage is partly inhibited by the consecutive oxidative destruction of NDMA in the incubation mixture.

Chemistry of a β-nitrosaminoaldehyde

The aldehyde 2-(*N*-nitroso-*N*-4-chlorophenyl)aminoethanal (NCAE) shown at the centre of Figure 4 was suspected to be a product of the nitrosation of *N*-4-chlorophenylpyrrolidine. It was synthesized independently and subjected to extensive spectroscopic characterization. NCAE is an extremely reactive material: it is unstable except when stored at $-10\,°C$ and is best purified by recrystallization from cold ether/hexane mixtures. Various chromatographic purification procedures led to decomposition of the aldehyde. The disappearence of NCAE in various reaction mixtures is easily monitored by following the disappearence of the very characteristic aldehyde proton (9.53 ppm) in its nuclear magnetic resonance (NMR) spectrum.

Fig. 4. Scheme showing chemical transformations of 2-(N-nitroso-N-4-chlorophenyl)aminotethanal (1); 2,β-naphthol; 3, dye; 4, N-nitrosodimethylamine; 5, p-chloroaniline; 6, p-chlorophenylmethylnitrosamine; 7, methyl hemiacetal.

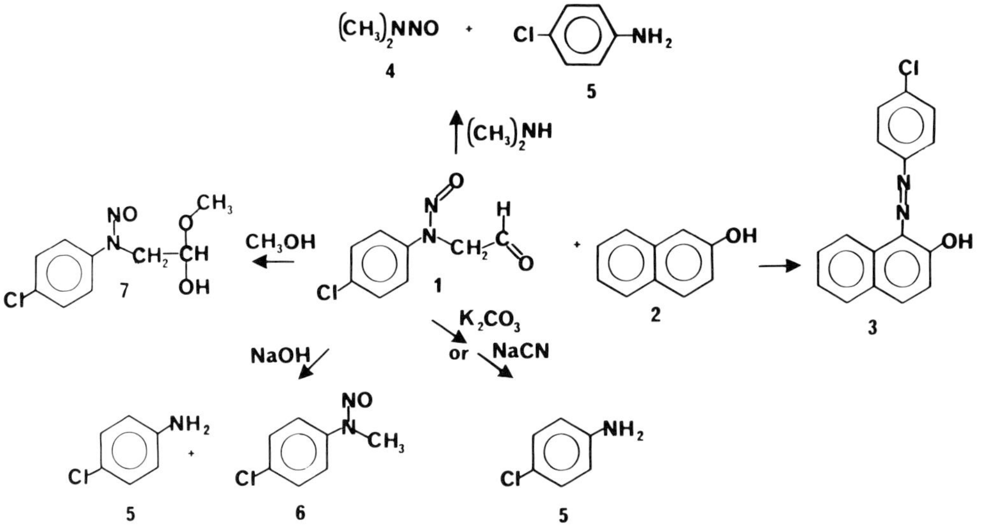

The various chemical transformations of NCAE (1) are summarized in Figure 4. All of these experiments were conducted in an argon atmosphere in the dark, and monitoring was performed by high-performance liquid chromatography and NMR. Mild heating (50 °C) of NCAE in chloroform results in its decomposition within 3 h. When the same experiment is performed with the addition of β-naphthol (2), several bright orange compounds are formed, along with a number of unidentified substances. Chromatography of this mixture permits the isolation and characterization of the dye (3) formed from the coupling of β-naphthol with the 4-chlorobenzenediazonium ion in a yield of 2.2% (see Fig. 4). This observation suggests that β-nitrosaminoaldehydes can form diazonium ions spontaneously.

Another very interesting feature of the chemistry of NCAE is its apparent activity as transnitrosating agent. Addition of 0.8 molar equivalents of dimethylamine to a chloroform solution of the aldehyde results in an 8% yield of NDMA (4) within 40 min. p-Chloroaniline (5) is also formed, in a yield of 33% at this time. Over the course of 10 h, the NDMA yield increased to 12.4%, while the yield of p-chloroaniline decreased to 27%. The reaction of NCAE with other bases (sodium hydroxide, potassium carbonate or potassium cyanide) also results in the formation of p-chloroaniline. In the case of the reaction with sodium hydroxide, p-chlorophenylmethylnitrosamine (6) is formed as well.

The extreme electrophilicity of the aldehyde group in NCAE is also noteworthy. NCAE forms the methyl hemiacetal (7) spontaneously when dissolved in deuterated methanol (NMR). This is a phenomenon shared by few other aldehydes (e.g. formaldehyde, trichloro-acetaldehyde).

The chemistry of this β-nitrosaminoaldehyde is extremely interesting and is of possible value in the area of chemical carcinogenesis. In addition to NCAE and Okada's N-butylnitrosaminoethanal, several other β-nitrosaminoaldehydes[1] have been reported to be

---

[1] Lijinsky, Hecht, personal communications

chemically unstable. We must consider therefore, that the instability and high reactivity of NCAE is a property not only of this specific molecule but of a compound which bears the β-nitrosaminoaldehyde structural unit. There are several possible explanations for this unusual chemical reactivity. In the simplest sense, both the aldehyde group and the *N*-nitrosamine function are known to be strong electron-withdrawing groups. The proximal positions of these functions within a molecule result in their interaction. The electron-withdrawing *N*-nitrosamine function confers on the aldehyde a high degree of electrophilicity, as is demonstrated by the extremely rapid formation of a hemiacetal (7). It is expected on the one hand that the aldehyde function will be unusually reactive toward nitrogen nucleophiles, such as an NH_2 group (perhaps that of adenine or guanine). On the other hand, the electron-withdrawing properties of the aldehyde could make the N-NO bond of the *N*-nitrosamide more labile. The *N*-nitrosamine could be considered to acquire more of the properties of an *N*-nitrosoamide, due to the electron-withdrawing effect of the attached CH_2CHO group. *N*-nitrosoamides are known to be much more effective transnitrosating agents than their *N*-nitrosamine counterparts. This could explain why NCAE is capable of affecting the nitrosation of dimethylamine.

We know that both the carbonyl and nitrosamine groups act to acidify the carbon-bound hydrogens of the CH_2 connecting them. The presence of trace amounts of acid or base should easily catalyse the self-condensation of β-nitrosaminoaldehyde and should also promote the enolization of aldehyde, to give not only an enol but an *N*-nitrosoeneamine. *N*-Nitroso-eneamines as well as enols are known to be quite reactive.

The arguments and rationale advanced above should apply to all aldehydes that contain electron-withdrawing groups in the β-position. The instability of NCAE and other β-nitrosamino aldehydes suggests that other factors may be involved. Our current working hypothesis centres on the idea that there is a covalent interaction between the *N*-nitroso oxygen and the aldehyde carbonyl carbon, as shown in Figure 5. This interaction should result in the production of a chemically very labile species. In Figure 5, it is shown how such an intermediate

Fig. 5. Scheme showing covalent interaction between the *N*-nitroso oxygen and the aldehyde carbonyl carbon of 2-(*N*-nitroso-*N*-4-chlorophenyl)aminoethanal.

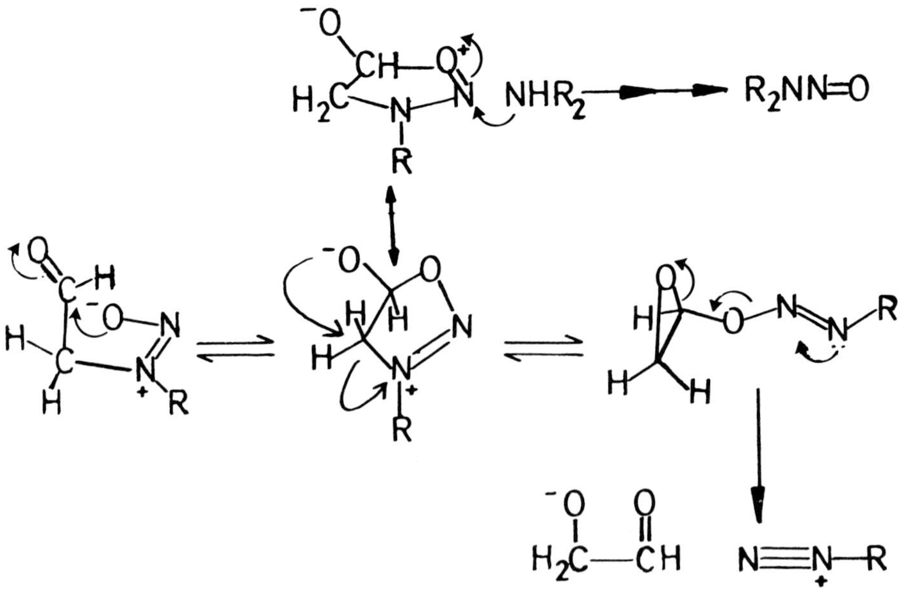

could give rise to a diazonium ion or produce the nitrosation of another amine. Okada's group has suggested this type of interaction for one of their β-nitrosamino esters. Moreover, it is known in sydnone formation (β-nitrosaminoacids), and Michejda's group has demonstrated that the *N*-nitroso oxygen can act through neighbouring group participation involving a five-membered ring to promote the ionization of a β-nitrosamino tosylate (Koepke *et al.*, 1979). Thus, both spectroscopic and chemical data suggest that the interaction between the *N*-nitroso oxygen and the carbonyl carbon may result in the chemical labilization of such molecules. More evidence must, of course, await further research on these very reactive compounds.

Extrapolation of the reactions described above to alkyl-β-nitrosaminoaldehydes suggests several ways in which these compounds could initiate the carcinogenic process directly. Spontaneous formation of diazonium ions, as has been demonstrated with NCAE, could result in the alkylation of nucleic acids and proteins. The extreme electrophilicity of the aldehyde group could result in its binding to these same macromolecules. The transnitrosating capacity of the β-nitrosaminoaldehyde could also produce carbonium ions from other cellular primary amines, which may bind or cross-link bioregulatory macromolecules, directly deaminate nucleic acid bases (somatic mutation) or produce other *N*-nitroso compounds which eventually produce cell damage. The two-carbon fragment from β-nitrosaminoaldehydes could also produce glyoxal or other reactive two-carbon fragments. In principle, any *N*-nitrosamine containing the $-N-C-CH_2OH$ group could be oxidized by an appropriate alcohol dehydrogenase or other oxidative enzyme-oxidation system to a β-nitrosaminoaldehyde. For example, the oxidation of NDELA to its monoaldehyde could result in its transformation into an effective alkylating or transnitrosating agent. Action by this latter mode (transnitrosation) could explain why no carbon fragment from NDELA has yet been found to be incorporated into nucleic acids after administration of NDELA to experimental animals.

CONCLUSION

The various experiments described above demonstrate that there are reasonable alternative modes for activating *N*-nitrosamines to proximate carcinogens, either without or in combination with β-oxidation. It is very likely that *N*-nitrosamine structure strongly influences the carcinogenic significance to these possible alternative routes of activation. Further research is obviously warranted.

ACKNOWLEDGEMENTS

The support of this research by the US National Cancer Institute under grant CA22289 is gratefully acknowledged.

REFERENCES

Archer, M.C. & Leung, K.H. (1981) *Mechanism of alkylation of DNA by* N-*nitrosodialkylamines*. In: Scanlan, R.A. & Tannenbaum, S.R., eds, N-*Nitroso Compounds,* Washington DC, American Chemical Society, pp. 39–47

Koepke, S.R., Kupper, R. & Michejda, C.J. (1979) Unusually facile solvolysis of primary tosylates. A case for participation by the *N*-nitroso group. *J. org. Chem., 44,* 2718–2722

Krüger, F.W. (1973) Metabolism of nitrosamines *in vivo.* II. On the methylation of nucleic acids by aliphatic di-*n*-alkyl-nitrosamines: The increased formation of 7-methylguanine after application of di-*n*-propylnitrosamine. *Z. Krebsforsch., 79,* 90–97

Lawson, T.A., Helgeson, A.S., Grandjean, C.J., Wallcave, L. & Nagel, D. (1981) The formation of *N*-nitrosomethyl(2-oxopropyl)amine from *N*-nitrosobis(2-oxopropyl)amine *in vivo*. *Carcinogenesis*, **2**, 845–849

Lethco, E.J., Wallace, W.C. & Brouwer, E. (1982) The fate of *N*-nitrosodiethanolamine after oral and topical administration to rats *Food Chem. Toxicol.*, **20**, 401–406

Loeppky, R.N. & Outram, J.R. (1982) *A biochemical retroaldol cleavage of β-hydroxynitrosamine*. In: Bartsch, H., O'Neill, I.K., Categnaro, M. & Okada, M., eds, N-*Nitroso Compounds: Occurrence and Biological Effects (IARC Scientific Publications No. 41)*, Lyon International Agency for Research on Cancer, pp. 459–472

Loeppky, R.N., Outram, J.R., Tomasik, W. & McKinley, W. (1981) *Chemical and biochemical transformations of β-oxidized nitrosamines*. In: Scanlan, R.A. & Tannenbaum, R.R., eds, N-*Nitroso Compounds*, Washington DC, American Chemical Society, pp. 21–37

Loeppky, R.N., McKinley, W.A., Hazlitt, L.G. & Outram, J.R., (1982) Base-induced fragmentation of β-hydroxynitrosamines. *J. org. Chem.*, **47**, 4833–4841

Preussmann, R., Habs, M., Habs, H. & Schmäl, D. (1982) Carcinogenicity of *N*-nitrosodiethanolamine in rats at five different dose levels *Cancer Res.*, **42**, 5167–5171

Singer, G.M., Lijinsky, W., Buettner, C. & McClusky, G.A. (1981) Relationship of rat urinary metabolites of *N*-nitrosomethyl-*N*-alkylamine to bladder carcinogenesis. *Cancer Res.*, **41**, 4942–4946

Suzuki, E. & Okada, M. (1979) Synthesis of *N*-nitrosamino aldehydes, metabolic intermediates possibly involved in the induction of tumors in rats by *N*-butyl-*N*-(ω-hydroxyalkyl)nitrosamine. *Chem. Pharm. Bull.*, **27**, 541–544

Suzuki, E., Iiyoshi, M. & Okada, M. (1980a) Nuclear magnetic resonance spectra of *N*-alkyl-*N*-(hydroxy-and-oxo-alkyl) nitrosamines and chromagraphic separation of their (Z)- and (E)-conformers. *Chem. Pharm. Bull.*, **28**, 979–983

Suzuki, E., Iiyoshi, M. & Okada, M. (1980b) Nuclear magnetic resonance spectra of *N*-alkyl-*N*-(ω-carboxylalkyl)nitrosamines and their esters, and chromatographic separation of the (Z)- and (E)- conformers of the esters. *Chem. Pharm. Bull.*, **28**, 1612–1618

α-HYDROXYLATION OF NITROGEN-15 LABELLED N-NITROSAMINES BY ISOLATED HEPATOCYTES

S.R. KOEPKE, M.B. KROEGER-KOEPKE, Y. TONDEUR, J.G. FARRELLY, M. STEWART & C.J. MICHEJDA

LBI-Basic Research Program, Chemical Carcinogenesis Program, Frederick Cancer Research Facility, Frederick, MD 21701, USA

SUMMARY

The principal pathway of nitrosamine metabolism has long been considered to be α-hydroxylation. For N-nitrosodialkylamines, this hypothesis requires that a molecule of molecular nitrogen be released for every molecule of nitrosamine that is α-hydroxylated. Thus, the quantitative determination of nitrogen formation should provide a measure of the importance of this pathway. This method was applied earlier to the doubly-labelled nitrogen-15 compounds, N-nitrosodimethylamine (NDMA), N-nitrosomethylphenylamine (NMPhA) and N-methyl-N-nitrosourea (MNU), using both a 9 000 × g supernatant fraction of liver and the intact animal as metabolic systems. The in-vitro results were quite different from those obtained *in vivo*. The majority of the NDMA (67%) and the MNU (88%) were converted to nitrogen *in vivo*, while NMPhA gave considerably less nitrogen (52%). These results differed by a factor of approximately two from those obtained *in vitro* (NDMA, 33%; NMPhA, 18.8% and MNU, 96%). Since such differences may be a result of the loss of cellular architecture, we have extended the work to include isolated hepatocytes.

It had been shown previously that isolated hepatocytes constitute a practical alternative to in-vivo systems, even though the correlation with in-vivo metabolism appears to depend on the substrate analysed. The values obtained using this system (NDMA, 47%; NMPhA, 23%; and MNU 105%) reconfirm that metabolism may be substrate dependent. As in our previous studies, no mixed nitrogen ($^{15}N^{14}N$) or labelled nitrogen oxides were found. The data are all consistent with the hypothesis that at least one demethylase for each of the nitrosamine substrates is associated with a cell membrane. This activity, furthermore, is subject to disruption when the integrity of the membrane is disturbed.

INTRODUCTION

The α-hydroxylation reaction has long been considered to be the principal pathway of nitrosamine metabolism. This hypothesis requires the production of one molecule of nitrogen for every molecule of N-nitrosodialkylamine so metabolized. We devised a system to measure α-hydroxylation *versus* total substrate loss and exploited it, using an in-vitro liver metabolic system (S9) and intact rats, with N-nitrosodimethylamine (NDMA), N-nitrosomethyl-phenylamine (NMPhA) and N-methyl-N-nitrosourea (MNU) (Kroeger-Koepke *et al.*, 1981; Michejda *et al.*, 1982). The results indicated an approximately two-fold difference in nitrogen production between the in-vivo and in-vitro cases. In order to elucidate possible explanations for these differences, it was decided to investigate other more realistic in-vitro systems.

Isolated hepatocytes have been widely used as a model system. They possess intact cellular membranes and the ability to perform sequential metabolic reactions (Henderson & Dedwaide, 1969; McMahon, 1980). They do not, however, constitute a perfect system. Their metabolism of drugs in many cases correlates well with in-vivo metabolism, but this correlation does not appear to depend on the substrate analysed (Billings *et al.*, 1977).

It has been reported that nitrosamines are metabolized to alkylating agents (Umbenhauer & Pegg, 1981a, b) and carbon dioxide (Farrelly *et al.*, 1982) by isolated hepatocytes. These results indicate that hepatocytes should be a good model system for studies with nitrosamines.

MATERIALS AND METHODS

Materials

The ^{15}N-labelled nitrosamines were prepared as reported previously (Kroeger-Koepke *et al.*, 1981). Dr Peter Magee (Fels Research Institute, Philadelphia, PA, USA) generously provided the labelled MNU. Trypan blue and Hank's balanced salt solution were obtained from Flow Laboratories (McLean, VA, USA). N-Nitrosodiethylamine (NDEA) and other reagents were purchased from Sigma Chemical Corporation (St Louis, MO, USA). All animals used in these experiments were 10–12-week old male Fischer F-344 rats, obtained from the NCI-FCRF animal breeding farm (Frederik, MD, USA).

Incubation procedure

Hepatocytes were prepared as described previously (Farrelly *et al.*, 1982). Yields of $1-3 \times 10^8$ cells per liver, with viabilities of 84–90%, were obtained from different preparations. A typical reaction employs 6 mL of hepatocytes (3×10^7 cells) and 1.5 mL of 5 mmol/L substrate (final concentration, 1 mmol/L) in a 25-mL gas bulb, equipped with a vacuum stopcock. The introduction of the reaction atmosphere, 5% CO_2 and 0.5% Ne in O_2 (Matheson, Dorsey, MD, USA), was performed as described previously (Kroeger-Koepke *et al.*, 1981). Control experiments determined that there was no loss of viability during the degassing procedure. After incubation at 37 °C for 2 h in a water-bath shaker, the gaseous contents were transferred at 0 °C (*via* a Toeppler pump) for mass spectrometric analysis. The aqueous portion was retained for subsequent substrate analysis.

Nitrogen determinations

(A more generalized and detailed account of the development of this procedure will be published in *Biomedical Mass Spectrometry*). The quantification of ^{15}N$_2$ was performed using an internal standard. Neon was chosen for this purpose because of its low natural abundance and its proximity in mass to ^{15}N$_2$. The absolute quantity of Ne added to each reaction could be calculated, since the volume of the reaction vessel was known.

The gas samples were expanded into a 75-mL chamber, equipped with a molecular leak, allowing the gas to penetrate the ion source of a VG Micromass ZAB-2F mass spectrometer. The Peak Matching Unit was used to monitor the two masses (^{20}Ne at m/z 19.9924 and ^{15}N$_2$ at m/z 30.0002) by voltage sweep corresponding to a mass window size equal to three peak widths (i.e., 200 ppm) and a dwell time of 6 sec. The instrument was operated in the electron-impact mode at a resolution of 15 000, using 70 eV electrons, 100 μA trap current and a source temperature of 200 °C. The energy of the ^{20}Ne ions was 8 KeV. The response factors were obtained by measuring the relative intensities of the Ne and $^{15}N_2$ signals on a chart pen recorder, using the 100 mv full-scale-deflection (FSD) sensitivity range. The recorder range was adjusted so that the most intense signal was at least 50% FSD.

Known volumes of primary standards of 0.5% Ne and 0.5% $^{15}N_2$ in O_2 and 0.5% Ne in O_2 were mixed to provide secondary standards. These were used to calibrate the mass spectrometer in order to eliminate differences in mass discrimination and ionization efficiencies. The same gas volume and pressure were used for all the standards and for the gas reaction mixtures. In all experiments, the $^{14}N_2$ peak was measured to ensure that there was not an unexpected excess of naturally-occurring $^{15}N_2$, resulting from a leak during incubation or gas transfer.

The primary standard of 0.5% $^{15}N_2$ and 0.5% Ne in O_2 was examined just before each secondary standard or sample. Ten measurements of each ion intensity ($^{15}N_2$ and Ne) were averaged, and the ratios of $^{15}N_2$ to Ne were determined. These ratios were then normalized to the primary standard ($^{15}N_2$/Ne) ratio. The normalized ratios were plotted *versus* the percentage of $^{15}N_2$ in the secondary standards to form the calibration curve.

Determination of nitrosamine loss

Following the transfer of gas for mass spectrometric analysis, 3.75 mL of a saturated solution of barium hydroxide were added to the reaction bulbs. Hepatocytes were disrupted by sonication for 15 sec, after which 375 μL of 2.7 mmol/L NDEA (used as an internal standard for chromatographic analysis) and 3.75 mL zinc sulfate were added to precipitate the protein (Somogyi, 1945; Farrelly *et al.*, 1982). After cooling to 0 °C, the precipitate was removed by centrifugation at 8 000 × g for 10 min.

The filtrates were analysed immediately by high-pressure liquid chromatography (HPLC) for loss of substrate, using a Whatman Partisil PXS 10/25 ODS 10-μm column with a Laboratory Data Control (LDC) pumping system; the column elution conditions depended on the substrate analysed. For NDMA, the column was developed at 1 mL/min with water:acetonitrile (85:15, v/v). Under these conditions, the retention time was 4.6 min for NDMA and 6.9 min for NDEA. When NMPhA was the substrate, the column was eluted at 1 mL/min with a 12-min linear gradient from 100% water to 100% acetonitrile. In this case, the retention time was 8.6 min for NDEA and 12.5 min for NMPhA. Samples were introduced through a 100-μL loop, and compounds were detected by ultra-violet absorbance at 254 nm, using an LDC UVII detector. Analytical data were processed with a Hewlett-Packard 3354 data system, interfaced to the instrument through an HP 18652A A/D converter. For each sample, two or three injections were used to determine the area of the nitrosamine peak. The ratio of the areas of the NDEA standard of the control and hepatocyte reactions was determined and was multiplied by the areas of substrate after the 2-h reaction. The fraction of metabolism was then determined by subtracting the hepatocyte reaction area (after 2 h) from the control reaction area and dividing by the latter.

RESULTS

The extent of substrate metabolism was monitored by HPLC on a standard reversed-phase column. As in our previous studies, this measurement involved the largest source of error: the precision was found to vary by 11% in the worst case. The data for each observation of

Table 1. Analysis of hepatocyte metabolism of labelled nitrosamines

Substrate	Hepatocyte[a] viability	Substrate loss (μmol)	Substrate metabolism (%)	$^{15}N_2$ produced (μmol)	% of substrate metabolized yielding $^{15}N_2$
NDMA	85	1.74	23.1	0.900	51.9
	85	1.79	23.8	0.917	51.3
	92	2.00	26.7	0.652	32.6
	92	1.59	21.2	0.647	40.8
	91	1.31	17.4	0.629	41.8
	88	1.14	15.3	0.711	62.0
	88	1.06	14.1	0.648	61.2
	88	1.37	18.3	0.524	38.2
	88	1.30	17.4	0.529	40.6
NMPhA	89	4.33[b]	27.1	1.03[b]	23.6
	89	3.79[b]	23.7	1.26[b]	33.3
	84	2.17	29.0	0.56	25.8
	84	2.18	29.0	0.49	22.5
	86	2.52	33.6	0.29	11.5
	85	2.58[c]	20.6	0.52[c]	20.2
	85	2.49[c]	19.9	0.52	20.9
MNU	91	8.25	100	8.58	104.0
	88	8.25	100	8.70	105.5

[a] As determined by trypan blue exclusion

[b, c] The incubation volumes of these reaction mixtures were 16.0 ml and 12.5 ml, respectively; all other volumes were 7.5 ml

NDMA, *N*-nitrosodimethylamine; NMPhA, *N*-nitrosomethylphenylamine; MNU, *N*-methyl-*N*-nitrosourea

substrate loss are shown in Table 1. The average percent metabolism was 19.7 ± 4.2 for NDMA and 26.1 ± 5.0 for NMPhA.

The quantity of labelled molecular nitrogen produced in each incubation was determined mass spectrometrically, using a known amount of Ne gas. The ratio of the intensities of the labelled nitrogen and neon peaks was found to be directly proportional to the concentration of labelled nitrogen, using standard gas mixtures.

The data for the reaction measurements are listed in Table 1. The amount of labelled nitrogen produced was 47.4 ± 10.2% of the theoretical maximum for NDMA and 22.5 ± 6.6% for NMPhA. A positive control, using doubly-labelled MNU, yielded 104.8 ± 1.0% of the theoretical amount. Incubation of MNU was carried out in a manner analogous to that employed for the other substrates. The 2-h incubation period is approximately equivalent to ten half-lives of the nitrosourea under the reaction conditions (Garrett *et al.*, 1965). Negative control experiments containing only media and labelled nitrosamine yielded virtually no detectable labelled nitrogen.

The gaseous products for all reactions were also examined for the presence of any of the labelled nitrogen oxides or for any isotopically mixed nitrogen ($^{14}N^{15}N$). No labelled gas other than nitrogen-30 was detected.

DISCUSSION

It was evident from our previous work (Kroeger-Koepke *et al.*, 1981, Michejda *et al.*, 1982) that a better model than the liver S9 fraction was necessary for comparison with the whole animal. Isolated hepatocytes, with their enhanced capacity to metabolize nitrosamines

(NDMA, 20%; NMPhA, 26%), appear to constitute an excellent system. When the amounts metabolized are compared on a μmol/g liver per h basis (using median values of 2×10^8 cells/4 g liver per animal), hepatocytes show an approximately two-fold increase per unit when compared with the S9 reaction.

The positive control substrate, MNU, was cleanly decomposed to labelled nitrogen under the conditions of the incubation, as shown by the results presented in Table 1. The data also revealed that isolated hepatocytes metabolized only 47% (NDMA) and 23% (NMPhA) of the substrates to molecular nitrogen. The remainder of the reaction presumably occurred by some pathway other than α-hydroxylation. The value for NMPhA is in good agreement with the data previously obtained with the S9 reaction (19%), but quite different from that found *in vivo* (52%). In the case of NDMA, the value falls approximately half-way between that obtained with S9 (33%) and that obtained *in vivo* (67%).

This divergence from a clear comparative pattern between the data obtained with hepatocytes for the two nitrosamines and that obtained with either S9 or the intact animal is not without precedent (Billings *et al.*, 1977). The type of enzyme activity assayed also seems to play a role in the correlation. For example, for isolated hepatocytes, *N*-demethylating activity is about 100%, hydroxylating activity 25% and glucuronidating activity 50% of that of the crude homogenate (Billings *et al.*, 1978). When the ability of NDMA to alkylate DNA was examined, it was found that alkylation occurred seven to ten times less in hepatocytes than in the intact animal (Umbenhauer & Pegg, 1981a). This difference was not due to the ability of the hepatocytes to metabolize the NDMA.

A number of studies have indicated that multiple enzyme pathways may be involved in the metabolism of nitrosamines, not all of them necessarily P-450-dependent processes. From product studies, some of these pathways appear not to be compatible with the α-hydroxylation hypothesis. Our data are in agreement with these findings. The results also indicate that at least some of the α-hydroxylation activities are associated with membrane-bound enzymes. The activity for NDMA in particular appears to be very sensitive to changes in the membrane. The nature and function of the other pathways, which become the major routes of metabolism when the α-hydroxylation path is disrupted, remain to be elucidated.

ACKNOWLEDGEMENTS

Research sponsored by the National Cancer Institute, DHHS, under contract No. NO1-CO-23 909 with Litton Bionetics, Inc. The contents of this publication do not necessarily reflect the views or policies of the Department of Health and Human Services, nor does mention of trade names, commercial products, or organizations imply indorsement by the US Government.

REFERENCES

Billings, R.E., McMahon, R.E., Ashmore, J. & Wagle, S.R. (1977) The metabolism of drugs in isolated rat hepatocytes. *Drug Metab. Dispos., 5*, 518–526

Billings, R.E., Murphy, P.J., McMahon, R.E. & Ashmore, J. (1978) Aromatic hydroxylation of amphetamine with rat liver microsomes, perfused liver, and isolated hepatocytes. *Biochem. Pharmacol., 27*, 2525–2529

Farrelly, J.G., Stewart, M.L. & Hecker, L.I. (1982) The metabolism of nitrosopyrrolidine by hepatocytes from Fischer rats. *Chem.-biol. Interact., 41*, 341–351

Garrett, E.R., Goto, S. & Stubbins, J.F. (1965) Kinetics of solvolyses of various *N*-alkyl-*N*-nitrosoureas in neutral and alkaline solutions. *J. pharm. Sci.,* **54,** 119–123

Henderson, P.Th. & Dedwaide, J.H. (1969) Metabolism of drugs in isolated hepatocytes. *Biochem. Pharmacol.,* **18,** 2087–2094

Kroeger-Koepke, M.B., Koepke, S.R., McClusky, G.A., Magee, P.N. & Michejda, C.J. (1981) α-Hydroxylation pathway in the *in vitro* metabolism of carcinogenic nitrosamines: *N*-nitrosodimethylamine and *N*-nitroso-*N*-methylaniline. *Proc. natl Acad. Sci. USA,* **78,** 6489–6493

McMahon, R.E. (1980) The metabolism of drugs and other foreign compounds in suspensions of isolated rat hepatocytes. *Ann. N.Y. Acad. Sci.,* **394,** 46–66

Michejda, C.J., Kroeger-Koepke, M.B., Koepke, S.R., Magee, P.N. & Chu, C. (1982) *Nitrogen formation during* in-vivo *and* in-vitro *metabolism of* N-*nitrosamines.* In: Magee, P.N., ed., *Nitrosamines and Human Cancer (Banbury Report No. 12),* Cold Spring Harbor, NY, Cold Spring Harbor Laboratory, pp. 69–85

Somogyi, M. (1945) Determination of blood sugar. *J. biol. Chem.,* **160,** 69–73

Umbenhauer, D.R. & Pegg, A.E. (1981a) Metabolism of dimethylnitrosamine and subsequent removal of O^6-methylguanine from DNA by isolated rat hepatocytes. *Chem.-biol. Interact.,* **33,** 229–238

Umbenhauer, D.R. & Pegg, A.E. (1981b) Alkylation of intracellular and extracellular DNA by dimethylnitrosamine following alkylation by isolated rat hepatocytes. *Cancer Res.,* **41,** 3471–3474

METABOLIC INACTIVATION OF *N*-NITROSAMINES BY CYTOCHROME P-450 *IN VITRO* AND *IN VIVO*

K.E. APPEL, C.S. RÜHL & A.G. HILDEBRANDT

Max von Pettenkofer Institute, Federal Health Office, 1000 Berlin (West) 33

SUMMARY

Nitrite was formed on incubation of *N*-nitrosamines with both microsomal systems and a reconstituted system consisting of cytochrome P-450 and NADPH P-450 reductase from pig liver. Nitrite was not obtained when the nitrosamines were incubated with NADPH P-450 reductase alone or when molecular oxygen or NADPH was omitted. Various inhibitors of the microsomal monooxygenase decreased nitrite generation. Furthermore, nitrite and a substantially higher amount of nitrate could be found in the urine of rats given *N*-nitrosodiphenylamine. Diphenylamine was also detected. From in-vitro studies, it is concluded that denitrosation of *N*-nitrosamines is a cytochrome P-450-dependent process, which also occurs *in vivo*.

INTRODUCTION

Carcinogenic *N*-nitrosamines are thought to be converted after an initial cytochrome P-450 (P-450)-dependent oxidative dealkylation to unstable reactive metabolites (Magee & Farber, 1962; Magee *et al.*, 1976). Studies have shown the existence of an additional detoxifying pathway apart from this metabolic activation. Nitrite was a metabolic product when nitrosamines were aerobically incubated with rat or mouse liver microsomes (Appel *et al.*, 1979, 1980). From studies of spectral data and metabolism, it was suggested that nitrosamines are reductively denitrosated by the catalytic action of P-450 (Appel *et al.*, 1979; Appel & Graf, 1982).

The present study was carried out to investigate the assumed participation of P-450 in the denitrosation reaction. In addition to microsomal incubations, we used a reconstituted system consisting of purified P-450 and NADPH P-450 reductase. In particular, we wished to know whether NADPH P-450 reductase alone would be able to catalyse this metabolic step. We also looked for metabolic products of the denitrosation reaction *in vivo*. For this purpose, *N*-nitrosodiphenylamine (NDPhA) was administered orally to rats. The urine was analysed for nitrite, nitrate and diphenylamine (DPhA).

MATERIALS AND METHODS

Chemicals

N-Nitrosamines were generous gifts from Dr Frank and Dr Wiessler, Institute of Toxicology and Chemotherapy, German Cancer Research Center, Heidelberg, or were obtained from Sigma Chemie, Munich. NADPH was obtained from Boehringer, Mannheim. All other chemicals were of reagent grade and were commercially available.

In-vitro incubations and measurement of nitrite

Preparation of microsomes and microsomal incubations were performed as described elsewhere (Appel *et al.*, 1980). Cytochrome P-450 and NADPH P-450 reductase were isolated from microsomes of phenobarbital-pretreated pigs according to the method of Graf *et al.* (1979, 1980). The complete monooxygenase system, as well as the P-450-free system, was reconstituted from its components, P-450 PLM IV and/or NADPH P-450 reductase and 1,2-dimyristeroyl-L-α-glycero-3-phosphatidylcholine, solubilized in 0.1 mol/L HEPES buffer, pH 7.6, containing 1% sodium cholate. The detergent was removed prior to use, as described by Graf *et al.* (1979, 1980).

Generally, the incubations were performed in the dark at 37 °C under aerobic conditions. The enzymatic reactions were stopped by addition of equal volumes of 20% zinc sulfate solution, followed by saturated barium hydroxide solution. After centrifugation, the clear supernatant was diluted with diazoreagent (equal volumes of 1 mmol/L β-naphthylethylenediamine in 3 mol/L hydrochloric acid and 0.1 mol/L sulfanilamide in 3 mol/L hydrochloric acid.

The amount of azo dye was determined photometrically at 564 nm.

Determination of denitrosation metabolites in the urine of rats

One dose of NDPhA (1 g/kg bw) dissolved in corn oil was fed to female Wistar rats by gastric intubation. Control rats received corn oil only. The urine was sampled over a period of 36 h by keeping the rats in metabolic cages. Aliquots of the urine were taken and filtered through a Millipore filter of 0.22 μm pore-width. The filtered urine was then pressed through a C-18 cartridge (Waters, Königstein, FRG). Aliquots were then diluted with the elution buffer (2.8 mmol/L sodium bicarbonate/2.24 mmol/L sodium carbonate) and analysed using a DIONEX high-performance liquid chromatography (HPLC) Ion-Chromatograph with a conductive detector. The anions nitrite and nitrate were quantified by means of a Hewlett Packard integrator, 3390A.

For the detection of DPhA, urine was extracted three times with dichloromethane, and the organic phases were concentrated to 1 mL. An aliquot was analysed by the HPLC system, using a reversed-phase column and a Hewlett Packard UV/Vis detector, HP 1040 A. Another aliquot was used for conversion of the amine to its trifluoroacetyl (TFA) derivative. The TFA derivative was detected by gas chromatography (GC), using an OV-101 column and a Thermal Energy Analyzer (TEA) (N) detector (Thermo Electron Corp., Waltham, MA, USA).

RESULTS AND DISCUSSION

Table 1 shows the inhibition of denitrosation of *N*-nitrosodimethylamine (NDMA) in a microsomal incubation system. By using various inhibitors of the microsomal monooxygenase system, e.g., piperonyl butoxide and metyrapone, nitrite generation was inhibited by about

Table 1. Formation of nitrite from 35 mmol/L N-nitrosodimethylamine in mouse liver microsomes

	Nitrite formed in 50 min (nmol/mg protein)	Percent inhibition
Complete system	8.3 $\pm$ 1.3	
Boiled microsomes	0.02 $\pm$ 0.01	99
Minus NADPH	0.05 $\pm$ 0.03	99
CO/O$_2$ (8/2)	5.4 $\pm$ 0.5	34
Anaerobic (N$_2$)	0.07 $\pm$ 0.03	99
Piperonylbutoxide 0.2 mmol/L	3.8 $\pm$ 0.3	54
Metyrapone 0.1 mmol/L	4.7 $\pm$ 0.5	43

Table 2. Metabolic nitrite formation from N-nitrosamines by a reconstituted monooxygenase system. The complete system contained 5 nmol P-450 PLM IV, 4 nmol NADPH P-450 reductase and 1 nmol 1,2-dimyristeroyl-L-α-glycero-3-phosphatidylcholine in 1 mL Tris/KCl buffer, as described in Materials and Methods. Concentration of substrate was 5 mmol/L; that of NADPH was 1 mmol/L. Formation of nitrite was linear with time over a period of 20 min. Blanks measured at zero time were subtracted

	(nmol nitrite/min)/nmol P-450			
	Complete system	Minus NADPH	Minus P-450	Anaerobic (N$_2$)
N-Nitrosodiethylamine	0.2	0.014	0.02	0.01
N-Nitrosodi-n-propylamine	1.4	0.0	0.0	0.0
N-Nitrosodi-n-butylamine	2.0	0.0	0.0	0.0
N-Nitrosodiphenylamine	0.18	0.0	0.0	0.04
N-Nitrosomorpholine	1.7	0.02	0.02	0.0

50% in control microsomes. Nitrite formation could not be observed under a nitrogen atmosphere or when NADPH was omitted. Similar experiments have already been performed with N-nitrosomorpholine (NMOR) as substrate (Appel et al., 1980).

Table 2 compares the nitrite formation observed when various nitrosamines were incubated with a complete reconstituted system. This system consisted of P-450 PLM IV, NADPH P-450 reductase and synthetic phospholipid. With longer alkyl chains, i.e., with higher lipophilicity, a higher rate of nitrite formation was generally obtained. When molecular oxygen, NADPH or P-450 was omitted from this system, nitrite was not generated from any of the nitrosamines tested. Figure 1 demonstrates the time-dependent formation of nitrite when NMOR or N-nitrosodi-n-propylamine (NDPA) was incubated with the reconstituted microsomal monooxygenase system. Incubation with NADPH P-450 reductase and NADPH, without P-450, did not result in the formation of nitrite. It is therefore concluded that NADPH P-450 reductase alone is not able to catalyse nitrite formation (Table 2, Fig. 1). This demonstrates that the haemoprotein is necessary for this metabolic process. Previous studies have shown that nitrosamines may bind to ferric P-450 either as ligands or as substrates (Appel et al., 1979). After reduction of the haem moiety with dithionite or NADPH, the specific optical and electron spin resonance spectra obtained could be interpreted as being derived from a hexa-coordinated NO-P-450 complex. Under aerobic conditions, nitric oxide is displaced by molecular oxygen and subsequently converted to nitrite in an aqueous medium (Appel & Graf, 1982).

In order further to substantiate this in-vitro model reaction, urine was analysed for metabolic products generated by the denitrosation reaction *in vivo*. NDPhA is an important industrial

Fig. 1. Kinetics of nitrite formation from *N*-nitrosomorpholine (a) and *N*-nitrosodipropylamine (b) in the reconstituted monooxygenase system. Substrate concentration was 30 µmol/L. The concentration of P-450 PLM IV was 2.07 µmol/L; that of NADPH P-450 reductase was 0.75 µmol/L; that of NADPH was 1 nmol/L. (●——●) represents the complete reconstituted system (P-450, P-450 reductase, NADPH); (△——△) represents the system without P-450 (only NADPH P-450 reductase and NADPH)

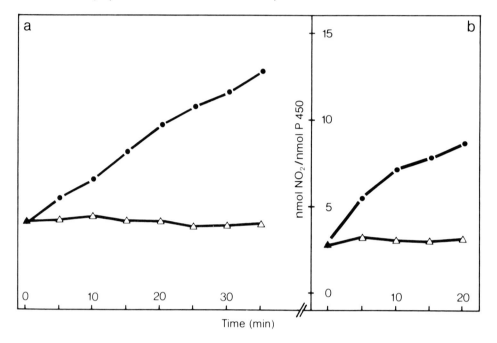

Time (min)

chemical used in the vulcanization of rubber. On the basis of earlier studies in rats and mice, NDPhA had been classified as a non-carcinogen (Argus & Hoch-Ligeti, 1961; Druckrey *et al.*, 1967; Boyland *et al.*, 1968). However, more recent studies showed that it induces transitional-cell carcinomas in the bladder of Fischer 344 rats (Cardy *et al.*, 1979). In in-vitro studies, NDPhA failed to induce DNA repair in rat hepatocytes, was non-mutagenic in both mammalian and microbial cells and did not induce transformation in mammalian cells (Yahagi *et al.*, 1977; Kuroki *et al.*, 1977; Brouns *et al.*, 1979; Jones & Huberman, 1980). However, it was shown recently that NDPhA is active in the induction of morphological transformation of hamster embryo cells *in vitro* (Schuman *et al.*, 1981). In addition, it could be demonstrated that NDPhA is mutagenic to *Salmonella typhimurium* TA98 when norharman (β-carboline) is present (Nagao & Takahashi, 1981; Wakabayashi *et al.*, 1981). Further investigations by Wakabayashi *et al.* (1982) indicated that enzymatic denitrosation of NDPhA is necessary for the production of a mutagenic effect. This conclusion was supported by the fact that diphenylamine (DPhA) was also mutagenic when norharman was present. For the detection of metabolites generated by denitrosation *in vivo*, NDPhA was administered orally to rats. The urine was sampled over a period or 36 h and immediately analysed for nitrite and nitrate by ion chromatography and for DPhA by GC and HPLC.

Figure 2 shows the chromatographic pattern of anion analyses of the urine from control and NDPhA-treated rats. In the latter case, both nitrite and nitrate could be detected. However, the concentration of nitrate was unexpectedly high compared with the nitrite concentration

Fig. 2. Chromatograph obtained by ion analysis of rat urine; (a) urine from control rats; (b) urine from rats treated with N-nitrosodiphenylamine

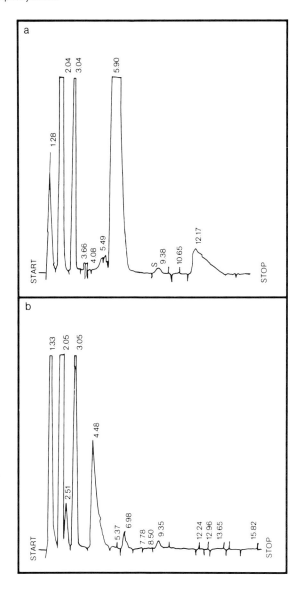

(Table 3). If we assume that nitrite is also generated *in vivo* by denitrosation of NDPhA, it can be concluded that substantial amounts are oxidized to nitrate in the organism. Two mechanisms may account for this observation. One site of nitrite conversion to nitrate is the erythrocyte, as demonstrated when nitrite is added to blood and the conversion of oxyhaemoglobin to methaemoglobin occurs. However, the biochemical pathway of this toxicologically important transformation is not fully understood. Furthermore, normal

Table 3. Urine analysis for nitrite, nitrate and diphenylamine (DPhA) after administration of 1 g/kg bw (5 mmol/kg body weight) *N*-nitrosodiphenylamine (NDPhA) or 850 mg/kg (5 mmol/kg) DPhA to rats. Phenobarbital (PB) was added to the drinking water (0.1%) over 5 days. Metyrapone (100 mg/kg body weight) was given 15 min before NDPhA by intraperitoneal injection. Values represent means from 2–4 experiments with 2 animals each

Test group	Nitrite	Nitrate	DPhA
	(μmol/rat)/36 h		
Control	<1.5	<9.0	<0.002
NDPhA	14.0	248.0	0.022
PB	<1.0	<9.0	<0.002
NDPhA + PB	15.7	165.0	0.018
NDPhA + PB + metyrapone	14.8	153.9	0.008
DPhA	<1.0	<9.0	0.050

Fig. 3. Gas chromatograph of rat urine; (a) urine from control rats; (b) urine from rats treated with *N*-nitrosodiphenylamine; the peak at 3.79 represents the TFA-derivative of diphenylamine

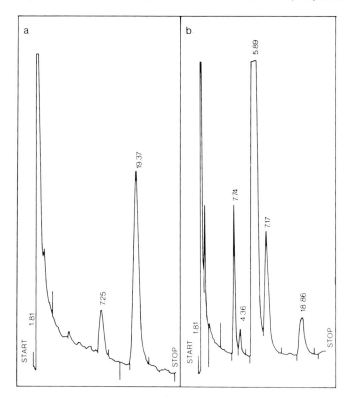

spontaneous autoxidation of oxyhaemoglobin in erythrocytes produces superoxide ion and methaemoglobin (Misra & Fridovich, 1972). The O_2^- is converted by superoxide dismutase to hydrogen peroxide. This in turn forms a catalase-hydrogen peroxide complex, for which nitrite may act as substrate, as has been shown to occur in erythrocytes by Cohen *et al.* (1964). Chance (1950) demonstrated that nitrite reacts rapidly with the catalase-peroxide complex

Fig. 4. Proposed scheme of metabolic activation and deactivation of N-nitrosamines by cytochrome P-450

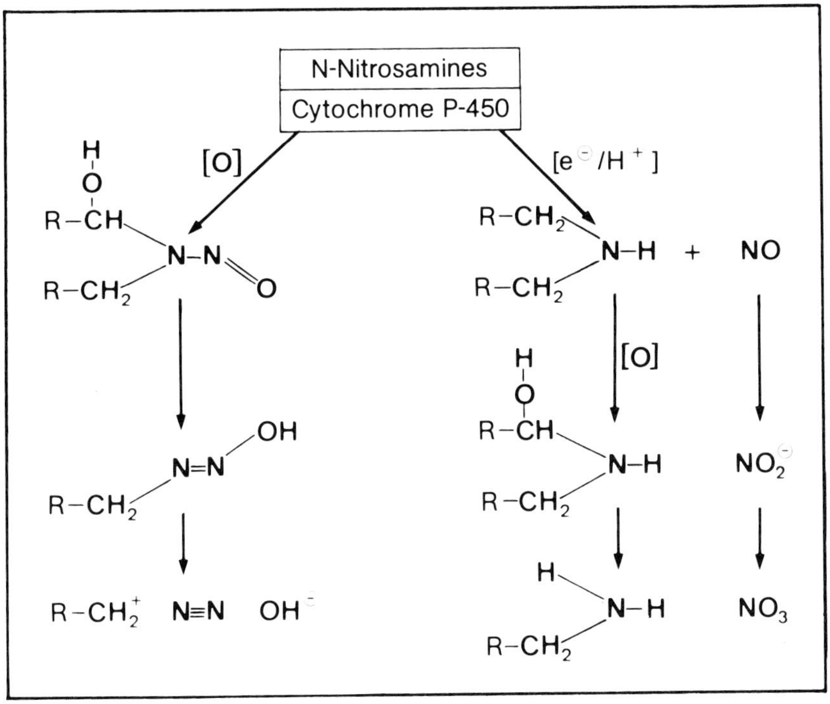

under physiological conditions and postulated a mechanism for the oxidation of nitrite to nitrate. Parks *et al.* (1981) hypothesized that *in vivo* with dosages up to 100 ng/kg body weight of nitrite this mechanism occurs preferentially.

DPhA was also detected when urine was extracted with organic solvents and the organic phase analysed by HPLC or GC (Fig. 3). Generally, the amounts were relatively low. It must be considered that further metabolites, e.g., hydroxy- and/or conjugated products of DPhA, can be generated. Wakabayashi *et al.* (1982) found DPhA as a denitrosation product in in-vitro incubation systems with liver microsomes. Rowland and Grasso (1975) have described a similar pathway in bacteria, where nitrite and the corresponding amines were formed from different nitrosamines. The enzymic mechanism involved was not further clarified or discussed. Very early work by Heath and Dutton (1958) showed that methylamine, but not dimethylamine, was a metabolic product in the urine of NDMA-treated rats. No substantial amount of nitrite was found. Haussmann *et al.* (1983) have observed a hydroxy radical-mediated oxidative decomposition of NDMA in an in-vitro xanthine/xanthine oxidase system in the presence of Fe^{3+}-EDTA. Both formation of nitrite and formaldehyde were obtained. However, the relevance of this in-vitro reaction *in vivo* is not clear.

From in-vitro data, it is concluded that the P-450-dependent monooxygenase system catalyses both 'activation' and 'inactivation' of carcinogenic N-nitrosamines (Fig. 4). The balance between activation and inactivation seems to depend on differences between the various forms of P-450 in a given target tissue. NDPhA possesses no oxidizable hydrogen on the carbon atoms alpha to the N-nitroso function, rendering the molecule unsusceptible to activation to form an alkylating moiety. As the aromatic amine DPhA exhibits mutagenic activity in the presence of norharman and is generated by denitrosation *in vivo,* this novel pathway suggests an activation mechanism rather than an inactivation of NDPhA.

ACKNOWLEDGEMENTS

The authors thank Mrs Jauer for her technical assistance and Dr Eva Schlede for helpful discussions.

REFERENCES

Appel, K.E., Ruf, H.H., Mahr, B., Schwarz, M., Rickart, R. & Kunz, W. (1979) Binding of nitrosamines to cytochrome P-450 of liver microsomes. *Chem.-biol. Interact., 28,* 17–33

Appel, K.E., Schrenk, D., Schwarz, M., Mahr, B. & Kunz, W. (1980) Denitrosation of *N*-nitrosomorpholine by liver microsomes; possible role of cytochrome P-450. *Cancer Lett., 9,* 13–20

Appel, K.E. & Graf, H. (1982) Metabolic nitrite formation from *N*-nitrosamines: evidence for a cytochrome P-450 dependent reaction. *Carcinogenesis, 3,* 293–296

Argus, M.F. & Hoch-Ligeti, C. (1961) Comparative study of the carcinogenic activity of nitrosamines. *J. natl Cancer Inst., 27,* 695–701

Boyland, E., Carter, R.L., Gorrod, J.W. & Roe, F.J.C. (1968) Carcinogenic properties of certain rubber additives. *Eur. J. Cancer, 4,* 233–239

Brouns, R.E., Poot, M., de Vrind, R., Hoek-Kon, T.V. & Henderson, P.T. (1979) Measurement of DNA-excision repair in suspension of freshly isolated rat hepatocytes after exposure to some carcinogenic compounds. *Mutat. Res., 64,* 425–432

Cardy, R.H., Lijinsky, W. & Hildebrandt, P.K. (1979) Neoplastic and non-neoplastic urinary bladder lesions induced in Fischer 344 rats and B6C3E hydrid mice by *N*-nitrosodiphenylamine. *Ecotoxicol. environ. Saf., 3,* 29–35

Chance, B. (1950) On the reaction of catalase peroxides with acceptors. *J. biol. Chem., 182,* 640–658

Cohen, G., Martinez, M. & Hochstein, P. (1964) Generation of hydrogen peroxide during the reaction of nitrite with oxyhemoglobin. *Biochemistry, 3,* 901–908

Druckrey, H., Preussmann, R., Ivankovic, S. & Schmähl, D. (1967) Organotrope carcinogene Wirkungen bei 65 verschiedenen *N*-nitroso-Verbindungen und BD-Ratten. *Z. Krebsforsch., 69,* 103–201

Graf, H., Nagel, R., Tsuji, H., Kremers, P. & Ullrich, V. (1979) In: *XIth International Congress of Biochemistry, Toronto,* abstract

Graf, H., Schramm, W., Nagel, R., Ullrich, V. & Kremers, P. (1980) *Characterization of multiple forms of cytochrome P-450 of pig liver microsomes.* In: Coon, M.J., Conney, A.H., Estabrook, R.W., Gelboin, H.V., Gilone, J.R. & O'Brien, P.J., eds, *Microsomes and Drug Oxidations and Chemical Carcinogenesis,* New York, Academic Press, pp. 615–618

Hausmann, H.J., Kuthan, H. & Werringloer, J. (1983) Hydroxyl radical mediated oxidative decomposition of *N*-nitrosodimethylamine. *Naunyn-Schmiedeberg's Arch. Pharmacol., Suppl. 322,* R 107

Heath, D.F. & Dutton, A. (1958) The detection of metabolic products from dimethylnitrosamine in rats and mice. *Biochemistry, 70,* 619–626

Jones, C.A. & Huberman, E. (1980) A sensitive hepatocyte assay for the metabolism of nitrosamines to mutagens for mammalian cells. *Cancer Res., 40,* 406–411

Kuroki, T., Drevon, C. & Montesano, R. (1977) Microsome mediated mutagenesis in V79 Chinese hamster cells by various nitrosamines. *Cancer Res., 37,* 1044–1050

Magee, P.N. & Farber, E. (1962) Toxic liver injury and carcinogenesis. Methylation of rat liver nucleic acids by dimethylnitrosamine *in vivo. Biochem. J., 83,* 114–124

Magee, P.N., Montesano, R. & Preussmann, R. (1976) N-*Nitroso compounds and related carcinogens.* In: Searle, C.E., ed., *Chemical Carcinogenesis (Am. Chem. Soc. Monogr. Ser., No. 173),* Washington, D.C., American Chemical Society, pp. 491–625

Misra, H.P. & Fridovich, I. (1972) The generation of superoxide radical during the autoxidation of hemoglobin. *J. biol. Chem., 247*, 6960–6962

Nagao, M. & Takahashi, Y. (1981) *Mutagenic activity of 42 coded compounds in the* Salmonella/microsome assay. In: de Serres, F. & Ashby, J., eds, *Evaluation of Short-Term Tests for Carcinogens,* New York, Elsevier, pp. 302–313

Parks, N.F., Krohn, A.K., Mathis, A.C., Chasko, J.H., Geiger, K.R., Gregor, M.E. & Peek, N.F. (1981) Nitrogen-13-labeled nitrite and nitrate: Distribution and metabolism after intratracheal administration. *Science, 212*, 58–60

Rowland, I.R. & Grasso, P. (1975) Degradation of *N*-nitrosamines by intestinal bacteria. *Appl. Microbiol., 29*, 7–12

Schuman, R.F., Lebherz, W.B. & Pienta, R.J. (1981) Induction of morphological transformation of hamster embryo cells *in vitro* by diphenylnitrosamine. *Carcinogenesis, 2*, 679–682

Wakabayashi, K., Nagao, M., Kawachi, T. & Sugimura, T. (1981) Comutagenic effect of norharman with *N*-nitrosamine derivatives. *Mutat. Res., 80*, 1–7

Wakabayashi, K., Nagao, M., Kawachi, T. & Sugimura, T. (1982) *Mechanism of appearance of mutagenicity of* N-*nitrosodiphenylamine with norharman.* In: Bartsch, H., O'Neill, I.K., Castegnaro, M. & Okada, M., eds, N-*Nitroso Compounds: Occurrence and Biological Effects (IARC Scientific Publications No. 41),* Lyon, International Agency for Research on Cancer, pp. 695–707

Yahagi, T., Nagao, M., Seino, Y., Matsushima, T., Sugimura, T. & Okada, M. (1977) Mutagenicities of *N*-nitrosamines on *Salmonella. Mutat. Res., 48*, 121–130

EVIDENCE FOR PENETRATION OF THE NUCLEAR ENVELOPE BY N-NITROSOMETHYLHYDROXYMETHYLAMINE

B. GOLD & L. HINES

Eppley Institute for Research in Cancer and Department of Biomedicinal Chemistry, University of Nebraska Medical Center, 42nd and Dewey Avenue, Omaha, Nebraska 68105, USA

SUMMARY

The metabolic activation of N-nitrosamines to alkylating agents is mediated by the hydroxylation of the carbon adjacent to the N-nitroso moiety. The resulting N-nitroso-α-hydroxy-amines are unstable and decompose to an aldehyde or ketone and a *syn*-alkane diazotic acid, the latter species being responsible for the carbenium ion reactions associated with nitrosamine-induced alkylation of DNA. Since this chain of events is thought to be initiated in the cytoplasm, there must be a 'transportable' metabolite that can diffuse through the cytoplasm, penetrate the nuclear envelope and alkylate the DNA therein. The 'transportability' of N-nitrosomethylhydroxymethylamine, the putative proximate metabolite of N-nitroso-dimethylamine, has been assessed by incubating N-nitroso-([^{14}C]-methyl)-methylacetoxy-methylamine with intact rat liver nuclei in the presence and absence of esterase. The results obtained demonstrate the ability of the in-situ-generated N-nitroso-α-hydroxyamine to penetrate the nuclear envelope and confirm that these unstable metabolites are 'transportable' proximate carcinogens.

INTRODUCTION

Nitrosamines constitute a class of potent carcinogens (Druckrey *et al.*, 1976; Magee *et al.*, 1976) that require metabolic activation to initiate the oncogenic process (Magee *et al.*, 1976). It is well-documented that an enzyme-mediated hydroxylation adjacent to the N-nitroso functionality affords a proximate carcinogenic structure (Druckrey *et al.*, 1961; Magee & Barnes, 1967; Keefer *et al.*, 1973; Dagani & Archer, 1976; Hecht *et al.*, 1978; Kroeger-Koepke *et al.*, 1981), which then spontaneously cleaves to form a *syn*-alkane diazotic acid (Gold & Linder, 1979) that eventually leads to alkylation of nucleic acids and proteins *via* carbenium ion-type intermediates. The α-hydroxylation step is assumed to occur in the cytoplasm (Magee & Barnes, 1967; Bartsch *et al.*, 1975), and the resulting N-nitroso-α-hydroxyamine is assumed to be sufficiently stable to diffuse through the cytoplasm, penetrate the nuclear envelope and decompose to the 'ultimate' electrophilic form that affords covalent adducts of DNA. The aim of the present investigation is to demonstrate whether or not an N-nitroso-α-hydroxyamine, generated *in situ* by the porcine liver esterase-catalysed hydrolysis of the corresponding

N-nitroso-α-acetoxyamine, can penetrate and eventually bind to the DNA of isolated, intact rat liver nuclei. The hydroxylated compound employed is *N*-nitrosomethyl-hydroxymethylamine (NMHMA).

MATERIALS AND METHODS

Di-isopropyl fluorophosphate (DFP) was purchased from Aldrich Chemical Co. (Milwaukee, WI, USA) and porcine liver esterase, Type II, from Sigma Chemical Co., (St Louis, MO, USA). Female Sprague-Dawley rats used in this study were purchased from Sasco Inc. (Omaha, NE, USA). *N*-Nitrosomethylacetoxymethylamine (NMAcMA) and *N*-nitroso [^{14}C-methyl]-methylacetoxymethylamine were prepared by the methods of Wiessler (1974, 1975) and Roller *et al.* (1981), respectively.

Preparation of intact rat liver nuclei

Rat liver nuclei were isolated by a modification of the procedure of Berezney *et al.* (1972). Female Sprague-Dawley rat (6-8 weeks old) were sacrificed by guillotine. Their livers were excised, rinsed in ice-cold 0.25 mol/L sucrose-TKM (50 mmol/L Tris hydrochloric acid, 25 mmol/L potassium chloride, 5 mmol/L magnesium chloride) buffer and weighed. The livers were minced and homogenized in three volumes of 0.25 mol/L sucrose-TKM, using five strokes of a loose Dounce homogenizer, followed by five strokes of a power-driven Teflon pestle homogenizer. The homogenate was filtered sequentially through two, four and eight layers of gauze to remove connective tissue and centrifuged at 0-5°C for 20 min at 1 085 × *g*. The supernatant was discarded and the pellet washed twice with 20 mL of 0.25 mol/L sucrose-TKM, using one or two strokes with a loose Dounce, and repelleted by centrifugation at 0-5°C for 5 min at 500 × *g*. The pellet was resuspended in 45 mL of 2.2 mol/L sucrose-TKM, using a loose Dounce, and the resulting nuclei suspension was centrifuged at 80 250 × *g* for 20 min at 0-5°C in four separate cellulose-nitrate tubes with metal sleeve caps. The supernatants were carefully discarded and the pellets combined into two tubes and washed once with 0.25 mol/L sucrose-TKM. One pellet was resuspended in 7.0 mL of 1.7 mol/L sucrose-TKM and layered into two 5-ml cellulose nitrate tubes over 1.5 mL of 2.2 mol/L sucrose-TKM. The other pellet was suspended in 1.7 mol/L sucrose-TKM which contained sufficient DFP to afford a final concentration of 1.0 mmol/L. This was then layered into two 5-ml cellulose-nitrate tubes. The discontinuous gradients were centrifuged at 0°-5°C for 45 min at 52 000 × *g*. The final nuclei pellets were washed once with 0.25 mol/L sucrose-TKM and resuspended in 1.0 mL of 0.25 mol/L sucrose-TKM containing 0.1 mL glycerol. An aliquot of the purified nuclei (control and DFP-treated) was counted using a Neubauer haemacytometer, after staining with 0.04% Trypan blue, then stored in liquid nitrogen until use. This preparation yielded 3-4 × 10^8 nuclei/mL, corresponding to ~ 10 mg/mL of protein, as determined by the Lowry assay (Lowry *et al.*, 1951)

Incubation of isolated intact nuclei with N-nitroso-[^{14}C-methyl]-methylacetoxymethylamine (NMAcMA)

Control and DFP-treated purified rat liver nuclei (3-4 × 10^7 nuclei) were incubated for 15 min at 37°C in 1.0 mL of 0.05 mol/L Tris-hydrochloric acid buffer (pH 7.0) containing 1-2 μmol NMAcMA (specific activity, 0.916 mCi/mmol). In certain experiments, 20 units of porcine liver esterase were added after the NMAcMA other studies, control and DFP-treated nuclei were disrupted by sonication before adding the NMAcMA.

Before, during and after incubation, the nuclei were examined by light microscopy, using Trypan blue stain. The integrity of the nuclear membrane was monitored by transmission electron microscopy. No appreciable loss or change occurred in the nuclei during the 15-min incubation.

After incubation, DNA was isolated by a modified Kirby-phenol extraction (Kirby, 1957). To each incubation was added 0.5 mL of TIPNS reagent (28 mmol/L tri-iso-propyl-naphthalenesulfonic acid sodium salt, 280 mmol/L *p*-aminosalicylic acid sodium salt, 6.0% butan-2-ol). Next, 1.0 mL of saturated phenol reagent was added and, after mixing for 15 min, the tubes were centrifuged (27 125 × *g*, 0-5°C) for 20 min. The aqueous top layer containing nucleic acids was removed, combined with 0.10 mL brine and re-extracted with 1.0 mL phenol reagent. This mixture was then centrifuged for 15 min at 27 125 × *g*. The aqueous top layer (∼ 1.0 mL) was pipetted off and combined with two volumes of ethanol:*m*-cresol (9:1, v/v) in 15-mL conical glass centrifuge tubes. The nucleic acids were precipitated by gently inverting the tube until a thread-like precipitate appeared. After precipitation overnight, the precipitate was collected, washed three times with 2% sodium acetate in 75% ethanol, resuspended in 0.1 mol/L sodium acetate and brought up to 4 mol/L with sodium chloride. This mixture was centrifuged to remove RNA and excess salt. The DNA was re-precipitated with an equal volume of ethoxyethanol and washed with 2% sodiuim acetate in 75% ethanol until the washings were at the radioactive background level. The DNA was then dissolved in a small volume of water (∼ 0.2 mL) and transferred to glass-fibre discs (Whatman GF/A), which were dried, placed in scintillation vials containing 2 mL Omnifluor (NEN) and counted in a Beckman Scintillation Counter (LS-335). The discs were then removed from the vials and washed with toluene. The DNA was hydrolysed in 1 mol/L perchloric acid at 70°C for 60 min and quantified using diphenylamine reagent (Burton, 1956).

RESULTS AND DISCUSSION

Metabolic activation of *N*-nitrosodialkylamines to alkylating agents is mediated by hydroxylation on the carbon adjacent to the *N*-nitroso moiety (Druckrey *et al.*, 1961; Magee & Barnes, 1967; Keefer *et al.*, 1973; Dagani & Archer, 1976; Hecht *et al.*, 1978; Kroeger-Koepke, 1981). The resulting *N*-nitroso-α-hydroxyamines are unstable and cleave at the hydroxylated C-N bond to yield an aldehyde or ketone and *syn*-alkane diazotic acid (Gold & Linder, 1979). The latter species rapidly reacts to give products associated with carbenium ion intermediates (White & Woodcock, 1968). Since this chain of events is thought to be initiated in the cytoplasm, there must be a transportable metabolite that can diffuse through the cytoplasm, penetrate the nuclear envelope and alkylate the DNA therein. We have previously shown that *N*-nitroso-α-hydroxyamine is the only possible candidate (Gold & Linder, 1979).

Theoretically, the transportability of an *N*-nitroso-α-hydroxyamine can be assessed by incubating the corresponding radio-labelled *N*-nitroso-α-acetoxyamine with intact nuclei and esterase. Esterase rapidly hydrolyses the α-acetoxy compound to the a-hydroxy compound. The amount of binding, measured as labelled nuclear DNA, can be used to quantify the extent of exonuclear-generated *N*-nitroso-α-hydroxy-penetration of the nuclear envelope.

Such a study is complicated experimentally by esterase activity on the nuclear membrane of isolated liver nuclei (Böcking, 1975; Deimling & Böcking, 1976), because this activity predominates over that of added exogenous esterase. Thus, hydrolysis of the NMAcMA to NMHMA occurs specifically on the nuclear envelope and the addition of exogenous esterase is unnecessary. Results of incubation of ^{14}C-labelled NMAcMA with isolated intact nuclei are shown in Table 1; these clearly demonstrate the ability of the in-situ-generated *N*-nitroso-α-hydroxyamine to diffuse through the nuclear envelope. Covalent binding of the ^{14}C-label to nuclear DNA is 97% inhibited by pretreating nuclei with DFP, a potent esterase inhibitor (Aldridge & Reiner, 1972) (Table 1). Binding to DNA when exogenous porcine liver

Table 1.   DNA binding resulting from the incubation of N-nitroso-[¹⁴C-methyl]-methylacetoxymethyl-amine[a] with isolated intact and sonicated rat liver nuclei

Conditions[b]	Specific activity of DNA (dpm/μg)[c]	Number of experiments
Intact nuclei	6.42 ± 1.33[g,h,i]	8
DFP[d]-inhibited intact nuclei	0.20 ± 0.11[g]	10
DFP-inhibited intact nuclei + 10 units esterase[e]	2.84 ± 0.64[h]	3
DFP-inhibited intact nuclei + 20 units esterase	2.85 ± 1.17[i]	12
Sonicated nuclei	5.03 ± 0.93[j,k]	5
DFP-inhibited sonicated nuclei	0.24 ± 0.05[j]	4
DFP-inhibited sonicated nuclei + 20 units esterase	2.84 ± 1.10[k]	6

[a] Specific activity, 0.916 mCi/mmol
[b] All incubations carried out for 15 min at 37 °C in 0.05 mol/L Tris-hydrochloric acid buffer (pH 7.4)
[c] Values normalized to 5×10^6 dpm/incubation. Control studies show that binding is linear with the concentrations used
[d] DFP, + diisopropyl fluorophosphate
[e] Porcine liver esterase (Sigma Type I)
[f] Sonication for 30 sec at 0 °C was shown by light and electron microscopy to disrupt nuclear envelope completely. [g,h,i,j,k] Significantly different (p < 0.01) from value with the same superscript

esterase is added to an incubation of DFP-inhibited nuclei and ¹⁴C-NMAcMA is also shown in Table 1. The binding to DNA in this case is only 50% of that observed in uninhibited control nuclei. This recovery is not sensitive to a two-fold increase in esterase concentration (Table 1).

We interpret these results to mean that binding to DNA is most efficient when the 'transportable' N-nitroso-α-hydroxyamine is generated on the nuclear envelope, because it must diffuse only through a lipophilic membrane. Mochizuki et al. (1980) have reported a shorter half-life for N-nitroso-α-hydroxyamines in an aqueous, rather than a non-polar, medium. The N-nitroso-α-hydroxyamine generated in the aqueous incubation buffer must diffuse further through an aqueous environment to reach the nuclear DNA.

The results with nuclei disrupted by sonication (Table 1) do not differ from those observed with intact nuclei. It is conceivable that the DNA adheres to the membrane fragments bearing the esterase activity, but this is only speculation.

Recently, Umbenhauer and Pegg (1981) and Kim et al. (1981) have provided evidence for the transportability of a pro-alkylating species derived from NDMA. The former paper reported that a potential alkylating agent could diffuse out of a hepatocyte and alkylate exogenous DNA. Binding to DNA was, interestingly, decreased by a factor of 30 when the hepatocytes were lysed. In our model, no significant difference was seen between intact and sonicated nuclei (Table 1). Kim et al. (1981) observed binding to protein of intact human erythrocytes when the erythrocytes were incubated with rat liver microsomes, NADPH and NDMA. Erythrocytes, themselves, cannot activate nitrosamines, again indicating the formation of a transportable alkylating agent during metabolism of NDMA.

A study to determine the partitioning of the reactive alkane diazotic acid intermediate, eventually formed from NMAcMA, into diazoalkane demonstrated that a yield of less than 1% of diazoalkane is obtained at pH 7.4. The failure to detect appreciable diazoalkane formation from NMAcMA at pH 7.4 is consistent with previous in-vivo binding experiments which showed all DNA alkylation, upon administration of NDMA, to result from carbenium ion intermediates (Lijinsky et al., 1968; Ross et al.,1971). Therefore the diazo compound cannot be responsible for the binding.

In conclusion, the present results reconfirm that *N*-nitroso-α-hydroxyamines are sufficiently stable to diffuse from the cytoplasm into the nuclei of the same cell, and perhaps into that of proximate cells which may not be capable of metabolizing nitrosamines, but which are susceptible to nitrosamine carcinogenesis.

REFERENCES

Aldridge, W.N. & Reiner, E. (1972) *Enzyme Inhibitors as Substrates. Interactions of Esterases with Esters of Organophosphorus and Carbamic Acids*, Amsterdam, North Holland

Bartsch, H., Malaveille, C. & Montesano, R. (1975) *In vitro* metabolism and microsome-mediated mutagenicity of dialkyl-nitrosamines in rat, hamster and mouse tissues. *Cancer Res., 35*, 644–651

Berezney, R., Macaulay, L.K. & Crane, F.L. (1972) The purification and biochemical characterization of bovine liver nuclear membranes. *J. biol. Chem., 247*, 5549–5561

Böcking, A. (1975) Esterase. XIX. Biochemical and ultrahistochemical investigations of the non specific esterase in nuclei from mouse liver. *Histochemistry, 41*, 313–321

Burton, K. (1956) a study of the conditions and mechanism of the diphenylamine reaction for the colorimetric estimation of deoxyribonucleic acid. *Biochem. J., 62*, 315–323

Dagani, D. & Archer, M.C. (1976) Brief communication: Deuterium isotope effect in the microsomal metabolism of dimethylnitrosamine. *J. natl Cancer Inst., 57*, 955–957

Deimling, O.V. & Böcking, A. (1976) Esterases in histochemistry and ultrahistochemistry. *Histochem. J., 8*, 215–252

Druckrey, H., Preussmann, R., Ivankovic, S. & Schmähl, D. (1967) Organotrope carcinogenic Wirkung bei 65 verschiedenen *N*-nitroso-Verbindungen and BD-Ratten. *Z. Krebsforsch., 69*, 103–201

Druckrey, H., Preussmann, R., Schmähl, D. & Muller, M. (1961) Chemische Konstitution und carcinogene Wirkung bei Nitrosaminen. *Naturwissenschaften, 48*, 134–135

Gold, B. & Linder, W.B. (1979) α-hydroxynitrosamines: Transportable metabolites of dialkylnitrosamines. *J. Am. chem. Soc., 101*, 6772–6773

Hecht, S.S., Chen, C.B. & Hoffmann, D. (1978) Evidence for metabolic α-hydroxylation of *n*-nitrosopyrrolidine. *Cancer Res., 38*, 215–218

Keefer, L.K., Lijinsky, W. & Garcia, H. (1973) Deuterium isotope effect on the carcinogenicity of dimethylnitrosamine in rat liver. *J. natl Cancer Inst., 51*, 299–302

Kim, S., park, W.K., Choi, J., Lotlikar, P.D. & Magee, P.N. (1981) Microsome-dependent methylation of erythrocyte proteins by dimethylnitrosamine. *Carcinogenesis, 2*, 179–182

Kirby, K.S. (1957) A new method for the isolation of deoxyribonucleic acids; evidence on the nature of bonds between deoxyribonucleic acid and protein. *Biochem. J., 66*, 495–504

Kroeger-Koepke, M.B., Koepke, S.R., McClusky, G.A., Magee, P.N. & Michejda, C.J. (1981) α-Hydroxylation pathway in the *in vitro* metabolism of carcinogenic nitrosamines: *N*-Nitrosodimethylamine and *N*-nitroso-*N*-methylaniline. *Proc. natl Acad. Sci. USA, 78*, 6489–6493

Lijinsky, W., Loo, J. & Ross, A.E. (1968) Mechanism of alkylation of nucleic acids by nitrosodimethylamine. *Nature, 218*, 1174–1175

Lowry, O.H., Rosebrough, N.J., Farr, A.L. & Randall, R.J. (1951) Protein measurements with folin reagent. *J. biol. Chem., 193*, 265–275

Magee, P.N. & Barnes, J.M. (1967) Carcinogenic nitroso compounds. *Adv. Cancer Res., 10*, 164–246

Magee, P.N., Montesano, R. & Preussmann, R. (1976) N-*Nitroso compounds and related carcinogens*. In Searle, C.E., ed., *Chemical Carcinogens (ACS Monograph 173)*, Washington DC, American Chemical Society, pp. 491–625

Mochizuki, M., Anjo, T. & Okada, M. (1980) Isolation and characterization of *N*-alkyl-*N*-(hydroxymethyl)nitrosamines from *N*-alkyl-*N*-(hydroperoxymethyl)nitrosamines by deoxygenation. *Tetrahedron Lett., 21*, 3693–3696

Roller, P.P., Keefer, L.K., Bradford, III. W.W. & Reist, E.J. (1981) Synthesis, analysis and stability studies of ¹⁴C-methyl(acetoxymethyl)nitrosamine. *J. Labelled Compd Radiopharmaceut., 18*, 1261–1272

Ross, A.E., Keefer, L. & Lijinsky, W. (1971) Alkylation of nucleic acids of rats liver and lung by deuterated *N*-nitrosodiethylamine *in vivo*. *J. natl Cancer Inst., 47*, 789–795

Umbenhauer, D.R. & Pegg, A.E. (1981) Alkylation of intracellular and extracellular DNA by dimethylnitrosamine following activation by isolated rat hepatocytes. *Cancer Res., 41,* 3471–3474

White, E.H. & Woodcock, D.J. (1968) *Cleavage of the carbon-nitrogen bond,* In Patai, S. ed., *The Chemistry of the Amino Group,* New York, Wiley-Interscience, pp. 440–483

Wiessler, M. (1974) Syntheses α-funktioneller nitrosamine. *Angew. Chem., 68,* 817–818

Wiessler, M. (1975) Chemie der Nitrosamine. II. Synthese α-funktioneller dimethylnitrosamine. *Tetrahedron Lett., 16,* 2575–2578

URINARY METABOLITES OF SOME ALICYCLIC NITROSAMINES

G.M. SINGER & W.A. MACINTOSH

LBI-Basic Research Program, Chemical Carcinogenesis Program, NCI-Frederick Cancer Research Facility, Frederick, Maryland 21701, USA

SUMMARY

We have studied the urinary metabolites of N-nitrosopiperidine, 3- and 4-hydroxy-N-nitrosopiperidine, N-nitroso-4-piperidone, N-nitrosohexamethyleneimine and N-nitroso-heptamethyleneimine. The N-nitrosopiperidines induce primarily oesophageal tumours in rats; N-nitrosohexamethyleneimine induces oesophageal and liver tumours and N-nitroso-heptamethyleneimine induces oesophageal and lung tumours. The products were identified by gas chromatographic comparison with standards, where possible, and by gas chromatography-mass spectrometry. The percentage of the dose excreted as metabolites in the urine increased with ring size. Hydroxy and ketone derivatives of all three of the N-nitrosoalicyclic amines were found. Pimelic acid was the major metabolite ($\simeq 25\%$) of N-nitrosoheptamethyleneimine; adipic acid was identified as a metabolite of N-nitroso-hexamethyleneimine, but no glutaric acid was found from N-nitrosopiperidine.

INTRODUCTION

Alicyclic nitrosamines are potent carcinogens in experimental animals, but each induces a different spectrum of tumours. The urinary metabolites of these compounds should indicate the general metabolic pathways which these compounds follow and thus may provide some insight into the chemistry involved in tumour induction. The metabolism of N-nitroso-pyrrolidine (NPYR) has been thoroughly investigated, but the larger alicyclic nitrosamines have received much less attention.

We have now examined the urinary metabolites of N-nitrosopiperidine (NPIP), N-nitro-sohexamethyleneimine (NHEX) and N-nitrosoheptamethyleneimine (NHEPT) in Fischer F344 rats, which were given equimolar doses comparable to those that were used in chronic toxicity studies of the compounds (Taylor & Nettesheim, 1975; Lijinsky & Reuber, 1981).

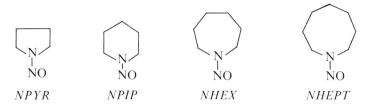

NPYR   NPIP   NHEX   NHEPT

MATERIALS AND METHODS

Chemicals

NPIP, NHEX, NHEPT and the substituted piperidines were available from previous studies and were shown by gas chromatography (GC) to be free of impurities. 2,7-^{14}C-NHEX and 2,8-^{14}C-NHEPT were also available from previous studies (Snyder *et al.*, 1977). Both compounds were purified by high-performance liquid chromatography before use (μ-Bondapak-C_{18}, 50% MeOH-H_2O). β- and λ-hydroxy- and γ-keto-NHEPT were kindly provided by Dr J. Saavedra. Glutaric, adipic and pimelic acids and their dimethyl esters, 5-hydroxypentanatal and valerolactone were obtained from the Aldrich Chemical Co. ε-Caprolactone (Aldrich Chemical Co.) was distilled before use.

Heptanolactone

This lactone was prepared in 45% yield by Baeyer-Villiger oxidation of cycloheptanone.

Metabolic experiments

Treatment of the animals and isolation of most of the metabolites were carried out as described previously (Singer *et al.*, 1981). The doses used were equal to that which each animal received weekly in the chronic carcinogenicity assays: NPIP, 11.4 mg/rat; NHEX, 12.6 mg/rat; NHEPT, 10.0 mg/rat. Identification and quantification was carried out by GC, GC/thermal energy analysis and GC/mass spectrometry (MS) on vitreous silica (VS) capillary columns, DB-5 and Durawax-1 (J. & W., Inc.), using the cold on-column injection technique in chromatographs equipped with SGE, Inc., OCI-2 or OCI-3 injectors. The distribution of metabolites was determined by the use of 2-^{14}C-NHEX and -NHEPT.

Isolation of aldehydes/ketones

Urine (1.0 mL) was diluted with ethanol (3.0 mL), vortexed for 30 sec and centrifuged at low speed for 4 min. The supernatant was removed. 2,4-Dinitrophenylhydrazine (DNPH) reagent (0.40 mL) and isooctane (1.0 mL) were added, and the solution was vortexed for 30 sec. The isooctane was removed and extracted with acetonitrile (0.20 mL) by vortexing for 30 sec. The acetonitrile solution was analysed by high-performance liquid chromatography (Waters Associates, μ-Bondapak-C_{18}, 1.5 mL/min).

Isolation of amines

An aliquot of urine (1.0 ml) was made basic (pH 11) with sodium hydroxide and treated with *p*-toluenesulfonyl chloride as previously described (Singer & Lijinsky, 1976). After boiling under reflux for one hour, the solution was cooled, acidified and continuously extracted with ether. The ether solution was evaporated under a nitrogen stream and the residue was dissolved in ethanol for GC analysis (DB-5 VS capillary, J. & W., Inc.).

RESULTS

The overall pattern of distribution of metabolites was determined by measuring the radioactivity (^{14}C) of the 24- and 48-h urine, the radioactivity extracted with neutral or acid metabolites and that left unextracted. The results are shown in Table 1. The overall excretion

Table 1. Recoveries of radioactivity (percentage of ^{14}C administered)

Compound[a]	Dose (mg/rat)	24-h total	Neutrals	Acids	Unextracted	48-h total	Neutrals	Acids	Un-extracted
NHEX	12.6	31%	4	17	11	18%	3	4	12
NHEPT	10.0	53%	8.8	27	16	3.9%	0.66	1.3	1.9
NHEPT[b]	10.0	29%	3.3	12	11	2.5%	0.2	0	0.8

[a] NHEX, N-nitrosohexamethyleneimine; NHEPT, N-nitrosoheptamethyleneimine
[b] 2-^{14}C-NHEPT administered on day 4 of a 5-day feeding experiment, with unlabelled nitrosamine

Table 2. Metabolites as percentage of dose, in 24 h

Compound[a]	Starting material	$(CH_2)_{n-2}^{(t,\ u)}(COOH)_2$	β-Alcohol	β-Ketone	γ-Alcohol	γ-Ketone	δ-Alcohol	δ
NPIP	0.49	ND[a]	0.09	ND	0.93	0	–	δ
NHEX	0.99	2.7	0.65	0.33	6.11	ND	–	–
NHEPT	0.40	23	ND	ND	3.49	ND	0.60	trace

[a] NPIP, N-nitrosopiperidine; NHEX, N-nitrosohexamethyleneimine; NHEPT, N-nitrosoheptamethyleneimine
ND, not detected

of NHEX metabolites (31%) agrees well with Granjean's finding of 37% (Grandjean, 1976). For both NHEX and NHEPT, more radioactivity was found in the fractions containing the acids than in the other fractions. In the case of NHEPT, most of the radioactivity in the fraction containing the acids can be accounted for by the 23% of the administered dose that was excreted as pimelic acid. Only 2.7% of NHEX was found as adipic acid, and NPIP gave no detectable glutaric acid.

The quantitative results for the identified neutral metabolites from the three alicyclic nitrosamines are given in Table 2. The identities of the derivatives of NPIP and NHEX were readily determined by GC and GC/MS comparisons with available standards. The molecular formulae of the derivatives of NHEPT were determined by GC-MS, both by accurate mass electron-impact and chemical ionization MS but the assignments of the positional isomers were made by extrapolation of GC retention time behavior from NPIP and NHEX.

In addition to identifying and quantifying known metabolites, we also sought evidence for several other plausible products: the appropriate α,ω-alkane diols, lactams, lactones and amines. With the exception of 1,5-pentanediol, reasonable recoveries of all these compounds were made readily. Nevertheless, we found no evidence of any of the aforementioned compounds in the urine of the treated rats.

DISCUSSION

The general pattern of metabolism of the alicyclic nitrosamines appears to be similar for all members of the series. A small amount ($< 1\%$) of the nitrosamine is excreted unchanged. Small amounts of ($< 1\%$) of β-oxidized derivatives are found, as well as somewhat larger amounts of γ-oxidized products and (from NHEPT) the δ-alcohol (0.6%). Aliquots of urine from rats fed each of the three nitrosamines were treated with glucuronidase, but no additional metabolite was found.

The major identified metabolite from NHEPT was pimelic acid (23%), a product of ring opening and oxidation of both α-carbons. A smaller amount of adipic acid (2.5%) was found from NHEX, but no glutaric acid was detected in the urine of rats fed NPIP. The latter results are not surprising, since these acids would be expected to be metabolized further by the usual pathways of intermediary metabolism. Analogous products have been found as major metabolites of N-nitrosonornicotine and N-nitrosanabasine (Hecht & Young, 1982). From the former, the product is 4-oxo-4-(3-pyridyl)butanoic acid, a keto-acid, since the presence of the pyridine ring precludes oxidation to a dicarboxylic acid.

In addition to identifying and quantifying as many metabolites as possible, we have also demonstrated the absence of a number of plausible metabolites. We were able to demonstrate that no denitrosated amine was present in the urine of rats fed any of the three nitrosamines. We used the sensitive tosylamide procedure already described (Singer & Lijinsky, 1976), by which we could have detected less than 0.05%. There was also no indication of the formation of lactams or lactones. In these cases as well, we could have detected as little as 0.05% of the metabolite produced, except for valero-lactam (0.1%).

Decarboxylation of the α,ω-dicarboxylic acids could lead to ω-hydroxycarboxylic acids with two fewer carbons, but we found no evidence of these. In fact, we were unable to demonstrate the presence of any ω-hydroxycarboxylic acid as a metabolite of the three heterocyclic nitrosamines. We sought these since we knew that 4-hydroxybutyric acid was produced by liver microsomes or hepatocyte metabolism of N-nitrosopyrrolidine (Hecker et al., 1979; Farrelly et al., 1982) and that 6-hydroxyhexanoic acid was the major microsomal metabolite of N-nitrosohexamethyleneimine (Hecker & McClusky, 1982).

No ω-hydroxyaldehyde was detected, although these have been found from hepatocyte and microsomal metabolism of NPYR (Hecker *et al.*, 1979; Farrelly *et al.*, 1982), NPIP (Leung *et al.*, 1979) and NHEX (Hecker & McClusky, 1982).

We assume that the absence in urine of compounds known to be produced by hepatocyte and microsomal metabolism is due to further metabolism of these compounds by other organs in the intact animal. Such metabolism probably also leads to the eventual formation of adipic acid from NHEX and pimelic acid from NHEPT.

The overall pattern of metabolism of NPIP, NHEX, NHEPT and NPYR as far as can be inferred from the identified excreted metabolites, appears to be very similar. Apparently, the differences in tumorigenic potency and organotropy must be due to rather subtle differences in metabolism, which remain to be investigated.

ACKNOWLEDGEMENTS

Research sponsored by the National Cancer Institute, DHHS, under contract No. NO1-CO-23 909 with Litton Bionetics, Inc. The contents of this publication do not necessarily reflect the views or policies of the Department of Health and Human Services, nor does mention of trade names, commercial products, or organizations imply endorsement by the US Government.

REFERENCES

Farrelly, J.G., Stewart, M.L. & Hecker, L.I. (1982) The metabolism of nitrosopyrrolidine by hepatocytes from Fischer rats. *Chem. -biol. Interact.*, *41*, 341–351

Grandjean, C.J. (1976) Metabolism of N-nitrosohexamethyleneimine. *J. natl cancer Inst.*, *57*, 181–185

Hecht, S.S. & Young, R. (1982) Regiospecificity in the metabolism of the homologous cyclic nitrosamines, *N'*-nitrosonornicotine and *N'*-nitrosoanabasine. *Carcinogenesis, 3*, 1195–1199

Hecker, L.I. & McClusky, G.A. (1982) Comparison of the in-vitro metabolism of N-nitroso-hexamethyleneimine by rat liver and lung microsomal fractions. *Cancer Res.*, *42*, 59–64

Hecker, L.I., Farrelly, J.G., Smith, J.H., Saavedra, J.E. & Lyon, P.A. (1979) Metabolism of the liver carcinogen *N'*-nitrosopyrrolidine by rat liver microsomes. *Cancer Res.*, *39*, 2679–2686

Leung, K.-H., Park, K.K. & Archer, M.C. (1978) Alpha-hydroxylation in the metabolism of N-nitro-sopiperidine by rat liver microsomes: Formation of 5-hydroxypentanal. *Res. Commun. Chem. Pathol. Pharmacol.*, *19*, 201–211

Lijinsky, W. & Reuber, M.D. (1981) Carcinogenic effect of nitrosopyrrolidine, nitrosopiperidine and nitrosohexamethyleneimine in Fischer rats. *Cancer Lett.*, *12*, 99–103

Singer, G.M. & Lijinsky, W. (1976) Naturally occurring nitrosatable compounds. I. Secondary amines in foodstuffs. *J. Agric. Food Chem.*, *24*, 550–553

Singer, G.M., Lijinsky, W. Buettner, L. & McClusky, G.A. (1981) Relationship of rat urinary metabolites of N-nitrosomethyl-N-alkylamine to bladder carcinogenesis. *Cancer Res.*, *41*, 4942–4946

Snyder, C.M., Farrelly, J.G. & Lijinsky, W. (1977) Metabolism of three cyclic nitrosamines in Sprague-Dawley rats. *Cancer Res.*, *37*, 3530–3532

Taylor, H.W. & Nettesheim, P. (1975) Influence of administration route and dosage schedule on tumor response to nitrosoheptamethyleneimine in rats. *Int. J. Cancer*, *15*, 301–307

CONJUGATES OF *N*-NITROSO-*TERT*-BUTYLMETHYLAMINE IN URINE

M. WIESSLER, G. ROSSNAGEL & B. RUGEWITZ-BLACKHOLM

Deutsches Krebsforschungszentrum, Institut für Toxikologie und Chemotherapie,
Im Neuenheimer Feld 280, D-6900 Heidelberg, FRG

SUMMARY

The glucuronide (α-anomer) and the mercapturic acid of *N*-nitroso-*tert*-butyl-hydroxymethylamine were synthesized. An analytical procedure was developed using high-performance liquid chromatography, which allowed the detection of both conjugates in a single run. A new and efficient synthesis of *N*-nitroso-*tert*-butyl-^{14}C-methylamine was developed, based on ^{14}C-formaldehyde. After subcutaneous administration of 23 mg/kg to a rat, the nitrosamine was metabolized to a high degree, and two conjugates were excreted in the urine.

INTRODUCTION

Conjugation reactions (phase II reactions) are effective detoxification mechanisms for foreign compounds in the organism. Besides sulfates and acetates and, in some special cases, phosphates (Boyland *et al.*, 1961; Capel *et al.*, 1974), glucuronides and mercapturic acids (formed by enzymatic degradation of glutathione adducts) are the most important conjugates excreted in urine or by the gall-bladder. The formation of such conjugates has been proven for many carcinogens (aromatic hydrocarbons, aromatic amines, aflatoxins). In a few cases, such conjugates are transport forms of the active metabolites or are biologically active themselves, but most of them seem to be detoxification products in the proper sense.

Only β- and γ-hydroxylated conjugates of *N*-nitrosodialkylamines are known (Suzuki & Okada, 1980; Suzuki *et al.*, 1981a, b; Archer *et al.*, 1981). These conjugates have not yet been found for α-hydroxylated nitrosamine, *in vivo* or *in vitro*. It may be asked if the stability of the α-hydroxylated nitrosamines is such as to allow conjugation reactions. Two arguments for the existence of the conjugates can be advanced. First, the half-lives of α-hydroxylated nitrosamines can be estimated, in spite of their high reactivity (Gold & Linder, 1979, Mochizuki *et al.*, 1980). Second, the UDP-glucuronyltransferase and the glutathiontransferase systems (Morgenstern *et al.*, 1979; Lee & McKinney, 1982) are located in the membranes of the endoplasmatic reticulum near the nitrosamine-activating monooxygenases; therefore the conjugation of α-hydroxylated nitrosamines seems possible (Fig. 1). In recent years, we developed chemical methods to synthesize such conjugates and have studied their peculiarities. These synthetic compounds should enable us to develop an analytical procedure for the

Fig. 1. Metabolism of *N*-nitroso-*tert*-butylmethylamine and formation of conjugates.

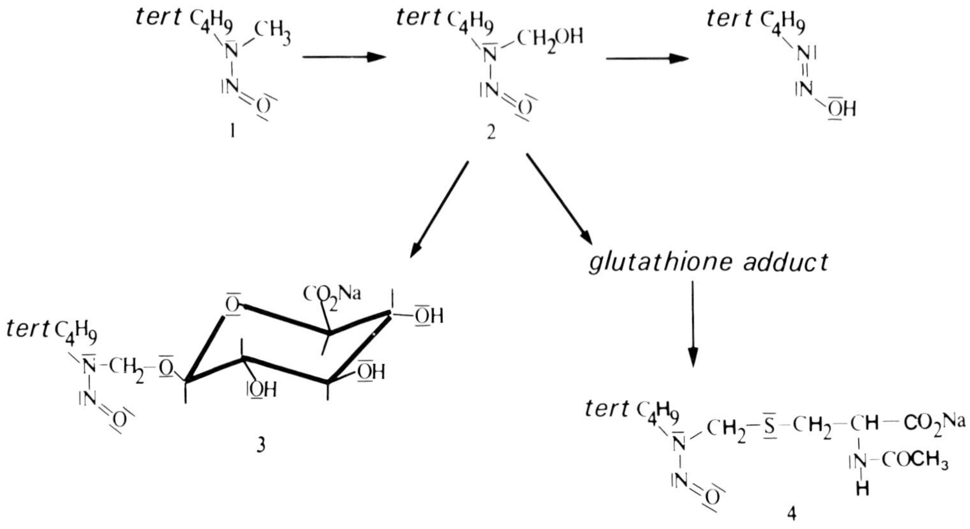

detection of conjugates of α-hydroxynitrosamines in urine. We began our studies with the non-carcinogenic *N*-nitroso-*tert*-butylmethylamine (Gold *et al.*, 1981) because it is easier to handle and less toxic than other nitrosamines.

MATERIAL AND METHODS

Compounds

All commercial chemicals were of analytical grade. The synthesis of glucuronide methyl esters of α-hydroxylated *N*-nitrosodialkylamines has already been described (Braun & Wiessler, 1980).

Conversion to the sodium salt was accomplished by reaction with sodium hydroxide and neutralization with DOWEX H$^\oplus$ and subsequently DOWEX Na$^\oplus$. Evaporation released 3 (Fig. 1) as a white powder. The chemical synthesis provides only the α-anomer and not the biologically relevant β-isomer. It can be assumed that the difference in retention times of the α- and β-anomers on high-performance liquid chromatography (HPLC) is not significant.

Fig. 2. Synthetic scheme for the preparation of *N*-nitroso-*tert*-butyl-^{14}C-methylamine.

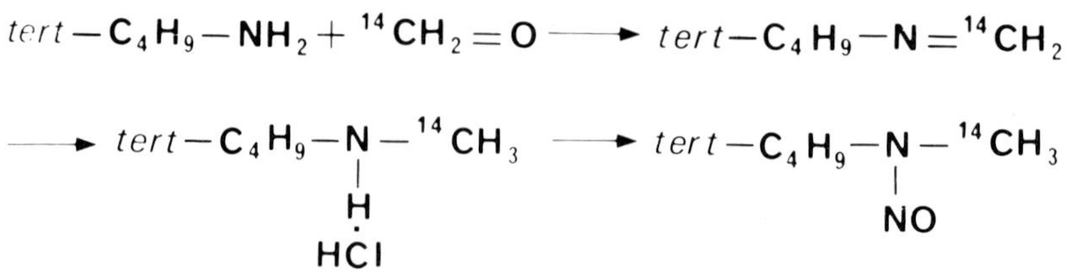

The mercapturic acid sodium salt, 4 (Fig. 1), was synthesized by reacting α-chloro-nitrosamines, created by addition of nitrosyl chloride to the double bond in the imine, 5 (Fig. 2) with *N*-acetylcysteinemethylester in the presence of pyridine or triethylamine. Chromatography on silica gel (methylene chloride:methanol, 9:1) yielded the mercapturic acid methylester, which was converted to the sodium salt by the same reaction sequence as described for 3.

Radioactive synthesis

The synthesis of *N*-nitroso-*tert*butyl-^{14}C-methylamine was based on $^{14}CH_2 = O$, as outlined in Figure 2. (Amersham, UK; 1–3% aqueous solution, 15.1 mCi/mmol specific activity).

The reaction of formaldehyde with *tert*-butylamine yielded the imine 5 (Fig. 2), which was hydrogenated by platinum hydrogen in aqueous solution. The ^{14}C-*tert*-butylmethylamine was isolated as the hydrochloride in 85–90% yield. Nitrosation was performed with nitrosyl tetrafluoroborate in acetonitrile in presence of pyridine. *N*-Nitroso-*tert*-butyl-^{14}C-methylamine was isolated in an over-all yield of 70–75%, based on ^{14}C-formaldehyde. Purity was checked by gas chromatography (GC) (Pye Unicam 104, 1-m column, 15% Carbowax 20M, 90 °C; flame-ionization detector temperature 350 °C).

The isolation of conjugates, *tert*-butanol and intact parent compound was performed as follows: organs or urine were distilled under reduced pressure at room temperature. The distillate was collected by cooling with liquid nitrogen and analysed for *N*-nitroso-*tert*-butylmethylamine and *tert*-butanol (Pye Unicam 104; 2.5-m column; 15% Carbowax 20M; 180 °C; flow rate, 25 mL N$_2$/min; injection temperature, 230 °C; flame-ionization detector temperature, 350 °C). Ten mL methanol were added to the non-volatile residue and the mixture stored at −28 °C for 15 h. After filtration, the clear methanolic solution was concentrated to 1 mL and analysed for conjugates by HPLC (Beckmann 110A Pump; 250-mm Shandon ODS; Hypersil 5 μ + 40 mm pre-column; UV detection at 235 nm with an LDC Spectromonitor III). Recovery experiments showed that all substances could be isolated quantitatively.

Animal experiments

Six μL (6 mg) *N*-nitroso-*tert*-butyl-^{14}C-methylamine (23 mg/kg, specific activity 0.41 mCi/mmol, corresponding to 21.4 μCi) were injected subcutaneously into a 257-g Sprague-Dawley rat. The rat was housed in a Metabowl Jencons Metabolic Cage and $^{14}CO_2$ was measured in an exhalation chamber (Frieseke & Hoepfner, Erlangen, FRG). ^{14}C-Radioactivity was measured in a Mark III Liquid Scintillation counter (Searle Analytic Inc.). $^{14}CO_2$ exhalation was measured and urine collected for 24 h. After sacrifice, organs and serum were analysed as described.

RESULTS AND DISCUSSION

Conjugates of α-hydroxylated nitrosamines have not been detected *in vitro* or *in vivo* until now (Hemminki, 1982). The successful synthesis of glucuronide 3 and mercapturate 4 demonstrates the chemical stability of such compounds (Fig. 1). The recovery experiments showed that both compounds are stable in rat urine and can be re-isolated with very high yields. The synthetic materials were found to be homogeneous.

The synthetic scheme for the preparation of the ^{14}C-labelled nitrosamine is shown in Figure 2. The keystep is the formation of the imine 5 and its catalytic reduction to the secondary amine-hydrochloride. This procedure is very efficient and can be done very easily, in contrast to reduction with metal hydrides.

Tabel 1 shows the amount of $^{14}CO_2$ exhaled in 24 h after subcutaneous administration of *N*-nitroso-*tert*-butyl-^{14}C-methylamine. The high yield of $^{14}CO_2$ in our experiment, in contrast to the data of Heath (1962), is due to the 12-fold lower dosage used here (Table 1). This result suggests a very efficient metabolism of low doses of *N*-nitroso-*tert*-butylmethylamine. The distribution of radioactivity in urine, blood, kidney, spleen and liver confirmed this hypothesis. Only in urine (residue and distillate) were measurable amounts of radioactivity found. All other organs contained only about 0.1% of the applied radioactivity, with the exception of the liver 'residue', which contained 0.46% (Table 2). GC analysis of the urine distillate showed that unchanged *N*-nitroso-*tert*-butylmethylamine was the only radioactive component (Fig. 3); none could be found in any other fluid or organ (Table 2).

tert-Butanol, a possible metabolite, could not be detected by GC. It is known from the literature (Smith & Williams, 1954) that, after application of *tert*-butanol, considerable amounts are excreted as a glucuronide. It thus seems possible that the amount of *tert*-butanol produced by the low dose of *N*-nitroso-*tert*-butylmethylamine given here was completely conjugated. Furthermore, *tert*-butanol can also be metabolized as shown *in vitro* by Cederbaum and Cohen (1980).

The analytical procedure based on HPLC allows the simultaneous estimation of both conjugates 3 and 4 in the same run (Fig. 4). This very efficient analytical method employed tetrabutylammonium salts in ion-pair HPLC (Bidlingmeyer, 1980; Hart *et al.*, 1981). The retention time of mercapturic acid could be varied from 10.10 min to 43.10 min by changing the mobile phase only slightly, as can be seen in the first column in Table 3. These results are important for the validation of our in-vivo experiments.

After subcutaneous administration of *N*-nitroso-*tert*-butyl-^{14}C-methylamine, the residue after distillation of the urine (24 h) contained 5.9% of the applied radioactivity and all the possible conjugates (Table 2). Treatment of the residue as described, followed by HPLC

Table 1.   Exhalation of $^{14}CO_2$ after administration of ^{14}C-*N*-nitroso-*tert*-butylmethylamine to rats (24 h)

Dose (mg/kg)	$^{14}CO_2$ (% of administered activity)	Animals
23	74	male Sprague-Dawley rats, 254 g
300[a]	11	female rats, albino
100[a]	5.5[b]	Porton Strain, 165–185 g

[a] Data of Heath (1962)
[b] 12 h 50 min

Fig. 3. High-performance liquid chromatograms of *N*-nitroso-*tert*-butylmethylamine; (A) standard, (B) urine distillate; mobile phase: 0.01 mol/L $TBA^+Na^+SO_4^{2-}$, 5% ethanol, 5% propanol-2; flow rates 1.5 mL/min.

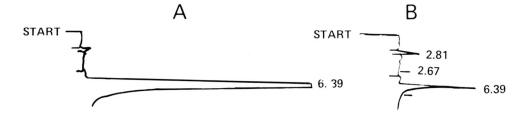

Table 2. Distribution of radioactivity in distilled rat urine, blood and organs after administration of [14]C-*N*-nitroso-*tert*-butylmethylamine

Sample[a]	Radioactivity	
	(μCi)	(% of administered dose)
urine r	1.26	5.9
urine d	0.336	1.57
blood (total activity in 7 ml)	0.03	0.14
kidney r	0.024	0.11
kidney d	–	–
spleen r	0.005	0.02
spleen d	–	–
liver r	0.1	0.46
liver d	–	–
other organs	(no radioactivity was detected)	

[a] r, distillation residue, extracted with methanol; d, distillate

Fig. 4. High-performance liquid chromatograms of glucuronide 3 (A), mercapturate, 4 (B), and urine distillation residue, (C), (recovery experiments); mobile phase: 0.01 mol/L TBA$^+$Na$^+$SO$_4^{2-}$, propanol-2; flow rate, 1.5 mL/min.

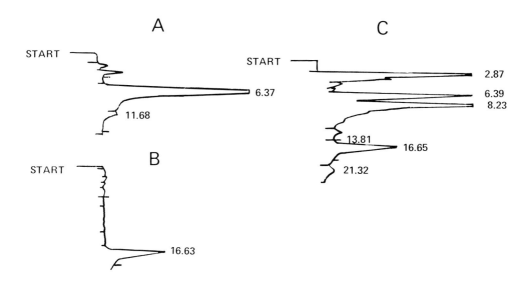

analysis, gave two radioactive peaks. Whereas one radioactive peak co-chromatographed with the sodium glucuronate 3 in different solvent systems, this does not hold for the second peak. It may be assumed that this unknown metabolite, the detailed structure of which is unknown, has a character similar to that of 4.

This work demonstrates that it should be possible to verify the concept of conjugation of α-hydroxylated nitrosamines.

Table 3. Comparison of retention times of compound 4 (Fig. 1) and
of a radioactive metabole using different compositions of mobile phase

Mobile phase[a] (aqueous solutions)	Retention time	
	Standard[b] (min)	Radioactive peak (min)
0.01 mol/L TBA⁺Na⁺SO₄²⁻ 8% ethanol, 5% propanol-2	10.10	10
0.01 mol/l TBA⁺Na⁺SO₄²⁻ 5% propanol-1	19.35	17
0.01 mol/l TAB⁺Na⁺SO₄²⁻ 20% methanol	30.30	23
0.004 mol/l TBA⁺Cl⁻ 0.005 mol/l H₃BO₃ 24% methanol	43.40	39

[a] TBA⁺, $(C_4H_9)_4N^+$ ion
[b] Compound 4, Fig. 1

REFERENCES

Archer, M.C. & Leung, K. (1981) *Mechanisms of alkylation of DNA by N-nitrosodialkylamines.* In: Scanlan, R.A. & Tannenbaum, S.R., eds, N-*Nitroso Compounds (Am. Chem. Soc. Symp. Ser. No. 174),* Washington DC, American Chemical Society, pp. 39–47

Bidlingmeyer, B.A. (1980) Separation of Ionic compounds by reversed high pressure liquid chromatography. An update of ion-pairing techniques. *J. chromatogr. Sci., 18,* 525–539

Boyland, E., Kinder, C.H. & Manson, D. (1961) The biochemistry of aromatic amines. 8. Synthesis and detection of di-(2-aminonaphthyl)hydrogen phosphate. A metabolite of 2-naphthylamine in dogs. *Biochem. J., 78,* 175–179

Braun, H. & Wiessler, M. (1980) α-D-Glucuronides of a-(N-alkyl-N-nitrosamino) alkylalcohols. *Angew. Chem. intern., Engl. Ed., 19,* 400–401

Capel, I.D., Millburn, P. & Williams, R.T. (1974) Monophenylphosphate, a new conjugate of phenol in the cat. *Biochem. Soc. Trans., 2,* 305–306

Cederbaum, A.I. & Cohen, G. (1980) Oxidative demethylation of tert butanol by rat liver microsomes. *Biochem. biophys. Res. Commun., 97,* 730–736

Gold, B. & Linder, W.B. (1979) α-hydroxynitrosamines: transportable metabolites of dialkylnitrosamines. *J. Am. chem. Soc., 101,* 6772–6773

Gold, B., Salamasi, S., Linder, W. & Althoff, J. (1981) Biological and chemical studies involving methyl-*tert*-butylnitrosamine, a non-carcinogenic nitrosamine. *Carcinogenesis, 2,* 529–532

Hart, S.J., Tontodonati, R. & Calder, I.C. (1981) Reversed phase chromatography of urinary metabolites of paracetanol using ion supression and ion pairing. *J. Chromatogr., 225,* 387–405

Heath, D.F. (1962) The decomposition and toxicity of dialkylnitrosamines in rats. *Biochem. J., 85,* 72–91

Hemminki, K. (1982) Dimethylnitrosamine adducts excreted in rat urine. *Chem.-biol. Interact., 39,* 139–148

Lee, G.C. & McKinney, J.I. (1982) Identity of microsomal glutathione-S-transferases. *Mol. cell. Biochem., 48,* 91–96

Mochizuki, M., Anjo, T. & Okada, M. (1980) Isolation and characterization of N-alkyl-N-(hydroxymethyl)nitrosamines from N-alkyl-N-(hydroperoxymethyl)-nitrosamines by deoxygenation. *Tetrahedron Lett., 21,* 3693–3696

Morgenstern, R., DePierre, J.W. & Ernster, L. (1979) Activation of microsomal glutathione-S-transferase activity by sulfhydryl reagents. *Biochem. biophys. Res. Commun., 87,* 657–663

Smith, J.N. & Williams, R.T. (1954) Studies in detoxication. 58. The metabolism of aliphatic alcohols. The glucuronic acid conjugation of chlorinated and some unsaturated alcohols. *Biochem. J., 56,* 618–621

Suzuki, E. & Okada, M. (1980) Metabolic fate of N,N-dibutylnitrosamine in the rat. *Gann, 71*, 856–862, 863–870

Suzuki, E., Jiyoshi, M. & Okada, M. (1981a) Metabolic fate of N-butyl N-(4-hydroxybutyl) nitrosamine homologs in the rat, in relation to their organotropic carcinogenicity to the urinary bladder. *Gann, 72*, 113–122

Suzuki, E., Jiyoshi, M. & Okada, M. (1981b) Metabolic fate of N-alkyl-N-(3-hydroxypropyl and 2-hydroxyethyl) nitrosamines in the rat in relation to the induction of bladder cancer by N-butyl-N-(4-hydroxybutyl)-nitrosamine and its homologs. *Gann, 72*, 254–258

Wiessler, M. (1974) Synthese α-funktioneller Nitrosamine. *Angew. Chem., 86*, 817–818

TISSUE AND SPECIES SPECIFICITY OF THE MICROSOMAL METABOLISM OF N-NITROSOMETHYLBENZYLAMINE

R. MEHTA, G.E. LABUC[1] & M.C. ARCHER[2]

Department of Medical Biophysics, University of Toronto, Ontario Cancer Institute, 500 Sherbourne Street, Toronto, Ontario M4X 1K9, Canada

SUMMARY

The microsomal activation of N-nitrosomethylbenzylamine (NMBzA) by oxidation at the methylene carbon atom was examined in various organs of a number of species to determine the role of metabolism in the organ-specificity of tumour induction by NMBzA. In Sprague-Dawley rats, NMBzA was metabolized by microsomes from liver, lung and oesophageal mucosa. In Fischer F-344 rats and in rabbits, metabolic activity was present in both liver and oesophageal mucosa, the only tissues studied in those species. In contrast, in Syrian hamsters and in BALB/cBYJ mice, no NMBzA metabolism was detectable in the oesophagus, but it occurred at relatively high rates in liver, lung and kidney. The forestomach mucosa exhibited undetectable levels of activity in all species except the hamster in which it was present at a very low level. In human oesophageal mucosal microsomes from six patients, rates of metabolism of NMBzA were either undetectable or approximately 70 times lower than those in the Sprague-Dawley rats. A comparison of NMBzA metabolism in the different species with the known carcinogenicity of the nitrosamine in rats and rabbits, and our preliminary data on the acute toxicity of NMBzA in hamsters and mice suggests that, in the oesophagus at least, metabolic activation of NMBzA is necessary to elicit its toxic and/or carcinogenic effect. However, in the liver,which in all species has high metabolic activity but which is also resistant to the toxic and carcinogenic effects of NMBzA, other factors besides metabolic activation must be involved.

INTRODUCTION

N-Nitrosomethylbenzylamine (NMBzA), one of the most potent of the carcinogenic nitrosamines, is highly selective in inducing tumours of the pharynx and oesophagus in rats after both oral and systemic administration (Druckrey *et al.*, 1967; Stinson *et al.*, 1978). Oesophageal tumours have also been induced in rabbits by oral treatment with sodium nitrite

---

[1] Present address: 41 Chadstone Road, Chadstone, Victoria, Australia 3148
[2] To whom correspondence should be addressed

and *N*-methylbenzylamine (Iizuka *et al.*, 1977). In NMRI mice, however, the route of administration influences the organ specificity of NMBzA: oral administration causes tumours of the oesophagus and forestomach, whereas subcutaneous injection induces forestomach carcinomas and lung adenomas (Sander & Schweinsberg, 1973).

We have shown previously (Labuc & Archer, 1982) that microsomes prepared from rat oesophageal mucosa metabolize NMBzA at a high rate, principally to benzaldehyde and a methylating agent, in a cytochrome P-450-dependent reaction. Furthermore, studies of DNA methylation in rats and NMRI mice have indicated that the capacity of tissues to activate NMBzA may influence its organ specificity for tumour induction (Hodgson *et al.*, 1980; Kleihues *et al.*, 1981).

In the present study we investigated the metabolism of NMBzA (NMBzA debenzylase) in microsomes prepared from various organs of Sprague-Dawley rats, Fischer F-344 rats, New Zealand white rabbits, BALB/cBYJ mice and Syrian golden hamsters to determine whether a relationship exists between the capacity of an organ to activate NMBzA and the toxic or carcinogenic action of the nitrosamine in that organ. Since the carcinogenicity of NMBzA in Syrian hamsters and BALB/cBYJ mice is not known, we present some preliminary data on the acute toxicity of NMBzA in those species. In order to evaluate the susceptibility of the human oesophagus to possible carcinogenic effects of NMBzA, we have also measured the metabolic activity of microsomes prepared from a numer of surgical specimens.

EXPERIMENTAL

Male Sprague-Dawley rats (21–23 days old), male Syrian golden hamsters (21–23 days old) and male Fischer F-344 rats (28–30 days old) were purchased from Charles River Inc. (Laprairie, Quebec, Canada). Male BALB/cBYJ mice (21–28 days old) were purchased from Jackson Laboratories (Bar Harbor, Maine, USA). These animals were maintained on a Teklad 6% fat rat-mouse diet *ad libitum*. Male New Zealand white rabbits (9–10 weeks old), purchased from Riemens Fur Ranches Ltd (St Agatha, Ontario, Canada), were maintained on a Teklad Rabbit diet *ad libitum*. After 5–10 days of acclimatization, animals were sacrificed by carbon dioxide asphyxiation.

Disease-free specimens of human oesophagus, obtained from patients undergoing surgery for either oesophageal cancer (HE 1: male, age 58; HE 2: female, age 60; HE 3: male, age 72; HE 4: male, age 53; HE 5: female, age 72) or a chronic penetrating ulcer (HE 6: male, age 80), were immersed immediately in saline and kept at 4 °C. Microsomes from the mucosa, dissected free from the muscle and submucosal layers, were usually prepared within 3 h of resection, except for specimen HE 4 which was processed after 16 h.

Microsomes from the liver and from the oesophageal mucosa of all species were prepared as described previously (Labuc & Archer, 1982). Lung and kidney were homogenized in three volumes of buffer (1.15% potassium chloride, 50 mmol/L Tris-hydrochloric acid, pH 7.4) with 30 passes of a motor-driven Duall all-glass homogenizer (lung) or 12 passes of a motor-driven Potter-Elvehjem homogenizer with a Teflon pestle (kidney). Forestomachs were slit open along the greater curvature, cleared of contents and rinsed in homogenizing buffer. The mucosa was scraped off with a scalpel then homogenized in the same way as oesophageal mucosa. Microsomes from all tissues were prepared as described for liver and oesophageal mucosa (Labuc & Archer, 1982). For each microsomal preparation, tissues were pooled from the following number of animals: for liver, 3 animals; lung and kidney, 3 rats, 10 hamsters or 10 mice; for forestomach and oesophageal mucosa, 10 rats, 20 hamsters or 80 mice. In the case of rabbits, both liver and oesophageal mucosa were pooled from 2 animals.

Incubations were carried out at 37 °C for 20 min (or 60 min for human oesophageal microsomes) in the presence of 5 mmol/L NMBzA, approximately 0.5 mg of microsomal protein, an NADPH-generating system and semicarbazide, exactly as described previously (Labuc & Archer, 1982). Benzaldehyde semicarbazone, benzyl alcohol and benzoic acid were determined by high-performance liquid chromatography (Labuc & Archer, 1982).

Protein was estimated by the method of Lowry *et al.,* as described by Colowick and Kaplan (1957), with bovine serum albumin as standard.

RESULTS AND DISCUSSION

The rates of formation of benzaldehyde, benzyl alcohol and benzoic acid after incubation of NMBzA with different tissues of various species are summarized in Table 1.

In Sprague-Dawley rats, NMBzA was metabolized to benzaldehyde by microsomes from either liver or oesophageal mucosa at rates similar to those observed previously (Labuc & Archer, 1982). Benzyl alcohol, arising principally from enzymatic reduction of benzaldehyde, and to a small extent from reaction with water of the benzylating agent produced by oxidation of NMBzA at the methyl group, was also formed in the presence of liver but not oesophageal microsomes (Labuc & Archer, 1982). A significant level of NMBzA debenzylase activity was detected in lung microsomes from Sprague-Dawley rats, although the activity was about a quarter that in the oesophagus. These findings follow the same pattern found by Hodgson *et al.* (1980) for Wistar rats treated with NMBzA, in which the highest level of DNA methylation, after liver and oesophagus, occurred in lung. These authors also detected low levels of DNA methylation in forestomach and kidney of Wistar rats; and the presence of NMBzA debenzylase activity in the forestomach of female SIV50 rats has been reported by Schweinsberg and Kouros (1979). We were, however, unable to detect any metabolism of NMBzA in either forestomach or kidney of Sprague-Dawley rats, suggesting strain and/or sex differences. Both the hepatic and oesophageal metabolic profiles in the F-344 rats were the same as in the Sprague-Dawley rats, although there were inter-strain differences in both tissues with respect to rates of metabolism.

With rabbit liver microsomes, benzaldehyde was produced at a rate similar to that for F-344 rats, although benzyl alcohol formation was diminished. With oesophageal microsomes from rabbits, NMBzA was metabolized at about a quarter of the rate of that seen with Sprague-Dawley rats. Unlike the situation in rats, however, both hepatic and oesophageal microsomes of rabbits produced benzoic acid at a significant rate. The benzoic acid presumably arises *via* oxidation of benzaldehyde.

With liver microsomes from Syrian hamsters and BALB/cBYJ mice, very high levels of NMBzA debenzylase activity were observed, with formation of benzaldehyde, benzyl alcohol and benzoic acid. In contrast to rats and rabbits, NMBzA was not metabolized by oesophageal microsomes from either hamsters or mice. Lung and kidney microsomes from both hamsters and mice, however, metabolized NMBzA at rates significantly higher than microsomes from these tissues in rats. A low level of NMBzA metabolism was also observed in microsomes from the forestomach mucosa of hamsters but not mice.

Following intraperitoneal administration of NMBzA to female NMRI mice, the highest levels of DNA methylation were observed in liver, followed by lung, forestomach, oesophagus and kidney (Kleihues *et al.,* 1981). Schweinsberg and Kouros (1979) also found detectable levels of NMBzA debenzylase activity in the forestomach of female NMRI mice. While our metabolic data on liver, lung and kidney from BALB/cBYJ mice parallel the relative extents of DNA methylation observed in the same tissues in NMRI mice, the lack of enzyme activity in forestomach and oesophageal mucosa in our studies suggests sex and/or strain differences. Neither metabolic activation nor carcinogenicity of NMBzA have been studied in Syrian hamsters, although *N*-nitrosodimethylamine and *N*-nitrosodiethylamine are metabolized by

Table 1. Metabolism of *N*-nitrosomethylbenzylamine by microsomes prepared from different tissues of various species

Species	Metabolite	Rate of metabolism (nmol/min per mg protein)				
		Liver	Oesophageal mucosa	Lung	Kidney	Forestomach mucosa
Sprague-Dawley rat	Benzaldehyde	1.415±0.150 (8)[a]	0.580±0.080 (6)	0.155±0.025 (12)	≤0.005 (6)	≤0.005 (11)
	Benzyl alcohol	2.73 ±0.32 (8)	≤0.10	≤0.10	≤0.10	≤0.10
	Benzoic acid	≤0.03	≤0.03	≤0.03	≤0.03	≤0.03
F-344 rat	Benzaldehyde	0.890±0.020 (14)	1.065±0.090 (11)	ND[c]	ND	ND
	Benzyl alcohol	2.46 ±0.10 (14)	≤0.10			
	Benzoic acid	≤0.03	≤0.03			
Rabbit	Benzaldehyde	0.880±0.155 (16)	0.145±0.030 (17)	ND	ND	ND
	Benzyl alcohol	1.38 ±0.13 (16)	≤0.10			
	Benzoic acid	0.26 ±0.04 (16)	0.17 ±0.02 (17)			
Syrian hamster	Benzaldehyde	4.525±0.175 (12)	≤0.005 (6)	0.355±0.015 (12)	0.310±0.025 (6)	0.010±0.010 (8)
	Benzyl alcohol	5.17 ±0.19 (12)	≤0.10	≤0.10	≤0.10	≤0.10
	Benzoic acid	0.54 ±0.04 (12)	≤0.03	0.10 ±0.03 (12)	≤0.03	0.09 ±0.04 (8)
BALB/cBYJ mouse	Benzaldehyde	3.745±0.145 (14)	≤0.005 (6)	2.340±0.110 (12)	0.070±0.010 (12)	≤0.005 (12)
	Benzyl alcohol	4.67 ±0.15 (14)	≤0.10	2.94 ±0.08 (12)	0.19 ±0.08 (12)	≤0.10
	Benzoic acid	0.17 ±0.02 (14)	≤0.03	≤0.03	≤0.03	≤0.03
Man[b]	Benzaldehyde	ND	0.010±0.005 (15)	ND	ND	ND
	Benzyl alcohol		≤0.1			
	Benzoic acid		≤0.03			

[a] Mean±S.E. Numbers in parentheses are numbers of determinations. Three or four experiments were carried out for each tissue, each experiment consisting of two to five determinations

[b] Data from six patients

[c] Not determined

liver, kidney, respiratory tract, oesophagus and small intestine of this species (Montesano & Magee, 1974).

In comparison with rat oesophagus, an extremely low level of benzaldehyde formation was detected when NMBzA was incubated with microsomes from human oesophageal mucosa. The rate of benzaldehyde formation in the human samples ranged from undetectable (< 0.005 nmol/min per mg protein) to 0.015 nmol/min per mg protein. Our results are in agreement with those of Autrup and Stoner (1982), which showed that methylation of DNA by NMBzA in rat oesophageal cultures was about 100-fold higher than in cultures of human oesophagus.

Although the livers of all species exhibited a high level of metabolic activity for NMBzA, no liver tumours have been observed in Sprague-Dawley rats, F-344 rats or rabbits (Druckrey et al., 1967; Iizuka et al., 1977; Fong et al., 1978; Stinson et al., 1978). In BALB/cBYJ mice and Syrian hamsters, in which the carcinogenicity of NMBzA is unknown, our preliminary studies have indicated no evidence of toxicity in the liver 48 h after intraperitoneal or oral administration of the nitrosamine. These observations suggest that, while metabolic activation may be the necessary first step in toxigenesis or carcinogenesis by nitrosamines, it is not sufficient to elicit these effects.

Our results indicate that the ability of the oesophageal mucosa to activate NMBzA plays an important role in determining its toxigenicity and carcinogenicity. Thus, Sprague-Dawley rats, F-344 rats and rabbits, in which there was significant metabolic activity, are all susceptible to oesophageal carcinogenesis by NMBzA. While it is difficult to compare the potency of NMBzA as an oesophageal carcinogen in these animals, because of differences in experimental design, for nitrosopiperidine-induced oesophageal tumours, F-344 rats are certainly more sensitive than Sprague-Dawley rats (Lijinsky et al., 1981). Our results show that microsomes from oesophageal mucosa of F-344 rats metabolize NMBzA at a greater rate than those from Sprague-Dawley rats. Furthermore, our preliminary observations indicate that NMBzA has negligible acute toxicity in the oesophagus of hamsters and mice in comparison with rats, again suggesting a correlation between metabolic activity in this tissue and the biological effects of the nitrosamine. The extremely low level of NMBzA debenzylase activity that we detected in microsomes prepared from human oesophageal mucosa suggests that NMBzA may not cause human oesophageal cancer.

The low but significant rate of NMBzA activation by rat lung microsomes also parallels its weak toxic and tumorigenic effects in that organ (Stinson et al., 1978; Kraft & Tannenbaum, 1980). Whether NMBzA has toxic and/or carcinogenic effects on the lung and kidney of hamsters or mice, in which we found comparatively high levels of activity, remains to be evaluated.

ACKNOWLEDGEMENTS

This research was supported by the Ontario Cancer Treatment and Research Foundation and grant MT 7025 from the Medical Research Council of Canada.

REFERENCES

Autrup, H. & Stoner, G.D. (1982) Metabolism of N-nitrosamines by cultured human and rat oesophagus. Cancer Res., 42, 1307–1311

Colowick, S.P. & Kaplan, N.O., eds (1957) Methods in Enzymology, Vol. 3, New York, Academic Press, pp. 448–450

Druckrey, H., Preussmann, R., Ivankovic, S. & Schmähl, D. (1967) Organotrope carcinogene Wirkungen bei 65 verschiedenen N-nitrosoverbindungen an BD-Ratten. Z. Krebsforsch., 69, 103–201

Fong, L.Y.Y., Sivak, A. & Newberne, P.M. (1978) Zinc deficiency and methylbenzylnitrosamine-induced oesophageal cancer in rats. *J. natl Cancer Inst., 61*, 145–150

Hodgson, R.M., Wiessler, M. & Kleihues, P. (1980) Preferential methylation of target organ DNA by the oesophageal carcinogen *N*-nitrosomethylbenzylamine. *Carcinogenesis, 1*, 861–866

Iizuka, T., Ichimura, S., Kawachi, T., Hirota, T. & Itabashi, M. (1977) Carcinoma of the oesophagus of rabbits induced with *N*-methylbenzylamine and sodium nitrite. *Gann, 68*, 829–835

Kleihues, P., Veit, C., Wiessler, M. & Hodgson, R.M. (1981) DNA methylation of *N*-nitrosomethylbenzylamine in target and non-target tissues of NMRI mice. *Carcinogenesis, 2*, 897–899

Kraft, P.L. & Tannenbaum, S.R. (1980) Distribution of *N*-nitrosomethylbenzylamine evaluated by whole-body radioautography and densitometry. *Cancer Res., 40*, 1921–1927

Labuc, G.E. & Archer, M.C. (1982) Esophageal and hepatic microsomal metabolism of *N*-nitrosomethylbenzylamine and *N*-nitrosodimethylamine in the rat. *Cancer Res., 42*, 3181–3186

Lijinsky, W., Singer, G.M. & Reuber, MD. (1981) The effect of 4-substitution on the carcinogenicity of nitrosopiperidine. *Carcinogenesis, 2*, 1045–1048

Montesano, R. & Magee, P.N. (1974) *Comparative metabolism* in vitro *of nitrosamines in various animal species including man.* In: Montesano, R. & Tomatis, L., eds, *Chemical Carcinogenesis Essays (IARC Scientific Publications No. 10)*, Lyon, International Agency for Research on Cancer, pp. 39–56

Sander, J. & Schweinsberg, F. (1973) Tumorinduction bei Mäusen durch *N*-methylbenzylnitrosamin in niedriger Dosierung. *Z. Krebsforsch., 79*, 157–161

Schweinsberg, F. & Kouros, M. (1979) Reactions of *N*-methyl-*N*-nitrosobenzylamine and related substrates with enzyme-containing cell fractions isolated from various organs of rats and mice. *Cancer Lett., 7*, 115–120

Stinson, S.F., Squire, R.A. & Sporn, M.B. (1978) Pathology of esophageal neoplasms and associated proliferative lesions induced in rats by *N*-methyl-*N*-benzylnitrosamine. *J. natl Cancer Inst., 61*, 1471–1475

METABOLISM AND ACTIVATION OF 1,1-DIMETHYLHYDRAZINE AND METHYLHYDRAZINE, TWO PRODUCTS OF N-NITROSODIMETHYL-AMINE REDUCTIVE BIOTRANSFORMATION

H.M. GODOY, M.I. DÍAZ GÓMEZ & J.A. CASTRO[1]

Centro de Investigaciones Toxicológicas (CEITOX), CITEFA/CONICET, Zufriategui y Varela, 1603 Villa Martelli, Province of Buenos Aires, Argentina

SUMMARY

N-Nitrosodimethylamine (NDMA) and two of its metabolites, monomethylhydrazine (MMH) and 1,1-dimethylhydrazine (UDMH) were metabolized to carbon dioxide by rat liver slices. Under these conditions, NDMA and MMH, but not UDMH, produced reactive metabolites that bound covalently to nucleic acids. Rat liver microsomes or $9\,000 \times g$ supernatants were able to transform NDMA, MMH and UDMH to formaldehyde. In the case of MMH and UDMH, enzymatic and non-enzymatic pathways of formaldehyde formation were present in both liver microsomes and $9\,000 \times g$ supernatants. NDMA, MMH and UDMH led to covalent binding in incubation mixtures containing either microsomes or $9\,000 \times g$ supernatants. In the case of NDMA, the process was enzymatic and required NADPH in both cellular fractions. In the case of MMH, the process was enzymatic in microsomes, and required NADPH and oxygen when using UDMH or MMH and $9\,000 \times g$ supernatants; interactions of a non-enzymatic nature leading to covalent binding to proteins were dominant.

These results suggest that part of the carbon dioxide produced during NDMA metabolism might derive from UDMH and MMH. Similarly, a significant part of the covalent binding of NDMA metabolites to proteins in incubation mixtures containing microsomes or $9\,000 \times g$ supernatants might derive from enzymatic and non-enzymatic reactions of UDMH or MMH. Also, a minor part of the covalent binding of NDMA reactive metabolites to nucleic acids might be due to further biotransformation of MMH to reactive metabolites. It may be concluded from the present results that biotransformation of NDMA to UDMH and MMH might not be a detoxication process, as previously thought, but one related to some of the toxic effects of NDMA

INTRODUCTION

We previously reported the existence of metabolic pathways of reductive metabolism and activation of N-nitrosodimethylamine (NDMA) in rat liver microsomes and $9\,000 \times g$

---

[1] To whom correspondence should be sent.

supernatants (Godoy *et al.,* 1978, 1980; Díaz Gómez *et al.,* 1981). Moreover, a correlation between a reductive process leading to NDMA-reactive metabolites that bind covalently to 9 000 × *g* supernatant proteins and NDMA-induced acute liver injury was suggested (Godoy *et al.,* 1980; Díaz Gómez *et al.,* 1981). This correlation was found to hold for rat liver preparations, but not for those from the other species investigated (Godoy *et al.,* 1982; Díaz Gómez *et al.,* 1983).

Studies by Lin and Fong (1980) confirmed and extended our finding of a reductive pathway of NDMA metabolism and activation in rat liver.

Grilli and Prodi (1975) had reported previously that monomethylhydrazine (MMH) and 1,1-dimethylhydrazine (UDMH) were produced by reduction of NDMA, catalysed by microsomal and cellular soluble enzymes.

In the present work, we analyse the possible contribution of the biotransformation of UDMH or MMH to the production of carbon dioxide and formaldehyde and to the NDMA-induced covalent binding of reactive metabolites to nucleic acids or proteins, under similar experimental conditions.

MATERIALS AND METHODS

Chemicals

NDMA, MMH and UDMH (Gold-label grade, Aldrich Chemical Co., Milwaukee, WI, USA) and ^{14}C-NDMA (54.2 mCi/mmol) (New England Nuclear, Boston, MA, USA) were obtained as indicated. Dimethylsulfate (^{14}C-methyl) 14.8 mCi/mmol, (New England Nuclear) was used to prepare ^{14}C-MMH and ^{14}C-UDMH, according to the method described by Shank (1979). The radioactive hydrazines obtained, ^{14}C-MMH (7.4 mCi/mmol) and UDMH (14.8 mCi/mmol), were dissolved in water.

Animals

Sprague-Dawley male rats (200–250 g) were used throughout. The animals were fasted for 12–14 h before use.

Methods

Radioactive ^{14}C-carbon dioxide and covalent binding to nucleic acids in liver slices were determined as described previously (Godoy *et al.,* 1978), except that ^{14}C-NDMA, ^{14}C-MMH or ^{14}C-UDMH (0.15 mmol/L final concentration, 7.1 × 10^5 dpm/mL) was used. The in-vitro metabolism to formaldehyde and the activation of NDMA, MMH or UDMH to reactive metabolites by 9 000 × *g* supernatants or microsomes were measured as described by Godoy *et al.* (1978), but ^{14}C-NDMA (0.15 mmol/L, 2 × 10^6 dpm/μmol), ^{14}C-MMH (0.15 mmol/L, 7.73 × 10^5 dpm/μmol) or ^{14}C-UDMH (0.15 mmol/L, 5.75 × 10^5 dpm/μmol) was used. The nitrogen used for anaerobic incubations was freed of oxygen as described elsewhere (Godoy *et al.,* 1978).

Statistics

The significance of the difference between two mean values was assessed by Student's t-test (Bancroft, 1960).

RESULTS AND DISCUSSION

As previously observed in our own and many other laboratories (Magee & Barnes, 1967; Godoy *et al.*, 1978, 1980; Lai & Arcos, 1980; Pegg, 1980; Díaz Gómez *et al.*, 1981; Godoy *et al.*, 1982; Díaz Gómez *et al.*, 1983), NDMA was transformed in incubation mixtures containing liver tissue slices to carbon dioxide and to reactive metabolites that bound covalently to nucleic acids. Incubation mixtures containing microsomes or 9 000 × *g* supernatants and NADPH also formed formaldehyde and reactive metabolites that bound covalently to proteins under anaerobic conditions. Furthermore, as previously reported (Godoy *et al.*, 1978, 1980), NDMA led to the formation of formaldehyde and to metabolites that bound covalently to proteins under anaerobic conditions when using microsomes or 9 000 × *g* incubation mixtures.

We now report that, under the experimental conditions employed here, both MMH and UDMH were metabolized to carbon dioxide and that only MMH led to reactive metabolites that bound covalently to nucleic acids (Table 1). This is in agreement with earlier studies by others (Dost *et al.*, 1966; Kruger *et al.*, 1970; Shank, 1979). Previous studies by Grilli and Prodi (1975) showed that both MMH and UDMH are produced *in vivo* during metabolism of NDMA by liver microsomes or 9 000 × *g* supernatant preparations.

Dougherty *et al.* (1977) also found evidence for the formation of both hydrazines from NDMA *in vivo*. The present results suggest that a part of the carbon dioxide formed from NDMA in the tissue slice experiments might derive from MMH and UDMH. Also, part of the covalent binding to nucleic acids observed when NDMA was incubated with liver slices might derive from MMH. The extent of the contribution of NDMA to carbon dioxide formation *via* MMH or UDMH biotransformation or to the formation of reactive metabolites that bind covalently to nucleic acids does not, however, appear to be important.

Under experimental conditions similar to those employed to show NDMA transformation to formaldehyde by microsomal or 9 000 × *g* supernatant preparations, we also find transformation of both MMH and UDMH to formaldehyde (Table 2). Previous studies by other workers showed that MMH and UDMH are demethylated oxidatively to yield formaldehyde by rat liver microsomal preparations in the presence of NADPH (Wittkop *et al.*, 1969; Prough *et al.*, 1981). In the present studies, however, we found that, in addition to these microsomal pathways of an oxidative nature, there are other non-negligible sources of formaldehyde formation from MMH and UDMH. One is of a non-enzymatic nature, since it is observed even in heated preparations of both microsomes and 9 000 × *g* supernatants. These processes occur to a greater extent under aerobic than under anaerobic conditions, except for the case of MMH and microsomal suspensions. In the presence of liver microsomes or 9 000 × *g* supernatants (but in the absence of NADPH), the amount of formaldehyde formed is usually less than that in heated preparations. This fact probably reflects the existence of

Table 1.   Carbon dioxide formation and covalent binding of nucleic acids

Compound[a]	Amount of compound transformed to CO_2 (nmol/g liver) $\pm$ SD	Amount of compound bound to nucleic acids (nmol/g liver) $\pm$ SD
MMH	4.7 $\pm$ 1.1	0.72 $\pm$ 0.13
UDMH	4.4 $\pm$ 0.9	0.03 $\pm$ 0.008
NDMA	80 $\pm$ 17	1.81 $\pm$ 0.38

[a]For experimental conditions, see Materials and Methods section; MMH, monomethyl-hydrazine; UDMH, 1,1-dimethylhydrazine; NDMA, *N*-nitrosodimethylamine

Table 2. Monomethylhydrazine (MMH), 1,1-dimethylhydrazine (UDMH) and N-nitrosodimethylamine (NDMA) metabolism to formaldehyde in liver microsomes and 9 000 × g supernatant under aerobic or anaerobic conditions[a]

	NDMA	MMH	UDMH
	(nmol CH_2O/g liver/10 min) $\pm$ SE		
AEROBIC			
− Microsomes			
Heated	1.8 ± 0.06	23.0 ± 1.4	41.3 ± 6.2
− NADPH	3.0 ± 0.9[b]	21.5 ± 2.4	39.0 ± 1.3
+ NADPH	33.6 ± 8.3[b]		
− 9 000 × g sup.			
Heated	0.75 ± 0.15	51.6 ± 6.2	68.4 ± 8.5
− NADPH	3.0 ± 1.1[b]	41.5 ± 4.4	31.7 ± 2.5[b]
+ NADPH	46.0 ± 8.9[b]	41.5 ± 5.2	41.9 ± 1.7[b]
ANAEROBIC			
− Microsomes			
Heated	1.8 ± 0.3	24.7 ± 3.6	9.5 ± 0.7
− NADPH	3.8 ± 0.6[b]	16.9 ± 3.7[b]	14.3 ± 1.8[b]
+ NADPH	13.9 ± 2.8[b]	24.2 ± 0.4	16.2 ± 3.6[b]
− 9000 × g sup			
Heated	0.95 ± 0.23	16.9 ± 1.3	18.1 ± 1.0
− NADPH	3.5 ± 1.0[b]	40.8 ± 0.1[b]	17.9 ± 1.9

[a] For experimental conditions, see Materials and Methods section.
[b] p < 0.05 compared to 'heated' control

enzymatic pathways of further formaldehyde biotransformation (e.g., aldehyde dehydrogenase and others). There are, however, two exceptions in which formaldehyde formation in liver preparations in the absence of NADPH is greater than in heated mixtures. One of these involves MMH and 9 000 × g supernatants under anaerobic conditions. The other, less important, is observed with microsomes and UDMH anaerobically (Table 3). No NADPH-dependent source of formaldehyde other than those which are microsomal and oxygen-dependent was found for MMH or UDMH. It is apparent that further metabolism of MMH and UDMH might contribute to a considerable extent to formaldehyde production when NDMA is metabolized. The present observations might also explain why we previously observed formaldehyde formation under anaerobic conditions when NDMA was incubated with microsomes or 9 000 × g supernatants (Godoy *et al.*, 1980). Formaldehyde, in this case, might derive from NDMA reductive metabolism to MMH and UDMH, which either enzymatically or non-enzymatically would produce formaldehyde.

In the case of MMH, we observed an activation process of an enzymatic nature leading to covalent binding to proteins. The process was NADPH-dependent and required oxygen, and the enzyme was present in the microsomal fraction. In all the other cases, interactions of a non-enzymatic nature leading to covalent binding to proteins were dominant.

Moreover, there are enzymatic processes in liver microsomes which decrease the intensity of the covalent binding of both MMH and UDMH to proteins. They are NADPH-dependent and non-dependent. Similar inactivating processes are also observed in preparations of 9 000 × g supernatants. It is not unlikely that the hydrazines produced during reductive metabolism of NDMA (Grilli & Prodi, 1975; Dougherty, 1977) account for a major part of the binding to proteins produced by NDMA during its biotransformation by microsomal or 9 000 × g preparations. This is particularly so in the case of MMH.

Table 3. Covalent binding of reactive metabolites of *N*-nitrosodimethylamine (NDMA), monomethylhydrazine (MMH) or 1,1-dimethylhydrazine (UDMH) to liver microsomal or $9\,000 \times g$ supernatant proteins under aerobic or anaerobic conditions[a]

	NDMA	MMH	UDMH
	(pmol/g liver/10 min)$\pm$SE		
AEROBIC			
− Microsomes			
Heated	130 ± 20	$6\,200\pm 200$	$8\,800\pm 800$
− NADPH	20 ± 30^{b}	$5\,300\pm 200^{b}$	$6\,000\pm 600^{b}$
+ NADPH	220 ± 30^{b}	$41\,500\pm 2\,300^{b}$	$6\,500\pm 800^{b}$
− $9\,000 \times g$ sup			
Heated	237 ± 24	$20\,500\pm 2\,700$	$26\,400\pm 800$
− NADPH	150 ± 30^{b}	$23\,700\pm 4\,600^{b}$	$12\,400\pm 1\,100^{b}$
+ NADPH	910 ± 290^{b}	$15\,300\pm 2\,000^{b}$	$8\,000\pm 900^{b}$
ANAEROBIC			
− Microsomes			
Heated	231 ± 62	$12\,600\pm 1\,300$	$15\,000\pm 2\,100$
− NADPH	40 ± 20^{b}	$6\,900\pm 800^{b}$	$11\,000\pm 200^{b}$
+ NADPH	370 ± 70^{b}	$8\,000\pm 1\,200^{b}$	$6\,200\pm 1\,200^{b}$
− $9\,000 \times g$ sup			
Heated	282 ± 52	$14\,000\pm 1\,100$	$20\,200\pm 2\,000$
− NADPH	90 ± 80^{b}	$11\,000\pm 3\,200$	$11\,200\pm 1\,300^{b}$
+ NADPH	690 ± 90^{b}	$9\,100\pm 1\,100^{b}$	$11\,900\pm 1\,600^{b}$

[a] The incubation mixtures are the same as in Table 2.
[b] $p < 0.05$ compared to 'heated' control

It is important to consider that both hydrazines may lead to covalent binding to proteins and that this binding by reactive chemicals usually correlates with various toxic manifestations (Gillete *et al.*, 1974). This fact and the covalent binding reported here and previously shown by others of MMH reactive metabolites to nucleic acids (Dost *et al.*, 1966; Kruger *et al.*, 1970) should warn against the assumption that NDMA metabolism to hydrazines is a detoxication reaction, as postulated by Appel *et al.* (1979).

ACKNOWLEDGEMENT

This work was supported in part by Public Health Service Grant AM-13195-14 from the National Institute of Arthritis, Metabolism and Digestive Diseases.

REFERENCES

Appel, K.E., Schwarz, M., Rickart, R. & Kunz, W. (1979) Influences of inducers and inhibitors of the microsomal monooxigenase system on the alkylating intensity of the dimethylnitrosamine in mice. *J. Cancer Res. clin. Oncol.*, **94**, 47–61

Bancroft, H. (1960) *Introducción a la Bioestadística*, Buenos Aires, Eudeba

Díaz Gómez, M.I., Godoy, H.A. & Castro, J.A. (1981) Further studies on dimethylnitrosamine metabolism, activation and its ability to cause liver injury. *Arch. Toxicol.*, **47**, 159–168

Díaz Gómez, M.I., Godoy, H.M., Villarruel, M.C. & Castro, J.A. (1983) No response of pigeon liver to dimethylnitrosamine acute effects. *Cancer Lett., 18,* 157–162

Dost, F.N., Reed, D.J. & Wang, C.H. (1966) The metabolic fate of monomethylhydrazine and unsymmetrical dimethylhydrazine. *Biochem. Pharmacol., 15,* 1325–1332

Dougherty, J.P., Clapp, N.K., Zehfus, M.H. & Brock, S.E. (1977) Radioactive components in the acid-soluble fraction of mouse liver cytosol after dimethylnitrosamine (methyl-^{14}C) administration. *Gann, 68,* 697–701

Gillette, J.R., Mitchell, J.R. & Brodie, B.B. (1974) Biochemical mechanisms of drug toxicity. *Ann. Rev. Pharmacol., 14,* 271–288

Godoy, H.M., Díaz Gómez, M.I. & Castro, J.A. (1978) Mechanism of dimethylnitrosamine metabolism and activation in rats. *J. natl Cancer Inst., 61,* 1285–1289

Godoy, H.M., Díaz Gómez, M.I. & Castro, J.A. (1980) Relationship between dimethylnitrosamine metabolism or activation and its ability to induce liver necrosis in rats. *J. natl Cancer Inst., 64,* 533–538

Godoy, H.M., Díaz Gómez, M.I., Marzi, A., de Ferreyra, E.C., de Fenos, O.M. & Castro, J.A. (1982) Chicken resistance to dimethylnitrosamine acute effects on the liver. A comparative study with other species. *J. natl Cancer Inst., 69,* 687–692

Grilli, S. & Prodi, G. (1975) Identification of dimethylnitrosamine metabolites in vitro. *Gann, 66,* 473–480

Kruger, F.W., Weissler, M. & Rucker, W. (1970) Investigation of the alkylating action of 1,1-dimethylhydrazine. *Biochem. Pharmacol., 19,* 1825

Lai, D.Y. & Arcos, J.C. (1980) Dialkylnitrosamine bioactivation and carcinogenesis. *Life Sci., 27,* 2149–2165

Lin, H.J. & Fong, L.Y.Y. (1980) Effects of oxygen depletion on in vitro metabolism of dimethylnitrosamine in microsomes from rat liver and human tissues. *J. natl Cancer Inst., 65,* 877–883

Magee, P.N. & Barnes, J.M. (1967) Carcinogenic nitroso compounds. *Adv. Cancer Res., 10,* 163–246

Pegg, A.E. (1980) *Metabolism of N-nitrosodimethylamine.* In: Montesano, R., Bartsch, H. & Tomatis, L., eds, *Molecular and Cellular Aspects of Carcinogen Screening Tests) (IARC Scientific Publications No. 27),* Lyon, International Agency for Research on Cancer, pp. 3–22

Prough, R.A., Freeman, P.C. & Hines, R.N. (1981) The oxydation of hydrazine derivatives catalysed by the purified liver microsomal FAD-containing monooxygenase. *J. biol. Chem., 256,* 4178–4184

Shank, R.C. (1979) *Comparative Metabolism of Propellant Hydrazines (AMRL-Tr-79-57),* Aerospace Medical Research Laboratory, Springfield, VA, National Technical Information Service

Wittkop, J.A., Prough, R.A. & Reed, D.J. (1969) Oxidative demethylation of *N*-methylhydrazines in rat liver microsomes. *Arch. Biochem. Biophys., 134,* 308–315

METABOLISM OF N-NITRODIALKYLAMINES

E. SUZUKI, M. MOCHIZUKI, N. SEKIGUCHI & M. OKADA

Tokyo Biochemical Research Institute, Tokyo, Japan

SUMMARY

The in-vitro and in-vivo metabolism of N-nitramines was investigated to compare it with that of N-nitrosamines. N-Nitrodibutylamine and N-nitrodiethylamine were incubated with rat liver microsomes and hepatocytes, and the products were analysed by high-performance liquid chromatography and gas-liquid chromatography. The in-vitro metabolic pattern of these N-nitramines was similar to that of the corresponding N-nitrosamines, except that N-nitromonoalkylamines (produced by α-hydroxylation) were isolated and identified after incubation of N-nitrodialkylamines. Seven N-nitramines, including glucuronides, were isolated and identified from urine of rats given N-nitrodibutylamine, produced by ω, ω-1, and α oxidations of the N-nitramine.The in-vivo metabolic pattern of N-nitrodibutylamine was also similar to that of N-nitrosodi-n-butylamine except that N-nitromonobutylamine (a product of α-hydroxylation) was isolated and identified.

N-Nitramines were mutagenic to *Escherichia coli* WP2 *hcr*⁻, but not to *Salmonella typhimurium* TA1535. N-Nitrodibutylamine and N-nitrodiethylamine were mutagenic only in the presence of hepatic microsomes, while N-nitromonobutylamine and N-nitromonoethylamine were direct mutagens. Thus, the N-nitrodialkylamine is also metabolically activated to a mutagen through an α-hydroxylation.

INTRODUCTION

N-Nitramines can be produced as atmospheric pollutants when nitrogen oxides react with secondary amines. The carcinogenic and other biological activities of N-nitramines were reported to be much lower than those of the corresponding N-nitrosamines. α-Hydroxylation has been shown to be a key step in the metabolic activation of N-nitrosamines (Mochizuki *et al.*, 1982), however, little is known about the metabolism and metabolic activation of N-nitramines. We have investigated the in-vitro metabolism of N-nitrodibutylamine (NO$_2$DBA) and N-nitrodiethylamine (NO$_2$DEA) by rat liver microsomes, with regard to their metabolic activation to mutagens and their metabolism by rat hepatocytes. In-vivo metabolism of NO$_2$DBA was also studied and compared with that of N-nitrosodi-n-butylamine (NDBA).

MATERIALS AND METHODS

Syntheses of N-*nitramines*

NO$_2$DBA and NO$_2$DEA were synthesized by the oxidation of NDBA and *N*-nitrosodiethylamine (NDEA), respectively, with trifluoroacetic acid and hydrogen peroxide (Emmons & Ferris, 1953). *N*-Nitro-*N*-(2-hydroxyethyl, 2-carboxyethyl and 3-carboxy-propyl)butylamines(NO$_2$HEBA, NO$_2$CEBA and NO$_2$CPBA) were synthesized similarly in good yields (60–98%). NO$_2$CEBA and NO$_2$CPBA were treated with diazomethane in the usual way, to give the corresponding methyl esters. The methyl esters of *N*-nitro-*N*-(carboxymethyl)-butylamine (NO$_2$CMBA), *N*-nitro-*N*-(1-acetoxybutyl)butylamine and *N*-nitro-*N*-(1-acetoxy-ethyl)ethylamine were prepared from the corresponding *N*-nitrosamines in hexane by photolysis in the presence of oxygen (yield, 50–60%) (Suzuki *et al.*, unpublished data). *N*-Nitro-*N*-(3-hydroxybutyl)butylamine (NO$_2$HBBA-3) was obtained by the alkaline hydrolysis of *N*-nitro-*N*-(3-acetoxybutyl)butylamine, which was prepared by the photolysis of the corresponding *N*-nitrosamine (overall yield, 47%). *N*-Nitromonobutylamine (NO$_2$BA) and *N*-nitromonoethylamine (NO$_2$EA) were synthesized by the method of Emmons and Freeman (1955).The structures of these *N*-nitramines were confirmed by their nuclear magnetic resonance and infra-red spectra, and by elemental analyses.

Assay for microsomal metabolism

Microsomes were obtained from livers of male Sprague-Dawley rats (six weeks old), treated with 0.1% sodium phenobarbital in the drinking-water for one week; and the microsomal oxidation of NO$_2$DBA and NO$_2$DEA (each 2 mmol/L) was carried out as described for NDBA (Suzuki *et al.*, 1983). After precipitation of proteins in the incubation mixture, aldehydes were determined by high-pressure liquid chromatography (HPLC) as described elsewhere (Suzuki *et al.*, 1983). NO$_2$BA, NO$_2$HBBA-3, NO$_2$DEA and NO$_2$EA were also determined by HPLC (LiChrosorb RP-8, 5 μ, eluting with 40% acetonitrile), while NO$_2$DBA was determined by gas-liquid chromatography (GLC) (1.5% OV-17 on Chromosorb W), after extracting it from the aqueous supernatant into ethyl acetate.

Metabolism by hepatocytes

Hepatocytes were isolated by collagenase perfusion from livers of male Sprague-Dawley rats (six to eight weeks old) (Seglen, 1976). The hepatocytes, finally suspended in a Leibovitz L-15 medium, were incubated with NO$_2$DBA and NO$_2$DEA (each 2 mmol/L) at 37°C under O$_2$:CO$_2$ (95:5, v/v). The products were analysed by HPLC and GLC, as described for microsomal metabolism.

In-vivo metabolism of N-*nitrodibutylamine (*NO$_2$DBA)

After an overnight fast, two male Sprague-Dawley rats (eight weeks old) received a total of 1 690 mg (820 mg and 870 mg/rat) of NO$_2$DBA by gastric intubation. Urine collection, urine fractionation by solvent extraction and β-glucuronidase hydrolysis were performed as described earlier (Suzuki & Okada, 1980). Each extract was analysed by thin-layer chromatography (TLC), HPLC (LiChrosorb SI-100, 5 μ, elution with hexane-ether [1:1, v/v] and hexane:ether:dichloromethane [8:3:2, v/v]; LiChrosorb RP-8, 5 μ, eluting with 40% acetonitrile) and GLC/flame thermionic detector (1.5% OV-17 on Chromosorb W). Acidic metabolites were analysed by GLC as their methyl esters, after treating the extract with diazomethane.

Mutation assay

The mutation test was carried out as described previously, in the absence of microsomes (Mochizuki *et al.*, 1979) and in the presence of phenobarbital-treated microsomes (Suzuki *et al.*, 1983) using *Salmonella typhimurium* TA1535 and *Escherichia coli* WP2 *hcr⁻*.

RESULTS

Metabolism by microsomes

The formation of NO$_2$BA, butyraldehyde and NO$_2$HBBA-3 from NO$_2$DBA was estimated to represent 31.2 ± 1.2, 29.8 ± 1.3 and $9.9 \pm 0.8\%$, respectively, of the NO$_2$DBA incubated in the case of phenobarbital-treated microsomes, and 10.5 ± 0.6, 5.2 ± 0.6 and $4.3 \pm 0.5\%$, respectively, of the NO$_2$DBA in the case of untreated microsomes. Incubation of *N*-nitro-*N*-(1-acetoxybutyl)butylamine (1 mmol/L) with microsomes gave NO$_2$BA (96%) and butyraldehyde (104%). This indicates that NO$_2$BA and butyraldehyde were produced from NO$_2$DBA through α-hydroxylation, followed by spontaneous degradation.

Fig. 1. Metabolism of *N*-nitrodibutylamine (NO$_2$DBA) *in vivo* and *N*-nitrodiethylamine (NO$_2$DEA) *in vitro* in the rat. Percentage of dose given in parentheses; G, β-D-glucopyranosiduronic acid residue; *, characterized as a metabolite *in vitro*

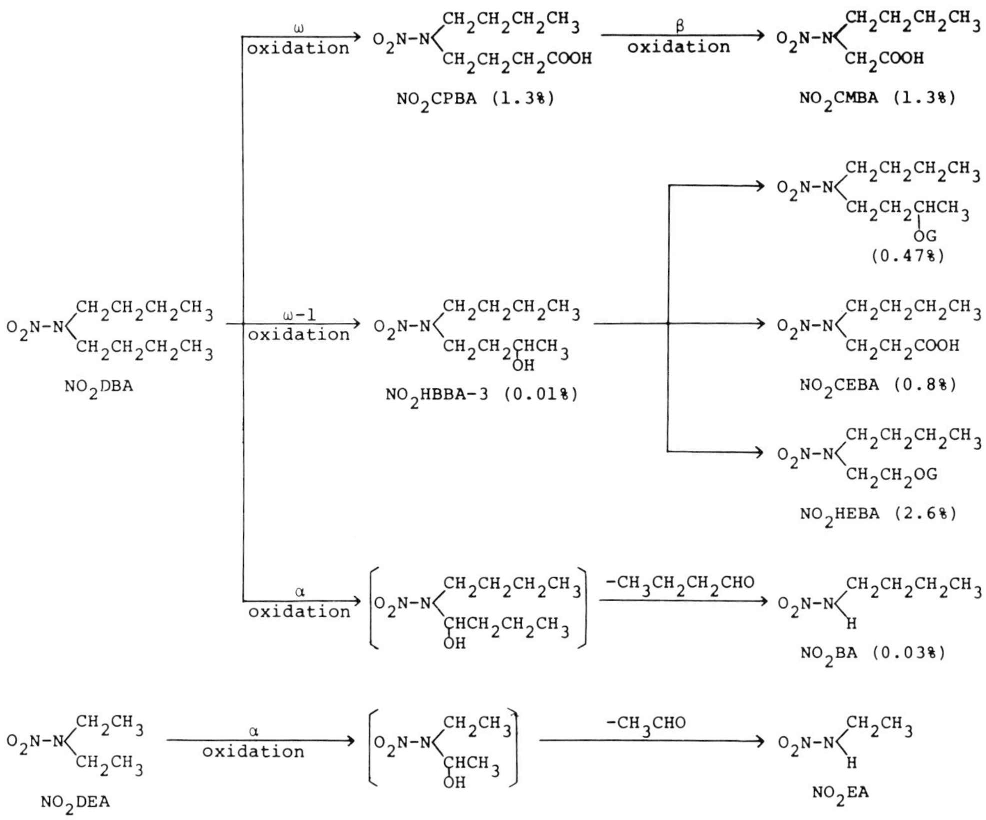

The formation of NO$_2$EA and acetaldehyde from NO$_2$DEA represented 12.2 ± 0.7 and 12.0 ± 0.5%, respectively, of the NO$_2$DEA incubated with treated microsomes, and 1.8 ± 0.2 and 2.9 ± 0.6%, respectively, of the NO$_2$DEA incubated with untreated microsomes. Quantitative production of NO$_2$EA (96%) and acetaldehyde (96%) was also demonstrated from N-nitro-N-(1-acetoxyethyl)ethylamine (1 mmol/L). The recovery of NO$_2$DBA (or NO$_2$DEA) in the incubation, expressed as the total of the products and the unchanged N-nitramine, amounted to more than 92%, indicating that α-oxidation is the main metabolic pathway for these N-nitramines.

Metabolism by hepatocytes

On the basis of a preliminary study, NO$_2$DBA and NO$_2$DEA (each 2 mmol/L) were incubated with hepatocytes (1 × 10^7 cells /mL) at 37 °C for 1 h. When hepatocytes from untreated rats were used, the major metabolites isolated were NO$_2$BA (9.0 ± 1.7%) and NO$_2$HBBA-3 (7.3 ± 1.1%) from NO$_2$DBA, and NO$_2$EA (5.1 ± 0.6%) from NO$_2$DEA.

Urinary metabolites of N-nitrodibutylamine (NO$_2$DBA) in the rat

Urinary metabolites of NO$_2$DBA in the rat are illustrated in Figure 1. ω-Oxidation of one butyl group produced NO$_2$CPBA and NO$_2$CMBA, while ω-1 oxidation resulted in the formation of NO$_2$HBBA-3, NO$_2$CEBA and NO$_2$HEBA. NO$_2$HBBA-3 was identified as such, and as the glucuronic acid conjugate, while NO$_2$HEBA was identified as the glucuronide. α-Oxidation led to the formation of NO$_2$BA. Approximate percentages of dose for these metabolites are indicated in the figure. No metabolite with an N-nitroso group, corresponding to these N-nitramine metabolites, could be detected.

Fig. 2. Mutagenicity of N-nitrodibutylamine (NO$_2$DBA), N-nitrodiethylamine (NO$_2$DEA) and related compounds in *Escherichia coli* WP2 *hcr* ⁻ in the presence (●, ▲) and absence (O) of hepatic microsomes from rats.

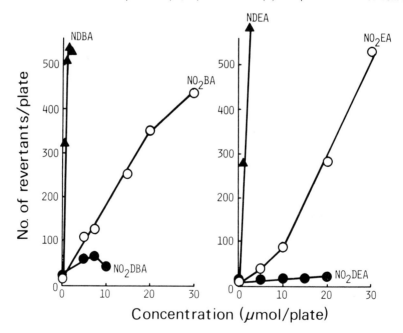

Mutagenicity of N-*nitramines*

NO$_2$DBA, NO$_2$DEA, NO$_2$BA and NO$_2$EA showed mutagenic activity toward *E. coli* WP2 *hcr*$^-$, but were inactive in *S. typhimurium* TA1535. The *N*-nitrodialkylamines (NO$_2$DBA, NO$_2$DEA) were far less mutagenic than the corresponding *N*-nitrosamines (NDBA, NDEA) in the presence of microsomes, while the *N*-nitromonoalkylamines (NO$_2$BA, NO$_2$EA) were found to be active in the absence of microsomes (Fig. 2).

DISCUSSION

The results of these investigations of in-vitro metabolism of NO$_2$DBA by hepatic microsomes and hepatocytes have shown that NO$_2$DBA is metabolized mainly through α and ω-1 oxidations. The metabolic pattern and the extent of these oxidations of NO$_2$DBA on incubation with treated and untreated liver microsomes were similar to those of NDBA (Suzuki *et al.*, 1983). A marked difference, however, is that the actual identity of the intermediary metabolite in the case of NO$_2$DBA has been established. Thus, NO$_2$BA has been separated and identified, but the identification of *N*-nitrosomonobutylamine as such, following incubation of NDBA, has not yet been accomplished, due to the extreme instability of the *N*-nitrosomonoalkylamine.

NO$_2$EA was also identified as a major metabolite of NO$_2$DEA after microsomal oxidation. A metabolic study of NO$_2$DEA in hepatocytes has shown that the α-oxidation is also a principal metabolic pathway for this *N*-nitramine.

An in-vivo metabolic study of NO$_2$DBA has revealed that ω and ω-1 oxidations are the major pathways. The metabolic pattern of NO$_2$DBA was similar to that of NDBA, except that the monodealkylated product, NO$_2$BA, was isolated and identified as a urinary metabolite. However, its excretion rate was much lower than expected, indicating that this compound undergoes further metabolic transformation *in vivo*. Reductive conversion of the *N*-nitramines to *N*-nitrosamines has not been demonstrated.

It has been shown that NDBA and NDEA are far more sensitive to *E. coli* WP2 *hcr*$^-$ than to *S. typhimurium* TA1535 in the presence of a metabolic activation system (Mochizuki *et al.*, 1982). No appreciable mutagenicity of NO$_2$DEA was observed in *S. typhimurium* TA1530 or TA100 (Khudoley *et al.*, 1981). In accordance with these findings, NO$_2$DBA and NO$_2$DEA did not show mutagenic activity toward *S. typhimurium* TA1535. They showed a weak mutagenicity activity toward *E. coli* WP2 *hcr*$^-$ in the presence of microsomes, while NO$_2$BA and NO$_2$EA were directly mutagenic toward this bacterial strain. Thus, the weak mutagenicity of the *N*-nitrodialkylamines (NO$_2$DBA, NO$_2$DEA) may be due to the metabolic formation of *N*-nitromonoalkylamines (NO$_2$BA, NO$_2$EA) through α-hydroxylation.

ACKNOWLEDGEMENTS

This work was supported in part by Grants-in-Aid for Cancer Research from the Ministry of Education, Science and Culture, and from the Ministry of Health and Welfare, Japan.

REFERENCES

Emmons, W.D. & Ferris, A.F. (1953) Oxidation reactions with pertrifluoroacetic acid. *J. Am. chem. Soc.,* **75**, 4623–4624

Emmons, W.D. & Freeman, J.P. (1955) Alkaline nitration. I. The nitration of amines with cyanohydrine nitrates. *J. Am. chem. Soc., 77*, **77**, 4387–4390

Khudoley, V., Malaveille, C. & Bartsch, H. (1981) Mutagenicity studies in *Salmonella typhimurium* on some carcinogenic *N*-nitramines *in vitro* and in the host-mediated assay in rats. *Cancer Res.,* **41,** 3205–3210

Mochizuki, M., Suzuki, E., Anjo, T., Wakabayashi, Y. & Okada, M. (1979) Mutagenic and DNA-damaging effects of *N*-alkyl-*N*-(α-acetoxyalkyl)nitrosamines, models for metabolically activated *N,N*-dialkylnitrosamines. *Gann, 70,* 663–670

Mochizuki, M., Anjo, T., Takeda, K., Suzuki, E., Sekiguchi, N., Huang, G.-F. & Okada, M. (1982) *Chemistry and mutagenicity of α-hydroxynitrosamines.* In: Bartsch, H., O′Neill, I.K., Castegnaro, M. & Okada, M., eds, N-*Nitroso Compounds: Occurrence and Biological Effects (IARC Scientific Publications No. 41),* Lyon, International Agency for Research on Cancer, pp. 553–559

Seglen, P.O. (1976) Preparation of isolated rat liver cells. *Methods Cell Biol., 13,* 29–83

Suzuki, E. & Okada, M. (1980) Metabolic fate of *N,N*-dibutylnitrosamine in the rat. *Gann, 71,* 863–870

Suzuki, E., Mochizuki, M., Wakabayashi, Y. & Okada, M. (1983) *In vitro* metabolic activation of *N,N*-dibutylnitrosamine in mutagenesis. *Gann, 74,* 51–59

BIOCHEMICAL AND BIOLOGICAL PROPERTIES OF PROSPECTIVE N-NITRODIALKYLAMINE METABOLITES AND THEIR DERIVATIVES

E. FREI, B.L. POOL, W. PLESCH & M. WIESSLER

Institute of Toxicology and Chemotherapy, German Cancer Research Center, Im Neuenheimer Feld 280, D-6900 Heidelberg, Federal Republic of Germany

SUMMARY

The metabolic conversion of N-nitrodimethylamine and of N-nitrosodimethylamine was compared *in vitro*. The biochemical properties of the two compounds were nearly identical; however, the biological activities (carcinogenicity, mutagenicity and toxicity) of the nitramine are many times less potent. N-Nitrodimethylamine was found to be mutagenic to *Salmonella typhimurium* TA100 when applied at above 200 μmol/plate with metabolic activation. Its suggested metabolite, N-nitromethylamine, was not mutagenic. N-Nitromethylhydroxymethylamine, N-nitromethylacetoxymethylamine and formaldehyde were mutagenic only to *S. typhimurium* TA100 at low concentrations and toxic above 2 μmol/plate. The evidence suggests that formaldehyde is the intermediate responsible for the mutagenicity of the nitramine derivatives and of the parent compound, N-nitrodimethylamine.

INTRODUCTION

The structural relationship between N-nitrodialkylamines and N-nitrosodialkylamines, as well as their concomitant formation in the atmosphere (Challis *et al.*, 1982) have prompted us to investigate some biological properties of N-nitrodimethylamine (NTDMA). Reports in the literature indicate that NTDMA is many times less carcinogenic (Mirvish *et al.*, 1980), toxic (Andersen & Jenkins, 1978) and mutagenic (Khudoley *et al.*, 1981) than N-nitrosodimethylamine (NDMA). The studies concerning the mutagenicity of NTDMA by Khudoley *et al.* (1981) indicate that the compound must be metabolically activated to yield a mutagenic intermediate. When postulating a pathway similar to that suggested for the bioactivation of NDMA, the products N-nitromethylhydroxymethylamine (NTMHMA), formaldehyde and N-nitromethylamine (NTMA) should be formed from NTDMA. NTMA, however, is chemically stable and therefore may not act as a direct alkylating agent, as does its N-nitroso analogue. In order to clarify the in-vitro metabolic pathway of bioactivation, studies of the biochemical and mutagenic properties of NTDMA and its suggested metabolites have been carried out. Further comparative studies are presented with N-nitromethyl-acetoxymethylamine (NTMAcMA) which, in analogy with the N-nitrosodialkylamino-acetates (Pool & Wiessler, 1981), is a model compound and may be cleaved by esterases to yield NTMHMA.

MATERIALS AND METHODS

Chemicals and synthesis

All chemicals used were of analytical grade (Merck Darmstadt, or Boehringer, Mannheim, FRG), except for the following substances, which were synthesized according to published methods: NDMA, NTDMA (Bamberger & Kirpal, 1895), NTMA (Franchimont & Klobbie, 1888), NTMHMA (Gaarev *et al.,* 1971) and NTMAcMA (Denkstein & Kaderabek, 1960).

All nitramines were checked for nitrosamine contamination by gas chromatographic analysis on a 3% Carbowax 20 M column (Pye Unicam 104); less than 0.05% contamination was detected, using a flame-ionization detector.

In-vitro metabolism

Incubations were performed with male Sprague-Dawley rat liver microsomes (60 min at 100 000 $\times$ *g* pellet), as described elsewhere (Bertram *et al.,* 1982). Briefly, in 6 mL 0.06 mol/L phosphate buffer (pH 7.4), 4 mg microsomal protein, 0.5 mmol/L NADP, 5.0 mmol/L glucose-6-phosphate, 5 IU glucose-6-phosphate dehydrogenase, 20 mmol/L magnesium chloride and 10 mmol/L semicarbazide-hydrochloric acid were incubated at 37 °C. For some experiments supernatant of 9 000 $\times$ *g* for 10 min (S9) was used instead of microsomes. Substrate concentrations are indicated in the legends to the figures. Blanks without substrate and blanks without enzyme source were used. Formaldehyde generated in the incubations was determined according to Nash (1953).

The kinetics of formate production from formaldehyde or NTMHMA were determined using 3-ml cuvettes containing 1 mmol/L reduced glutathione, 0.67 mmol/L NAD, 5.8 mg 'cytosolic' (100 000 $\times$ *g* for 60 min supernatant) protein and 0.2–1.2 mmol/L substrate. $\varepsilon_M = 6620$ cm^{-1} at 340 nm was used to calculate the amount of formaldehyde oxidized (Uotila & Koivusalo, 1974).

Mutagenicity assays

The mutagenicity assays were performed with the histidine auxotrophic *Salmonella typhimurium* strains TA1535 and TA100, supplied by B.N. Ames of Berkeley, CA, USA. The tests for their reversion to prototrophy were performed with the plate incorporation assay, as well as with the preincubation modification (60 min at 37 °C) described by Ames *et al.* (1975). The metabolizing mixture was that which had been found sensitive for the detection of the mutagenicity of *N*-nitroso compounds (Preussmann *et al.,* 1981): it contained 0.5 ml S9 mix (6 mg protein), 1–2 $\times$ 10^8 cells in 0.1 mL medium and the test compounds dissolved in 10–20 µl dimethyl sulfoxide. The sources of S9 were livers of either untreated, Aroclor- or sodium phenobarbitone-pretreated, male Sprague-Dawley rats.

RESULTS

The in-vitro metabolism of NTDMA and NTMA was compared to that of NDMA by monitoring the amount of formaldehyde produced. Figure 1 shows a slightly higher V_{max} for NTDMA than for NDMA. NTMA was a poor substrate, even at concentrations below 0.5 mmol/L. Diethyldithiocarbamate, an inhibitor of NDMA demethylase, also inhibited the demethylation of NTDMA. The inhibitor concentration yielding half maximal enzyme activity was 0.05 mmol/L diethyldithiocarbamate at 2 mmol/L substrate concentration for both

Fig. 1. Yield of formaldehyde from *N*-nitrodimethylamine, ■; *N*-nitrosodimethylamine, ○; *N*-nitromethylamine, ▽, in the microsomal incubation system after 30 min.

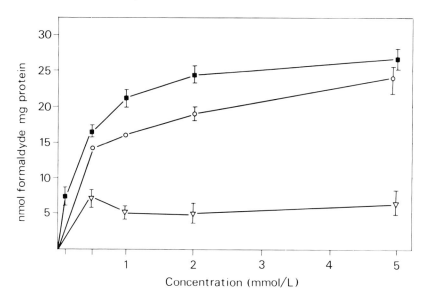

compounds. The time dependence of demethylation was also similar for both compounds. Formaldehyde production reached a plateau after 60 min incubation. The observed characteristics of NTDMA metabolism are probably not due to the formation of NDMA: less than 0.01% nitrosamine was detected in dichloromethane extracts of incubations of NTDMA with microsomes and cofactors (analysis by gas chromatography-thermal energy analysis).

In the nitrosamine-sensitive strain, *S. typhimurium* TA1535, NTDMA and NTMA were not mutagenic at concentrations of up to 50 μmol/plate with preincubation and S9 mix. NTMHMA was toxic, with and without S9, at a concentration above 4 μmol/plate. At higher concentrations, NTDMA was mutagenic to *S. typhimurium* TA100 after metabolic activation by S9 from livers of sodium phenobarbitone- and particularly of Aroclor-treated rats (Fig. 2). In TA1535, only borderline mutagenicity was observed with 350 μmol NTDMA per plate. NTMA was non-mutagenic or slightly toxic under all conditions tested.

The metabolism of NTDMA and of NTMA was compared using S9 from control animals and S9 from Aroclor-pretreated rats. The S9 composition used for testing their mutagenicity was also employed in these determinations. Aroclor pretreatment resulted in a doubling of NTDMA demethylase activity above 10 mmol/L substrate concentration. With 200 mmol/L NTDMA, 108 nmol formaldehyde were released per 6 mg S9 protein.

NTMHMA was mutagenic to *S. typhimurium* TA100 in a very narrow concentration range, without metabolic activation by S9, and was toxic to the bacteria at concentrations above 1 μmol/plate. Without metabolic activation, NTMAcMA was not mutagenic; with S9 preincubation, its mutagenicity was comparable to that of the hydroxy compound. The source of S9 (livers from Aroclor- or phenobarbitone-pretreated or untreated rats) was not relevant to the mutagenicity of these two compounds, but omission of the NADPH generating system resulted in a higher yield of revertants at lower concentrations.

Other possible metabolites of NTDMA were also tested. Nitrite was slightly mutagenic in both *Salmonella* strains at levels above 25 μmol/plate, and nitrate was not mutagenic.

Fig. 2. Mutagenicity of *N*-nitrodimethylamine, ● ○, and *N*-nitromethylamine, ■ □, in *Salmonella typhimurium* TA 100 (filled symbols) and TA 1535 (empty symbols) after preincubation with liver S9 from Aroclor-pretreated rats.

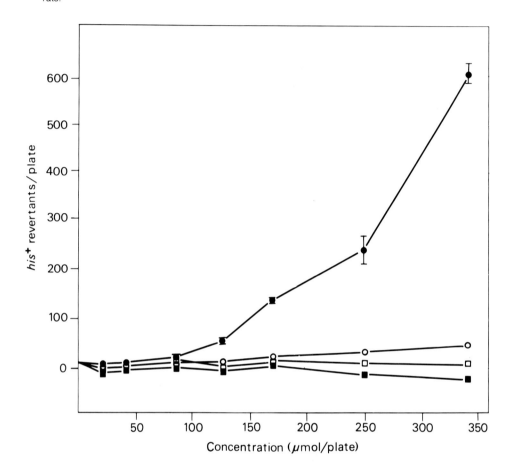

Formaldehyde showed the same kinetics as NTMHMA and NTMAcMA. It was mutagenic to *S. typhimurium* TA100 in a narrow concentration range (up to 0.5 μmol/plate) and became toxic at higher concentrations. The use of S9 without cofactors also provided the most sensitive condition to detect the mutagenicity of formaldehyde. In Figure 3, the relative mutagenic activities of NTMHMA, NTMAcMA, and formaldehyde are shown under these conditions. Formaldehyde is not mutagenic to TA1535 (Pool & Wiessler, 1981), nor are the other two compounds.

The amount of formaldehyde liberated from NTMHMA could not be determined directly using colorimetric methods because the compound is labile in acid. Indirect analysis of generated NADH, in the presence of reduced glutathione and cytosolic formaldehyde dehydrogenase (Uotila & Koivusalo, 1974), gave the same change in absorption per min as formaldehyde itself. Apparently, formaldehyde is liberated from NTMHMA at the same rate at which it is oxidized to formate. In nuclear magnetic resonance analysis in water, an equilibrium was observed between the hydroxy compound, NTMA and formaldehyde.

Fig. 3. Mutagenicity of *N*-nitromethylhydroxymethylamine, ○; *N*-nitromethylacetoxymethylamine, ▼; and formaldehyde, ●, in *Salmonella typhimurium* TA 100 after preincubation with liver S9 from Aroclor-pretreated rats without NADPH-generating cofactors.

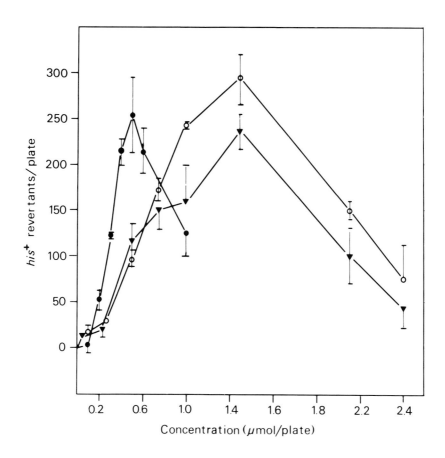

DISCUSSION

The metabolism of NTDMA to formaldehyde, at substrate concentrations up to 5 mmol/L, showed the same kinetics and time dependence as the low K_m form of NDMA demethylase (Arcos *et al.*, 1977). The resulting NTMA is stable and is a poor substrate for further demethylation. The studies reported in this paper were performed to determine which metabolite is responsible for the biological effects exerted by nitramines.

NTMHMA, the first reaction product after γ-C-hydroxylation, was the most active metabolite that still contained the N-NO$_2$ group. NTMA, its suggested degradation product, is not mutagenic. The mutagenicity of NTMAcMA was dependent on the presence of S9, but not on that of a NADPH generating system. The spectrum of NTMAcMA mutagenicity was similar to that of NTMHMA. The only common metabolite of the three mutagenic compounds tested, which itself was mutagenic, is formaldehyde. Reports concerning the mutagenicity of formaldehyde in *S. typhimurium* strains are very scarce (Turner, 1981) and controversial (Pool & Wiessler, 1981). While this work was going on, Connor *et al.* (1983) found formaldehyde to be mutagenic in the Ames test in *S. typhimurium* TA100 at concentrations similar to those reported here.

We suggest that the mutagenic effect of NTDMA in *S. typhimurium* TA100, observed in our experiments and in those of Khudoley *et al.* (1981), is due to the formation of formaldehyde. Pretreatment of rats with Aroclor resulted in a doubling of NTDMA demethylase activity in S9 at high substrate concentrations, and the amount of formaldehyde generated could account for the observed induction of *S. typhimurium* T100 *his*[+] revertants.

The other potential metabolites of NTDMA (nitrate and NTMA) were non-mutagenic. NDMA or nitrite, which, it could be argued, arise from NTDMA reduction (we detected less than 0.05%), cannot be responsible for the mutagenicity of nitramine. Substantial formation would also give rise to mutagenicity in *S. typhimurium* TA1535.

The in-vivo activities of NTDMA (liver tumours and toxicity) cannot yet be explained. They may not be due to formaldehyde, since the latter is rapidly oxidized to formate and carbon dioxide (Uotila & Koivusalo, 1974) and in the intact animal liver. A carcinogenicity experiment with NTDMA and NTMA is in progress. To date, no animal has shown any ill effects after one year of treatment with as much as 1 mmol/kg per week.

ACKNOWLEDGEMENT

This work was supported by the Deutsche Forschungsgemeinschaft.

REFERENCES

Ames, B.N., McCann, J. & Yamasaki, E. (1975) Methods for detecting carcinogens and mutagens with the *Salmonella*/mammalian-microsome mutagenicity test. *Mutat. Res., 31*, 347–364

Andersen, M.E. & Jenkins, L.J., Jr (1978) The toxicity of single doses of *N*-nitrodimethylamine in rodents. *Drug Chem. Toxicol., 1*, 363–371

Arcos, J.C., Davies, D.L., Brown, C.E.L. & Argus, M.F. (1977) Repressible and inducible forms of dimethylnitrosamine-demethylase. *Z. Krebsforsch., 89*, 181–199

Bamberger, E. & Kirpal, A. (1895) Nitration of aliphatic bases (in German). *Berichte, 28*, 535 ff

Bertram, B., Schuhmacher, J., Frei, E., Frank, N. & Wiessler, M. (1982) Effects of disulfiram on mixed function oxidase system and trace element concentration in the liver of rats. *Biochem. Pharmacol., 31*, 3613–3619

Challis, B.C., Shuker, D.E.G., Fine, D.H., Goff, E.U. & Hoffmann, C.A. (1982) *Amine nitration and nitrosation by gaseous nitrogendioxide.* In: Bartsch, H., O'Neill, I.K., Castegnaro, M. & Okada, M., eds, *N-Nitroso Compounds: Occurrence and Biological Effects (IARC Scientific Publications No. 41)*, Lyon, International Agency for Research on Cancer, pp. 11–20

Connor, T.H., Barrie, M.D., Theiss, J.L., Matney, T.S. & Ward, J.B., Jr (1983) Mutagenicity of formalin in the Ames assay. *Mutat. Res., 119*, 145–149

Denkstein, J. & Kaderabek, V. (1960) Synthesis of nitramines I. *N*-Acetoxymethylnitramines (in French). *Coll. Czech. Chem. Commun., 25*, 2334–2340

Franchimont, A. & Klobbie E. (1888) Some nitramines and their preparation (in French). *Rec. Trav. chim., 7*, 343 ff

Gaarev, G.A., Cheskashina, V.A., Matveev, V.A. & Danilova, T.A. (1971) Preparation of 2-nitro-2-aza-1-propanol (in Russian). *Zh. org. Khim, 7*, 623–624 (translation, p. 631)

Khudoley. V., Malaveille, C. & Bartsch, H. (1981) Mutagenicity studies in *Salmonella typhimurium* on some carcinogenic *N*-nitramines *in vitro* and in the host-mediated assay in rats. *Cancer Res., 41*, 3205–3210

Mirvish, S.S., Bulay, O., Runge, R.G. & Patil, K. (1980) Study of the carcinogenicity of large doses of dimethylnitramine, *N*-nitroso-L-proline and sodium nitrite administered in drinking water to rats. *J. natl Cancer Inst., 64*, 1435–1440

Nash, T. (1953) The colorimetric determination of formaldehyde by means of the Hantzsch reaction. *Biochem. J.*, **55**, 416–421

Pool, B.L. & Wiessler, M. (1981) Investigations on the mutagenicity of primary and secondary acetoxynitrosamines with *Salmonella typhimurium:* activation and deactivation of structurally related compounds by S–9. *Carcinogenesis*, **2**, 991–997

Preussmann, R., Habs, M., Pool, B.L., Stummeyer, D., Lijinsky, W. & Reuber, M.D. (1981) Fluoro substituted *N*-nitrosamines. 1. Inactivity of *N*-nitroso-bis(2,2,2-trifluorethyl)amine in carcinogenicity and mutagenicity tests. *Carcinogenesis*, **8**, 753–756

Turner, L., ed. (1981) *The Mutagenic Potential of Formaldehyde* (*Technical Report No. 2*), ECOTOC (European Commission on the Evaluation of Toxic Chemicals), Brussels

Uotila, L. & Koivusalo, M. (1974) Formaldehyde dehydrogenase from human liver. *J. biol. Chem.*, **249**, 7653–7663

MODIFIERS OF METABOLISM AND CARCINOGENICITY OF *N*-NITROSO COMPOUNDS

EFFECT OF ETHANOL ON NITROSAMINE METABOLISM AND DISTRIBUTION. IMPLICATIONS FOR THE ROLE OF NITROSAMINES IN HUMAN CANCER AND FOR THE INFLUENCE OF ALCOHOL CONSUMPTION ON CANCER INCIDENCE

P.F. SWANN

Courtauld Institute of Biochemistry, Middlesex Hospital Medical School, London, UK

SUMMARY

For reasons that have never been explained, the consumption of alcohol is associated with an increase in the incidence of human cancer, notably that of the oesophagus. The effect of ethanol on nitrosamine metabolism and carcinogenicity is reviewed, together with new work on pharmacokinetics. This work shows that small quantities of ethanol alter the distribution and metabolism of small oral doses of N-nitrosodimethylamine and N-nitrosodiethylamine in rats, to increase by several fold the alkylation of DNA in organs that are particularly susceptible to their carcinogenic effect. It is shown that in the case of N-nitrosodimethylamine this is the result of prevention of first-pass clearance of the nitrosamine as it travels in the blood draining the gut through the liver before entering the general circulation. There is evidence that the same happens in man. These results explain the findings from various experiments in animals and they lend credence to the observation that nitrosamines occur in human blood after high-nitrate meals are taken with alcohol. The results have led to the hypothesis that the influence of alcohol consumption on human cancer may be mediated through the effect of ethanol on the pharmacokinetics of nitrosamines derived from diet, from tobacco smoke and from endogenous synthesis. The evidence for this hypothesis and its wider implications are discussed.

INTRODUCTION

A primary objective of research into chemical carcinogenesis is to delineate the role of chemicals in human cancer. Cancer incidence in the developed world is influenced in particular by tobacco smoking, alcohol consumption and some ill-defined aspects of diet (Doll & Peto, 1981). The exact mechanism by which these factors exert their influence is still unknown, but investigation of any one of them might throw light upon the general mechanism of cancer induction in man and provide a basis for an intelligent approach to cancer prevention. Of these influences, alcohol consumption is well established and particularly interesting. It is responsible for only 3% of human cancer deaths, but the disease is so common that this small percentage represents 12 000 deaths each year in the USA alone (Tuyns, 1979; Doll & Peto, 1981). An increase in the incidence of laryngeal and oesophageal cancer, in which alcohol and tobacco smoking apparently act synergistically (Tuyns *et al.*, 1977; Wynder *et al.*, 1977), is the best documented effect, but there have also been reports that alcohol consumption is associated with increases in the incidence of cancers of the colon and rectum and of the liver consequent to cirrhosis (for reviews, see Pollack *et al.*, 1984; National Academy of Science, 1982). These effects, which seem to be caused by ethanol itself, have never been explained, since alcohol, wine and spirits have not been found to be carcinogenic in experiments in animals (Schmähl *et al.*, 1965; Griciute *et al.*, 1981). Thus, ethanol presumably acts either by increasing the susceptibility of tissues to some other carcinogen; or, by catalysing the endogenous synthesis of carcinogens; or by increasing the effectiveness of carcinogens by altering their pharmacokinetics.

None of the previous explanations of the effect of alcohol (for review, see National Academy of Science, 1982) has received widespread acceptance. However, recent experiments show that, in animals, ethanol can increase the effectiveness of some carcinogenic nitrosamines by altering their metabolism and distribution. Although the evidence is still incomplete, alcohol appears to have a similar effect on the pharmacokinetics of these nitrosamines in man. This finding has led to the hypothesis (Swann, 1982) that the influence of alcohol consumption of human cancer is mediated through its effect on the metabolism and distribution of nitrosamines derived from the diet, from tobacco smoke, and from endogenous synthesis. If this hypothesis is correct it would imply that nitroso compounds are not only involved in alcohol-related cancer but play a significant role in cancer in general. This article summarizes and discusses this evidence.

THE INFLUENCE OF ETHANOL ON THE METABOLISM OF NITROSAMINES *IN VITRO* AND IN LABORATORY ANIMALS

A number of experiments have now been reported on the influence of ethanol on nitrosamines: it changed the rate of synthesis of nitrosamines *in vitro* (Pignatelli *et al.*, 1976; Kurechi *et al.*, 1980); induced the activity of drug-metabolizing enzymes, including those which metabolize nitrosamines (Maling *et al.*, 1975; McCoy *et al.*, 1979; Schwarz *et al.*, 1980; Peng *et al.*, 1982); and inhibited those enzymes (Phillips *et al.*, 1977; Schwarz et al., 1982; Peng *et al.*, 1982). Furthermore, ethanol increased the carcinogenicity of nitrosamines and altered their organotropism in some experiments (Gibel, 1967; Griciute *et al.*, 1981, 1982), although not in others (Schmähl *et al.*, 1965; Habs & Schmähl, 1981).

At first sight these results seem isolated and conflicting, but recently it has been possible to piece together some of the observations on the effect of alcohol on the metabolism and carcinogenicity of *N*-nitrosodimethylamine (NDMA) and *N*-nitrosodiethylamine (NDEA), and, although much is still unexplained, it is possible to gain a blurred picture of the overall effect of alcohol on these nitrosamines in animals and to begin to understand what effect alcohol might have on these and other nitrosamines in man.

Influence of ethanol on the pharmacokinetics of NDMA and NDEA

Nitrosamines are carcinogenic because they form metabolites which alkylate DNA. The metabolites of the simple, water-soluble nitrosamines, NDMA and NDEA, are so unstable that they cannot pass from organ to organ; thus, the amount of alkylation in any one organ depends upon the amount of nitrosamine metabolized in it. This amount depends upon the activity of the nitrosamine-metabolizing system, the availability of the nitrosamine (which in turn depends upon its distribution), and on the K_m of the enzyme system. When large doses of NDMA are given they are uniformly distributed, the metabolizing enzymes are saturated, and the amount of methylation in each organ reflects the amount of metabolizing enzyme in it. However, as the dose is decreased, distribution of the nitrosamine begins to play a crucial role. Distribution is particularly important if NDMA is given by mouth, for, after absorption from the gut, the nitrosamine passes in the portal blood through the liver before entering the general circulation. As the dose is decreased, the liver is able to remove an increasing proportion of the nitrosamine on this first pass (first-pass clearance), until, at very low oral doses – equal to or less than 30 μg/kg body weight in the rat – the liver removes virtually all the NDMA, and very little passes to the other organs (Diaz Gomez *et al.*, 1977; Pegg & Perry, 1981).

The effect of this lowering the dose of NDMA on the methylation of liver and kidney DNA is shown in Figures 1 and 2. Whereas methylation in the liver is directly proportional to dose over the range 1 μg to 1 mg/kg body weight (Fig. 1), methylation in the kidney (Fig. 2) falls disproportionately as the dose decreases, until, at less than 30 μg/kg body weight, it can no longer be detected with ^{14}C-NDMA of the specific activity used (64 mCi/mmol). This disproportionate fall occurs only after oral administration and has been ascribed to first-pass clearance (Diaz Gomez *et al.*, 1977; Pegg & Perry, 1981). To conclude from Figure 1 that, with very small doses, the liver removes all the NDMA and that the other organs are *completely* protected may not be correct, since experiments with ^{3}H-NDMA (specific radioactivity, 12 Ci/mmol) have shown that a little methylation of kidney DNA occurs with doses of only 0.09 μg NDMA/kg body weight. The latter findings suggests that the liver can clear doses of around 10 μg/kg body weight more effectively than much lower doses. These results cannot be accepted entirely without reservation, for there is a hydrogen isotope effect on first-pass clearance of NDMA (Swann *et al.*, 1983), and these studies with tritiated NDMA may not reflect accurately the fate of unlabelled material. However, this result is discussed again below since it may be relevant to understanding the source of the small amounts of nitrosamine found in the peripheral blood of normal and untreated people (Lakritz *et al.*, 1980).

Consumption of a very small quantity of ethanol, equivalent to a man's drinking less than 0.5 L of beer, prevented this first-pass clearance of NDMA by the liver. When NDMA was given in ethanol (1 mL; 5% v/v), instead of water, the disproportionate fall in methylation of kidney DNA did not occur (Fig. 2). Using ^{3}H-NDMA, it was possible to show that this effect of ethanol was maintained for doses of NDMA down to 0.09 and 0.27 μg/kg, which, after distribution, would give a concentration of NDMA in the blood similar to that which Fine *et al.*, (1977) found in man.

Fig. 1 Extent of methylation of rat liver DNA (measured as μmol 7-methylguanine/mol DNA-guanine produced by each unit dose of 1 μg NDMA/kg body weight) with different doses of *N*-nitrosodimethylamine, ○, in water; ●, in 1 mL 5% ethanol.

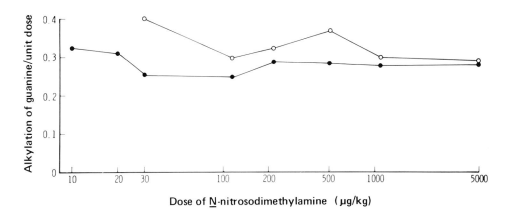

Dose of N-nitrosodimethylamine (μg/kg)

Fig. 2 Extent of methylation of rat kidney DNA produced (measured as μmol 7-methylguanine/mol DNA-guanine produced by each unit dose of 1 μg NDMA/kg body weight) with different doses of *N*-nitrosodimethylamine. ○, in water; ●, in 1 mL 5% ethanol.

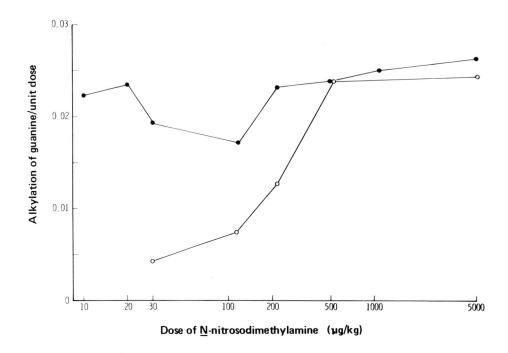

Prevention of first-pass clearance has a dramatic effect on the methylation of kidney DNA. When large doses were given, methylation was similar whether the rats received the NDMA in water or in dilute ethanol; but, as the dose decreased, the values diverged until, with 30μg/kg, methylation of the kidney DNA of the ethanol-treated rat was five times that in the control. Lower doses of ^{14}C-NDMA produced methylation in the kidney of the ethanol-treated rat, but none was detectable in the control; and, although methylation was detected in the control with very much lower doses of tritiated NDMA (0.09 and 0.27 μg/kg), the amount was still increased by about three fold by ethanol.

It has been known for several years that ethanol inhibits NDMA metabolism (Phillips *et al.*, 1977), but an important contribution to our understanding was made by Peng *et al.* (1982) who showed that inhibition by ethanol of a rat liver microsomal NDMA metabolizing system is competitive, with very low K_i. Similar results are obtained with liver slices (Fig. 3.): the apparent K_m (23 μmol/L) is lower than that reported for microsomal metabolism (56 μmol/L) (Peng *et al.*, 1982), but the K_i for ethanol is almost identical (0.5 mmol/L in slices; 0.32 mmol/L in microsomes). The amount of ethanol in which the NDMA was administered (1 mL/ 5%) would, after distribution, give a concentration in the rat of 8–9 mmol/L. This is so much greater than the K_i (0.5 mmol/L) that the prevention of first-pass clearance could be explained as a consequence of the inhibition of metabolism.

The study of NDMA metabolism *in vitro* has been so bedevilled by technical problems and by confusing and conflicting results (Lai & Arcos, 1980) that it is necessary to compare critically any in-vitro result with established measurements of NDMA metabolism in the intact animal. In this case, the K_m and rate calculated from Figure 2 are consistent with results from studies in whole animals (Heath, 1962). Since the liver is the predominant site of NDMA metabolism,

Fig. 3 Lineweaver-Burk plot of metabolism of *N*-nitrosodimethylamine (NDMA) by liver slices, and its inhibition by ethanol. Slices of liver ($\simeq$ 100 mg) were incubated in Warburg flasks containing 2 mL buffer in an atmosphere of oxygen. After equilibration, ^{14}C-NDMA was added and the incubation continued for exactly 10 min. the ^{14}C-carbon dioxide was trapped in sodium hydroxide. The figure shows the rate of transformation of NDMA to carbon dioxide. An average factor for converting these numbers to the actual amount of NDMA metabolized was found by extracting the remaining NDMA from the incubation mixture with dichloromethane and comparing it with blank samples. The K_i was calculated from the ratio of the slopes of the lines. K_m, 25 µmol/L; ●, with I mmol/L ethanol; ○, control.

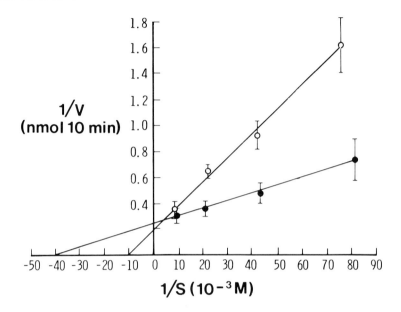

the rate *in vitro* should approximate that in intact rats. Not all NDMA is metabolized to carbon dioxide, but the rate of production of carbon dioxide from NDMA by liver slices (Fig. 3) can be converted to the actual amount of NDMA metabolized by using a conversion factor of 3.5 ($\pm$ 0.4 SEM) (details are given in the legend to Fig. 3) to give a V_{max} of 18 nmol/min per 100 mg tissue. The liver represents about 5% of the body weight, so that the livers of 1 kg of rats would, on the basis of this figure, be expected to metabolize a maximum of 4 mg NDMA/kg body weight per hour. This admittedly fairly inexact number compares favourably with the rate of 5.4 mg/kh per hour metabolized by whole rats (Heath, 1962) and justifies extrapolation of results obtained with this slice system to the whole animal. Slices have been used successfully in measuring the metabolism of other nitrosamines (see, e.g., Castonguay *et al.*, 1983).

NDMA produces cancer in the liver, kidney and nasal cavity of rats; but, in man, alcohol consumption is linked predominantly to cancer of the oesophagus. For this reason, studies of DNA alkylation were also done with NDEA, which produces oesophageal cancer in rats. The results are shown in Figure 4. A relatively high degree of ethylation of DNA was observed in the oesophagus, particularly with low doses of NDEA. This effect does not depend upon intimate contact with the nitrosamine during dosing, because it occured to an equal extent after intramuscular injection. Ethanol increased the ethylation of oesophageal DNA by 1.8 to 4.6 times, but it decreased the ethylation of kidney DNA. The mechanism of these changes is not yet clear, but, as they also occur with intramuscular administration, it is unlikely that first-pass clearance plays any significant role. The results are tentatively interpreted as being the consequence of organ-selective inhibition of NDEA metabolism. The change with dose in the

Fig. 4 Influence of ethanol on the ethylation (measured as 7-ethylguanine) of DNA in kidney (□), oesophagus ■ and lung ([▨]) relative to that in the liver. Ethanol was given orally by tube as 1 mL 5% ethanol with 20 μg/kg *N*-nitrosodimethylamine (NDEA) or as 0.5 mL 30% ethanol with 2.8 mg/kg NDEA. The nitrosamine was either dissolved in the ethanolic solution and given orally or given separately by intramuscular (i.m.) injection.

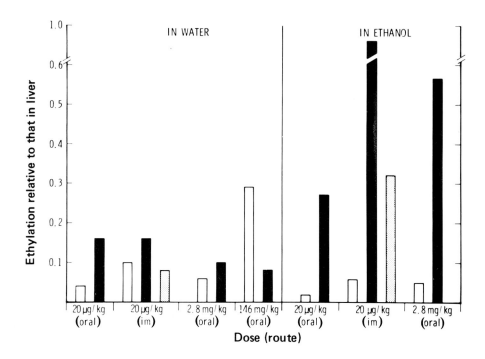

relative metabolism of NDEA between liver, kidney and oesophagus would also suggest that the enzymes of these organs differ in their K_m and would support the postulate that they differ in K_i. In preliminary experiments, we have found that ethanol inhibits the metabolism of NDEA to carbon dioxide by rat kidney slices but does not inhibit metabolism by oesophageal epithelium.

RELATIONSHIP BETWEEN EFFECT OF ETHANOL ON NDMA AND NDEA METABOLISM, AND ITS EFFECT ON CARCINOGENESIS BY THESE NITROSAMINES

To what extent do the experiments above explain the results of tests for carcinogenesis? Prevention of first-pass clearance, and the changes in relative metabolism towards the sensitive organs, would be expected to alter the organotropism of these nitrosamines. In addition, as it seems likely that the liver is less sensitive than other organs to the carcinogenic action of nitrosamines, first-pass clearance, and the concentration of metabolism in the liver, act to protect not only the internal organs but also the whole animal. Since nitrosamines are characteristically hepatocarcinogens, the statement that the liver is 'less sensitive' might seem ridiculous; however, studies have shown clearly that the liver is less sensitive than the brain, kidney or lung of rats to single doses of nitrosamines or nitrosamides. The relative sensitivity of each organ to prolonged administration of these compounds is less clear, because the liver almost invariably receives a much greater proportion of the dose than any other organ; but it is less sensitive than most other organs.

As could be predicted, ethanol produces a change in organotropism and an increase in the carcinogenic effectiveness of nitrosamines in animal experiments. Oral administration of NDEA in 30% ethanol rather than water increased the incidence of oesophageal tumours in rates by three fold (Gibel, 1967). In mice, oral administration of NDMA in water produced only liver tumours but administration in 40% ethanol produced slightly fewer liver tumours with a 36% incidence of tumours in the nasal cavity (Griciute *et al.,* 1981). Griciute *et al.,* (1982) and McCoy *et al.* (1982) also found that ethanol increased tumour incidence and changed the organotropism of *N*-nitrosopyrrolidine.

In contrast to the report by Gibel (1967), Habs and Schmähl (1981) found that ethanol had no effect on the oesophageal carcinogenicity of NDEA. This difference may be explained by the pharmacokinetic studies reported above. Although the half-life of small doses of NDEA in rats has not been measured, it would be expected to be in the order of 10 min; in the experiment of Habs and Schmähl, the ethanol was given after the nitrosamine and possibly did not reach sufficient concentration soon enough to affect the metabolism of NDEA. Schmähl (1976) also found that ethanol had no effect on the carcinogenicity of *N*-nitrosophenylmethylamine. Although the experimental details given in that report are insufficient to allow discussion, the conclusion that ethanol does not affect all nitrosamines in the same way would be supported by the observation that ethanol does not change the carcinogenicity of *N'*-nitrosonornicotine (McCoy *et al.,* 1981, 1982).

If the explanation given above to resolve the contrast between the results of Gibel (1967) and of Habs and Schmähl (1981) with NDEA is correct, an important conclusion can be drawn. The induction of nitrosamine – (McCoy *et al.,* 1979; Peng *et al.,* 1982) and other carcinogen – metabolizing enzymes by chronic administration of ethanol has been suggested to be the mechanism by which ethanol affects cancer incidence (for a review, see National Academy, 1982). If this explanation were correct, it would not be necessary to give the carcinogen and ethanol at the same time; however, at least in the case of NDEA in rats, the ethanol and nitrosamine must be given simultaneously for there to be an effect on carcinogenicity. This is consistent with the hypothesis that ethanol inhibits nitrosamine metabolism, but is not consistent with the hypothesis that the effect of ethanol on the carcinogenicity of this nitrosamine depends upon the induction of drug-metabolizing enzymes. Enzyme induction undoubtedly plays some role, but it does not seem to be an essential one.

The experiments on the effects of ethanol on the metabolism of NDMA and NDEA provide a reasonable explanation for the results of these carcinogenicity experiments. They emphasize that the relationship between metabolism and carcinogenesis is dynamic, and that measurements of the activity of nitrosamine-metabolizing enzymes in specific organs in isolation, using high concentrations of substrate, are insufficient to predict the situation in animals and may be misleading. The amount of reaction with nucleic acids depends upon distribution (itself a complex relationship between blood flow, vascular anatomy and metabolism), the K_m as well as V_{max} of the enzyme systems and the *relative* effectiveness of the inhibitor in each organ. When small doses of nitrosamine are given, the rate of metabolism does not depend directly upon the amount of enzyme present. For example, the half-life of small doses of NDMA depends only on the blood flow to the liver (Gough *et al.,* 1983).These simple nitrosamines are not excreted unchanged in significant amounts, and they circulate in the animal until they are metabolized. Because of its size and metabolic activity, the liver dominates nitrosamine metabolism, and changes that alter by several fold the amount of nitrosamine metabolized in extrahepatic organs do not produce a significant change in alkylation in the liver – the alkylation may take longer to occur but eventually the same amount is produced. Therefore, chronic administration of ethanol, which induces the activity of nitrosamine-metabolizing enzymes (Maling *et al.*, 1975; McCoy *et al.*, 1979; Garro *et al.*, 1981), does not affect host-mediated mutagenesis (Glatt *et al.*, 1981) or alkylation of liver DNA (Belinsky *et al.*, 1982). The experiments described above show that the absolute activity of nitrosamine-metabolizing enzymes is not important; what is important is the relationship of metabolism in one organ to that in another. Leaving aside the special case of first-pass clearance, if inhibitors (or inducers) of enzyme activity are selective, they will alter that relationship and affect carcinogenesis and organotropism; if they are not selective, and everything changes in concert, then the outcome will be unchanged. Fortunately, measurements of alkylation of DNA give a realistic view of the situation in the whole animal; studies of nitrosamine metabolism *in vitro* must include estimates of K_m and K_i for a number of organs before they can be used to predict events *in vivo*.

EFFECT OF ETHANOL ON NITROSAMINE METABOLISM IN MAN, AND ITS POSSIBLE RELATIONSHIP TO THE EPIDEMIOLOGICAL LINK BETWEEN ALCOHOL CONSUMPTION AND HUMAN CANCER

For this hypothesis to be acceptable, it must explain the effect of ethanol on the carcinogenicity of nitrosamines in animals, there must be evidence that the same effect might occur in man, and it must be consistent with the epidemiology of human cancer. It has been shown above that, in general terms, the hypothesis is consistent with the results of animal experiments. In the following section, the relationship between these results, observations in man, and epidemiological results are discussed.

Comparison of the excretion of NDMA in man and rats suggests that ethanol has the same effect on first-pass clearance in both species. As would be expected from the experiments discussed above, no part of an oral dose of NDMA is excreted in the urine of rats if it is given in water, but there is a small but appreciable excretion if first-pass clearance is prevented by ethanol. The same happens in man; NDMA was excreted in urine after it had been drunk in beer, but not after it had been drunk in orange juice (Spiegelhalder *et al.*, 1982).

These experiments may also resolve several conflicting reports on the transient appearance, or rise in concentration, of NDMA in human blood after a meal high in nitrate. Concurrent administration of an inhibitor of first-pass clearance (e.g., ethanol) is essential to allow the nitrosamine to pass without loss from the gut to the peripheral blood. Thus, reports of an increase in NDMA concentration in blood after a meal taken with beer (Fine *et al.*, 1977; Gough *et al.*, 1983) are not invalidated by the failure of others to confirm the observation with similar meals taken without alcohol (Yamamoto *et al.*, 1980; Melikian et al., 1981; Ellen *et al.*, 1982). It should be noted, however, that Kowalski *et al.* (1980) did not consistently find nitrosamines in blood, even after a high-nitrate meal taken with alcohol. Claims that these small amounts of nitrosamines are present cannot be accepted without reservation until the analytical difficulties have been resolved and the possibility of artefactual formation of nitrosamines during analysis conclusively ruled out. Experiments with alcohol and NDMA in rats confirm these measurements in humans and they are given further support by the demonstration of endogenous nitrosation of ingested proline (Ohshima & Bartsch, 1981). Furthermore, the tentative conclusion from studies with ^{3}H-NDMA that first-pass clearance of very small doses of NDMA is incomplete may be relevant to an assessment of the validity of reports that the blood of untreated people also contains very small amounts of NDMA (Lakritz *et al.*, 1980), even though these findings have been dismissed as artefacts (Fine, 1982). This dismissal was based in part upon calculations of the probable synthesis of nitrosamines *in vivo*, from which the conclusion was reached that there would be insignificant endogenous synthesis of volatile nitrosamines in humans (Challis *et al.*, 1982). The calculations provide figures that are completely at variance with the observation of nitrosamines in blood, and it is important to discover whether the calculations, or the observations, are correct. One aspect of the calculations that seems to have escaped notice is that they ignore the physiological process by which amines are recycled and concentrated from the blood into the stomach (Shore *et al.*, 1957). In the case of strong bases, the concentration in the stomach is limited only by gastric blood flow; in some studies in dogs, the concentration in the stomach was 40 times greater than that in the blood. Uncertainly over the validity of reports that volatile nitrosamines are synthesized in humans suggests that the excretion of nitrosamines in human urine after ingestion of ethanol should be examined more extensively. The proportion of an ingested dose of NDMA found in human urine (0.5–2.4%) was greater than that found in rats (0.18%) (Spiegelhalder *et al.*, 1982), and greater than that which would be expected. This finding suggests that the level of NDMA given in the beer might have been augmented by nitrosamine synthesized *in vivo* and that the nitrosamine excreted was derived from both sources. Even though the single urine sample from a person who had taken ethanol without added NDMA did not contain the nitrosamine, it is clear that a more extensive examination of the urinary excretion of nitrosamines is needed.

This discussion on nitrosamines in blood should not be allowed to give a false perspective on the influence of alcohol on human cancer. Although alcohol consumption alone does increase cancer incidence, the effect of alcohol is greatly augmented by a synergism with smoking (Tuyns *et al.*, 1977). The mechanism of this synergism is not known, but it would be consistent with this hypothesis if it were the result of an influence of ethanol on tobacco-specific nitrosamines (Hoffmann *et al.*, 1982), analogous to its effect on simple nitrosamines in rats, or if it were a superimposition of the effect of tobacco-specific carcinogens onto the ethanol-augmented effect of nitrosamines from other sources. In this context, it should be noted that ethanol inhibits the metabolism of at least some cyclic nitrosamines (Johansson-Brittebo & Tjälve, 1979; McCoy *et al.*, 1982). Similarly, the hypothesis could be extended to explain the high incidences to oesophageal cancer in Iran and the People's Republic of China (Li *et al.*, 1980; Yang, 1980), where an epidemiological connection with alcohol consumption has not been established if, in these areas, some other agent were found which had an effect similar to that of ethanol in increasing the effectiveness of the relevant nitrosamines (Yang, 1982). Ethanol is not the only treatment that selectively inhibits nitrosamine metabolism: protein-free diet selectively reduces the ability of the liver to metabolize NDMA (Swann & McLean, 1971), and as a consequence increases the incidence of kidney tumours produced by that nitrosamine; other such inhibitors will certainly be found.

The hypothesis cannot explain why there is an apparent excess of cancer of the large bowel in beer drinkers in particular (Pollack *et al.*, 1984), but it is consistent with two other aspects of the epidemiological evidence. An essential aspect of this hypothesis is that alcohol should affect only circulating carcinogens: it should not affect the carcinogenicity of locally acting carcinogens that are applied topically. In this respect, it is consistent with the observation that ethanol increases the incidence of oesophageal cancer in smokers but does not alter the incidence of lung cancer (Doll & Peto, 1981). Furthermore, the hypothesis suggests that the outcome depends upon the amount of nitrosamine produced in the gut which depends upon diet and upon temporal relationships between eating and drinking, which depend upon social customs. Thus, it is generally consistent with the observation that there is a strong geographical element in the effectiveness of alcohol in increasing cancer incidence.

Ethanol increases the effectiveness of NDMA (Griciute *et al.*, 1981) and NDEA (Gibel, 1967) probably because it diverts the nitrosamine from the liver to other organs that are more sensitive to these carcinogens. The resistance of the liver has been associated with the presence in it of a protein which removes the O^6-alkylguanine that the carcinogen produces in DNA (Goth & Rajewsky, 1974). If this is correct, human liver should be also be resistant, because the concentration of this protein is ten times greater than that in rat liver (Pegg *et al.*, 1982).

Thus, a diversion of nitrosamines from the liver to other organs would be expected to increase the effectiveness of these carcinogens in humans also.

These experiments with ethanol, NDEA and NDMA, therefore make plausible the hypothesis that the influence of ethanol on human cancer incidence is mediated through its effect on the pharmacokinetics of nitrosamines derived from the diet, from tobacco smoke and from endogenous synthesis. The hypothesis has broad implications, for if ethanol acts merely by modulating the effectiveness of nitrosamines, then nitrosamines must play a significant and perhaps central role in human cancer. If this is proven to be correct, it would solve one of the central problems in cancer research and allow an intelligent approach to cancer prevention. It is clear that a great amount of work, for example on the metabolism of nitrosamines by human organs, is needed to support this hypothesis, but its greatest weakness is its total dependence on the premise that humans synthesize, or take in, sufficient amounts of nitrosamine to cause cancer. There is at present inadequate evidence to support this, or any other, hypothesis linking nitrosamines to cancer in the general population.

ACKNOWLEDGEMENTS

I am most grateful for the generous support of the Cancer Research Campaign and for the invaluable help of Mr Raymond Mace.

REFERENCES

Belinsky, S.A., Bedell, M.A. & Swenberg, J.H. (1982) Effect of chronic ethanol diet on the replication, alkylation, and repair, of DNA from hepatocytes and non-parenchymal cells following dimethylnitrosamine administration. *Carcinogenesis, 3*, 1293–1297

Castonguay, A., Tjälve, H. & Hecht, S.S. (1983) Tissue distribution of the tobacco specific carcinogen 4-(methylnitrosamino)-1-(3-pyridyl)-1-butanone and its metabolites in F344 rats. *Cancer Res., 43*, 630–638

Challis, B.C., Lomas, S.J., Rzepa, H.S., Bavin, P.M.G., Darkin, D.W., Viney, N.J. & Moore, P.J. (1982) *A kinetic model for the formation of gastric N-nitroso compounds.* In: Magee, P.N., ed., *Nitrosamines and Human Cancer (Banbury Report No. 12),* Cold Spring Harbor, NY, Cold Spring Harbor Laboratory, pp. 243–253

Diaz Gomez, M.I., Swann, P.F. & Magee, P.N. (1977) The absorption and metabolism in rats of small oral doses of dimethylnitrosamine. *Biochem. J., 164*, 497–500

Doll, R. & Peto, R. (1981) The causes of cancer. *J. natl Cancer Inst., 66*, 1191–1308

Ellen, G., Schuller, P.L., Froeling, P.G.A.M. & Bruijns, E. (1982) No volatile *N*-nitrosamines detected in blood or urine from patients ingesting daily large amounts of ammonium nitrate. *Food Chem. Toxicol., 20*, 879–882

Fine, D.H. (1982) *Presence of nitrosamines in human beings.* In: Magee, P.N., ed., *Nitrosamines and Human Cancer (Banbury Report No. 12),* Cold Spring Harbor, NY, Cold Spring Harbor Laboratory, pp. 271–276

Fine, D.H., Ross, R., Rounbehler, D.P., Silvergleid, A. & Song, L. (1977) Formation *in vivo* of volatile *N*-nitrosamines in man after ingestion of cooked bacon and spinach. *Nature, 265*, 753–754

Garro, A.J., Seitz, H.K. & Lieber, C.S. (1981) Enhancement of dimethylnitrosamine metabolism and activation to a mutagen following chronic alcohol consumption. *Cancer Res., 41*, 120–124

Gibel, W. (1967) Experimentelle Untersuchungen zur Synkarzinogenese beim Oesophaguskarzinom. *Arch. Geschwulstforsch., 30*, 181–189

Glatt, H., de Balle, L. & Oesch, F. (1981) Ethanol or acetone pretreatment of mice strongly enhances the bacterial mutagenicity of dimethylnitrosamine in assays mediated by liver subcellular fractions, but not in host mediated assays. *Carcinogenesis, 2*, 1057–1061

Goth, R. & Rajewsky, M.F. (1974) Persistence of O^6-ethylguanine in rat brain DNA. *Proc. natl Acad. Sci. USA*, **71**, 639–643

Gough, T.A., Webb, K.S. & Swann, P.F. (1983) An examination of human blood for the presence of volatile nitrosamines. *Food Chem. Toxicol.*, **21**, 151–156

Griciute, L., Castegnaro, M. & Bereziat, J.-C. (1981) Influence of ethyl alcohol on carcinogenesis with *N*-nitrosodimethylamine. *Cancer Lett.*, **13**, 345–352

Griciute, L., Castegnaro, M. & Bereziat, J.-C. (1982) *Influence of ethyl alcohol on the carcinogenic activity of* N-*nitrosodi*-N-*propylamine*. In: Bartsch, H., O'Neill, I.K., Castegnaro, M. & Okada, M., eds, N-*Nitroso Compounds: Occurrence and Biological Effects (IARC Scientific Publications No. 41)*, Lyon, International Agency for Research on Cancer, pp. 643–647

Habs, M. & Schmähl, D. (1981) Inhibition of the hepatocarcinogenic activity of diethylnitrosamine (DENA) by ethanol in rats. *Hepato-gastroenterology*, **28**, 242–244

Heath, D.F. (1962) The decomposition and toxicity of dialkylnitrosamines in rats. *Biochem. J.*, **85**, 72–91

Hoffmann, D., Brunnemann, K.D., Adams, J.D., Rivenson, A. & Hecht, S.S. (1982) N-*Nitrosamines in tobacco carcinogenesis*. In: Magee, P.N. ed., *Nitrosamines and Human Cancer (Banbury Report No. 12)*, Cold Spring Harbor, NY, Cold Spring Harbor Laboratory, pp. 211–220

Johansson-Brittebo, E., & Tjälve, H. (1979) Studies on the distribution and metabolism of *N*-[^{14}C]nitrosopyrrolidine in mice. *Chem-biol. Interactions*, **25**, 243–253

Kowalski, B., Miller, C.T. & Sen, N.P. (1980) *Studies on the in vivo formation of nitrosamines in rats and humans after ingestion of various meals*. In: Walker, E.A., Griciute, L., Castegnaro, M. & Börzsönyi, M., eds, N-*Nitroso Compounds: Analysis, Formation and Occurrence (IARC Scientific Publications No. 31)*, Lyon, International Agency for Research on Cancer, pp. 609–612

Kurechi, T., Kikugawa, K. & Kato, T. (1980) Effect of alcohol on nitrosamine formation. *Food Cosmet. Toxicol.*, **18**, 591–595

Lai, D.Y. & Arcos, J.C. (1980) Dialkylnitrosamine bioactivation and carcinogenesis. *Life Sci.*, **27**, 2149–2165

Lakritz, L., Simenhoff, M.L., Dunn, S.R. & Fiddler, W. (1980) *N*-Nitrosodimethylamine in human blood. *Food Cosmet. Toxicol.*, **18**, 77–79

Li, M., Li, P., & Li, B. (1980) Recent progress in research on oesophageal cancer in China. *Adv. Cancer Res.*, **33**, 173–249

Maling, H.M., Stripp, B., Sipes, I.G., Highman, R., Saul, W. & Williams, M.A. (1975) Enhanced hepatotoxicity of carbon tetrachloride, thioacetamide, and dimethylnitrosamine by pretreatment of rats with ethanol and some comparisons with potentiation by isopropanol. *Toxicol. appl. Pharmacol.*, **33**, 291–308

McCoy, G.D., Chen, C.G., Hecht, S.S. & McCoy, E.C. (1979) Enhanced metabolism and mutagenesis of nitrosopyrrolidine in liver fractions isolated from chronic ethanol consuming hamsters. *Cancer Res.*, **39**, 793–796

McCoy, G.D., Hecht, S.S., Katayama, S. & Wynder, E.L. (1981) Differential effect of chronic ethanol consumption on the carcinogenicity of *N'*-nitrosopyrrolidine and *N*-nitrosonornicotine in male Syrian golden hamsters. *Cancer Res.*, **41**, 2849–2854

McCoy, G.D., Katayama, S., Young, R., Wyatt, M. & Hecht, S. (1982) *Influence of chronic ethanol consumption on the metabolism and carcinogenicity to tobacco-related nitrosamines*. In: Bartsch, H., O'Neill, I.K., Castegnaro, M. & Okada, M., eds, N-*Nitroso Compounds: Occurrence and Biological Effects (IARC Scientific Publications No. 41)*, Lyon, International Agency for Research on Cancer, pp. 635–642

Melikian, A.A., LaVoie, E.J., Hoffmann, D. & Wynder, E.L. (1981) Volatile nitrosamines: analysis in breast fluid and blood of non lactating women. *Food Cosmet. Toxicol.*, **19**, 757–759

National Academy of Science (1982) *Report of the Committee on Diet, Nutrition, and Cancer*, Washington DC, National Academy Press, pp. 1–11; 11–1, 11–15; 17–1, 17–39

Ohshima, H. & Bartsch, H. (1981) Quantitative estimation of endogenous nitrosation in humans by monitoring *N*-nitrosoproline excreted in urine. *Cancer Res.*, **41**, 3658–3662

Pegg, A.E. & Perry, W. (1981) Alkylation of nucleic acids and metabolism of small doses of dimethylnitrosamine in the rat. *Cancer Res.*, **41**, 3128–3132

Pegg, A.E., Roberfroid, M., von Bahr, C., Foote, R.S., Mitra, S., Bresil, H., Likhachev, A. & Montesano, R. (1982) Removal of O^6-methylguanine from DNA by human liver fractions. *Proc. natl Acad. Sci. USA*, **79**, 5162–5165

Peng, R., Tu, Y.Y. & Yang, C.S. (1982) The induction or competitive inhibition of a high affinity microsomal nitrosodimethylamine demethylase by ethanol. *Carcinogenesis., 3,* 1457–1461

Phillips, J.C., Lake, B.G., Gangolli, S.D., Grasso, P. & Lloyd, A.G. (1977) Effect of pyrazole and 3-amino-a, 2, 4-triazole on the metabolism and toxicity of dimethylnitrosamine in the rat. *J. natl Cancer Inst., 58,* 629–633

Pignatelli, B., Castegnaro, M. & Walker, E.A. (1976) *Effects of gallic acid and of ethanol on formation of nitrosodiethylamine.* In: Walker, E.A., Bogovski, P. & Griciute, L., eds, *Environmental N-Nitroso compounds Analysis and Formation (IARC Scientific Publications No. 14),* Lyon, International Agency for Research on Cancer, pp. 173–178

Pollack, E.S., Nomura, A.M.Y., Heilbrun, L.K., Stemmermann, G.N. & Green, S.B. (1984) Prospective study of alcohol consumption and cancer. *New Engl. J. Med., 310,* 617–621

Schmähl, D. (1976) Investigations on esophageal carcinogenicity by methylphenylnitrosamine and ethyl alcohol in rats. *Cancer Lett., 1,* 215–218

Schmähl, D., Thomas, C., Sattler, W. & Scheld, G. (1965) Experimentelle Untersuchungen zur Syncarcinogenese. 3. Mitteilung: Versuche zur Krebserzeugung bei Ratten bei gleichzeitiger Gabe von Diäthylnitrosamin und Tetrachlorkohlenstoff bzw. Aethylalkohol, zugleich ein experimenteller Beitrag zur Frage der Alkoholcirrhose. *Z. Krebsforsch., 66,* 526–532

Schwarz, M., Appel, K.E., Schrenk, D. & Kunz, W. (1980) Effect of ethanol on microsomal metabolism of dimethylnitrosamine. *J. Cancer Res. clin. Oncol., 97,* 233–240

Schwarz M., Wiesbeck, G., Hummel, J. & Kunz, W. (1982) Effect of ethanol on dimethylnitrosamine activation and DNA synthesis in rat liver. *Carcinogenesis, 3,* 1071–1075

Shore, P.A., Brodie, B.B. & Hogben, C.A.M. (1957) The gastric secretion of drugs: a pH partition hypothesis. *J. Pharmacol. exp. Ther., 119,* 361–369

Spiegelhalder, B., Eisenbrand, G. & Preussmann, R. (1982) *Urinary excretion of N-nitrosamines in rats and humans.* In: Bartsch, H., O'Neill, I.K., Castegnaro, M. & Okada, eds, N-*Nitroso Compounds: Occurrence and Biological Effects (IARC Scientific Publications No. 41),* Lyon, International Agency for Research on Cancer, pp. 443–449

Swann, P.F. (1982) *Metabolism of nitrosamines: observations on the effect of alcohol on nitrosamine metabolism and on human cancer.* In: Magee, P.N. ed., *Nitrosamines and Human Cancer (Banbury Report No. 12),* Cold Spring Harbor, NY, Cold Spring Harbor Laboratory, pp. 53–68

Swann, P.F. & McLean, A.E.M. (1971) Cellular injury and carcinogenesis. The effect of a protein-free high-carbohydrate diet on the metabolism of dimethylnitrosamine in the rat. *Biochem. J., 124,* 283–288

Swann, P.F., Mace, R., Angeles, R.M. & Keefer, L.K. (1983) Deuterium isotope effect on metabolism of N-nitrosodimethylamine *in vivo* in rats. *Carcinogenesis, 4,* 821–825

Tuyns, A.J. (1979) Epidemiology of alcohol and cancer. *Cancer Res., 39,* 2840–2843

Tuyns, A.J., Pequignot, G. & Jensen, O.M. (1977) Le cancer de l'oesophage en Ille-et-Vilaine en fonction des niveaux de consommation d'alcool et de tabac. Les risques se multiplient. *Bull. Cancer, 64,* 45–60

Wynder, E.L., Mushinski, M.H. & Spivak, J.C. (1977) Tobacco and alcohol consumption in relation to the development of multiple primary cancers. *Cancer, 10,* 1872–1878

Yamamoto, M., Yamada, T. & Tanimura, S. (1980) Volatile nitrosamines in human blood before and after a meal containing high concentrations of nitrate and secondary amines. *Food Cosmet. Toxicol., 18,* 297–299

Yang, C.S. (1980) Research on oesophageal cancer in China: a review. *Cancer Res., 40,* 2633–2644

Yang, C.S. (1982) *Nitrosamines and other etiological factors in the esophageal cancer in Northern China.* In: Magee, P.N., ed., *Nitrosamines and Human Cancer (Banbury Report No. 12),* Cold Spring Harbor, NY, Cold Spring Harbor Laboratory, pp. 487–499

QUANTITATIVE MEASUREMENT OF THE EXHALATION RATE OF VOLATILE N-NITROSAMINES IN INHALATION EXPERIMENTS WITH ANAESTHETIZED SPRAGUE-DAWLEY RATS

R.G. KLEIN & P. SCHMEZER

Institute of Toxicology and Chemotherapy, German Cancer Research Center, 6900 Heidelberg, Federal Republic of Germany

SUMMARY

Volatile N-nitrosamines have been detected in the human environment – in work places, such as the rubber, leather and chemical industries, in tobacco smoke and also inside new cars. In order to make risk assessments on the basis of inhalation experiments with animals at dose levels relevant to the human situation, it is important to know the actual absorption rate in the respiratory tract. In this study, 63 female Sprague-Dawley rats were exposed to four nitrosamines (N-nitrosodimethylamine, N-nitrosodiethylamine, N-nitrosopyrrolidine and N-nitrosomorpholine) in air. Respiratory parameters were monitored by pneumotachography. After 10 min of inhalation, the exhaled air was collected for 10 min in steps of 2 min intervals and analysed for its content of nitrosamines with a Thermal Energy Analyzer. Inhalation and exhalation were maintained by endotracheal intubation under narcosis with Thalamonal. The influence of this anaesthetic on the urinary excretion of N-nitrosodimethylamine after gavage and inhalation was tested: in comparison with unanaesthetized animals and with a group under ether narcosis, the excretion of the nitrosamine by the Thalamonal-anaesthetized animals was drastically reduced (factor of 20 to 60). Independent of the concentration of inhaled nitrosamine, ranging from 1–450 µg/L in air, the relative amounts of exhaled substance 10 min after inhalation were 0.9% N-nitrosodimethylamine, 0.4% N-nitrosodiethylamine, 6% N-nitrosopyrrolidine and 5% N-nitrosomorpholine. Extrapolation of these data back to the first exhalation (i.e., following the last inhalation) revealed that a remarkable amount of substance may be exhaled (up to 30% N-nitrosodimethylamine).

INTRODUCTION

Exposure to nitrosamines and their precursors can occur in certain working places (Fine *et al.*, 1975; Rounbehler *et al.*, 1981; Spiegelhalder & Preussmann, 1981). In general, the major route of absorption into the organism is inhalation of these volatile substances. In order to carry out risk estimations on the basis of dose level and length of exposure, it is important to assess the actual absorption rate in the respiratory tract under conditions similar to those in the human situation. Depending on the physico-chemical structure of the substance and its biological behaviour in the respiratory tract, a considerable amount of the inhaled substance may be exhaled. For our measurements with rats, we therefore used a method of inhalation which by-passes the filtering effect of the nasal region and thus introduces the inhaled vapours directly into the trachea and the deeper regions of the lung. In this paper, we describe the use of endotracheal intubation to deliver controlled amounts of four volatile nitrosamines into the respiratory tract of rats. The data show that a significant proportion of these substances is not immediately absorbed by the animal and that, as a result, exposure to carcinogens, which has previously been assumed to be 100%, may be greatly overestimated.

MATERIALS AND METHODS

Animals

Female Sprague-Dawley rats (Medizinische Hochschule, Hannover, FRG), weighing 320 ± 50 g, were housed in Makrolon cages under standard conditions and were provided with water and food (Altromin pellets) *ad libitum*. Food was removed the day before an experiment.

Anaesthesia

The most suitable narcosis for endotracheal intubation of rats was found to be obtained with Thalamonal (Droperidol/Fentanyl, H. Janssen, Düsseldorf, FRG). Ten minutes after injection of the narcotic, Levallorphan (1,3-hydroxy-N-allylmorphinantartrate, Hoffmann-LaRoche) was given to overcome the Thalamonal-induced reduction in respiration.

Pneumotachography

The principle of this method for measuring the tidal volume in breathing was first reported by Fleisch (1925). We used a glass tube with an inner diameter of 0.8 mm and a length of 10 cm, which was connected to a membrane capacitor (MKS Baratron, type 223A) and to the intubated animal. The pressure differences caused by the breathing of the animal through the glass tube were amplified (MKS Baratron, PDR-5B) and recorded over 20 breathing cycles. Each breath could be monitored, and the peak area was equivalent to the volume of inhaled or exhaled air. The apparatus was initially calibrated by injecting 0.5–5 cm^3 of air through a precision pipette (Gilson, France) at the same rate as the normal breathing cycle in rats. A calibration curve was obtained using linear regression.

Nitrosamine evaporator

The nitrosamine evaporator (Klein, 1982) comprised a thermostatted cabinet containing a glass flask with three necks, for a laboratory thermometer (graduated in tenths of degrees), a Teflon stirrer for the gas phase and a thin glass tube. The 4-L flask contained 200 mL of an aqueous solution of the nitrosamine. The gas-liquid equilibrium of the nitrosamine vapour was made constant before inhalation. After intubation, the animal was attached to the thin glass tube by a short silicon tube. The animal's environment was controlled thermostatically at a temperature just above that of the condensation temperature of breath. The animal remained in this position for 10 min, during which it was observed and its breathing frequency recorded.

Inhalation procedure

The animal was fixed on an inclined plane, as described by Saffiotti *et al.* (1968). The tube was introduced gently through the epiglottis with the aid of transillumination (Lany *et al.*, 1980) and then fixed slightly by a small ribbon around the animal's neck and forelimbs. The pneumotachogram was taken in order to monitor the level of breathing from the moment of intubation until steady state, which was usually reached after 30 min. The rat was then housed in the thermostatted chamber and attached to the flask with the defined concentration of the nitrosamine vapour. The rat inhaled the atmosphere of the flask for 10 min and was then detached as quickly as possible from the inhalation apparatus and connected to the exhalation tube, whereupon it was allowed to inhale fresh air (which had been verified as being free from nitrosamines). All exhaled air was collected into ThermoSorb tubes (Thermo Electron Corp., Waltham, MA, USA). The absorption tubes were exchanged at intervals of 2 min in order to measure the kinetics of exhalation. The higher concentrations of nitrosamine vapours were fully absorbed in up to five tubes. The contents were eluted with methanol:dichloromethane, 20:80 (v/v) and the nitrosamines analysed in a Thermal Energy Analyzer.

Exhalation procedure

A larger tube ($\varnothing$ 10 mm), which allowed the by-pass of fresh air for inhalation, bore two connections: one from the animal's tube and the other from the ThermoSorb tube and the pump (Rotheroe & Mitchell, type L2SF). All exhaled air was collected by the pump. The rat, all connecting tubes and the ThermoSorb tube with the pump were contained inside the thermostatted box to avoid condensation of the moisture associated with expired air. The laboratory air, the tubes and the endotracheal tubes were tested continuously for traces of nitrosamines. The amount of substance absorbed for analysis was calculated against standards.

Urinary excretion

The influence of Thalamonal narcosis on the excretion of N-nitrosodimethylamine (NDMA) was compared with that of diethyl ether. Groups of eight rats (four male and female) received 350 µg NDMA either orally (groups 1–3) or by inhalation (group 4); group 1 remained unanaesthetized; group 2 was anaesthetized with ether and groups 3 and 4 with Thalamonal. Urine was collected from rats held in metabolic cages and analysed over 24 h (Spiegelhalder *et al.*, 1982).

RESULTS AND DISCUSSION

At least three concentrations of each nitrosamine, in the range of 1–400 µg/L were tested (Table 1). The standard error in the exhalation rates was in the range of 5–30%. The exhalation curves, with a logarithmic mass ordinate and a linear time axis, as exemplified with the highest concentration of NDMA (354 µg/L) (Fig. 1), shows clearly the decrease in nitrosamine with time. By extrapolating back to zero time, it was possible to assess the amount of nitrosamine exhaled as a percentage of the mass inhaled (last column, Table 1). The uptake of nitrosamine by an animal was calculated from the formula:

$$\text{tidal volume (L/min)} \times \text{duration of inhalation (min)} \times \text{concentration (µg/L)} = \text{uptake (µg)}$$

The tidal volume was taken from the plethysmographic traces and the observed breathing frequency during inhalation and was compared with a body weight correlation table (Gaddum, 1959; Stahl, 1967). The agreement with body weight was satisfactory, despite the enlarged respiratory resistance due to plethysmography. During inhalation, the thermometer neck had to be raised for pressure equilibration. The nitrosamine concentration inside the flask remained

Table 1.   Amounts of nitrosamines inhaled and exhaled by 5 animals per nitrosamine concentration after 10 min of inhalation, and percentages of exhaled and inhaled substance extrapolated from the kinetic analysis (see Fig. 1)

Nitrosamines	Concentration inhaled (µg/L)	Calculated amount inhaled (µg)	Concentration exhaled (ng)	Percentage exhaled (extrapolated from graph)
NDMA	354	630	6 000	
	12.8	21	265	10–30
	0.98	1.8	11	
NDEA	332	550	1 600	
	10	18	84	3–10
	0.75	1.3	7	
NPYR	450	850	44 000	
	7.2	12	360	
	0.9	1.6	170	10–30
	0.25	0.44	33	
NMOR	341	520	20 000	
	9.6	15	800	5–15
	1	1.5	90	

[a] NDMA, N-nitrosodimethylamine; NDEA, N-nitrosodiethylamine; NPYR, N-nitrosopyrrolidine; NMOR, N-nitrosomorpholine

Fig. 1. Exhalation rate of N-nitrosodimethylamine (354 µg/L) in 2-min intervals after a 10-min inhalation period

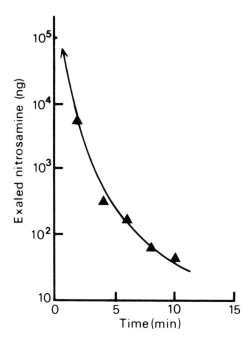

constant within 1%, as controlled before, during and after inhalation by ultra-violet spectrometry (Zeiss PQM) at 230 nm of an aqueous solution and compared with a calibration curve.

A considerable decrease in the elimination of NDMA was seen in the 24-h urine of animals anaesthetized with Thalamonal (0.009% *per os* and 0.006% by inhalation) when compared to those anaesthized with ether (0.59%) or those without anaesthesia (0.15%). The amounts of NDMA eliminated were similar in groups given Thalamonal orally and in those that received it by inhalation. The amount inhaled was calculated on the basis of the length of exposure and concentration. The excreted mass of the substance was 0.03 ± 0.014 μg for oral and 0.021 ± 0.009 μg for inhalation exposure. The differences are in the range of the standard deviation.

No significant difference was found between male and female rats in their excretion ratio. As stated previously (Spiegelhalder *et al.*, 1982), the control group without narcosis eliminated a smaller amount of NDMA (0.51 μg ± 0.2) than those anaesthetized with ether (2.07 ± 1.0 μg).

These results indicate that the main loss of nitrosamine in rats occurs on exhalation. In order to overcome the problem of having to extrapolate the kinetic data of the summed mass exhaled to zero time just after inhalation, we are trying to reduce the dead volume of a small glass valve that controls the air stream in order to obtain measurements of the exhaled concentration of the compound. This value may be corrected additionally by calculating the proportion of the known dead volume of the valve to the dimensions of the rat's trachea.

ACKNOWLEDGEMENTS

We thank Miss C. Kamphausen and Miss B. Rech for excellent technical assistance and Mr G. Wuertele for carrying out the analysis. The editorial assistance of Dr P. Bedford is gratefully acknowledged.

REFERENCES

Fine, D.H., Lieb, D. & Rufeh, F. (1975) Principle of operation of the Thermal Energy Analyzer for the trace analysis of volatile and non-volatile N-nitroso compounds. *J. Chromatogr.*, **107**, 351–357

Fleisch, A. (1925) Der Pneumotachograph: ein Apparat zur Geschwindigkeitsregistrierung der Atemluft. *Pfluegers Arch.*, **209**, 715–716

Gaddum, J.H. (1959) *Pharmocology*, 5th ed., London, Oxford University Press

Klein, R.G. (1982) Calculations and measurements on the volatility of N-nitrosamines and their aqueous solutions. *Toxicology*, **23**, 135–147

Lany, J., Wesely-Lany, L. & Klein, R.G. (1980) A simple method for exact intratracheal instillation in small laboratory rodents. *Cancer Lett.*, **10**, 91–94

Rounbehler, D.P., Reisch, J.W., Coombs, J.R. & Fine, D.H. (1981) Nitrosamine air sampling sorbents compared for quantitative collection and artifact formation. *Anal. Chem.*, **52**, 273–276

Saffiotti, U., Cefis, C. & Kolb, L.H. (1968) A method for the experimental induction of bronchogenic carcinoma. *Cancer Res.*, **28**, 104–124

Spiegelhalder, B. & Preussmann, R. (1982) *Nitrosamines and rubber*. In: Bartsch, H., O'Neill, I.K., Castegnaro, M. & Okada, M., eds, N-*Nitroso Compounds: Occurence and Biological Effects (IARC Scientific Publications No. 41)*, Lyon, International Agency for Research on Cancer, pp. 231–243

Spiegelhalder, B., Eisenbrand, G. & Preussmann, R. (1982) *Urinary excretion of* N-*nitrosamines in rats and humans*. In: Bartsch, H., O'Neill, I.K., Castegnaro, M. & Okada, M., eds, N-*Nitroso Compounds: Occurence and Biological Effects (IARC Scientific Publications No. 41)*, Lyon, International Agency for Research on Cancer, pp. 443–449

Stahl, W.R. (1967) Scaling of respiratory variables in mammals. *J. appl. Physiol.*, **22**, 453–460

INFLUENCE OF DISULFIRAM
ON THE METABOLISM OF *N*-NITROSODIETHYLAMINE

N. FRANK & M. WIESSLER

*Institute of Toxicology and Chemotherapy, German Cancer Research Center Heidelberg,
Federal Republic of Germany*

D. HADJIOLOV

Center of Oncology Sofia, Bulgaria

SUMMARY

The effect of disulfiram (DSF) on the biological activity of *N*-nitrosodiethylamine (NDEA) was studied *in vivo*. We determined its influence on NDEA level, on NDEA-induced DNA damage and on DNA alkylation in the liver and oesophagus.

It was found that 500 mg/kg DSF given 2 h before a single dose of 28 mg/kg NDEA inhibited the metabolism and increased the concentrations of NDEA in the organs, especially in the oesophagus. Consequently, DNA damage and the alkylation of DNA are inhibited in both the liver and the oesophagus.

INTRODUCTION

It is well known that disulfiram (DSF) inhibits single-strand breaks (Hadjiolov *et al.*, 1977) and alkylation of liver DNA (Frank *et al.*, 1980) induced by chronic application of NDEA. The carcinogenic activity of NDEA is also influenced: when NDEA is given in combination with DSF, the predominant site of carcinogenesis is shifted from the liver to the oesophagus (Schmähl *et al.*, 1976). In order to elucidate the mechanisms of DSF activity, we investigated the metabolism of NDEA in liver and oesophagus, with and without DSF pretreatment. We determined the elimination of unchanged NDEA from organs after oral and intraperitoneal application of the nitrosamine. We also studied the influence of DSF on NDEA-induced DNA damage and on DNA alkylation in the liver and oesophagus.

MATERIALS AND METHODS

Compounds

DSF (Merck, Darmstadt, FRG).
NDEA was synthesized by nitrosation of diethylamine hydrochloride with sodium nitrite. ^{14}C-labelled NDEA was synthesized from 1-^{14}C-acetic acid sodium salt (Amersham, Braunschweig, FRG; 58.7 mCi/mmol) according to standard methods.
All commercial chemicals were of analytical grade.

Animal treatment

Male Sprague Dawley rats (120-200 g) received 500 mg/kg DSF in 4% starch solution (by gavage) 2 h before receiving the carcinogen. The controls were fed starch solution alone. The NDEA dose was 28 mg/kg, applied in 0.9% sodium cloride solution *per os* or intraperitoneally. The ^{14}C-labelled NDEA was diluted with inactive material to 2 mCi/28 mg.

Elimination of NDEA from organs

Six animals in each group received NDEA with and without DSF pretreatment. After 0.5, 2, 4, 8 and 24 h, the animals were sacrificed. Liver, kidney, lung and oesophagus were isolated and homogenized 1 : 10 in dichloromethane (Ultraturrax homogenizer). The oesophagi from three animals were pooled; all other organs were treated individually. The organic phases were analysed by gas chromatography (GC) (Hewlett Packard HP 7620A) on a Carbowax 20M TPA column, using a nitroso-specific thermal energy analyser detector (Thermo Electron, Waltham, USA).

Analysis of single-strand breaks

The livers and oesophagi were isolated from three animals per group, 4 h after the application of 28 mg/kg NDEA. The size of the DNA was measured by sedimentation in alkaline sucrose gradients, as described earlier (Hadjiolov et al., 1977). The DNA content in gradient fractions was determined fluorimetrically (Kissane & Robins, 1958). Sucrose gradients were calibrated using DNA from T_4 and T_7 phages as markers. Each experiment was repeated at least three times.

Analysis of DNA alkylation

Each group of 10 animals received 28 mg/kg ^{14}C-labelled NDEA (2 mCi/kg) *per os,* with and without DSF pretreatment. The animals were killed 4 h after NDEA application. Liver and oesophageal DNA was isolated by phenolic extraction (Frei & Lawley, 1975), hydrolysed with 0.1 mol/L hydrochloric acid for 30 min at 70 °C and separated on an ion-exchange column (Aminex A6, Uziel et al., 1968). Unlabelled O^6-ethylguanine and ^7N-ethylguanine were added as internal markers.

RESULTS AND DISCUSSION

Figure 1 shows the concentration of unchanged NDEA extracted from liver, kidney, lung and oesophagus at different times. It can be seen that after oral application (Fig. 1A), as well as after intraperitoneal application (Fig. 1B), the concentrations of NDEA in the organs of the

Fig. 1. Time-dependent distribution of *N*-nitrosodiethylamine (NDEA) concentrations in different organs. Each column represents the median value (with range) of six individual determinations (liver, kidney, lung) or two determinations (oesophagus). Chart A shows the distributions after oral application, chart B after intraperitoneal treatment with 28 mg/kg NDEA in each case. The hatched columns indicate the carcinogen-treated groups, the empty columns represent the NDEA concentrations after pretreatment with 500 mg/kg disulfiram (DSF)

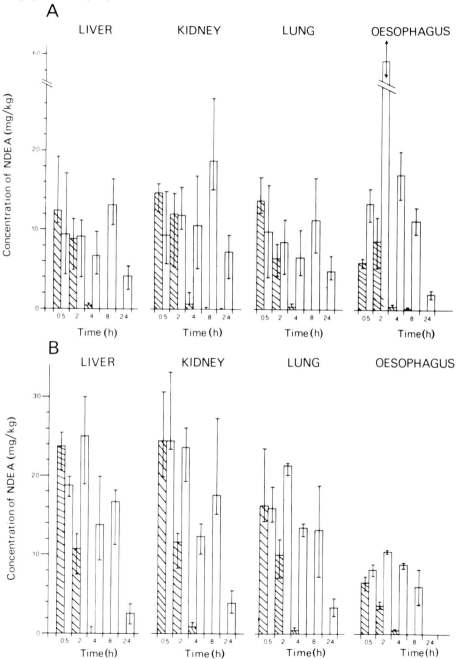

control animals (28 mg/kg NDEA) decreased to zero within 4–8 h. In contrast, NDEA persists in the organs of the experimental groups (500 mg/kg DSF + 28 mg/kg NDEA) for a period of over 24 h. In the first 8 h after intraperitoneal administration, the mean NDEA concentration in liver, kidney and lung of the control and experimental groups is higher than the respective concentrations after gavage.

With DSF pretreatment, it is conspicuous that the concentration of NDEA in the oesophagus is drastically increased 2 h after oral application of NDEA. Since this effect occurs only after oral, but not after intraperitoneal, administration, we suggest that NDEA may exert a local influence on the oesophageal epithelium. However, at 0.5 h after administration (oral and intraperitoneal), the NDEA concentration in the oesophagus is higher in the DSF-treated group than in the controls. Therefore, in addition to the strong local effect, a general tendency for NDEA enrichment in the oesophagus after DSF pretreatment can be observed up to 2 h after NDEA application.

The administration of a single dose of 28 mg/kg NDEA produced DNA damage in liver cells and in oesophageal epithelial cells. The results presented in Figure 2 show that after 4 h of NDEA treatment, fragmentation of oesophageal DNA is greater than fragmentation of liver DNA. By reducing the metabolism, DSF consequently inhibits the massive induction of DNA single-strand breaks in both the liver and oesophageal mucosa for at least 4 h.

The results of the alkylation experiments with liver and oesophageal DNA after a single dose of 28 mg/kg ^{14}C-labelled NDEA, with and without DSF pretreatment, are listed in Table 1. Both in the liver and the oesophagus, alkylation is inhibited by DSF. The decrease of the O^6:^{7}N

Fig. 2. Sedimentation profiles of oesophageal DNA (part A) and liver DNA (part B) in alkaline sucrose gradients, 4 h after an oral application of 28 mg/kg *N*-nitrosodiethylamine (NDEA) (●–●) and 500 mg/kg disulfiram (DSF) 2 h before the carcinogen (○–○). The horizontal lines indicate the position of DNA of untreated controls

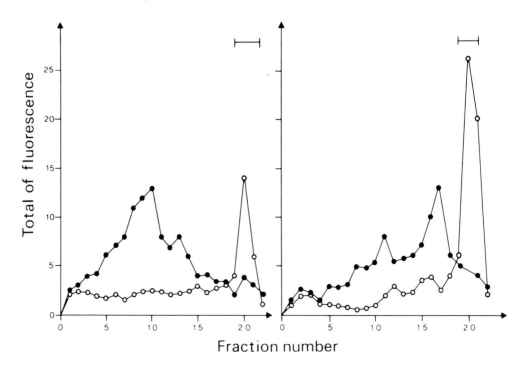

Table 1. Radioactivity and its distribution as O^6-ethylguanine and ^{7}N-ethylguanine in DNA of rat liver and oesophagus 4 h after a single oral dose of ^{14}C-*N*-nitrosodiethylamine (NDEA)

Treatment	Organ	Total activity (dpm 10 mg DNA)	^{7}-N-ethylguanine:O^6-ethylguanine		Ratio O^6:^{7}N
			(mol/10^6 mol guanine)	(mol/10^6 mol guanine)	
28 mg/kg NDEA	Liver	17 873	43.2	22.4	0.52
	Oesophagus	8 481	1.5	0.7	0.50
500 mg/kg disulfiram + 28 mg/kg NDEA	Liver	2 691	3.6	0.6	0.17
	Oesophagus	3 328	n.d.[a]	n.d.	–

[a] Not detected

ratio in the liver from 0.52 to 0.17 may be caused by a more effective repair, since the actual concentration of metabolized NDEA is reduced by DSF.

In conclusion, it may be stated that the metabolism of NDEA is strongly inhibited by DSF. This is supported by our findings, which show that relatively higher concentrations of unchanged NDEA are present in various organs after DSF pretreatment. Also, we have shown that DSF inhibits single-strand breaks and DNA alkylation in liver and in oesophagus. Our previous experiments (Hadjiolov *et al.*, 1977; Frank *et al.*, 1980) had shown that NDEA produces little damage when the protecting effect of DSF is over. Furthermore, the oesophagus shows a higher tendency to incorporate NDEA after DSF pretreatment than do other organs. The repair of NDEA-induced single-strand breaks in the oesophagus is lower than in the liver (Hadjiolov *et al.*, unpublished results). These observations may therefore explain the shift of organotropism from liver to oesophagus during carcinogenesis after DSF pretreatment.

ACKNOWLEDGEMENTS

The authors thank Mrs Knauft, Mr Klokow and Mr Würtele for excellent technical assistance and Dr B. Pool for correcting the manuscript.

REFERENCES

Frank, N., Hadjiolov, D., Bertram, B. & Wiessler, M. (1980) Effect of disulfiram on the alkylation of rat liver DNA by nitrosodiethylamine. *J. Cancer Res. clin. Oncol.*, **97**, 209–212

Frei, J.V. & Lawley, P.D. (1975) Methylation of DNA in various organs of C57Bl mice by a carcinogenic dose of *N*-methyl-*N*-nitrosourea and stability of some methylation products up to 18 hours. *Chem.-biol. Interact.*, **10**, 413–427

Hadjiolov, D., Frank, N. & Schmähl, D. (1977) Inhibition of diethylnitrosamine-induced strand breaks in liver DNA by disulfiram. *Z. Krebsforsch.*, **90**, 107–109

Kissane, J. & Robins, E. (1958) The fluorometric measurement of deoxyribonucleic acid in animal tissues with special reference to the central nervous system. *J. biol. Chem.*, **233**, 184–188

Schmähl, D., Krüger, F.W., Habs, M. & Diehl, B. (1976) Influence of disulfiram on the organotropy of the carcinogenic effect of dimethylnitrosamine and diethylnitrosamine in rats. *Z. Krebsforsch.*, **85**, 271–276

Uziel, M., Koh, C.K. & Cohn, W.E. (1968) Rapid ionexchange chromatographic microanalysis of ultraviolet absorbing material and its application to nucleosides. *Anal. Biochem.*, **25**, 77–98

EFFECT OF DISULFIRAM ON *N*-NITROSO-*N*-METHYLBENZYLAMINE METABOLISM. BIOCHEMICAL ASPECTS

F. SCHWEINSBERG, I. WEISSENBERGER, B. BRÜCKNER & E. SCHWEINSBERG

Hygiene Institute of the University of Tübingen

V. BÜRKLE & H. WITTENBERG

Department of Pathology, University of Tübingen

H.-J. REINECKE

Isotopenlabor, University of Tübingen, Federal Republic of Germany

SUMMARY

The present biochemical experiments show that disulfiram inhibits *N*-nitroso-*N*-methylbenzylamine metabolism in the rat. More *N*-nitroso-*N*-methylbenzylamine may therefore reach extrahepatic tissues. The pathological lesions observed in the lungs in the present system can be explained by the finding that alkylation of lung DNA is increased and repair processes are impaired by enhanced cell proliferation in this organ.

INTRODUCTION

It has been shown that disulfiram (DSF) strongly influences the carcinogenicity of a number of chemicals occurring in the human environment (for a review, see Fiala, 1981). With respect to *N*-nitrosamines, the observed effects of DSF are conflicting: decrease of tumour development in various target organs and shifts in the organotropic carcinogenic action have been reported (Schmähl *et al.*, 1976; Irving *et al.*, 1979).

In an earlier study in our laboratory, administration of DSF with *N*-nitroso-*N*-methylbenzylamine (NMBzA) accelerated the formation of oesophageal tumours and, in addition, induced pathological lesions in the tracheal system of the rat (Schweinsberg & Bürkle, 1981; Schweinsberg *et al.*, 1982). Because of this dramatic increase in carcinogenicity, elucidation of the biochemical mechanism responsible for these effects appeared to be worthwhile. The process of activation of the carcinogen was therefore investigated at different stages.

MATERIALS AND METHODS

Chemicals

NMBzA was obtained from EMKA-Chemie (Markgroningen, FRG); [methyl-^{14}C]-NMBzA from LKB (Karlsruhe, FRG); DSF from Fluka (Buchs, Switzerland); incubation reagents, NADP$^+$, sodium isocitrate, isocitrate dehydrogenase (ICDH) from Boehringer (Mannheim, FRG); derivatization agents, 2,4-dinitrophenylhydrazine from Merck (Darmstadt, FRG) and dansylhydrazine (DnsH) from Fluka (Buchs, Switzerland).

Animals

Female SIV 50 rats (Ivanovas, Kisslegg, FRG) were used for the experiments. If not otherwise indicated, a standard diet (ALMA^R, Botzenhardt, Kempten, FRG) and tap water were given *ad libitum*.

NMBzA in blood

Five rats (220 g body weight) were pretreated for one week with DSF (0.2 g/kg diet). The control group received the standard diet. Thereafter, all animals were kept without drinking water for one day. After this they were allowed to drink water containing 75 mg NMBzA/L for 10 min (about 10 mL/animal). Subsequently, animals were sacrificed at time intervals ranging from 20–180 min, and blood was collected from the vena cava (about 7 mL/animal). The blood was extracted with ether. After centrifugation (2 000 × *g*, 10 min), the organic layer was concentrated under nitrogen to 2 mL. Aliquots of this solution (2 μL) were subjected to gas-liquid chromatography (GLC) analysis (Hewlett-Packard 5710A, equipped with a nitrogen-specific flame-ionization detector; 1.83 m glass column, 3% Carbowax 20M on Chrom. W HP 100; column temperature: 130 °C; carrier gas: helium).

Exhalation of CO_2

Pretreatment was as described above. Two rats per experiment were allowed to drink water containing 75 mg [^{14}CH$_3$]-NMBzA/L (0.5 mCi/mmol; about 7 mL/animal) for 10 min. The expired $^{14}CO_2$ was determined as described by Hodgson *et al.* (1980).

Microsomal reactions

Enzyme preparation: Microsomes were prepared from organs of control rats and those subjected to pretreatment as above (body weight, 200–300 g). Thereafter, the animals were sacrificed by decapitation and allowed to bleed. The preparation procedure was carried out as described earlier (Schweinsberg & Kouros, 1979) and employed an ice-cooled saccharose-EDTA-Tris-HCl (Mic I) buffer system. The final microsomal fraction was rehomogenized and centrifuged in potassium chloride-Tris-hydrochloric acid (Mic II) buffer (pH 7.4) and kept frozen at −20 °C. The protein content of the microsomal suspension for the metabolism studies was determined by the method of Lowry *et al.* (1951), using bovine serum albumin as a standard, and was diluted to a concentration of 5–8 mg protein/mL, using homogenizing buffer.

Incubation conditions: Incubation mixtures contained, in a total volume of 3.0 mL, 10 mg NMBzA (0.067 mmol), a NADPH-generating system (0.005 mmol NADP$^+$, 0.04 mmol sodium isocitrate, 0.04 mmol magnesium chloride, 0.4 units of ICDH) in potassium chloride/Tris-hydrochloric acid buffer (120 mmol/L potassium chloride, 50 mmol/L Tris, pH 7.4), and 0.5 mL microsomal suspension with 2.5–4 mg protein.

The incubation reaction was carried out in covered, 25-mL, Erlenmeyer flasks in a shaking water bath at 37 °C: NMBzA was dissolved in ether (100 mg/10 mL), and 1 mL of the solution was delivered to the flask and evaporated by shaking in the dark, in order to distribute the nitrosamine uniformly on the bottom of the flask. The reaction was then started by adding preincubated microsomes and incubation reagents in Mic II buffer. After 20 min, the reaction was terminated by transferring the mixture to 1.5 mL of an ice-cold solution of zinc sulfate (20% w/v) in a centrifuge tube and adding 1.5 mL saturated barium hydroxide solution (Labuc & Archer, 1982). In order to avoid nonenzymatic benzaldehyde formation, it is very important to use a *neutral* deproteinization reaction and to complete the procedure as quickly as possible in absence of light. After leaving the deproteinizing mixture on ice for 1 h, it was centrifuged for 10 min at 2 000 × *g,* and the clear supernatant was used for the determination of benzaldehyde, benzyl alcohol and benzoic acid.

Metabolite analysis: Benzaldehyde was assayed by derivatization with dansylhydrazine, using a modification of the DNPH-method of Selim (1977). Dansylhydrazone determination permitted a more selective and sensitive estimation using fluorometric detection after high-performance liquid chromatography (HPLC) separation.

In a glass-joint reaction tube, 3 mL (of a total of 6 mL) deproteinized reaction mixture were mixed with 3 mL water and 0.2 mL DnsH reagent (2 mg dansylhydrazine in 1 mL of a solution of 50% ethanol and 12.5% hydrochloric acid). After standing for 20 min in the dark, the mixture was extracted with 1 mL dichloromethane. The dichloromethane extracts were kept frozen at –20 °C until HPLC analysis of the DnsH derivatives on a Beckman Model 110 A, equipped with an Altex Ultrasil-ODS column (25 cm × 4.6 mm i.d.). Eighty percent aqueous methanol solution was used for elution, at a flow rate of 2.5 mL/min. Fluorescence of the eluate was measured with a Gilson Spectra/Glo fluorometer (excitation filter, 330–400 nm; emission filter, 460–600 nm).

Benzyl alcohol and benzoic acid were analysed directly from the deproteinized aqueous solution, which was acidified with 100% acetic acid (20 μL/0.5 mL) and subjected to HPLC. The two products were separated from each other on an Ultrasil-ODS column (25 cm × 4.6 mm i.d.), eluted with 40% aqueous methanol and detected at 223 nm, using a Hitachi Model 100-10 spectrophotometer.

Alkylation of DNA in various organs

Animals were treated for one week with drinking water containing 10 mg NMBzA/L and a diet containing 0.2 g DSF/kg. The controls also received water containing 10 mg NMBzA/L. Subsequently, the animals were kept without drinking water for one day. After this treatment, they were allowed to drink water containing 100 mg [^{14}CH$_3$]-NMBzA/L for 10 min (20 mCi/mmol; about 7 mL/animal). After 4, 8 and 12 hours, the animals were sacrificed by exsanguination under thiogenal anaesthesia. Isolation of DNA and the determination of alkylated purine bases was performed according to Hodgson *et al.* (1980).

RESULTS AND DISCUSSION

NMBzA in blood

Up to 20 min after oral administration of NMBzA, a sharp increase in the concentration of NMBzA in blood was observed. Quantitative documentation of this effect is difficult to obtain because the method of administration allowed the animals to ingest the carcinogen over

a 10-min period. As can be seen in Figure 1, DSF had only a slight effect on the resorption
of NMBzA from the intestinal tract (Fig. 1, blood concentration after 20 min). Subsequently,
NMBzA disappeared quickly from the blood in both groups; this effect was clearly slowed by
DSF. At any time, the NMBzA concentrations were approximately twice as high in the animals
pretreated with DSF.

Exhalation of $^{14}CO_2$

   As depicted in Figure 2, about 50% of the administered dose of labelled NMBzA was expired
as $^{14}CO_2$ within 12 h in untreated animals. The inhibiting effect of DSF on carcinogen
metabolism could be seen clearly in pretreated animals. Not only was CO_2 exhalation delayed,
but also the overall amount of labelled CO_2 was reduced to 40%. Thus, it can be concluded
that DSF inhibits NMBzA metabolism.

Fig. 1. Variation in concentration of *N*-nitroso-*N*-methylbenzylamine (NMBzA) in blood with time following oral
       administration of 3.4 mg/kg body weight to rats. [], NMBzA; [], NMBzA + disulfiram

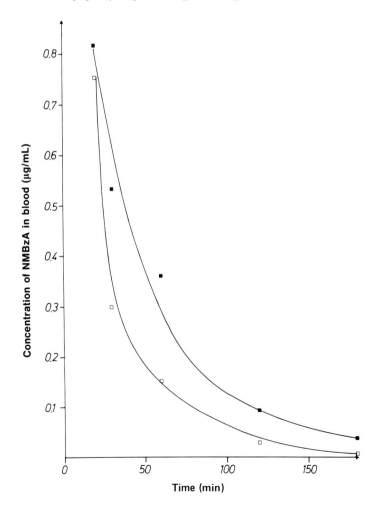

Fig. 2. Cumulative exhalation of carbon dioxide after oral administration of [$^{14}CH_3$]-*N*-nitroso-*N*-methylbenzylamine (NMBzA). ■, NMBzA; ●, NMBzA + disulfiram

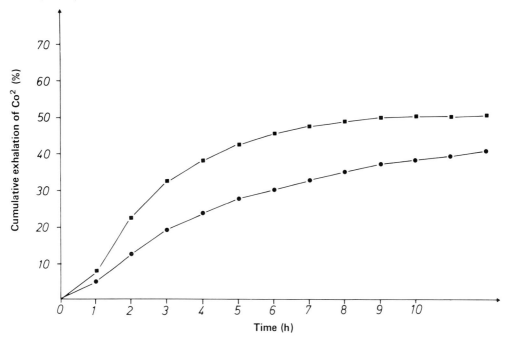

Microsomal reactions in vitro

The results of these experiments are recorded in Table 1. Microsomal preparations from rat liver converted NMBzA to benzaldehyde and benzyl alcohol, in agreement with results reported by Labuc and Archer (1982). Benzyl alcohol is formed by reduction of benzaldehyde, demonstrated when benzaldehyde was used as a substrate in the same assay. The extent of

Table 1. Influence of disulfiram (DSF) on *N*-nitroso-*N*-methylbenzylamine (NMBzA) metabolism by microsomes isolated from rat liver and lungs

Organ	DSF pretreatment	Metabolite (nmol/mg protein[a])	
		Benzaldehyde	Benzylalcohol
Liver	+[b]	4.11 ± 0.36[c]	32.10 ± 0.65
	−	10.49 ± 3.24	31.92 ± 7.37
Lung	+	5.22 ± 0.37	ND[d]
	−	ND	ND

[a] Values were calculated from 4 replicate assays; reaction time was 20 min.
[b] Pretreated rats were fed 200 mg DSF/kg diet for 8 days prior to experiment.
[c] Mean ± SE
[d] ND, not detected (detection limits: benzaldehyde, 0.1 µg/mg protein; benzylalcohol, 1 µg/mg protein)

SCHWEINSBERG *ET AL.*

Table 2. Effect of disulfiram (DSF) on methylation and labelling of guanine in DNA of various rat tissues at different time intervals, following a single oral dose of $^{14}CH_3$-N-nitroso-N-methylbenzylamine (NMBzA)

Time after application (h)	treatment DSF mg/kg diet	NMBzA mg/kg b.w.	Liver[a] 7-MeG[c]	O⁶-MeG[c]	G[d]	Lung[b] 7-MeG	O⁶-MeG	G	Oesophagus[b] 7-MeG	O⁶-MeG
4	200	1.5	33	0.5	23	8	1.7	346	261	22
	0	1.8	45	ND	40	8	ND	544	230	16
8	200	1.8	51	ND	95	33	3.8	1 150	–	–
	0	2.2	104	0.5	96	18	1.8	498	–	–
12	200	2.7	68	0.8	160	69	6.9	728	–	–
	0	2.8	105	0.8	627	28	2.1	336	–	–

[a] DNA collected from five animals
[b] DNA collected from 11 animals
[c] Expressed as $10^6 \times$ fraction of guanine (G)
[d] Incorporation of ^{14}C in guanine (G) (dpm/μmol)
ND, not detected

benzyl alcohol formation *in vivo* is, of course, not clear. Kraft *et al.* (1980) found in in-vivo experiments that NMBzA is metabolized predominantly to hippuric acid, which is formed from benzoic acid. No benzoic acid, however, was detected in the present in-vitro experiments. In livers from DSF-treated rats, benzaldehyde formation was slightly reduced.

Lung microsomes of rats that had not been pretreated did not contain reaction products of NMBzA, whereas microsomes of rats subjected to DSF pretreatment contained benzaldehyde. This finding can be interpreted to indicate that, despite DSF inhibition of overall (essentially hepatic) NMBzA metabolism, a specific concomitant induction of enzyme activity occurs in the lungs. Therefore, the pathological lesions that have been seen in the lungs (Bürkle *et al.*, this volume, p. 533) can be explained by the present biochemical finding that DSF pretreatment permits increased amounts of NMBzA to reach the lungs and be activated there to toxic metabolites.

Fig. 3. Effect of disulfiram (open symbols) on the formation of 7-methylguanine in DNA of liver and lungs at various times after administration of a single oral dose of 2.0 mg [$^{14}CH_3$]-*N*-nitroso-*N*-methylbenzylamine per kg body weight

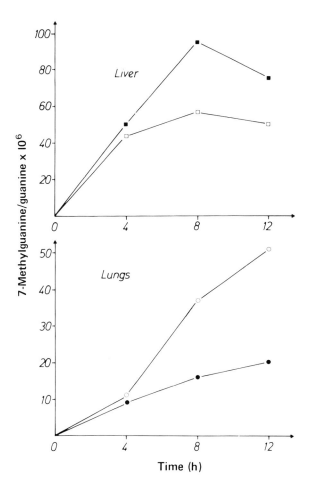

Alkylation of DNA in various organs

It can be seen from Table 2 that, 4 h after administration alkylation was highest in the oesophagus, the primary target organ of NMBzA in rats. This is in agreement with experiments of Hodgson *et al.* (1980) after intravenous injection of NMBzA. Pretreatment with DSF inhibited the degree of alkylation in the liver at all the time intervals investigated. No effect of DSF was apparent in the lungs 4 h after application of the carcinogen; 8 and 12 h after application, however, DSF induced a significant increase in DNA alkylation in this organ. This is displayed in Figure 3 for 7-methylguanine, in which the degree of alkylation in the lungs surpasses that in the liver after 12 h.

The enhanced incorporation of ^{14}C into guanine of lung DNA *via* the C_1 pool (8 h and 12 h, Table 2) can be explained by enhanced cell proliferation in this organ, as is convincingly demonstrated by morphological findings (see Bürkle *et al.*, this volume p. 533). The increased cell proliferation is presumably crucial for the carcinogenic process, for it fixes precancerous lesions, e.g., purine alkylation. As shown in Figure 3, alkylation in the liver decreases between 8 and 12 h after administration; this may be attributable to repair processes.

ACKNOWLEDGEMENT

This work was partly supported by the Deutsche Forschungsgemeinschaft, and Übelmesser-Passera-Stiftung. The authors thank Prof. P. Kleihues for stimulating discussions.

REFERENCES

Fiala, E.S. (1981) *Inhibition of carcinogen metabolism and action by disulfiram, pyrazole, and related compounds.* In: Zedeck, M.S. & Lipkin, M., eds, *Inhibition of tumor induction and development.* New York, Plenum Press, pp. 23–69

Hodgson, R.M., Wiessler, M. & Kleihues, P. (1980) Preferential methylation of target organ DNA by the oesophageal carcinogen *N*-nitrosomethylbenzylamine. *Carcinogenesis, 1,* 861–866

Irving, C.C., Tice, A.J. & Murphy, W.M. (1979) Inhibition of *N-n*-butyl-*N*-(4-hydroxy-butyl)nitrosamine-induced urinary bladder cancer in rats by administration of disulfiram in the diet. *Cancer Res., 39,* 3040–3043

Kraft, P.L., Skipper, P.L. & Tannenbaum, S.R. (1980) In vivo metabolism and whole-blood clearance of *N*-nitrosomethylbenzylamine in the rat. *Cancer Res., 40,* 2740–2742

Labuc, G.E. & Archer, M.C. (1982) Esophageal and hepatic microsomal metabolism of *N*-nitrosomethylbenzylamine and *N*-nitrosodimethylamine in the rat. *Cancer Res., 42,* 3181–3186

Lowry, O.H., Rosebrough, N.J., Farr, A.L. & Randall, R.J. (1951) Protein measurement with the Folin phenol reagent. *J. biol. Chem., 193,* 265–275

Schmähl, D., Krüger, F.W., Habs, M. & Diehl, B. (1976) Influence of disulfiram on the organotropy of the carcinogenic effect of dimethylnitrosamine and diethylnitrosamine in rats. *Z. Krebsforsch. klin. Onkol., 85,* 271–276

Schweinsberg, F. & Bürkle, V. (1981) Wirkung von Disulfiram auf die Toxizität von *N*-methyl-*N*-nitrosobenzylamin bei Ratten. *J. Cancer Res. clin. Oncol., 102,* 43–47

Schweinsberg, F. & Kouros, M. (1979) Reactions of *N*-methyl-*N*-nitrosobenzylamine and related substrates with enzyme-containing cell fractions isolated from various organs of rats and mice. *Cancer Lett., 7,* 115–120

Schweinsberg, F., Weissenberger, I. & Bürkle, V. (1982) *The effect of disulfiram on the carcinogenicity of nitrosamines.* In: Bartsch, H., O'Neill, I.K., Castegnaro, M. & Okada, M., eds, N-*Nitroso Compounds: Occurrence and Biological Effects (IARC Scientific Publications No. 41),* Lyon, International Agency for Research on Cancer, pp. 649–656

Selim, S. (1977) Separation and quantitative determination of traces of carbonyl compounds as their 2,4-dinitrophenylhydrazones by high-pressure liquid chromatography. *J. Chromatogr., 136,* 271–277

ROLE OF THE RESPIRATORY SYSTEM IN METABOLISM OF *N*-NITROSAMINES AFTER SIMULTANEOUS APPLICATION OF DISULFIRAM

V. BÜRKLE & H. WITTENBERG

Pathologisches Institut der Universität, Liebermeisterstrasse 8, 74, Tübingen, FRG

F. SCHWEINSBERG, I. WEISSENBERGER, E. SCHWEINSBERG & B. BRÜCKNER

Hygiene Institut der Universität, Liebermeisterstrasse 8, 74, Tübingen, FRG

SUMMARY

Subsequent to modification of *N*-nitrosamine metabolism by disulfiram, mucus-producing cells and Clara cells in the respiratory tract are involved increasingly in detoxification as well as in bioactivation of *N*-nitroso-*N*-methylbenzylamine and *N*-nitrosodibutylamine. Overtaxing of these cells or local concentration of antigenic metabolites leads to cytolytic defects in tracheal, bronchial and bronchiolar epithelium, in addition to toxic degenerative lesions. The resulting continuous stimulation of proliferation leads to basal-cell hyperplasia, squamous-cell metaplasia and squamous papillomas. In areas with insufficient differentiation, due to cell proliferation, there is an increased probability that focal mutation, subsequent to alkylation of purine bases, will be passed from one cell generation to the next, with subsequent formation of tumours in the bronchiolo-alveolar region.

INTRODUCTION

One possible means of inhibiting toxification of cancer noxae to their ultimate carcinogenic form is to modify their enzyme-dependent metabolism. The inhibitory action of disulfiram (tetraethylthiuramdisulfide, DSF), used commercially in processing of natural and synthetic rubbers and medically in the treatment of alcoholism, is well documented (Fiala, 1981). Reduced tumour formation in the respective target organs and alterations of the carcinogenic organotropic effect have been reported as a result of the simultaneous application of DSF with *N*-nitrosodimethylamine or *N*-nitrosodiethylamine (Schmähl *et al.*, 1976), *N*-nitroso-*n*-butyl(4-hydroxybutyl)amine (Irving *et al.*, 1979), *N*-nitrosomethylacetoxymethylamine (Habs *et al.*, 1981) and *N*-nitrosodibutylamine (NDBA) (Schweinsberg *et al.*, 1982). Our own observations indicate that the toxicity of *N*-nitroso-*N*-methylbenzylamine (NMBzA) is increased by the simultaneous oral application of DSF. We found, furthermore, that toxic-degenerative lesions and numerous proliferative, metaplastic and dysplastic alterations were produced in the respiratory tract of the rat (Schweinsberg & Bürkle, 1981). Peripheral lung tumours are induced in the rat by the simultaneous application of *N*-nitrosodibutylamine and DSF (Schweinsberg *et al.*, 1982). It thus appears likely that the respiratory tract plays an essential role in nitrosamine metabolism, subsequent to administration of DSF. In the present paper, the morphological evidence for this notion is collected, analysed histogenetically and integrated into an overall concept of pathogenesis.

MATERIALS AND METHODS

Chemicals

DSF was obtained from Fluka, Buchs (Switzerland); NMBzA from EMKA-Chemie, Markgröningen (FRG) and NDBA from Serva, Heidelberg (FRG).

Animals and treatment

A total of 142 female, SIV-50 rats (Ivanovas, Kisslegg, FRG) were used. DSF was administered simultaneously to 87 animals with one of the carcinogens, NMBzA or NDBA, as shown in Table 1.

Preparation and examination

The respiratory organs of animals that died spontaneously were filled *in situ* with buffered 4% formaldehyde solution *via* the trachea and subsequently dissected in a block. Regular histological processing was performed on 3–5 μm whole-ring segments of the upper, middle and lower trachea, extrapulmonary stem bronchi and on several longitudinal sections of the left lung. Staining was carried out using haematoxylin-eosin, periodic acid-schiff, Giemsa and Evans blue.

Each week after the onset of treatment, four animals from group A were killed with an overdose of Thiogenal[R] and exsanguinated *via* the abdominal aorta. The pressure-controlled perfused organs (2 % glutaraldehyde solution in 0.1 mol/L cacodylate buffer; pH 7.4; 180 mosm) were dissected as a block and further immersed (glutaraldehyde/formaldehyde mixture; pH 7.4). The respiratory organs were prepared as described above. In addition, regions of the trachea and stem bronchi selected under the macroscope (Zeiss, Tessovar) were examined by Raster electron microscopy (Leitz, AMR 1000). Regions of interest were embedded in Araldite[R]. One-μm thick sections were prepared and examined, subsequent to staining with toluidine-blue and haematoxylin-eosin.

Table 1.   Treatment of animals

Group	Number of effective animals	Dosage of *N*-nitros-amine in drinking-water (mg/L)	Dosage of disulfiram in diet (mg/kg)
A	44	10 (NMBzA)	200
B	8	5 (NMBzA)	200
C	8	2,5 (NMBzA)	200
D[a]	30	–	200
E[a]	25	750 (NDBzA)	–
F[a]	27	750 (NDBzA)	200

[a] As reported by Schweinsberg *et al.* (1982)

RESULTS

The animals of Group A (NMBzA and DSF) were killed at the intervals designated above, after the onset of simultaneous administration. The animals of group B and C (reduced dosage of NMBzA) were killed after eight months. Oesophageal tumours were found in all animals. The death rate and alterations in the primary target organs of NDBA in the rat have already been reported (Schweinsberg *et al.*, 1982).

Group A

Macroscopic lesions were not apparent before three weeks after the onset of simultaneous administration of NMBzA and DSF. Light microscopy showed alterations in the trachea, stem bronchi and lobar bronchi. In these regions of the respiratory tract, increasingly fewer mucus-producing cells were encountered, and the rest of the epithelium became thinner. Adjacent to dilatated capillaries in the lamina propria, focal intercellular contact was abolished, although most epithelia still adhered to the basal lamina. Individual cell necrosis caused expansion of intraepithelial cavities, which were sealed off from the lumen in an arched-shaped fashion by pleomorphic epithelia (Figs 1 and 2). Part of the basal lamina disappeared, subsequent to an oedema and infiltration by mononuclear and polymorphonuclear cells of subepithelial and peribronchial tissue. Focal microerosions and tiny ulcerations appeared in areas with reduced thickness of epitehelium. In the immediate vicinity of such lesions, as well as in areas low in goblet cells, we found basal cells with frequent mitotic figures, followed by focal basal-cell proliferation. Transitional-cell hyperplasia, nonkeratinizing, and later keratinizing, squamous metaplasias occurred as early as the third week of exposure in the pars membranacea, then later in the entire trachea and the proximal bronchial branches. Micropapillary folding of metaplastic epithelium and squamous papillomas were observed at week 4 and up to the end of the experiment (Fig. 3).

Subsequent to the expanded metaplastic alterations in proximal bronchi, cubic epithelium of small bronchial branches was replaced by thicker hyperplastic epithelium. In addition, an

Fig. 1. Circumscript vacuolar degeneration in bronchial epithelium; *N*-nitroso-*N*-methylbenzylamine + disulfiram; haematoxylin and eosin

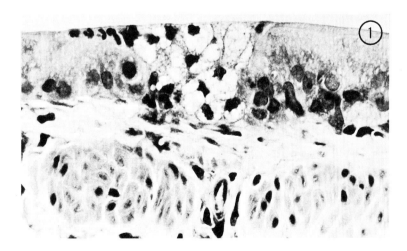

536   BÜRKLE *ET AL.*

Fig. 2. Dissociation of necrobiotic cells in bronchial epithelium and infiltration by inflammatory cells; *N*-nitroso-*N*-methylbenzylamine + disulfiram; semi-thin section; haematoxylin and eosin

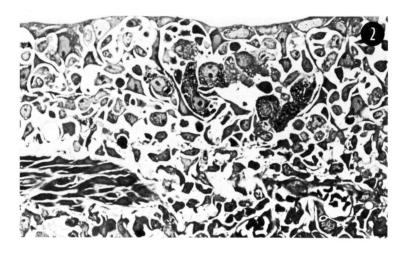

Fig. 3. Papilloma formation in the trachea and squamous metaplasia; *N*-nitroso-*N*-methylbenzylamine + disulfiram; Raster electron microscopy; x 170

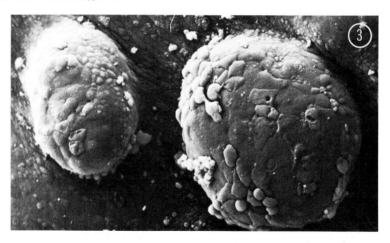

increase in goblet cells, partly with bizarrely-clumped periodic acid-Schiff positive contents and bloated cell bodies, appeared, as well as intraepithelial mucus cysts after destruction of their cell borders (Fig. 4). There was also an expansion of peribronchial lymphatic tissue, ending at the level of the most distally situated mucus-producing cell. Basal cells proliferated progressively to individual bronchioles. Squamous metaplasias, sometimes with disturbed polarity and stratification of cells and with chromatin-dense heteromorphic nuclei, followed. Proliferation of basal cells and squamous epithelium raised intact ciliated cells and forced them into the lumen (Fig. 5). Mucus backed up into the bronchioles and in some cases overflowed

Fig. 4. Intraepithelial mucus-cyst formation; *N*-nitroso-*N*-methylbenzylamine + disulfiram; haematoxylin and eosin

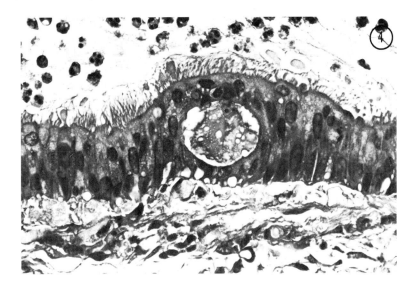

Fig. 5. Basal-cell proliferation raising intact epithelium; *N*-nitroso-*N*-methylbenzylamine + disulfiram; haematoxylin and eosin

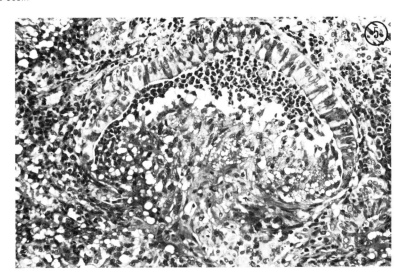

into the alveolar space. The epithelial lining of the terminal bronchioles remained intact for a long time, although Clara-cell hyperplasia appeared to develop. Toward the end of the experiment, cell vacuolization increased; necrobiotic cells were ejected into the lumen. Fibrolast-like cells, collagen fibres and inflammatory cells budded into the resulting defects and obliterated many bronchiolar lumens (Fig. 6). The capillary-rich connective tissue frequently cut off metaplastically altered islands of epithelium. In the vicinity of small pulmonary vessels, pervasive inflammatory infiltration occurred occasionally during the first week of exposure, and began in the seventh experimental week in all animals.

Fig. 6. Obstructive bronchiolitis; *N*-nitroso-*N*-methylbenzylamine + disulfiram; haematoxylin and eosin

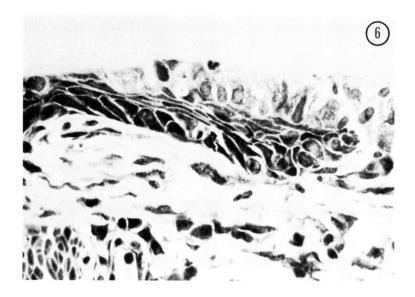

Fig. 7. Centrally necrotic squamous-cell carcinoma

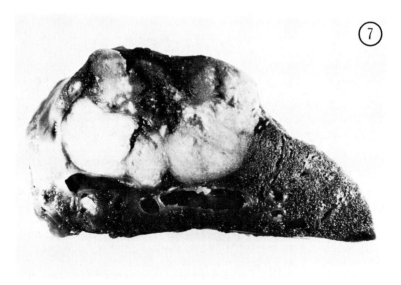

Groups B and C

The characteristic findings in the proximal airways, subsequent to simultaneous application, were less pronounced than in the earlier experiment (Schweinsberg & Bürkle, 1981). In contrast, mucus-producing cell hyperplasia progressed well into bronchioles. In addition to severely obstructive bronchiolitis, numerous infected bronchiectases were observed.

Groups D, E and F

Group F (NDBA and DSF) revealed alterations similar to those observed in group A. Besides squamous-cell papillomas in the trachea and extended squamous-cell metaplasias in the bronchi, well delimited nodes or poorly-defined masses within a lobe were observed in the bronchiolo-alveolar regions (Fig. 7). They were identified histologically as variously differentiated squamous-cell carcinomas, adenomas or adenocarcinomas. Individual tumours consisted of both adenoid and squamous structures. With the exception of slight peribronchial lymphatic tissue hyperplasia, the respiratory organs in group D (DSF) appeared normal. Animals in group E (NDBA) revealed no alterations in the respiratory organs.

DISCUSSION

NMBzA selectively induces oesophageal and pharyngeal tumours in rats. Application of NDBA leads to tumour formation in the liver, bladder and oesophagus (Druckrey *et al.*, 1967). The organ-specific effect of NMBzA has been attributed to a preference for bioactivation in the oesophagus (Schweinsberg & Kouros, 1979; Hodgson *et al.*, 1980; Labuc & Archer, 1982). Comparable mechanisms may be assumed with regard to the metabolism of NDMA, as is the case with most *N*-nitrosamines (Preussmann, 1981; Weisburger & Williams, 1982). Activation to the ultimate carcinogen is carried out partly by cytochrome-P-450-dependent mixed-function oxidases (MFO). DSF depresses this activity, in microsomes.

The amount of aldehyde formed, exhalation studies and determinations of the biological half-life of NMBzA indicate that the metabolism of NMBzA in the liver is inhibited by DSF (Schweinsberg *et al.*, this volume p. 525). Furthermore, four hours after administration of [$^{14}CH_3$]-NMBzA simultaneously with DSF, less N7-methylguanine and O^6-methylguanine is found in liver tissue than is the case when the *N*-nitrosamine is administered alone.

The alterations in the respiratory tract are strong indications that modification of hepatic metabolism increases the demands placed on organs subsequently involved in the metabolism and elimination of the carcinogen and its metabolites, and in particular on the respiratory tract. Indeed. the amount of N7- and O^6-methylguanine increases eight hours after application of labelled NMBzA in pulmonary tissue under the influence of DSF (Schweinsberg *et al.*, this volume, p. 525). Since mucus-producing cells and Clara cells are the apparent site of cytochrome-P-450-dependent monooxygenase activity (Boid, 1977; Reznik-Schüller & Hague, 1981), the increased demands placed on them lead to their hyperplasia after the beginning of exposure. Local accumulation of alkylation products and of aldehyde, which are produced in equimolar amounts leads to the cell necroses described above. Comparable alterations and squamous carcinomas in the perinasal sinuses of the rat were induced by inhalation of high concentrations of formaldehyde (Swenberg *et al.*, 1980; Boreiko *et al.* 1982). Schmähl *et al.* (1976) also observed tumours in this region under the influence of *N*-nitrosodiethylamine, of *N*-nitrosodimethylamine and DSF, Furthermore, as in all lymphoepithelial structures, hyperplasia of the peribronchial lymphatic system goes hand in hand with 'dedifferentiation' of the associated epithelium. When hyperplasia is excessive, undifferentiated cells appear at the points of intersection with epithelium, and like numerous mucus-producing cells, they also succumb to vacuolar degeneration and subsequent cytolytic necrosis. Potential inducers of hyperplasia could be antigenic components and products of mucus-producing cells. This notion is also supported by the observation of hilifugal extension of goblet cells and the confluent hyperplastic lymph follicules. A certain amount of modified mucus is produced even after the application of DSF alone, because expansion of the 'lung tonsil' is also observed in this experimental group. The extension of mucus-producing cells to the bronchioles, histologically detectable modification of mucus production and the metaplasia-induced reduction of ciliated cells lead to disturbed mucociliary clearance. The result is development of bronchiectases. Reparative-regeneratory proliferation of basal cells occurs in response to epithelial micronecroses. Continued stimulation of proliferation leads to the development of excessive basal-cell and squamous metaplasias, as well as squamous papillomas in proximal airways. When the necrosis extends distally beyond the basal membrane, alterations typical of obstructive bronchiolitis develop in the periphery. The proliferative alterations represent cell populations with reduced ability to eliminate alkylated DNA bases, and thus the probability of passing mutations on to the following cell generations is increased. These alterations probably play the role of a 'promoting environment', because lung tumours develop in some of these regenerative regions.

The present work reveals that *N*-nitrosamines can exert a carcinogenic effect on the lungs subsequent to modification of the metabolism of those carcinogens by xenobiotics. The significance of these findings seems to be worthy of discussion, because of the increasing rate of bronchial carcinomas in man.

ACKNOWLEDGEMENT

This work was supported by the Deutsche Forschungsgemeinschaft.

REFERENCES

Boreiko, C.J., Couch, D.B. & Swenberg, J.A. (1982) *Mutagenic and carcinogenic effects of formaldehyde.* In: Tice, R.R., Costa, D.L. & Schaich, K.M., eds, *Genotoxic Effects of Airborne Agents*, New York, Plenum Press, pp. 353–367

Boyd, M.R. (1977) Evidence for the Clara cell as a site of cytochrome P 450-dependend mixed-function oxidase activity in the lungs. *Nature, 269*, 713–715

Druckrey, H., Preussmann, R., Ivankovic, S. & Schmähl, D. (1967) Organotrope carcinogene Wirkungen bei 65 verschiedenen *N*-Nitrosoverbindungen an BD-Ratten. *Z. Krebsforsch., 69*, 103–201

Fiala, E.S. (1981) *Inhibition of carcinogen metabolism and action by disulfiram, pyrazole, and related compounds.* In: Zedeck, M.S. & Lipkin, M., eds, *Inhibiton of Tumor Induction and Development*, New York, Plenum Press, pp. 23–69

Habs, M., Schmähl, D. & Kretzer, H. (1981) Effect of disulfiram on acetoxy-methyl-methyl-nitrosamine-induced tumors in rats. *Oncology, 38*, 18–22

Hodgson, R.M., Wiessler, M. & Kleihues, P. (1980) Preferential methylation of target organ DNA by the oesophageal carcinogen *N*-nitrosomethyl-benzylamine. *Carcinogenesis, 1*, 861–866

Irving, C.C., Tice, A.J. & Murphy, W.M. (1979) Inhibition of *N-n*-butyl-*N*-(4-hydroxybutyl)-nitrosamine-induced urinary bladder cancer in rats by administration of disulfiram in the diet. *Cancer Res., 39*, 3040–3043

Labuc, G.E. & Archer, M.C. (1982) Esophageal and hepatic microsomal metabolism of *N*-nitroso-methylbenzylamine and *N*-nitrosodimethylamine in the rat. *Cancer Res., 42*, 3181–3186

Preussmann, R. (1981) *Pharmakologie und biochemischer Wirkmechanismus chemischer Cancerogene.* In: Schmähl, D., ed., *Maligne Tumoren. Entstehung, Wachstum, Chemotherapie*, Aulendorf, Editio Cantor, pp. 221–250

Reznik-Schüller, H.M. & Hague, B.F., Jr (1981) Autoradiographic study of the distribution of bound radioactivity in the respiratory tract of Syrian hamsters given N-^{3}H-nitrosodiethylamine. *Cancer Res.*, *41*, 2147–2150

Schmähl, D., Krüger, F.W. Habs, M. & Diehl, B. (1976) Influence of disulfiram on the organotropy of the carcinogenic effect of dimethylnitrosamine and diethylnitrosamine in rats. *Z. Krebsforsch.*, *85*, 271–276

Schweinsberg, F. & Bürkle, V. (1981) Wirkung von Disulfiram auf die Toxizität und Carcinogenität von N-Methyl-N-nitrosobenzylamin bei Ratten. *J. Cancer Res. clin. Oncol, 102*, 43–47

Schweinsberg, F. & Kouros, M. (1979) Reactions of N-methyl-N-nitrosobenzylamine and related substrates with enzyme-containing cell fractions isolated from various organs of rats and mice. *Cancer Lett., 7*, 115–120

Schweinsberg, F., Weissenberger, I. & Bürkle, V. (1982) *The effect of disulfiram on the carcinogenicity of nitrosamines.* In: Bartsch, H., O'Neill, I.K., Castegnaro, M. & Okada, M., eds, N-*Nitroso Compounds: Occurrence and Biological Effects (IARC Scientific Publications No. 41)*, Lyon, International Agency for Research on Cancer, pp. 649–657

Swenberg, J.A., Kerns, W.D., Mitchell, R.I., Gralla, E.J. & Pavkov, k.L. (1980) Induction of squamous cell carcinomas of the rat nasal cavity by inhalation exposure to formaldehyde vapor. *Cancer Res., 40*, 3398–3402

Weisburger, J.h. & Williams, G.M. (1982) *Metabolism of chemical carcinogens.* In: Becker, F., ed., *Cancer I: A Comprehensive Treatise*, 2nd ed., New York, Plenum Press, pp. 241–333

N-NITROSODIMETHYLAMINE-INDUCED FORESTOMACH TUMOURS IN MALE SPRAGUE-DAWLEY RATS FED A ZINC-DEFICIENT DIET

L.Y.Y. FONG[1]

Department of Biochemistry, University of Hong Kong, Hong Kong

W.L. NG

Department of Pathology, University of Hong Kong, Hong Kong

P.M. NEWBERNE

Department of Nutrition and Food Science, Massachusetts Institute of Technology, Cambridge, MA, USA

SUMMARY

Fifty-one zinc-deficient rats and 46 zinc-sufficient, pair-fed controls were administered N-nitrosodimethylamine intragastrically at a dose level of 2 mg/kg body weight, twice weekly for three weeks, followed by 4 mg/kg body weight of the same carcinogen twice weekly for another five weeks. After 45 weeks, none of the control rats had developed epithelial abnormalities in the oesophagus or forestomach or any lesion in other tissues. Oesophageal epithelial hyperkeratosis was detected in all zinc-deficient rats, but no tumour was found. Hyperkeratosis and acanthosis were found in the forestomach of 100% and 88%, respectively, of the zinc-deficient rats; 63% of the zinc-deficient rats also developed squamous papillomas in the forestomach.

INTRODUCTION

We demonstrated earlier that dietary zinc-deficiency increased the incidence of and shortened the lag time of N-nitroso-N-methylbenzylamine (NMBzA)-induced oesophageal tumours in rats (Fong *et al.*, 1978). Furthermore, we showed that zinc-deficient rats fed only the precursors of the carcinogen NMBzA also had a higher incidence of oesophageal-forestomach tumours (Fong *et al.*, 1982). Dietary zinc deficiency *per se* is known to cause hyperplasia and parakeratosis in the oesophagus (Diamond & Hurley, 1970; Follis, 1966); however, oral administration of NMBzA and endogenously-formed NMBzA from precursors have been found to induce only oesophageal tumours (Sander *et al.*, 1968; Stinson *et al.*, 1978). It is not known if this dietary deficiency has a strictly organ-specific effect. The present communication reports preliminary data on the effect of dietary zinc deficiency on tumour induction by a non-oesophageal carcinogen, N-nitrosodimethylamine (NDMA) in rats.

---

[1] To whom correspondence should be addressed

EXPERIMENTAL

Animals and diet

Male, non-inbred, Sprague-Dawley rats (21 days old, Laboratory Animal Unit, University of Hong Kong) were distributed randomly in plastic cages. They were given deionized water and fed either an EDTA-washed, soya bean-protein based zinc-deficient diet containing approximately 7 mg/kg of diet zinc or a control diet supplemented with 100 mg/kg of diet zinc (Fong *et al.*, 1978). The deficient diet resulted in a chronic rather than acute lethal deficiency. Treated rats were fed the deficient diet *ad libitum*, while the control rats were pair-fed the zinc-sufficient diet with the deficient rats. They were given their respective diets for five weeks before NDMA treatment.

Tumorigenesis studies

Beginning at eight weeks of age, 51 zinc-deficient and 46 pair-fed, control rats were administered six doses of NDMA (Tokyo Kasie Kogyo Co. Ltd, Tokyo) dissolved in deionized water, intragastrically at a dose of 2 mg/kg body weight, twice weekly, followed by a dose of 4 mg/kg body weight, twice weekly for another five weeks. The rats were killed when moribund. The first death occurred at the tenth week and all the rats were killed at week 45. One control rat was always sacrificed when a zinc-deficient rat was killed. Complete necropsies were performed; the major organs were fixed in 10% neutral buffered formalin and processed for pathohistological examination.

RESULTS AND DISCUSSION

None of the rats in the pair-fed control group developed significant epithelial abnormalities in the oesophagus or the forestomach, and no lesion was seen elsewhere.

Epithelial changes, in the form of mild to moderate hyperkeratosis, were present in the oesophagi of all animals in the zinc-deficient group. In addition, mild to moderate acanthosis was observed in 24 animals and focal parakeratosis on 16 animals. None, however, showed an oesophageal epithelial tumour. Significant epithelial lesions, as detailed in Table 1, were present in the forestomachs of the experimental animals; these included epithelial hyperkeratosis, acanthosis, parakeratosis, dyskeratosis, mucosal erosions and ulcerations. Squamous papillomas were found in the forestomachs of 32 animals, located most commonly along the junctions between the fore- and glandular stomachs, where they appeared as warty discontinuous lesions (Fig. 1). In 12 animals, nodular papillomas were also seen in the more proximal parts of the forestomach (Fig. 2). Histologically, verrucous and fibroepithelial types of squamous papillomas were identified (Fig. 3). The former corresponded to the warty lesions found along the junctions and the latter to more peripheral nodular lesions. Focal mild epithelial dysplastic changes were also seen in 13 verrucous papillomas. There was, however, no evidence of malignancy. Apart from multiple mesenchymal hamartomas seen in both kidneys of one animal, there was no significant change in other organs of these animals.

These findings demonstrate that NDMA, at a total dose of 52 mg/kg body weight administered intragastrically, was tumorigenic to zinc-deficient rats after 45 weeks but not to pair-fed, zinc-sufficient controls. Another interesting result of our investigation is that NDMA, a non-oesophageal, non-forestomach carcinogen in rats (Magee *et al.*, 1976), when administered by this regimen and route, produced only squamous papillomas in the forestomach of the zinc-deficient rats.

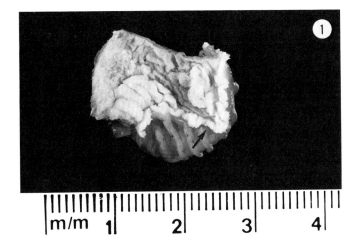

Fig. 1. Forestomach of zinc-deficient eat fed N-nitrosodimethylamine, showing irregular warty
papillomatous lesion (arrow)
along junction between fore-
and glandular stomachs

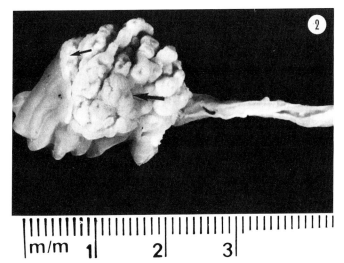

Fig. 2. Forestomach of zinc-deficient rat fed N-nitrosodimethylamine, showing discontinuous
junctional warty papillomatous
lesion (short arrow) and peripheral nodular lesion (long arrow)

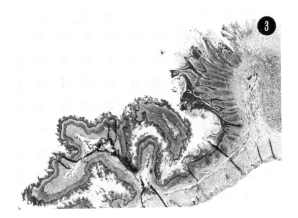

Fig. 3. Forestomach of zinc-deficient rat fed
N-nitrosodimethylamine, showing junctional
verrucous squamous papilloma and more
peripheral fibroepithelial squamous papilloma
(haematoxylin and eosin, × 17,5)

Table 1. Histopathology of forestomach of zinc-deficient rats Fed *N*-nitrosodimethylamine

Lesion	Number of rats (%)
Epithelial changes	
hyperkeratosis	51 (100)
acanthosis	45 (88)
focal parakeratosis	9 (18)
focal dyskeratosis	5 (10)
erosion/ulceration	9 (18)
Tumours	
junctional	19
junctional & other areas	13
Total	32 (63)

In view of the fact that dietary zinc deficiency occurs in several populations among whom there is a high incidence of oesophageal cancer, as in certain parts of South Africa (van Rensburg, 1981), our data are of more than routine interest.

ACKNOWLEDGEMENT

This work was supported by a research grant from the University of Hong Kong, and by Hoffmann-La Roche of Nutley, NJ, USA.

REFERENCES

Diamond, I. & Hurley, L.S. (1970) Histopathology of zinc-deficient fetal rats. *J. Nutr., 100,* 325–329

Follis, R.H., Jr (1966) *The pathology of zinc deficiency.* In: Prasad, A.S., ed., *Zinc Metabolism,* Springfield, IL, C.C. Thomas, pp. 129–141

Fong, L.Y.Y., Sivak, A. & Newberne, P.M. (1978) Zinc Deficiency and methylbenzylnitrosamine-induced esophageal cancer in rats. *J. natl Cancer Inst., 61,* 145–150

Fong, L.Y.Y., Lee, J.S.K., Chan, W.C. & Newberne, P.M. (1982) *Zinc deficiency and the induction of oesophageal tumours in rats by benzylmethylamine and sodium nitrite.* In: Bartsch, H., O'Neill, I.K., Castegnaro, M. & Okada, M., eds, N-*Nitroso Compounds: Occurrence and Biological Effects (IARC Scientific Publications No. 41).* Lyon, International Agency for Research on Cancer, pp. 679–683

Magee, P.N., Montesano, R. & Preussmann, R. (1976) N-*Nitroso compounds and related carcinogens.* Searle, C.E., ed., *Chemical Carcinogens (ACS Monograph No. 173),* Washington, DC, American Chemical Society, pp. 491–625

van Rensburg, S.J. (1981) Epidemiological and dietary evidence for a specific nutritional predisposition to esophageal cancer. *J. natl Cancer Inst., 67,* 243–251

Sander, J., Schweinsberg, F. & Menz, H.P. (1968) Untersuchungen über die Entstehung cancerogener Nitrosamine im Magen. *Hoppe-Seyler's Z. physiol. Chem., 349,* 1691–1697

Stinson, S.F., Squire, R.A. & Sporn, M.B. (1978) Pathology of esophageal neoplasms and associated proliferative lesions induced in rats by *N*-methyl-*N*-benzylnitrosamine. *J. natl Cancer Inst., 61,* 1471–1475

EFFECT OF ASCORBIC ACID AND SOME REDUCING AGENTS ON N-NITROSOPIPERIDINE METABOLISM BY LIVER MICROSOMES

M. NAKAMURA & Y. HORIGUCHI

Department of Food and Drug Science, Kanagawa Prefectural Public Health Laboratory, 52-2 Nakao-cho, Asahi-ku, Yokohama 241, Japan

T. KAWABATA

Department of Biomedical Research on Food, National Institute of Health, 2-10-35 Kamiosaki, Shinagawa-ku, Tokyo 141, Japan

SUMMARY

The effect of ascorbic acid on the oxidation of N-nitrosopiperidine by a microsomal preparation obtained from guinea-pig liver has been examined. The metabolites from the oxidation of N-nitrosopiperidine were found to be 5-hydroxypentanal (about 1.93%), N-nitroso-3-hydroxypiperidine (about 0.02%), and N-nitroso-4-hydroxypiperidine (about 0.15%). With microsomes separated from the liver of guinea-pigs pretreated with phenobarbital and 3-methylcholranthrene, the yields of N-nitroso-3-hydroxypiperidine and N-nitroso-4-hydroxypiperidine were found to decrease upon increasing the concentration of ascorbic acid in the reaction mixture. In the presence of small amounts of ascorbic acid, the yields of these compounds with untreated liver microsomes apparently increased, while the presence of larger amounts of ascorbic acid caused a decrease in the yields of these metabolites. In contrast with the yields of N-nitroso-3-hydroxypiperidine and N-nitroso-4-hydroxy-piperidine, that of 5-hydroxypentanal decreased with increasing amounts of ascorbic acid.

INTRODUCTION

N-Nitrosopiperidine (NPIP) is known to be a potent carcinogen, causing tumours of the oesophagus, pharynx and nasal cavity in the rat when administered intravenously and subcutaneously, and of the liver and oesophagus of the rat when added to its drinking-water. In the hamster, it causes tumours of the lung when administered subcutaneously. In the presence of rat liver metabolic activating systems, NPIP has been shown to be mutagenic towards *Salmonella typhimurium* (Rao *et al.*, 1977). Metabolism of NPIP by a microsomal preparation from rat liver was shown to yield 5-hydroxypentanal (Leung *et al.*, 1978) or N-nitroso-4-hydroxypiperidine (4-OH-NPIP) Rayman *et al.*, 1974). Gilbert *et al.* (1982) have shown that 5-hydroxypentanal was immediately metabolized by cytosolic enzymes into

5-hydroxy-pentanoic acid and 1,5-pentanediol. However, Guttenplan (1977) reported that bacterial mutation by *N*-methyl-*N'*-nitro-*N*-nitrosoguanidine and *N*-nitrosodimethylamine was inhibited by ascorbate and other biological compounds. The aim of the present study was to investigate the rate of biotransformation of NPIP into 5-hydroxypentanal, *N*-nitroso-3-hydroxypiperidine (3-OH-NPIP) and 4-OH-NPIP in the presence of a liver microsome fraction obtained from guinea-pigs which cannot synthesize ascorbic acid (AsA) and to investigate the effect of AsA and some reducing agents on the metabolism of NPIP.

MATERIALS AND METHODS

Chemicals

NPIP, 3-OH-NPIP and 4-OH-NPIP were synthesized by nitrosation of the corresponding secondary amines, as described by Rayman *et al.* (1974). 5-Hydroxypentanal was obtained from Aldrich Chemical Co., while monosodium glucose-6-phosphate, disodium NADP and glucose-6-dehydrogenase (grade 1) were obtained from Boehringer Mannheim, Co. (FRG). All other reagents were of the purest grades available.

Treatment of animals

Male guinea-pigs (Hartley, 250–300 g) were used and maintained on a commercial feed (Nippon Crea Co. Ltd, Tokyo) and water *ad libitum*. Cytochrome P-450-dependent enzymes were induced by a five-day pretreatment with 0.1% sodium phenobarbital (PB) in the drinking-water, and a single intraperitoneal injection of 80 mg/kg 3-methylcholanthrene (MC) in corn oil. Control animals received tap water or corn oil (5 mg/kg) instead of the PB or MC, respectively, received by the test group.

Preparation of microsomes

All animals were killed by decapitation 24 h after the last treatment. After bleeding, livers were rapidly removed, washed and minced in ice-cold 1.15% potassium chloride (buffered with 0.1 mol/L potassium phosphate buffer, pH 7.4), then homogenized with three volumes of potassium chloride solution in a Potter-Elvehjem homogenizer. The homogenate was centrifuged at $9\,000 \times g$ for 20 min, and the supernatant was recentrifuged at $105\,000 \times g$ for 60 min. The pellet was washed with ice-cold 0.1 mol/L potassium phosphate buffer (pH 7.4) and re-sedimented ($105\,000 \times g$, 60 min). This microsomal fraction was suspended in a small amount of buffer solution and stored at $-80\,°C$ until use.

The protein content was determined according to the method of Lowry *et al.* (1951). Cytochrome P-450 was determined by the method of Omura and Sato (1964) using the CO-difference spectra of dithionite-reduced microsomes (450–490 nm) and an absorption coefficient of 91 cm²/μmol.

Incubation

Incubation was carried out at 37 °C for 120 min under air in stopped conical flasks. Each flask contained the following components in a final volume of 20 mL: 0.9 mL microsomal suspension (3 g wet-weight liver); 0.1 mol/L potassium phosphate buffer, pH 7.4, and a NADPH-generating system consisting of 60 μmol magnesium chloride, 120 μmol niacin, 12 μmol monosodium NADP, 120 μmol monosodium glucose-6-phosphate and 12 Units of glucose-6-phosphate dehydrogenase. To start the reaction, 20 mg (0.175 mmol) NPIP and various reducing agents were added. To ensure reaction throughout the incubation, the microsome and co-factors were added in these equal portions, at the start of incubation and then at 30 and 60 min. As a control, the microsomal preparation was boiled for 10 min prior to the experiment. After 120 min, reaction was terminated by the addition of 3 mL 20% zinc sulfate, followed by 3 mL saturated barium hydroxide and centrifugation at 2 500 × *g* for 10 min. The supernatant was extracted with ethyl acetate (3 × 30 mL). The combined extracts, concentrated to 1.0 mL, were examined by gas chromatography (GC) and gas chromatography-mass spectrometry (GC-MS).

Identification and determination of metabolites

GC-MS was performed with a Shimadzu LKB-9000-type mass spectrometer. Metabolites were identified by GC-MS (by comparison with authentic 4-OH-NPIP and 5-hydroxypentanal), followed by thin-layer chromatography of 2,4-dinitropenylhydrazone derivatives. The very small amounts of 3-OH-NPIP and 4-OH-NPIP were determined by MS monitoring at m/z = 130, 100, 71 and 30, and at 130, 113, 100 and 30, respectively. The absence of a peak at m/z = 113 was used as an aid to the identification of 3-OH-NPIP, GC-MS operating conditions were as follows: column, 2 m × 3 mm id, packed with 3% silicon OV-17 on Uniport HP (80–100 mesh); column temperature, 150 °C; injection temperature, 210 °C; separator temperature, 250 °C; ion source temperature, 270 °C; carrier gas (He) flow rate, 40 mL/min; electron energy, 70 eV.

The spectrum of 5-hydroxypentanal was monitored at m/z = 102, 101 and 84. GC-MS operating conditions were the same as described above, except for the column packing (2% PEG 20M on Chromosorb, WHP, 80–100 mesh) and the column temperature (80 °C). The fairly large amounts of 5-hydroxypentanal formed by metabolism were determined by GC. The GC operating conditions employed were almost the same as those for GC-MS.

In order to confirm the presence of 5-hydroxypentanal, the protein-free incubate mixture was reacted with 2,4-dinitrophenylhydrazine to yield the 2,4-dinitrophenylhydrazone derivative, as described by Leung *et al.* (1978). The 2,4-dinitrophenylhydrazone derivative formed was extracted with ethyl acetate and concentrated under reduced pressure. The product was examined by thin-layer chromatography with a pre-coated plate (silica gel 60 F_{254}, Merck) which was developed in toluene : ethyl acetate (75:25 and 1:1). The 2,4-dinitrophenylhydrazone derivative was identified directly by its yellow colour or under ultraviolet light at 254 nm.

RESULTS AND DISCUSSION

As shown in Table 1, 5-hydroxypentanal, 3-OH-NPIP and 4-OH-NPIP were detected as metabolites of NPIP with guinea-pig liver microsomes as well as with rat liver microsomes. In guinea-pig, 5-hydroxypentanal was the major metabolite (about 1.93%), and the yields of 3-OH-NPIP and 4-OH-NPIP were 0.02% and 0.15%, respectively. The amount of 3-OH-NPIP in rats was 5.7 times greater than that found with the guinea-pig microsomes.

PB and MC, enzyme inducers, increased the cytochrome P-450 concentration of the liver microsomes. The cytochrome P-450 content of the liver microsomes induced by PB was found to be greater than that induced by MC. While the levels of 5-hydroxypentanal and 4-OH-NPIP tended to increase in liver microsomes of guinea-pigs treated with PB, the 3-OH-NPIP content tended to decrease. It was also found that 5-hydroxypentanal and 3-OH-NPIP tended to increase in liver microsomes of guinea-pigs treated with MC. Furthermore, the amount of

4-OH-NPIP detected was as high as in microsomes of untreated guinea-pigs; however, there was no significant correlation between the content of induced cytochrome P-450 and the rate of formation of metabolites by enzymatic hydroxylation of NPIP.

As shown in Figure 1A, the higher the AsA concentration in uninduced liver microsomes, the greater the observed inhibition of 5-hydroxypentanal formation from NPIP. The rate of 5-hydroxypentanal formation from NPIP by liver microsomes treated with PB was greater than

Table 1.   Comparison of *N*-nitrosopiperidine (NPIP) metabolism by liver microsomes induced by pheno-barbital (PB) and 3-methylcholanthrene (MC) [a]

Animal	Inducer	Cytochrome P-450 content (nmol/mg protein)	Yield of metabolites of NPIP (%)		
			5-Hydroxy-pentanal	3-OH-NPIP	4-OH-NPIP
Guinea-pig (Hartley, ♂)	none [b]	0.58	1.93	0.020	0.145
	PB	1.34	2.40	0.017	0.196
	corn oil [c]	0.54	1.95	0.021	0.138
	MC	0.76	2.27	0.027	0.150
Rat (Wistar, ♂)	none	0.51	1.65	0.113	0.199

[a] See Materials and Methods section for experimental conditions.
[b] Water, control for PB
[c] Control for MC

Fig. 1. Effect of varying the concentration of ascorbic acid on the enzymatic hydroxylation of *N*-nitrosopiperidine by liver microsomes (see Materials and Methods, section for experimental conditions). A, yield of 5-hydroxypentanal;   B, yield of *N*-nitroso-hydroxypiperidine (3-OH-NPIP);   C, yield of *N*-nitroso-4-hydroxypiperidine (4-OH-NPIP);   ●,   control   (water);   ○,   phenobarbital-treated   microsomes;   △, 3-methylcholanthrene-treated microsomes.

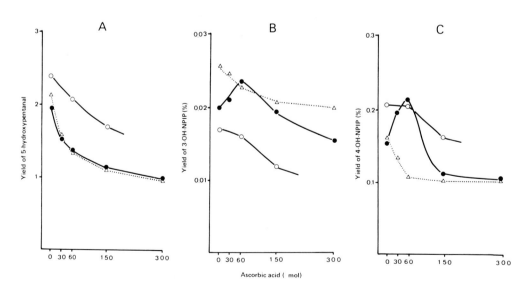

those from untreated and MC-treated microsomes, but cytochrome P-450 in liver microsomes of animals untreated and treated with PB and MC showed a similar effect of AsA on enzymatic α-oxidation of NPIP.

As shown in Figures 1B and 1C, the yields of 3-OH-NPIP and 4-OH-NPIP in the presence of small amounts (30–60 μmol) of AsA significantly increased in untreated liver microsomes, whereas the presence of larger amounts, such as 150–300 μmol AsA, apparently inhibited the formation of these compounds. In the microsomes treated with MC and PB, greater inhibition of the oxidation of NPIP was observed with higher concentrations of AsA. The inhibition patterns for β and γ-oxidation of NPIP by AsA in PB- and MC-treated microsomes were very similar. These results imply that AsA may act on β-oxidation enzymes as well as on γ-oxidation enzymes. Cytochrome P-450 induced by PB or MC is known to be fairly homogeneous (Werrigloer & Estabrook, 1975; Fujii *et al.*, 1982; Yamazoe, 1982), while cytochrome P-450 of untreated liver microsomes consists of many isozymes. This increase of β- and γ-oxidation of NPIP at low concentrations of AsA may have occurred as a result of the effect of several cytochrome P-450s, rather than of one cytochrome P-450. Both 3-OH-NPIP and 4-OH-NPIP have been reported to be mutagens which require activation with the rat liver enzymes in a 9 000 × *g* supernatant fraction (Rao *et al.*, 1977), suggesting that 3-OH-NPIP and 4-OH-NPIP may be metabolized further by those enzymes, although no data are yet available. The increased yields of these compounds in the presence of low concentrations of AsA may be due to inhibition of their further metabolism.

Table 2 shows the effects of various reducing agents, in rather large amounts, on NPIP metabolism by untreated liver microsomes. L-Cysteine, glutathione and sodium hydrogen sulfite have similar effects on the enzymatic oxidation of NPIP. Those compounds strongly inhibited α-oxidation, slightly inhibited γ-oxidation, but had no effect on β-oxidation. Sodium hydrosulfite strongly inhibited the γ-oxidation of NPIP (the yield of 4-OH-NPIP decreased to one-quarter that of control), but inhibited α- and β-oxidation only a little. An entirely different effect from that of AsA was observed in the liver microsomal oxidation of NPIP when reducing agents such as L-cysteine, glutathione, sodium bisulfite and sodium hydrosulfite were employed. However, the amount of unmetabolized NPIP was found to be about 96% in the mixture without reducing agents and about 87% with reducing agents. Although the amounts of oxidation products were decreased by the addition of reducing agents, the amount of unmetabolized NPIP was not increased.

The results obtained in this study indicate that AsA plays a complicated role in NPIP metabolism by guinea-pig liver microsomes.

Table 2. Effects of various reducing agents on *N*-nitrosopiperidine (NPIP) metabolism by guinea-pig liver microsomes[a]

Reducing agent (150 μmol)	Yield of metabolite (%)			Remaining NPIP (%)
	5-Hydroxy-pentanal	3-OH-NPIP	4-OH-NPIP	
None	1.93	0.020	0.145	95.6
Ascorbic acid	1.13	0.020	0.122	85.2
L-Cysteine	0.24	0.019	0.129	89.2
Glutathione	0.42	0.019	0.113	87.2
Sodium hydrosulfite	1.63	0.017	0.040	87.0
Sodium bisulfite	0.35	0.022	0.115	84.6

[a] See Materials and Methods section for experimental conditions.

REFERENCES

Fujii-Kuriyama, Y., Mizukami, Y., Kawajiri, K., Sogawa, K. & Muramatsu, M. (1982) Primary structure of a cytochrome P-450: Coding nucleotide cytochrome P-450 cDNA from rat liver. *Proc. natl Acad. Sci. USA, 79,* 2793–2797

Gilbert, P.J., Rollman, B., Rondelet, J., Mercier, M. & Poncelet, F. (1982) Mutagenicity and α-hydroxylation of *N*-nitrosopyrrolidine and *N*-nitrosopiperidine: a possible correlation. *Toxicology, 22,* 345–352

Guttenplan, J.B. (1977) Inhibition by L-ascorbate of bacterial mutagenesis induced by two *N*-nitroso compounds. *Nature, 268,* 368–370

Leung, K.H., Park, K.K. & Archer, C. (1978) Alpha-hydroxylation in the metabolism of *N*-nitrosopiperidine by rat liver microsomes: formation of 5-hydroxypentanal. *Res. Comm. Chem. Pathol. Pharmacol., 19,* 201–211

Lowry, O.H., Rosenbrough, H.J., Farr, A.L. & Randell, R.I. (1951) Protein measurement with the folin phenol reagent. *J. biol. Chem., 193,* 265–275

Omura, T. & Sato, R. (1964) The carbon monoxide-binding pigment of liver microsomes. 1. Evidence for its hemoprotein nature. *J. biol. Chem., 239,* 2370–2378

Rao, T.K., Hardigree, A.A., Young, J.A., Lijinsky, W. & Epler, J.L. (1977) Mutagenicity of *N*-nitrosopiperidine with *Salmonella typhimurium*/microsomal activation system. *Mutat. Res., 56,* 131–145

Rayman, M.P., Challis, B.C., Cox, P.J. & Jarman, M. (1974) Oxidation of *N*-nitrosopiperidine in the Udenfriend model system and its metabolism by rat-microsomes. *Biochem. Pharmacol., 24,* 621–626

Werringloer, J. & Estabrook, R.W. (1975) Heterogenicity of liver microsomal cytochrome P-450: the spectral characterization of reactants with reduced cytochrome P-450. *Arch. Biochem. Biophys., 167,* 270–286

Yamazoe, Y. (1982) Induction and inhibition of drug metabolizing enzymes (cytochrome P-450s) by various chemicals. *Mutagens Toxicol., 5,* 408–435

EFFECTS OF FLUORINATION ON IN-VITRO METABOLISM AND BIOLOGICAL ACTIVITY OF N-NITROSODIALKYLAMINES

C. JANZOWSKI & G. EISENBRAND

Department of Food Chemistry and Environmental Toxicology,
University of Kaiserslautern, 6750 Kaiserlautern, FRG

J. GOTTFRIED & R. PREUSSMANN

Institute of Toxicology and Chemotherapy, German Cancer Research Center,
6900 Heidelberg, FRG

SUMMARY

Substitution of N-nitrosodialkylamines with fluorine at specific sites inhibits oxidative metabolism at the respective carbon atoms. The results of in-vitro metabolism studies with N-nitrosodiethylamine (NDEA), N-nitrosodibutylamine (NDBA) and their fluorinated analogues, N-nitroso-2,2,2-trifluoroethyl-ethylamine (NDEA-F_3), N-nitroso-bis(2,2,2-trifluoroethyl)amine (NDEA-F_6), N-nitroso-4,4,4-trifluorobutyl-butylamine (NDBA-F_3), N-nitroso-bis(4,4,4-trifluo-robutyl)amine (NDBA-F_6) and N-nitroso-bis(2,2,3,3,4,4,4-heptafluorobutyl)-amine (NDBA-F_{14}), showed effects of fluorination on biotransformation which can explain results of carcinogenicity and mutagenicity experiments; NDEA-F_6 and NDBA-F_{14} were practically not metabolized by microsomal fractions, even though no decrease in binding affinity to cytochrome P450 was observed. Both compounds were not biologically active and were exhaled unchanged in high proportions after oral administration to the rat. Biologically active analogues, NDEA, NDBA, NDBA-F_3 and NDBA-F_6, were found to be dealkylated at the unfluorinated alkyl chains and, to a lesser extent, at the ω-fluorinated alkyl chains.

Detection of corresponding alcohols as hydrolysis products confirmed the generation of electrophilic intermediates by α-C-hydroxylation. However, trifluorethanol was detected only in very small proportions from dealkylation of NDEA-F_3, although dealkylation occurred almost exclusively at the unfluorinated site.

INTRODUCTION

Selective fluorination of N-nitrosodialkylamines (Fig. 1) was found to inhibit metabolic oxidations at adjacent, non-fluorinated positions as well. Fluorination of N-nitroso-diethylamine (NDEA) and N-nitrosodibutylamine (NDBA) at all positions except α-C giving N-nitroso-bis(2,2,2-trifluoroethyl)amine (NDEA-F_6) and N-nitroso-bis(2,2,3,3,4,4,4-hepta-fluorobutyl)amine (NDBA-F_{14}) results in compounds that are not metabolized by microsomal

Fig. 1 Fluorinated N-nitrosodialkylamines

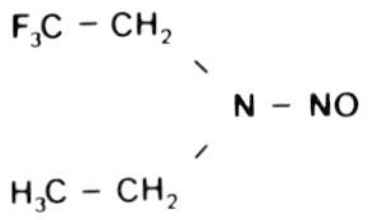

$F_3C - CH_2$
$H_3C - CH_2$
N – NO

N – Nitroso – 2,2,2 –
trifluoroethyl – ethylamine
(NDEA-F$_3$)

$F_3C - CH_2$
$F_3C - CH_2$
N – NO

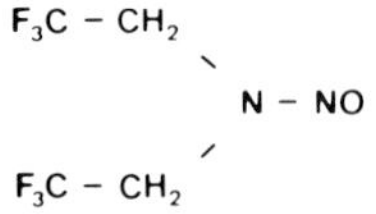

N – Nitroso – bis (2,2,2 –
trifluoroethyl) amine
(NDEA-F$_6$)

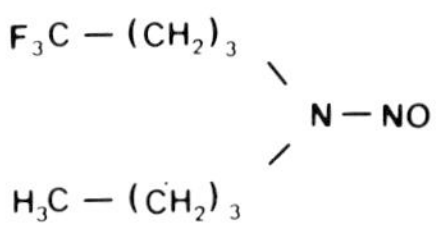

$F_3C - (CH_2)_3$
$H_3C - (CH_2)_3$
N — NO

N – Nitroso – 4,4,4 –
trifluorobutyl – butylamine
(NDBA-F$_3$)

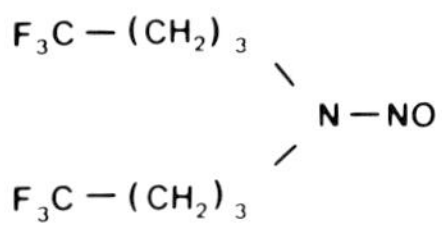

$F_3C - (CH_2)_3$
$F_3C - (CH_2)_3$
N — NO

N – Nitroso – bis (4,4,4 –
trifluorobutyl) amine
(NDBA-F$_6$)

$F_3C - (CF_2)_2 - CH_2$
$F_3C - (CF_2)_2 - CH_2$
N — NO

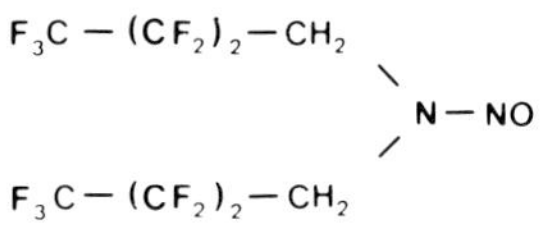

N – Nitroso – bis (2,2,3,3,4,4,4 –
heptafluorobutyl) amine
(NDBA – F$_{14}$)

enzymes in vitro (Janzowski et al., 1982a,b) and which are not mutagenic (Pool et al., 1982) or carcinogenic (Preussmann et al., 1981). In the case of N-nitroso-2,2,2-trifluoroethyl-ethylamine (NDEA-F$_3$), N-nitroso-4,4,4-trifluorobutyl-butylamine (NDBA-F$_3$), and N-nitroso-bis(4,4,4-trifluorobutyl)amine(NDBA-F$_6$), metabolism at the fluorinated alkyl chains was also inhibited to some extent (Janzowski et al., 1982a,b).

NDEA, NDBA, NDEA-F$_3$, NDBA-F$_3$ and NDBA-F$_6$ were carcinogenic and mutagenic; the mutagenicity of NDEA-F$_3$, however, was only marginal (Druckrey et al., 1967; Preussmann et al., 1982, 1983)[1].

To study further the effect of fluorination on the biotransformation of dialkylnitrosamines, binding to cytochrome P450 and in-vitro formation of alcohols from electrophilic intermediates after incubation with microsomal fractions, were investigated. In order to elucidate the fate of the biologically-inactive congeners, NDEA-F$_6$ and NDBA-F$_{14}$, possible accumulation and/or excretion of the intact compounds was investigated in vivo. These studies are reported below.

MATERIALS AND METHODS

Chemicals

NDEA-F$_3$, NDEA-F$_6$, NDBA-F$_3$, NDBA-F$_6$ and NDBA-F$_{14}$ were synthesized as described elsewhere (Preussmann et al., 1981, 1982, 1983). Other nitrosamines were obtained from laboratory stocks. 4,4,4-Trifluorobutanol was synthesized according to the method of McBee et al. (1950). 2,4-Dinitrophenylhydrazones were synthesized from the corresponding aldehydes. All other chemicals were obtained commercially.

---

[1] Also, Preussmann et al., in preparation

Preparation of microsomal fractions

Microsomal fractions were prepared from male BD-VI rats, pretreated with sodium phenobarbital (PB), as described previously (Janzowski *et al.*, 1982).

In-vitro metabolism

Nitrosamines (NDEA, 10 mmol/L; NDEA-F_3, 10 mmol/L; NDBA, 3 mmol/L; NDBA-F_3, 3 mmol/L, NDBA-F_6, 3 mmol/L) were incubated with microsomal fractions and an NADPH generating system (Janzowski *et al.*, 1982a,b). For the preparation of incubation mixture, standard solutions of *N*-nitrosamines in buffer, methanol or ethanol were used. Control experiments were performed without *N*-nitrosamines, without the NADPH generating system or with added aldehydes and alcohols.

Aldehydes were determined by high-performance liquid chromatography (HPLC), after reaction to the corresponding 2,4-dinitrophenylhydrazones (Janzowski *et al.*, 1982a,b).

Alcohols were determined by gas chromatography-mass spectrometry (GC-MS), after precipitation of proteins with barium hydroxide and zinc sulfate (gas chromatograph, Pye Unicam 105; mass spectrometer LKB 9000; carrier gas (helium) flow-rate, 20 mL/min; electron energy, 70 eV). For determination of butanol-(1) and butanol-(2), the aqueous filtrate (1 µL) was injected directly (glass column, 2,8 m × 2,2 mm i.d.; GP60/80 Carbopack B/5% Carbowax 20M; column temperature, 180 °C) and analysed by specific ion monitoring (butanol-(1) m/z 56; butanol-(2) m/z 59).

4,4,4-Trifluorobutanol was determined by GC-MS after extraction into ethyl formiate (glass column, 2,8 m × 2,2 mm i.d.; 80/100 Carbopack C/0.3% Carbowax 20M; column temperature, 180 °C; m/z 78; 1 µL injected). Ethanol was determined in the aqueous filtrate. For determination of 2,2,2-trifluoroethanol, the filtrate (10 mL) was concentrated by distillation. The first mL of distillate, containing 70% of the total amount of alcohol, as confirmed by recovery experiments, was used for GC-MS analysis (glass column, 2.8 m × 2.2 mm i.d.; 80/100 Carbopack C/O, 2% Carbowax 1500; Column temperature for ethanol, 90 °C, m/z 45; column temperature for 2,2,2-trifluoroethanol, 140 °C, m/z 51, 1 µL injected).

Control experiments with the respective alcohols, added as pure compounds to the incubation mixtures, resulted in 90–100% recoveries.

Optical difference spectra

Liver microsomal fractions were diluted to a protein concentration of 2 mg/mL in buffer of pH 7.5 (used for preparation of microsomal fractions, Appel *et al.*, 1980).

Spectral changes after addition of increasing amounts of *N*-nitrosamine to the microsomal mix were followed (350-600 nm), compensating for the absorption of the *N*-nitroso chromophore by a suitable cuvette arrangement (Shimazu UV 300 spectrophotometer).

Optical spectra (450-325 nm)

λ_{max} and ε of NDEA, NDEA-F_3, NDEA-F_6, NDBA, NDBA-F_3 and NDBA-F_6 were determined in hexane and water:methanol (1:1). Spectra were recorded on a Zeiss DMR 21 spectrophotometer.

Exhalation and tissue storage of NDEA-F_6 and NDBA-F_{14} in rats

Male Sprague-Dawley rats (approximately 400 g body weight) were given NDEA-F_6 (30 mg/kg) and NDBA-F_{14} (59 mg/kg) orally in equimolar concentrations. The animals were then placed in a desiccator for 24 h. Air (16 L/h) was drawn through the desiccator, then through two cooling traps (2 °C), filled with ethyl acetate for experiments with NDEA-F$_6$ and with ethyl propionate for experiments with NDBA-F$_{14}$. The content of the traps was directly analysed for unchanged *N*-nitrosamine by GC-Thermal Energy Analyzer (TEA) [gas chromatograph: Hewlett Packard 5880A; glass column, 2.8 m × 2.2 mm, i.d.; 15% Carbowax 20 M TPA; carrier gas (helium) flow-rate, 30 mL/min; column temperature, 90 °C].

Control experiments were performed by placing in the desiccator a petri dish containing *N*-nitrosamine standard solution (0.7-14 mg/200 µL iso-octane) in 10 mL water.

The rats were killed after 24 h and dissected; organs and tissues were separated, homogenized and extracted with ethyl formiate (NDEA-F$_6$) or ethyl propionate (NDMA-F$_{14}$). The extracts were analysed by GC-TEA for NDEA-F$_6$ and NDBA-F$_{14}$, as described above.

RESULTS

The amounts of aldehydes and alcohols generated by incubation of NDEA, NDEA-F$_3$, NDBA, NDBA-F$_3$ and NDBA-F$_6$ with microsomal fractions are shown in Table 1. Ethanol was generated from NDEA in amounts that accounted for 85% of the generated acetaldehyde, However, only very small amounts of trifluoroethanol were detected after incubation of NDEA-F$_3$ accounting for only 5% of the quantity acetaldehyde generated.

From NDBA and its fluorinated analogues (NDBA-F$_3$ and NDBA-F$_6$), alcohols were formed in amounts of 84-100% of the corresponding amounts of aldehydes. Two isomers of butanol were detected, butanol-(1) - the more abundant - and butanol-(2).

Optical difference spectra with phenobarbital-induced microsomal fractions were obtained for all *N*-nitrosamines. NDEA showed a mixed spectrum; NDEA-F$_3$, NDBA, NDBA-F$_3$ and NDBA-F$_6$, as well as NDEA-F$_6$ and NDBA-F$_{14}$, were found to be type I substrates, with characteristic minima of absorption between 420 and 425 nm. The maxima of absorption at 380-390 nm, which are also characteristic for type I substrates, were partially superimposed on the absorption of the *N*-nitrosamines, resulting from differences in absorption spectra in aqueous and lipophilic microsomal media. These differences in the optical absorption spectra

Table 1.   Amounts of aldehydes and corresponding alcohols formed from *N*-nitrosodiethylamine (NDEA), *N*-nitroso-2,2,2-trifluoroethyl-ethylamine (NDEA-F$_3$), *N*-nitrosodibutylamine (NDBA), *N*-nitroso-4,4,4-trifluorobutyl-butylamine (NDBA-F$_3$) and *N*-nitroso-bis(4,4,4-trifluorobutyl)amine (NDBA-F$_6$) on incubation with microsomal fractions[a]

Compound (mmol/L)	Aldehydes formed (nmol/mL incubation mixture in 60 min); x̄ (min; max)	Alcohols formed (nmol/mL incubation mixture in 60 min); x̄ (min; max)	Ratio of alcohol to corresponding aldehyde (%)
NDEA (10)	Acetaldehyde 693 (691; 695)	Ethanol 581 (541; 628)	84
NDEA-F$_3$ (10)	Acetaldehyde 251 (245; 260)	Trifluoroethanol 10 (5; 15)	4
NDBA (3)	Butyraldehyde 364 (300; 398)	Butanol-(1) 207 (194; 231)	57
		Butanol-(2) 99 (76; 118)	27
NDBA-F$_3$ (3)	Butyraldehyde 268 (247; 302)	Trifluorobutanol-(1) 246 (223; 268)	92
	Trifluorobutyraldehyde 157 (150; 166)	Butanol-(1) 85 (72; 107)	54
		Butanol-(2) 67 (50; 91)	43
NDBA-F$_6$ (3)	Trifluorobutyraldehyde 239 (231; 248)	Trifluorobutanol-(1) 257 (252; 262)	107

[a] Incubation time: 60 min; protein concentration, 0.67 mg/mL incubation mixture; number of experiments, 3–6

Table 2. Optical absorption spectra of N-nitrosodiethylamine (NDEA), N-nitrosodibutylamine (NDBA) and of fluorinated analogues

Compound[a]	Solvent, water:methanol (1:1)		Solvent, n-hexane	
	λ_{max} (nm)	ε(min/max)[b]	λ_{max} (nm)	ε(min/max)[b]
NDEA	342	88 (88/89)	365	108 (107/109)
NDEA-F$_3$	355	86 (84/88)	370	101 (98/102)
NDEA-F$_6$	368	90 (85/96)	371	104 (103/107)
NDBA	343	88 (87/89)	365	97 (93/101)
NDBA-F$_3$	347	92 (87/98)	366	97 (93/101)
NDBA-F$_6$	348	87 (86/88)	368	100 (98/104)
NDBA-F$_{14}$	–[c]	–	371	100 (99/100)

[a] NDEA-F$_3$, N-nitroso-2,2,2-trifluoroethyl-ethylamine; NDEA-F$_6$, N-nitroso-bis(2,2,2-trifluoro-ethyl)amine; NDBA-F$_3$, N-nitroso-4,4,4-trifluorobutyl-butylamine; NDBA-F$_6$, N-nitroso-bis(4,4,4-trifluorobutyl)amine; NDBA-F$_{14}$, N-nitroso-bis(2,2,3,3,4,4,4-heptafluorobutyl)amine
[b] Number of experiments, 2–4
[c] Not soluble in water:methanol (1:1)
ε, extinction coefficient

of NDEA, NDBA and the fluorinated analogues are shown in Table 2. Increasing fluorination of the N-nitrosamine side chains caused bathochromic shifts of the λ_{max}. Changing from polar water:methanol to nonpolar n-hexane also causes a shift to longer wavelength for all compounds, in agreement with the results of Layne et al. (1963) .

Our first in-vivo experiments show that after oral administration to rats, high percentages of NDEA-F$_6$ and NDBA-F$_{14}$ are excreted unchanged by exhalation. In organs, tissues, urine and faeces, only traces of unchanged NDEA-F$_6$ were detected (< 2% of dose ingested).

DISCUSSION

After incubation of NDEA in liver microsomal fractions, acetaldehyde, formed by enzymatic dealkylation, and ethanol, formed from hydrolysis of electrophiles liberated after loss of acetaldehyde, were found in corresponding amounts. Also, similar ratios of aldehydes and corresponding alcohols were found after incubation of NDBA, NDBA-F$_3$ and NDBA-F$_6$. Two isomeric forms of butanol, butanol-(1) and butanol-(2), were detected, confirming the results of Park et al. (1977) and Suzuki et al. (1983) These high proportions of alcohols formed, which are indicative of the generation of alkylating intermediates, correlate well with the respective mutagenic and carcinogenic effects of these compounds. In contrast, NDEA-F$_3$ yielded only very small amounts of trifluoroethanol after incubation. This result was unexpected, since the formation of substantial amounts of acetaldehyde from NDEA-F$_3$ suggests normal dealkylation of NDEA-F$_3$ at the non-fluorinated ethyl chain.

Optical binding spectra with phenobarbital-induced microsomal fractions show that all N-nitrosamines bind to cytochrome P450. For NDEA-F$_6$ and NDBA-F$_{14}$, two congeners which have been found not to be metabolized by cytochrome P450-dependent monooxygenases, even higher maximal absorptions were found than for compounds that were metabolically activated. This may be due to the higher lipophilicity of these highly-fluorinated compounds (Janzowski et al., 1982a,b).

NDEA-F$_6$ and NDBA-F$_{14}$, which are not metabolized by microsomal fractions in vitro and which are not mutagenic/carcinogenic, are excreted in large amounts via exhalation, because of their high volatility. There was no indication of an accumulation in specific organs or tissues.

In conclusion, selective fluorination of dialkyl nitrosamines had diverse effects on biotransformation: at non-fluorinated alkyl chains, microsomal metabolism appears to be enhanced; this may be due to the higher lipophilicity and a higher binding affinity to cytochrome P450 of the fluorinated analogues. The inhibition of metabolism by cytochrome P450-mediated monooxygenases at adjacent molecular positions may be explained by the electron-withdrawing effect of the fluorine substituents, which reduces the electron density of the non-fluorinated CH_2-groups. A cleavage of the C-H bond by a radical mechanism, which is discussed as a possible mechanism of hydroxylation reaction by Ullrich (1978), may therefore be inhibited. The failure to detect equivalent amounts of trifluoroethanol from NDEA-F_3, although the compound is dealkylated at a considerable rate (as measured by acetaldehyde formation), remains unexplained at present. We are currently investigating this problem.

ACKNOWLEDGEMENTS

We thank Ms I. Hofmann for competent technical assistance and Ms R. Haubner for performing the GC-MS analysis. This work was supported by the Deutsche Forschungsgemeinschaft.

REFERENCES

Appel, K.E., Schrenk, D., Schwarz, M., Mahr, B. & Kunz, W. (1980) Denitrosation of *N*-nitrosomorpholine by liver microsomes; possible role of cytochrome P-450. *Cancer Lett., 9*, 13-20

Drückrey, H., Preussmann, R., Ivankovic, S. & Schmähl, D. (1967) Organotrope carcinogene Wirkungen bei 65 verschiedenen *N*-nitroso-Verbindungen an BD-Ratten. *Z. Krebsforsch., 69*, 103-201

Janzowski, C., Pool., B.L., Preussmann, R. & Eisenbrand, G. (1982a) Fluoro-substituted *N*-nitrosamines. 2. Metabolism of *N*-nitrosodiethylamine and of fluorinated analogues in liver microsomal fractions. *Carcinogenesis, 3*, 155-159

Janzowski, C., Gottfried, J., Eisenbrand, G. & Preussmann, P. (1982b) Fluoro-substituted *N*-nitrosamines. 3. Microsomal metabolism of *N*-nitrosodibutylamine and of fluorinated analogues. *Carcinogenesis, 3*, 777-780

Layne, W.S., Jaffé, H.H. & Zimmer, H. (1963) Basicity of *N*-nitrosamines I. Non-polar solvents. *J. Am. chem. Soc., 85*, 435-438

Mc Bee, E.T., Kelley, A.E. & Rapkin, E. (1950) Compounds derived from 3-halo-1,1,1-trifluoropropane. *J. Am. chem. Soc., 72*, 5071-5073

Park, K.K., Wishnok, J.S. & Archer, M.C. (1977) Mechanism of alkylation by *N*-nitroso compounds: detection of rearranged alcohol in the microsomal metabolism of *N*-nitrosodi-*n*-propylamine and base-catalysed decomposition of *N*-*n*-propyl-*n*-nitrosourea, *Chem. biol. Interact., 18*, 349-354

Pool., B.L. Janzowski, C., Eisenbrand, G. & Preussmann, R. (1982) Fluoro-substituted *N*-nitrosamines. 4. Comparative genotoxic activities of *N*-nitrosodibutylamine and three fluorinated analogues in two bacterial system. *Carcinogenesis, 3*, 781-784

Preussmann, R., Habs, M., Pool, B., Stummeyer, D., Lijinsky, W. & Reuber, M.D. (1981) Fluoro-substituted *N*-nitrosamines 1. Inactivity of *N*-nitroso-bis(2,2,2-trifluoroethyl)amine in carcinogenicity and mutagenicity tests. *Carcinogenesis, 2*, 753-756

Preussmann, R., Habs, M., Habs, H. & Stummeyer, D. (1982) Fluoro-substituted *N*-nitrosamines. 5. Carcinogenicity of *N*-nitroso-bis-(4,4,4-trifluoro-n-butyl)amine in rats. *Carcinogenesis, 3*, 1219-1222

Preussmann, R;., Habs, M., Habs, H. & Stummeyer, D. (1983) Fluorosubstituted *N*-nitrosamines. 6.Carcinogenicity of *N*-nitroso-(2,2,2-trifluoroethyl)-ethylamine in rats. *Carcinogenesis, 4*, 755-757

Suzuki, E., Mochizuki, M., Wakabayashi, Y. & Okada, M. (1983). In vitro metabolic activation of *N,N*-dibutylnitrosamine in mutagenesis. *Gann, 74*, 51-59

Ullrich, V. (1978) *Cytochrome P-450 and biological hydroxylation reactions.* In: Boschke, F.L., ed., *Topics in Current Chemistry*, Berlin, Springer, pp. 67-104

DNA REPAIR AND DETECTION OF ALKYLATED MACROMOLECULES

ENZYMOLOGY OF REPAIR OF DNA ADDUCTS PRODUCED BY N-NITROSO COMPOUNDS

R.B. SETLOW, E.H. CAO & N.C. DELIHAS

Biology Department, Brookhaven National Laboratory, Upton, NY, USA

SUMMARY

The biological effects of DNA adducts depend on their nature, and on their half-lives relative to the rates of DNA replication and transcription. Their half-lives are determined by the rates of spontaneous decay, such as depurination, and the rates of enzymatic repair of the adducts or their decay products. The principal modes of repair of methylating and ethylating agents are by glycosylase-catalysed depurination of 7-alkylguanine and 3-alkyladenine and by the dealkylation of O^6-alkylguanine. The latter repair is accomplished by the transfer of the alkyl group to cysteine residues of acceptor proteins in a stoichiometric reaction. Repair by dealkylation cannot be detected by the standard methods used to measure DNA repair, but it is easy to estimate the acceptor activity in cell extracts by measuring the transfer of radioactive O^6-alkyl groups in an exogenous DNA to protein. In extracts of cells treated with alkylating agents, the activity is depressed because the endogenous DNA is rapidly dealkylated, using up the acceptor activity. In many cell types, the decrease in activity is followed by an increase to the normal constitutive level. In other cells, there is no such adaptive response. We may catalogue the cell strains and lines investigated into three classes: (1) high constitutive activity (30 000–100 000 acceptor sites per cell) and rapid adaptive response (several hours), (2) high constitutive activity and very slow adaptive response, and (3) low constitutive activity. The cytotoxicity of methylating agents is highest for the last and lowest for the first class. Differences in constitutive levels of methyl accepting activity in extracts of human lymphocytes and in the acceptor activity in lung macrophages from smokers (low activity) and nonsmokers (high activity) have been observed.

INTRODUCTION

Directly acting alkylating agents react with macromolecules, in particular DNA, and produce a variety of products (Singer & Kusmierek, 1982). The distributions of products among the various bases of DNA are similar to those produced by agents which need enzymatic activation to alkylating species, such as N-nitrosamines and N-methyl-N'-nitro-N-nitrosoguanidine (MNNG) and N-ethyl-N'-nitro-N-nitrosoguanidine, which are activated by thiols. The biological effects of alkylating agents – cytotoxicity, mutagenicity and presumably the initiation steps in carcinogenesis – depend on many aspects of the agents' pharmacokinetics relative to the rates of replication and transcription of DNA (Hoel & Kaplan, 1983). An additional important kinetic parameter is the lifetime of the adducts in DNA: a short half-life resulting from chemical instability or enzymatic repair could tend to render a particular adduct relatively innocuous.

Because of the enzymatic or chemical activation steps needed to convert many compounds to alkylating agents, the external concentration in µmol/L or mg/kg of body weight may be greatly different from the internal dosimetry in cells or tissues. The difference between internal and external dosimetry is certainly relevant to *N*-nitrosamines, which are activated primarily in the liver (Pegg & Perry, 1981a), and is even true for MNNG acting on cells in culture (see below).

There are a number of pathways for repairing alkylation damage to DNA. One might wonder, from an evolutionary point of view, why such pathways exist. A possible explanation lies in observations that there are endogenous reactions that can alkylate DNA. For example, *S*-adenosylmethionine is able to alkylate DNA *in vitro* (Barrows & Magee, 1982; Rydberg & Lindahl, 1982; Naeslund *et al.*, 1983), and the repair of damage from this essential cellular compound may be the reason for the repair of alkylation damage in cells.

MODELS OF ALKYLATION REPAIR

Figure 1 is a diagram of various possibilities for repairing alkylation damage (Lindahl, 1982; Setlow, 1982). Pathway (a) is the simplest to understand, in that it represents the removal of an alkyl group from DNA without affecting the DNA backbone. This is the major pathway for the repair of O^6-methylguanine (O^6-meG) or O^6-ethylguanine (O^6-eG). No unscheduled DNA synthesis or strand breakage is associated with this repair system. Pathways (b) and (c) involve the action of glycosylases which remove altered purines from the polynucleotide. Subsequent steps and repair are aimed at replacing the removed purines by the proper ones. In scheme (b), a new purine is inserted directly into the polynucleotide. Such a pathway would not show unscheduled DNA synthesis, as measured by ^{3}H-thymidine incorporation, or any strand break unless the breaks are measured in alkali which labilizes the backbone of the chain at apurinic sites. The existence of the insertase mechanism of repairing an apurinic site has been questioned as a major pathway of repair in bacteria (Kataoka & Sekiguchi, 1982) and in mammalian cells in culture (Wintersberger, 1982). Pathway (c) involves an apurinic endonuclease following the glycosylase and results in a strand break and further incorporation to repair any nucleotides removed during this phase of the enzymatic action. Hence, such repair will give rise to unscheduled DNA synthesis and to the appearance of single strand breaks in DNA and their disappearance as repair is completed.

Which lesions are important

Determination of the biological effects of particular DNA adducts is a real problem (Setlow, 1980). It cannot be done by an analysis of the shape of dose-response curves, since the ratios of the yields of various products usually do not change with dose. The solution to the problem necessitates, among other things, knowing how various adducts change the template activity of polynucleotides (Singer & Kusmierek, 1982; Miyaki *et al.*, 1983) as well as the persistence of the products. For example, the product O^6-eG arising from the treatment of animals with *N*-ethyl-*N*-nitrosourea (ENU) is known to code for thymine as well as for cytosine. It is removed rapidly from the liver of neonatal rats but persists in brain for long periods of time. Hence, this product of ENU is implicated in brain carcinogenesis (Goth & Rajewsky, 1974; Müller & Rajewsky, 1983). However, such an argument is not foolproof, because a number

Fig. 1. Schematic illustration of various possibilities for base excision repair. Circles represent pyrimidines and squares, purines. The solid square is an altered purine (perhaps an alkylated one). The solid line in pathway c represents repair replication or unscheduled DNA synthesis

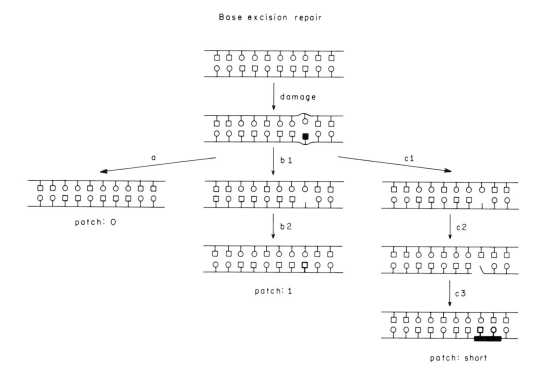

of other minor O-ethyl products are removed almost as effectively as is O^6-eG (Singer *et al.*, 1981). Nevertheless, products such as O^6-eG that are biologically important (but not necessarily the only important ones) are repaired rapidly in many tissues (see below). High doses of ENU can saturate this repair pathway and would be expected to result in dose-response curves that have an apparent threshold. Indeed, this is what is observed for specific locus mutations in mice injected with ENU (Russell *et al.*, 1982a, b).

Two other techniques are used in attempts to identify particular products with biological effects. In one (Connell & Medcalf, 1982), the effects of alkylating agents such as N-methyl-N-nitrosourea and dimethyl sulfate are compared at equitoxic doses in terms of sister chromatid exchanges (SCE). At such doses, equal levels of SCE are observed. This means that O^6-meG cannot be correlated with SCE production, since the two alkylating agents produce completely different levels of this product, and no specific alkylation product can be held accountable for the formation of SCE. A second approach is to grow cells in culture medium containing DNA precursors, such as O^6-meG. Kaina *et al.* (1983) observed appreciable numbers of mutations and SCE in Chinese hamster V79 cells following growth in O^6-meG medium but not in cells grown in 3-methyladenine or 7-methylguanine. Such observations are not necessarily at variance with those of Connell and Medcalf (1982), because the amounts of O^6-meG in the latter experiments were probably much less than in the former, and, although O^6-meG in DNA appears to result in the formation of SCE, the amount of O^6-meG in DNA of cells treated with alkylating agents may be too low to increase significantly the background level of SCE.

Repair of O⁶-meG in DNA

We have outlined above several reasons for supposing that O^6-meG is important in mutagenesis and carcinogenesis, although the cytotoxic effects of methylating agents on bacteria are associated more closely with 3-methyladenine and 3-methylguanine (Evensen & Seeberg, 1982; Karran *et al.*, 1982). However, the ability of cells to remove O^6-meG is correlated strongly with high survival of cells after MNNG treatment and with the ability of cells to reactivate adenovirus 5 treated with MNNG (Day *et al.*, 1980). The latter cells are called Mer⁺; those cells unable to reactivate treated virus are designated Mer⁻. Lymphoblastoid cells resistant to MNNG are called Mex⁺, and those that are sensitive are called Mex⁻ (Sklar & Strauss, 1981).

The repair of O^6-meG or O^6-eG falls into the special category outlined in Figure 1, in which repair is accomplished by the simple removal of the alkyl group. In bacteria (Olsson & Lindahl, 1980; Sedgwick & Lindahl, 1982). Rodent (Bogden *et al.*, 1981; Mehta *et al.*, 1981) and human cells (Pegg *et al.*, 1982; Waldstein *et al.*, 1982a), the removal is accompanied by the transfer to a cysteine group of an acceptor protein. The reaction is a stoichiometric one and is a suicide reaction, in that the acceptor protein is no longer available to accept additional alkyl groups. Characteristics of repair by treatment of mammalian cells with radioactive alkylating agents cannot be measured at high concentrations since the acceptor protein would rapidly be used up. As a result, large numbers of cells must be used at low concentrations of alkylating agents to obtain sufficient O^6-meG or O^6-eG for analysis. Many fewer cells are needed if the acceptor activity is assayed in cell extracts or in partially purified extract, because the activity of the extract may be estimated in terms of its ability to remove O^6-meG from an exogenous DNA or polynucleotide.

Table 1 outlines three different assays we have used. In the first method, the loss of O^6-meG from exogenous DNA is determined by high-performance liquid chromatography of depurinated DNA. In the second method, the amount of ³H-methyl transferred to protein is

Table 1. Comparison of three assays[a] for the repair of
O^6-methylguanine (O^6-meG) in DNA

Tissue[b]	fmol removed/200 µg protein		
	Method 1	Method 2	Method 3
A	384	390	408
	379	383	428
B	34	36	53
	32	32	64

[a] Sonicated extracts (Waldstein *et al.*, 1982c) containing 200 µg protein were incubated for 1 h at 37°C with DNA containing O^6-[³H-methyl]guanine (~600 fmol). The repair of O^6-meG was measured in duplicate assays by three methods: (1) the DNA was depurinated and the loss in O^6-meG measured by high-performance liquid chromatography; (2) the protein in the extract was degraded by proteases (Waldstein *et al.*, 1982b), and the ³H in the acid soluble fraction was measured; (3) the DNA was depurinated, and the ³H in the acid-insoluble fraction (protein) was measured (Delihas & Setlow, unpublished data)
[b] A, frozen baboon liver; B, frozen human liver. These tissues, obtained from R. Cutler of the National Institute on Aging, were used as examples of high and low activity and are not necessarily representative of baboons or humans

determined by digesting the protein with proteases and measuring the radioactivity liberated into the acid-soluble fraction of the reaction mixture (Waldstein et al., 1982b). In the third method, the amount of ^{3}H transferred to protein is determined after depurination of the DNA by measuring the amount of radioactivity in an acid precipitate[1]. The three assays give similar results; however, the third assay is the most convenient to use since it measures directly the transfer of small amounts of radioactivity to protein and is not affected by nucleases in tissue or cell preparations that may act during the long protease digestion used in the second method. Moreover, it does not require the use of an exogenous substrate depleted of methylated purines other than O^6-meG.

The assays described above have been used to estimate activity in human peripheral lymphocytes (Waldstein et al., 1982c). The measurements indicate variation of several fold in O^6-meG acceptor activity among humans. The variation is not sex- or age-dependent. There are at present no good data indicating that the magnitude of the variation observed in lymphocytes would be similar to that observed in other tissues; but a reasonably large variation has been reported in the acceptor activity obtained from human livers (Pegg et al., 1982). It is an attractive hypothesis that the variation in repair activity could be associated with an individual's susceptibility to mutagenesis or carcinogenesis by simple alkylating agents. Such a hypothesis derives most of its support from the big difference in sunlight-induced cancer between xeroderma pigmentosum patients and normal individuals. The prevalence of skin cancer in the patients is approximately 10^4-fold greater than that in the average population (Setlow, 1982), but the average repair defect is only approximately 80%. Hence, in the case of sunlight-induced cancer, a five-fold decrease in repair activity results in an increase in cancer susceptibility of 10^4, indicating that relatively small differences in repair could have large effects on the sensitivity of individuals to exogenous or endogenous carcinogenic agents (Setlow, 1983).

Recent measurements of acceptor activity in lung macrophages from smokers and non-smokers indicate that cells from nonsmokers have high activities – approximately 80 fmol removed per 200 µg of protein – whereas the macrophages from smokers have an activity between 0 and 20 fmol per 200 µg of protein[2]. Mixing experiments indicate that the low activity in the cells from smokers' lungs is not the result of a diffusable inhibitor in such cells. There are no data indicating whether these results on lung macrophages can be extrapolated to lung tissue itself.

The levels of O^6-meG repair activity in human cells in culture has been used to explain differences among them in the cytotoxic effects of MNNG or its killing effects on viruses used to infect them (Day et al., 1980). However, before discussing such results in more detail it is useful to digress and consider two other aspects of the effects of alkylating agents on tissues and on cells in culture. The first is the relationship between internal and external dosimetry and the second is the ability of cells or tissue to adapt to low levels of alkylating agents.

Internal versus *external dosimetry*

External dosing in µg/kg or in concentration in culture medium is a useful start to dosimetry, but it is not sufficient because of the many metabolic steps often needed before alkylation takes place. The best measure is one in which the numbers of the different alkylation products per cell are estimated directly by use of radioactive alkylating agents. Such procedures are used extensively in work with animals and with large numbers of cells in culture. A second convenient way of converting from external to relative internal dosimetry is to determine the

---

[1] Delihas & Setlow, unpublished data
[2] Cao, Setlow & Janoff, unpublished data

Table 2.   Comparison of effects of N-methyl-N'-nitro-N-nitrosoguanidine (MNNG) on five HeLa cell lines

Line [a]	Single-strand breaks per 10⁸ daltons [b]	D_{10} [c]	Constitutive activity [d]	Resynthesis time ($\frac{1}{2}$) [e]
229 (ATCC)	10.0	9.4	240	200
2 (ATCC)	15.2	9.7	190	200
2 (BNL)	5.0	9.7	180	75
S3 (ATCC)	5.6	6.0	210	>200
S3 (BNL)	5.0	6.0	400	>200
MR (Day)	10.9	0.12	0	

[a] ATCC, American Type Culture Collection; BNL, Brookhaven National Laboratory; Day, R.S. Day, III
[b] Cells treated with 6 µmol/L MNNG in serum-containing medium; breaks determined by the method of Abbondandolo et al. (1982)
[c] Concentration in µmol/L to give 10% colony forming survival
[d] Activity in fmol of O^6-methylguanine repaired per 200 µg protein
[e] Cells were treated for 5 min with 0.5–1.5 µmol/L MNNG, and the time in min for the activity to return halfway to the constitutive level was estimated; >200 indicates no detectable increase in 3 h (Waldstein et al., 1983)

number of phosphotriesters per unit length of DNA by the lability of the triesters in alkali (Snyder & Regan, 1981; Abbondandolo et al., 1982). This technique works well for cells in culture and demonstrates that even in such a simple situation the ratio of internal to external dosimetry of MNNG varies among cell lines (Table 2). Differences in internal dosimetry presumably arise because of different sulfhydryl levels in different cells. A knowledge of the numbers of triesters and the distribution of the products resulting from particular alkylating agents (Singer & Kusmierek, 1982) permits estimation of the numbers of particular alkylation products per cell.

Adaptation

In a number of instances, biological systems exposed to low chronic doses of alkylating agents are able to resist exposure to a single, high challenging dose. This phenomenon, called 'adaptation', has been observed in systems as diverse as rat liver and *Escherichia coli*. In the latter case, cells exposed to low doses of MNNG are resistant to the mutagenic effects of subsequent high challenging doses (Cairns, 1980). The cells were shown to adapt during administration of chronic doses by making appreciable amounts of new acceptor protein for O^6-meG which protected them against the challenging dose (Robins & Cairns, 1979). Adaptation is also observed for the cytotoxic effects of MNNG on *E. coli*, but this adaptation is associated with an increase of glycosylases capable of repairing 3-methyladenine and 3-methylguanine (Evensen & Seeberg, 1982; Karran et al., 1982). Thus, in bacteria, adaptation has several facets.

The ability of rat liver following chronic exposure of animals to N-nitrosodimethylamine to remove O^6-meG from cells also shows an adaptive response (Montesano et al., 1980; Margison, 1982). Since a similar response is observed to follow treatment with agents such as aflatoxin that kill liver cells or following partial hepatectomy, it is possible that adaptation in rat liver is associated with cell division in the damaged liver rather than with the increase in the number of acceptor molecules per cell (Chu et al., 1981; Pegg & Perry, 1981b). However, a kinetic analysis of the appearance of enhanced O^6-meG acceptors in rats treated with N-nitrosodimethylamine makes the above explanation improbable (Margison, 1982). If the latter point of view is correct, adaptation in rat liver is similar to that in bacteria and involves synthesis of new protein in the affected cells. The trigger for the adaptation is not well understood. In any event, the adaptive phenomenon cannot be generalized to species other than rat since it is not observed in mice (Maru *et al.*, 1982), hamsters (Smith & Margison, 1981) or gerbils (Bamborschke *et al.*, 1983).

Some mammalian cell strain and lines in culture can also adapt to low doses of MNNG and show fewer SCE (Samson & Schwartz, 1980). Chinese hamster cells show less mutation and greater survival after a subsequent challenge dose than do cells not exposed to initial small doses (Kaina, 1982; Laval & Michel, 1983).

Adaptation in terms of the appearance of new O^6-meG acceptor activity is also observed in a number of human cell strains (Waldstein *et al.*, 1982d). In order to appreciate how such experiments are done, using any one of the assays outlined in Table 1, one must remember that the reaction of the acceptor protein with O^6-meG is very rapid (Shiloh & Becker, 1981; Sklar *et al.*, 1981; Waldstein *et al;* 1982d), and, as a result, treatment of cells with MNNG will lead to depletion of acceptor activity in extracts prepared after treatment. The depletion of acceptor activity is also observed if extracts of cells are treated with MNNG. In this case, the depletion is the result of the action of the alkylating agent on DNA and not on the acceptor protein itself, because digestion of the majority of the DNA by nucleases renders the acceptor activity in extracts relatively insensitive to treatment with MNNG[1]. The depletion of activity occurs rapidly after treatment with an alkylating agent, and in some cell strains or lines the activity returns to the normal constitutive level in a few hours. The return to normal is inhibited by cycloheximide, indicating that new protein must be synthesized for such an adaptive response.

EFFECTS ON CELLS IN CULTURE

The cytotoxic effects on human cells of externally applied MNNG depend on a number of parameters, including internal dosimetry, constitutive levels of repair activity and the ability to adapt to single doses of the chemical by resynthesis of O^6-meG acceptor activity from its depleted to its normal levels. The roles of these relative factors are well illustrated with different HeLa cell lines (Table 2). The lines fall into three distinct groups, among which there is no clear correlation between differences in external and internal dosimetry. However, there is a strong correlation between cytotoxicity and the constitutive level of repair for O^6-meG and its adaptive response. The most resistant group is made up of cell strains with high constitutive levels and a rapid ability to adapt. A somewhat more sensitive group, HeLa S3, is made up of cells with a normal level of constitutive activity but a negligible ability to adapt. The third group, HeLa MR, is extraordinarily sensitive to the cytotoxic effects of MNNG and has a negligible amount of constitutive activity. The magnitude of the cytotoxic effects among these three groups is in inverse proportion to the numbers of O^6-meG that can be repaired within several hours.

CONCLUSIONS

The cytotoxic, mutagenic and presumed carcinogenic effects of alkylating agents are dependent to a large extent on the ability to repair alkylation products in treated cells or tissues. The magnitude of repair depends markedly on two parameters – the constitutive level of repair

---

[1] Delihas & Setlow, unpublished data

activities and the ability to adapt to low levels of alkylating agents. Cells with high constitutive activity and high adaptibility are the most resistant. Most of the analyses that have been carried out emphasize the role of O^6-meG because it seems to be one of the more important lesions resulting from treatment with methylating agents. Other O^6-alkyl products are also important but have not been analysed as carefully. There are wide differences in repair activity among different cells from the same animal and among similar tissues from different species. In some instances, it has been possible to correlate carcinogenic susceptibility to alkylating agents with a low level of repair. The wide differences in ability to repair O^6-meG observed among humans have not been correlated with susceptibility to disease resulting from endogenous or exogenous alkylating agents, but there are good experimental grounds for supposing that more rapid repair is to be preferred to slow or absent repair. It will take an elaborate prospective study to determine whether the variances in alkylation repair among humans have any relation to susceptibility to disease.

ACKNOWLEDGEMENT

This work was support by the United States Department of Energy.

REFERENCES

Abbondandolo, A., Gugliotti, E., Lohman, P.H.M. & Berends, F. (1982) Molecular dosimetry of DNA damage caused by alkylation. I. Single-strand breaks induced by ethylating agents in cultured mammalian cells in relation to survival. *Mutat. Res., 92,* 361–377

Bamborschke, S., O'Connor, P.J., Margison, G.P., Kleihues, P. & Maru, G.B. (1983) DNA methylation by dimethylnitrosamine in the Mongolian gerbil (*Meriones unguiculatus*): Indications of a deficient inducible hepatic repair system for O^6-methylguanine. *Cancer Res., 43,* 1306–1311

Barrows, L.R. & Magee, P.N. (1982) Nonenzymatic methylation of DNA by S-adenosylmethionine *in vitro. Carcinogenesis, 3,* 349–351

Bogden, J.M., Eastman, A. & Bresnick, E. (1981) A system in mouse liver for the repair of O^6-methylguanine lesions in methylated DNA. *Nucl. Acids Res., 9,* 3089–3103

Cairns, J. (1980) Efficiency of the adaptative response of *Escherichia coli* to alkylating agents. *Nature, 286,* 176–178

Chu, Y.H., Craig, A.W. & O'Connor, P.J. (1981) Repair of O^6-methylguanine in rat liver DNA is enhanced by pretreatment with single or multiple doses of aflatoxin B_1. *Cancer, 43,* 850–855

Connell, J.R. & Medcalf, A.S.C. (1982) The induction of SCE and chromosome aberrations with relation to specific loss methylation of DNA in Chinese hamster cells by *N*-methyl-*N*-nitrosourea and dimethyl sulfate. *Carcinogenesis, 3,* 385–390

Day, R.S., III, Ziolkowski, C.H.J., Scudiero, D.A., Meyer, S.A., Luminiecki, A.S., Girardi, A.J., Galloway, S.M. & Bynum, G.D. (1980) Defective repair of alkylated DNA by human tumor and SV40-transformed human cell strains. *Nature, 288,* 724–727

Evensen, G. & Seeberg, E. (1982) Adaptation to alkylation resistance involves induction of a DNA glycosylase. *Nature, 296,* 773–775

Goth, R. & Rajewsky, M.F. (1974) Molecular and cellular mechanisms associated with pulse-carcinogenesis in the rat nervous system by ethylnitrosourea: ethylation of nucleic acids and elimination rates of ethylated bases from the DNA of different tissues. *Z. Krebsforsch., 82,* 37–64

Hoel, D.G. & Kaplan, N.L. (1983) Implication of nonlinear kinetics on risk estimation in carcinogenesis. *Science, 219,* 1 032–1 037

Kaina, B. (1982) Enhanced survival and reduced mutation and aberration frequencies induced in V79 Chinese hamster cells pre-exposed to low levels of methylating agents. *Mutat. Res., 93,* 195–211

Kaina, B., Heindorff, K. & Aurich, O. (1983) 0^6-Methylguanine, but not N^7-methylguanine or N^3-methyladenine, induces gene mutation, sister chromatid exchanges, and chromosomal aberrations in Chinese hamster cells. *Mutat. Res., 108,* 279–292

Karran, P., Hjelmgren, T. & Lindahl, T. (1982) Induction of a DNA glycosylase for N-methylated purines is part of the adaptive response to alkylating agents. *Nature, 296,* 770–773

Kataoka, H. & Sekiguchi, M. (1982) Are purine bases enzymatically inserted into depurinated DNA in *Escherichia coli? J. Biochem., 92,* 971–973

Laval, F. & Michel, S. (1983) Adaptive DNA repair process in CHO cells. *J. cell. Biochem., Suppl. 7B,* 197

Lindahl, T. (1982) DNA repair enzymes. *Ann. Rev. Biochem., 51,* 61–87

Margison, G.P. (1982) Chronic or acute administration of various dialkylnitrosamines enhances the removal of O^6-methylguanine from rat liver DNA *in vivo. Chem-biol. Interactions, 38,* 189–201

Maru, G.B., Margison, G.P., Chu, Y.-H. & O'Connor, P.J. (1982) Effects of carcinogenesis and partial hepatectomy upon the hepatic O^6-methylguanine repair system in mice. *Carcinogenesis, 3,* 1247–1254

Mehta, J.R., Ludlum, D.B., Renard, A. & Verly, W.G. (1981) Repair of O^6-methylguanine in DNA by a chromatin fraction from rat liver: Transfer of the ethyl group to an acceptor protein. *Proc. natl Acad. Sci. USA, 78,* 6766–6770

Miyaki, M., Suzuki, K., Aihara, M. & Ono, T. (1983) Misincorporation in DNA synthesis after modification of template or polymerase by MNNG, MMS and UV radiation. *Mutat. Res., 10,* 203–218

Montesano, R., Brésil, H., Planche-Martel, G., Margison, G.P. & Pegg, A.E. (1980) Effect of chronic treatment of rats with dimethylnitrosamine on the removal of O^6-methylguanine from DNA. *Cancer Res., 40,* 452–458

Müller, R. & Rajewsky, M.F. (1983) Elimination of O^6-methylguanine from the DNA of brain, liver, and other rat tissues exposed to ethylnitrosourea at different states of prenatal development. *Cancer Res., 43,* 2897–2904

Naeslund, M., Segerbaeck, D. & Kolman, A. (1983) S-Adenosylmethionine, and endogenous alkylating agent. *Mutat. Res., 119,* 229–232

Olsson, M. & Lindahl, T. (1980) Repair of alkylated DNA in *Escherichia coli*. Methyl group transfer from O^6-methylguanine to a protein cystein residue. *J. biol. Chem., 255,* 10569–10571

Pegg, A.E. & Perry, W. (1981a) alkylation of nuclei acids and metabolism of small doses of dimethylnitrosamine in the rat. *Cancer Res., 41,* 3128–3132

Pegg, A.E. & Perry, W. (1981b) Stimulation of transfer of methyl groups from O^6-methylguanine in DNA to protein by rat liver extracts in response to hepatotoxins. *Carcinogenesis, 2,* 1195–1200

Pegg, A.E., Roberfroid, M., von Bahr, C., Foote, R.S., Mitra, S., Brésil, H., Likhachev, A. & Montesano, R. (1982) Revoval of O^6-methylguanine from DNA by human liver fractions. *Proc. natl Acad. Sci. USA, 79,* 5162–5165

Robins, P. & Cairns, J. (1979) Quantitation of the adaptive response to alkylating agents. *Nature, 280,* 74–76

Russell, W.L., Hunsicker, P.R., Raymer, G.D., Steele, M.H., Stelzner, K.F. & Thompson, H.M. (1982a) Dose-response curve for ethylnitrosourea-induced specific-locus mutations in mouse spermatogonia. *Proc. natl Acad. Sci. USA, 79,* 3589–3591

Russell, W.L., Hunsicker, P.R., Carpenter, D.A., Cornett, C.V. & Guinn, G.M. (1982b) Effect of dose fractionation on the tethylnitrosourea induction of specific-locus mutations in mouse spermatogonia. *Proc. natl Acad. Sci. USA, 79,* 3592–3593

Rydberg, B. & Lindahl, T. (1982) Nonenzymatic methylation of DNA by the intracellular group donor S-adenosyl-L-methionine is a potentially mutagenic reaction. *Eur. mol. Biol. org. J., 1,* 211–216

Samson, L. & Schwartz, J.L. (1980) Evidence for an adaptive repair pathway in CHO and human skin fibroblast cell lines. *Nature, 287,* 861–863

Sedgwick, B. & Lindahl, T. (1982) A common mechanism for repair of O^6-methylguanine and O^6-ethylguanine in DNA. *J. mol. Biol., 154,* 169–175

Setlow, R.B. (1980) Damages to DNA that result in neoplastic transformation. *Adv. Biol. Med. Phys., 17,* 99–108

Setlow, R.B. (1982) DNA repair, aging, and cancer. *Natl Cancer Inst. Monogr., 60,* 249–255

Setlow, R.B. (1983) *Variations in DNA repair among people.* In: Harris, C.C. & Autrup, H.N., eds, *Humans Carcinogenesis,* New York, Academic Press, pp. 231–252

Shiloh, Y. & Becker, T. (1981) Kinetics of O^6-methylguanine repair in normal and ataxia telangiectasia cell lines and correlation of repair capacity with cellular sensitivity to methylating agents. *Cancer Res., 41,* 5 114–5 120

Singer, B., Spengler, S. & Bodell, W.J. (1981) tissue dependent enzyme-mediated repair or removal of O-ethyl pyrimidine and ethyl purines in carcinogen-treated rats. *Carcinogenesis, 2,* 1 069–1 073

Singer, B. & Kusmierek, J.T. (1982) Chemical mutagenesis. *Ann. Rev. Biochem.,* **52,** 655–693

Sklar, R. & Strauss, B. (1981) Removal of O^6-methylguanine from DNA of normal and xeroderma pigmentosum-derived lymphoblastoid lines. *Nature, **289,** 417–420*

Sklar, R., Brady, K. & Strauss, B. (1981) Limited capacity for the removal of O^6-methylguanine and its regeneration in a human lymphoma line. *Carcinogenesis, **2,** 1 293–1 298*

Smith, R.S. & Margison, G.P. (1981) Effect of dialkylnitrosamine administration on alkylguanine removal from Syrian golden hamster liver DNA. *Br. J. Cancer, **44,** 27–31*

Snyder, R.D. & Regan, J.D. (1981) Quantitative estimation of the extent of alkylation of DNA following treatment of mammalian cells with non-radioactive alkylating agents. *Mutat. Res., **91,** 307–314*

Waldstein, E.A., Cao, E.H., Miller, M.E., Cronkite, E.P. & Setlow, R.B. (1982a) Extracts of chronic lymphocytic leukemia lymphocytes have a high level of repair activity for O^6-methylguanine. *Proc. natl Acad. Sci. USA, **79,** 4786–4790*

Waldstein, E.A., Cao, E.H. & Setlow, R.B. (1982b) Direct assay for O^6-methylguanine-acceptor protein in cell extracts. *Anal. Biochem., **126,** 268–272*

Waldstein, E.A., Cao, E.H., Bender, M.A. & Setlow, R.B. (1982c) Abilities of extracts of human lymphocytes to remove O^6-methylguanine from DNA. *Mutat. Res., **95,** 405–416*

Waldstein, E.A., Cao, E.H. & Setlow, R.B. (1982d) Adaptive resynthesis of O^6-methylguanine-accepting protein can explain the differences between mammalian cells proficient and deficient in methyl excision repair. *Proc. natl Acad. Sci. USA, **79,** 5115–5121*

Waldstein, E.A., Cao, E.H. & Setlow, R.B. (1983) *Constitutive levels and resynthesis of O^6-methylguanine acceptor activity in mammalian cells.* In: Friedberg, E.C. & Bridges, B.R., eds, *Cellular Responses to DNA Damage,* New York, Alan R. Liss, pp. 279–283

Wintersberger, E. (1982) Methods for the detection of single-strand breaks in DNA under neutral conditions and their application in a study on the mechanism of repair of *N*-methylated purines in mouse cells. *Eur. J. Biochem., **125,** 151–156*

REPAIR AND REPLICATION OF DNA CONTAINING O^6-METHYLGUANINE IN FETAL AND ADULT ANIMAL TISSUES IN RELATION TO THEIR SUSCEPTIBILITIES TO CANCER INDUCTION BY N-NITROSO-N-ALKYLUREAS

V.M. CRADDOCK

Toxicology Unit, MRC Laboratories, Woodmansterne Road, Carshalton, Surrey, UK

SUMMARY

Experimental evidence and basic concepts support the view that replication of DNA containing the mispairing base O^6-alkylguanine is an essential event in the initiation of cancer by simple alkylating agents. The likelihood of induction of cancer in a particular organ would depend on three factors: (1) the initial level of alkylation of DNA in that organ, (2) the rate of removal of O^6-alkylguanine from DNA and (3) the extent of DNA replication during the critical period in which O^6-alkylguanine is present. In systems in which the initial level of alkylation is approximately uniform in different organs, their relative susceptibilities to cancer would depend on their abilities to remove O^6-methylguanine from DNA, and on the rates of replication of DNA after treatment with the carcinogen.

To test this concept, repair and replication were studied in tissues with very different susceptibilities to induction of cancer by a low dose of N-methyl-N-nitrosourea, i.e., rat and mouse brain and lung, and rat brain at different stages of fetal and postnatal development. The ability of the tissue to remove O^6-methylguanine from DNA was determined by incubation of tissue extracts with extraneously methylated DNA. Replication was studied by measurements of incorporation of ^{3}H-thymidine into DNA. The outstandingly high level of replication of alkylated DNA in mouse thymus correlates with its outstanding susceptibility to cancer induction by N-methyl-N-nitrosourea (MNU). The result of comparing repair ability and DNA replication in rat and mouse brain and lung suggest that unknown factors are involved in the resistance of the nontarget organs. Experiments with fetal and postnatal rat brain and liver support the idea that replication of DNA containing O^6-methylguanine is a necessary event in carcinogenesis.

INTRODUCTION

Evidence strongly supports the concept that an essential event in the induction of cancer by N-nitroso-N-methyl compounds is the replication of DNA containing O^6-methylguanine (O^6-MG). The extent of replication of alkylated DNA depends on the level of initial alkylation, the rate of removal of O^6-MG by repair processes, and the extent of replication of DNA which occurs after treatment with the carcinogen before the O^6-MG has been removed. When the level of DNA alkylation in different rodent organs is approximately uniform, as after intraperitoneal injection of a low dose of MNU (Swann, & Magee, 1968), the susceptibility of the different organs to carcinogenesis depends on their relative abilities to remove O^6-MG from DNA, and on the relative rates of DNA replication during the critical period when O^6-MG is present in DNA.

There are many systems in which this concept can be tested. After treatment of adult rats with low doses of MNU, cancer is induced specifically in the brain (Swenberg et al., 1975). In mice, lung and lymphoid tissues are the most susceptible organs (Frei, 1970). A second exploitable situation is provided by the fact that the incidence of brain cancer induced in rats by a single injection of N-ethyl-N-nitrosourea varies markedly with age (Ivankovic & Druckrey, 1968). Treatment of pregnant rats at day 12 of gestation does not induce brain cancer in the offspring, but susceptibility increases to a maximum in the perinatal period, and then decreases. The liver of rats apparently is not susceptible at any age. DNA replication and capacity for removal of O^6-MG were studied in various tissues and at different stages in fetal development and postnatal growth.

Until recently, work on repair of alkylated DNA in rodents has been done using in-vivo techniques (Goth & Rajewsky, 1974); however, with these methods, alkylated DNA is diluted out by newly synthesized DNA, especially in those tissues which divide rapidly in adult and fetal tissues. This would appear as a loss of O^6-MG, and differences in rates of replication between different tissues would affect measurements of repair of DNA. As the methyl group is transferred stoichiometrically from the O^6-position of guanine to a cysteine residue in a specific alkyl acceptor protein (Olsson & Lindahl, 1980), we determined the ability of the tissues to repair alkylated DNA by incubating tissue extracts with extraneously methylated DNA and determining the amount of S-methylcysteine formed.

Surprisingly, the effect of MNU on DNA replication in the relevant organs has not previously been reported.

MATERIALS AND METHODS

Female Wistar rats, 195–205 g, and C57Bl x 10 mice, 20 g, were used, except when otherwise stated. MNU was given by intraperitoneal injection of 20 mg/kg body weight. Fetal livers and brains or whole heads were placed in liquid nitrogen before storage for a few days at −70 °C. DNA replication was studied by measuring incorporation of ^{3}H-TdR given by intraperitoneal injection (1 μCi/g body weight, 0.2 μCi/mmol), and the animals were killed after 60 min. The ability of tissues to remove O^6-MG from DNA was measured as described previously (Craddock et al., 1982).

RESULTS

The ability of a tissue to repair DNA is most meaningfully expressed on a per-nucleus basis. Liver of rats and mice possessed the highest repair activities of the organs studied (Table 1), although rat spleen was more active on a per-g tissue basis. In both species, brain and lung had low levels of activity. DNA replication in rat and mouse brain was inhibited to approximately 50% and lung to 30% of control values by 24 h after MNU treatment. No appreciable recovery was apparent in these organs by two days after treatment.

Table 1. Ability of rodent organs to repair O^6-methylguanine-DNA and rates of DNA replication after treatment with 20 mg/kg body weight N-methyl-N-nitrosourea (MNU)

Species	Organ	Repair capacity[a]	Replication 24 h after MNU[b]	Susceptibility of adult animals to low dose of MNU[c]
Rat	liver	4.5	62 613	−
	spleen	0.7	10 645	−
	thymus	0.3	2 633	(+)
	lung	0.5	6 494	−
	brain	0.2	1 679	+ + + +
Mouse	liver	2.6	40 747	−
	spleen	0.2	4 146	−
	thymus	0.1	26 082	+ + +
	lung	0.3	8 220	+ + + +
	brain	0.2	3 932	−

[a] Repair capacity is expressed as pmol S-methylcysteine formed per mg DNA in the tissue sample from which the extract was prepared
[b] Replication is expressed as dpm ^{3}H-TdR incorporated per mg DNA
[c] Susceptibility of organs to carcinogenesis: rat, Swenberg et al. (1975); mouse, Frei (1970)

Table 2. Levels of alkyl acceptor protein in rat liver and brain at different stages of fetal and postnatal development

Age	pmol S-methylcysteine per mg DNA in extracted tissue sample		pmol S-methylcysteine per g tissue		mg DNA per g tissue	
	liver	brain	liver	brain	liver	brain
8 weeks	3.3	0.1	8.2	0.2	2.7	1.9
19 days	2.3	0.3	9.0	0.5	3.7	1.9
10 days	1.9	0.2	9.4	0.3	4.9	2.2
1 day	1.0	0.1	5.2	0.3	6.8	3.3
20-day fetus	0.7	0.2	9.8	1.0	13.7	5.1
18-day fetus	0.8	0.3[a]	12.7	1.5[a]	14.6	4.7[a]
16-day fetus	0.8	0.4[a]	−	−	−	−
12-day fetus	(0.8)[b]	1.0[a]	−	−	−	−

[a] Indicates that whole fetal head was used instead of brain
[b] Value for whole fetus

Repair activity in rat brain was highest in 12-day fetuses (whole head) (Table 2), decreased during fetal development, and remained low in adults. The liver in 12-day fetuses is a primordial bud; during fetal development it possessed a higher level of activity than brain, but this did not begin to increase to adult levels until after birth. Incorporation of ^{3}H-TdR into liver DNA was greater than into brain DNA at all stages of fetal and postnatal development.

DISCUSSION

The outstanding result is the high degree of replication of alkylated DNA in mouse thymus, which correlates with the outstanding susceptibility of this organ to cancer induction by MNU. However, the low abilities of rat and mouse brain and lung to remove O^6-MG from DNA, and the similar extents of replication of DNA following MNU treatment, suggest that replication of DNA containing O^6-MG does not occur more extensively in the target organs, i.e., rat brain and mouse lung, than in less susceptible organs, i.e., rat lung and mouse brain. Replication of alkylated DNA may be necessary for induction of cancer, but carcinogenesis does not inevitably ensue. Comparison of levels of repair and replication of alkylated DNA in rat brain and liver during development, however, shows a good correlation with carcinogenesis. Thus, in the 12-day fetal brain, the replication rate is high, but repair activity is high also. Around birth, repair ability is low, and DNA replication is rapid; while in the adult repair ability remains low, but replication is low also. Replication is greater in liver than in brain at all ages, but repair ability is higher also. These experiments therefore support the concept that replication of alkylated DNA is an initiating event in carcinogenesis.

ACKNOWLEDGEMENTS

The author would like to acknowledge the assistance of A.R. Henderson and S. Gash.

REFERENCES

Craddock, V.M., henderson, A.R. & Gash, S. (1982) Nature of the constitutive and induced mammalian O^6-methylguanine DNA repair enzyme. *Biochem. biophys. Res. Commun., 107,* 546–553

Frei, J.V. (1970) Toxicity, tissue changes, and tumor induction in inbred Swiss mice by methylnitrosamine and amide compounds. *Cancer Res., 30,* 11–17

Goth, R. & Rajewsky, M. (1974) Persistence of O^6-ethylguanine in rat brain DNA; correlation with nervous system-specific carcinogenesis by *N*-ethyl-*N*-nitrosourea. *Proc. natl Acad. Sci. USA, 71,* 639–643

Ivankovic, S. & Druckrey, H. (1968) Transplacental induction of malignant tumors of the nervous system. 1. *N*-Nitroso-*N*-ethylurea in BD-IX rats. *Z. Krebsforsch., 71,* 320–360

Olsson, M. & Lindahl, T. (1980) Repair of alkylated DNA in *E. coli;* methyl group transfer from O^6-methylguanine to a protein cysteine residue. *J. biol. Chem., 255,* 10569–10571

Swann, P.F. & Magee, P.N. (1968) Nitrosamine induced carcinogenesis. *Biochem. J., 110,* 39–47

Swenberg, J.A., Koestner, A., Wechsler, W., Brunden, M.N. & Abe, H. (1975) Differential oncogenic effects of *N*-methyl-*N*-nitrosourea. *J. natl Cancer Inst., 54,* 89–96

PROPERTIES OF THE O^6-ALKYLGUANINE-DNA REPAIR SYSTEM OF MAMMALIAN CELLS

A.E. PEGG

Department of Physiology and Cancer Research Center,
The Milton S. Hershey Medical Center,
The Pennsylvania State University, Hershey, PA 17033, USA

SUMMARY

O^6-Alkylguanine is an important lesion produced in DNA after exposure to N-nitrosodimethylamine or *N*-nitrosodiethylamine and may lead to mutagenesis or carcinogenesis if unrepaired. Repair of this product is accomplished by a unique DNA-repair activity which resides in a single protein. This protein catalyses the transfer of the alkyl group from the guanine O^6-position to a cysteine residue. The cysteine acceptor site appears to be present on the same protein and is not regenerated. There is, therefore, a stoichiometric relationship between the amount of this protein and the number of O^6-alkylguanine residues that can be repaired. The protein has been partially purified from rat liver and from a number of human tissues. The rodent and human O^6-alkylguanine-DNA alkyltransferases have similar properties and a molecular weight of about 23 000. The protein is specific for O^6-alkylguanine in DNA, prefers double-stranded DNA as substrate and binds tightly to double-stranded DNA, whether alkylated or not. Both methyl and ethyl groups are removed, although the rate of removal of the ethyl groups is four times slower. Liver has the highest content of this protein among all tissues tested from both rats and humans, but all human tissues have substantially higher levels than the equivalent rodent tissue. O^6-Alkylguanine-DNA alkyltransferase was found in all primary human tumours and tissues tested (including brain, which in rodents has very little activity). It is concluded that human tissues are likely to be able to repair O^6-alkylguanine but that the capacity of repair is tissue-specific and linked to the level of this protein.

INTRODUCTION

A number of potent *N*-nitroso carcinogens, including *N*-nitrosodimethylamine (NDMA) and *N*-nitrosodiethylamine (NDEA) are thought to act by virtue of their decomposition to form simple alkylating agents. These alkylating species react with at least 12 sites in DNA, but there is suggestive evidence that alkylation of the exo-oxygen atoms of the bases may be critical in carcinogenesis and mutagenesis (Pegg, 1977; Montesano, 1981; Singer & Kushmierek, 1982; Pegg, 1983). The major lesion of this type produced by NDMA is O^6-methylguanine, and there is substantial evidence (see reviews cited above) that this product or its ethyl equivalent may initiate neoplastic growth if not repaired before cell division and DNA synthesis. The properties and capacity of the enzymatic system capable of removing this product from DNA are, therefore, of particular interest and are the subject of this article.

MATERIALS AND METHODS

Rats were treated with NDMA and NDEA, and nucleic acids were isolated from the liver and analysed for the content of alkylated bases, as described previously (Pegg & Balog, 1979; Pegg & Perry, 1981a). The rates of removal of O^6-alkylguanine were then calculated as described by Scicchitano and Pegg (1982). The activity of O^6-alkylguanine-DNA alkyltransferase was assayed as described by Pegg et al. (1983), and tissue extracts containing this activity were prepared as described by Pegg et al. (1982).

RESULTS

Removal of O^6-*alkylguanine from DNA* in vivo

When rats were treated with NDMA or NDEA and the content of alkylated bases present in the liver DNA determined, it was found that small (less than 2 mg/kg) doses of these nitrosamines given by oral or intravenous administration were very rapidly metabolized. The production of 7-alkylguanine in DNA could be used as an index of metabolism, since this adduct is lost relatively slowly and it is a major product which is easily quantitated (Pegg, 1983). Formation of 7-alkylguanine, and hence activation of the nitrosamine, was complete within less than 1 h, and no significant decline in 7-alkylguanine was seen during the next 4 h. Since it is known that O^6-alkylguanine is formed in DNA in amounts equal to 0.11 times the 7-alkylguanine content for NDMA and to 0.67 times the 7-alkylguanine content for NDEA, the amounts of O^6-alkylguanine formed could be calculated. However, even a few minutes after treatment, substantially less O^6-alkylguanine was actually found than was calculated to have been formed. Also, the actual O^6-alkylguanine content declined rapidly with time, and virtually all was lost within 3 h after administration of doses of NDMA of 5–500 µg/kg. By subtracting the amount of O^6-methylguanine found from that formed, as calculated from the 7-methylguanine content, it was found that half of the O^6-methylguanine was removed within 15 min and more than 80% within 1 h (Scicchitano & Pegg, 1982). A similar analysis of the loss of O^6-ethylguanine from DNA after administration of NDEA, using the data of Pegg and Balog (1979), indicated that O^6-ethylguanine was lost about four times more slowly than O^6-methylguanine, when comparisons were made after doses of the nitrosamines which produce approximately similar amounts of the O^6 adduct.

When larger doses of the nitrosamines were given, the percentage of O^6-alkylguanine that could be removed during the first 4 h after treatment declined, indicating that the repair system had a limited capacity to carry out this reaction. With normal Sprague-Dawley rats which had not been pre-exposed to NDMA or other factors which induce the system (Montesano, 1981; Pegg, 1983), the capacity for removal was such that the damage produced by about 0.5–1.0 mg/kg NDMA could be rapaired almost completely. This corresponds to about 30–60 000 molecules/cell.

Removal of O⁶-alkylguanine from DNA in vitro

Extracts of rat liver were found to catalyse the loss of O^6-methylguanine from DNA. The protein responsible for this reaction was purified more than one thousand-fold starting from rat liver isolated during regeneration after partial hepatectomy (Pegg *et al.*, 1983). Partial hepatectomy results in six- to seven-fold increase in the concentration of this protein (Pegg *et al.*, 1981). The protein was found to have a molecular weight of about 23 000 and did not require cofactors for activity but was much more stable if isolated and stored in the presence of dithiothreitol. As shown in Table 1, only O^6-methylguanine was lost from DNA when double-stranded calf thymus DNA, which had been methylated by reaction with N-[³H]methyl-N-nitrosourea, was incubated with the protein. In this experiment, 96% of the O^6-methylguanine present in the DNA was removed by the liver protein without significant removal of any other adduct. (Small losses of 7-methyladenine, 3-methylguanine and other N-methyl purines was also seen when bovine serum albumin was substituted for the liver protein; this is due to spontaneous depurination of these adducts.)

It should be noted that it is possible that the liver protein can remove other adducts with a much lower affinity and rate than that for O^6-methylguanine. Since the protein is used up in the reaction (see below), it may be consumed in reaction with O^6-methylguanine and, therefore, not be available for other less favoured substrates. Experiments with a very large excess of the protein would be needed to rule out this possibility, and these have not yet been carried out. At present, only O^6-alkylguanine is known to be attacked. The protein is also able to repair O^6-ethylguanine, but at a rate about four times slower than for O^6-methylguanine, and can also act (even more slowly) on hydroxyethyl, chloroethyl and propyl groups attached to the O^6 position (A.E. Pegg, unpublished data).

The protein greatly prefers double-stranded DNA as a substrate. It acts much more slowly on single-stranded DNA, and reaction with O^6-methylguanine in RNA was too slow to be detected (Pegg *et al.*, 1983). It is important to note that the rate of reaction depended on the extent of alkylation of the substrate DNA. Substrates containing a high level of replacement of guanine with O^6-methylguanine (one part in 2 000) were repaired much faster than those containing only one part in 500 000 (Scicchitano & Pegg, 1982). Therefore, comparisons of rates of repair of different alkyl groups must be carried out with substrates alkylated to similar extents.

Table 1. Specific removal of 0⁶-methylguanine from methylated DNA by rat liver protein

Methylated adduct in DNA	Radioactivity (dpm × 10⁻¹) present in adduct shown		
	Prior to incubation	After incubation for 1 h[a]	
		Plus bovine serum albumin	Plus liver protein
7-Methylguanine	5 485	5 238 (95%)	5 307 (97%)
3-Methylguanine	66	55 (83%)	60 (91%)
3-Methyladenine	572	516 (90%)	520 (91%)
7-Methyladenine	102	73 (72%)	80 (78%)
1-Methyladenine	48	40 (83%)	42 (88%)
0⁶-Methylguanine	603	600 (100%)	23 (4%)
Methylated pyrimidines plus methylphosphate triesters	1 149	1 102 (96%)	1 119 (97%)

[a]The values in parentheses represent the percentage of the adduct shown still present in DNA after incubation for 60 min with purified liver protein or an equal amount of bovine serum albumin. The analysis was carried out as described by Pegg *et al.* (1983)

The loss of O^6-methylguanine from DNA brought about by the rat liver protein is paralleled by the production of equivalent amounts of guanine in the DNA and by the formation of S-methylcysteine in the protein. This stoichiometry, and the fact that the protein is consumed in the reaction which halts unless more protein is added, indicates that the mechanism of repair is the transfer of the methyl group to a cysteine-acceptor residue which is not regenerated. This mechanism is similar to that found by Lindahl and colleagues for a protein from *Escherichia coli* (Olsson & Lindahl, 1980; Demple *et al.*, 1982), which has a molecular weight of 18 500 and is slightly smaller than the mammalian O^6-alkylguanine-DNA alkyltransferase, although in all other respects they appear to be similar. The bacterial protein has been purified to homogeneity, and it is therefore certain that the acceptor site and the transferase activity reside in the same molecule. This is probably also true for the mammalian protein, since these functions have not yet been separated; however, the liver protein is not homogeneous, and the existence of a separate acceptor molecule, although unlikely, is not totally ruled out.

Comparisons of O^6-alkylguanine-DNA alkyltransferase activity in different organs and species

Measurement of the amount of O^6-alkylguanine-DNA alkyltransferase in rat tissues indicated that liver has the highest activity, followed by oesophagus and kidney. Lower levels of activity were found in lung and colon, and the activity in brain was so low that accurate measurement was difficult (Table 1). The activity in the liver could be increased to about 220 fmol/mg by chronic treatment with NDMA and to almost 500 fmol/mg by partial hepatectomy (Montesano, 1981; Pegg & Perry, 1981b; Pegg *et al.*, 1981).

Estimations have now been made of the amount of O^6-alkylguanine-DNA alkyltransferase in a number of human tissues (Table 1). The human samples show considerable individual variations, with a five-fold range for samples from different individuals; but this variation is not unexpected in view of the diverse genetic background of the subjects and is strikingly lower than the 50–150-fold range in the activities of carcinogen activating enzymes (Harris *et al.*, 1982). In all cases, the activity found for human tissues was substantially greater than that for the equivalent rat tissues, with mean values of five to twenty times higher, depending on the tissue. As with rats, liver was the most active tissue and brain the least, but activity was easily measurable even in the brain samples. Detailed characterization of the protein and the reaction catalysed has been carried out for human liver (Pegg *et al.*, 1982), brain (Wiestler, Kleihues and Pegg, unpublished data), lung and colon proteins (Grafstrom *et al.*, 1983). In all cases, the reaction was catalysed by a protein with a molecular weight of 20–25 000 and was similar to that mediated by the rat liver protein in producing stoichiometric amounts of S-methylcysteine and guanine in the DNA.

We have also measured the O^6-alkylguanine-DNA alkyltransferase activity of about 30 primary human tumours, mainly originating in the brain but including some gastrointestinal neoplasms. All of these samples had detectable activity, which was equal to or greater than that in the normal tissues from which the tumours were derived.

DISCUSSION

Although it is certainly possible that other DNA repair processes exist which can remove O^6-alkylguanine from DNA, there is good reason to believe that the alkyltransferase described in the present paper is the major factor in the rapid removal of this adduct. There is a reasonable agreement between the results of in-vivo experiments, in which the organ specificity of rate of repair of this product has been measured, and the levels of the alkyltransferase described in Table 2. For example, O^6-alkylguanine is removed most rapidly from liver and very slowly from DNA of rat brain (Pegg, 1977, 1983). Most of the O^6-alkylguanine-DNA alkyltransferase

Table 2. Levels of 0⁶-alkylguanine-DNA alkyltransferase present in rat and human tissues

Tissue	0⁶-Alkylguanine-DNA alkyltransferase activity (fmol/mg protein)	
	Rat (mean)	Human (mean and range)
Liver	86	873 (411–1 795) [a]
Regenerating liver	494	ND
Lung	29	122 (41–194) [b]
Colon	21	261 (135–413) [b]
Oesophagus	54	217 (184–282) [b]
Brain	∼ 15	76 (37–122) [c]
Kidney	41	ND

[a] From Pegg et. al. (1982)
[b] From Grafstrom et al. (1983)
[c] From Wiestler, Kleihues and Pegg (unpublished data)
ND, not determined

present in rat liver is actually in the hepatocytes, which are much better able to remove O^6-methylguanine from their DNA *in vivo* than the nonparenchymal cells (Swenberg *et al.*, 1982). The level present in hepatocytes amounts to about 60 000 molecules per cell, which is in reasonable agreement with the number of O^6-methylguanine molecules that can be removed rapidly before repair becomes saturated. Finally, the rate of repair of O^6-methylguanine and the slower rate of repair of O^6-ethylguanine seen *in vitro* with DNA substrates alkylated to extents of one to five O^6 adducts per million guanines agree quite well with the rate at which these lesions are lost from the liver *in vivo* after treatment with NDMA and NDEA.

The higher levels of O^6-alkylguanine-DNA alkyltransferase protein found in human tissue extracts than in the equivalent rodent tissue are consistent with the findings of several other groups that certain human cell lines in culture have relatively high levels of this protein (30 000–150 000 molecules/cell), whereas rodent cell lines have very low activities (Foote *et al.*, 1983a, b; Pegg, 1983; Yarosh *et al.*, 1983). One apparent exception is the report by Waldstein *et al.* (1982) that hamster V79 and CHO cells contain about 100 000 molecules/cell; but this report is directly contradictory to findings by Foote *et al.* (1983a) and by Grafstrom *et al.* (1983) that these cell lines contain less than 1 000 molecules/cell. The explanation for this discrepancy is not clear but may relate to incorrect identification of the cell lines, as subsequent work on *mer⁻* cell lines studied by Waldstein *et al.* (1982) now indicates that these lines were actually *mer⁺* (Foote *et al.*, 1083a, b; Yarosh *et al.*, 1983). The division of human tumour cell lines into two classes (those competent to support the growth of adenovirus damaged by alkylating agents, which are designated *mer⁺*, and those unable to do this, which are designated *mer⁻*) is supported by experiments from several laboratories (see Yarosh *et al.*, 1983 and Pegg, 1983). The *mer⁻* classes are more sensitive to alkylating agents and lack the O^6-alkylguanine-DNA alkyltransferase activity. A substantial number of the human tumour cell strains tested were found to be *mer⁻* However, it is not yet known whether the expression of the O^6-alkylguanine-DNA transalkylase protein is lost during culture or is part of the phenotype of the primary tumour. It has been suggested that the absence of the O^6-alkylguanine-DNA alkyltransferase be exploited for therapy, because *mer⁻* cells are more sensitive to drugs such as 1-(2-chloroethyl)nitrosourea, and the alkyltransferase may protect against cross-linking by such agents (Yarosh *et al.*, 1983). However, our finding that of 30 human tumours tested all were positive for this activity suggests that the *mer⁻* phenotype may be a consequence of culture; if this is the case, such attempts are likely to be unsuccessful.

ACKNOWLEDGEMENTS

This research was supported by grants CA-18137 and 1P30-CA-18450. The author wishes to thank Mrs Bonnie Merlino for preparation of this paper.

REFERENCES

Demple, B., Jacobsson, A., Olsson, M., Robins, P. & Lindahl, T. (1982) Repair of alkylated DNA in *Escherichia coli*. Physical properties of O^6-methylguanine-DNA methyltransferase. *J. biol. Chem., 257,* 13 776–13 780

Foote, R.S., Pal, B.C. & Mitra, S. (1983a) Quantitation of O^6-methylguanine-DNA methyltransferase in HeLa cells. *Mutat. Res., 119,* 221–228

Foote, R.S., Hsie, A.W., Pal, B.C. & Mitra, S. (1983b) O^6-Methylguanine-DNA methyltransferase in mammalian cells. *J. cell. Biochem., Suppl. 7B,* 195

Grafstrom, R.C., Pegg, A.E. & Harris, C.C. (1983) Formaldehyde inhibits O^6-methylguanine excision repair in human bronchial cells. *Proc. Am. Assoc. Cancer Res.* (in press)

Harris, C.C., Grafstrom, R.C., Lechner, J.F. & Autrup, H. (1982) *Metabolism of N-nitrosamines and repair of DNA damage in cultured human tissues and cells.* In: Magee, P.N., ed., *Nitrosamines and Human Cancer, (Banbury Report 12),* Cold Spring Harbor, NY, Cold Spring Harbor Laboratories, pp. 121–140

Montesano, R. (1981) Alkylation of DNA and tissue specificity in nitrosamine carcinogenesis. *J. Supramol. Struct., 17,* 259–273

Olsson, M. & Lindahl, T. (1980) Repair of alkylated DNA in *Escherichia coli. J. biol. Chem., 255,* 10569–10571

Pegg, A.E. (1977) Formation and metabolism of alkylated nucleosides: possible role in carcinogenesis by nitroso compounds and alkylating agents. *Adv. Cancer Res., 25,* 195–267

Pegg, A.E. (1983) Alkylation and subsequent repair of DNA after exposure to dimethylnitrosamine and related compounds. *Rev. Biochem. Toxicol., 5,* 83–133

Pegg, A.E. & Balog, F. (1979) Formation and subsequent excision of O^6-ethylguanine from DNA of rat liver following administration of diethylnitrosamine. *Cancer Res., 39,* 5 003–5 009

Pegg, A.E. & Perry, W. (1981a) Alkylation of nucleic acids and metabolism of small doses of dimethylnitrosamine in the rat. *Cancer Res., 41,* 3128–3132

Pegg, A.E. & Perry, W. (1981b) Stimulation of transfer of methyl groups from O^6-methylguanine in DNA to protein by rat liver extracts in response to hepatotoxins. *Carcinogenesis, 2,* 1195–1200

Pegg, A.E., Perry, W. & Bennett, R.A. (1981) Partial hepatectomy increases the ability of rat liver extracts to catalyze removal of O^6-methylguanine from alkylated DNA. *Biochem. J., 197,* 195–201

Pegg, A.E., Roberfroid, M., von Bahr, C., Foote, R.S., Mitra, S. Bresil, H., Likhachev, A. & Montesano, R. (1982) Removal of O^6-methylguanine from DNA by human liver fractions. *Proc. natl. Acad. Sci. (USA), 79,* 5162–5165

Pegg, A.E., Wiest, L., Foote, R.S., Mitra, S. & Perry, W. (1983) Purification and properties of O^6-methylguanine-DNA transmethylase from rat liver. *J. biol. Chem., 258,* 2327–2333

Scicchitano, D. & Pegg, A.E. (1982) Kinetics of repair of O^6-methylguanine in DNA by O^6-methyl-guanine-DNA methyltransferase *in vitro* and *in vivo. Biochem. biophys. Res. Commun., 109,* 995–1001

Singer, B. & Kushmierek, J.T. (1982) Chemical mutagenesis. *Ann. Rev. Biochem. 51,* 655–693

Swenberg, J.A., Bedell, M.A., Billings, K.C., Umbenhauer, D.R. & Pegg, A.E. (1982) Cell-specific differences in O^6-alkylguanine DNA repair activity during continuous exposure. *Proc. natl. Acad. Sci. (USA), 79,* 5499–5502

Waldstein, E.A., Cao, E.-H. & Setlow, R.B. (1982) Adaptive resynthesis of O^6-methylguanine-accepting protein can explain the differences between mammalian cells proficient and deficient in methyl excision repair. *Proc. natl Acad. Sci. (USA), 79,* 5117–5121

Yarosh, D.B., Foote, R.S., Mitra, S. & Day, R.S., III (1983) Repair of O^6-methylguanine in DNA by demethylation is lacking in *Mer⁻* human tumor cell strains. *Carcinogenesis, 2,* 199–205

HIGH-AFFINITY MONOCLONAL ANTIBODIES FOR THE SPECIFIC RECOGNITION AND QUANTIFICATION OF DEOXYNUCLEOSIDES STRUCTURALLY MODIFIED BY *N*-NITROSO COMPOUNDS

J. ADAMKIEWICZ, O. AHRENS, N. HUH, P. NEHLS & M.F. RAJEWSKY

Institut für Zellbiologie (Tumorforschung), Universität Essen(GH), Hufelandstrasse 55, D-4300 Essen 1, FRG

E. SPIESS

Institut für Zell- und Tumorbiologie, Deutsches Krebsforschungszentrum, Im Neuenheimer Feld 280, D-6900 Heidelberg 1, FRG

SUMMARY

The applicability of conventional radiochromatographic procedures to the detection and quantification of specific, carcinogen-induced structural modifications in the DNA of mammalian cells is limited by the necessity of using radioactively labelled agents and by the relatively large amounts of DNA required for analysis of low levels of DNA modification. Recently developed immunoanalytical methods have improved this situation considerably. High-affinity monoclonal antibodies (MAB), in combination with radio- and enzyme-immunoassays, now permit the sensitive detection of alkyldeoxynucleosides in small samples of hydrolysed DNA from tissues and cultured cells exposed previously to non-radioactive (e.g., environmental) alkylating *N*-nitroso carcinogens. Furthermore, MAB can be used to quantify by direct immunofluorescence (and with the aid of computer-based image analysis of electronically intensified fluorescence signals) specific alkylation products in the DNA of individual cells. With this method, the present detection limit for, e.g. O^6-ethyl-2'-deoxyguanosine (O^6-EtdGuo) is of the order of 7×10^2 O^6-EtdGuo molecules per diploid genome. Therefore, cells (e.g. from biopsy material) can now be monitored directly for the presence of specific carcinogen-DNA adducts, or with respect to their capacity to remove enzymatically such modified structures from DNA. In combination with transmission electron microscopy, MAB also permit the direct visualization of specific carcinogen-modified sites in DNA. Thus, O^6-EtdGuo can be localized in double-stranded DNA molecules by the binding of a MAB specifically directed against this ethylation product.

INTRODUCTION

The majority of chemical carcinogens and many chemical agents used in cancer therapy cause structural alterations in the DNA of target cells. A precise structural characterization is still lacking for the DNA adducts of many chemical agents known to react with DNA. However, the various types of DNA modifications resulting from exposure of cells to alkylating *N*-nitroso compounds (alkylnitrosamines, alkylnitro-nitrosoguanidines, alkylnitrosoureas) have to a large extent been identified (Lawley, 1976; Pegg, 1977; Grover, 1979; Kohn, 1979; O'Connor *et al.*, 1979; Singer, 1979; Rajewsky, 1980). In cells exposed to DNA-reactive chemicals at toxicologically tolerable dose levels, the respective reaction products in DNA are generally formed at low frequencies. Therefore, highly sensitive methods are required for their detection and quantification in studies on DNA repair, mutagenesis and carcinogenesis, and for the dosimetry of cellular DNA damage.

Conventional radiochromatography (Beranek *et al.*, 1980) has until recently been the method of choice for the analysis of DNA modified structurally by chemical agents. However, the sensitivity of radiochromatographic techniques is limited by the specific radioactivity of the respective ^{3}H- or ^{14}C-labelled compounds, and by the relatively large amounts of DNA (cells) needed for analysis. The detection of specific carcinogen-DNA adducts in (e.g., human) tissues and cells exposed to low doses of non-radioactive (e.g., environmental) agents is not possible except when ^{32}P 'post-labelling methods' can be used (Gupta *et al.*, 1982). Recently developed immunoanalytical procedures, especially those involving high-affinity MAB directed against specific carcinogen-modified components of DNA, have changed this situation considerably (Rajewsky *et al.*, 1980; Poirier, 1981; Adamkiewicz *et al.*, 1982; Müller *et al.*, 1982). Since immunoglobulins possess an exceptional capability to recognize subtle alterations of molecular structure, both the specificity and the sensitivity of immunoanalysis are extremely high. Equally important, the antigens (i.e., in the case of carcinogen-modified nucleosides, the haptens coupled to carrier proteins for immunization) need not be radioactively labelled.

On the basis of the original work of Erlanger, Plescia, Stollar and others, immunological assays have during the past years been established to quantify a number of specific carcinogen-DNA adducts in hydrolysed DNA, notably for deoxynucleosides modified by *N*-nitroso compounds, acetylaminofluorene, benzo[*a*]pyrene and aflatoxin B$_1$ (for references, see reviews by Müller & Rajewsky, 1981; Müller *et al.*, 1982). As part of a research programme on molecular and cellular mechanisms in chemical carcinogenesis, we have developed (and are further expanding) a collection of high-affinity MAB directed against specific alkyldeoxynucleosides produced in the DNA of mammalian cells exposed to *N*-nitroso compounds (Rajewsky *et al.*, 1980; Adamkiewicz *et al.*, 1982). This collection presently includes MAB specific for O^6-methyl-2'-deoxyguanosine (O^6-MedGuo), O^6-EtdGuo, O^6-n-butyl-2'-deoxyguanosine (O^6-BudGuo), O^6-isopropyl-2'-deoxyguanosine (O^6-iProdGuo) and O^4-ethyl-2'-deoxythymidine (O^4-EtdThd). These MAB are currently used for immunoanalysis of hydrolysed DNA by radioimmunoassay (RIA) or enzyme-linked immunosorbent assay (Müller & Rajewsky, 1978, 1980), direct immunofluorescence in individual cells (using computer-based image analysis of electronically intensified fluorescence signals (Adamkiewicz *et al.*, 1983), and immune electron microscopy (Nehls *et al.*, 1983).

EXPERIMENTAL

O^6- and O^4-Alkylribonucleosides were used as the haptens coupled to carrier protein for immunization (Müller & Rajewsky, 1978, 1980). The synthesis of all alkylribo- and alkyldeoxyribonucleosides, with the exception of O^6-*n*-butylguanosine which was a gift from Dr R. Saffhill (Paterson Labs, Manchester, UK), of other alkylated nucleic acid constituents used for cross-reactivity tests, and of high specific ^{3}H-activity tracers for the competitive RIA has been described by Müller and Rajewsky (1978, 1980), Rajewsky *et al.* (1980) and Adamkiewicz *et al.* (1982).

For immunization, alkylribonucleosides were coupled to keyhole limpet haemocyanin (KLH) (Calbiochem, Marburg, FRG; molecular weight, $\sim$ 800 000), the binding ratio being

~ 100 hapten molecules per molecule of KLH (Erlanger & Beiser, 1964; Müller & Rajewsky, 1980). Adult female rats of the inbred BDIX-strain (Druckrey, 1971) were immunized by multiple intracutaneous injections of the hapten-KLH conjugate, as described by Rajewsky *et al.* (1980) and Adamkiewicz *et al.* (1982). The animals were 'boosted' five and eight weeks later, and spleen cells were collected three to four days after the last booster injection for fusion with cells of the hypoxanthine-aminopterine-thymidine (HAT)-sensitive rat myeloma cell line Y3-Ag.1.2.3. (Galfré *et al.*, 1979) *in vitro*. The protocol for cell fusion, and the culturing, cloning and recloning of rat x rat hybridoma cells secreting anti-alkyldeoxynucleoside MAB have been described in detail by Rajewsky *et al.* (1980) and Adamkiewicz *et al.* (1982). Culture supernatants were tested for the presence of specific antibodies by ELISA, and aliquots of positive clones were either injected into Pristan-pretreated, X-irradiated (4 Gy) BDIX-rats for growth and antibody production in the ascites, or cultured *in vitro* for antibody secretion into the cell culture fluid. Isotype analysis of MAB was carried out by immunoprecipitation in agar, using anti-rat-isotype antisera (Miles, Frankfurt am Main, FRG). MAB concentrations in cell culture or ascites fluid and antibody affinity constants were calculated from the data obtained by competitive RIA, according to Müller (1980). MAB were isolated with the use of the respective specific haptens coupled to epoxy-activated Sepharose 6B (Pharmacia, Uppsala, Sweden) at acid or alkaline pH (Müller & Rajewsky, 1980; Rajewsky *et al.*, 1980).

As previously described (Müller & Rajewsky, 1980), DNA isolated from tissues or cultured cells was hydrolysed enzymatically to deoxynucleosides with DNase I (Boehringer Mannheim, Mannheim, FRG), snake venom phosphodiesterase (Boehringer), and grade 1 alkaline phosphatase (Boehringer). Adenosine deaminase was sometimes used to convert deoxyadenosine to deoxyinosine in the DNA hydrolysates. Deoxyguanosine (dGuo) and deoxythymidine (dThd) concentrations in the DNA hydrolysates were determined by peak integration after separation by high-performance liquid chromatography (HPLC). When necessary, HPLC was also used for the separation of different alkyldeoxynucleosides from the same DNA sample prior to analysis by RIA (Adamkiewicz *et al.*, 1982). The competitive RIA and the ELISA were performed as described in detail by Müller and Rajewsky (1978, 1980) and Adamkiewicz *et al.* (1982).

RESULTS AND DISCUSSION

In contrast to antisera raised in animals, MAB are, by definition, uncontaminated with unrelated antibodies that would cause reduced specificity in immunological assay procedures. They represent, therefore, analytical tools of unmatched precision for the detection of subtle differences in the structure of biological macromolecules such as DNA. The detection limit of a competitive RIA for a given alkyldeoxynucleoside is primarily dependent on the affinity constant of the respective MAB. However, the specificity of the MAB (i.e., a low cross-reactivity with other DNA constituents) becomes a most important factor, too, when DNA hydrolysates are to be analysed that contain both unmodified deoxynucleosides and various other alkylation products. Furthermore, even when highly specific MAB with very high affinity constants are used in a competitive RIA, the limit of detection of a given deoxynucleoside still remains dependent on the specific radioactivity of the tracer, which cannot be raised above a certain value. The detection limit of the RIA can, however, be lowered substantially if the level of cross-reactants is further reduced or if the cross-reactants are completely removed from the DNA hydrolysate. The latter can be achieved by separating the alkylation products in question from the complete DNA hydrolysate by HPLC prior to analysis, thus permitting larger samples of DNA with a low level of modification to be analysed by RIA (Adamkiewicz *et al.*, 1982).

The best of our presently available anti-alkyldeoxynucleoside MAB have affinity constants in the range of 1–2×10^{10} L/mol (Table 1). A number of these MAB cross-react with normal deoxynucleosides to only a very low degree; i.e., they require more than seven orders of magnitude greater amounts of the corresponding unaltered deoxynucleosides to inhibit tracer-antibody binding in a competitive RIA by 50%. In some cases, 50% inhibition of tracer-antibody binding is not reached at all by the normal deoxynucleosides at concentrations up to the limit of their solubility in the RIA samples. However, only a fraction of the MAB in our collection exhibit this extreme specificity, and it is therefore recommended to produce and characterize a sufficient number of MAB directed against a given structurally modified DNA component if maximum specificity and affinity are required.

As indicated in Table 1, the MAB that recognize O^6-alkyl-2'-deoxyguanosines detect, at 50% inhibition of tracer-antibody binding in the competitive RIA, 40–250 fmol of the respective products in a 100 µL RIA sample. In a probability grid used to transform the sigmoidal inhibition curves into straight lines (Müller & Rajewsky, 1980), accurate readings are usually possible at inhibition values $< 50\%$. Reading at 20% inhibition, for example, will lower the limit for detection of O^6-EtdGuo by MAB ER-6 from ~ 40 fmol (at 50% inhibition) to ~ 10 fmol in a 100 µL RIA sample. In the competitive RIA, MAB ER-6 thus detects O^6-EtdGuo at an O^6-EtdGuo:dGuo molar ratio as low as $\sim 3 \times 10^{-7}$ in a hydrolysate of 100 µg DNA (equivalent to the DNA of $\sim 1.6 \times 10^7$ diploid cells). This O^6-EtdGuo:dGuo molar ratio is equivalent to ~ 700 O^6-EtdGuo molecules per diploid genome.

One of the important applications of MAB directed against structurally altered components of cellular DNA will be the direct detection and quantification of specific DNA modifications in individual cells with the aid of immunostaining procedures. Among the numerous applications of this approach will be the unequivocal demonstration of the presence, and the monitoring of the concentration, of specific DNA adducts (e.g., resulting from exposure to carcinogens or chemotherapeutic agents) in small samples of (e.g., human) cells or biopsy material. Furthermore, comparative measurements may be made in different types of cells at different stages of differentiation and development, with respect to their capacity for the enzymatic activation of chemicals to their respective DNA binding derivatives, the elimination of specific adducts from their DNA, and DNA repair. This might, for example, facilitate the detection of individuals with hereditary defects in DNA repair enzymes (risk groups in terms of carcinogen exposure), as well as the prediction of individual response to cancer chemotherapy. A further important problem that may be approached using immunostaining techniques is the determination within defined cell populations and tissues of the relative frequencies of cells that are deficient in their capacity for enzymatic removal and repair of specific DNA lesions.

Our attempts to use MAB for the direct demonstration of carcinogen-DNA adducts in individual cells by immunofluorescence are still in their beginning. However, promising results have already been obtained. Thus, we have recently established a standardized procedure for the quantification of specific alkyldeoxynucleosides in the nuclear DNA of individual cells by direct immunofluorescence. Staining with tetramethylrhodamine isothiocyanate-labelled MAB is used in combination with computer-based image analysis of electronically intensified fluorescence signals (Adamkiewicz *et al.*, 1983, 1984). Using an anti-(O^6-EtdGuo) MAB, the present limit of detection for O^6-EtdGuo in the nuclei of cells previously exposed to an ethylating *N*-nitroso compound (e.g., *N*-ethyl-*N*-nitrosourea), corresponds to ~ 700 O^6-EtdGuo molecules per diploid genome, i.e., a value equivalent to an O^6-EtdGuo:dGuo molar ratio in DNA of $\sim 3 \times 10^{-7}$. With the same O^6-EtdGuo:Guo molar ratio in their DNA, $\sim 1.6 \times 10^7$ diploid cells would be required for the quantification of O^6-EtdGuo by competitive RIA (see above). When used in immune electron microscopy (in conjunction with a protein-free DNA spreading technique), MAB also permit the direct visualization of specific

Table 1. High-affinity monoclonal antibodies (MAB) specific for deoxynucleosides structurally modified by N-nitroso compounds

Alkyldeoxy-nucleoside	Immunogen	Designation of MAB (isotype)	Antibody affinity constant (L/mol)	Radioactive tracer in RIA (specific ^{3}H-activity)	Detection limit of RIA (pmol/100-µL RIA sample)[a]	Cross-reactivity with hydrolysate of unmodified DNA
O^6-MedGuo	O^6-EtGuo-KLH	ER-7 (IgG1)	1.2×10^9	O^6-Me-(8,5'-^{3}H) dGuo (~25 Ci/mmol)	0.25	6×10^5 [c]
O^6-EtdGuo	O^6-EtGuo-KLH	ER-6 (IgG2b)	2.0×10^{10}	O^6-Et-(8,5'-^{3}H) dGuo (~27 Ci/mmol)	0.04	2.5×10^6 [d]
O^6-BudGuo	O^6-EtGuo-KLH	ER-11 (ND)	9.1×10^9	O^6-n-Bu-(8,5'-^{3}H) dGuo (~22 Ci/mmol)	0.06	2.5×10^6 [d]
O^6-iProdGuo	O^6-iProGuo-KLH	ER-05 (IgG2a)	1.2×10^{10}	O^6-iPro-(8,5'-^{3}H) dGuo (~17 Ci/mmol)	0.05	2.4×10^6 [d]
O^4-EtdThd	O^4-EtThd-KLH	ER-01 (IgG2a)	1.3×10^9	O^4-Et-(6-^{3}H) dThd (~17 Ci/mmol)	0.24	1.3×10^6 [e]

Me, methyl; Et, ethyl; Bu, butyl; iPro, isopropyl; KLH, keyhole limpet haemocyanin; RIA, competitive radioimmunoassay; ND, not determined

[a] Value determined at 50% ITAB (inhibition of tracer-antibody binding in the RIA)

[b] Multiple of the value for 50% ITAB by the respective alkyldeoxynucleoside. For cross-reactivity determinations, either adenosine deaminase-treated DNA hydrolysates were used, or a mixture of dGuo, 2'-deoxyinosine, 2'-deoxycytidine, and dThd, at the molar ratios for rat DNA

[c] Value given for 50% ITAB

[d, e] Value given for 10–15% ITAB (d) or <10% ITAB (e), respectively, because the ITAB curve did not reach a value of 50% within the range of DNA hydrolysate concentrations tested in the RIA samples

alkyldeoxynucleosides in individual DNA molecules (Nehls *et al.*, 1983, 1984). O^6-EtdGuo sites can thus be localized in double-stranded DNA molecules by the binding of MAB ER-6 (Table 1) without a requirement for a second antibody carrying an electron-dense label. The latter type of analysis is currently being used to investigate the problem of the distribution of specific carcinogen-DNA adducts in the DNA of cellular chromatin in general, and in defined nucleotide sequences in particular.

ACKNOWLEDGEMENTS

Research supported by the Deutsche Forschungsgemeinschaft (SFB 102/A9), by the Commission of the European Communities (ENV-544-D, B), and by the Wilhelm und Maria Meyenburg Stiftung.

REFERENCES

Adamkiewicz, J., Drosdziok, W., Eberhardt, W., Langenberg, U. & Rajewsky, M.F. (1982) *High-affinity monoclonal antibodies specific for DNA components structurally modified by alkylating agents.* In: Bridges, B.A. Butterworth, B.E. & Weinstein, I.B., eds, *Indicators of Genotoxic Exposure (Banbury Report 13)* Cold Spring Harbor, NY, Cold Spring Harbor Laboratory, pp. 265–276

Adamkiewicz, J. Ahrens, O., Huh, N. & Rajewsky, M.F. (1983) Quantitation of alkyl-deoxynucleosides in the DNA of individual cells by high-affinity monoclonal antibodies and electronically intensified, direct immunofluorescence. *J.Cancer Res. clin. Oncol, 105,* A15

Adamkiewicz, J., Ahrens, O. & Rajewsky, M.F. (1984) *High-affinity monoclonal antibodies specific for deoxynucleosides structurally modified by alkylating agents: Applications for immunoanalysis.* In: Eisert, W.G. & Mendelsohn, M.L., eds, *Biological Dosimetry,* Berlin-Heidelberg, Springer-Verlag, pp. 325–334

Beranek, D.T., Weis, C.C. & Swenson, D.H. (1980) A comprehensive quantitative analysis of methylated and ethylated DNA using high pressure liquid chromatography. *Carcinogenesis, 1,* 595–606

Druckrey, H. (1971) Genotypes and phenotypes of ten inbred strains of BD-rats. *Arzneimittel-Forsch., 21,* 1274–1278

Erlanger, B.F. & Beiser, S.M. (1964) Antibodies specific for ribonucleosides and ribonucleotides and their reaction with DNA. *Proc. natl Acad. Sci. USA, 52,* 68–74

Galfré, G., Milstein, C. & Wright, B. (1979) Rat x rat hybrid myelomas and a monoclonal anti-Fd portion of mouse IgG. *Nature, 277,* 131–133

Grover, P.L., ed (1979) Chemical Carcinogens and DNA, Boca Raton, FL, CRC Press

Gupta, R.C. Reddy, M.V. & Randerath, K. (1982) ^{32}P-postlabeling analysis of non-radioactive aromatic carcinogen-DNA adducts. *Carcinogenesis, 3,* 1081–1092

Kohn, K.W. (1979) DNA as a target in cancer chemotherapy: Measurements of macromolecular DNA damage produced in mammalian cells by anticancer agents and carcinogens. *Meth. Cancer Res., 16,* 291–345

Lawley. P.D. (1976) *Carcinogenesis by alkylating agents.* In: Searle, C.E., ed., *Chemical Carcinogens (ACS Monograph No. 173),* Washington DC, American Chemical Society, pp. 83–244

Müller, R. (1980) Calculation of average antibody affinity in anti-hapten sera from data obtained by competitive radioimmunoassay. *J. Immunol. Meth., 34,* 345–352

Müller, R. & Rajewsky, M.F. (1978) Sensitive radioimmunoassay for detection of O^6-ethyldeoxyguanosine in DNA exposed to the carcinogen ethylnitrosourea *in vivo* or *in vitro. Z. Naturforsch., 33c,* 897–901

Müller, R. & Rajewsky, M.F. (1980) Immunological quantification by high-affinity antibodies of O^6-ethyldeoxyguanosine in DNA exposed to *N*-ethyl-*N*-nitrosourea. *Cancer Res., 40,* 887–896

Müller, R. & Rajewsky, M.F. (1981) Antibodies specific for DNA components structurally modified by chemical carcinogens. *J. Cancer Res. clin. Oncol., 102,* 99–113

Müller, R., Adamkiewicz, J. & Rajewsky, M.F. (1982) *Immunological detection and quantification of carcinogen-modified DNA components.* In: Bartsch, H. & Armstrong, B., eds, *Host Factors in Human Carcinogenesis (IARC Scientific Publications No. 39),* Lyon, International Agency for Research on Cancer, pp. 463–479

Nehls, P., Spiess, E. & Rajewsky, M.F. (1983) Visualization of O^6-ethylguanine in ethylnitrosourea-treated DNA by immune electron microscopy. *J. Cancer Res. clin. Oncol., 105,* A23

Nehls, P., Rajewsky, M.F., Spiess, E. & Werner, D. (1984) Highly sensitive sites for guanine-O^6 ethylation in rat brain DNA exposed to *N*-ethyl-*N*-nitrosourea *in vivo. EMBO J., 3,* 327–332

O'Connor, P.J., Saffhill, R. & Margison, G.P. 91 979) *N-Nitroso compounds:Biochemical mechanisms of action.* In: Emmelot, P. & Kriek, E., eds, *Environmental Carcinogenesis,* Amsterdam, Elsevier/North-Holland Biomedical Press, pp. 73–96

Pegg, A.E. (1977) Formation and metabolism of alkylated nucleosides: Possible role in carcinogenesis by *N*-nitroso compounds and alkylating agents. *Adv. Cancer Res., 25,* 195–269

Poirier, M.C. (1981) Antibodies to carcinogen-DNA adducts. *J. natl Cancer Inst., 67,* 515–519

Rajewsky, M.F. (1980) *Specificity of DNA damage in chemical carcinogenesis.* In: Montesano, R., Bartsch, H. & Tomatis, L., eds, *Molecular and Cellular Aspects of Carcinogen Screening Tests (IARC Scientific Publications No. 27),* Lyon, International Agency for Research on Cancer, pp. 41–54

Rajewsky, M.F., Müller, R., Adamkiewicz, J. & Drosdziok, W. (1980) *Immunological detection and quantification of DNA components structurally modified by alkylating carcinogens (ethylnitrosourea).* In: Pullman, B.,Ts'o, P.O.P. & Gelboin, H., eds, *Carcinogenesis: Fundamental Mechanisms and Environmental Effects,* Dordrecht, Boston, London, Reidel Publishers, pp. 207–218

Singer, B. (1979) *N*-nitroso alkylating agents: Formation and persistence of alkyl derivatives in mammalian nucleic acids as contributing factors in carcinogenesis. *J. natl Cancer Inst., 62,* 1329–1339

METHYLATION OF PROTEIN AND NUCLEIC ACIDS *IN VIVO*: USE OF TRIDEUTEROMETHYLATING AGENTS OR PRECURSORS

D.E.G. SHUKER, E. BAILEY, & P.B. FARMER

MRC Toxicology Unit, Medical Research Council Laboratories, Carshalton, Surrey SM5 4EF, UK

SUMMARY

Dose-dependent excretion of 7-(d_3-methyl)guanine in rat urine was observed following administration by gavage of d_6-aminopyrine and nitrite. Preliminary experiments showed that S-(d_3-methyl)cysteine in haemoglobin is formed under the same dosing conditions that result in 7-(d_3-methyl)guanine excretion in the urine.

INTRODUCTION

Exposure to alkylating agents can be assessed by monitoring the resulting alkyl adducts of macromolecules.

In rats, the presence of *S*-methylcysteine residues in haemoglobin is a good indicator of exposure to methylating agents (Segerbäck *et al.*, 1978; Bailey *et al.*, 1981). Similarly, methylation of DNA bases occurs *in vivo*. Craddock and Magee (1967) showed that urinary 7-methylguanine (7-MeG), derived from radioactively-labelled *N*-nitrosodimethylamine, resulted from the alkylation of intact DNA and that the excretion of labelled 7-MeG occurs exclusively *via* the urine (Craddock *et al.*, 1968).

However, in most animals there are significant background levels of protein *S*-methylcysteine (Bailey *et al.*, 1981), and background levels of urinary 7-MeG occur in rats (Mandel *et al.*, 1966) and man (Weissmann *et al.*, 1957).

In order to circumvent this problem and to increase the sensitivity of our existing methods, we decided to use tri-deuteromethyl (d_3-Me) compounds. For example, using a gas chromatographic-mass spectrometric (GC-MS) procedure already described (Farmer *et al.*, 1980), small amounts of *S*-(d_3-methyl)cysteine (S-d_3MeCys) could be determined in the presence of a large excess of *S*-methylcysteine in haemoglobin.

This paper describes some of our results concerning the alkylation of haemoglobin and DNA (by urinary excretion of 7-MeG) *in vivo*, using a combination of d_6-aminopyrine (d_6-AP) as a model compound, and sodium nitrite (Lijinsky & Greenblatt, 1972).

MATERIALS AND METHODS

d$_3$-Methyl iodide (99+%, Aldrich) and d$_6$-dimethyl sulfate (99+%, Aldrich) were used as supplied. Mass spectra were recorded on a VG 7070 double-focussing mass spectrometer, operating with a 70 eV ionizing electron beam. 7-MeG was supplied by Sigma Chemical Co. 7-Ethylguanine (7-EtG) was a gift of Dr M Jarman, Institute of Cancer Research, Sutton, UK.

d$_6$-AP

d$_6$-AP (Fig. 1) was prepared from 4-aminoantipyrine by a modification of a method for the preparation of *N,N*-dimethylanilines (Johnstone *et al.*, 1969). CD$_3$I (5 g, Aldrich 99+%) and *N*-trifluoroacetyl-4-aminoantipyrine (2.6 g, prepared from 4-aminoantipyrine and trifluoroacetic anhydride) in dry acetone (50 mL) were treated with powdered potassium hydroxide (1.94 g) and heated to reflux for 10 min. After cooling, 50 mL of water were added and the mixture was heated to reflux for another 10 min. After cooling, acetone was removed on a rotary evaporator, and the aqueous residue was extracted with chloroform (3 × 50 mL). The combined organic fraction was dried over anhydrous sodium sulfate and evaporated to dryness. The residue was dissolved in petroleum ether (80–100 fraction) and treated with charcoal, filtered and concentrated until crystallisation began; yield, 0.5 g of crude product, plus an additional 0.3 g, obtained from the mother liquor. The product was purified in 0.3-g portions on a 2 mm-thick, rotating, preparative thin-layer chromatography plate of silica gel (Chromatotron Model 7924, Harrison Research), using dichloromethane : ethanol (90 : 10, v/v) as eluant. Bands corresponding to aminopyrine were collected, combined and evaporated to give a residue which was recrystallized from hexane; yield, 0.5 g (25%) m.p. 104–105 °C nuclear magnetic resonance δ (CCl$_4$), 2.12 (3H,s,CH$_3$–C), 2.87 (3H,s,CH$_3$–N), 7.1-7.45 (5H,m,C$_6$H$_5$–), no peak was observed at 2·7 ppm, indicating that the (CD$_3$)$_2$N-group was present. M/Z(70 eV) 237 (M$^+$,85) 118(18) 100(40) 77(14) 56(100)[1]; purity(gas chromatography) ≥ 99·9%.

N-7-d$_3$-methyl-guanine (7-d$_3$MeG)

7-d$_3$MeG was prepared from guanosine and d$_6$-dimethyl sulfate (Jones & Robins, 1963) M/Z (70 eV) 168(M$^+$, 100), 127(17), 126(11), 71(27), 70(11).

Alkylation in vivo *in rats*

Female rats (150–200 g, LAC:P strain, Carshalton, Surrey) were housed in polycarbonate metabolism cages and allowed food (MRC 41B powdered diet) and water *ad libitum*. Urine was

Fig. 1. Structure of deuterated aminopyrine (d$_6$-AP)

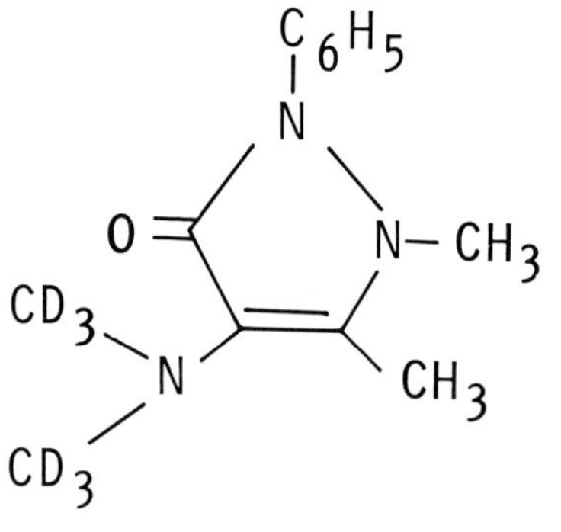

---

[1] Relative ionic intensities are given in parentheses.

Fig. 2. Gas chromatogram(flame-ionization detector) of an extract from rat urine (1 mL) containing 7-ethylguanine (7-EtG) (5 µg) as internal standard. Conditions: 20 m × 0.3 mm SE52, fused-silica capillary column, 100 °C for 3 min then programmed at 30 °C/min to 280 °C. He carrier gas. Split-injection mode. 7-MeG, 7-methylguanine

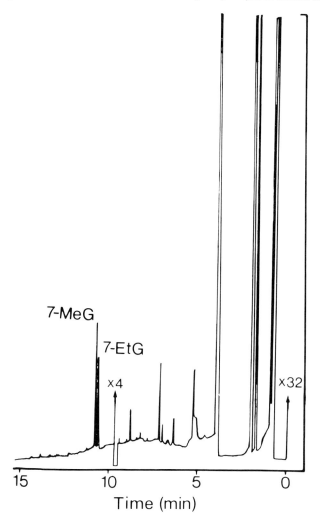

collected over 24-h periods and frozen immediately. Alkylating agents or precursors were administered by gavage as freshly prepared aqueous solutions.

Globin was obtained from blood as described previously (Farmer *et al.*, 1980).

Analysis of urinary 7-d_3MeG

The volume of 24-h urines was standardized to 10 mL. One-mL aliquots of these urines were analysed by GC-MS with multiple-ion detection. A new method has been employed for the extraction and analysis of urinary 7-MeG (Shuker *et al.*, 1984). Briefly, 7-MeG is extracted from urine as an ion-pair, using a reversed-phase Sep-pak. The dried extract is treated first with heptafluorobutyric anhydride, then with pentafluorobenzyl bromide *via* extractive alkylation, to give *N*-2-heptafluorobutyryl-*O*^{6}-pentafluorobenzyl-*N*-7-methylguanine, which has good GC properties.

Levels of 7-MeG were determined by capillary-GC, using 7-EtG as an internal standard (Fig.2). 7-d$_3$MeG was determined by GC-MS, using multiple-ion detection of the molecular ions (7-MeG, M/Z 541; 7-d$_3$MeG, M/Z 544).

Analysis of S-d$_3$MeCys

S-d$_3$MeCys levels in rat globin were determined as described elsewhere (Bailey *et al.*, 1981).

RESULTS

Rats were dosed with d$_6$-AP (5 mg/rat) in conjunction with sodium nitrite (0–10 mg/rat). Figure 3 shows the amount of 7-d$_3$MeG excreted in the urine, as a function of nitrite dose, during the 24 h after dosing. With no nitrite, no measurable urinary 7-d$_3$MeG was observed. Each point represents a value obtained for an individual rat.

With higher doses, the excretion in the urine of some rats was measured for several days after dosing. Figure 4 shows the daily excretion of 7-d$_3$MeG in two of the high-dose rats, following coadministration of d$_6$-AP and sodium nitrite.

Fig. 3. Urinary excretion of deuterated 7-methylguanine (7-d$_3$MeG) for a fixed dose of d$_6$-aminopyrine (d$_6$-AP) (5 mg/rat) and varying doses of sodium nitrite

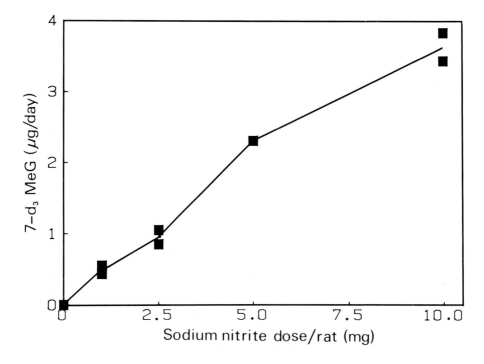

Fig. 4. Urinary excretion of deuterated 7-methylguanine (7-d$_3$MeG) as a function of time after dosing. ●, d$_6$-aminopyrine, 5 mg/rat; sodium nitrite, 10 mg/rat; ▲ d$_6$-aminopyrine, 5 mg/rat; sodium nitrite, 5 mg/rat

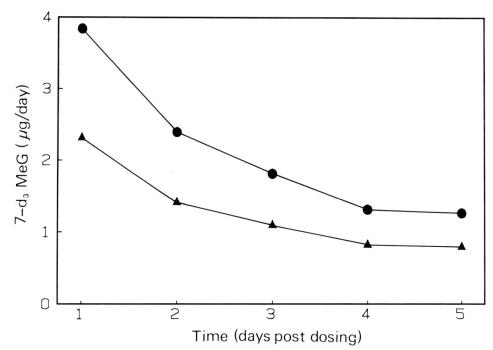

Coadministration of d$_6$-AP (5mg/rat) and sodium nitrate(50 mg/rat) produced no measurable excretion of 7-d$_3$MeG (data not shown).

No measurable rise in the total levels of urinary 7-MeG could be seen with any of the doses of aminopyrine and nitrite employed (data not shown).

In preliminary experiments, both urinary 7-d$_3$MeG and globin S-d$_3$MeCys were observed after a given dose of d$_6$-AP plus sodium nitrite. Thus, coadministration of d$_6$-AP (20 mg/rat) and sodium nitrite (20 mg/rat) resulted in S-d$_3$MeCys (28 ng/10 mg globin) and 7-d$_3$MeG (7.75 μg/24 h). d$_6$-AP (20 mg/rat) alone did not give rise to any detectable incorporation of d$_3$-methyl groups. Further studies on the relationship between the levels of DNA and protein alkylation are in progress.

DISCUSSION

The results presented in this paper clearly show that a model compound d$_6$-AP, which is a precursor of *N*-nitroso-d$_6$-dimethylamine, gives rise to dose-dependent d$_3$-methylation of DNA *in vivo* when administered in conjunction with nitrite. The analytical method allows selective observation of d$_3$-methyl incorporation resulting from intact methyl group transfer *in vivo* (Lijinsky *et al.*, 1968), characteristic of *N*-methyl-*N*-nitrosamine metabolism.

Clearly, this technique could be applied to any compounds that might be expected to give rise to alkylating agents *in vivo*. We are currently looking at a number of substances that are potential methylating agents, in particular those derived from *N*-methyl-*N*-nitroso compounds.

ACKNOWLEDGEMENTS

We would like to thank Sue Gorf and Richard Verschoyle for their expert help with animal experiments, John Lamb for GC-MS measurements and Alan Brooks for GC analyses.

REFERENCES

Bailey, E., Connors, T.A., Farmer, P.B., Gorf, S.M. & Rickard, J (1981) Methylation of cysteine in haemoglobin following exposure to methylating agents. *Cancer Res., 41,* 2514–2517

Craddock, V.M. & Magee, P.N. (1967) Effects of administration of the carcinogen dimethylnitrosamine on urinary 7-methylguanine. *Biochem. J., 104,* 435–440

Craddock, V.M., Mattocks, A.R. & Magee, P.N. (1968) The fate of 7[^{14}C]-methylguanine after administration to the rat. *Biochem. J., 109,* 75–78

Farmer, P.B., Bailey, E., Lamb, J.H. & Connors, T.A. (1980) Approach to the quantitation of alkylated amino acids in haemoglobin gas chromatograph/mass spectrometry. *Biomed. Mass Spectrom., 7,* 41–46

Johnstone, R.A.W. Payling, D.W. & Thomas, C. (1969) A rapid method for the N-alkylation of amines. *J.chem. Soc. (C),* 2223–2224

Jones, J.N. & Robins, R.K. (1963) Purine-nucleosides. III. Methylation studies of certain naturally occurring purine nucleosides. *J. Am. chem. Soc., 85,* 193–201

Lijinsky, W. & Greenblatt, M. (1972) Carcinogen dimethylnitrosamine produced *in vivo* from nitrite and aminopyrine. *Nature (New Biol.) 236,* 177–178

Lijinsky, W., Loo, J. & Ross, A.E. (1968) Mechanism of alkylation of nucleic acids by nitrosodimethylamine. *Nature, 218,* 1174–1175

Mandel, L.R., Srinivasan, P.R. & Borek, E. (1966) Origin of urinary methylated purines. *Nature, 209,* 586–588

Segerbäck, D., Calleman, C.J., Ehrenberg, L., Löfroth, G. & Osterman-Golkar, S. (1978) Evaluation of genetic risks of alkylating agents. IV: Quantitative determination of alkylated amino acids in haemoglobin as a measure of the dose after treatment of mice with methyl methane sulfonate. *Mutat. Res., 49,* 71–82

Shuker, D.E.G., Bailey, E., Gorf, S.M., Lamb, J. & Farmer, P.B. (1984) Determination of N-7-[^{2}H$_{3}$]methylguanine in rat urine by gas chromatography–mass spectrometry following administration of trideuteromethylating agents or precursors. *Anal. Biochem.* (in press)

Weissmann, B., Bromberg, P.A. & Gutman, A.B. (1957) The purine bases of human urine. I. Separation and identification. *J. biol. Chem., 224,* 407–422

DNA METHYLATION BY *N*-NITROSOMETHYLBENZYLAMINE IN TARGET AND NON-TARGET TISSUES OF LABORATORY RODENTS. COMPARISON WITH CARCINOGENICITY

O.D. WIESTLER & A. UOZUMI

Division of Neuropathology, Department of Pathology, University of Freiburg, 7800 Freiburg, FRG

P. KLEIHUES

Division of Neuropathology, Department of Pathology, University of Zürich, 8091 Zürich, Switzerland

SUMMARY

Following oral or systemic (subcutaneous) administration to rats, *N*-nitroso-methylbenzylamine (NMBzA) causes a high incidence of oesophageal tumours. Methylation of DNA purines by a single oral dose of [^{14}C-methyl]-NMBzA was most extensive in the oesophagus, followed by liver, forestomach and lung. After a single intravenous injection, alkylation levels were also highest in oesophageal DNA, followed by liver, lung and forestomach. These differences in the extent of alkylation were found to correlate with the autoradiographic distribution of tissue-bound ^{14}C-radioactivity in in-situ preparations of the upper gastrointestinal tract following oral exposure to [^{14}C-methyl]-NMBzA.

In mice, systemic administration of NMBzA leads to the development of forestomach and lung tumours; in this species, DNA methylation after intraperitoneal injection of NMBzA is highest in liver, followed by lung and forestomach. Administration of [^{14}C-methyl]-NMBzA to mice in the drinking-water led to very high concentrations of alkylated DNA bases in both oesophagus and forestomach. This finding is in good agreement with carcinogenicity studies, which showed 100% carcinoma incidence at these sites.

Autoradiographic studies indicate that in rats and mice the metabolism of NMBzA in the oesophagus is largely restricted to the mucosa, whereas in lung, bioactivation occurs predominantly in the bronchial epithelium. In autoradiographs from liver, tissue-bound radioactivity showed a patchy distribution, with predominant reaction in the centrilobular region.

In Mongolian gerbils, methylation of lung DNA by a similar subcutaneous dose of [^{14}C-methyl]-NMBzA was greater than in rats and mice, whereas in the remaining tissues, levels of methylated purines were comparatively low. Chronic subcutaneous administration of NMBzA to gerbils caused no tumour within an observation period of two years.

INTRODUCTION

There is increasing evidence that environmental factors are involved in human oesophageal carcinogenesis (Yang, 1980; Lu & Lin, 1982). Many investigations have focused on high-risk areas in Northern China, where humans and domestic fowls frequently develop tumours of the pharynx and the oesophagus. *N*-Nitrosamines have been isolated from corn bread and traditional food preparations in these geographic regions (Cheng *et al.*, 1980; Lu *et al.*, 1980). Fungi, which accelerate the nitrosative formation of *N*-nitrosomethylbenzylamine (NMBzA) and related compounds from their chemical precursors (Hsia *et al.*, 1981), frequently colonize the oesophageal mucosa of patients with premalignant or malignant lesions. However, a causal relationship between exposure to nitrosamines and tumours of the oesophagus in humans and chickens has not yet been proven.

In rats and mice, NMBzA causes a high incidence of oesophageal neoplasms following its oral administration in the drinking-water. We report here experiments which indicate a close correlation between the initial extent of DNA methylation and organ-specific tumour induction by NMBzA.

MATERIALS AND METHODS

Animals

Adult male Wistar rats (150 g body weight), adult female NMRI mice (average body weight, 20 g) and adult male gerbils (average body weight, 65 g) were given a standard laboratory diet and water *ad libitum*.

Chemicals

[^{14}C-methyl]-NMBzA (specific radioactivity, 52 mCi/mmol) was purchased from NEN (Boston, MA, USA). Unlabelled NMBzA was added to lower the specific activity to 18 mCi/mmol. Radiochemical purity, as checked by high-performance liquid chromatography, was greater than 95%. The unlabelled NMBzA was synthesized by Dr M. Wiessler, German Cancer Research Centre, Heidelberg, FRG.

DNA alkylation in vivo

Following 20 h of water deprivation, the animals received a single dose of [^{14}C-methyl]-NMBzA (60 mg/L; 2.5 mg/kg; 18 mCi/mmol) in the drinking-water. After 5 h, DNA was isolated from pooled organs by phenolic extraction, as described earlier (Margison & Kleihues, 1975). Acid hydrolysates were adjusted to pH 5–6 and analysed on a Sephasorb HP column (Hodgson *et al.*, 1980).

Autoradiographic studies

Following a 20-h period of water deprivation, animals were allowed to drink an aqueous solution containing [^{14}C-methyl]-NMBzA (60 mg/L; 2.5 mg/kg; 18 mCi/mmol) and were killed 4 h later. Oesophagus, forestomach, glandular stomach and duodenum were removed, opened longitudinally and pinned out flat on a cork plate. After rinsing with saline, tissue was fixed in buffered formaldehyde (5%) and dried by gently pressing between sheets of filter paper. Some organs (oesophagus, liver, spleen, lung, jejunum, colon) were removed, fixed in buffered formaldehyde (5%), embedded in paraffin and cut into 2-μm sections. Exposure (2–4 weeks) was carried out in X-ray cassettes using an LKB 3H-Ultrofilm.

RESULTS AND DISCUSSION

The carcinogenicity of *N*-nitrosamines is dependent on their enzymatic conversion to alkylating metabolites. For NMBzA, this bioactivation proceeds *via* hydroxylation at the methylene bridge, leading to methyldiazoniumhydroxide as methylating intermediate and benzaldehyde. Alternatively, hydroxylation at the methyl group would yield benzyldiazonium hydroxide and formaldehyde. In in-vivo studies using NMBzA labelled with ^{14}C at the methylene bridge, however, no benzylated base was detectable (Hodgson *et al.*, 1982), indicating that NMBzA exerts its biological effects by methylation of nucleic acids.

In rats, NMBzA selectively induces a high incidence of oesophageal neoplasms after both oral and systemic (subcutaneous) administration (Druckrey *et al.*, 1967; Schweinsberg *et al.*, 1977; Stinson *et al.*, 1978). Following a single oral dose of [^{14}C-methyl]-NMBzA (2.5 mg/kg) in the drinking water, levels of methylated purine bases were by far the highest in the oesophagus, followed by liver, forestomach and lung DNA (Table 1). Four hours after administration of the same dose (2.5 mg/kg) by intravenous injection, methylation of DNA purines was again most extensive in oesophageal tissue, followed by liver, lung and forestomach. The concentration of the promutagenic base O^6-methylguanine was six times higher in oesophageal DNA than in lung and nine times higher than in hepatic DNA. Chromatographic analyses showed that the radioactivity in DNA hydrolysates was associated mainly with methylated purines, whereas metabolic incorporation of ^{14}C into normal DNA bases was minimal. We concluded, therefore, that under these conditions most of the tissue-bound radioactivity represents alkylation products with DNA, RNA and proteins. In order to visualize the ^{14}C-incorporation into these macromolecules, contact autoradiographs were made of the upper gastrointestinal tract of the rat following oral intake of [^{14}C-methyl]-NMBzA. These autoradiographs (Fig. 1) showed high levels of ^{14}C-radioactivity in the pharyngeal and oesophageal mucosa, whereas in forestomach, glandular stomach and duodenum the reaction was hardly detectable. There is a sharp transition between oesophagus and forestomach, although both tissues share an anatomically similar type of squamous epithelium. The autoradiographic pattern of tissue-bound radioactivity correlates closely with the concentrations of methylated DNA purines determined in the biochemical studies. These

Table 1.   DNA methylation by *N*-nitrosomethylbenzylamine (NMBzA) in rats and mice

Organ	Rat				Mouse			
	i.v.[a]		oral		i.p.[b]		oral	
	7-meG	O^6-meG	7-meG	O^6-meG	7-meG	O^6-meG	7-meG	O^6-meG
Oesophagus	*344.5*	*46.1*	*404.2*	*14.6*	18.3	1.5	289.1	39.1
Forestomach	10.3	ND	41.5	1.8	23.3	1.7	*291.1*	*29.2*
Glandular stomach	2.3	ND	5.2	0.3	2.5	ND	14.2	1.5
Small intestine	ND	ND	1.3	ND	ND	ND	3.4	ND
Liver	120.2	4.9	190.0	6.7	162.9	11.8	171.7	13.5
Lung	64.9	7.7	23.6	2.7	*46.1*	*4.8*	6.0	0.7

Male Wistar rats (120–150 g) or female NMRI mice (25 g) received a single i.v., i.p. or oral (60 mg/L in the drinking water) dose of [^{14}C-methyl]-NMBzA 2.5 mg/kg) and were killed 4 h later. Concentrations of methylated DNA purines are expressed as μmol/mol guanine. For each species and mode of administration, values of the respective target organ are underlined
meG, methylguanine; ND, not detectable
[a] Data from Hodgson *et al.* (1982)
[b] Data from Kleihues *et al.* (1981)

Fig. 1. Autoradiograph of rat upper gastrointestinal tract, following a single oral dose of [¹⁴C-methyl]-NMBzA (2.5 mg/kg; 18 mCi/mmol) in the drinking-water. Pharynx (a), oesophagus (b), forestomach (c), glandular stomach (d) and duodenum (e) were removed, opened longitudinally, fixed and exposed for 14 days with an LKB 3H-Ultrofilm. Copies were made directly onto photographic paper, i.e., the light areas on the autoradiographs represent high levels of radioactivity. Strong reaction in the pharynx and the oesophagus; in contrast, stomach and duodenum are nearly unlabelled.

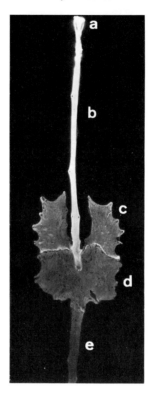

data suggest that, in the oesophageal epithelium of the rat, a cytochrome P-450 isozyme exists with a high capacity to metabolize NMBzA and related asymmetrical nitrosamines.

In mice, chronic oral administration of NMBzA in the drinking-water (20 mg/L) has been shown to result in a 100% tumour incidence in both oesophagus and forestomach. In contrast, multiple intraperitoneal injections (2.5 mg/kg/week) induce a high incidence of forestomach carcinomas and lung adenomas, but no oesophageal tumour (Sander & Schweinsberg, 1973). Following a single oral dose of [¹⁴C-methyl]-NMBzA, methylation of purine bases was most extensive in DNA of oesophagus and forestomach, the target organs for this route of application. Analysis of DNA alkylation by [¹⁴C-methyl]-NMBzA in various mouse tissues after intraperitoneal injection (2.5 mg/kg) showed highest concentrations of 7-methylguanine (7-meG) and O^6-meG in the liver, followed by the principal target tissues, lung and forestomach (Kleihues *et al.*, 1981). The observation that DNA methylation in the oesophagus was only 12% less than in forestomach suggests that the extent of initial DNA modification required for malignant transformation differs considerably between these two tissues, despite their morphological similarity. The very high DNA alkylation levels in oesophagus and forestomach

Fig. 2. Histoautoradiographs from liver (a), lung (b) and oesophagus (c) of rat (A) and mouse (B) following a single oral dose of [¹⁴C-methyl]-NMBzA (2.5 mg/kg; 18 mCi/mmol) in the drinking-water. After 4 h, the organs were removed, fixed, embedded in paraffin and cut in 2-μm sections. Exposure was carried out in X-ray cassettes for 2–4 weeks using an LKB 3H-Ultrofilm.

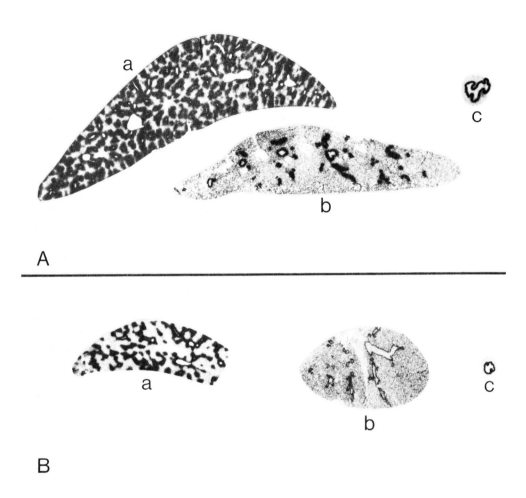

after oral intake are probably due to direct uptake of NMBzA from the drinking-water.

In order to localize target cell populations in different tissues, we carried out histoautoradiographic investigations (Fig. 2). In the oesophagus of rats and mice, tissue labelling by [¹⁴C-methyl]-NMBzA following a single oral dose occurs predominantly in the mucosa, in contrast to the remaining layers of the oesophageal wall, which incorporate radioactive intermediates to only a very low extent. The livers of rats and mice showed a markedly inhomogeneous distribution of radioactivity, due to a compartmentation of the hepatic nitrosamine metabolism, with predominant reaction in the centrilobular region. In the lung, the binding of methylating intermediates is largely confined to the bronchial walls. It is known that after inhibition by disulfiram of NMBzA bioactivation in the liver, rats develop not only oesophageal carcinomas but also tumours of the tracheobronchial system (Schweinsberg & Bürkle, 1981).

In gerbils, methylation of lung DNA by a single subcutaneous injection of [^{14}C-methyl]-NMBzA (2.5 mg/kg) was greater than in rats and mice, whereas in the remaining tissues levels of methylated purine bases were comparatively low (Bamborschke *et al.*, 1982). One would, therefore, expect that systemic administration of NMBzA is most likely to induce pulmonary neoplasms in these animals. We carried out a chronic carcinogenicity study in gerbils using 20 weekly subcutaneous injections (2.5 mg/kg each). After a two-year observation period, no tumour was observed. This treatment would induce a high incidence of oesophageal tumours in rats and of forestomach and lung tumours in mice. Similarly, we were unable to induce any tumour in 25 chickens which received NMBzA (25 mg/L) continuously in the drinking-water for six months. These animals are known to develop pharyngeal and oesophageal neoplasms in high-risk areas for humans in China. We are currently investigating the metabolism of NMBzA in this species.

CONCLUSIONS

These studies were performed to elucidate biochemical mechanisms which underly the organ-specific tumour induction by NMBzA in experimental animals. The following points can be summarized:

(1) In laboratory rodents, the incidence and location of tumours induced by NMBzA correlates with the initial extent of DNA alkylation. This was found particularly for the promutagenic base O^6-meG. However, the concentration of methylated purine bases required to induce neoplastic transformation differs between animal species and tissues.

(2) The induction of oesophageal, forestomach and lung tumours by NMBzA in rats and mice results from a preferential bioactivation of the carcinogen in the target tissue.

(3) The distribution of NMBzA-metabolizing enzymes in different organs is inhomogeneous. In the oesophagus, bioactivation occurs in the mucosa; in the lung, it is largely restricted to the bronchial epithelium; in the liver, there is evidence for a regional compartmentation of *N*-nitrosamine metabolism in both rats and mice.

ACKNOWLEDGEMENTS

This work was supported by the Deutsche Forschungsgemeinschaft (SFB 31) and Bundesministerium für Forschung und Technologie (CMT 15).

REFERENCES

Bamborschke, S., Shoji, M. & Kleihues, P. (1982) Metabolism of *N*-nitrosomethylbenzylamine in the Mongolian gerbil *(Meriones unguiculatus)*. *Anticancer Res., 2*, 241–244

Cheng, S.-J., Sala, M., Li, M.H., Wang, M.-Y., Pot-Deprun, J. & Chouroulinkov, J. (1980) Mutagenic, transforming and promoting effect of pickled vegetables from Linxian county, China. *Carcinogenesis, 1*, 685–692

Druckrey, H., Preussmann, R., Ivankovic, S. & Schmähl, D. (1967) Organotrope carcinogene Wirkungen bei 65 verschiedenen *N*-nitroso-Verbindungen an BD-Ratten. *Z. Krebsforsch., 69*, 103–201

Hodgson, R.M., Wiessler, M. & Kleihues, P. (1980) Preferential methylation of target organ DNA by the oesophageal carcinogen *N*-nitrosomethylbenzylamine. *Carcinogenesis, 1*, 861–866

Hodgson, R.M., Schweinsberg, F., Wiessler, M. & Kleihues, P. (1982) Mechanism of esophageal tumor induction in rats by *N*-nitrosomethylbenzylamine and its ring-methylated analog *N*-nitrosomethyl(4-methylbenzyl)amine. *Cancer Res., 42*, 2836–2840

Hsia, C.-C., Sun, T.-T., Wang, U.-U., Anderson, L.M., Armstrong, D. & Good, R.A. (1981) Enhancement of formation of the esophageal carcinogen benzylmethylnitrosamine from its precursors by *Candida albicans. Proc. natl Acad. Sci. USA, 78*, 1878–1881

Kleihues, P., Veit, C., Wiessler, M. & Hodgson, R.M. (1981) DNA methylation by *N*-nitrosomethylbenzylamine in target and non-target tissues of NMRi mice. *Carcinogenesis, 2*, 897–899

Lu, S.H. & Lin, P. (1982) Recent research on the etiology of esophageal cancer in China. *Z. Gastroenterol., 20*, 361–367

Lu, S.H., Camus, A.-M., Ji, C., Wang, Y.L., Wang, M.Y. & Bartsch, H. (1980) Mutagenicity in *Salmonella typhimurium* of *N*-3-methylbutyl-*N*-1-methylacetonylnitrosamine and *N*-methyl-*N*-benzylnitrosamine, *N*-nitrosation products isolated from corn-bread contaminated with commonly occurring moulds in Linshien county, a high incidence area for oesophageal cancer in Northern China. *Carcinogenesis, 1*, 867–870

Margison, G.P. & Kleihues, P. (1975) Chemical carcinogenesis in the nervous system. Preferential accumulation of O^6-methylguanine in rat brain deoxyribonucleic acid during repetitive administration of *N*-methyl-*N*-nitrosourea. *Biochem. J., 148*, 521–525

Sander, J. & Schweinsberg, F. (1973) Tumorinduktion bei Mäusen durch *N*-Methylbenzyl-nitrosamin in niedriger Dosierung. *Z. Krebsforsch., 79*, 157–161

Schweinsberg, F. & Bürkle, V. (1981) Wirkung von Disulfiram auf die Toxizität und Carcinogenität von *N*-Methyl-nitrosobenzylamin bei Ratten. *J. Cancer Res. clin. Oncol., 102*, 43–47

Schweinsberg, F., Schott-Kollat, P. & Bürkle, G. (1977) Veränderung der Toxizität und Carcinogenität von *N*-Methyl-*N*-nitrosobenzylamin durch Methylsubstitution am Phenylrest bei Ratten. *Z. Krebsforsch., 88*, 231–236

Stinson, S.F., Squire, R.A. & Sporn, M.B. (1978) Pathology of esophageal neoplasms and associated proliferative lesions induced in rats by *N*-methyl-*N*-benzylnitrosamine. *J. natl Cancer Inst., 6*, 1471–1475

Yang, C.S. (1980) Research on esophageal cancer in China: a review. *Cancer Res., 40*, 2633–2644

INVOLVEMENT OF THIOLS IN GASTRIC CANCER INDUCED BY N-METHYL-N'-NITRO-N-NITROSOGUANIDINE: BIOCHEMICAL AND AUTORADIOGRAPHIC STUDIES

P. KLEIHUES

Division of Neuropathology, Department of Pathology, University of Zürich, 8091 Zürich, Switzerland

O.D. WIESTLER

Division of Neuropathology, Department of Pathology, University of Freiburg, 78 Freiburg, Federal Republic of Germany

SUMMARY

Chronic administration of N-methyl-N'-nitro-N-nitrosoguanidine (MNNG) in drinking water causes a high incidence of carcinomas of the glandular stomach in rats (Sugimura & Fujimura, 1967). Following a single oral dose of [^{14}C-methyl]-MNNG (80 mg/L; 2.5 mg/kg b.w.), the extent of DNA methylation in the glandular stomach was 9 and 21 times higher than in forestomach and oesophagus, respectively. These differences were found to correlate with regional variations in the concentration of cellular thiols, which are known to accelerate the heterolytic decomposition of MNNG. When [^{14}C-methyl]-MNNG was given intragastrically together with the thiol-blocking agent, N-ethylmaleimide, covalent binding of ^{14}C-radioactivity to forestomach, glandular stomach and duodenum was almost completely abolished.

INTRODUCTION

Several methylating carcinogens have been shown to induce carcinomas selectively in different segments of the gastrointestinal tract. Although the mechanisms underlying this organ specificity are not yet completely understood, data from our laboratory and from other authors indicate that the initial extent of DNA methylation by these agents is among the most important factors in determining the site of tumour development. Preferential DNA alkylation in certain organs of the gastrointestinal tract is produced by a variety of mechanisms, some of which have been clarified during recent years. In rats, N-nitrosomethylbenzylamine selectively induces tumours of the pharynx and oesophagus, and this has been shown to be caused by a very high capacity of the oesophageal mucosa to metabolize this nitrosamine and related asymmetric nitrosamines (Hodgson *et al.*, 1980). Intraperitoneal administration of

N-nitrosomethyl(acetoxymethyl)amine induces a high incidence of carcinomas in the small and large intestine, due to rapid activation by esterases in the abdominal cavity (Kleihues, 1979). Induction of colonic tumours by 1,2-dimethylhydrazine correlates with its preferential metabolism by the large-bowel mucosa (Swenberg *et al.*, 1979). In the present paper, we report experiments which indicate strongly that the selective induction of glandular stomach carcinomas by *N*-methyl-*N*'-nitro-*N*-nitrosoguanidine (MNNG) (Sugimura & Fujimura, 1967; Sugimura *et al.*, 1969) is mediated by high thiol concentrations in the target tissue.

MATERIALS AND METHODS

Animals

Adult female Wistar rats (150-200 g body weight) were obtained from Zentralinstitut für Versuchstiere, Hannover, FRG. Animals were fed a standard laboratory diet with water *ad libitum*.

Chemicals

[(^{14}C-methyl])-MNNG (specific radioactivity, 10–15 mCi/mmol) was purchased from NEN Chemicals (Dreieich, FRG). The radiochemical purity was checked by high-performance liquid chromatography and proved to be greater than 95%. In some experiments, nonradioactive MNNG was added to lower the specific activity to 5 mCi/mmol.

DNA alkylation in vivo

After 20 h of water deprivation, female Wistar rats received a single oral dose of [^{14}C-methyl]-MNNG (80 mg/L; 2.5 mg/kg b.w.; 5 mCi/mmol) in their drinking water. Following a survival time of 5 h, DNA was isolated from the pooled organs of eight animals by phenolic extraction, as described earlier (Margison & Kleihues, 1975). After mild acid hydrolysis in 0.1 mol/L hydrochloric acid for 20 h (37°C), the pH of the hydrolysates was adjusted to 5–6, and they were analysed on a Sephasorb HP column (Hodgson *et al.*, 1980).

Autoradiographic studies

Following a 20-h period of water deprivation, female Wistar rats received a single oral dose of [^{14}C-methyl]-MNNG in their drinking water (80 mg/L; 2.5 mg/kg b.w., 10 mCi/mmol) or by gastric intubation (2.5 mg/kg; 15 mCi/mmol) and were killed 5 h later. Oesophagus, forestomach, glandular stomach and duodenum were removed, opened longitudinally and pinned out flat on a cork plate. After rinsing with saline, tissues were fixed in buffered formaldehyde (5%) and dried by gentle pressing between sheets of filter paper. Exposure (14–21 days) was carried out in X-ray cassettes, using an LKB 3H-Ultrofilm.

Determination of thiol concentrations

Free thiol concentrations were determined in trichloroacetic acid-soluble supernatants of different rat organs using the Ellman procedure (Ellman, 1959). Briefly, tissues were homogenized in 10 volumes of cold 50 g/L trichloroacetic acid and centrifuged for 10 min at 1500 g. The supernatant was diluted with phosphate buffer (0.1 mol/L, pH 8, mixed with 5,5'-dithiobis-(2-nitrobenzoic acid) and the ultra-violet absorption measured at 412 nm. Mean values were calculated from determinations on groups of five to seven animals.

RESULTS AND DISCUSSION

Evidence has accumulated to show that both the mutagenicity and the carcinogenicity of MNNG and related carcinogens result from a methylation of DNA bases (Pegg, 1977; Singer, 1979). We therefore determined the extent of DNA alkylation in various rat tissues following a single oral exposure to [^{14}C-methyl]-MNNG in drinking water (2.5 mg/kg, 80 mg/L). After a survival time of 5 h, methylated purines were determined by radiochromatography in acid DNA hydrolysates. Concentrations of methylpurines in glandular stomach and duodenum greatly exceeded those in other segments of the gastrointestinal tract and the liver (Table 1). In the glandular stomach, the concentration of 7-methylguanine was 9 and 20 times higher than in DNA of forestomach and oesophagus, respectively. O^6-Alkylation of guanine is considered to be a critical event in the initiation of malignant transformation by alkylating agents (Singer, 1979; Newbold et al., 1980), and this DNA modification was present in detectable amounts only in glandular stomach and duodenum. This finding correlates with those of carcinogenicity studies which show that, after the glandular stomach, the duodenum is the preferred site for tumour induction by MNNG (Sugimura & Fujimura, 1967; Sugimura et al., 1969). Chromatographic analyses showed that the radioactivity in DNA hydrolysates was mainly associated with methylated purines, whereas metabolic incorporation of ^{14}C into normal DNA bases was minimal. We concluded that under these experimental conditions most of the tissue-bound radioactivity represents alkylation products with DNA, RNA and proteins.

In order to determine the extent of ^{14}C-incorporation into these macromolecules autoradiographically, in-situ preparations were made of the upper gastrointestinal tract following intake of approximately 5 mL of an aqueous solution containing [^{14}C-methyl]-MNNG (2.5 mg/kg, 80 mg/L; 5-h survival time). The autoradiographic distribution of ^{14}C radioactivity (Fig. 1) corresponded well with the extent of DNA methylation: low levels of alkylation in oesophagus and forestomach and high levels in glandular stomach and duodenum. There was a sharp transition between alkylation levels in forestomach and glandular stomach. Hence, the distribution of tissue-bound radioactivity correlates closely with the preferential site of tumour induction.

Table 1. DNA alkylation by N-methyl-N'-nitro-N-nitrosoguanidine and thiol concentrations in various tissues (means from 5–7 rats)

Organ	Methylated DNA purine (µmol/mol guanine)		Thiol concentration (µmol/g tissue ± SD)
	7-Methylguanine	O^6-Methylguanine	
Oesophagus	9.9	ND	0.279 ± 0.069
Forestomach	22.2	ND	0.119 ± 0.038
Glandular stomach	204.7	9.0	1.249 ± 0.098
Duodenum	169.8	6.7	2.149 ± 0.253
Jejunum	16.0	ND	2.659 ± 0.359
Ileum	ND	ND	1.834 ± 0.406
Liver	5.7	ND	5.003 ± 0.466

ND, not detectable

Fig. 1. Autoradiographs of the upper gastrointestinal tract, following a single exposure to [^{14}C-methyl]-N-methyl-N'-nitro-N-nitrosoguanidine (MNNG); oesophagus (a), forestomach (b), glandular stomach (c) and duodenum (d). (A) Following a 20-h period of water deprivation, a female Wistar rat was allowed to drink approximately 5 mL of an aqueous solution containing ^{14}C-MNNG (80 mg/L; 2.5 mg/kg b.w.; 10 mCi/mmol) and was killed 5 h later; (B, C) female Wistar rats (WIS/HAN) received a single intragastric dose of [^{14}C-methyl)-MNNG (50 µCi in 0.6 mL aqueous solution; 15 mCi/mmol) alone (B) or together (C) with the thiol blocking agent, N-ethylmaleimide (50 mg/kg) and were killed 2 h later

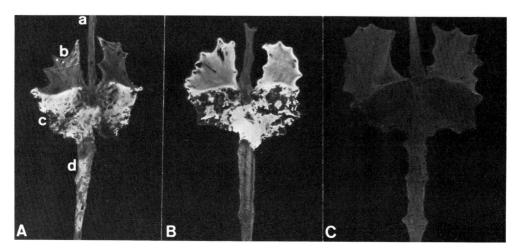

Several factors have been discussed that might contribute to the organ-specific carcinogenicity of MNNG, including differences in its uptake by the intestinal mucosa, pH and gastrin (Tahara *et al.*, 1982). Since animal experiments revealed that tumour induction also occurs in the adjacent duodenum, we considered it unlikely that local factors, which differ greatly between glandular stomach and duodenum, were responsible. However, it is known that the heterolytic breakdown of MNNG is greatly accelerated in the presence of thiols. The guanidine moiety of MNNG rapidly binds to SH groups of compounds such as glutathione and cysteine, leading to the formation of thiazoline derivatives (Schulz & McCalla, 1969; Lawley & Thatcher, 1970; Wheeler & Bowdon, 1971). During this thiol-mediated decomposition, methyldiazonium hydroxide is released, which subsequently reacts with cellular macromolecules. We determined the concentration of free thiols in various rat tissues (Table 1) and found considerable differences within the upper gastrointestinal tract, with values in the glandular stomach five and ten times higher than those in the oesophagus and forestomach, respectively. This suggests that the lack of susceptibility of oesophagus and forestomach to tumour induction might be due to their low thiol content. Thus, after oral administration, MNNG would be bioactivated to a significant extent only upon reaching the glandular stomach. A significant fraction of the carcinogen passes the stomach but decomposes in the duodenum, leaving the lower intestinal segments (jejunum, ileum, colon) unexposed.

In order to exclude a coincidental correlation between high thiol concentrations and extensive DNA alkylation by MNNG in glandular stomach, we carried out additional experiments using a thiol blocking agent, N-ethylmaleimide. This compound was found to inhibit completely the thiol-mediated decomposition of MNNG *in vitro* (data not shown). Since rats do not readily drink solutions containing this inhibitor, we used stomach gavage as an alternative route of administration. The autoradiograph in Fig. 1B shows the distribution of ^{14}C-MNNG-derived radioactivity following a single intragastric dose of MNNG alone (3 mg/kg; 15 mCi/mmol): in contrast to the distribution following MNNG administration in drinking water (Fig. 1A), significant covalent binding occurred in both the glandular stomach and the forestomach, possibly due to extended period of exposure. This correlates well with the observation that after intragastric instillation of MNNG, rats develop both adenocarcinomas of the glandular stomach and squamous-cell carcinomas of the forestomach (Schoental, 1966; Hirono & Shibuya, 1972). When MNNG was given intragastrically together with N-ethylmaleimide (50 mg/kg), covalent binding to forestomach, glandular stomach and upper duodenum was almost completely abolished (Fig. 1C). This dose of N-ethylmaleimide had been found previously to reduce gastric thiol concentrations to about 10% of that in control animals.

In conclusion, our experiments demonstrate that the initial extent of DNA methylation is a significant factor in organ-specific tumour induction by MNNG and that, after oral administration in drinking water, its preferential reaction with DNA of glandular stomach and duodenum is mediated by high thiol concentrations in those target tissues.

ACKNOWLEDGEMENTS

This work was supported by a grant from the Deutsche Forschungsgemeinschaft (SFB 31).

REFERENCES

Ellman, G.L. (1959) Tissue sulfhydryl groups. *Arch. Biochem. Biophys., 82*, 70–77

Hirono, I. & Shibuya, C. (1972) *Induction of stomach cancer by a single. dose of* N-*methyl*-N′-*nitro*-N-*nitrosoguanidine through a stomach tube*. In: Nakahara, W., Takayama, S., Sugimura, T. & Odashima, S., eds, *Topics in Chemical Carcinogenesis,* Tokyo, University of Tokyo Press, pp. 121–132

Hodgson, R.M., Wiessler, M. & Kleihues, P. (1980) Preferential methylation of target organ DNA by the oesophageal carcinogen N-nitrosomethylbenzylamine. *Carcinogenesis, 1*, 861–866

Kleihues, P., Doerjer, G., Keefer, L.K., Rice, J.M., Roller, P.P. & Hodgson, R.M. (1979) Correlation of DNA methylation by methyl(acetoxymethyl)nitrosamine with organ-specific carcinogenicity in rats. *Cancer Res., 39*, 5136–5140

Lawley, P.D. & Thatcher, C.J. (1970) Methylation of deoxyribonucleic acid in cultured mammalian cells by N-methyl-N′-nitro-N-nitrosoguanidine: The influence of cellular thiol concentrations on the extent of methylation and the 6-oxygen atom of guanine as a site of methylation. *Biochem. J., 116*, 693–707

Margison, G.P. & Kleihues, P. (1975) Chemical carcinogenesis in the nervous system. Preferential accumulation of O^6-methylguanine in rat brain deoxyribonucleic acid during repetitive administration of N-methyl-N-nitrosourea. *Biochem. J., 148*, 521–525

Pegg, A.E. (1977) Formation and metabolism of alkylated nucleosides: Possible role in carcinogenesis by nitroso compounds and alkylating agents. *Adv. Cancer Res., 25*, 195–269

Schoental, R. (1966) Carcinogenic activity of N-methyl-N′-nitro-N-nitrosoguanidine. *Nature, 209*, 726–727

Schulz, U. & McCalla, D.R. (1969) Reactions of cysteine with N-methyl-N-nitroso-p-toluenesulfonamide and N-methyl-N′-nitro-N-nitrosoguanidine. *Can. J. Chem., 47*, 2021–2027

Singer, B. (1979) N-Nitroso alkylating agents: Formation and persistence of alkyl derivatives in mammalian nucleic acids as contributing factors in carcinogenesis. *J. natl Cancer Inst., 62*, 1229–1239

Sugimura, T. & Fujimura, S. (1967) Tumour production in glandular stomach of rat by N-methyl-N′-nitro-N-nitrosoguanidine. *Nature, 216*, 943–944

Sugimura, T., Fujimura, S., Kogure, K., Baba, T., Saito, T., Nagao, M., Hosoi, H., Shimosato, Y. & Yokoshima, T. (1969) Production of adenocarcinomas in glandular stomach of experimental animals by N-methyl-N′-nitro-N-nitrosoguanidine. *Gann Monogr., 8*, 157–196

Swenberg, J.A., Cooper, H.K., Bücheler, J. & Kleihues, P. (1979) 1,2-Dimethylhydrazine-induced methylation of DNA bases in various rat organs and the effect of pretreatment with disulfiram. *Cancer Res., 39,* 465–467

Tahara, E., Shimamoto, F., Taniyama, K., Ito, H., Kosako, Y. & Sumiyoshi, H. (1982) Enhanced effect of gastrin on rat stomach carcinogenesis induced by *N*-methyl-*N'*-nitro-*N*-nitrosoguanidine. *Cancer Res., 42,* 1781–1787

Wheeler, G.P. & Bowdon, B.J. (1971) Comparison of the effects of cysteine upon the decomposition of nitrosoureas and of 1-methyl-3-nitro-1-nitrosoguanidine. *Biochem. Pharmacol., 21,* 265–267

Wiestler, O., von Deimling, A., Kobori, O. & Kleihues, P. (1983) Location of *N*-methyl-*N'*-nitro-*N*-nitrosoguanidine-induced gastrointestinal tumors correlates with thiol distribution. *Carcinogenesis, 4,* 879–883

UNSCHEDULED DNA SYNTHESIS IN HUMAN LEUCOCYTES AFTER A FISH (AMINE SOURCE) MEAL WITH OR WITHOUT SALAD (NITRITE SOURCE)

C.T. MILLER[1]

Health Protection Branch, Food Directorate, Health & Welfare, Canada

SUMMARY

Increased unscheduled DNA synthesis (UDS) was observed previously in leucocytes from human volunteers after various meals containing nitrite from cured meats and vegetables. To explore further the role of ingested nitrite, UDS response was measured in human leucocytes after a meal of bread, butter and cod fish alone (amine source) or bread, butter and cod fish plus a salad of lettuce, radish and spinach (nitrite source). A cross-over design was used so that all subjects (10 male, 10 female) were tested after both meals. Salad (nitrite source) had no effect on the level of UDS after the meal; however, UDS increased after the meal with or without salad for trial 1, but decreased for trial 2. The difference between trials could not be accounted for by sources of variation such as differences between individuals or experimental technique. The factor(s) responsible for this significant difference between trials must be associated with the non-salad components of the meal.

INTRODUCTION

There is evidence to suggest that *N*-nitroso compounds can be formed by the interaction of nitrite and secondary or tertiary amines *in vivo*. However, it is not clear whether formation of detrimental amounts actually takes place in man after ingesting a 'normal diet' containing the necessary precursors. Fine *et al.* (1977) reported elevated levels of *N*-nitrosodimethylamine in blood after a meal of bacon and raw spinach. A previous study in our laboratory (Kowalski *et al.*, 1980) confirmed this observation, but to a lesser extent. Our study also included an assay of unscheduled DNA synthesis (UDS) in leucocytes from the volunteers.

UDS is a well-documented cellular response to DNA damage by a variety of agents administered *in vitro* or *in vivo* (eg., McQueen & Williams, 1982). Many nitrosamines and nitrosamides are metabolized very quickly or react chemically under physiological conditions, yielding biologically active products which form adducts with nuclear and/or mitochondrial

---

[1] Present address: Priority Issues Directorate, Environmental Protection Service, Environment Canada, Place Vincent Massey, Hull, Québec KIA IC8

DNA. A sensitive UDS assay should detect repair synthesis in response to even short-lived DNA-damaging agents which do not persist long enough for chemical detection. In our previous study, UDS was significantly increased in leucocytes from 6/10 volunteers after a variety of meals consisting of cured meats or fish and vegetables. The present study explores the role of ingested nitrite in the induction of UDS in leucocytes. Volunteers consumed a meal of bread, butter, and codfish alone (amine source) or bread, butter and codfish, plus a salad of lettuce, radish and spinach (nitrite source).

METHODS

Hydroxyurea-resistant unscheduled DNA synthesis (UDS) in human leucocytes was assayed as described previously in the cat (Miller *et al.,* 1979). This procedure recovers both nuclear and mitochondrial DNA, with RNA and protein removed.

To assess the sources of variation in the UDS assay, a preliminary study was conducted. Blood samples were taken at 7:30 (fasting) or 10:30 in the morning from volunteers (10 male and 10 female), four times, at intervals of one week. Leucocytes separated from whole blood (Coulson & Chalmers, 1964) were cultured with hydroxyurea, to detect UDS induced *in vivo,* and without hydroxyurea to observe total DNA synthesis. At weeks 1 and 2 only, additional cultures were challenged with methylmethanesulfonate (MMS), 10^{-3} mol/L to test for individual variations in DNA repair capacity in response to a standard insult. All cultures were performed in duplicate. Analysis of variance (Searle, 1971) was performed to determine the effects of sex, day of observation, time of observation, person-to-person variation and replication error.

On the third week, after the morning blood sample had been taken, half of the volunteers (five male, five female allocated at random) were given a lunch consisting of baked codfish (150 g), obtained frozen from a local retailer, bread and butter. The remaining volunteers were given the same lunch plus a salad of lettuce, radish and spinach (200 g). Comparable meals were homogenized and assayed for nitrite and volatile nitrosamines. On the basis of previous observations (Kowalski *et al.,* 1980), two hours post-meal was the optimum time to detect peak UDS levels in most volunteers, Leucocytes obtained two hours after the meal were cultured with hydroxyurea (HU) for 18 h to detect continuing UDS. Uninhibited cultures without HU were also prepared. All cultures were prepared in duplicate.

On the fourth week, the procedure was repeated with a cross-over of meals, so that all volunteers were tested after both meals. Analysis of variance was conducted using synthesized F-tests (Sokal & Rohlf, 1969) to determine effects attributable to the meal, the day of observation, sex, person-to-person variation and variation among replicates.

Volunteers were asked to record every item of food or drink consumed on the day preceding each blood sampling day, to indicate consumption of vitamin supplements, and to indicate whether they were a smoker or non-smoker. The study was approved by the human studies committee.

RESULTS

UDS was measured in leucocytes form pre-meal blood samples from 20 volunteers (10 male and 10 female) at four weekly intervals (Table 1). There was no statistically significant effect attributable to the week of observation, sex or volunteer. However, leucocytes obtained at 10:30 in the morning (after breakfast) displayed higher UDS than fasting samples. Fasting levels of UDS in leucocytes were remarkably reproducible under the conditions employed.

Table 1. Assays of ^{3}H-thymidine incorporation into leucocytes from pre-meal blood samples

		Unscheduled DNA synthesis (+HU) ^{3}H-Thymidine (cpm/µg DNA)	Total DNA synthesis (−HU)	Response to MMS (+HU+MMS)
Week 1				
7:30 am	Male	43 + 1	146 + 30	475 + 31
Fasting	Female	41 + 1	130 + 10	407 + 38
Week 2				
7:30 am	Male	39 + 3	198 + 45	467 + 31
Fasting	Female	41 + 1	215 + 21	476 + 36
Week 3				
10:30 am	Male	50 + 6	128 + 37	
	Female	53 + 4	131 + 23	
Week 4				
10:30 am	Male	63 + 4	151 + 56	
	Female	56 + 6	112 + 12	

Source of variation	F-test (degrees of freedom)		
Week observed	2.08 (2,2)	10.05^a (2,2)	1.09 (1,1)
Hour observed	10.72^a (1,2)	1.66 (1,2)	not applicable
Sex	0.12 (1,2)	0.20 (1,1)	1.15 (1,1)
Person-to-person	1.19 (18,18)	23.29^a (18,18)	0.93 (18,18)

^{a} $p < 0.05$
HU, hydroxyurea; MMS, methylmethanesulfonate

Cultures from pre-meal blood samples without HU to suppress any semi-conservative DNA synthesis (Table 1) demonstrated a significant person-to-person variation ($F = 23.3$, d.f = 18,18). They also varied from week to week. [It is of peripheral interest that three individuals were detected statistically as outliers with high levels of DNA synthesis in circulating leucocytes. Autoradiographs of lymphocytes show high levels of extra-nuclear ^{3}H-thymidine incorporation, localized in one quadrant of the cytoplasm – possibly attributable to mitochondria surrounding the cytopore.]

The ability of leucocytes from fasting blood samples to respond to a standard insult with MMS was comparable regardless of the individual, the sex, or the week of observation (Table 1).

Assays of DNA synthesis in leucocytes from blood sampled after the two test meals are summarized in Table 2. There was no effect of the salad (nitrite source) on UDS observed after the meal for males or females, trial 1 or trial 2. However, results for the two trials were quantitatively different ($F = 193$, d.f = 1,14). In trial 1 (week 3), levels of UDS after the meal (with and without salad) were significantly lower than those observed in trial 2 (week 4), and were even lower than fasting levels. There was no difference between trials in the total amount of DNA synthesis without hydroxyurea.

Levels of nitrate and nitrite in typical salads varied from about 100 to 600 mg sodium nitrate, and 1 to 6 mg sodium nitrite per 200 g serving. Nitrosamine levels in the fish samples did not exceed 2 µg/kg.

Three volunteers took a multivitamin preparation daily, and four volunteers were habitual smokers. In neither case did UDS responses deviate significantly from the mean.

Table 2.   Assays of ³H-thymidine incorporated into leucocytes after a
meal of fish (F) of fish and salad (F & S)

		Unscheduled DNA synthesis (+ HU)	Total DNA synthesis (− HU)
		³H-thymidine (cpm/μg DNA)	
Trial 1 Male	F	28 + 5	121 + 15
Week 3	F & S	37 + 3	113 + 6
Female	F	34 + 1	181 + 9
	F & S	31 + 2	170 + 10
Trial 2 Male	F & S	60 + 2	213 + 51
Week 4	F	56 + 5	141 + 20
Female	F & S	55 + 1	156 + 16
	F	57 + 3	114 + 12
Source of variation		Unscheduled DNA synthesis (+ HU)	Total DNA synthesis (− HU)
		F-test (degrees of freedom)	
Week observed		192.9[a] (1,14)	0.2 (1,1)
Sex		0.2 (1,2)	2.5 (1,2)
Meal (F *versus* F + S)		1.5 (1,14)	0.02 (1,14)
Person-to-person		1.4 (18,14)	1.53[a] (18,14)

[a] $p < 0.05$
HU, hydroxyurea

CONCLUSIONS

Ingested nitrite had no effect on the level of UDS in circulating leucocytes after consumption of an amine-containing meal. Thus, although the UDS sometimes observed after a meal may be associated with DNA damage induced by nitroso compounds formed *in vivo*, dietary nitrite is not implicated.

The difference between trials could not be accounted for by known sources of variation, such as differences between individuals or experimental technique. The factor(s) responsible for this significant difference between trials were associated with the non-salad components of the meal.

Analysis of the sources of variation in the DNA synthesis assays indicated that, while total DNA synthesis (including semi-conservative replication) varied between individuals and over time, the fasting level of UDS was remarkably reproducible. Furthermore, the capacity to respond to a standard insult to DNA did not vary significantly between individuals. The assay described is therefore well-suited to the study *in vivo* of human exposure to suspected genotoxic agents.

REFERENCES

Coulson, A.S. & Chalmers, D.G. (1964) Separation of viable lymphocytes from human blood. *Lancet, i,* 468–481

Fine, D.H., Ross, R. Rounbehler, D.P., Silvergleid, A. & Song, L. (1977) Formation *in vivo* of volatile *N*-nitrosamines in man after ingestion of cooked bacon and spinach. *Nature, 265,* 753–755

Kowalski, B., Miller, C.T. & Sen, N.P. (1980) *Studies on the* in vivo *formation of nitrosamines in rats and humans after ingestion of various meals.* In: Walker, E.A., Griciute, L. Castegnaro, M. & Börszönyi, M., eds, N-*Nitroso Compounds: Analysis, Formation and Occurrence (IARC Scientific Publications No. 31),* Lyon, International Agency for Research on Cancer, pp. 609–617

McQueen, C.A. & Williams, G.M. (1982) *Determination of host genetic susceptibility to genotoxic chemicals in hepatocyte cultures.* In: Bartsch, H. & Armstrong, B., eds, *Host Factors in Human Carcinogenesis (IARC Scientific Publications No. 39),* Lyon, International Agency for Research on Cancer, pp. 413–420

Miller, C.T., Zawidzka, Z., Nagy, E. & Charbonneau, S.M. (1979) Indicators of genetic toxicity in leucocytes and granulocytic precursors after chronic methylmercury ingestion by cats. *Bull. environ. Contam. Toxicol., 21,* 296–303

Searle, S.R. (1971) *Linear Models,* New York, John Wiley & Sons

Sokal, R. & Rohlf, F. (1969) *Biometry,* San Francisco, W.H. Freeman & Co.

BIOLOGICAL EFFECTS: CARCINOGENICITY AND MUTAGENICITY

CONTRASTING RESPONSES OF RATS AND SYRIAN HAMSTERS TO ORALLY ADMINISTERED N-NITROSO COMPOUNDS

W. LIJINSKY

LBI-Basic Research Program, Chemical Carcinogenesis Program, NCI-Frederick Cancer Research Facility, Frederick, MD 21701, USA

INTRODUCTION

In the past 25 years of study of the carcinogenic actions of N-nitroso compounds, emphasis has been placed on the chemical structure of the nitroso compound in determining its carcinogenic activity. This was clearly the outcome of the extensive study by Druckrey *et al.* (1967) of the carcinogenicity of N-nitroso compounds in BD-IX rats. The work of Magee and many others has emphasized the significance of conversion of N-nitroso compounds to the oraalkylating agents able to alkylate cellular DNA in the induction of neoplasia. Of increasing importance recently has been the role of differential repair of DNA damage produced by alkylating agents in various organs, which seems to be related to the specificity with which tumours are induced in some organs and not in others (Pegg, 1977). Thus, it has been observed that DNA ethylation produced in rat brain by N-nitrosoethylurea is eliminated much more slowly than DNA ethylation produced in the liver of the same rat, which is linked to the failure of N-nitrosoethylurea to induce liver tumours in rats, whereas this nitrosamide induces tumours of the nervous system in that species. However, the ethylation produced in the DNA of rat liver by N-nitrosodiethylamine is related to the induction of liver tumours, because this nitrosamine is a potent liver carcinogen in rats (Druckrey *et al.*, 1967).

It seems clear that many of the differences in the carcinogenic effectiveness of a given nitrosamine between one species and another, both in potency and in target organ, could be explained by differences in pathways of metabolic activation between species. This matter is being studied extensively in many laboratories. However, in the case of nitrosoalkylamides, which are directly acting carcinogens requiring no metabolic activation, the difference in metabolic activation should be unimportant. Yet there are instances in which directly acting N-nitroso compounds induce quite different tumours in different species. For example, N-nitrosoethylurethane induced forestomach tumours in rats, but cholangiocarcinomas in the livers of guinea-pigs (Lijinsky & Reuber, 1982a); N-nitroso-N-methylurea induced tumours of the nervous system in rats (Druckrey *et al.*, 1967) but not in guinea-pigs or gerbils.

A most important question in understanding carcinogenesis by chemicals is the extent to which the properties of the cells exposed to the chemical determine the induction of tumours. A comparison of the carcinogenic effects of a single compound in several species is insufficient to provide an answer, because of the enormous complexity of the animal body and the paucity of knowledge of the mechanism of carcinogenesis within any cell, as distinct from knowledge of simple reactions of the carcinogen. It seemed that a more informative impression would be gained by examination of the tumours induced by a number of closely related carcinogenic N-nitroso compounds and a comparison of the spectrum of tumours in one species with that in another species induced by the same compounds. Since there is a large store of information about the carcinogenicity of more than 150 N-nitroso compounds in Fischer F344 rats of our laboratory, we selected many of these compounds for a parallel series of chronic toxicity studies in Syrian golden hamsters. The compounds were administered to both species by the oral route.

RESULTS AND DISCUSSION

Nitrosoalkylamides

It is simplest to describe first the results with nitrosoalkylamides, which are assumed to be directly acting compounds and therefore do not suffer the diversity of activating enzymes between species, which might play a vital role in determining target organ specificity of nitrosamines.

With few exceptions, all nitrosoalkylamides are carcinogenic, whereas there are many noncarcinogenic nitrosamines which, presumably, are not converted by activating enzymes to carcinogenic intermediates. The nitrosoalkylamides examined in both rats and hamsters include a number of nitrosoalkylureas. In Table 1 are given the target organs in rats and hamsters, the approximate total dose received by each animal and the median time to death with tumours. In addition, two nitrosotrialkylureas are listed, which require metabolic activation. In rats, the carcinogenic actions of the various nitrosoalkylamides were often quite different, whereas in the hamsters their effects were all very similar in the target organs affected, although they differed in potency. N-Nitroso-2-hydroxyethylurea induced a great variety of tumours in rats, including several rarely induced by N-nitroso compounds, such as in colon, duodenum, glandular stomach, bone and kidney (Lijinsky & Reuber, 1983). The homologous N-nitroso-2-hydroxypropylurea induced the equally unusual leukaemia of the thymus, but only tumours of the forestomach and a few of the duodenum that were in common with those induced by N-nitroso-2-hydroxyethylurea. Both compounds at comparable doses induced almost exclusively tumours of the forestomach and haemangiosarcomas of the spleen in hamsters; N-nitroso-2-hydroxyethylurea led to earlier death of hamsters with tumours than did N-nitroso-2-hydroxypropylurea, while the converse was true in the rat. The non-directly acting N-nitrosotriethylurea and N-nitrosomethyldiethylurea, which induced, respectively, mammary carcinomas and tumours of the central nervous system in rats (and these are tumours induced by the directly acting N-nitrosomonoalkylureas in rats), induced tumours of the forestomach and angiosarcomas of the spleen in hamsters, together with a small number of pancreas-duct tumours. As in rats, the disposition of tumours induced by N-nitrosotrialkylureas was not very different from that with the N-nitrosomonoalkylureas. An intriguing question is why nitrosoalkylureas induce angiosarcomas in the spleen of hamsters, but not in rats, yet do not cause tumours to develop in endothelial cells of other organs of the hamster, other than a few in liver. Furthermore, several nitrosamines induce angiosarcomas of the liver, but not of the spleen, in hamsters.

Cyclic nitrosamines

A second group of N-nitroso compounds of interest are the cyclic nitrosamines, which require metabolic activation and might, therefore, be expected to evoke different responses in rats and hamsters, because metabolic activation could well differ between the two species.

Table 1. Carcinogenicity of nitrosoalkylureas in rats and hamsters

Nitroso-	Dose rate (μmol/week)	Median week of death	Total dose/kg (mmol)	Tumours in rats (%)	Tumours in hamsters (%)
triethylurea	95	33	12	mammary carcinomas (95) forestomach (40) uterus (30) brain (10)	
	52	30	10		spleen haemangiosarcoma (85) forestomach (75) pancreas (5)
diethylmethylurea	95	32	12	brain (55) spinal cord (60)	
	50	29	10		spleen haemangiosarcoma (75) forestomach (85) liver (35) pancreas (20)
2-hydroxyethylurea	40	51	3	lung (55) forestomach (25) thyroid (25) colon (15) bone (10) duodenum (15) bladder (15) glandular stomach (10) lymphosarcoma (10)	
	21	24	4		spleen haemangiosarcoma (80) liver (40) forestomach (25)
2-hydroxypropylurea	40	32	3	thymus leukaemia (65) forestomach (15) lung (10) duodenum (5)	
	22	36	4.5		spleen haemangiosarcoma (75) forestomach (80) liver (30) lymphosarcoma (20)

Table 2. Carcinogenicity of cyclic nitrosamines in rats and hamsters

Nitroso-	Dose rate (μmol/week)	Median week of death	Total dose/kg (mmol)	Tumours in rats (%)	Tumours in hamsters (%)
azetidine	200 115	53 64	40 50	liver carcinomas (100)	liver adenomas (30)
morpholine	35	52	7	liver carcinomas (85) liver angiosarcomas (80) oesophagus (60)	
	45	35	10		nasal carcinomas (90) tracheal adenomas (30)
2-methylmorpholine	35	27	3.5	liver angiosarcomas (95) liver carcinomas (55) oesophagus (50) tongue (20)	
	42	34	10		nasal carcinomas (75) liver angiosarcomas (5) lung (55) trachea (30) forestomach (40)
2,6-dimethylmorpholine	35	23	3	oesophagus (100) forestomach (15)	
	42	34	10		liver angiosarcoma (90) pancreas (95) lung (100) nasal carcinomas (60) forestomach (20)
oxazolidine	35	53	7	liver carcinomas (95) liver angiosarcomas (85)	
	45	43	12		liver cholangiocarcinomas (75) liver carcinomas (25) forestomach (10)
5-methyloxazolidine	35	85	7	liver carcinomas (95) liver angiosarcomas (40)	
	25	35	8		liver angiosarcomas (40) liver cholangiocarcinomas (5) liver carcinomas (25) liver adenomas (60) pancreas (15)

3,4,5-trimethylpiperazine	70	27	7	thymic leukaemia (90)	lung (85) forestomach (70) liver angiosarcoma (20) trachea (10)
	38	59	14	nasal carcinomas (30)	
Dinitroso-2,6-dimethyl-piperazine	70	27	5.5	oesophagus (35) nasal carcinomas (25) forestomach (10)	forestomach (45) lung (20) liver angiosarcoma (10) trachea (10)
	40	67	12		

Table 3. Carcinogenicity of acyclic nitrosamines in rats and hamsters

Nitroso-	Dose rate (μmol/week)	Median week of death	Total dose/kg (mmol)	Tumours in rats (%)	Tumours in hamsters (%)
n-hexylmethylamine	88	31	6	liver angiosarcoma (90) liver carcinoma (30) oesophagus (95) lung (45) forestomach (10)	
	43	56	24		forestomach (90) lung (70) bladder (35)
methyl-oxopropylamine	86	23	4.5	liver angiosarcomas (75) oesophagus (95) nasal carcinomas (65) trachea (30)	
	17	20	2.5		liver angiosarcoma (40) liver cholangiocarcinoma (65) nasal carcinoma (20)
methyl-2-hydroxypropylamine	86	29	4.5	oesophagus (100) lung (60)	
	17	25	3		liver angiosarcoma (50) liver cholangiocarcinoma (50) liver adenoma (35) pancreas (45) lung (50)
bis-oxopropylamine	35	61	7	liver carcinoma (60) liver angiosarcoma (45) lung (75)	
	15	25	3		liver cholangiocarcinoma (100) pancreas (50) lung (20)
bis-hydroxypropylamine	135	42	23	oesophagus (80) nasal carcinoma (35)	
	120	32	32		pancreas (50) liver (20) lung (30) nasal carcinoma (80)
hydroxypropyloxopropylamine	35	41	5.5	liver carcinoma (80) oesophagus (90) lung (65) nasal carcinoma (30)	nasal carcinoma (80)

	38	27	6	liver cholangiocarcinoma (55) liver adenoma (50) pancreas (70) lung (10)
dihydroxypropyloxopropylamine	35	26	3	oesophagus (100) forestomach (45) tongue (40) lung (25)
	37	38	13	forestomach (95) pancreas (40) liver (25)
allyloxopropylamine	35	74	7	liver carcinoma (75) oesophagus (35) forestomach (10) nasal carcinoma (10)
	43	50	13	liver adenoma (30) nasal carcinoma (20)

Indeed, it is well known that hamster liver microsomes are more effective in activating nitrosamines to bacterial mutagens than are rat liver microsomes (Raineri *et al.*, 1981). Of all the cyclic nitrosamines tested in rats, only a few were selected for study in hamsters and were administered by gavage at doses similar to those given to rats (Table 2). *N*-Nitrosoazetidine had only a weakly carcinogenic effect, the tumours induced being mainly hepatocellular adenomas, with a few carcinomas of the liver; several animals did not develop tumours at all. *N*-Nitrosomorpholine induced tumours of the liver and a few in the oesophagus and forestomach of the rat, but no liver tumours, and, instead, tumours of the nasal cavity and trachea in hamsters. *N*-Nitroso-2-methylmorpholine gave rise to tumours of the oesophagus and liver in rats, but in hamsters induced angiosarcomas of the liver together with tumours of the lung, trachea and forestomach, but not in the nasal cavity. *N*-Nitroso-2,6-dimethylmorpholine induced only oesophageal tumours in rats, whether given by gavage or drinking water, whereas in hamsters it induced a high incidence of ductal carcinomas of the pancreas and angiosarcomas of the liver, as well as tumours of the lung and nasal cavity. The reason for these profound differences, particularly between the rat and hamster in response to *N*-nitroso-2,6-dimethylmorpholine is probably related to differences in metabolism in the two species, and this is being explored (Underwood & Lijinsky, 1982). The carcinogenic effect of *N*-nitrosomorpholine and of its lower homologue *N*-nitroso-1,3-oxazolidine, is almost identical in rats (Lijinsky & Reuber, 1982b), but in the hamster the homologue induced mainly cholangiocarcinomas and adenomas in the liver but few liver-cell carcinomas. Whereas 5-methylnitrosooxazolidine is considerably less potent than the parent compound as a liver carcinogen in rats, in the hamster the 5-methyl derivative is considerably more potent than *N*-nitrosooxazolidine and induces angiocsarcomas in the liver as well as cholangiocarcinomas, adenomas and hepatocellular carcinomas; there were also a few tumours of the pancreatic duct. These differences suggest that the mechanisms of activation of this type of nitrosamine might be quite different in the rat and the hamster.

Two derivatives of *N*-nitrosopiperazine were studied in the hamster, and they had quite different carcinogenic effects from those seen in rats. *N*-Nitroso-3,4,5-trimethylpiperazine induced a high incidence of thymic leukaemia and tumours of the nasal cavity in rats. In hamsters, however, mainly tumours of the forestomach and of the lung, together with a few angiosarcomas of the liver were induced. Dinitroso-2,6-dimethylpiperazine was a more potent carcinogen in the rat than *N*-nitrosotrimethylpiperazine, whereas in the hamster the reverse was true. Dinitrosodimethylpiperazine induced tumours similar to those observed with *N*-nitrosotrimethylpiperazine in hamsters, but the incidence was smaller, and there were very few lung tumours.

Acyclic nitrosamines

The acyclic nitrosamines have been studied in hamsters more extensively than cyclic nitrosamines. A great similarity between rats and hamsters was observed following treatment with *N*-nitrosomethyl-*n*-dodecylamine, which induced transitional-cell carcinomas of the bladder in both species. It can probably be assumed that the mechanism suggested by Okada *et al.* (1976) for the induction of bladder tumours by this and similar compounds is common to both species, namely β oxidation of the long chain to form *N*-nitrosomethyl-3-carboxypropylamine, which is a bladder carcinogen in rats (Lijinsky *et al.*, 1983). *N*-Nitroso-*n*-hexylmethylamine is a potent carcinogen in rats, inducing tumours of the liver, oesophagus, forestomach and lung, but no bladder tumours; but, in hamsters it is much less potent and induces tumours of the lung, forestomach and bladder, but no oesophageal tumours (Table 3). This suggests that, while the mechanisms of activation of *N*-nitrosododecylmethylamine to proximate carcinogenic forms might be similar in rats and hamsters, this is clearly not the case for *N*-nitrosohexylmethylamine, with its broader tumour spectrum.

Most of the other acyclic nitrosamines that have been examined in both rats and hamsters have the specificity of nitrosoalkyl-2-oxopropylamines for the pancreatic duct of the Syrian hamster (Krüger et al., 1974). They are all hydroxyalkylnitrosamines or the corresponding ketones. They tend to be more potent carcinogens in hamsters than in rats, and they induce quite different patterns of tumours in the two species. The principal target organ in the rat is the oesophagus, with the liver also being a common site for tumour induction. In the hamster, the pancreas is a common target and the liver is even more common, but they rarely, if ever, develop tumours of the oesophagus. Tumours of the pancreatic duct are never induced in rats by these nitrosamines.

There were marked differences in potency between many of the compounds, whether compared in rats or in hamsters. In general, nitroso derivatives of alkyloxopropylamines were quite potent and had the liver as the main target organ, although frequently also inducing pancreatic tumours in hamsters. An exception was N-nitrosomethyl-2-oxopropylamine, which has been reported to be a potent inducer of pancreatic ductal tumours in hamsters (Pour et al., 1980), but which in our experiments induced only a few pancreatic tumours at a variety of doses. All of these 2-oxopropylamine derivatives induced liver tumours in rats, and often tumours of the oesophagus also. Derivatives of alkyldihydroxypropylnitrosamines were generally weak carcinogens in hamsters and produced mainly tumours of the forestomach, together with some pancreatic tumours; in rats, all except N-nitrosodihydroxypropylethanol-amine were very potent carcinogens and induced mainly tumours of the oesophagus.

Nitroso derivatives of alkyl-2-hydroxypropylamines were very similar to the corresponding ketones in their carcinogenic action in both rats and hamsters, although they were less potent. In hamsters they induced tumours of the liver and pancreas and in rats tumours of the liver and oesophagus.

The effects of allyl groups, which were assumed to resist metabolism and, therefore, to accentuate the carcinogenic activity of the other alkyl substituent, were variable. Frequently, the action of the allyl group was to increase carcinogenic potency, but sometimes the target organs were changed, both in hamsters and in rats. In rats, the main effect of the presence of the allyl group was to decrease carcinogenic potency.

CONCLUSION

The conclusion to be drawn from these comparisons of the action of N-nitroso compounds in rats and hamsters is that no firm deduction can be made about the mechanisms of action of these compounds in inducing tumours in either species. However, it does appear that certain patterns of tumours are induced in rats and other patterns in hamsters. The oesophagus is the most common target organ in rats, followed by the liver; while in hamsters the oesophagus is very rarely, if ever, the target, and liver and pancreas often are. Further, the pancreas is almost never the target of N-nitroso compounds in rats. These results suggest that, in addition to the chemical properties of the nitroso compound in determining its carcinogenic action, the biological properties of specific organs, or types of cell within them, are also influential and vary from species to species. It is these biological properties which are probably responsible for the pronounced organ specificity seen in nitrosamine carcinogenesis.

ACKNOWLEDGEMENTS

Research sponsored by the National Cancer Institute, DHHS, under contract No. NO1-CO-23909 with Litton Bionetics, Inc. The contents of this publication do not necessarily reflect the views or policies of the Department of Health and Human Services, nor does mention of trade names, commercial products, or organizations imply endorsement by the US Government.

REFERENCES

Druckrey, H., Preussmann, R., Ivankovic, S. & Schmähl, D. (1967) Organotrope carcinogene Wirkungen bei 65 verschiedenen *N*-Nitroso-Verbindungen an BD-Ratten. *Z. Krebsforsch., 69*, 103–201

Krüger, F.W., Pour, P. & Althoff, J. (1974) Induction of pancreas tumours by diisopropanolnitrosamine. *Naturwissenschaften, 61*, 328

Lijinsky, W. & Reuber, M.D. (1982a) Studies of a deuterium isotope effect in carcinogenesis by *N*-nitroso-*N*-alkylurethanes in rats. *Cancer Lett., 16*, 273–279

Lijinsky, W. & Reuber, M.D. (1982b) Comparative carcinogenesis by nitrosomorpholines, nitrosooxazolidines and nitrosotetrahydrooxazine in rats. *Carcinogenesis, 3*, 911–915

Lijinsky, W. & Reuber, M.D. (1983) Carcinogenicity of hydroxylated alkylnitrosoureas and nitrosooxazolidones by mouse skin painting and by gavage in rats. *Cancer Res., 43*, 214–221

Lijinsky, W., Reuber, M.D., Saavedra, J.E. & Singer, G.M. (1983) Carcinogenesis in F344 rats by nitrosomethyl-*n*-propylamine derivatives. *J. natl Cancer Inst., 70*, 959–963

Okada. M., Suzuki, E. & Mochizuki, M. (1976) Possible important role of urinary *N*-methyl-*N*-(3-carboxypropyl)nitrosamine in the induction of bladder tumors in rats by *N*-methyl-*N*-dodecylnitrosamine. *Gann, 67*, 771–772

Pegg, A.E. (1977) Formation and metabolism of alkylated nucleosides: possible role in carcinogenesis by nitroso compounds and alkylating agents. *Adv. Cancer Res., 25*, 195–267

Pour, P., Gingell, R., Langenbach, R., Nagel, D., Grandjean, C., Lawson, T. & Salmasi, S. (1980) Carcinogenicity of *N*-nitrosomethyl(2-oxopropyl)amine in Syrian hamsters. *Cancer Res., 40*, 3585–3590

Raineri, R., Poiley, J.A., Andrews, A.W., Pienta, R. & Lijinsky, W. (1981) Greater effectiveness of hepatocyte and liver S9 preparations from hamsters than rat preparations in activating *N*-nitroso compounds to metabolites mutagenic to *Salmonella. J. natl Cancer Inst., 67*, 1117–1122

Underwood, B. & Lijinsky, W. (1982) Comparative metabolism of 2,6-dimethylnitrosomorpholine in rats, hamsters and guinea pigs. *Cancer Res., 42*, 54–58

NITROSAMINE CARCINOGENESIS IN 5120 RODENTS: CHRONIC ADMINISTRATION OF SIXTEEN DIFFERENT CONCENTRATIONS OF NDEA, NDMA, NPYR AND NPIP IN THE WATER OF 4440 INBRED RATS, WITH PARALLEL STUDIES ON NDEA ALONE OF THE EFFECT OF AGE OF STARTING (3, 6 OR 20 WEEKS) AND OF SPECIES (RATS, MICE OR HAMSTERS)[1]

R. PETO & R. GRAY

ICRF Cancer Studies Unit, Nuffield Department of Clinical Medicine, Radcliffe Infirmary, Oxford OX2 6HE, UK

P. BRANTOM & P. GRASSO

British Industrial Biological Research Association (BIBRA), Woodmansterne Road, Carshalton, Surrey, UK

SUMMARY

A Weibull analysis is presented of the dose and time relationships for the effects on 4 080 inbred rats of chronic ingestion in the drinking water of 16 different doses of N-nitrosodimethylamine (NDMA) and of N-nitrosodiethylamine (NDEA). The sites chiefly affected were the liver (by both agents) and the oesophagus (by NDEA only). Since the experiment continued into extreme old age, effects became clearly measurable even at a dose of only 0.01 mg/kg per day, which is an order of magnitude lower than previously achieved. (After only two years of treatment, however, the 'TD$_{50}$' doses needed to halve the proportion of tumourless survivors would have been about 0.06 mg/kg per day of NDEA and about 0.12 mg/kg per day of NDMA.) The general pattern of response was that the log probability of remaining tumourless was given by the product of two terms, the first (the 'Weibull b-value') depending on the dose-rate but not on the duration of exposure, and the second depending not on dose at all but on (approximately the seventh power of) duration.

For oesophageal tumours, the 'Weibull b-value' was approximately proportional to the cube of the dose-rate of NDEA (males 21 d^3, females 11 d^3, where d = dose-rate in mg/kg adult body weight/day, and the background incidence was unmeasurably low. For liver tumours

---

[1] This experiment was commissioned by the Ministry of Agriculture, Fisheries and Food (MAFF) in consultation with the Department of Health and Social Security (DHSS), and was executed at the British Industrial Biological Research Association and analysed at Oxford.

induced by NDEA, the b-value was approximately proportional to the fourth power of dose-rate + 0.04 mg/kg per day (males, 19 $(d+0.04)^4$; females, 32 $(d+0.04)^4$), although the relationships were slightly different for the different subsites of liver tumour. This one formula implies both approximate linearity at low doses and an approximately cubic relationship within the higher range of doses that was studied. For liver tumours induced by NDMA, the Weibull b-value was approximately proportional to the sixth power of dose rate + 0.1 mg/kg per day (males, 37 $(d+0.1)^6$; females, 51 $(d+0.1)^6$), again with variation between liver subsites, and again implying approximate linearity at low doses. The difference between the latter two relationships may represent differences in the induction of particular DNA repair enzymes by NDMA and NDEA, or in the effects of those enzymes on methylated and on ethylated DNA. These formulae should, of course, be trusted only in the range of doses from which they were derived, and particularly not for those above it. If that for NDMA is extrapolated to lower doses, it suggests that the tumour risks from two years' chronic exposure of such rats to low dose-rates of this agent would, in the absence of other causes of death, be of the order of 0.03% (males) and 0.04% (females) per µg/kg per day. Similar extrapolation using the formula for NDEA suggests that at low dose levels the oesophageal cancer risk would become much less important than the liver tumour risk, and that the latter might be about 0.06%(males) or 0.1% (females) per µg/kg per day. (This is compatible with the observation that, at those low dose-levels at which its effects are measurable, NDEA appears to be about two or three times as potent as NDMA.) But, among animals allowed to live out their natural lifespan (some of which would die before completing two years of treatment but some of which would survive substantially longer and therefore suffer higher tumour onset rates), the absolute risks produced by continuous treatment from six weeks of age onwards might be about seven times as great, i.e., averaging the two sexes, about 0.24% for each µg/kg NDMA and about 0.58% for each µg/kg NDEA. No direct estimate is obtained, of course, of the net effects of these agents on humans.

In addition, various smaller experiments on a total of 1040 more rodents were undertaken, in which three further questions were addressed.

(1) Studies of 16 different concentrations of *N*-nitrosopyrrolidine (NPYR) and *N*-nitroso-piperidine (NPIP) given from age six weeks onwards to small groups of rats yielded dose-response relationships for the effects of NPYR on inducing liver tumours and for those of NPIP on inducing tumours of the liver and upper gastrointestinal tract that resembled those seen with NDMA and NDEA, respectively, except that NPYR and NPIP were less potent (the respective $TD_{50}s$, i.e., the dose-rates needed to halve the proportion of tumourless survivors after two years of treatment, being approximately 0.4 (males) and 0.6 (females) mg/kg adult body weight per day (ABWD) for each agent). Alternatively, it was estimated that the risks from lifelong exposure to 1 µg/kg ABWD of each agent might be about 0.1%, and that the risk *to rats* from lower doses would be proportionately less.

(2) Studies of 16 different concentrations of NDEA on small groups of female mice and female hamsters yielded the types of dose-response relationships that would be expected for upper gastrointestinal tract tumours, liver-cell tumours and Kupffer-cell tumours in mice (no other type of liver tumour being produced, in contrast to previous reports) and for tracheal and liver-cell tumours in hamsters (no clear effect on upper gastrointestinal tract tumours being apparent in hamsters). The dose-rates needed to halve the proportion of tumourless survivors after two years of treatment were approximately 0.3 mg/kg ABWD, i.e., five times that for the same agent in rats. In part, however, this may be because treatment started at an older age in these species (see below).

(3) Studies were undertaken of the effects on oesophageal and liver tumorigenesis of starting treatment of rats with NDEA at three or at 20 weeks of age instead of at six weeks of age (as in the main experiment). Earlier treatment resulted in slightly greater dosage-rates, if dosage was measured in mg/kg per day, and hence in a correspondingly more rapid yield of oesophageal tumours, but the effect was not large. By contrast, an earlier start to treatment resulted, after a fixed duration of treatment, in a three-fold higher incidence rate of liver tumours, while a later start resulted in a two-fold decrease. (The effects at a fixed age would, of course, be even greater.) This indicates a profound influence of nitrosamine treatment of the liver during the first few weeks of life on subsequent tumour onset rates, due to some temporary factor(s) that greatly enhances the sensitivity of the organ to NDEA.

All but one of the dose-response relationships studied in these ancillary experiments involved a decrease in the median time to tumour with increasing dose-rate, approximately according to the general rule

$$(\text{dose-rate}) \times (\text{median})^{2.3 \text{ or so}} = \text{constant}.$$

The chief exception was tumours of the bile-duct in hamsters, for which the median varied much more slowly than this.

INTRODUCTION

A large dose-response experiment on a total of 5120 rodents (mice, hamsters and rats) was undertaken, details of which are provided in Table 1. The design was fairly standard, except that (a) nitrosamine concentrations were constant in ppm of the water, and so varied in mg/kg per day, and (b) the duration of observation was unusually long [except that (c) some animals were sacrificed at 12 or 18 months]; so only selected details of the methods follow. A fuller report was drafted recently for the UK government departments that sponsored this study.

SELECTED DETAILS OF THE EXPERIMENTAL METHODS

Interim sacrifices

One-tenth of the original animals were scheduled for sacrifice after 12 months and after 18 months of treatment, but the remaining eight-tenths were scheduled to live their normal lifespan, with no terminal sacrifice. As a result, the experiment involved just over three years of treatment for some animals.

Context of observation (fatal/incidental)

At routine post-mortem examination, tumours were sought in the usual ways, but with special attention to the liver and oesophagus. When possible, liver tumours were then subdivided histologically as to subsite of origin (see below). For animals with tumours at any particular site (or subsite), an attempt was made to determine whether such tumours had been observed in a 'fatal' context – i.e., had contributed directly or indirectly to the death of the host – or in an 'incidental' context[1]. Doubtful cases were classified as 'probably fatal' or 'probably

---

[1] As discussed by the IARC (1980), such contexts of observation are required not to determine the biological nature of the lesions – that is chiefly sought histologically, of course – but merely to determine which denominator to relate them to statistically. For any reasonably short age range, the appropriate denominator for the fatal tumours found in it is the number of animals still alive and thus at risk of death from tumours. Conversely, the appropriate denominator for the incidental tumours found in it is the number of deaths from unrelated causes that bring animals to post-mortem examination and thereby enable incidental tumours to be discovered.

Table 1. Experimental design

	Parallel studies						Main experiment			
Species	Colworth rats	Colworth rats	C57-BO mice	Syrian hamster	Colworth rats	Colworth rats	Colworth rats	Colworth rats	Colworth rats	Colworth rats
Age at start of treatment (weeks)	6	6	12	20	3	20	6	6	–	6
Scheduled date of sacrifice	2½ yrs	2½ yrs	25 mths[c]	22 mths	2½ yrs	2½ yrs	Never[a]	Never[a]	Never[a]	Never[a]
Group size (male & female)	6M 6F	6M 6F	10F only	10F only	6M 6F	6M 6F	48M[a] 48F[a]	48M[a] 48F[a]	192M[a] 192F[a]	48M[a] 48F[a]
Agent	NPYR	NPIP	NDEA	NDEA	NDEA	NDEA	NDEA		Control	NDMA
MW (Daltons)	100.2	114.2	102.1	102.1	102.1	102.1	102.1		–	74.1
Density	1.085	1.063	0.942	0.942	0.942	0.942	0.942		–	1.006
ppm v/v[b] in group 1	–	–	zero			–	–		zero	–
2	0.56	0.18	0.033			0.033	0.033		–	0.033
3	1.12	0.36	0.066			0.066	0.066		–	0.066
4	2.24	0.73	0.132			0.132	0.132		–	0.132
5	4.49	1.45	0.264			0.264	0.264		–	0.264
6	8.98	2.90	0.528			0.528	0.528		–	0.528
7	17.95	5.81	1.056			1.056	1.056		–	1.056
8	26.93	8.71	1.584			1.584	1.584		–	1.584
9	35.90	11.62	2.112			2.112	2.112		–	2.112
10	44.88	14.52	2.640			2.640	2.640		–	2.640
11	53.86	17.42	3.168			3.168	3.168		–	3.168
12	71.81	23.23	4.224			4.224	4.224		–	4.224
13	89.76	29.04	5.280			5.280	5.280		–	5.280
14	107.71	34.85	6.336			6.336	6.336		–	6.336
15	143.62	46.46	8.448			8.448	8.448		–	8.448
16	287.23	92.93	16.896			16.896	16.896		–	16.896

[a] In addition, numbers one-eighth as large were scheduled for sacrifice at 6 and at 12 months

[b] Conversion to mg/kg adult body weight per day (ABWD) requires multiplication of the concentration v/v by the density and by the water intake in adult life, in mL/kg ABWD. For rats, this was approximately 41 for males and 72 for females. For female mice and hamsters, it was approximately 290 and 110.

[c] The mouse experiment was terminated at 28 months, but due to an administrative error all records relating to the last 3 months were lost.

incidental'. The total proportion that fell into these two indeterminate classes was, however, only about 6% (IARC, 1980); so, separate analysis of them was not necessary, and the 'fatal' category was extended to include 'probably fatal', while the 'incidental' category was extended to include 'probably incidental'. For the few livers or oesophaguses that were autolysed, cannibalized or otherwise lost to histology, there is no record of the presence or absence of incidental tumours, but in some such cases observations by the animal-house technicians could be used to indicate whether or not the animal was likely to have died of a neoplasm at one of those sites. When such judgements were available they were accepted (and the lesions assumed to have been malignant, which would probably have been correct in most such instances).

Histology

All tumours from which sections were examined were classified simply as 'benign' or 'malignant'; and if an animal had more than one tumour at some site (or, for the liver, subsite: see below), only the most malignant one was utilized. Sub-categorization of the grade of malignancy was attempted, but in the view of the histologist (P.G.) this sub-categorization was not consistent or reliable, so no use has been made of it. The site of origin of the liver tumours has been further subdivided into 'liver cell', 'bile duct', 'mesenchymal' (i.e., blood vessels), 'Kupffer' and 'not known' (due to autolysis, cannibalism or loss of tissues). Analyses have been undertaken for the above four specific sites, and for 'any liver'.

Survival

Age-specific rates of death from the aggregate of all causes other than tumours of the liver and oesophagus were not significantly related to treatment. Consequently, most animals given the lowest eight dose levels survived well into old age (median, 31 months of treatment for males and 28 for females, i.e., approximately 33 and 30 months of age), while most of those given the top eight dose levels died of tumours.

Units of time

These are measured (generally in years) from the start of chronic treatment at age six weeks, not from birth.

Units of dosage

These are constant in the unusual units of ppm (v/v) in the water, but for uniformity with other reports they will be described in (approximate) mg/day per kg *adult* body weight, calculated on the approximation that adult males and females consumed about 41 and 72 mL/day per kg adult body weight, respectively. Although water and food were available *ad libitum,* water intake and body weight were not materially affected by treatment.

Statistical methods for determining affected sites

Unbiased correction for the effects of intercurrent mortality on expected tumour yields is advisable in many long-term carcinogenesis experiments, and is particularly important in the present one because (*a*) the dependence of longevity on treatment is unusually strong, and (*b*) the numbers are unusually large, so that for tumours other than of the liver or oesophagus even small residual biases in the statistical method might change what should be a non-significant result into a highly significant one, or *vice versa*. The statistical methods required for such data have recently become standardized (IARC, 1980). For each tumour type of interest, separate analyses are first performed of the Observed and Expected numbers of (*a*) fatal and (*b*) incidental such lesions. These two separate analyses are then combined to yield total Observed and Expected numbers of tumour-bearing animals.

Tests of statistical significance involve calculating T, a measure of the trend with respect to nitrosamine concentration of the (O-E) values for each treatment group; z, the number of its standard errors by which T exceeds zero; and lP, an estimate of the one-tailed P-value associated with z. (The methods of estimation used for lP allow for the possible skewness and kurtosis of z, and so should be somewhat more reliable than a standard normal approximation.)

Statistical methods for describing dose-response relationships: 'double Weibull' distributions

For one particular type of tumour, in the absence of other causes of death and other tumours, the probability of being Alive and Tumourless (AAT) after t years of treatment would, under a Weibull distribution (Peto & Lee, 1973), be given by

$$\log \text{AAT} = -0 \cdot 3 \ t^7 / \text{med}^7$$

where 'log' denotes the common – i.e., base 10 - logarithm, and 'med' is the group-specific Weibull median. Alternatively, if b, the Weibull constant of proportionality, is defined by the relationship

$$b = 0.69 / \text{med}^7,$$

then an equivalent way of writing the first equation above can be shown to be

$$\text{CI} = b.t^7,$$

where 'CI' denotes the Cumulative Incidence after t years of treatment. The need is therefore to describe how 'med' – or, equivalently, b – depends on treatment, i.e., on the daily dose-rate of nitrosamine (which will be written 'mg/kg ABWD' to denote 'estimated mg/kg ABWD'), and to be able to fit Weibull distributions unbiasedly to both the fatal and the incidental tumours in a group. This is done by the use of a dose-independent 'fatality factor' (see Fig.1). The physical meaning of various Weibull medians is illustrated in Figure 1B.

Advantages of using double Weibull distributions

The fact that only the Weibull median depends on treatment simplifies the complex problem of describing the ways in which differences in dose between one group and another affect the pattern of times at which animals die from or with the tumour type of interest – a problem that may be made still more complex by the prior deaths of some animals from other dose-related conditions. For, this can be reduced to the far simpler problem of describing how the dose in each group relates to the Weibull median in each group, perhaps by a simple plot of dose *versus* 'med'; once 'med' is known, the Weibull formula completely specifies the distribution of tumour times.

Although these Weibull formulae may at first sight appear to be somewhat removed from reality, they can thus provide a remarkably economical summary of a large mass of experimental data. Moreover, the summary that they provide is likely (Peto, 1977) to be more

Fig. 1 Statistical methods: double Weibull distributions

A. Example of a 'double Weibull' distribution, with log alive and tumourless (AAT = -0.3 (t/1.5)^7 and log alive (A) = -0.34 × 0.3(t/1.5)^7. N.B. The proportion of tumourless animals among the survivors at 21 months (see vertical line) is AAT/A, and in general the log of the proportion of the survivors that are tumourless is -0.66 × 0.3(t/1.5)^7, which is itself a Weibull distribution.

B. Example of the dose-response relationship predicted by Weibull distributions for a hypothetical 10-group experiment in animals with a three-year lifespan, where groups 1-5 (the high-dosed groups) have Weibull medians of med = 0.5, 1, 1.5, 2 and 2.5 years, while groups 6-10 (the low-dosed groups) have Weibull medians of med = 3, 3.5, 4, 4.5, and 5 years. In the high-dosed groups, treatment affects the mean time to disease onset much more than it affects the proportion of affected animals. In the low-dosed groups, however, the opposite is true, and treatment has a strong effect on the number of affected animals but no appreciable effect whatever on the mean (or median) time to tumour onset of those animals that actually develop tumours.

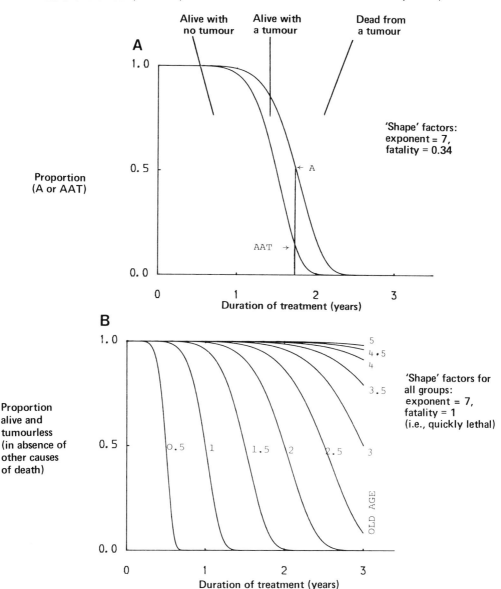

directly related to the rates at which the actual cellular processes of carcinogenesis operate than are conventional summary statistics such as 'percentage of tumour-bearing animals', 'mean (or median) latency of the observed tumours', etc.

RESULTS FOR TUMOURS AT SITES OTHER THAN THE LIVER OR OESOPHAGUS

Figure 2A describes mortality in NDEA-exposed males from the aggregate of all diseases except of the oesophagus or liver (and, of course, except for scheduled sacrifice, or sacrifice on suspicion of a palpable liver lump). As for females and for NDMA-treated males (data not shown), no clear treatment-related trend is evident. Likewise, no significant treatment-related trend is evident in mortality from the aggregate of all remaining tumours other than of the liver or oesophagus, or in the prevalence of these remaining tumours among animals that died of non-neoplastic causes (or of liver or oesophageal neoplasms). Neither body weight nor water intake was clearly related to treatment (Fig 2B, 2C, 2D).

Fig. 2 Survival, body weight and water intake
A. Mortality from diseases other than of liver or oesophagus, by NDEA dose: males. Based on Kaplan-Meier estimates of the percentages that would have remained alive at various times if deaths from scheduled sacrifice, oesophageal disease or liver disease (including sacrifice following palpation of an apparent liver abnormality) were prevented. Groups 2-5, 6-9, 10-13 and 14-16 have been pooled.

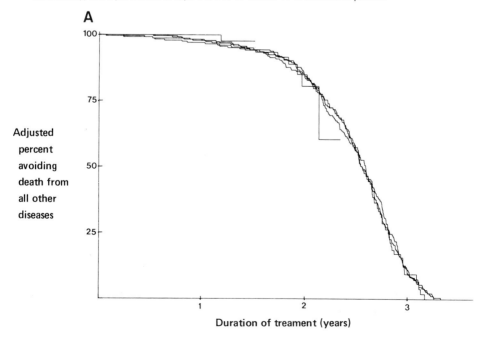

Fig. 2 B. Mean body weight per survivor, by treatment group and sex. Animals were weighed weekly, but data were key-punched only for weeks 9, 19, 29, etc. △, control (group 1); ▽, NDEA (2-5); ◇, NDEA (6-9); ⊠, NDEA (10-13); ⊗, NDEA (14-16); □, NDMA (2-5); ○ NDMA (6-9); ⊕, NDMA (10-13); ✳, NDMA (14-16)

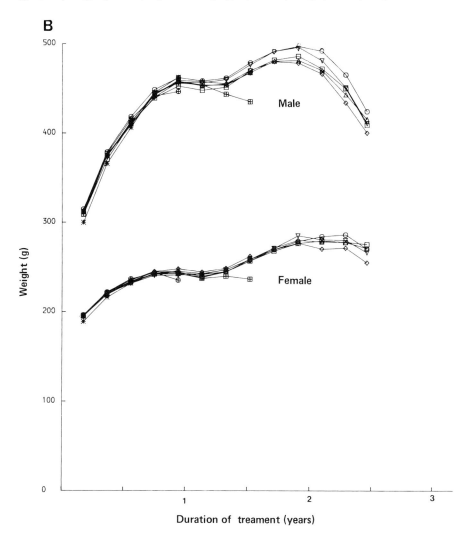

The individual sites for which the pooled z-value achieves a value of at least 2.0 (either for 'malignant neoplasms' or for 'any neoplasms') are listed in Table 2. The only site for which the trend is so overwhelmingly strong that it cannot reasonably be suggested that the apparent association might be a 'false positive' is the nasopharynx, which appears (like the oesophagus) to be clearly affected by NDEA but not by NDMA.

Fig. 2 C. Mean water intake in mL/survivor, by treatment group and sex. Intake per cage was estimated directly from weekly changes in bottle contents, as spillage and wastage by animals was thought to amount to no more than a few percent of total usage. △, control (group 1); ▽, NDEA (2-5); ◇, NDEA (6-9); ⊞, NDEA (10-13); ⊕, NDEA (14-16); □, NDMA (2-5); ○, NDMA (6-9); ✛, NDMA (10-13); ✳, NDMA (14-16)

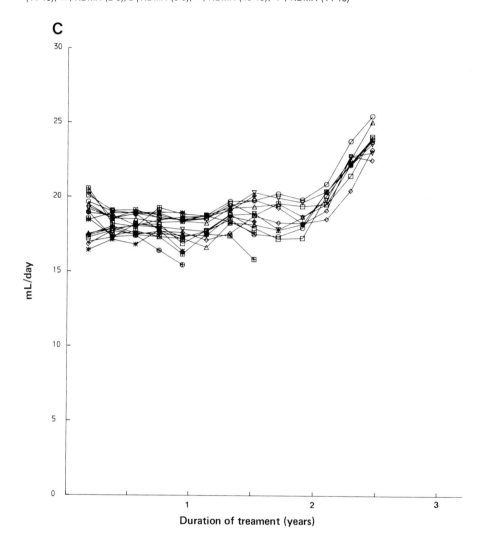

For some of the remaining sites the 'statistically significant trend' with respect to one type of nitrosamine that is noted in Table 2 appears (on comparison with the onset rates in the aggregate of all animals treated with the other type of nitrosamine, for which no trend was evident) to be due chiefly to a shortage of affected animals at the lower dose-levels rather than to an excess at the higher dose-levels.

The only two NDMA associations in Table 2 that have the characteristics one might expect of a real cause-and-effect relationship are those of NDMA with the seminal vessels and the lungs. Although the former has no obvious biological rationale, and so may be a somewhat extreme artefact of chance, the latter is more plausible: NDMA, if given by a route that reaches

Fig. 2 D. Mean water intake in mL/kg bodyweight per day, by treatment group and sex. △, control (group 1); ▽, NDEA (2-5); ◇, NDEA (6-9); ⊞, NDEA (10-13); ⊕, NDEA (14-16); □, NDMA (2-5); ○, NDMA (6-9); ⊕, NDMA (10-13); ✳, NDMA (14-16)

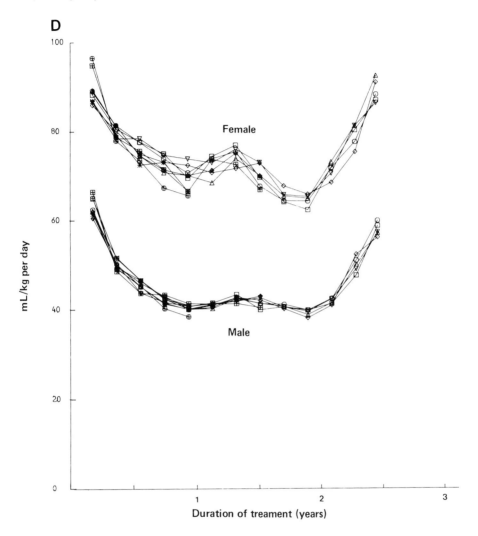

the lungs, has previously been shown to be a lung carcinogen, and in the present experiment at least some NDMA must reach the lungs simply by inhalation.

Thus, of the apparent effects listed in Table 2, only that of NDEA on the nasopharynx and, perhaps, that of NDMA on the lungs can be regarded as established by this experiment. However, although the remaining effects are not of themselves convincing, that does not prove that they are not real; and if these associations were independently supported by other such studies – or if a significant degree of alkylation by the appropriate nitrosamines were reported at some such site(s) – then judgement as to the most plausible interpretation of these findings might change. This would be particularly true for tumours of the lower jaw (and, perhaps, the stomach) in relation to NDEA, as the cell types involved are rather similar to those involved

Table 2.   Sites (other than liver or oesophagus) at which a suggestively[a] positive trend was observed

Site of neoplasm	Trend with NDEA[b]			Trend with NDMA[b]		
	No.[c]	z	1P	No.[c]	z	1P
Nasopharynx	8	4.62	<0.1%	1	−0.25	NS
Lower jaw, etc.	36	2.05	3.0%	47	−0.49	NS
Stomach	8	2.92	0.8%	12	0.65	NS
Lung, etc.	3	−0.32	NS	8	3.09	0.4%
Kidney	8	1.93	4.7%	15	0.08	NS
Skin, etc.	12	0.94	NS	13	2.60	1.1%
Bladder or ureter	11	1.42	NS	10	0.61	NS
Ovaries	8	2.28	3.8%	12	0.29	NS
Seminal vessels, etc.	3	2.21	4.0%	8	3.21	0.4%
Lymphatic/haematopoietic	82	0.71	NS	78	2.00	3.2%

[a] i.e., z ≥ 2.0 in the pool of the analyses of males and of females for any of (1) NDEA, malignant neoplasms, (2) NDEA, any neoplasms, (3) NDMA, malignant neoplasms, or (4) NDMA, any neoplasms
[b] The tabulated analyses are for any neoplasm (i.e., benign or malignant), and derive from the pool of the analyses of males and of females
[c] No. of affected animals in control group + groups treated with specified agent
NS = Not significant (1P > 0.05)

in the effects of NDEA on the oesophagus; moreover, this agent can undoubtedly cause stomach tumours in mice. Finally, NPIP, another nitrosamine that, like NDEA, strongly affects the oesophagus, definitely causes tumours of the lower jaw in Colworth rats (see below).

RESULTS FOR OESOPHAGEAL TUMOURS

Results will be presented first for the oesophagus and then for the liver. The oesophageal analyses are easier to present because:

(*a*) the spontaneous background rate of oesophageal tumours is so low – no controls developed oesophageal tumours, while 29 developed liver tumours – that the question of how to allow for the background does not arise;

(*b*) whereas the liver tumours represent four anatomically distinct categories of neoplasm – liver-cell, bile-duct, mesenchyme and Kupffer-cell – the dose-response relationships of which must be examined separately, no such subcategorization of the oesophageal neoplasms exists; and, finally,

(*c*) whereas NDMA and NDEA both affect the liver, only NDEA affects the oesophagus, so only one dose-response relationship – that for NDEA – need be examined for oesophageal tumours.

The Weibull medians for oesophageal tumours are plotted against the NDEA dose-rates (mg/kg ABWD) in Figure 3C. The plotted medians in Figure 3C define a reasonably straight line of slope, approximately −1/2.33.

Although there is, of course, some uncertainty as to the effects of dose-rates less than 0.01 mg/kg ABWD, since they are so small that they cannot be measured reliably, a reasonably simple characterization of the effects of treatments in the dose-range 0.02 to 1 mg/kg ABWD has been achieved, viz:

$$\text{females: } = \log_{10} \text{AAT} -4.8\ d^3\ t^7$$
$$\text{males: } = \log_{10} \text{AAT} -9.2\ d^3\ t^7,$$

where d denotes the dose-rate, in units of mg/kg ABWD, t denotes the duration, in years, of treatment, $\log_{10}$ denotes common logarithms, and AAT denotes the proportion that would be alive and tumourless in the absence of other tumours or other causes of death.

Fig. 3   Combined analyses. Combination of the analysis of benign oesophageal tumours (Fig. 3A) with that of malignancies (Fig. 3B) yields an overall analysis of all oesophageal neoplasms in NDEA-treated rats (Fig. 3C). Solid circles denote males, open ones females, and vertical lines represent approximate 95% confidence limits. Combination is by direct addition of the corresponding b-values, a procedure that can be shown always to produce a combined median that is less than 10% more extreme than the more extreme of the two medians that are being combined. Thus, for example, in the group of females that received over 1 mg/kg per day, the Weibull median for benign tumours was about 0.7 years (Fig. 3A: this corresponds to a b-value of about $0.69/0.7^7$, or 8.4), the Weibull median for malignant tumours was about 0.8 years (Fig. 3B: this corresponds to a Weibull median of about $0.69/0.8^7$, or 3.3), and addition of the two corresponding b-values yielded a total of about 11.7 (corresponding to a Weibull median of about $(0.69/11.7)^{1/7}$ years, i.e., about 0.66 years), as in Fig. 3C.
A. Benign oesophageal tumours (analysed with f = 0.065). The 'maximum likelihood' lines of preselected slope -3/7 (i.e., -1/2.33) cross the two-year mark at dosage levels that suggest 'TD$_{50}$' values for males and females of 0.072 and 0.086 mg/kg ABWD.

A

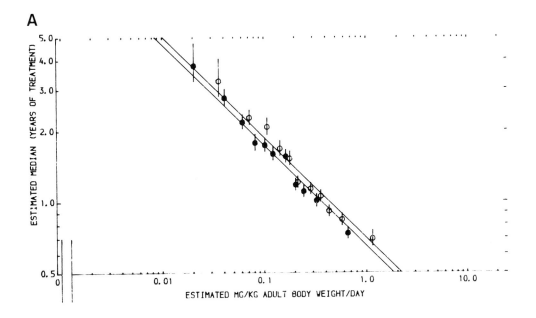

Fig. 3 B. Malignant oesophageal tumours (analysed with f = 0.46). The 'maximum likelihood' lines of preselected slope -3/7 (i.e., -1/2.33) cross the two-year mark at dosage levels that suggest 'TD$_{50}$' values for males and females of 0.093 and 0.127 mg/kg ABWD.
C. Combined analysis of benign and malignant oesophageal tumours, derived *via* addition of the b-values corresponding to the Weibull medians in Figs 3A and 3B. The 'maximum likelihood' lines of preselected slope -3/7 (i.e., -1/2.33) cross the two-year mark at dosage levels that suggest 'TD$_{50}$' values for males and females of 0.063 and 0. 079 mg/kg ABWD.

B

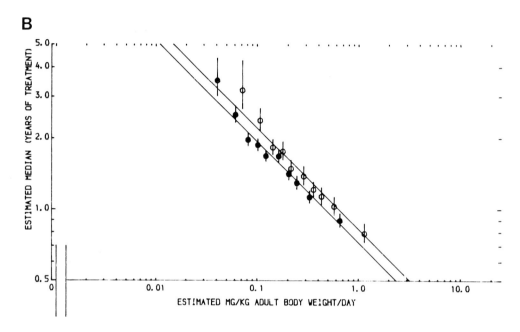

C

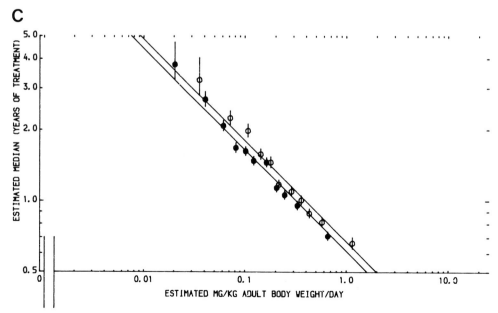

RESULTS FOR LIVER TUMOURS (Figs 4–11)

These are somewhat less simple to describe than were the results for oesophageal tumours, because there is an appreciable spontaneous liver tumour onset rate. This means that the data cannot be adequately described by any unmodified formula of the type

Weibull constant of proportionality, b,

is proportional to some power of dose.

It may, however, be possible to describe the b-values adequately by a modified formula, such as 'value among controls *plus* a term proportional to some power of dose' (Figs 6B and 9B) or 'some power of the sum of the effective background dose and the applied dose' (Figs 6A and 9A)

Fig. 4 Effects of NDEA on tumour induction in various different parts of the liver: (A) liver cell, (B) bile duct, (C) mesenchyme, and (D) Kupffer cell, with data for groups 2-5 pooled for statistical stability. Solid circles: males, open circles: females. Small circles denote groups of about 60 animals each, while large circles denote groups of 240 animals. Lines of slope -1/2.3 are plotted for comparison. For the three less common types of tumour (in Figs B, C and D), several groups have no such tumours, and so are not plotted. Hence, the plotted points are a biased sample, and a line through them will tend to over-estimate the effects of treatment. Despite this, it is noteworthy that in the range 0.02-1.0 mg/kg ABWD the four graphs have strikingly similar slopes. A. NDEA, liver-cell tumours, calculated with f = 0.63 (malignant) and 0.09 (benign). The 'maximum likelihood' lines of preselected slope -3/7 (i.e., -1/2.33) cross the two-year mark at dosage levels that suggest 'TD$_{50}$' values for males and females of 0.091 and 0.069 mg/kg ABWD.

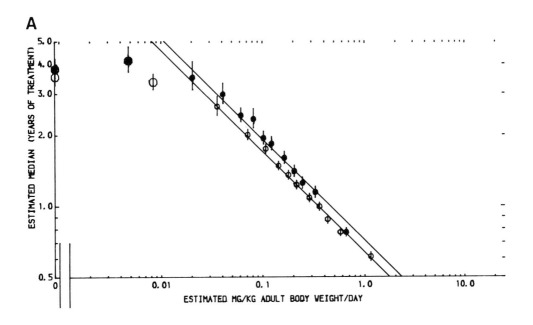

Fig. 4 B. NDEA, bile-duct tumours, calculated with f = 0·11 irrespective of malignancy. The 'maximum likelihood'
        lines of preselected slope -3/7 (i.e., -1/2.33) cross the two-year mark at dosage levels that suggest 'TD$_{50}$' values
        for males and females of 0.20 and 0.21 mg/kg ABWD.
        C. NDEA, mesenchymal tumours, calculated with f = 60, irrespective of malignancy. The 'maximum likelihood'
        lines of preselected slope -3/7 (i.e., -1/2.33) cross the two-year mark at dosage levels that suggest 'TD$_{50}$' values
        for males and females of 0.181 and 0.310 mg/kg ABWD.

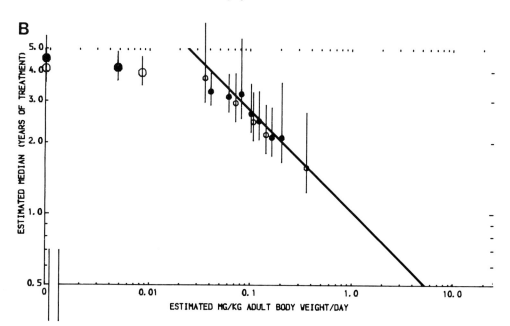

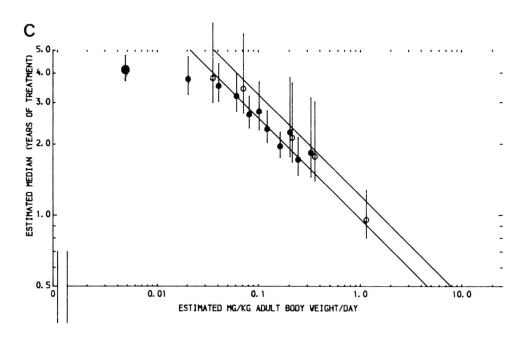

Fig. 4 D. NDEA, Kupffer-cell tumours, calculated with f = 0.65, irrespective of malignancy. The 'maximum likelihood' lines of preselected slope -3/7 (i.e., -1/2.33) cross the two-year mark at dosage levels that suggest 'TD$_{50}$' values for males and females of 0.29 and 0.46 mg/kg ABWD.

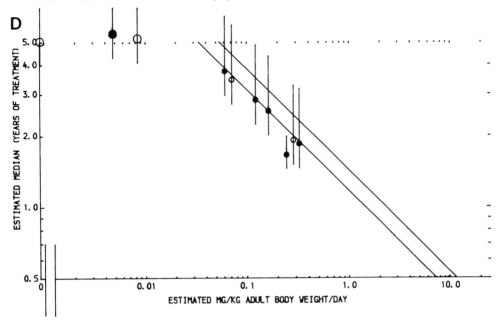

Fig. 5 Effects of NDEA on liver tumour induction (all sub-sites). A, direct plot; B as Fig. 5A but with bottom four dose groups merged for statistical stability.

A. NDEA, all liver tumours, calculated with f = 0.08 (benign) and 0.63 (malignant). The 'maximum likelihood' lines of preselected slope -3/7 (i.e., -1/2.33) cross the two-year mark at dosage levels that suggest 'TD$_{50}$' values for males and females of 0.084 and 0.067 mg/kg ABWD. (See, however, Fig. 6A for somewhat improved estimates of these 'TD$_{50}$' values).

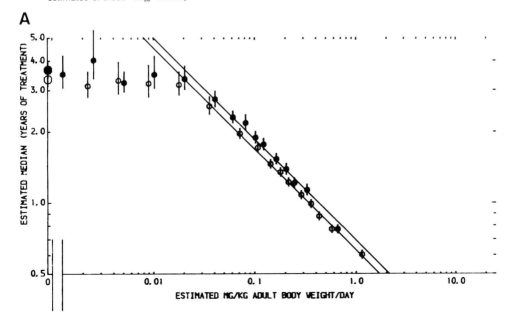

Fig. 5 B. As Fig. 5A but with the bottom four dose groups pooled for statistical stability. (Lines of slope -3/7 (-1/2.33),
as in Fig. 6A)

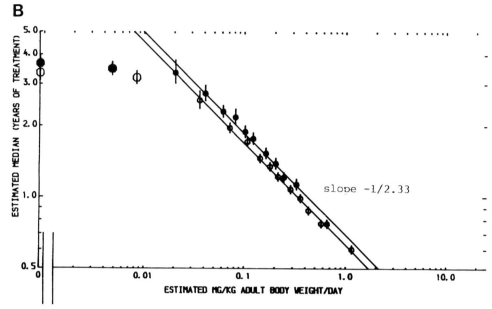

Fig. 6 Effects of NDEA on liver tumour incidence (all sub-sites from Fig. 5B), re-plotting (A) risks *versus* dose-rate
plus 0.04 mg/kg ABWD, and (B) excess risks *versus* dose-rate. (N.B. The excess risks in Fig. 6B were
estimated by subtraction of the control b-values from the b-values for the treated groups.)
A. NDEA, all liver tumours: risk *versus* dose-rate plus 0.04 mg/kg. The 'maximum likelihood' lines of
preselected slope -4/7 (i.e., -1/1.75) cross the two-year mark at dosage levels that suggest 'TD$_{50}$' values for
males and females of 0.090 and 0.074 mg/kg ABWD. Because the fit of the straight lines in this graph is better
than that in Fig. 5, these TD$_{50}$ values are likely to be more reliable than those suggested by the lines in
Fig. 5.

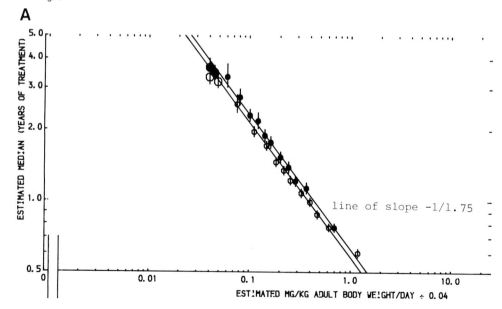

Fig. 6 B. NDEA, all liver tumours: excess risk *versus* dose-rate. The line that is plotted is an arbitrary one of slope
-3/7 (i.e., -1/2.33), plotted near to the points merely for visual comparison with the slope suggested by them.
It is not a line that has been formally fitted to the points.

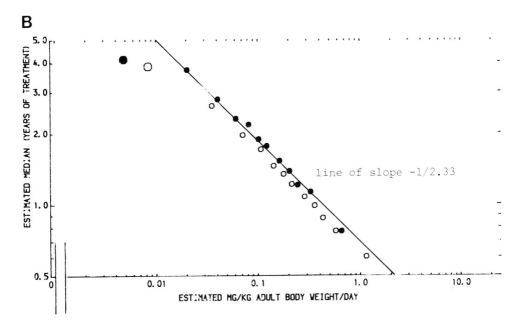

Comparison of hepatocellular dose-response curves for NDEA and NDMA (Figs 4A and 7A)

Except for the existence of a measurable background risk at zero dose, for NDEA the shape of the dose-response relationship for hepatocellular tumours (Fig. 4A) appears fairly similar to that for oesophageal tumours (Fig. 3C), albeit perhaps with some slight downward curvature. Still, throughout the dose-range above 0.02 mg/kg ABWD, both these graphs do have a fairly simple structure defining an approximately straight line of slope, approximately $-1/2.33$. When we examine the dose-response relationship for the effects of NDMA on hepatocellular tumorigenesis (Fig. 7A), however, this simplicity of shape is no longer seen. Instead of the straight line for NDEA in the dose-range above 0.02 mg/kg ABWD, a 'shoulder' is seen for NDMA, involving a shallower slope below than at above 0.1 mg/kg ABWD.

The Weibull medians that are plotted in Figures 4A and 7A provide a reasonably satisfactory visual format for describing the effects of high dose-rates (above 0.1 mg/kg ABWD), but they provide a much less satisfactory visual format for describing the effects of the lower doses. As already noted, however, there exists an alternative format that may be preferred for describing the dose-response relationship at low doses, *viz.* use of Weibull 'b-values' rather than Weibull medians. Logically the two are equivalent[1], but at low dose-levels the b-value is approximately proportional to the number of affected animals, while the median is not. Figure 10 is a plot of the first few of these b-values against dose using an ordinary, non-logarithmic scale to see whether the risks appear to be proportional to dose at low dose-rates.

---

[1] Given one, the other can readily be calculated from the relationship b = 0.69/median[7].

Examination of Figure 10, coupled with comparison of Figure 4A with Figure 7A, indicates that although at dose-rates of around 1 mg/kg ABWD NDEA and NDMA have similar effects, at dose-rates of around 0.1 mg/kg ABWD the effects of NDMA are substantially smaller than those of NDEA. Indeed, the effects of 0.1 mg/kg ABWD of NDMA appear to be similar to those of barely half as much NDEA. So, on a *molar* basis, in this central dose-range, NDMA (with a molecular weight of 74.1) appears to be only about a third as potent as NDEA (with a molecular weight of 102.1). In contrast, at higher doses (of about 1 mg/kg ABWD), the two substances appear to be approximately equipotent on a molar basis. Unfortunately, it is not possible to determine reliably how the ratio of their relative potencies varies at doses below 0.01 mg/kg ABWD, because of the statistical problems that are introduced by random errors when small numbers of extra tumours are to be counted in the presence of an appreciable background.Thus, the ratio of their molar potencies might increase, decrease or remain at about one-third at dose-rates progressively lower than 0.01 mg /kg ABWD.

Fig. 7   Effects of NDMA on tumour induction in various parts of the liver: (A) liver cell, (B) bile duct, (C) mesenchyme, (D) Kupffer cell, with data from groups 2-5 pooled for statistical stability. Solid circles: males, open circles: females. Small circles denote groups of 60 animals each, while large circles denote groups of 240 animals. Lines of slope -1/2.3 are plotted for comparison, but in no case (except perhaps Fig. 4D, where there are insufficient data to tell) do they appear to provide a good fit to the data at high doses.
A. NDMA, liver-cell tumours, calculated with f = 0.61 (malignant) and f = 0.07 (benign). Although 'maximum likelihood' lines of slope -3/7 (i.e., -1/2.33) are plotted, they fit the data so poorly that the TD_{50} values they suggest cannot be accepted: see Fig. 9A for a more satisfactory set of TD_{50} estimates.

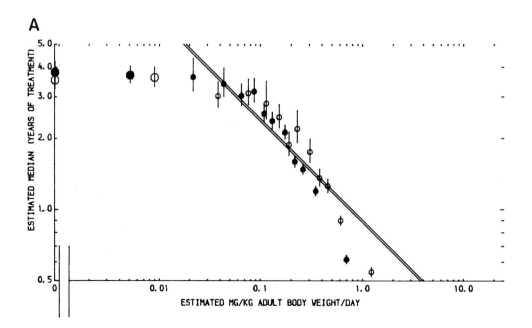

Fig. 7 B. NDMA, bile-duct tumours (nearly all of which were benign), calculated with f = 0.21, irrespective of malignancy. As with Fig. 7A, the fit of the 'maximum likelihood' lines of slope -3/7 to the data is not satisfactory.
C. NDMA, mesenchymal tumours (nearly all of which were malignant), calculated with f = 0.92, irrespective of malignancy. As with Fig. 7A, the fit of the 'maximum likelihood' lines of slope -3/7 to the data is not satisfactory.

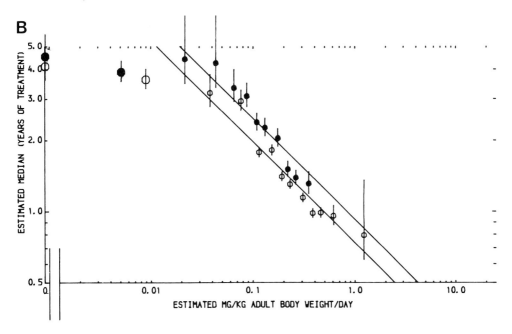

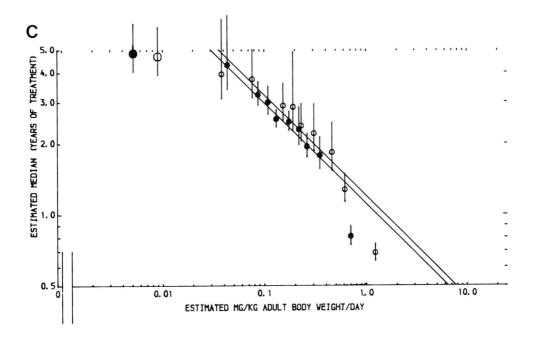

Fig. 7 D. NDMA, Kupfer-cell tumours (all of which were malignant), calculated with f = 0.87. The data are too
sparse to check on the quality of fit of the 'maximum likelihood' lines of slope -3/7. (The apparently poor fit
is not informative, and arises merely because groups in which no such tumours arose pull the lines upwards.)

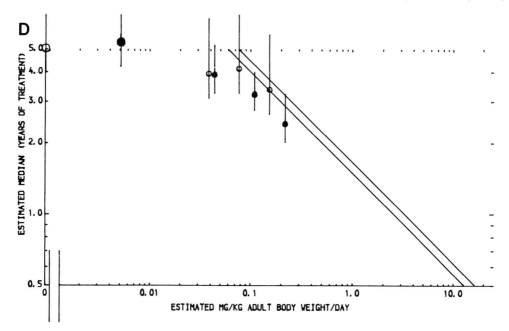

Fig. 8   Effects of NDMA on liver tumour induction (all subsites). A, direct plot; B as Fig. 8A but with bottom four dose
groups merged for statistical stability.
A. NDMA, all liver tumours, calculated with f = 0.16 (benign) and 0.71 (malignant). Although 'maximum
likelihood' lines of slope -3/7 (i.e., -1/2.33) are plotted, they fit the data so poorly that the TD_{50} values they
suggest cannot be accepted: See Fig. 9A for a more satisfactory set of TD_{50} estimates.

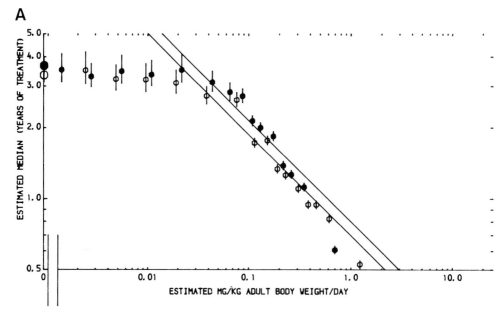

Fig. 8 B. As Fig. 8A but with the bottom four dose-groups merged for statistical stability. (The plotted lines of slope -3/7 cannot be trusted: see above.)

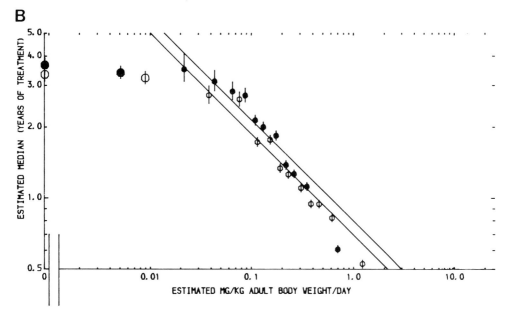

Fig. 9   Effects of NDMA on liver tumour incidence (all subsites, from Fig. 8B), re-plotting (A) risks *versus* dose-rate + 0.1 mg/kg ABWD, and (B) excess risks *versus* dose-rate (estimated by subtraction of the Weibull b-value for the corresponding control group from those for the treated groups).
A. NDMA, all liver tumours: risk *versus* dose-rate + 0.1 mg/kg. The 'maximum likelihood' lines of preselected slope -6/7 (i.e., -1/1.17) cross the two-year mark at dosage levels that suggest 'TD$_{50}$' values of 0.129 (male) and 0.117 (female) mg/kg ABWD. Because the fit of these lines to the data appears better than that of the lines in Figs 7 and 8, the TD$_{50}$ values that it suggests are likely to be more reliable than those suggested by the earlier figures.

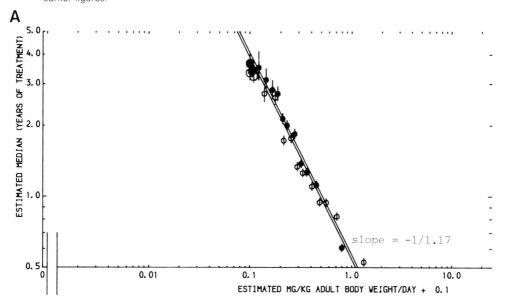

Fig. 9 B. NDMA, all liver tumours: excess risk *versus* dose-rate. The line that is plotted is an arbitrary one of slope -4/7 (i.e., -1/1.75), plotted near the points merely for visual comparison with the slope suggested by them. It is not a line that has been formally fitted to the points.

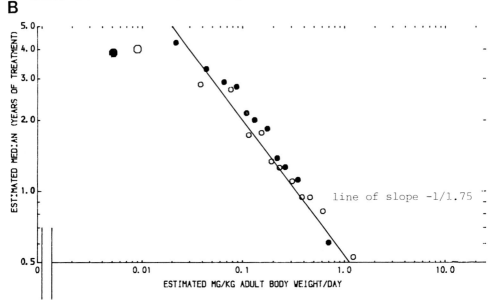

Fig. 10 Weibull b-values comparing the effects of low doses of NDEA and NDMA on hepatocellular tumorigenesis in (A) males and (B) females. (Note: For each sex, the lowest four non-zero dose-levels are pooled, for statistical stability.)

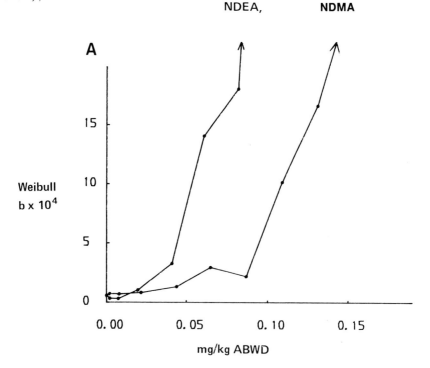

Fig. 10 (contd)

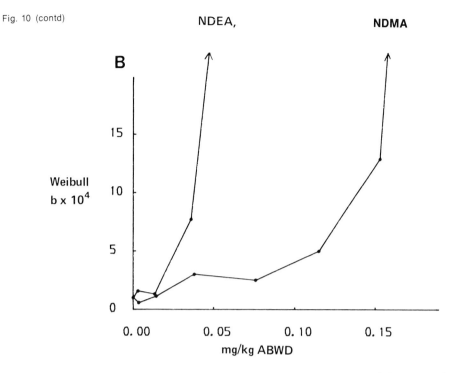

Fig. 11 Weibull b-values comparing the effects of NDEA and NDMA on the aggregate of all liver tumours in (A) males and (B) females

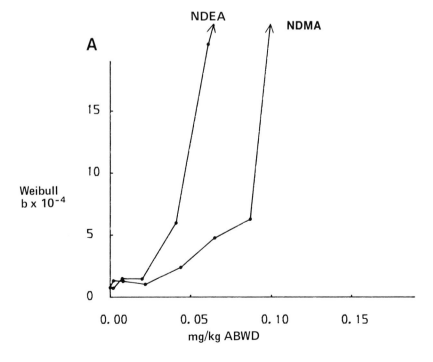

Fig. 11 (contd)

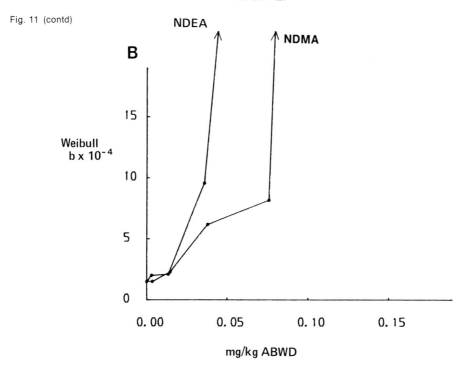

mg/kg ABWD

In summary, the molar ratio of the potencies of NDMA to NDEA for hepatocellular tumour induction is about unity at around 1 mg/kg ABWD, but decreases to about one-third at around 0.1 mg/kg ABWD. Why? There is no obvious reason why the ratio of the transport to the target cells of these two nitrosamines should vary in a dose-dependent way, nor why there should be dose-dependent variation in the ratio of the extent to which, once there, they alkylate the DNA. There are, however, some reasons why the degree of persistence of relevant DNA methylation and ethylation might differ importantly from one dose-level to another in a manner that is different for methylation and for ethylation. For, one of the nitrosamine-induced DNA lesions that is particularly suspected of being importantly involved in carcinogenesis is alkylation of the O^6 position on guanine. This DNA alkylation is potentially miscoding, since it can lead to misreading of guanine as adenine during DNA replication. Perhaps because of this, an unusually rapid system to repair it is available, consisting of a transalkylase that covalently transfers alkyl (ethyl or methyl) groups from O^6-alkylguanine onto its own active site. This corrects the DNA lesion but destroys one molecule of the repair enzyme in the process. This repair enzyme certainly acts more rapidly on methyl than on ethyl groups, which might account for the carcinogenicity of NDEA being greater than that of NDMA at moderate dose rates. In addition, the enzyme is known to be induced when DNA synthesis begins; but although it is possible that other circumstances can also induce it, there is as yet no clear evidence as to exactly what those 'other circumstances' may be, nor whether they would be produced more readily by methylating than by ethylating agents.

Comparison of the effects of NDEA and NDMA on the remaining types of liver tumour (mesenchyme, Kupffer cells and bile ducts)

Among the 1 800 NDMA-treated animals, 94 developed a liver tumour that was classified histologically as 'mesenchymal', 11 developed tumours in the Kupffer cells, and 427 in the bile ducts, while among the 1 800 NDEA-treated animals the corresponding numbers were 42, 12 and 33, respectively. Superficially, this comparison suggests that NDMA has a greater carcinogenic effect on the non-parenchymal tissues than NDEA does. But, crude comparisons such as this cannot be trusted, for they do not take into account the fact that, except at the highest dose-level, the various NDMA-treated groups tended to live somewhat longer than did the corresponding NDEA-treated groups. (This was partly because the NDMA-treated animals had no oesophageal tumour, and partly because, except for the highest dose-level, a given concentration of NDMA tended to have less effect than did a similar concentration of NDEA on hepatocellular tumours.) When the longer survival is allowed for, the results are approximately as follows.

For any particular NDMA (MW 74.1) dose-rate of around 0.1-0.5mg/kg ABWD, the dose-rate of NDEA (MW 102.1) required to produce the same age-specific onset rate of bile-duct tumours would be approximately equimolar; that required to produce the same age-specific onset rate of mesenchymal (and, perhaps, Kupffer-cell) tumours would be about 0.7 of the NDMA molarity; and that required to produce the same age-specific onset rate of hepatocellular tumours would be about 0.3 of the NDMA molarity. Due to random fluctuations, the ratios for lower doses are not known reliably, and, in view of the odd findings in the highest dose group (at about 1 mg/kg ABWD), neither are the ratios for higher doses.

DISCUSSION OF EFFECTS OF NDMA AND NDEA

This experiment has included the range of moderately high doses studied by Druckrey (1967), and in that range the dose-response relationship (dose-rate $\times$ median$^{2.3}$ $\simeq$ constant) that he reported has been nicely confirmed, at least for NDEA. But, among animals given any one particular dose-level, the extraordinarily sharp dependence of tumour onset times on duration of exposure that Druckrey described in that dose-range has been replaced in the present study by a more ordinary 'Weibull' distribution, in which at a given dose-level the disease onset rate is proportional to only about the seventh power of the duration of exposure.

The present experiment has also included a range of moderately low dose-rates, lower than those studied by Druckrey. In this lower range, some significant carcinogenic effects have been picked up, but for liver tumours these are not what would have been predicted by simple extrapolation downwards of the dose-response relationships that are found at higher doses both in Druckrey's and in the present experiment.

The overall relationships observed in the present experiment were approximately:

Site	Sex	Agent	Cumulative incidence[a]
Oesophagus	F	NDEA	11.16 d^3 t^7
Oesophagus	M	NDEA	21.17 d^3 t^7
Liver (all sites)	F	NDEA	32.09 $(d + 0.04)^4$ t^7
Liver (all sites)	M	NDEA	18.70 $(d + 0.04)^4$ t^7
Liver (all sites)	F	NDMA	51.45 $(d + 0.1)^6$ t^7
Liver (all sites)	M	NDMA	37.43 $(d + 0.1)^6$ t^7

[a] Approximate cumulative incidence observed after administration of d mg/kg ABWD for t years (N.B. It can be shown that -$\log_e$ AAT is equal to the cumulative incidence.)

For oesophageal tumours, the background is unmeasurably low (probably less than 1 in 1 000, since no oesophageal tumour developed among the 480 controls, the 480 animals given NDEA at dose-levels 2–5, or the 1 800 NDMA-treated animals). Consequently, although low-dose linearity is certainly consistent with the oesophageal dose-response relationship (Fig. 3), there is no strong evidence for it, and no useful estimate of its likely magnitude is available.

For liver tumours, however, the background rate is appreciable, with 6% of the controls affected (or 8% if the animals undergoing scheduled sacrifice after only 12 or 18 months are excluded). The existence of this background makes low-dose linearity more probable, at least in the range of doses that produce extra effects that do not greatly exceed this background. For NDEA, the data shown in Figures 10 and 11 provide a non-significant suggestion of low-dose linearity, and for NDMA they provide clear evidence of approximate linearity in the dose-range below 0.1 mg/kg ABWD. Moreover, a significant increase in the incidence of liver lesions is produced by a dose of only 0.3 ppm v/v (note the change of units; 0.3 ppm is approximately 0.02 mg/kg per day). Even among the four lowest dose-levels (of zero, 0.033, 0.066 and 0.132 ppm v/v), a positive trend in the proportions of animals with liver cancer is apparent that just attains statistical significance (1P = 1.7%: see Table 3). This provides for the first time direct evidence of the carcinogenicity for the rat liver of a dose of only about 0.1 ppm (less than 0.01 mg/kg per day) of these agents.

Table 3.   Pooled trend in four lowest dose groups. This table gives an analysis, stratified for sex, of the numbers of liver-tumour bearing animals, pooling the NDEA-treated and the NDMA-treated animals at each dose level. It is obtained by combining a death-rate analysis of the fatal liver tumours and a prevalence analysis of the incidental liver tumours. (N.B. At these four dose levels no animal was found to have any hyperplastic or neoplastic lesion of the oesophagus, and no liver neoplasm was found at the scheduled sacrifices at 12 or at 18 months.)

Treatment group	Nitrosamine concentration (NDEA/NDMA)	Initial group size	No. not scheduled for sacrifice	Numbers with any liver neoplasm		
				Observed (O)	Expected (E)	Ratio, O/E
1	0 ppm	480	384	29	35.9	0.81
2	0.033 ppm [a]	240	192	19	19.6	0.97
3	0.066 ppm [a]	240	192	19	18.1	1.05
4	0.132 ppm [a]	240	192	23	16.4	1.40
Total (all doses)		1200	960	90	90	1.00

[a] A concentration of 0.132 ppm corresponds to an approximate dose-rate (in mg/kg ABWD) of 0.007 (0.005 for NDEA-treated males, 0.009 for NDEA-treated females, 0.005 for NDMA-treated males and 0.010 for NDMA-treated females).

Summary: The best estimate of the likely carcinogenic effects on Colworth rats of very low doses of NDMA and NDEA is that (1) their effects on the liver will exceed their effects on all other sites, and that (2) in the absence of other causes of death, in a two-year experiment starting at six weeks of age, their effects per μg/kg ABWD would probably be to produce, respectively, liver tumour risks of about 0.03–0.04% (NDMA) and about 0.06–0.1% (NDEA). In the presence of other causes of death, lifelong exposure from week 6 onwards (not truncated after two years of treatment) would probably yield risks about seven times as large as these.

Public health implications of low-dose extrapolations

What is really wanted, of course, is not the lifelong risk per μg/kg per day for Colworth rats, but rather the corresponding lifelong risk for humans in a heterogeneous, wild population. This cannot, however, be inferred directly from the present experiment. For rats, lifelong risks of about 0.4% per µg/kg per day have been demonstrated; but, although the lifelong human risks might happen to be similar to this, they might easily be a few orders of magnitude[1] different from it in either direction. The reasons for this uncertainty, and possible approaches to the control of cancer in the light of it, are discussed by Doll and Peto (1981), sections 4.2 *et seq.*

RESULTS: THE EFFECT OF THE CHOICE OF NITROSAMINE, THE SPECIES STUDIED AND THE AGE OF STARTING EXPOSURE

Various smaller, parallel studies took place concurrently with the major study, and involved a total of 1 040 extra animals (Table 1). The aims of these parallel studies were:

(1) To compare the separate effects on the oesophagus and on the liver of starting treatment of rats with NDEA at six weeks (as described above) with the effects of starting at three weeks or at 20 weeks of age.

(2) To compare the effects on rats of treatment with NDEA and NDMA (as described above) with the effects of treatment with NPIP and NPYR instead. These agents are found in many foodstuffs, and in tobacco smoke (IARC, 1978), and were already known (IARC, 1978) to induce tumours of the liver (both agents), oesophagus (NPIP only) and respiratory system (NPIP only), although detailed dose-response data were not available.

(3) To compare the effects of NDEA treatment of rats (as described above) with those of NDEA treatment of mice and hamsters. NDEA was already known to induce a variety of neoplasms in mice (liver, oesophagus, forestomach and lung: IARC, 1978) and in Syrian hamsters (liver and respiratory tract, especially trachea: IARC, 1978).

Effects of NPYR and NPIP on Colworth rats

NPYR has clear effects only on the liver, and on no other site. Although its effects on the nasopharynx, and on nervous and lymphatic tissues, are moderately significant, some moderately significant effects must be expected to arise in data as extensive as these purely by the play of chance; the observation of such effects should therefore be regarded merely as a data-generated hypothesis, to be borne in mind when viewing any related material (although the clear effects of NDEA and NPIP on nasopharyngeal tumours make it plausible that the moderately significant effect on this site seen with NPYR may be real). Moreover, even in the liver, its effects appear to be limited to the parenchymal cells and the bile ducts, for, no apparent effect whatever is seen on the blood vessels or Kupffer cells.

The median times to liver tumour development in the absence of other causes of death are given in Figure 12. Despite the small size of the groups, a reasonable characterization of the dose-response relationship appears to have been achieved, in which dose-rates of about 0.4 mg/kg ABWD (females) or 0.6 mg/kg ABWD (males) would be needed to halve the proportion of liver-tumour-free survivors after two years of treatment, suggesting that 0.5 mg/kg ABWD is a reasonable estimate of the TD_{50} (i.e., that daily dose-rate required to halve the proportion of tumourless survivors after two years of treatment). This figure is nearly an order of magnitude larger than that estimated for NDEA.

---

[1] This is because in order for humans to avoid cancer throughout their large bodies throughout their long lifespan means that they require controls on the processes of carcinogenesis that are millions of times stricter than those required by small, short-lived rodents. This figure derives chiefly from consideration of our lifespan, which is about 30 times that of rats. Since cancer onset rates rise as at least the fourth or fifth power of duration of exposure, we need protection by a factor of $30^{4 \text{ or } 5}$ throughout our large bodies: for discussion, see Doll and Peto (1981), section 4.2.

Fig. 12 Rats: effect of NPYR concentration on estimated median time from start of treatment to development of any tumour of liver of bile ducts, calculated with f = 0.04 (benign) and 0.34 (malignant); ●, males; ○ females

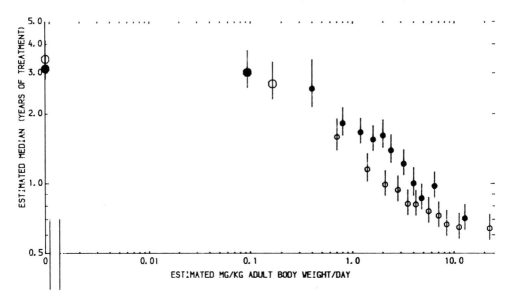

Fig. 13 Rats: effect of NPIP concentration on estimated median time from start of treatment to development of any tumour of liver or bile ducts, calculated with f = 0.07 (benign) and 0.48 (malignant); ●, males ○, females

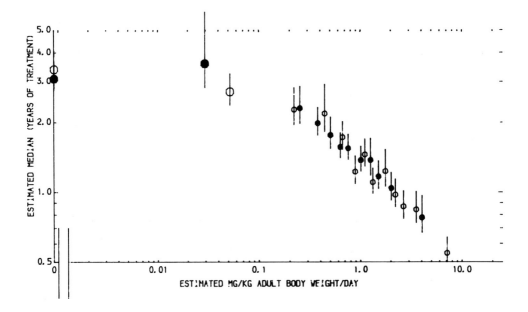

Fig. 14 Rats: effect of NPIP concentration on estimated median time from start of treatment to development of any tumour of the oesophagus, calculated with f = 0.01 (benign) and 0.54 (malignant); ●, males; ○, females

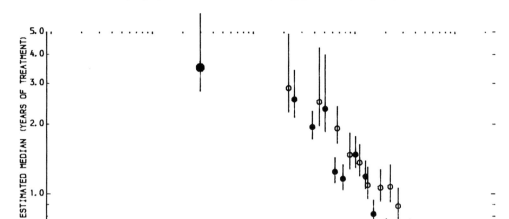

By contrast, NPIP has highly significant effects on all parts of the liver, on the oesophagus and on the lower jaw (P < 0.001). The cell types affected in the lower jaw are, moreover, similar to those affected in the oesophagus, so the former association is undoubtedly real. These clear effects of NPIP on the incidence of tumours of the lower jaw reinforce the moderately significant effect of NDEA on the incidence of tumours of the lower jaw (see above); it appears that the spectrum of sites affected by the two agents is very similar, both affecting the liver, oesophagus, lower jaw and nasopharynx.

The median times to liver tumour development are plotted against dose in Figure 13, and the median times to oesophageal tumour development are presented in Figure 14. Despite some irregularities in Figure 14 due to small numbers, a reasonable characterization of both relationships appears to have been achieved. As with NPYR, doses of about 0.4 (females) and 0.6 (males) mg NPIP/kg ABWD would halve the proportion of liver-tumour-free survivors among animals of each sex, and would also produce a small risk of oesophageal cancer. Consequently, the TD_{50} is again about 0.5 mg/kg, for, although at higher dose-levels NPIP is a more potent liver carcinogen than NPYR, at these low-dose levels their effects on the liver appear to be rather similar.

Extrapolation to very low dose-levels of NPYR and NPIP

For reasons that are discussed by Peto (1978), the existence of a measurable background of liver tumour incidence means that at low doses the dose-response relationship for liver tumours is likely to become one of simple proportionality between excess risk and applied dose. Analogy with the effects of NDMA and NDEA that have been observed in the main experiment suggests that this will happen at doses just below the TD_{50}, and there is some indication in Figure 13 that this is indeed the case. Perhaps the best estimate of the low-dose effects of these agents, therefore, is that obtained by assuming that the ratios of their potencies, as assessed by the TD_{50}, to that of NDEA will be similar to the ratio of their low-dose potencies to that of NDEA. As already noted, the TD_{50}s for NPIP and NPYR were similar (0.4 and 0.6 mg/kg ABWD for females and for males, respectively), and were five or six times as large as those estimated for NDEA (0.074 and 0.090, respectively). The low-dose data for NDEA indicated that low dose-rates would produce extra risks of the order of 0.08% per µg/kg ABWD after two years of treatment, or 0.6% after lifelong treatment. Consequently, both for NPYR and for NPIP, the extra cancer risk per µg/kg ABWD in a standard two-year experiment on males and females starting from six weeks of age would presumably be of the order of 0.014%, in the absence of other causes of death. As discussed in the main experiment, however (see above), for the risks from *lifelong* exposure (during which some animals die of unrelated causes before completing two years of treatment, while others undergo treatment for substantially longer before they die), the absolute risks per µg/kg ABWD might be about seven times as big as two-year risks, *viz.* about 0.1%. Finally, it must always be emphasized that these are the estimated risks for rats, and that the risks for humans *may* well be some orders of magnitude different.

COMPARISON OF EFFECTS OF NDEA IN MAIN EXPERIMENT ON RATS WITH ITS EFFECTS ON FEMALE MICE AND HAMSTERS

Anatomic sites affected in mice and hamsters

For mice, the only sites clearly affected are the liver, oesophagus (Fig. 15) and stomach (Fig.16). The effect on the lung (Fig.17) is only moderately significant ($1P = 1.3\%$), but since similar effects have been reported by others (IARC, 1978), it can be accepted as real.

For hamsters, clear effects were seen on the liver and trachea (Fig. 18), but not on any other site. Particularly, no clear effect was seen on the nasopharynx, lower jaw, oesophagus or stomach, and, although when all of them were taken together a slight positive trend (based on eight tumours) existed, it was not statistically significant ($1P > 0.05$).

Effects of NDEA on the livers of mice

In contrast with the effects of NDEA in the livers of rats, there is clear evidence of an effect in the livers of mice only on the incidences of hepatocellular tumours and of Kupffer-cell tumours, the latter being much more numerous than in NDEA-treated rats. This finding is in marked contrast to the results reported in the literature reviewed by the IARC (1978), in which, apart from hepatocellular tumours, the chief type of liver tumour arising in mice appeared to be a haemangioendotheliomas, with no mention of any Kupffer-cell tumour.The overall results for the incidence of tumours of any part of the mouse liver are given in Figure 19, but due to the small group sizes and the numbers of animals dying of other tumours even this overall graph is rather irregular.

Effects of NDEA on the livers of hamsters

By contrast with the finding in mice, in hamsters NDEA appears to affect all parts of the liver *except* for the Kupffer cells. The data for hepatocellular tumours are illustrated in Figure 20, and the dose-response relationship is, in view of the smallness of the number of animals involved, reasonably similar to most other such relationships. For bile-duct tumours, however,

Fig. 15 Female mice: effect of NDEA concentration on estimated median time from start of treatment to development of any tumour of the oesophagus, calculated with f = 0.12 (benign) and 0.45 (malignant)

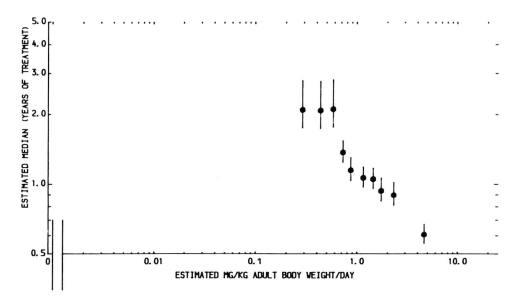

Fig. 16 Female mice: effect of NDEA concentration on estimated median time from start of treatment to development of any tumour of the stomach, calculated with f = 0.04, irrespective of malignancy

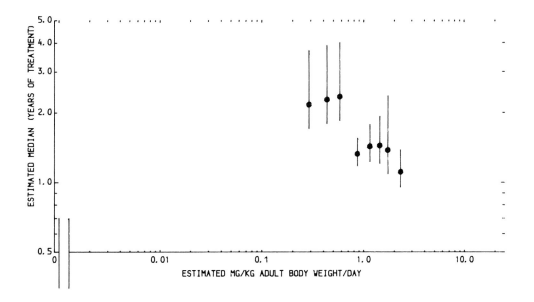

Fig. 17 Female mice: effect of NDEA concentration on estimated median time from start of treatment to development of any tumour of the bronchus (all of which were benign), calculated with f = 0.001

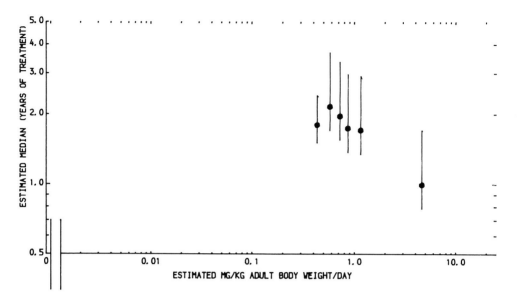

Fig. 18 Female hamsters: effect of NDEA concentration on estimated median time from start of treatment to development of any tumour of the trachea (nearly all of which were benign), calculated with f = 0.78, irrespective of malignancy

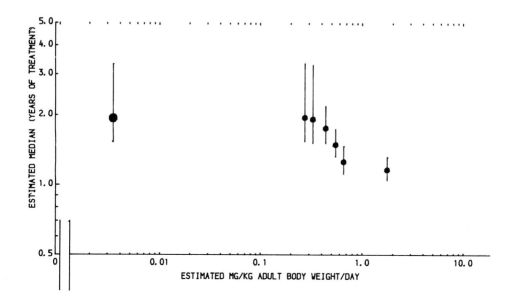

Fig. 19 Female mice: effect of NDEA concentration on estimated median time from start of treatment to development of any tumour of the liver, calculated with f = 0.02 (benign) and 0.48 (malignant)

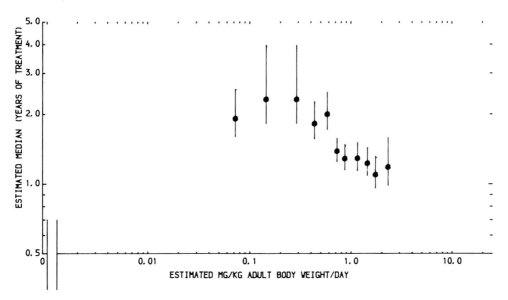

Fig. 20 Female hamsters: effect of NDEA concentration on estimated median time from start of treatment to development of any hepatocellular tumour (all of which were malignant), calculated with f = 0.10

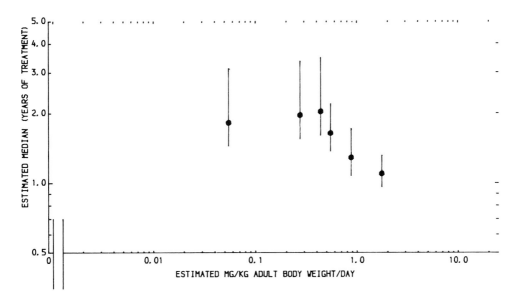

Fig. 21 Female hamsters: effect of NDEA concentration on estimated median time from start of treatment to development of any tumour of the bile ducts (all of which were benign), calculated with f = 0.15

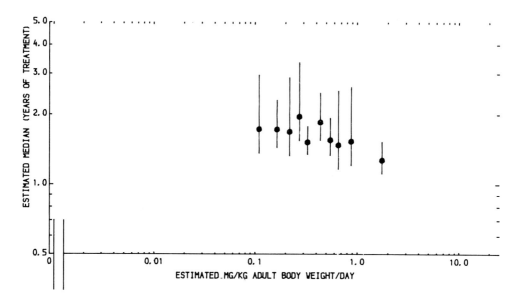

the pattern (Fig. 21) is quite different, and it appears that the onset rate is merely proportional to the first power of dose. It is not clear why hamsters should differ so markedly from mice and rats in this respect, but the reasons may be related to the far higher prevalence of bile-duct hyperplasia that is seen in these animals than in mice.

Effects of NDEA on the aggregate of all dose-related sites in mice and hamsters

For mice, the dose-response relationship suggests that a TD_{50} of about 0.3 mg NDEA/kg ABWD must be administered chronically for two years in order to halve the probability of tumour-free survival in the absence of other causes of death. By contrast, in hamsters, so few animals lived to the end of two years of treatment that no reliable estimate of the TD_{50} can be obtained, although comparison of the effects of the higher doses of NDEA in mice and hamsters suggests that the potency of this agent is similar for both.

For comparison, it may be noted that the TD_{50}s for NPYR and NPIP in rats were about 0.5 mg/kg ABWD – in other words, rather similar to the value of 0.3 mg NDEA/kg in mice – but that the TD_{50}s for NDEA and NDMA in rats were smaller (0.07 and 0.12 mg/kg, respectively), indicating greater potency. Part of the reason why the TD_{50}s were somewhat higher (indicating less carcinogenic effect) in mice and hamsters than in rats may have been because rats began treatment at six weeks of age (as against 12 weeks for mice and 20 for hamsters). When treatment of rats began instead at 20 weeks of age (see below), the yield of tumours after a given duration of treatment was lower.

ASSESSMENT OF EFFECTS OF AGE ON RESPONSE OF RATS TO NDEA

In parallel with the main experiment in which 1 800 rats were treated with various fixed concentrations of NDEA from the age of six weeks, experiments have been done with the same set of concentrations of NDEA (Table 1) in which treatment began at three weeks of age (180

Table 4. Effect on subsequent incidence[a] of neoplasms of the liver and oesophagus in rats when lifelong exposure to a given concentration of NDEA commences at 3, 6 or 20 weeks of age

Site	Age at first exposure (weeks)	No. of rats	Fatal lesions			Lesions found at autopsy in animals dying from unrelated causes			Combined fatal and 'incidental' analyses		
			Observed	Expected	O/E	Observed	Expected	O/E	Observed	Expected	O/E
LIVER (any subsite)	3	180	85	22.32	3.81	20	14.36	1.37	105	36.68	2.86
	6	1440	581	574.26	1.01	133	138.87	0.96	714	713.14	1.00
	20	180	53	122.42	0.43	23	22.76	1.01	76	145.18	0.52
1P-value[b]				c			9%			c	
OESOPHAGUS	3	180	18	16.17	1.11	59	46.37	1.27	77	62.55	1.23
	6	1440	250	243.05	1.03	413	423.87	0.97	663	666.92	0.99
	20	180	39	47.78	0.82	49	50.76	0.97	88	98.53	0.89
1P-value				7.4%			0.2%			0.3%	

[a] N.B. 'Incidence' refers to the incidence after a given *duration of treatment*, and not to the incidence at a given *age*.
[b] One-tailed P-value for trend of increasing subsequent incidence with earlier age at first exposure
[c] 1P < 0.0005

rats) and at 20 weeks of age (180 rats). For reasons that are reviewed by Peto *et al.* (1975), the aim is to see whether, after a fixed duration of treatment, the cumulative incidence among older animals exceeds that among younger animals. The results of standard (IARC, 1980) tests of statistical significance to see whether this was in fact the case are given in Table 4. It is clear that both for oesophageal tumours and especially for liver tumours exactly the opposite is the case: older animals are actually *less* subject to the processes of tumorigenesis than young animals are. Since water intake (in mL/kg per day) in young animals is 50% higher than in adult animals (Fig. 2), the daily dose-rate (in mg/kg per day) at each particular concentration of NDEA is likewise higher in young than in old animals; this could produce a slight difference in the mean dose in mg/kg per day between one group and another during the first few months of treatment. The difference, however, would cease to be appreciable after about six months of treatment, and prior to that it would probably involve less than a 10% difference between the groups that started at three and at six weeks of age, and about a 30% difference between the groups that started at six and at 20 weeks of age. Even though these differences operate only for the first few months of treatment, they could well provide a sufficient explanation for most or all of the moderate difference that is observed between the oesophageal tumour onset rates among animals starting treatment at three, six and 20 weeks of age. So, for oesophageal tumorigenesis it appears that age *per se* is of little relevance, and that all that matters is duration of chronic treatment.

The difference in liver tumour onset rates, however, is nearly six fold (Table 4), which is considerably more extreme than the moderate difference seen in the same table in oesophageal tumour onset rates. This six-fold difference cannot plausibly be ascribed to the slight differences in water intake/kg that existed during the first few months of treatment, and it must therefore point to a greater susceptibility of the liver in early life. These age-related effects on the susceptibility of the liver of the young rat to the effects of NDEA are remarkably large, especially when the groups starting treatment at three and six weeks are compared (Table 4).

For the rat liver, at least, the degree of nitrosamine exposure during the first weeks of life is an extremely important determinant of the response to nitrosamines in middle and old age, and there is no evidence whatever of any greater susceptibility of old animals – quite the reverse, in fact. So, no intrinsic effect of ageing can plausibly be invoked to help account for the extraordinarily high (seventh power) dependence of tumour onset rates on the duration of exposure found in the main experiment. There are mathematical ways of 'explaining' such seventh-power time relationships, by the use of suitable multistage models, but as yet they have only limited biological content (Peto, 1977) and so are not very satisfactory. Although the present results do not tell us what the underlying biological processes are that are involved in the rate-determining steps of carcinogenesis, they may assist in the search for them, either by emphasizing the importance of the first few weeks of life to nitrosamine carcinogenesis in the rat, or by emphasizing how large the number of rate-determining steps is that still awaits discovery.

ACKNOWLEDGEMENTS

This study was commissioned by the Ministry of Agriculture, Fisheries and Food (MAFF) in consultation with the Department of Health and Social Security (DHSS), and was executed at the British Industrial Biological Research Association (BIBRA) and analysed at Oxford by courtesy of the Oxford Computing Service, using programmes of Dr S. Richards. Dr R.F. Crampton, then director of BIBRA, originally devised the study, and Drs D. Conning, B. MacGibbon and W. Wintersgill have persistently encouraged its completion. The manuscripts were prepared by Jini Hetherington and Gale Mead.

REFERENCES

Doll, R. & Peto, R. (1981) The causes of cancer: quantitative estimates of avoidable risks of cancer in the United States today. *J. natl Cancer Inst.*, **66**, 1191–1308

Druckrey, H. (1967) *Quantitative aspects in chemical carcinogenesis.* In: *Potential Carcinogenic Hazards from Drugs (UICC Monograph Series, 7)*, Berlin, Springer-Verlag, pp. 60–78

IARC (1978) *IARC Monographs on the Evaluation of the Carcinogenic Risk of Chemicals to Humans*, Vol. 17, *Some N-Nitroso Compounds*, Lyon

IARC (1980) *IARC Monographs on the Evaluation of the Carcinogenic Risks of Chemicals to Humans*, Suppl. 2, *Long-term and Short-term Screening Assays for Carcinogens: A Critical Appraisal*, Lyon

Peto, R. (1977) *Epidemiology, multistage models and short-term mutagenicity tests.* In: Hiatt, H.H., Watson, J.D. & Winsten, J.A., eds, *Origins of Human Cancer*, Cold Spring Harbor, NY, Cold Spring Harbor Laboratory, pp.1403–1428

Peto, R. (1978) Carcinogenic effects of chronic exposure to very low levels of toxic substances. *Environ. Health Perspect.*, **22**, 155–159

Peto, R. & Lee, P.N.(1973) Weibull distributions for continuous carcinogenesis experiments. *Biometrics*, **29**, 457–470

Peto, R., Roe, F.J.C., Lee, P.N., Levy, L. & Clack, J. (1975) Cancer and ageing in mice and men. *Br. J. Cancer*, **32**, 411–425

ANIMAL FEEDING STUDY WITH NITRITE-TREATED MEAT

P. OLSEN, J. GRY, I. KNUDSEN, O. MEYER & E. POULSEN

Institute of Toxicology, National Food Institute, Søborg, Denmark

SUMMARY

In order to detect possible formation of carcinogenic N-nitroso compounds from nitrite and nitrosatable compounds in meat, studies were carried out with 70 male and 140 female F_0 rats, divided into six groups, and 60, 100, 70, 60, 60 and 66 of their male and female offspring. One control group received casein and other groups chopped pork as the sole protein source (45%, mass/mass) on a fresh basis, either salted (sodium chloride) or not. For test groups, nitrite was also added to the meat before autoclaving and storing the diet and represented mass fractions of 200, 1 000 and 4 000 mg/kg, as sodium nitrite.

The results do not demonstrate any effect on reproduction and no significant carcinogenic effect was revealed. However, an observed tendency toward an increased number of tumour-bearing rats in the highest dose group, plus the possible formation of carcinogenic N-nitroso compounds in nitrite-treated meat products, led to a recommendation to reduce the use of nitrite. Results from a concomitant study demonstrate that it is possible to produce many cured-meat products with the addition of only 50 mg/kg nitrite.

INTRODUCTION

Carcinogenic N-nitroso compounds in food, due to the use of nitrite, form a major contribution to total human intake. Exposure to volatile N-nitrosamines formed in food is estimated to be of the order of 0.5 µg per day per person (Gough *et al.,* 1978; Spiegelhalder *et al.,* 1980), whereas the amount of non-volatile N-nitroso compounds is unknown. It is also well established that N-nitroso compounds may be formed in the human body (Sander & Seif, 1969; Ohshima & Bartsch, 1981), but the extent and importance of such formation is difficult to evaluate.

Danish studies have been initiated in recent years in order to investigate a possible reduction of the use of nitrite and nitrate in meat and fish (Huss *et al.,* 1982; Gry *et al.,* 1983). These investigations have been carried out on a full commercial scale in factories, in cooperation between the Danish authorities and the food industry. The aim has been to give both a realistic picture of the health aspects and the technological aspects of a reduction in the use of nitrite and nitrate, especially with respect to nitrosamine content, microbial flora and organoleptic properties. Nitrite and nitrate-treated meat constitute a major source of preformed N-nitroso compounds in food.

In order to elucidate the importance of this contribution, toxicological investigations, including carcinogenicity, mutagenicity and teratogenicity studies, have been performed with a commercial meat product containing different amounts of nitrite (Gry *et al.,* 1982). The present paper reports the results of a two-generation carcinogenicity study.

MATERIALS AND METHODS

Meat products

These were prepared by adding curing mix to cut lean pork to obtain a meat product with an initial content of sodium chloride of 25 000 mg/kg and of potassium nitrite of 200, 1 000 and 4 000 mg/kg (expressed as sodium nitrite). The meat was chopped, vaccum-mixed, placed in cans and heated to 108 °C for 70 min. After being autoclaved, the cans were kept at room temperature for 1 month, to simulate storage in shops, and thereafter at 4 °C. The fresh canned meat for group 2 was stored at 4 °C immediately after being autoclaved. Determinations of nitrite in the prepared meat showed reductions to an average of 6, 47 and 580 mg/kg, respectively. The presence of volatile *N*-nitroso compounds was demonstrated only in meat to which 4 000 mg/kg nitrite had been added. Up to 30 μg/kg *N*-nitrosodimethylamine were found in these samples during the experiment.

Animals

SPF rats, Mol:Wistar, kept in stainless-steel wire cages, two animals/cage, under optimal condition of hygiene; temperature, 24 °C, relative humidity, 60%; air changed six to eight times per hour.

Diet

The canned meat was mixed in a ratio of 45% (mass/mass) with a balanced semisynthetic diet (Knudsen & Meyer, 1975). Except for one group fed the semisynthetic diet plus casein the meat was the only protein source (Table 1). The amino acid valine was added to make the meat diet nutritionally sufficient. The various diets were prepared once a week and stored under refrigeration until given to the rats daily, *ad libitum.* Analysis of nitrite content in the final diets showed 2, 2, 4, 4 and 94 mg/kg for groups 2 to 6, respectively, Tap-water acidified with citric acid (pH 3.5) was provided *ad libitum.*

Experimental design

The carcinogenicity study was performed over two generations. The F_0 rats, including 70 males and 140 females, were distributed into six groups and dosed as shown in Table 1 for 10 weeks before mating. Groups of 60, 100, 70, 60, 60 and 66 F_1 males and F_1 females, maintained on the respective F_0 diet, were formed at weaning. Group 3 was taken as the control group, and groups 1 and 2 served as controls for group 3. Weight again and clinical observations were recorded for the F_1 generation. Rats still alive after week 128 were sacrificed. The study was terminated at week 132. All rats, including those found dead and moribund animals killed during the experiment, were examined grossly. Tissues from liver, kidney, spleen, heart, aorta, lung, brain, spinal cord, peripheral nerve, pituitary gland, thyroid, parathyroid, thymus, pancreas, adrenal, testis, seminal vesicle, ovary, uterus, bladder, axillary and mesenteric lymph nodes, stomach, duodenum, caecum, colon, sternum, skeletal muscle, eye, Harderian gland, as well as samples from pathological changes found at autopsy, were fixed in buffered formalin. The tissues were embedded in paraffin and sections were stained with haematoxylin and eosin.

Table 1.   Protein source, mass fraction of potassium nitrite added (expressed as equivalent of sodium nitrite) and sodium chloride in the diet given to rats

Group	Protein	Nitrite added to meat (mg/kg)	NaCl in diet (g/kg)
1	casein	0	3.8
2	meat	0	3.8
3	meat	0	11.5
4	meat	200	11.5
5	meat	1 000	11.5
6	meat	4 000	11.5

Statistical methods

Weight gain data were analysed by Student's t test. Incidence of tumour and death rate were analysed statistically in accordance with guidelines recommended by Peto (Peto, 1974; IARC, 1980), using group 3 as control. The test for linear trend was performed according to Armitage (1955). When the number of specific tumours was less than five per group, Fisher's exact test was used. Time intervals for making up the number of tumour-bearing rats and rats with one, two and more than two tumours were: week 0–62 and periods of five weeks thereafter, ending at week 132. For calculating the incidence of tumour-bearing rats with benign or malignant tumours the time intervals were: week 0–107, 108–122 and 123–132; and for the mortality rate were: week 0–62, 63–92 and periods of 10 weeks thereafter, ending at week 132.

RESULTS

Growth, food intake and mortality

No difference in appearance or behaviour of test and control rats was noted in the F_0 generation. Reproduction data concerning pregnancy rate, litter size, mean pup weight and survival were comparable within groups, and no sign of any teratogenic effect was observed in F_1 rats.

Throughout the experiment, the F_1 rats in all groups exhibited normal appearance and behaviour. The mean body weights throughout the experiment are given in Table 2. The males in group 6 receiving the diet containing meat treated with 4 000 mg/kg nitrite had a significantly lower body weight in the first 50 weeks of the study, compared to group 3. The same tendency was found for group 6 females, but was less pronounced. During most of the experiment, group 5 females showed a significantly higher body weight. When comparing the control group 3 with dosed groups, no difference was noted in the mortality rate for male and female rats (Table 3).

Pathology

A tendency to increased incidence of specific tumours was found in male rats (squamous-cell carcinoma of the skin, Leydig-cell adenoma, subcutaneous fibroma, adenoma of the kidney) and in females (islet-cell adenoma, thymoma, fibroadenoma of the mammary gland) (Table 4). Using the Armitage-Cochran test for trend, no statistically significant difference at the 5% level was noted for the specific tumours in control and test groups, apart from a positive trend for adenomas in the male rat kidney. The latter was confirmed with Fisher's exact test at the 5% level, but only when using groups 2 and 3 pooled as control.

Table 2. Mean body weight of F, rats fed diets cited in Table 1

Group	Body weight (g) at different ages (weeks from birth)							
	3[a]	6	12	26	54	78	102	122
	Males							
1	43	115	284*	413*	531*	618*	659	628
2	42	131*[b]	326	463	596	701	728	710
3	42	116	326	453	584	679	692	655
4	44	123*	320	449	570	671	703	684
5	42	136*	332	462	593	686	696	668
6	42	113	303*	425*	565	665	691	683
	Females							
1	43	103	192*	244*	293*	356*	390	406
2	42	109	209	262	338*	425	465*	480
3	42	104	207	260	321	395	429	427
4	44	109	208	264	334	409	453	475
5	42	115*	218*	272	356*	437*	472*	452
6	42	100	198	248	317	386	426	416

[a] Recorded as mean pup weight at weaning
[b] Values marked with asterisks differ significantly from the controls at $p < 0.001$

Table 3. Cumulative mortality of F, rats fed diets cited in Table 1

Group	Initial group size	Weeks						Survivals at week 127 (%)
		62	92	102	112	122	127	
		No. of males						
1	60	0	11	13	19	30	46	23
2	100	11	27	34	43	59	69	31
3	70	14	22	28	39	50	55	21
4	60	7	12	19	31	41	47	22
5	60	5	17	24	34	46	48	20
6	66	8	17	25	34	44	55	17
		No. of females						
1	60	0	9	14	26	32	41	32
2	100	6	19	25	35	59	67	33
3	70	2	14	21	30	47	49	30
4	60	6	16	22	27	34	43	28
5	60	7	15	20	27	36	44	27
6	66	12	18	25	29	43	50	24

Table 4. Incidence of tumours in male and female rats fed diets cited in Table 1

Nitrite added to meat (mg/kg)	0		0		0		200		1 000		4 000	
Group	1		2		3		4		5		6	
Sex	♂	♀	♂	♀	♂	♀	♂	♀	♂	♀	♂	♀
No. of rats	60	60	100	100	70	70	60	60	60	60	66	66
BRAIN												
Glioma	–	2	5	1	4	–	4	–	2	1	2	–
Haemangiopericytoma	–	–	–	–	–	–	–	–	–	–	–	1

Table 4 (continued)

Nitrite added to meat (mg/kg)	0		0		0		200		1 000		4 000	
Group	1		2		3		4		5		6	
Sex	♂	♀	♂	♀	♂	♀	♂	♀	♂	♀	♂	♀
No. of rats	60	60	100	100	70	70	60	60	60	60	66	66
PITUITARY GLAND												
Adenoma	7	15	12	24	4	18	7	13	6	16	5	17
Adenocarcinoma	–	–	1	–	–	–	–	–	–	–	–	–
THYROID GLAND												
C-cell adenoma	1	2	2	1	2	1	3	–	1	2	2	2
Papillary adenoma	–	1	–	–	1	–	–	–	–	–	2	–
Follicular adenoma	–	–	1	1	–	–	–	–	–	1	–	–
Papillary carcinoma	–	–	–	–	1	–	–	–	–	–	–	–
Solid-cell carcinoma	–	–	–	1	–	–	–	–	–	1	–	–
PARATHYROID GLAND												
Adenoma	–	–	–	–	–	–	1	–	–	–	–	–
ADRENAL GLAND												
Cortical adenoma	–	–	–	–	1	1	–	–	–	–	–	1
Medullary adenoma	6	3	4	2	3	1	3	–	3	1	3	–
Neurofibroma	–	–	–	–	–	–	–	–	–	1	–	–
Malignant neuroblastoma	–	–	–	–	–	–	–	–	–	–	–	1
PANCREAS												
Islet-cell adenoma	2	–	13	2	5	2	7	1	4	1	8	4
Exocrine adenoma	7	2	5	–	3	–	2	2	3	–	3	2
Exocrine adenocarcinoma	–	1	–	–	–	–	–	–	–	–	–	–
TESTIS												
Leydig-cell adenoma	3		6		3		3		1		6	
OVARY												
Mesothelioma		–		1		–		–		–		–
Luteal-cell adenocarcinoma		–		–		–		–		–		1
Granulosa-cell adenocarcinoma		–		–		1		–		–		–
Theca-cell adenoma		–		–		1		–		–		–
Haemangiopericytoma		–		–		–		1		–		–
Blastoma		–		–		1		–		1		1
UTERUS												
Endometrial polyp		10		16		13		10		9		15
Endometrial adenoma		–		–		1		2		2		1
Fibroma		–		–		–		–		1		–
Fibrosarcoma		–		1		1		–		–		–
Adenocarcinoma		–		1		1		–		–		1
VAGINA												
Papilloma		–		2		–		–		–		1
Squamous-cell carcinoma		1		1		1		–		1		–
Leiomyosarcoma		–		–		–		–		1		–
URINARY BLADDER												
Papilloma	1	–	2	2	5	1	4	2	6	–	1	–
KIDNEY												
Tubular adenoma	–	–	–	–	–	–	2	–	–	–	4	–
Haemangiopericytoma	–	–	–	–	–	–	–	–	1	–	–	–
Lipoma	–	–	3	–	–	–	1	–	–	–	1	–
Hamartoma	–	–	1	–	–	–	–	–	–	–	–	–
ORAL CAVITY												
Papilloma	–	–	–	2	–	–	–	–	–	–	–	–
Squamous-cell carcinoma	–	–	–	–	–	1	–	1	–	–	–	–

Table 4   (continued)

Nitrite added to meat (mg/kg)	0		0		0		200		1 000		4 000	
Group	1		2		3		4		5		6	
Sex	♂	♀	♂	♀	♂	♀	♂	♀	♂	♀	♂	♀
No. of rats	60	60	100	100	70	70	60	60	60	60	66	66
STOMACH												
Papilloma	–	1	1	–	–	–	1	–	1	–	–	–
Fibrosarcoma	1	–	–	–	–	–	1	–	–	–	–	–
Adenocarcinoma	–	–	–	–	–	–	1	–	1	–	–	–
Squamous-cell carcinoma	–	–	1	–	–	–	–	–	–	–	–	–
Hamartoma	–	–	–	–	–	–	–	–	–	1	–	–
INTESTINE												
Fibrosarcoma	1	–	–	2	–	–	–	1	–	–	2	1
Adenocarcinoma	–	1	1	–	–	–	1	–	1	–	1	–
Leiomyosarcoma	–	–	–	–	–	–	–	–	–	–	–	1
LIVER												
Hepatocellular adenoma	–	–	1	1	–	–	1	–	–	–	–	–
Hepatocellular carcinoma	–	–	–	–	–	–	–	–	1	–	–	–
Haemangiosarcoma	–	–	1	–	–	–	–	–	–	–	–	–
Fibrosarcoma	–	–	–	–	–	–	–	–	–	1	–	–
LUNG												
Bronchogenic adenoma	–	–	–	–	–	–	–	–	1	–	–	–
Bronchogenic carcinoma	–	–	2	–	–	–	1	–	1	–	–	–
Unclassified carcinoma	1	1	–	–	–	1	–	–	1	–	–	–
Fibroma	–	–	1	–	–	–	–	–	–	–	–	–
THORACIC CAVITY												
Malignant mesothelioma	–	–	–	–	–	–	–	–	–	–	1	–
Mesothelioma	–	–	–	–	–	–	–	–	–	1	–	–
Fibroma	1	–	–	–	–	–	–	–	–	–	–	2
ABDOMINAL CAVITY												
Fibroma	–	–	1	–	–	–	–	1	–	–	–	–
Haemangioendothelioma	–	–	2	1	–	1	1	–	1	–	1	1
Fibrosarcoma	1	–	–	–	–	–	1	–	–	–	1	–
Unclassified sarcoma	–	–	–	–	–	–	–	–	–	3	–	–
Lipoma	–	–	–	–	–	–	–	–	–	1	–	–
BONE												
Fibroosteoma	–	–	–	1	1	–	–	–	–	–	–	–
Osteosarcoma	–	–	1	–	–	–	–	–	1	–	–	1
LYMPHORETICULAR SYSTEM												
Thymoma	–	1	1	10	–	4	–	2	–	2	2	5
Malignant thymoma	–	–	–	–	–	–	–	–	–	–	–	1
Haemangioendothelioma	–	–	5	1	4	–	4	1	–	–	2	–
Fibrosarcoma	–	1	1	1	–	–	–	–	–	–	–	–
Lymphosarcoma	1	–	–	3	2	1	1	3	2	–	1	2
Reticulum-cell sarcoma	–	–	3	–	–	–	–	–	–	–	3	–
SUBCUTANEOUS TISSUE												
Fibroma	4	1	7	1	2	–	2	–	2	1	5	–
Lipoma	–	–	2	2	–	–	2	–	1	–	1	–
Haemangioendothelioma	2	–	–	–	–	–	1	–	2	–	–	1
Haemangiosarcoma	–	–	–	–	1	–	–	–	–	–	–	1
Fibrosarcoma	1	–	3	1	–	3	1	1	–	–	1	–
Liposarcoma	–	–	–	–	–	1	–	–	–	–	–	–
Unclassified sarcoma	–	–	–	–	1	–	–	1	1	–	1	–

Table 4 (continued)

Nitrite added to meat (mg/kg)	0		0		0		200		1 000		4 000	
Group	1		2		3		4		5		6	
Sex	♂	♀	♂	♀	♂	♀	♂	♀	♂	♀	♂	♀
No. of rats	60	60	100	100	70	70	60	60	60	60	66	66
SKIN												
Squamous-cell papilloma	1	1	4	–	1	–	2	1	2	–	–	–
Keratoacanthoma	1	–	3	–	1	–	2	–	1	–	1	1
Trichoepithelioma	–	–	–	–	–	–	–	–	1	–	1	–
Sebaceous adenoma (Zymbal gland)	–	–	1	–	–	–	–	–	–	–	–	–
Squamous-cell carcinoma	3	4	4	4	3	1	2	1	2	1	7	1
Basal-cell carcinoma	–	–	–	–	–	–	–	–	–	–	1	–
Unclassified carcinoma	–	–	–	–	–	1	–	–	–	–	–	–
MAMMARY GLAND												
Fibroadenoma	–	7	–	32	–	16	–	16	–	13	–	18
Adenoma	–	5	–	2	–	–	–	2	–	3	–	2
Papillary cystadenoma	–	–	–	2	–	–	–	–	–	1	–	1
Adenocarcinoma	–	6	1	11	–	1	1	4	–	3	–	2
SALIVARY GLAND												
Adenoma	–	–	1	–	–	–	–	–	–	–	–	–
NASAL CAVITY												
Unclassified carcinoma	–	–	–	–	1	–	–	–	–	–	–	–
HEART												
Rhabdomyosarcoma	–	–	–	–	–	–	–	–	–	–	–	1
MISCELLANEOUS (UNKNOWN ORIGIN) EYE												
Squamous-cell carcinoma	–	–	1	–	–	–	–	–	–	–	–	–
Unclassified carcinoma	–	–	–	1	–	–	–	–	–	–	–	–
SEMINAL GLAND												
Squamous-cell carcinoma	–	–	1	–	–	–	–	–	–	–	–	–
MESENTERIC LYMPH NODE												
Adenocarcinoma	–	–	–	–	–	–	–	–	–	–	1	–
ABDOMINAL CAVITY												
Adenocarcinoma	1	–	–	–	–	–	–	–	–	–	–	–

Although a positive trend was noted for tumour-bearing male rats with malignant tumours (16 rats) in the highest dose group, this was not statistically significant at the 5% level when compared to the number in group 3 (nine rats) (Table 5). However, a statistically significant difference at the 5% level was found when comparing the total number of 20 malignant tumours in the high-dose group (6) to the nine tumours in the control group (3).

No statistically significant difference at the 5% level was found for the incidence of tumour-bearing male or female rats with benign and/or malignant tumours, or for rats bearing one, two or more than two tumours in groups 4, 5, 6, compared to the control group 3 alone or pooled with group 2 (Tables 5 and 6).

A variety of non-neoplastic lesions was observed in all groups in animals of both sexes. The incidences were not dose-related and fell within the normal range for Wistar rats.

Table 5.   Numbers of tumour-bearing male animals and tumours in male rats fed diets cited in Table 1

Nitrite added (mg/kg)	0	0	0	200	1 000	4 000
Group	1	2	3	4	5	6
No. of rats	60	100	70	60	60	66
Tumour-bearing rats	33	64	35	40	37	42
Tumour-bearing rats with benign tumours	27	55	29	36	30	33
Number of benign tumours	36	84	40	53	39	50
Tumour-bearing rats with malignant tumours	9	19	9	10	10	16
Number of malignant tumours	10	20	9	10	11	20
Tumour-bearing rats with multiple tumours	11	26	10	21	11	19
Tumour-bearing rats with one tumour	22	38	25	19	26	23
Tumour-bearing rats with two tumours	8	20	8	19	11	13
Tumour-bearing rats with more than two tumours	3	6	2	2	0	6

Table 6.   Numbers of tumour-bearing female animals and tumours in female rats fed diets cited in Table 1

Nitrite added (mg/kg)	0	0	0	200	1 000	4 000
Group	1	2	3	4	5	6
No. of rats	60	100	70	60	60	66
Tumour-bearing rats	43	83	44	38	41	48
Tumour-bearing rats with benign tumours	35	69	39	34	37	41
Number of benign tumours	51	106	61	54	59	75
Tumour-bearing rats with malignant tumours	15	25	13	12	11	14
Number of malignant tumours	16	27	15	12	11	15
Tumour-bearing rats with multiple tumours	18	40	19	22	19	26
Tumour-bearing rats with one tumour	25	38	25	16	22	22
Tumour-bearing rats with two tumours	13	26	12	17	11	16
Tumour-bearing rats with more than two tumours	5	14	7	5	8	10

DISCUSSION

A positive but not statistically significant trend at the 5% level, was demonstrated in male rats with squamous-cell carcinomas of the skin when using the Armitage-Cochran test. The number of male rats with malignant tumours of any kind showed a similar trend. However, no statistically significant difference was found using the method described by Peto. The significant increase observed in the total number of malignant tumours in males in the highest dose group is not considered to be an important effect, since the condition for using the Peto test – the statistical unit being the tumour-bearing rat – is not fulfilled (IARC, 1979; Ebbesen & Poulsen, 1981).

A statistically significant increase in number of dosed males with kidney adenomas was demonstrated. This finding is considered of minor importance, as no malignant tumour originating from the same tissues was seen (IARC, 1979; Ebbesen & Poulsen, 1981).

The evaluation of the two-generation carcinogenicity study does not reveal a significant carcinogenic effect of feeding rats nitrite-treated meat, nor does it demonstrate an effect on reproduction. Thus, the results of this study support those of van Logten et al., (1972), who fed nitrite-treated, canned meat to rats, but for only one generation. In another long-term study, rats were fed diets containing up to 25% cooked bacon without carcinogenic effects when compared to controls (Procter et al., 1977).

Due to the possible formation of carcinogenic N-nitroso compounds in nitrite-treated meat products, and to the tendency towards an increase in the number of tumour-bearing rats observed in the high-nitrite group in the present study, a reduction of nitrite addition to meat products is recommended.

In addition, recently published results demonstrate that it is commercially possible to produce many cured-meat products with good shelf life and organoleptic properties by the addition of only 50 mg/kg nitrite (Gry *et al.*, 1983). On the basis of these considerations, the health authorities have proposed a reduction of nitrite in most of the cured-meat products in Denmark.

REFERENCES

Armitage, P. (1955) Tests for linear trends in proportions and frequencies. *Biometrics, 11,* 375–386

Ebbesen, P. & Poulsen, E. (1981) *In-vivo tests for carcinogenic effect.* In: Cohr, K.-H., Danø, K., Ebbesen, P., Forchhammer, J., Møller-Jensen, O., Knudsen, I., Poulsen, E., Visfeldt, J. & Svane, O., eds, *Cancer and Chemical Substances,* Copenhagen, Danish Labor Inspection, pp. 39–46 (in Danish)

Gough, T.A., Webb, K.S. & Coleman, R.F. (1978) Estimate of the volatile nitrosamine content of UK food, *Nature, 272,* 161–163

Gry, J., Meyer, O., Olsen, P. & Poulsen, E. (1982) *Toxicological Investigations on Nitrite Treated Meat,* Søborg, National Food Institute, Institute of Toxicology (in Danish)

Gry, J., Damm Rasmussen, N.J., Kinth Jensen, W., Brandt, I.G. & Fabech, B. (1983) *Investigations on Effects of Nitrite in Commercially Prepared Danish Cured Meat Products,* Copenhagen and Søborg, The Federation of Danish Co-operative Bacon Factories and National Food Institute (in Danish)

Huss, H.H., Knöchel, S., Jensen, N.C. & Thomsen, J. (1982) *The Technological Effect of Nitrate in the Production of Sugar-Salted Herring,* Lyngby, Technological Laboratory, Ministry of Fisheries (in Danish)

IARC (1979) *IARC Monographs on the Evaluation of the Carcinogenic Risk of Chemicals to Humans,* Suppl. 1, *Chemicals and Industrial Processes Associated with Cancer in Humans, IARC Monographs, Volumes 1 to 20,* Lyon, International Agency for Research on Cancer

IARC (1980) *IARC Monographs on the Evaluation of the Carcinogenic Risk of Chemicals to Humans,* Suppl. 2, *Long-term and Short-term Screening Assays for Carcinogens. A Critical Appraisal,* Lyon, International Agency for Research on Cancer

Knudsen, I. & Meyer, O. (1975) Note on the use of a semisynthetic diet for SPF rodents in toxicological experiments. *Toxicology, 4,* 203–206

von Logten, M.J., den Tonkelaar, E.M., Kroes, R., Berkvens, J.M. & van Esch, G.J. (1972) Long-term experiment with canned meat treated with sodium nitrite and glucono-delta-lactone in rats. *Food Cosmet. Toxicol., 10,* 475–488

Ohshima, H. & Bartsch, H. (1981) Quantitative estimation of endogenous nitrosation in humans by monitoring N-nitrosoproline excreted in the urine. *Cancer Res., 41,* 3658–3662

Peto, R. (1974) Guidelines on the analysis of tumour rates and death rates in experimental animals. *Br. J. Cancer, 29,* 101–105

Procter, B.G., Grice, H.C., Sen, N.P., Chappel, C.J. & Rona, G. (1977) *A study of the potential carcinogenesis of cooked bacon fed to albino rats.,* In: *First International Congress on Toxicology (Abstracts), Toronto, 1977,* p. 32

Sander, J. & Seif, F. (1969) Bakterielle Reduktion von Nitrat im Magen des Menschen als Ursache einer Nitrosamin-Bildung. *Arzneim.-Forsch., 19,* 1091–1093

Spiegelhalder, B. Eisenbrand, G. & Preussmann, R. (1980) Volatile nitrosamines in food. *Oncology, 37,* 211–216

CARCINOGENIC ACTIVITY OF *N*-NITROSODIETHYLAMINE IN SNAKES (*PYTHON RETICULATUS*, SCHNEIDER)

D. SCHMÄHL & H.R. SCHERF

Institute of Toxicology and Chemotherapy, German Cancer Research Center,
Im Neuenheimer Feld 280, 6900 Heidelberg, FRG

SUMMARY

Fourteen snakes of the species *Python reticulatus* were randomized after one year's adaptation in our laboratory, i.e., at the age of 18 months. Groups of three animals (average body weight, 1 kg) were subjected to lifelong administration of 24, 12 or 6 mg/kg body weight of *N*-nitrosodiethylamine (NDEA) at fortnightly intervals. The NDEA-containing aqueous solution (0.3 ml/kg body weight) was administered by gavage. Five untreated animals served as controls. Snakes receiving 24 mg/kg NDEA died from toxic liver and kidney damage within the first year of experimentation. The three snakes receiving 12 mg/kg NDEA died within the last three months of the second year of treatment. These animals had developed multiple benign and malignant tumours in the liver and the kidney. The two animals that died last also developed tumours in the oral cavity and the trachea. Animals treated with 6 mg/kg NDEA died from tumours in the trachea.

INTRODUCTION

Comparative investigations of the effects of chemical carcinogens should be carried out in several animal species whenever a compound occurs ubiquitously in the environment and its activity cannot be detected epidemiologically in man. If such a compound is carcinogenic in several vertebrate species, this will increase the probability that it will also be a hazard to man (Schmähl *et al.*, 1978). These investigations, furthermore, may help to elucidate the diverse mechanisms of chemical carcinogenesis (dose-response relationship, dose-time relationship, organotropism).

N-Nitrosodiethylamine (NDEA) has so far been tested for carcinogenicity in 25 vertebrates. The compound was carcinogenic in 19 mammals, two bird species, one amphibian, and three fish species (Schmähl & Habs, 1980; Bogovski & Bogovski, 1981). Reptiles, however, have been missing in the spectrum of investigated species. We therefore decided to investigate NDEA for carcinogenic activity in the species *Python reticulatus* (Schneider). NDEA was administered at three different doses. The results permit a direct comparison with dose-response studies in small rodents.

MATERIALS AND METHODS

Fourteen snakes of the species *Python reticulatus,* born in the wild state, were randomized after one year's adaptation in our laboratory, i.e., at an age of about 18 months, when their body weight was about 1 kg. Three groups of three animals each were treated for life with 24, 12 and 6 mg/kg NDEA at fortnightly intervals. The aqueous NDEA solution (0.3 mL/kg) was administered by gavage via a 20-cm stomach tube. Animals were left under a hood for two days after treatment. They were at first kept in groups and later separately at 29 °C in polyvinyl chlorid terrariums, 80-cm high, 80-cm long and 50-cm deep. Each terrarium contained a Macrolon tank filled with water and was illuminated for 12 h a day by means of a 20W fluorescent tube (Truelight), giving light corresponding to normal daylight. The snakes were fed mice and, later on, rats. For histological examination, organs were fixed in formaldehyde or Carnoy's mixture and stained with haematoxylin-eosin for general specimens. Alcian blue was used to detect acid mucopolysaccharides and the periodic acid-Schiff reaction to 5 show glycogen and neutral mucopolysaccharides.

RESULTS

Animals treated fortnightly with 24 mg NDEA/kg body weight died within the first year of experimentation (animals 1–3, Table 1). Death was caused by the cytotoxic effect of NDEA on liver and kidneys. NDEA-induced parenchymatous necrosis in the liver resulted in regenerative processes. The hepatocytes exhibited relatively high mitotic activity. The necrotized parenchyma was replaced by mesenchymal connective tissue consisting partly of foci which were rich in cells and poor in fibres, and partly of foci which were rich in fibres and poor in cells. The latter always appeared together with basophilic dense hepatocyte foci or proliferating bile ducts. The kidneys of these animals were characterized by focally necrotic tubuli, surrounded by loose mesenchymal connective tissue. In animal no. 3, individual renal cysts had formed.

Snakes receiving 12 mg/kg NDEA every fortnight died within three months of the end of the second year of experimentation (animals 4–6, Table 1). All animals in this group had multiple benign and malignant tumours of hepatocellular and cholangiolar origin, besides

Table 1. Carcinogenic activity of *N*-nitrosodiethylamine (NDEA) in *Python reticulatus* (Schneider)

Animal no.	Individual dose[a] (mg/kg b.w.)	Total dose (mg/kg body weight)	Survival time (days)	Organs with neoplasms:			
				Liver	Kidney	Oral cavity	Trachea
1	24	384	218		+		
2	24	432	248		+		
3	24	552	317		+		
4	12	576	666	+	+		
5	12	588	693	+	+	+	+
6	12	636	749	+	+	+	+
7	6	372	857				+
8	6	372	861				+
9	6	384	899				+

[a] NDEA was administered at fortnightly intervals

Fig. 1. *Python reticulatus*, liver
    a. Liver (control animal), bar = 50 μ
    b. Liver with multiple tumours (snake no. 6) bar = 50 μ
    c. Cholangiolar adenoma (snake no. 6) bar = 50 μ
    d. Hepatocellular carcinoma (snake no. 6) bar = 50 μ

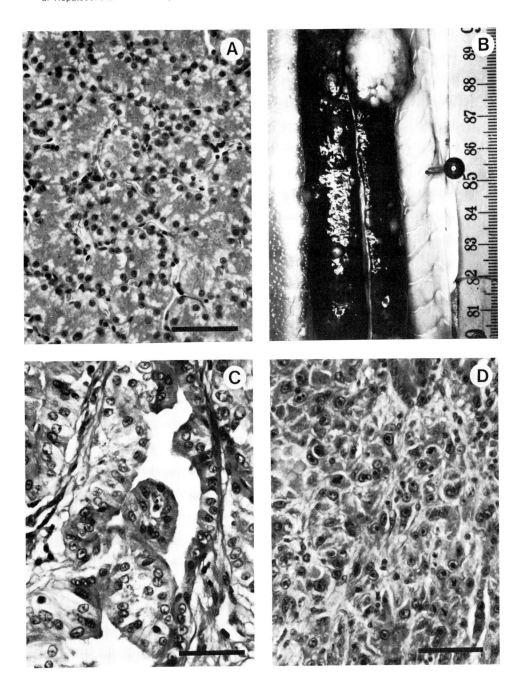

Fig. 2. *Python reticulatus*, kidney
 a. Kidney (control animal), bar = 50 μ
 b. Kidney with cystadenoma (snake no. 5) bar = 1 cm
 c. Proliferating mesenchyme with rests of epithelium of necrotized tubuli (arrows) (snake no. 5), bar = 50 μ
 d. Cystadenoma with confluent cysts (snake no. 5) bar = 50 μ

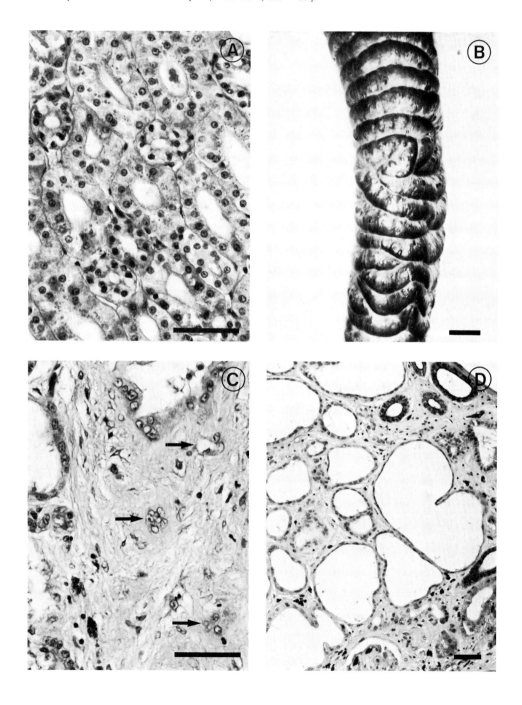

Fig. 3. *Python reticulatus*, trachea

    a. Endophytically growing papillary adenoma, trachea (snake no. 8), bar = 1 cm
    b. Adenocarcinoma of the trachea (snake no. 8), bar = 50 μ
    c. Epiphytically and endophytically growing adenocarcinoma, trachea (snake no. 9) bar = 1 cm
    d. Adenocarcinoma of the trachea (snake no. 9) bar = 50 μ

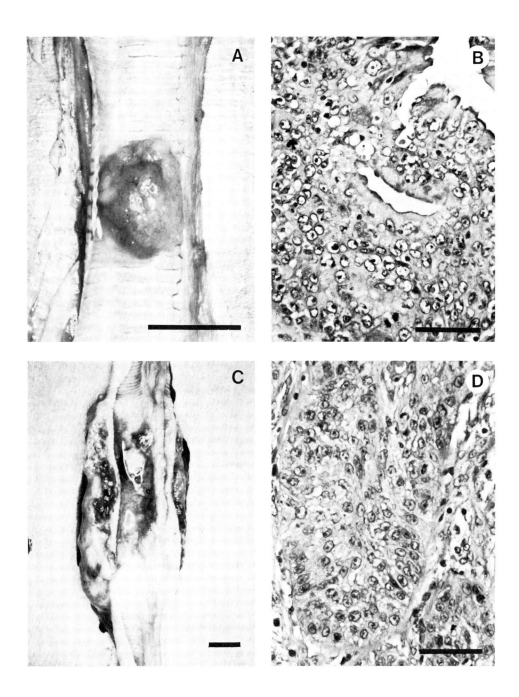

tissue changes that were also observed in animals of the high-dose group. All neoplasms derived from the bile ducts were surrounded by connective tissue. Growth of connective tissue and epithelial tissue was synchronous (Fig. 1). The mesenchymal connective tissue in the kidneys of animals of this group was highly multiplied. Cysts had formed all over the organ (Fig. 2). The two animals that died last (5 and 6) had, in addition, developed a tumour each in the trachea and in the oral cavity. Both tumour types originated in the mucosa of these organs.

Animals treated with the lowest dose of NDEA (animals 7–9, Table 1) died from multiple tracheal tumours at the beginning of the third year of experimentation. Here, too, the tumours originated in the tracheal mucosa. The tumours grew at first into the lumen and then broke through the tracheal wall to grow epiphytically (Fig. 3). Livers of these animals were characterized by uniformly disseminated foci of connective tissue which were rich in cells and indicated local parenchymatous necroses. The renal tissue was unchanged.

One control animal was killed after one year and another after two years. The remaining three control animals were sacrificed when all treated animals had died. No histologically detectable tissue change was seen in any control animal.

DISCUSSION

NDEA was as carcinogenic in snakes as in all the other animal species investigated to date. A total dose of about 600 mg/kg resulted in hepatomas in *Python reticulatus*. This is within the dose range that induced liver tumours in other animal species as well (Schmähl *et al.*, 1978). The multiplication of mesenchymal connective tissue in the kidneys is a NDEA-induced dose- and time-related reaction. Since alterations in the renal parenchyma (necroses, formation of cysts) manifest themselves only after proliferation of the connective tissue, the latter cannot be regarded as a regenerative process, but suggests a neoplastic proliferation of the mesenchyme. Tracheal tumours developed irrespective of the total dose administered (300–600 mg/kg). They were formed in snakes treated with 12 and 6 mg/kg NDEA within the relatively short time of 200 days.

The most prominent finding of our investigation is that the administration of relatively high doses of NDEA to snakes resulted in fatal liver and renal tumours, while animals receiving the low dose died from tracheal tumours. As in rats (Druckrey *et al.*, 1963), it has thus been demonstrated in this species that the organotropism of carcinogenic effects is determined substantially by the size of the individual doses.

REFERENCES

Bogovski, P. & Bogovski, S. (1981) Animal species in which *N*-nitroso compounds induce cancer. *Int. J. Cancer, 27*, 471–474

Druckrey, H., Schildbach, A., Schmähl, D., Preussmann, R. & Ivankovic, S. (1963) Quantitative Analyse der carcinogenen Wirkung von Diäthylnitrosamin. *Arzneimittel Forsch., 13*, 841–850

Schmähl, D., Habs, M. & Ivankovic, S. (1978) Carcinogenesis of *N*-nitrosodiethylamine in chickens and domestic cats. *Int. J. Cancer, 22*, 552–557

Schmähl, D. & Habs, M. (1980) Carcinogenicity of *N*-nitroso compounds. *Oncology, 37*, 237–242

PANCREATIC CARCINOGENIC NITROSAMINES IN SYRIAN HAMSTERS

P.M. POUR

The Eppley Institute for Research in Cancer and Allied Diseases and Department of Pathology and Laboratory Medicine

T. LAWSON

The Eppley Institute for Research in Cancer and Allied Diseases, University of Nebraska Medical Center, Omaha, NE 68105, USA

SUMMARY

Pancreatic neoplasms similar to those seen in humans have been induced by a group of related nitrosamines only in Syrian golden hamsters. Studies indicate a relationship between the structure of the carcinogens and their affinity for the pancreas: the presence of one keto or hydroxy group in the β-position on one of the aliphatic chains of alkyl nitrosamines is a prerequisite for their pancreatic carcinogenicity; addition of a second β-keto group significantly increases their activity on and specificity for the pancreas; replacement of one 2-oxo chain with a methyl group diminishes their specificity for the pancreas as does prolongation of the aliphatic chain. Carboxylation at the 3-position is associated with a complete loss of pancreatotropism. N-Nitrosomethyl(2-oxopropyl)amine appears to be a proximate carcinogenic metabolite of these compounds. The lack of tumour induction in the pancreas of rats correlates with the inability of this species to metabolize carcinogens to this metabolite, whereas all the pancreatic cells of the hamster (ductal/ductular, acinar and islet cells) have this ability. The results of in-vivo and in-vitro studies strongly suggest that the hamster pancreatic ductal and ductular cells are the most active unit of the organ in metabolizing the carcinogen and are also the progenitor cells of the induced pancreatic lesions.

INTRODUCTION

We have developed a model for pancreatic cancer in which the induced tumours are morphologically and biologically similar to the predominant form of human pacreatic cancer (Pour & Wilson, 1980). These tumours are induced by treating Syrian golden hamsters with one of several nitrosamines related to *N*-nitrosodi-*n*-propylamine. Our studies have established a relationship between the structure of carcinogens and their affinity for the pancreas. In this article, we report on the metabolism *in vivo* of several such compounds and propose a theory to explain their pancreaticotrophic effects.

MATERIALS AND METHODS

The carcinogens (Table 1) were synthesized in our laboratory. Equitoxic doses were given corresponding to 1-10, 1-10 and 1-40 of the LD_{50}, unless otherwise stated, Most were injected subcutaneously (s.c.); a few were also given *per os* (p.o.) or percutaneously (p.c.). In all studies, carcinogens were given to 8–10 week old hamsters either weekly or as a single dose. Experiments were carried out under defined laboratory conditions, and tumours were evaluated histopathologically each time by the same methods and by the same diagnostic criteria. Studies on the metabolism of these compounds (Gingell *et al.*, 1976, 1979, 1980; Gingell & Pour, 1978; Lawson *et al.*, 1981a) and on DNA alkylation (Lawson *et al.*, 1981b), damage and repair (Lawson *et al.*, 1982) were carried out by published methods. Pancreatic cell types were isolated by a modified method of Githens *et al.* (1980).

RESULTS AND DISCUSSION

The carcinogenicity of nitrosamines for the Syrian hamster pancreas is summarized in Table 1. Of these compounds, *N*-nitrosobis(2-oxopropyl)amine (ND2OPA) is the most specific for the pancreas, whereas the other carcinogens showed a broad tumour spectrum, even after a single dose (Pour & Raha, 1981). Of the postulated β-metabolites of *N*-nitrosodi-*n*-propylamine with a single carboxy or hydroxy group in the β-position, only *N*-nitrosopropyl-*n*-2-oxopropylamine (NP2OPA) affected the pancreas, whereas *N*-nitrosopropyl-*n*-2-hydroxypropylamine (NP2HPA) and *N*-nitrosomethyl-*n*-propylamine (NPMA) were not effective. Lower doses of NP2OPA induced more pancreatic tumours (55%) than did higher doses (5%), perhaps due to longer survival of hamsters, which had a reduced tumour incidence in organs other than the pancreas with low doses. However, later studies suggested that the metabolism of this class of nitrosamines is dose-dependent. The fact that different quantities of metabolites were produced when doses of 10 mg/kg and 40 mg/kg ND2OPA were given to hamsters (Lawson, unpublished data) might also contribute to the varying carcinogenicities of high and low doses of NP2OPA.

Table 1.   Nitrosamines tested for pancreaticotrophic effects (reviewed in Pour & Wilson, 1980)

Compound	Abbreviation	Route of administration	Pancreatic effect
N-Nitrosobis(2-acetoxypropyl)amine	ND2AcPA	s.c., p.c., p.o.	+ + +
N-Nitrosobis(2-hydroxypropyl)amine	ND2HPA	s.c., p.c., p.o.	+ + +
N-Nitrosobis(2-oxobutyl)amine	ND2OBA	s.c.	+ +
N-Nitrosobis(2-oxopropyl)amine	ND2OPA	s.c., p.c., p.o.	+ + +
N-Nitroso(2-hydroxypropyl) (2-oxopropyl)amine	N2HP2OPA	s.c., p.c., p.o.	+ + +
N-Nitroso(2-oxobutyl) (2-oxopropyl)amine	N2OB2OPA	s.c.	+ +
N-Nitrosomethyl(2-oxopropyl)amine	NM2OPA	s.c.	+ + +
N-Nitrosomethyl(2-oxobutyl)amine	NM2OBA	s.c.	+ +
N-Nitrosomethyl(3-oxobutyl)amine	NM3OBA	s.c.	−
N-Nitroso-2,6-dimethylmorpholine	NMOR-26DM	s.c.	+ +
N-Nitroso-2-methoxy-2,6-dimethylmorpholine	NMOR-2OM-26DM	s.c.	+ +
N-Nitrosopropyl-*n*-2-oxopropylamine	NP2OPA	s.c.	+
N-Nitrosopropyl-*n*-2-hydroxypropylamine	NP2HPA	s.c.	−
N-Nitroso-*n*-propylproprionamide	NPPAm	s.c.	(+)
N-Nitroso(1-acetoxypropyl)-*n*-propylamine	NPIAcPA	s.c.	(+)
N-Nitrosoethylvinylamine	NEVA	s.c.	(+)
N-Nitrosomethyl-*n*-propylamine	NPMA	s.c.	−
N-Nitrosodi-*n*-propylamine	NDPA	s.c.	−

Table 2. Concentration (μg/g tissue) of N-nitroso(2-hydroxypropyl)(2-oxopropyl)amine (N2HP2OPA) and its metabolites in tissues of Syrian golden hamsters given a single dose of 40 mg/kg sc

Tissue	Minutes after dosing	Concentration (μg/g tissue)[a]				
		ND2HPA	ND2OPA	N2HP2OPA	NM2HPA	NM2OPA
Liver[b]	15	8.7 ± 2.8	0.9 ± 0.7	18.9 ± 9.2	ND[c]	0.5 ± 0.2
	30	19.7 ± 7.5	0.6 ± 0.4	11.4 ± 5.0	ND	0.2 ± 0.2
	45	13.1 ± 5.9	0.6 ± 0.4	8.5 ± 2.2	ND	ND
	60	23.1 ± 13.2	0.2 ± 0.1	16.7 ± 7.5	ND	ND
Pancreas[b]	15	7.2 ± 4.1	3.7 ± 3.5	22.2 ± 7.8	ND	0.3 ± 0.2
	30	12.8 ± 5.6	2.3 ± 1.9	15.1 ± 3.3	ND	ND
	45	30.3 ± 4.3	10.9 ± 1.4	22.3 ± 9.9	1.4 ± 1.2	ND
	60	7.8 ± 3.3	1.7 ± 1.1	13.1 ± 4.8	ND	ND

[a] Mean ± SD of 9 animals; ND2HPA, N-nitrosobis(2-hydroxypropyl)amine; ND2OPA, N-nitrosobis(2-oxopropyl)amine; NM2HPA, N-nitrosomethyl(2-hydroxypropyl)amine; NM2OPA, N-nitrosomethyl(2-oxopropyl)amine
[b] About 1 g liver and 0.5 g pancreas were extracted
[c] ND = not detected

Oral administration of N-nitrosobis(2-acetoxypropyl)amine (ND2AcPA), N-nitrosobis(2-hydroxypropyl)amine (ND2HPA) and ND2OPA was less effective in producing tumours in the pancreas, but more carcinogenic to the liver; however, when ND2AcPA, ND2HPA and ND2OPA were painted on the skin, more pancreatic tumours than liver tumours were induced.

In hamsters, ND2OPA was metabolized to ND2HPA, N-nitroso(2-hydroxypropyl)(2-oxo-propyl)amine (N2HP2OPA), N-nitrosomethyl(2-hydroxypropyl)amine (NM2HPA) and NM2OPA (Gingell et al., 1976, 1979, 1980; Gingell & Pour, 1978; Pour et al., 1981a; Lawson et al., 1981a). Higher concentrations of ND2OPA metabolites, especially of NM2OPA and NM2HPA, were found in the pancreas than in the other tissues examined (liver, colon, salivary gland) (Pour et al., 1981a; Lawson et al., 1981a).

Since studies showed that ND2AcPA, ND2HPA, ND2OPA, N-nitrosodimethylamine (NDMA) and N-nitroso-2-methoxy-2,6-dimethylmorpholine (NMOR-20M-26DM) are metabolized to N2HP2OPA, it was felt that the latter represented a proximate pancreatic carcinogen (see Table 1). The cyclic structure of N2HP2OPA resembles the pyranose form of sugars and could cause the preferential uptake of N2HP2OPA pancreatic cells. However, N2HP2OPA given to hamsters (1 × 40 mg/kg sc) did not concentrate in the pancreas (Table 2) as did ND2OPA; very little or no NM2HPA or NM2OPA was found. This suggests that N2HP2OPA is not on the route of metabolism of ND2OPA to NM2OPA or NM2HPA and this favours strongly a one-step metabolism of ND2OPA to NM2OPA. Such a step could well be a de-acylation and perhaps involves acetyl coenzyme A, which would convert ND2OPA into NM2OPA (the latter could itself be reduced to NM2HPA by one of the NADPH-dependent reductases present in the cytoplasm). The finding of an acetyl derivative of dichlorothiophenol, when ND2OPA was metabolized by pancreas microsomes in its presence, (Lawson, unpublished data) supports this idea.

DNA alkylation studies showed that the specific activity of pancreatic DNA after administration of 2,3-[^{14}C]-ND2OPA was only 2% of that found when 1-[^{14}C]-ND2OPA was given (Lawson et al., 1981b). 7-Methylguanine (Lawson et al., 1981b) and O^6-methylguanine (Lawson, unpublished data) were found in hydrolysates of liver and pancreatic DNA. Nearly equal amounts of alkylation were produced in the liver when 1-[^{14}C]- and 2,3-[^{14}C]-ND2OPA were given and at least one-half of the radioactivity in the liver was associated with N-alkylated purine, whereas only 20% was in this form in the pancreas (Lawson et al., 1981b). The detection of methylated bases led us to look for methyl-containing metabolites of ND2OPA, such as NM2OPA and NM2HPA.

Investigations of DNA damage by alkaline sucrose gradient centrifugation revealed extensive damage in the pancreas (target tissue for ND2OPA), salivary glands (non-target tissue) and liver (intermediate tissue).

The damage was largely repaired by four weeks in the salivary gland, whereas in the liver and pancreas, some DNA damage persisted. When higher doses of ND2OPA (20 and 40 mg/kg, instead of 10 mg/kg bw) were used, considerable damage was still evident in the pancreas, but not in the liver at six weeks (Lawson et al., 1982).

These findings have been confirmed by the more sensitive alkaline elution technique (Lawson, unpublished data). The alkaline elution method was combined with a recently developed technique for isolating individual cell types from the pancreas to measure their responsiveness. Hamsters were given a single dose of ND2OPA (10 mg/kg sc) and were killed at various times thereafter. DNA in the duct cells was most damaged, and this also persisted longer than damage in the acinar cells: the half-life of DNA damage in acinar cells was about 100 h and that in duct cells 300 h. NM2OPA produced more DNA damage in the duct cells that ND2OPA at a much lower dose (0.005 mmol/L compared with 0.01 mmol/L for ND2OPA), which supports the idea that NM2OPA is a more proximate carcinogenic form of ND2OPA.

We have also demonstrated that all 3 pancreatic cell components (ductal, acinar and islet cells) metabolize ND2OPA when added to a culture medium at a concentration of 0.01 mmol/L. (A higher concentration was toxic.) The metabolic rate differed significantly between the three cell colonies: 0.4% for ductal cells, 1.5% for acinar cells and 6.0% for islet cells. It must be pointed out that the technique used did not separate acinar cells from centroacinar cells, which are derived from ductules and may be responsible for ND2OPA metabolism in acinar cell preparations.

Our data, in conjunction with that from other laboratories (Scarpelli et al., 1982) indicate that all pancreatic cell components metabolize pancreatic carcinogens and also demonstrate the existence of a significant relationship between the molecular structure of the nitrosamines and their affinity for the pancreas. The presence of at least one keto group in the β-position of the aliphatic chain appears to be a prerequisite for their pancreatic carcinogenicity. A second β-keto group in the chain significantly increases activity on and specificity for the pancreas, whereas replacement of one 2-oxopropyl or 2-oxobutyl chain by a methyl group diminishes their pancreatic specificity, as does prolongation of the aliphatic chain, i.e., in the case of a 2-oxobutyl compared to a 2-oxopropyl analogue. Carboxylation at the 3-position is associated with complete loss of pancreatotropism.

With regard to the mechanism of pancreatic carcinogenesis, the cyclic structure of N2HP2OPA, a common metabolite of pancreatic carcinogens, provided a basis for speculations that its glucose-like structure, which resembles that of the glucose moiety of the insulotropic carcinogen streptozotocin (SZ), may facilitate its uptake into the islet cells. Several observations supported this view. First, a high concentration of N2HP2OPA, NMOR-2OM-26DM, N-nitroso(2-oxobutyl)amine (N2OBA), N-nitroso(2-oxobutyl) (2-oxopropyl)amine (N2OB2OPA), all of which occur partially in a cyclic structure, causes islet-cell necrosis (Pour & Raha, 1981; Pour et al., 1981b), as does SZ. Second, in-vitro data show a significantly greater capacity of islet cells to metabolize the carcinogen compared with acinar cells. Further strong support stemmed from experiments that SZ inhibited pancreatic cancer induction by ND2OPA when administrered at the peak of alloxan-caused islet-cell necrosis (Pour et al., 1983). Complete destruction of islet cells by multiple doses of SZ one week prior to ND2OPA administration prevented formation of any hyperplastic or neoplastic pancreatic lesion, although ND2OPA was given weekly for 24 weeks (Bell et al., 1983). Also, ND2OPA, when administered at the peak of hypoglycaemia caused by exogenous insulin (known to inhibit islet-cell function), significantly lost its pancreatic carcinogenic effect (Pour *et al.*, unpublished data). Other results led us to postulate that islet cells are the principal pancreatic cells in which the carcinogen is metabolized. Since it has been shown that the blood supply of the exocrine pancreas is mediated largely by the efferent branches of the insular arteries (i.e., blood flows to the islets first and to exocrine cells later), we assumed that N2HP2OPA taken up preferentially by islet cells, due to its glucose-like structure, is metabolized to the more proximate carcinogen NM2OPA. After excretion by islet cells, NM2OPA reaches exocrine tissue by the above-mentioned insular-exocrine blood shunt (Pour *et al.*, 1981b, 1983). Strong support for the validity of this mechanism was the finding that initial development of most, if not all, hyperplastic and neoplastic lesions took place in immediately peri-insular regions in which NM2OPA concentrations would be highest. However, the fact that NM2OPA itself is a potent pancreatic carcinogen diminishes the importance of the cyclic structure of carcinogens as a prerequisite for their pancreatic carcinogenic effect. Moreoever, NO2OPA is a more specific pancreatic carcinogen than N2HP2OPA; and the results of metabolic studies described above make the cyclic theory less attractive. Nevertheless, the role of islets in metabolizing ND2OPA to NM2OPA (or NM2OPA to NDMA) remains of particular interest. Although we have not been able to demonstrate that NDMA is a ND2OPA metabolite, its formation cannot be entirely excluded, and studies are underway to clarify this matter. Hamster pancreatic microsomes metabolize NDMA efficiently: when NDMA (10 mmol/L) was incubated with hamster pancreas microsomes, 75% was metabolized in 10 min. Thus, NDMA might be difficult to detect in in-vitro metabolic studies of ND2OPA or NM2OPA.

The ability to metabolize ND2OPA or related carcinogens to NM2OPA (a process which seems to be unique to the hamster) appears to be important in pancreatic carcinogenesis, since rats, which are unresponsive to the pancreatic carcinogenic effect of ND2OPA and ND2HPA do not form NM2OPA (Lawson, unpublished data). Morphological and in-vivo and in-vitro studies indicate that ductal/ductular cells are targets for the carcinogen and are consequently the progenitor cells of induced pancreatic tumours.

CONCLUSION

These studies allow us to conclude that (i) addition of the oxo (or hydroxy) group β to the nitroso group is essential for pancreatic carcinogenicity of this group of nitrosamines; (ii) NM2OPA is a more proximate carcinogenic form of ND2OPA; (iii) islet cells may be involved in the metabolism of NM2OPA even though they are not its target cells; (iv) ductal/ductular cells are the ultimate target cells of these carcinogens.

ACKNOWLEDGEMENTS

The authors are indebted to Dr Jürgen Althoff, Dr Ulrich Mohr, the late Dr Friedrich W. Krüger, Dr Donald Nagel, Dr Ralph Gingell and Dr Lawrence Wallcave for their valuable contributions to the study, to Ms Katherine Stepan for her skilled technical assistant and to Ms Mardelle Susman for preparing the manuscript. These studies were supported by Public Health Service contract NO1 CP33278, by Program Project Grant NO1 PO1 CA25100 and by grant R26 CA20198 from the National Cancer Institute, NIH, USA.

REFERENCES

Bell, R.H., Sayers, H.J. & Strayer, D.S. (1982) Streptozotocin prevents development of pancreatic cancer in the hamster. *Surg. Forum, 33,* 437–439

Bell, R.H. & Strayer, D.L. (1982) *Preatment with streptozotocin prevents development of N-nitrosobis(2-oxopropyl)amine (BOP)-induced pancreatic cancer in the Syrian hamster.* Chicago, Pancreas Club, Inc. Annual Meeting

Gingel, R. & Pour, P. (1978) Metabolism of the pancreatic carcinogen *N*-nitrosobis(2-oxopropyl)amine after oral and intraperitoneal administration to Syrian hamsters: brief communication. *J. natl Cancer Inst., 60,* 911–913

Gingell, R., Wallcave, L., Nagel, D., Kupper, R. & Pour, P. (1976) Metabolism of the pancreatic carcinogens *N*-nitrosobis(2-oxopropyl)amine and *N*-nitrosobis(2-hydroxypropyl)amine in the Syrian hamster. *J. natl Cancer Inst., 57,* 1175–1178

Gingell, R., Brunk, G., Nagel, D. & Pour, P. (1979) Metabolism of three radiolabeled pancreatic carcinogenic nitrosamines in hamsters and rats. *Cancer Res., 39,* 4579–4583

Gingell, R., Brunk, G., Nagel, D., Wallcave, L., Walker, B. & Pour, P. (1980) Metabolism and mutagenicity of *N*-nitroso-2-methoxy-2,6-dimethylmorpholine in hamsters. *J. natl Cancer Inst., 64,* 157–161

Githens, S., Holmquist, D.R.G., Whelan, J.F. & Ruby J.R. (1980) Characterization of ducts isolated from the pancreas. *J. Cell Biol., 85,* 122–134

Lawson, T., Helgeson, A.S., Grandjean, C.J., Wallcave, L. & Nagel, D. (1981a) The formation of *N*-nitrosomethyl(2-oxopropyl)amine from *N*-nitrosobis(2-oxopropyl)amine *in vivo. Carcinogenesis, 2,* 845–849

Lawson, T.A., Gingell, R., Nagel, D., Hines L.A. & Ross, A. (1981b) Methylation of hamster DNA by the carcinogen *N*-nitrosobis(2-oxopropyl)amine. *Cancer Lett., 11,* 252–255

Lawson, T., Hines, L., Helgeson, S. & Pour, P. (1982) The persistence of DNA damage in the pancreas of Syrian golden hamsters treated with *N*-nitrosobis(2-oxopropyl)amine. *Chem. biol. Interactions, 38,* 317–323

Pour, P.M. & Raha, C. (1981) Pancreatic carcinogenic effect of *N*-nitrosobis(2-oxobutyl)amine and *N*-nitroso(2-oxobutyl)(2-oxopropyl)amine in the Syrian hamster. *Cancer Lett., 12,* 223–229

Pour, P.M. & Wilson, R. (1980) *Experimental pancreas tumors.* In: Moosa, A., ed., *Cancer of the Pancreas,* Baltimore, Williams & Wilkins, pp. 37–158

Pour, P.M., Runge, R.G., Birt, D., Gingell, R., Lawson, T., Nagel, D. & Wallcave, L. (1981a) Current knowledge of pancreatic carcinogenesis in the hamster and its relevance to the human disease. *Cancer, 47,* 1573–1587

Pour, P.M., Wallcave, L. & Nagel, D. (1981b) The effect of *N*-nitroso-2-methoxy-2,6-dimethylmorpholine on endocrine and exocrine pancreas in Syrian hamsters. *Cancer Lett., 13,* 233–240

Pour, P.M., Donnelly, K & Stepan, K. (1983) Modification of pancreatic carcinogenesis in the hamster model. 3. Inhibitory effect of alloxan. *Am. J. Pathol., 110,* 310–314

Scarpelli, D.G., Kokkinakis, D.M., Rao, M.S., Subbarao, V., Luetteke, N. & Hollenberg, P.F. (1982) Metabolism of the Pancreatic carcinogen *N*-nitroso-2,6-dimethylmorpholine by hamster liver and component cells of pancreas. *Cancer Res., 42,* 5089–5095

CHARACTERIZATION OF ALKYLDINITROGEN SPECIES IMPLICATED IN THE CARCINOGENIC, MUTAGENIC AND ANTICANCER ACTIVITIES OF *N*-NITROSO COMPOUNDS

J.W. LOWN, R.R. KOGANTY & S.M.S. CHAUHAN

Department of Chemistry, University of Alberta, Edmonton, Alberta, Canada

SUMMARY

The syntheses of certain specifically ^{15}N-labelled *E* and *Z* alkyldiazotates and alkylnitrosoamines, together with related dinitrogen species, including diazoalkanes, are reported. A study of their conformational and configurational equilibria by ^{15}N and ^{13}C nuclear magnetic resonance spectrometry has revealed: (1) corresponding pairs of *E* and *Z* alkyldiazotates do not interconvert at ambient temperatures in aprotic solvents; (2) a preferential *Z* conformer of the alkylnitrosamines; (3) a fast interchange of metal counterion between oxygen and nitrogen in the *Z*-diazotates, but a slow interchange of metal ion between oxygen and nitrogen in the corresponding *E* diazotates; (4) interconversion of *Z* aryldiazotates, *via* detectable *Z* and *E* diazohydroxides, to the *E* diazotates; and (5) rapid stereoelectronically-assisted decomposition of *Z*-alkyldiazotates to diazoalkanes, in contrast with the behaviour of the more stable *E* diazotates.

Self-Consistent Field calculations *ab initio* show that *Z* methyl diazohydroxide is the higher energy and more reactive form, while the carbon is relatively soft. In contrast, the *E* isomer is the more stable (by $\simeq 18.0$ kcal/mol) and the carbon harder. These data are in accord with the view that the *Z* form (from *N*-nitrosodimethylamine) attacks G–O_6 (softer center) preferentially by S_N1, while the *E* form prefers to react at the harder G–N_7 and by an S_N2 mechanism. These data provide a rationale for the known propylation of G–N_7 without rearrangement, for propylation of G–O_6 with rearrangement and possibly for the origin of the characteristic G–O_6 alkylation carcinogenic lesion.

INTRODUCTION

Alkyldiazotates and the corresponding alkyldiazohydroxides or alkyldiazonium ions have been implicated in the carcinogenic action of alkylnitrosamines (Magee & Barnes, 1967), in the mutagenic action of certain nitrosamides and in the anticancer action of certain nitrosoureas (Montgomery, 1976). These species appear to be primarily responsible for critical lesions in the cellular macromolecules DNA, RNA and proteins (Montgomery, 1976).

Since the site of DNA alkylation is crucial in terms of the biological response [e.g., O^6-guanine alkylation may correlate with carcinogenicity (Singer, 1976)], differences in chemical reactivity between, for example, Z and E alkyldiazohydroxides for such sites may ultimately determine in-vivo activity. We report the synthesis of certain ^{15}N-labelled Z and E alkyldiazotates, as well as ^{15}N and ^{13}C nuclear magnetic resonance (NMR) spectrometric studies of equilibration between these and other alkyldinitrogen species, and account for their site-selective DNA reactions in relation to the biological actions of N-nitroso compounds.

MATERIALS AND METHODS

Ammonium chloride ^{15}N (95–99%), sodium nitrite ^{15}N (96–99%) and potassium phthalimide ^{15}N (95–99%) were obtained from Merck Sharpe and Dohme (Pointe Claire, PQ, Canada). The specifically ^{15}N, ^{15}N$_2$-Z-alkyldiazotates were prepared by reaction of ^{15}N-labelled alkylnitrosoureas in 99% enrichment (Lown & Chauhan, 1981) under anhydrous conditions, with potassium *tert*-butoxide in butanol, according to equation 1. The E-alkyldiazotates (4) were prepared from the corresponding alkylhydrazines by treatment with two equivalents of potassium *tert*-butoxide, as shown in equation 2.

Authentic diazomethane ^{15}N$_1$, ^{15}N$_2$, was prepared by reaction of Z-methyldiazotate (2a) with two equivalents of potassium *tert*-butoxide in methanol-d$_4$ at $-80\,^\circ$C. ^{15}N-Nitrosylchloride was prepared by addition of hydrogen chloride to a 10% aqueous solution of Na^{15}NO$_2$.

RESULTS

Equation 1

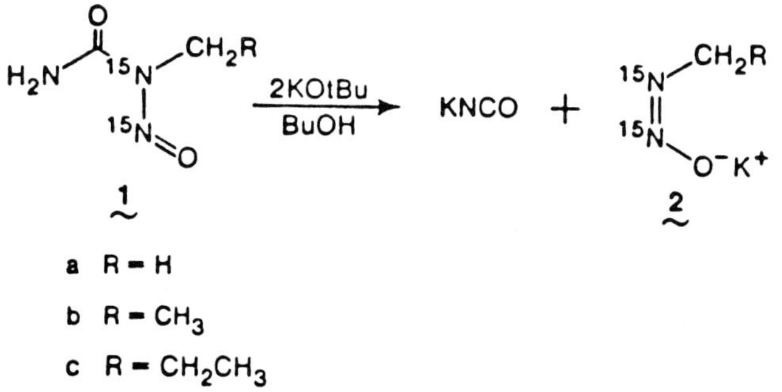

a R = H

b R = CH$_3$

c R = CH$_2$CH$_3$

Equation 2   RCH$_2$NHNH$_2$ $\xrightarrow{\text{nBuO}^{15}\text{NO}}$ RCH$_2$NNH$_2$ $\xrightarrow[\text{KOtBu}]{\text{nBuONO}}$ RCH$_2$—N

a R = H

b R = CH$_3$

c R = CH$_2$CH$_3$

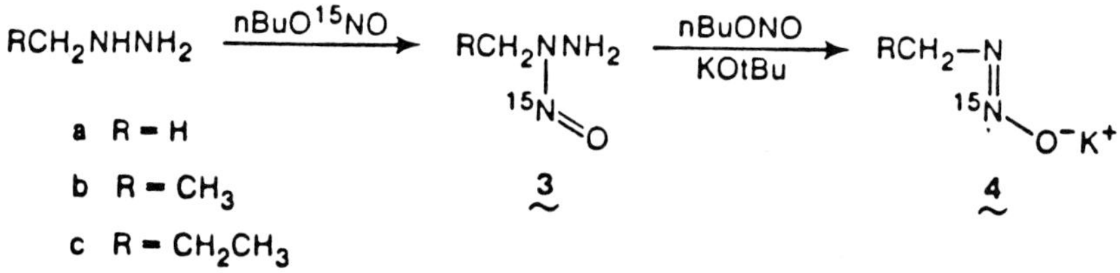

The corresponding pairs of Z and E alkyldiazotates (2 and 4) detected by ^{15}N-NMR (see Table 1) (Lichter & Roberts, 1971) are quite stable at ambient temperature in dimethyl sulfoxide-d$_6$ and do not interconvert. The Z-methyldiazotate (2a) is rapidly converted into diazomethane ^{15}N$_1$, ^{15}N$_2$ (7a), *via* (8a) (see Fig. 1) in the protic solvent, methanol-d$_4$, at room temperature. The corresponding E-alkyldiazotates in methanol-d$_4$ are stable at room temperature for up to 12 h and required treatment of a suspension of (4a) in diethylether with carbon dioxide to afford diazomethane ^{15}N (7a).

Table 1. ^{15}N-NMR chemical shifts and coupling constants for E and Z alkyldiazotates and related compounds[a]

Compound[b]	Solvent	^{15}N-nuclear magnetic resonance spectra			
		N_1	N_2	$^{1}J^{15}N\text{-}^{15}N(Hz)$	$^{3}J^{15}N\text{-}H(Hz)_2$
2a	DMSO-d_6	339.5	514.9	17.4	–
2b	DMSO-d_6	345.0	510.8	17.5	–
2c	DMSO-d_6	356.6	509.3	17.6	–
4aA	DMSO-d_6	–	539.8	–	4.5
4aB	DMSO-d_6	–	516.3	–	2.2
4a	CD$_3$OD	–	506.8	–	3.5
4cA	DMSO-d_6	–	535.4	–	3.5
4cB	DMSO-d_6	–	517.3	–	–
5aA	ether	–	553.62		
5aB	ether	–	395.34		
7a	CD$_3$OD	289.3	395.9	7.5	
7b	CD$_3$OD	305.4	427.3	9.5	
7c	CD$_3$OD	303.8	428.9	9.1	
9-E	DMSO-d_6	371.92	540.58	16.1	
9-Z	DMSO-d_6	351.8	501.8	19.5	
10-E	DMSO-d_6	372.35	555.38	16.4	
10-Z	DMSO-d_6	310.45	495.08	15.1	

[a] Proton coupled spectra were obtained with 1–4K scans at 20.283 MHz and are reported by using ammonia as standard and dimethylformamide as external reference
[b] As shown in equations 1 and 2 and Figure 1; 9, potassium benzene diazotate; 10, benzene diazohydroxide

Figure 1. Reactions of alkylnitroso compounds

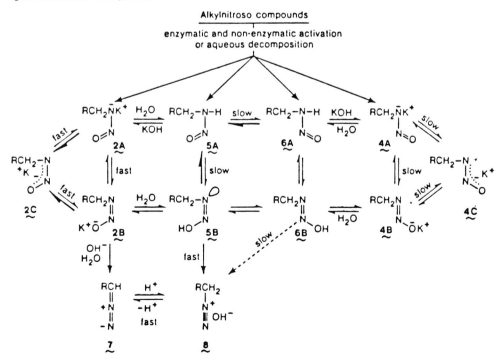

Treatment of benzene $^{15}N_1$, $^{15}N_2$ diazonium chloride with potassium hydroxide afforded potassium Z benzene $^{15}N_1$, $^{15}N_2$-diazotate, 9 (Table 1). Addition of 10% (v/v) water to this solution resulted in equilibration *via* the Z-benzenediazohydroxide 10, thence to the E-benzenediazohydroxide (10) and finally to the potassium benzenediazotate (9). The signals due to the more stable E forms gradually increased over the course of six hours at the expense of the Z isomers.

When methylamine was treated with ^{15}N-nitrosylchloride in anhydrous ether at $-50\,°C$, the proton-decoupled ^{15}N-NMR spectrum showed two signals at $\delta553.62$ and $\delta395.34$. The former signal is ascribed to Z monomethylnitrosamine (5aA) and the smaller peak at $\delta395.34$ is ascribed either to the Z methyldiazohydroxide (5aB) or to its decomposition product (7a).

Self-Consistent Field (SCF) calculations were made *ab initio* of energies and carbon electron densities, using full geometry optimization and STO-3G minimum basis sets on E and Z methyldiazohydroxides. The E had the lower energy ($-220.981587H$) and the Z the higher ($-220.953721H$), corresponding to a difference of $\simeq18.0$ kcal/mol. The E configuration had the shorter C–N bond (1.5029 Å), i.e., the softer carbon, while Z had a longer C–N bond (1.5090 Å), predicting this to be a harder centre on the Hard and Soft Acids and Bases (HSAB) treatment (Pearson, 1966).

DISCUSSION

The results demonstrate that the Z methyldiazotate is best represented by 2C (Fig. 1), which is in accord with X-ray diffraction evidence on Z-methyldiazotate (Müller *et al.*, 1963) and indicates rapid equilibration between species 2A and 2C. In contrast, the NMR data for the E methyldiazotate indicate two discrete species in dimethyl sulfoxide, with slow interconversion in which the potassium ion moves across the resonance hybrid of the N–N–O system (4A → 4C).

The more rapid conversion of the Z alkyldiazotates and diazohydroxides into diazoalkanes in proton-exchanging solvents (compared with the E forms) may be accounted for either by *syn* selectivity or stereoelectronic elimination of hydroxyl, due to participation of the *anti* N_1 lone pair.

The results (Fig. 1) indicate that, while the pathway 2aB → 5aB → 8a → 7a is plausible, a direct elimination of hydroxide from 2aB to give 7a is also possible. The evidence suggests a preferred Z conformation for the key carcinogen N-nitrosomethylamine (NMA) (5aA) when generated directly from methylamine. In contrast, the formation of E NMA (6aA) and E methyldiazohydroxide (6aB) has been inferred in the aqueous decomposition of acetoxynitrosamine (Wiessler, 1979). The barrier to rotation about the N–N bond in N-nitrosodimethylamine is about 23 kcal/mol, which may be compared with the calculated energy difference between Z and E of $\simeq18.0$ kcal/mol which, of course, neglects medium effects.

Evidence has been obtained for the lack of detectable rearrangement of the propyl group during alkylation of $G-N_7$ of DNA by N-nitrosodipropylamine (NDPA) (Park *et al.*, 1980). Recent studies have also showed that while alkylation of the $G-N_7$ by NDPA gives *n*-propylation, alkylation of $G-O_6$ gives the rearranged product (Scribner & Ford, 1982). These data suggest that the ultimate electrophile responsible for the carcinogenic action of nitrosamines, for the mutagenic action of nitrosamides or for the anticancer action of nitrosoureas is not primarily a carbenium ion (Magee & Barnes, 1967), but rather a species which may be subject to S_N2 attack. The results indicate this may be the alkyldiazohydroxide. A treatment based on the HSAB principle (Pearson, 1966) accounts for the observed site-selectivity of nitrosamine action on DNA. If NMA forms the Z methyldiazohydroxide, this species, which has a longer C–N bond and a softer carbon than the E isomer, will react preferentially with the softer $G-O_6$ centre. The greater reactivity of Z, with its longer C–N bond, also favours S_N1 attack to give the carcinogenic $G-O_6$ alkylation with rearrangement in the case of propylation, as observed. In contrast, acetoxynitrosamine gives the E methyldiazohydroxide (this may also be formed from nitrosamides and nitrosoureas) which, since it has a shorter C–N bond, has a harder carbon than the Z isomer. It would then prefer reaction at the $G-N_7$, which is a harder centre than $G-O_6$. In addition, the lower reactivity of E and its shorter C–N bond will favour an S_N2 mechanism, leading to an unrearranged product, again in accord with experimental observations. The HSAB treatment of intermediate alkyldiazohydroxides may therefore provide a rationale for the characteristic biological activity of N-nitroso compounds.

ACKNOWLEDGEMENTS

This work was supported by grant 1RO1 CA21488-01 awarded by the National Cancer Institute, DHHS, by the National Foundation for Cancer Research and by the Alberta Cancer Board.

REFERENCES

Lichter, R.L. & Roberts, J.D. (1971) ^{15}N-NMR of pyridine-^{15}N. *J. Am. chem. Soc.,* **93,** 5218–5224

Lown, J.W. & Chauhan, S.M.S. (1981) Synthesis of specifically ^{15}N and ^{13}C-labelled antitumor (2-haloethyl)nitrosoureas. *J. org. Chem.,* **46,** 5309–5321

Magee, P.N. & Barnes, J.M. (1967) Carcinogenic nitroso compounds. *Adv. Cancer Res.,* **10,** 163–238

Montgomery, J.A. (1976) Chemistry and structure-activity studies of the nitrosoureas. *Cancer Treat. Rep.,* **60,** 651–664

Müller, E., Hoppe, W., Hagenmaier, H., Huiss, H., Huber, R., Runder, W. & Suhr, H. (1963) Structure of isomeric diazotates: The Hantzsch methyldiazotate. *Chem. Ber.,* **96,** 1712–1716

Park, K.K., Archer, M.C. & Wishnok, J.S. (1980) Alkylations of nucleic acids by N-nitroso-n-propylamine. *Chem.-biol. Interact.,* **29,** 139–144

Pearson, R.G. (1966) Acids and bases. *Science,* **151,** 172–177

Scribner, J.D. & Ford, G.W. (1982) n-Propyldiazonium ion alkylates O^6 of guanine with rearrangement but alkylates N–7 without rearrangement. *Cancer Lett.,* **16,** 51–56

Singer, B. (1976) All oxygens in nucleic acids react with carcinogenic ethylating agents. *Nature,* **264,** 333–339

Wiessler, M. (1979) *Am. Chem. Soc. Symp. Ser. No. 101,* pp. 57–75

ANTICANCER NITROSOUREAS: INVESTIGATIONS ON ANTINEOPLASTIC, TOXIC AND NEOPLASTIC ACTIVITIES

G. EISENBRAND

*Department of Food Chemistry and Environmental Toxicology, University of Kaiserslautern,
6750 Kaiserslautern, FRG and Institute of Toxicology and Chemotherapy, German Cancer
Research Center, 6900 Heidelberg, FRG*

SUMMARY

Nitrosoureas are among the most effective antineoplastic drugs in experimental models. New water-soluble analogues have been tested extensively in preclinical studies, and the results show that new congeners, such as 1-(2-chloroethyl)-1-nitroso-3-(2-hydroxyethyl)urea (HECNU), are more effective antineoplastic agents in most model systems than are clinically used compounds, such as 1,3-bis(2-chloroethyl)-1-nitrosourea or chlorozotocin. In chronic toxicity studies in rats, however, HECNU was found to be considerably less toxic than its clinically used congeners and was also less carcinogenic. Carbamoylating and alkylating potential and glutathione reductase inhibition do not parallel its antitumour effectiveness, chronic toxicity or carcinogenic potential. Compounds with higher anti-tumour activity in preclinical trials also show a higher potential for DNA-DNA interstrand cross-link formation *in vivo*.

It is concluded that selection of analogues for clinical application should take into account not only antineoplastic effectiveness and acute toxicity, but also chronic toxicity and carcinogenicity.

INTRODUCTION

2-Chloroethyl-*N*-nitrosoureas (CNUs) are highly active anticancer agents with a broad antitumour spectrum in experimental systems. Their clinical application, however, is limited because they show delayed and cumulative toxic side effects, bone-marrow suppression being prevalent and dose-limiting. Much effort has been expended by many groups to obtain new analogues with higher effectiveness and/or lower toxicity; so far, however, these attempts have not been convincingly successful. The high experimental antitumour activity of many CNUs impedes rather than facilitates the selection of candidates for clinical trials. First-generation CNUs, like 1,3-bis(2-chloroethyl)-1-nitrosourea (BCNU), 1-(2-chloroethyl)-1-nitroso-3-cyclohexylnitrosourea (CCNU) and 1-(2-chloroethyl)-1-nitroso-3-(4-methyl) cyclohexyl-nitrosourea (Me-CCNU) (Fig. 1), were introduced in rapid succession because of their activity against Hodgkin's and non-Hodgkin's lymphomas, brain-tumours, gastrointestinal tumours and some other neoplasms. The clinical results, however, do not provide enough evidence to

Fig. 1. Structures of derivatives of 2-chloroethyl-*N*-nitrosoureas (CNUs)

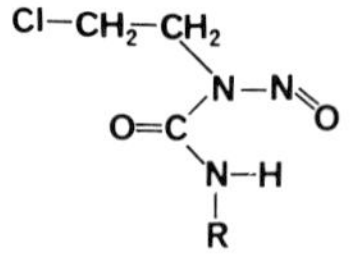

CNU derivative	— R
1,3-Bis (2-chloroethyl)-1-nitrosourea (BCNU)	$-CH_2-CH_2Cl$
1,2-(Chloroethyl)-1-nitroso-3-(2-hydroxyethyl) urea (HECNU)	$-CH_2-CH_2OH$
1-(2-Chloroethyl)-1-nitroso-3-(methylenecarboxamido) urea (Acetamido CNU)	$-CH_2-CONH_2$
[2-(3-Chloroethyl)-3-nitrosoureido]-D-desoxyglucopyranose (Chlorozotocin)	D-glucopyranose
1-(2-Chloroethyl)-1-nitroso-3-cyclohexylnitrosourea (CCNU)	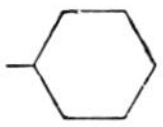
1-(2-Chloroethyl)-1-nitroso-3-(4-methyl)cyclohexylnitrosourea (MeCCNU)	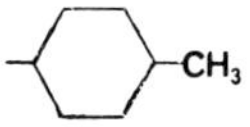

differentiate clearly between these analogues with regard to clinical antitumour spectrum and toxicity.

A second generation CNU is chlorozotozin, 2-[3-(2-chloroethyl)-3-nitrosoureido]-D-desoxyglucopyranose (CZT) (Fig. 1), the first water-soluble analogue tested clinically (Johnston *et al.*, 1975). CZT was less active in a series of experimental tumour systems than the first-generation CNUs (Zeller *et al.*, 1979; Fiebig *et al.*, 1980; Spreafico *et al.*, 1981); and clinically, it has therapeutic activity in non-Hodgkin's lymphomas and sarcomas and is less myelosuppresive than first generation CNUs (Talley *et al.*, 1981).

Part of our own work has been devoted to the synthesis of water-soluble analogues, with the aim of obtaining compounds that, unlike CZT, retain, as far as possible, their lipophilic properties. Lipophilicity is considered to be essential for the antineoplastic effectiveness of such compounds, especially against intracerebral tumours. By exchanging a chlorine atom in BCNU against a hydroxy group, a new analogue, 1-(2-chloroethyl)-1-nitroso-3-(2-hydroxyethyl)urea (HECNU), was obtained (Fig. 1). HECNU is about 30 times more water-soluble than BCNU but still has a high degree of lipophilicity, as exemplified by a log P (octanol/water) of 0.3 (Eisenbrand *et al.*, 1976).

MECHANISM OF ACTION

The molecular mechanisms by which CNUs exert their antitumour and toxic effects are not yet fully elucidated. They are monofunctional as well as bifunctional alkylating agents, and modification of DNA by alkylation and cross-linking is considered an important factor in their activity. Considerable evidence has been accumulated that a major pathway of CNU decomposition involves formation of 2-chloroethyldiazohydroxide or equivalent bifunctional electrophiles (2-chloroethyldiazotate, -diazonium or -carbenium ions) and an isocyanate (Fig. 2). Cross-linking of DNA is considered to proceed *via* direct and rapid transfer of 2-haloethyl groups to nucleophilic sites of DNA bases, followed by a slow secondary reaction by which the primary monofunctional adducts give rise to intra- and inter-strand cross-links between DNA bases (Lundlum & Tong, 1981). Other reaction pathways might also play a role, and detailed mechanistic in-vitro investigations suggest that formation of cyclic intermediates, such as 2-(alkylimino)-3-nitroso-2-oxazolidines (Montgomery, 1981; Lown & Chauhan, 1981) or 4,5-dihydro-1,2,3-oxadiazolium intermediates (Tong & Ludlum, 1979; Brundrett, 1980), can be envisaged (Fig. 2).

Such transient intermediates might be responsible, at least in part, for the formation of the 2-hydroxyethylated nucleosides found after reaction of CNUs with polynucleotides, either by direct nucleophilic reaction with the oxadiazolium intermediates (Tong & Ludlum, 1979; Brundrett, 1980; Tong *et al.*, 1981), or, alternatively, by reaction with 2-hydroxyethyl nitrosoureas or 2-hydroxyethyl diazotates as minor intermediates, formed in equilibrium with 3-nitroso oxazolidines (Lown & Chauhan, 1981) (Fig. 2). Such mechanistic concepts are supported by the finding that 2-hydroxyethyl derivatives of nucleosides do not arise from corresponding haloethyl derivatives (Tong & Ludlum, 1979; Tong *et al.*, 1981). After reaction of BCNU with DNA, two products have so far been identified that are considered to be the

Fig. 2. Possible reactions of derivatives of 2-chloroethyl-*N*-nitrosoureas *in vivo*

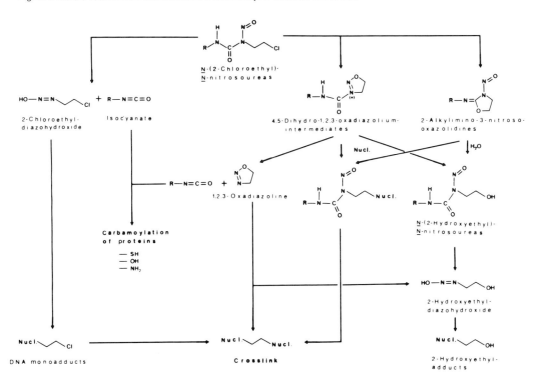

result of difunctional alkylation: 1.2-(diguan-7-yl)ethane (Tong & Ludlum, 1981) and 1-[N^3-deoxycytidyl]-2-[N^1-deoxyguanosinyl]ethane (Tong *et al.*, 1982), the former being attributed to intrastrand crosslinks and the latter to interstrand crosslinks.

In addition to alkylation, CNUs carbamoylate cellular macromolecules, because they give rise to isocyanates on decomposition (Bowden & Wheeler, 1971) (Fig. 2). Carbamoylation also induces a multiplicity of biomolecular effects. It has been shown, for instance, to inhibit the ligation of X-ray-induced DNA strand breaks (Fornace *et al.*, 1978), to inhibit repair of alkylated DNA (Heal *et al.*, 1979) and to inhibit excision repair of UV-irradiated DNA (Kann *et al.*, 1980). Moreover, reduction of glutathione levels in rodent liver (McConnell *et al.*, 1979), inhibition of glutathione-reductase in erythrocytes (Frisher & Ahmad, 1977; Babson & Reed, 1978), and other effects due to carbamoylation of proteins (Reed, 1981) have been described.

The biological significance of such carbamoylation reactions is uncertain. For instance, 1-(2-chloroethyl)-3-(β-D-glucopyranosyl)-1-nitrosourea (GANU), a sugar-linked CNU with high carbamoylating activity, inhibits the early removal of DNA alkylation in murine bone marrow, whereas CZT, which is only weakly carbamoylating, allows repair to proceed (Ahlgren *et al.*, 1982). Since both compounds display a similarly low degree of myelosuppresion, carbamoylating activity is not directly related to bone-marrow toxicity; the same is true for its therapeutic efficacy, which also does not appear to be influenced directly by carbamoylating potential. The validity of such interpretations is limited, however, because carbamoylating potential is normally measured in an in-vitro test towards lysine, and this might not be relevant for in-vivo situations (Reed, 1981).

ANTINEOPLASTIC ACTIVITY

During systematic structure-activity studies, a wide spectrum of CNU analogues was synthesized in our laboratory to investigate the influence of various substituents on the un-nitrosated urea-nitrogen of these analogues on biological activities (Eisenbrand *et al.*, 1981). Results obtained with two promising new analogues, HECNU and 1-(2-chloroethyl)-1-nitroso-3-methylenecarboxamido)urea (acetamido-CNU) are summarized below.

HECNU has been tested in a very wide spectrum of experimental rodent tumours, and in most cases the drug exhibited equal or superior activity to clinically used reference compounds (Spreafico *et al.*, 1981; EORTC[1]). High antineoplastic activity, frequently with high cure rates, was obtained in murine transplantation tumours, such as leukaemia L1210 and P388, TLX-9 lymphoma, Lewis lung carcinoma, C22-LR osteosarcoma, P815 mastocytoma, colon carcinoma 26, subcutaneous ependymoblastoma and glioma 26. The drug was also highly effective against B16 melanoma, mammary carcinomas 16, TM-2 and 3641/75, ovarian carcinoma M555, fibrosarcoma ICIG-1 and sarcoma 180. Results of primary screening in rat tumours were also very favourable, e.g., in leukaemia L5222, Yoshida sarcoma, Walker 256 carcinosarcoma, lymphatic leukaemia and anaplastic mammary carcinoma.

Log dose-response curves for BCNU, HECNU, acetamido-CNU and CZT against rat leukaemia L5222 (Fig. 3) demonstrate cytostatic efficacy, optimal dose and toxic dose range (Zeller *et al.*, 1979). HECNU and acetamido-CNU induced an 800% increase in life span (ILS) and effected high cure rates at several doses, whereas CZT was only marginally active.

Table 1 shows the LD_{50} values and the activity of these compounds against Walker 256 carcinosarcoma in rats (Fiebig *et al.*, 1980). BCNU was less active than HECNU and

---

[1] In preparation

Fig. 3. Antineoplastic activity of 2-chloroethyl-*N*-nitrosoureas against preterminal rat leukaemia L5222. Each point represents the mean of six animals; figures are numbers of cures observed. BCNU, 1,3-bis(2-chloroethyl)-1-nitrosourea; acetamido-CNU, 1-(2-chloroethyl)-1-nitroso-3-methylene-carboxamido-urea; HECNU, 1-(2-chloroethyl)-1-nitroso-3-(2-hydroxyethyl)urea; CZT, 2-[3-(2-chloroethyl)-3-nitrosoureido]-D-desoxyglucopyranose-(chlorozotozin). Nucl., nucleophile or nucleoside

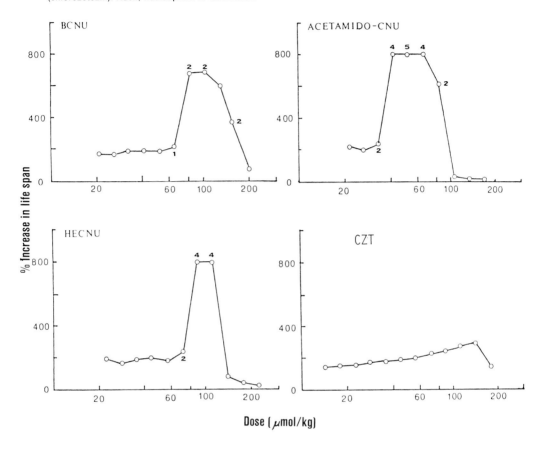

Dose (μmol/kg)

Table 1.   Comparative effectiveness of 2-chloroethyl-*N*-nitrosoureas against subcutaneously implanted Walker carcinosarcoma in the rat

Substance[a]	LD 50[b] (mg/kg)	ED 50[c] (mg/kg)	LD 50 / ED 50
BCNU	25	11.9	2.1
HECNU	25	8.6	2.9
CZT	27	not reached	–
Acetamido CNU	20	7.4	2.4

[a] BCNU, 1,3-bis(2-chloroethyl)-nitrosourea; HECNU, 1-(2-chloroethyl)-1-nitroso-3-(2-hydroxyethyl)urea; CZT, chlorozotozin 2-[3-(2-chloroethyl)-3-nitrosoureido]-D-desoxyglucopyranose)
[b] Period of observation, 60 days
[c] Dose that caused 50% inhibition of tumour weight gain

Table 2.   Antineoplastic effectiveness of 2-chloroethyl-N-nitrosoureas in transplantation tumours (optimal doses)

Substance[a]	Mouse-colon 26		Mouse-mammary Ca 16		Mouse-Lewis lung		% animals with metastases	% T/C
	dose mg/kg	% cures	dose mg/kg	% T/C[b]	dose mg/kg	% TW1[c]		
BCNU	40	35	30	178	40	61	55	203
Me-CCNU	40	60	40	181	30	75	35	>225
CZT	40	25	40	179	30	54	70	191
HECNU	20	55	20	187	20	69	50	215

[a] BCNU, 1,3-bis(2-chloroethyl)-1-nitrosourea; Me-CCNU, 1-(2-chloroethyl)-1-nitroso-3-(4-methyl)cyclohexylnitroso-urea; CZT, chlorozotozin (2-[3-(2-chloroethyl)-3-nitrosoureido]-D-desoxyglucopyranose); HECNU, 1-(2-chloroethyl)-1-nitroso-3-(2-hydroxyethyl)urea

[b] % increase in lifetime ($\frac{\text{test}}{\text{control}} \times 100$)

[c] % inhibition of tumour weight gain ($\frac{\text{control-treated}}{\text{control}} \times 100$)

acetamido-CNU; CZT did not reach the ED_{50} (dose that caused 50% inhibition of tumour weight gain) level of activity in this system. Similar differences in activity against murine transplantation tumours were seen for optimal doses of BCNU, Me-CCNU, CZT and HECNU (Table 2). For colon 26 and mammary 16 carcinoma, HECNU had the lowest optimal dose (20 mg/kg), displaying an activity about equal to that of the best clinically used analogue, Me-CCNU (40 mg/kg). In Lewis lung carcinoma, the optimal dose of Me-CCNU was again higher than that for HECNU (30 versus 20 mg/kg). As a further example, Table 3 shows a comparison of antimetastatic activities against anaplastic mammary carcinoma in the mouse[1]. HECNU and acetamido-CNU had the greatest antimetastatic effectiveness at the lowest optimal doses of all the substances tested.

HECNU has been found to be particularly active against intracerebrally implanted tumours, such as anaplastic mammary mouse carcinoma[1], murine ependymoblastoma[2] and astrocytoma HT60 in the rat (Fiebig & Schmähl, 1979). The superiority of HECNU in the treatment of intracerebrally implanted tumours is exemplified in Table 4. At a maximal nontoxic dose, HECNU had remarkably greater activity against murine leukaemias L1210-Cr (non-immunogenic) and L1210-Ha (highly immunogenic) after intraperitoneal or intracerebral inoculation; the same phenomenon was observed in the treatment of late intracerebrally implanted rat leukaemia L5222 (Zeller et al., 1978; Spreafico et al., 1981). For BCNU and Me-CCNU, the effectiveness was clearly better on the immunogenic line, whereas for HECNU and CZT, effectiveness appears to be independent of tumour immunogenicity (Spreafico et al., 1981).

Therapy with HECNU of human xenografts implanted subcutaneously into nude mice, yielded partial remissions for colon carcinoma 158, soft-tissue sarcoma 81 and Wilms' tumour 162. Complete remission was obtained with gastric carcinoma 97; colon carcinoma 280 was cured. Dose-response studies showed HECNU to be more active than another third-generation CNU, 1-(4-amino-2-methylpyrimidine-5-yl)-methyl-3-(2-chloroethyl)-3-nitrosourea hydrochloride (ACNU). Seven further colon carcinoma xenografts were resistant to CNU therapy (Fiebig, 1982).

[1] Radacic et al., in preparation
[2] Atassi et al., in preparation

Table 3. Antitumour effect of 2-chloroethyl-N-nitrosoureas on spontaneous lung metastases of murine anaplastic mammary carcinoma[a]

Substance[b]	Dose (mg/kg)	Number of lung metastases	Mean
HECNU	20	0; 0; 0; 0; 0; 0; 0; 1; 3; 9	1.3
BCNU	25	8; 8; 14; 17; 25; 29; 30; 50; 50; 50	36
CCNU	25	0; 4; 14; 18; 21; 23; 24; 36; 50; 50	24
Acetamido-CNU	15	0; 0; 0; 0; 1; 1; 1; 3; 3; 5	1.4
Cyclophosphamide	200	0; 1; 3; 6; 10; 12; 18; 21; 23	10.5
Control	–	6; 10; 14; 22; 23; 26; 34; 46; 50; 56	28.7

[a] Treatment on day 7 after inoculation. All animals were killed when untreated controls began to die (Radacic et al., in preparation)
[b] HECNU, 1-(2-chloroethyl)-1-nitroso-3-(2-hydroxyethyl)urea; BCNU, 1,3-bis(2-chloroethyl)-1-nitrosourea; CCNU, 1-(2-chloroethyl)-1-nitroso-3-(4-methyl)cyclohexylnitrosourea; Acetamido-CNU, 1-(2-Chloroethyl)-1-nitroso-3-methylene-carboxamidourea

Table 4. Antineoplastic activity of 2-chloroethyl-N-nitrosoureas against transplanted leukaemias

Substance[a]	Mouse dose (mg/kg)	L 1210 Cr.i.p. (% cures)	L 1210 Cr.i.c. (% cures)	L 1210 Ha.i.p. (% cures)	Rat dose (mg/kg)	L 5222 i.c. (% cures)
BCNU	30	55	50	85	10	37
Me-CCNU	30	40	35	60		
CZT	20	50	50	45		
HECNU	20	100	100	100	10	100
	10	55	40	55		

[a] BCNU, 1,3-bis(2-chloroethyl)-1-nitrosourea; Me-CCNU, 1-(2-chloroethyl)-1-nitroso-3-(4-methyl)cyclohexylnitrosourea; CZT, chlorozotozin (2-[3-(2-chloroethyl)-3-nitrosoureido]-D-desoxyglucopyranose); HECNU, 1-(2-chloroethyl)-1-nitroso-3-(2-hydroxyethyl)urea
i.p., intraperitoneally; i.c., intracerebrally

Autochthonous tumours are much more difficult models than transplantation tumours. Against 7,12-dimethylbenz[a]anthracene-induced acute leukaemia, HECNU effected significant prolongation of life span, whereas BCNU did not (Berger, 1979). HECNU was not tested against 7,12-dimethylbenz[a]anthracene-induced mammary carcinoma in the rat, but at equitoxic doses acetamido-CNU induced a higher remission rate than did CZT, BCNU or adriamycine (Fiebig et al., 1980). HECNU resulted in the greatest prolongation of life, in comparison with six other CNUs, including those applied clinically, in N-ethyl-nitrosourea-induced neurogenous rat tumours (Strobel, 1980).

LONG-TERM TOXICITY

A series of CNUs was tested comparatively in a life-time study by intravenous application, every six weeks for up to 10 applications, at individual doses of 9.5–150 mg/m², respectively. Treatment was discontinued when massive lethal toxicity became apparent or after the maximal total dose had been reached (Habs, 1980; Eisenbrand et al., 1981). Table 5 summarizes, as an example, results obtained for BCNU and the congeners HECNU, acetamido-CNU and CZT.

Table 5.   Long-term toxicity of nitrosoureas after repeated intravenous application to rats, every six weeks[a]

| | Individual dose (mg/m²) | | | |
	75	38	19	9.5
I. BCNU				
max. number of applications	4	10	10	10
med. total dose (mg/m²)	300	266	152	95
med. survival time (days)	164	263	314	568
(95% confidence range)	(157–211)	(230–312)	(295–410)	(514–588)
II. HECNU				
max. number of applications	10	10	10	10
med. total dose (mg/m²)	565	380	190	95
med. survival time (days)	331	541	572	558
(95% confidence range)	(294–456)	(518–627)	(522–617)	(492–606)
III. CHLOROZOTOCIN				
max. number of applications	–	10	10	10
med. total dose (mg/m²)	–	380	190	95
med. survival time (days)	–	474	590	583
(95% confidence range)	–	(436–513)	(518–613)	(565–638)
IV. ACETAMIDO-CNU				
max. number of applications	5	10	10	10
med. total dose (mg/m²)	375	380	190	95
med. survival time (days)	278	557	672	630
(95% confidence range)	(243–313)	(493–623)	(611–730)	(539–697)

[a] Male Wistar, 30 in groups I–III and 40 in group IV; 120 control animals; medium survivals of controls, 621 days (range, 579–674)

BCNU, 1,3-bis(2-chloroethyl)-1-nitrosourea; HECNU, 1-(2-chloroethyl)-1-nitroso-3-(2-hydroxyethyl)urea
CHLOROZOTOCIN, 2-[3-(2-chloroethyl)-3-nitrosoureido]-D-desoxyglucopyranose
ACETAMIDO-CNU, 1-(2-chloroethyl)-1-nitroso-3-methylene-carboxamido-urea

As can be seen from the median survival times (MST), BCNU had a very strong cumulative lethal toxicity. With 75 mg/m², treatment had to be discontinued after the fourth course because 6/30 animals were already dead at that point, and the MST of the remaining animals was only 164 days. Similar cumulative toxic effects were seen at doses down to 19 mg/m², as exemplified by strong and highly significant reductions in MST when compared with those of untreated controls. In most cases, the cause of death was infection, mainly bronchopneumonia, except in animals that died of tumours. There was no specific organ-related toxicity; in all groups, weight gain was considerably reduced; cachexia was observed with doses of 38 mg/m² and more.

Obviously, the new analogues are considerably less toxic than BCNU, HECNU being best tolerated. Only the highest dosage of HECNU (75 mg/m²) produced a significant reduction in MST; infections were again the most frequently diagnosed cause of death (Habs, 1980; Eisenbrand et al., 1981). Acetamido-CNU was more toxic than HECNU at a dose of 75 mg/m², but still significantly less toxic than BCNU. At lower doses, the reduction in toxicity of the new analogues remains impressive compared to that of BCNU; only at the lowest dose level (9.5 mg/m²) was no significant difference seen.

CZT could not be given repeatedly at doses exceeding 38 mg/m². Almost one-third of the animals receiving a single dose of 75 mg/m² died within 14 days, and about 80% of this group were dead by day 200. In all cases, haemorrhagic pneumonia was found to be lethal. At a dose of 38 mg/m², MST was significantly reduced; the most prominent toxic effect was nephrotoxocity, which was not seen to a comparable extent with any other of the compounds tested. Lungs showed infectious lesions similar to those found with the other compounds.

Table 6. Long-term toxicity of CNUs

Substance [a]/ Parameter	LD 50 [b] (μmol/kg)	Long-term toxicity [c] after repeated intravenous applications (mmol/m²)	DNA cross-linking potential in vivo (rad-equiv.) [d]	Inhibition of glutathione-reductase [e] (min)
BCNU	117	0.71	34	20
HECNU	128	2.89	156	60
Acetamido CNU	95	1.80	155	∞
CZT	87	1.22	24	∞

[a] BCNU, 1,3-bis(2-chloroethyl)-1-nitrosourea; HECNU, 1-(2-chloroethyl)-1-nitroso-3-(2-hydroxyethyl)urea; CZT, chlorozotozin (2-[3-(2-chloroethyl)-3-nitrosoureido]-D-desoxyglucopyranose); Acetamido CNU, 1-(2-chloroethyl)-1-nitroso-3-methylene-carboxamido-urea
[b] 60 days' observation, single dose i.p., rat
[c] Median total dose showing first significant decrease of median survival time when compared with that of untreated controls
[d] After 24 h in bone marrow, rats
[e] Human glutathione reductase, time required for 50% inhibition

These results show clearly that there are extreme differences in the long-term toxicities of CNUs after *repeated application*.

Some characteristic biological data for selected CNUs are summarized in Table 6. On a molar base, the single-dose, acute LD_{50} values show BCNU to be about as toxic as HECNU, the latter being less toxic than acetamido-CNU, and CZT being the most toxic. However, toxicity ranking is totally different when considering long-term toxicity after repeated application every 6 weeks (a dose schedule similar to the clinical situation): BCNU is by far the most toxic compound, followed by CZT and acetamido-CNU, HECNU being the least toxic.

Reliable biochemical parameters that might be of use for interpretation, and probably prediction, of toxicity to the host and of cytostatic effectiveness are not yet available. In-vitro carbamoylating activity towards lysine has been found to be high for BCNU, but negligible for HECNU, acetamido-CNU and CZT (Nakra, 1983). The relative alkylating potential, as measured by the 4-nitrobenzylpyridine method (Preussmann *et al.*, 1969), was 3.3 for BCNU, 2.1 for HECNU, 5.1 for acetamido-CNU and 4.9 for CZT (Nakra, 1983). Human erythrocyte glutathione reductase is strongly inhibited by BCNU; HECNU is much less inhibitory; and acetamido-CNU and CZT are not inhibitory[1] (Table 6).

A comparison of the kinetics of formation and removal of DNA-DNA interstrand cross-links in the bone marrow of rats after a single intraperitoneal dose of CNUs (100 μmol/kg) revealed strong differences between HECNU and acetamido-CNU on the one hand and BCNU and CZT on the other. The former agents were much more effective than the latter in inducing interstrand cross-links *in vivo* (Bedford & Eisenbrand, 1984). HECNU, found to be about one-fourth as toxic as BCNU in the long-term study, induced almost five times as many cross-links in the bone marrow than BCNU. Cross-linking in the bone marrow appears therefore to reflect to a greater extent differences in antileukaemic and antitumour effectiveness than acute or chronic toxicities (Bedford & Eisenbrand, 1984) (Table 6).

---

[1] Schirmer *et al.*, in preparation

NEOPLASTIC EFFECTS

All of the CNU derivatives tested in the long-term toxicity study displayed neoplastic effectiveness. However, with the exception of BCNU, the observed tumour incidences were rather low (Habs, 1980; Eisenbrand *et al.*, 1981). There was no common target organ in which all compounds tested increased the risk for neoplastic lesions, although a prevalence for lung and nervous tissue was recognizable, and for these two organs the neoplastic properties of the substances after repeated i.v. application can be regarded as proven.

In this study, BCNU was shown to be a relatively strong carcinogen, inducing a significantly increased risk for lung and neurogenous tumours. Although at a dose of 75 mg/m² it could be applied only four times – because of its strong and cumulative toxicity – within the very short MST of 164 days, malignant neoplasms were seen in the lung (five adenocarcinomas, lethal) and in the brain (one oligodendroglioma, lethal). There was a prevalence for carcinogenic effects in the lung because at all doses tumour incidence in the lungs was higher than that in controls, except for the group given 19 mg/m². Comparison of observed *versus* expected age-standardized tumour incidences and trend test statistics according to Peto *et al.* (1980) revealed a dose-related neoplastic effect on the lung at doses of $\geq$ 38 mg/m² ($p < 0.05$). Despite an inconsistency in the dose-response relationship at the dose 19 mg/m², there was already a significant tumorigenic effect at 9.5 mg/m² when compared with untreated controls (two-tailed $p < 0.0025$) (Habs, 1980).

HECNU was a considerably weaker carcinogen than BCNU, as evidenced by the much higher median total doses applied (Table 5) and longer induction times. Treatment increased the risk for malignant neurogenic tumours ($p < 0.025$). In the two highest dosage groups, incidental benign or pre-malignant lesions were seen in the lung (one bronchiologenic adenoma, three adenomatous hyperplasias), which were treatment-related ($p < 0.05$) (Habs, 1980; Eisenbrand *et al.*, 1981).

There was an indication with BCNU of a reduced incidence of spontaneously occurring pheochromocytomas ($p < 0.1$). For HECNU, a treatment-related decrease in neoplasms of haematopoetic and lymphatic tissue was observed ($p < 0.08$) in this study (Habs, 1980; Eisenbrand *et al.*, 1981).

Results of a further comparative life-time study are given in Table 7. BCNU and HECNU were applied repeatedly by intraperitoneal injection, once a week for up to 52 weeks, at doses of 0.2 and 1.0 mg/kg, respectively. In the higher dosage group, BCNU was again much more toxic (MST, 359 days) than HECNU (MST, 648 days). Although a much higher total dose was reached with the latter, no treatment-related induction of tumours was observed in the intraperitoneal cavity and the total tumour incidence was not higher than in the untreated controls. BCNU, however, showed a clear dose-related local carcinogenic effect, inducing a high yield of malignant neoplasms in the intraperitoneal cavity (Eisenbrand, 1979). In a similar lifetime study, after repeated intraperitoneal application of CZT at comparable doses, it was found to be a very potent carcinogen, inducing a high incidence of local tumours in the intraperitoneal cavity (Habs *et al.*, 1979).

Clinically, BCNU has been the most frequently used CNU derivative since the mid 1960s. It has been associated in case reports with the development of acute nonlymphocytic leukaemia following treatment of primary malignant diseases. However, in all these cases, BCNU was not administered as a single drug but in combination with other anticancer agents suspected or known to be carcinogenic as well. Therefore clear-cut epidemiological evidence to evaluate the carcinogenicity of BCNU in man is not available at present (IARC, 1981).

The experimental results reported here exemplify that within a series of close analogues, remarkable differences can exist with respect to cytostatic, long-term toxic and carcinogenic properties. BCNU was not only found in most experimental chemotherapy studies to be

Table 7. Carcinogenic activity of nitrosoureas after repeated intravenous application to Sprague-Dawley rats

Substance[a]	Number of animals	Individual dose (mg/kg/week)	MST[b] (days)	MTD[c]	Animals with tumours (%)	Local tumours in peritoneal cavity (%)
BCNU	39	0.2	703	0.2	45	30
	37	1.0	359	0.4	46	83
HECNU	35	0.2	682	0.2	15	–
	38	1.0	648	0.7	24	–
Control	37	–	803	–	23	25

[a] BCNU, 1,3-bis(2-chloroethyl)-1-nitrosourea; HECNU, 1-(2-chloroethyl)-1-nitroso-3-(2-hydroxyethyl)urea
[b] Median survival time
[c] Median total dose

inferior to newly developed analogues, such as HECNU, but also exhibited by far the strongest long-term toxic and carcinogenic effects.

In view of the very favourable experimental results obtained for HECNU, this compound was recently entered into a clinical phase I study. It was given intravenously every four to six weeks in doses of 7.5–150 mg/m². Treatment was well tolerated, delayed bone-marrow toxicity being the dose-limiting toxic side effect. Of 47 patients who could be evaluated for antitumour effectiveness (60–150 mg/m²), four went into partial remission, two had a minor regression and seven had no change. The partial remissions were 1/6 epidermoid carcinomas of the lung, 2/7 stomach carcinomas and 1/2 melanomas. Recommended maximal doses are 100 mg/m² for pretreated and 120 mg/m² for non-pretreated patients. Since antitumour effectiveness was observed with a dose as low as 60 mg/m², HECNU appears to have a high therapeutic index (Fiebig *et al.*, 1983).

In summary, these results demonstrate that antitumour activity can be dissociated from the chronic toxicity and carcinogenicity of such compounds. The selection of new candidates for clinical trial should be based, therefore, not only on antitumour activity and acute toxicity but also on the basis of chronic toxicity and carcinogenicity after repeated application.

ACKNOWLEDGEMENTS

Work summarized here was supported in part by the German Ministry for Research and Technology within the project "Drug development and testing for cancer chemotherapy" (BMFT subprojects PTB 8205, 8216, 8217, 8219). A substantial part of the preclinical testing was carried out by the EORTC-screening and pharmacology group.

REFERENCES

Ahlgren, J.D., Green, D.S., Tew, K.D. & Schein, P. (1982) Repair of DNA alkylation induced in L1210 leukemia and murine bone marrow by three chloroethylnitrosoureas. *Cancer Res., 42*, 2605–2608

Babson, J.R. & Reed, D.J. (1978) Inactivation of glutathione reductase by 2-chloroethyl nitrosourea-derived isocyanates. *Biochem. biophys. Res. Commun., 83*, 754–762

Bedford, P. & Eisenbrand, G. (1984) DNA damage and repair in the bone marrow of rats treated with four chloroethylnitrosoureas. *Cancer Res., 44*, 514–518

Berger, M. (1979) *Chemotherapie der Rattenleukämie L 5222 und von autochthonen Leukämien, die durch DMBA induziert wurden,* Thesis, University of Heidelberg

Bowden, B.J. & Wheeler, G.P. (1971) Reaction of 1,3-bis(2-chloroethyl)-1-nitrosourea (BCNU), with protein. *Proc. Am. Assoc. Cancer. Res., 12*, 67

Brundrett, R.B. (1980) Chemistry of nitrosoureas, intermediacy of 4,5-dihydro-1,2,3-oxadiazole in 1,3-bis(2-chloroethyl)-1-nitrosourea decomposition. *J. med. Chem., 23*, 1245–1247

Eisenbrand, G. (1979) Carcinogenic action of BCNU analogues after repeated application to SD rats. *Proc. Am. Assoc. Cancer Res., 20*, 46

Eisenbrand, G., Habs, M., Zeller, W.J., Fiebig, H., Berger, M., Zelesny, O. & Schmähl, D. (1981) *New nitrosoureas – Therapeutic and longterm toxic effect of selected compounds in comparison to established drugs.* In: Serrou, B., Schein, P.S. & Imbach, J.L., eds, *Nitrosoureas in Cancer Treatment (INSERM Symposium No. 19),* Paris, INSERM, pp. 175–191

Eisenbrand, G., Fiebig, H. & Zeller, W.J. (1976) Some new congeners of the anticancer agent 1,3-bis (2-chloroethyl)-1-nitrosourea (BCNU). Synthesis of bifunctional analogues and water soluble derivatives and preliminary evaluation of their chemotherapeutic potential. *Z. Krebsforsch., 86*, 279–286

Fiebig, H.H., Eisenbrand, G., Zeller, W.J. & Zentgraf, R. (1980) Anticancer activity of new nitrosoureas against Walker carcinosarcoma 256 and DMBA-induced mammary cancer of the rat. *Oncology, 37,* 177–183

Fiebig, H.H., Schmähl, D. (1979) Development of models for brain tumors in rats and their responsiveness to chemotherapy with nitrosoureas. *Proc. Am. Assoc. Cancer Res., 20,* 276

Fiebig, H.H. (1982) Wachstum und Chemotherapie menschlicher Tumoren in der thymusaplastischen Maus. *Habil-Schrift Med. Fak. Univ. Freiburg,* Federal Republic of Germany

Fiebig, H.H., Schuchhardt, C., Henss, H., Eisenbrand, G. & Löhr, G.-W. (1983) Phase I-study of the watersoluble nitrosourea 1-(2-hydroxyethyl)-3-(2-chloroethyl)-3-nitrosourea (HECNU). *Proc. Am. Assoc. Cancer Res., 24,* 139

Fornace, A.J., Jr, Kohn, K.W. & Kann, H.E. (1978) Inhibition of the ligasestep of excision repair by 2-chloroethyl isocyanate, a decomposition product of 1,3-bis (2-chloroethyl)-1-nitrosourea. *Cancer Res., 38,* 1064–1069

Frisher, H. & Ahmad, T. (1977) Severe generalized glutathione reductase deficiency after antitumour chemotherapy with BCNU [1,3-bis (2-chloroethyl)-1-nitrosourea]. *J. Lab. clin. Med., 89,* 1080–1091

Habs, M. (1980) *Experimentelle Untersuchungen zur Cancerogenen Wirkung zytostatischer Arzneimittel,* Habilitationsschrift, University of Heidelberg

Habs, M. Eisenbrand, G. & Schmähl, D. (1979) Carcinogenic activity in Sprague-Dawley rats of 2-[3-(2-chloroethyl)-3-nitrosoureido] D-glucopyranose (Chlorozotocin). *Cancer Lett., 8,* 133–137

Heal, J.W., Fox, P.A. & Schein, P.S. (1979) Effect of carbamoylation on the repair of nitrosourea-induced DNA alkylation damage in L 1210 cells. *Cancer Res., 39,* 82–89

IARC (1981) *IARC Monographs on the Evaluation of the Carcinogenic Risk of Chemicals to Humans,* Vol. 26, *Some Antineoplastic and Immunosuppressive Agents,* Lyon, pp. 79–95

Johnston, T.P., McCaleb, G.S. & Montgomery, I.A. (1975) Synthesis of chlorozotocin, the 2-chloroethyl analog of the anticancer antibiotic streptozotocin. *J. med. Chem., 18,* 104–106

Kann, H.E., Jr, Schott, M.A. & Petkas, A. (1980) Effects of structure and chemical activity on the ability of nitrosoureas to inhibit DNA repair. *Cancer Res., 40,* 50–55

Lown, J.W. & Chauhan, S.M.S. (1981) Mechanism of action of (2-haloethyl) nitrosoureas on DNA. *J. med. Chem., 24,* 270–279

Ludlum, D.P. & Tong, W.P. (1981) *Modification of DNA and RNA bases by the nitrosoureas.* In: Serrou, B., Schein, P.S. & Imbach, J.L., eds, *Nitrosoureas in Cancer Treatment, (INSERM Symposium No. 19),* Paris, INSERM, pp. 21–31

McConnell, W.R., Kari, P. & Hill, D.L. (1979) Reduction of Glutathione levels in livers of mice treated with *N,N'*-bis (2-chloroethyl)*N*-nitrosourea. *Cancer Chemother. Pharmacol., 2,* 221–223

Montgomery, J.A. (1981) *The development of the nitrosoureas: A study in congener synthesis.,* In: Prestayko, A.W., Baker, L.H., Crooke, S.T., Carter, S.K. & Schein, P.S. eds, *Nitrosoureas, Current Status and New Developments,* New York, Academic Press, pp. 3–8

Nakra, M. (1983) *Untersuchungen zu Struktur-Wirkungs-Beziehungen einiger heterocyclischer N-(2-chloroethyl)-N-nitrososemicarbazide und N-(2-chloroethyl)-N-nitrosoharnstoffe,* PhD Thesis, University of Heidelberg

Peto, R., Pike, M.C., Day, N.E., Gray, R.G., Lee, P.N., Parish, S., Peto, J., Richards, S. & Wahrendorf, J. (1980) *Guidelines for simple sensitive significance tests for carcinogenic effects in long-term animal experiments.* In: *IARC Monographs on the Evaluation of the Carcinogenic Risk of Chemicals to Humans,* Suppl. 2, *Long-term and Short-term Screening Assays for Carcinogens, a Critical Appraisal,* Lyon, pp. 311–426

Preussmann, R., Schneider, H. & Epple, F. (1969) Untersuchungen zum Nachweis alkylierender Agentien II. Der Nachweis verschiedener Klassen alkylierender Agentien mit einer Modifikation der Farbreaktion mit 4-(4-Nitrobenzyl)-pyridin (NBP). *Arzneimittel.-Forsch. (Drug. Res.), 19,* 1059–1073

Reed, D.J. (1981) *Metabolism of nitrosoureas.* In: Prestayko, A.W., Baker, L.H., Crooke, S.T., Carter, S.K. & Schein, P.S., eds, *Nitrosoureas, Current Status and New Developments,* New York, Academic Press, pp. 51–67

Spreafico, I., Filippeschi, S., Falautano, P., Eisenbrand, G., Fiebig, H.H., Habs, M., Zeller, W.J., Schmähl, D., van Putten, L.M. & Smink, T. (1981) *The development of novel nitrosoureas.* In: Prestayko, A.W., Crooke, S.T., Baker, L.H., Carter, S.K. & Schein, P.S., eds, *Nitrosoureas, Current Status and New Developments,* New York, Academic Press, pp. 175–191

Strobel, H. (1980) *Autochtone, chemisch induzierte, neurogene Tumoren der Ratte als Modelle für chemotherapeutische Studien,* Thesis, University of Heidelberg

Talley, R.W., Samson, M.K., Brownlee, R.W., Samhouri, A.M., Fraile, R.J. & Baker, L.H. (1981) Phase II evaluation of chlorozotocin (NSC-178248) in advanced human cancer. *Eur. J. Cancer,* **17,** 337–343

Tong, W.P. & Ludlum, D.B. (1979) Mechanism of action of the nitrosoureas. III. reaction of bis-chloroethyl nitrosourea and bis-fluoroethyl nitrosourea with adenosine. *Biochem. Pharmacol.,* **28,** 1175–1179

Tong, W.P., Kirk, M.C. & Ludlum, D.P. (1981) Molecular pharmacology of the haloethyl nitrosoureas: formation of 6-hydroxyethylguanine in DNA treated with BCNU. *Biochem. biophys. Res. Commun.,* **100,** 351–357

Tong, W.P., Kirk, M.C. & Ludlum, D.B. (1982) Formation of cross-link 1^1-[N^3-deoxycytidyl], 2-[N^1-deoxyguanosinyl]-ethane in DNA treated with *N,N′*bis(2-chloroethyl)-*N*-nitrosourea. *Cancer Res.,* **42,** 3102–3105

Zeller, W.J., Eisenbrand, G. & Fiebig, H.H. (1978) Chemotherapeutic activity of new 2-chloroethylnitrosoureas in rat leukemia L5222. Comparison of bifunctional and water-soluble derivatives with BCNU. *J. natl Cancer Inst.,* **60,** 345–348

Zeller, W.J., Eisenbrand, G. & Fiebig, H.H. (1979) Examination of four newly synthesized 2-chloroethylnitrosoureas in comparison with BCNU, CCNU, MeCCNU. Chlorozotocin and Hydroxyethyl-CNU in preterminal rat leukemia L 5222. *J. Cancer Res. clin. Oncol.,* **95,** 43–49

INTERACTION OF BIS- AND MONO-*N*-NITROSOUREAS WITH RAT LIVER CHROMATIN *IN VITRO*

K. MORIMOTO & T. YAMAHA

National Institute of Hygienic Sciences, Tokyo, 158, Japan

SUMMARY

The effects of nine *N*-nitrosoureas (three bis-*N*-nitrosoureas, five mono-*N*-nitrosoureas and chloroethyl-*N*-nitrosourea) on the template activity of rat liver chromatin and *Escherichia coli* DNA were compared. The template activity of rat liver chromatin was inhibited by some *N*-nitrosoureas that have relatively strong alkylating activity. The inhibitory effects with respect to *E. coli* DNA were stronger than those with respect to rat liver chromatin. The inhibitory effects had a tendency to decrease with increasing length of the alkyl chain. The template activity of rat liver chromatin was slightly increased by some *N*-nitrosoureas, potassium cyanate and some alkyl isocyanates. The chromatin reacting with 1,1′-ethylene-bis-(1-nitrosourea) was more sensitive than the control chromatin to DNase 1 and *Staphylococcal* nuclease. The solubility of chromatin carbamoylated by 1,1′-ethylene-bis-(1-nitrosourea) was clearly higher than that of control chromatin in the presence of magnesium or calcium ion.

INTRODUCTION

Since the biological activities of *N*-nitrosoureas are based principally on their abilities to alkylate and carbamoylate cell constituents, it is interesting to compare these biological effects in a series of bisureido-type nitrosoureas (bis-*N*-nitrosourea), which have antitumour activity, and in a series of monoureido-type nitrosoureas (mono-*N*-nitrosourea), which have both antitumour and carcinogenic activities.

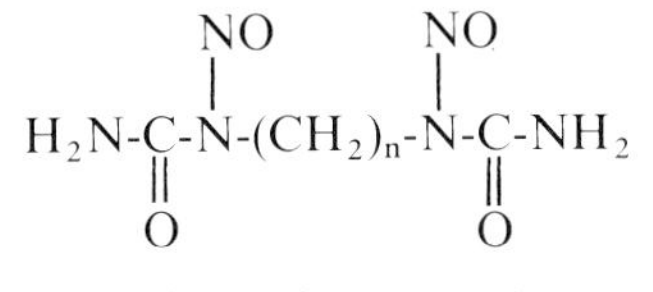

$$\begin{array}{ccccc} & NO & & NO & \\ & | & & | & \\ H_2N-C-N-(CH_2)_n-N-C-NH_2 \\ & \| & & \| & \\ & O & & O & \end{array}$$

(bis-*N*-nitrosourea)

The purpose of this paper is to summarize our recent observations (Morimoto & Yamaha, 1982a,b) on the interaction of *N*-nitrosoureas with rat liver chromatin *in vitro*.

MATERIALS AND METHODS

Materials

N-nitrosoureas: 1,1'-ethylene-bis(1-nitrosourea) (EDNU); 1,1'-propylene-bis(1-nitrosourea) (PDNU);1,1'-hexamethylene-bis(1-nitrosourea) (HxDNU); *N*-methyl-*N*-nitrosourea (MNU); *N*-ethyl-*N*-nitrosourea (ENU); *N*-propyl-*N*-nitrosourea (PNU); *N*-butyl-*N*-nitrosourea (BNU); *N*-isobutyl-*N*-nitrosourea (i-BNU); *N*-(2-chloroethyl)-*N*'-cyclohexyl-1-nitrosourea (CCNU) were obtained from Dr M. Nakadate of this Institute. Chromatin was prepared from rat liver (Wistar male, 150–200 g) by the intermediate ionic strength method (Garrard & Hancock, 1978). This chromatin was then sheared in a Dounce homogenizer (tight pestle) in 10 mmol/L Tris-hydrochloric acid or boric acid-borax buffer (pH 8.0) containing 0.2 mmol/L EDTA. The homogenate was centrifuged for 10 min at $1200 \times g$. The supernatant solution was used for chromatin determination.

Reaction of N-*nitrosoureas and related compounds with rat liver chromatin and* E. coli *DNA*

N-Nitrosoureas and related compounds were preincubated with chromatin or *E. coli* DNA (175–300 µg DNA per mL) at pH 8.0 and 37°C for 6.5 h. After dialysis against 10 mmol/L Tris-hydrochloric acid buffer (pH 8.0), the biological activity was assayed.

Determination of template activity

Template activity was determined by the method of Marushige (1976).

Digestion of chromatin

Digestion by DNase 1 (Grade 1, Boehringer Mannheim, GmbH; 3.5 units/mL) was performed in 10 mmol/L Tris-hydrochloric acid buffer (pH 8.0) and 0.3 mmol/L magnesium chloride, at 37°C. Digestion by *Staphylococcal* nuclease (Boehringer Mannheim, GmbH; 15 units/mL) was performed in 10 mmol/L Tris-hydrochloric acid buffer (pH 8.0) and 0.3 mmol/L calcium chloride, at 37° C. Percent digestion was determined by the method of Jahn and Litman (1979).

Solubility of rat liver chromatin reacted with N-*nitrosourea*

The chromatin was adjusted to the desired concentration in magnesium chloride or calcium chloride and centrifuged at 4°C for 10 min at $1500 \times g$. The absorbance of the supernatant at 260 nm was measured, and the value was expressed as percentage of total absorbance.

RESULTS AND DISCUSSION

Effects of N-*nitrosoureas and related compounds on template activity*

The inhibition of template activity of rat liver chromatin was dependent on the concentration of EDNU from 1 mmol/L to 4 mmol/L. This activity was inhibited by 4 mmol/L EDNU, PDNU, MNU, ENU and CCNU. The inhibitory effects had a tendency to decrease with increasing length of the alkyl chain (Fig. 1). The inhibitory effects with respect to *E.coli* DNA

Fig. 1. Effects of *N*-nitrosoureas on template activity of rat liver chromatin and *Escherichia coli* DNA
Template activity of control without *N*-nitrosourea was 100%. □, bis-*N*-nitrosourea; ■, mono-*N*-nitrosourea;
▨, chloroethyl-*N*-nitrosourea

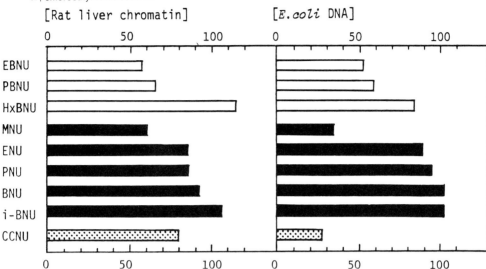

were greater than those of rat liver chromatin (Fig.1). In our previous work (Morimoto *et al.*, 1978), chemical stability, alkylating activity and lipophilicity of these *N*-nitrosoureas were compared. The inhibitory effects with respect to *E.coli* DNA coincided with the order of alkylating activity measured by the 4-(*p*-nitrobenzyl)pyridine method, except for CCNU. We have already reported that *E.coli* DNA was cross-linked by CCNU (Morimoto *et al.*, 1980). The high inhibition by CCNU might thus be due to cross-linking action.

Although the template activity of rat liver chromatin was slightly increased by HxDNU and i-BNU, that of *E. coli* DNA was not. We therefore investigated the effects of various kinds of acylating agents. Template activity was greatly increased by acetic anhydride and slightly increased by potassium cyanate and some alkyl isocyanates (methyl, ethyl, *n*-propyl and *n*-butyl). Marushige (1976) reported that the activity of calf thymus chromatin is markedly increased by modification of the histones with acetic anhydride. In our study as well, template activity was greatly increased by acetic anhydride. The order of binding to rat liver chromatin was acetic anhydride[1-^{14}C] >> EDNU[carbonyl-^{14}C] > ENU[carbonyl-^{14}C] > ^{14}C-potassium cyanate. The extent of modification of nuclear protein may be related to the increase of template activity. These results suggest that alkylation of DNA in chromatin decreases template activity, and carbamoylation of nuclear protein increases template activity. In most *N*-nitrosoureas, the effects of alkylation may be much stronger than those of carbamoylation, except for HxDNU and i-BNU.

Effects of nuclease sensitivity and solubility of N-*nitrosourea-treated chromatin*

The carbamoylating activity of EDNU for histone and poly-lysine was at least two-fold greater than that of MNU, ENU, and PNU (Morimoto *et al.*, 1979). N^6-Carbamoyllysine was the main reaction product of EDNU[carbonyl-^{14}C] and poly-lysine (Morimoto *et al.*, 1981), and EDNU was therefore chosen to study the effects of carbamoylation of rat liver chromatin.

Fig. 2. Digestion of rat liver chromatin treated with 1,1′-ethylenebis(1-nitrosourea) (EDNU) by DNase I and *Staphylococcal* nuclease. ●, control; □, EDNU (2 mmol/L); ■, EDNU (4 mmol/L)

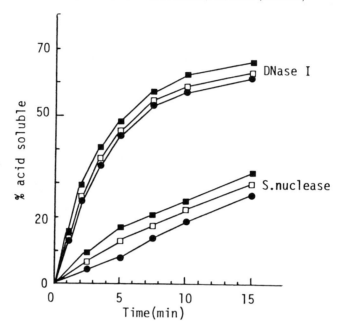

Fig. 3. Effects of magnesium chloride and calcium chloride on solubility of *N*-nitrosourea-treated chromatin. ●, control; □, 1,1′-ethylenebis (1-nitrosourea) (EDNU) (2 mmol/L); ■, EDNU (4 mmol/L); ○, *N*-ethyl-*N*-nitrosourea (ENU) (4 mmol/L)

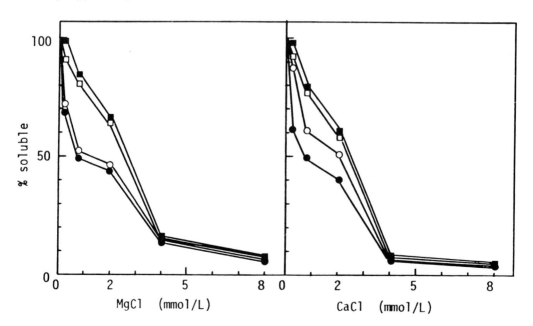

As shown in Figure 2, the sensitivity of chromatin to DNase and *Staphylococcal* nuclease was slightly increased after treatment with EDNU.

We also compared the solubility of control chromatin and EDNU- or ENU-reacted chromatin in various concentrations of magnesium chloride and calcium chloride (Fig. 3) The solubility of chromatin reacted with EDNU was clearly higher than that of the control chromatin. Wallace *et al.* (1977) reported that acetylation of rat liver chromatin has dramatic effects on magnesium solubility and nuclease sensitivity. Although the effect of carbomoylation is not as great as that of acetylation, the carbamoylation of nuclear protein might have a significant effect on DNA-histone interactions.

ACKNOWLEDGEMENTS

The authors wish to thank the Deputy Director, Dr I. Suzuki, and Dr A. Tanaka and Dr M. Nakadate, National Institute of Hygienic Sciences, and Professor Y. Kawazoe, Nagoya City University, for their valuable advice and encouragement.

This work was supported in part by a Grant-in-aid for Cancer Research from the Ministry of Education, Science and Culture, Japan.

REFERENCES

Garrard, W.T. & Hancock, R. (1978) Preparation of chromatin from animal tissues and cultured cells. *Meth.Cell Biol.*, *17*, 27–50

Jahn, C.L. & Litman, G.W. (1979) Accessibility of deoxyribonucleic acid in chromatin to the covalent binding of the chemical carcinogen benzo[a]pyrene. *Biochemistry*, *18*, 1442–1449

Marushige, K. (1976) Activation of chromatin by acetylation of histone side chains. *Proc. natl Acad. Sci., USA*, *73*, 3937–3941

Morimoto, K. & Yamaha, T. (1982a) Effects of EBNU and related compounds on template activity of rat liver chromatin. *Yakugaku-zasshi*, *102*, 452–457 (in Japanese)

Morimoto, K. & Yamaha, T. (1982b) Carbamoylation and biological change of rat liver chromatin by EBNU and related compounds. *Yakugaku-zasshi*, *102*, 859–865 (in Japanese)

Morimoto, K. Yamaha, T., Nakadate, M. & Suzuki I. (1978) Chemical stability, alkylating activity, and lipophilicity of EBNU and related compounds. *Gann*, *69*, 139–142

Morimoto, K., Tanaka, A. & Yamaha, T. (1979) Comparative binding studies on EBNU and some 1-alkyl-1-nitrosoureas with nucleic acids and proteins *in vitro*. *Gann*, *70*, 693–698

Morimoto, K., Yoshikawa, K. & Yamaha, T. (1980) Comparative studies on the mutagenicity of EBNU and related compounds in *Escherichia coli* in relation to the formation of DNA interstrand cross-links. *Gann*, *71*, 674–678

Morimoto, K., Tanaka, A., Sato, M. & Yamaha, T. (1981) Modification of poly-L-lysine by treatment with EBNU *in vitro*. *Gann*, *72*, 189–196

Wallace, R.B., Sargent, T.D., Murphy R.F. & Bonner, J. (1977) Physical properties of chemically acetylated rat liver chromatin. *Proc. natl Acad. Sci. USA*, *74*, 3244–3248

MUTAGENICITY OF α-HYDROXY N-NITROSAMINES IN V79 CHINESE HAMSTER CELLS

M. MOCHIZUKI, M. OSABE, T. ANJO, K. TAKEDA, E. SUZUKI & M. OKADA

Tokyo Biochemical Research Institute, Tokyo, Japan

SUMMARY

N-Nitrosodialkylamines are activated metabolically by α-hydroxylation. Chemical properties and bacterial mutagenicity of α-hydroxy N-nitrosamines have been reported previously. This paper describes potent and direct mutagenicity of four N-nitroso-N-(hydroxymethyl)alkylamines in V79 Chinese hamster cells, using ouabain resistance as an indicator. The mutagenic potency depended on the alkyl group, decreasing in the following order: methyl > ethyl > propyl, butyl. A similar order was observed for cytotoxicity. Mutagenic and cytotoxic potencies of these α-hydroxy N-nitrosamines in V79 cells were well correlated not only with those of model compounds (α-acetoxy and α-hydroperoxy N-nitrosamines), but also with their alkylating ability, measured by alkylation of thiophenol. The mutagenic activity of the α-hydroxy N-nitrosamines in V79 cells was shown to be parallel to that in *Salmonella typhimurium* TA1535 and to that of N-nitrosodialkylamines in V79 cells, after metabolic activation by rat hepatocytes. The results obtained here further support the conclusion that the α-hydroxy N-nitrosamine is the active species in the metabolic activation of carcinogenic and mutagenic N-nitrosodialkylamines.

INTRODUCTION

N-Nitrosodialkylamines are activated metabolically before they act as carcinogens and mutagens. α-Hydroxy N-nitrosamines are most probably the activated form. The synthesis of α-hydroxy N-nitrosamines (Mochizuki *et al.*, 1980) and their direct and potent mutagenicity in *Salmonella typhimurium* and *Escherichia coli* have been reported recently (Mochizuki *et al.*, 1982). In contrast, α-hydroperoxy and α-acetoxy N-nitrosamines are good models of unstable α-hydroxy N-nitrosamines, since they are easily converted to α-hydroxy compounds in biological systems. Mutagenicity and cytotoxicity of these two types of model compounds in V79 Chinese hamster cells have also been reported earlier (Huang *et al.*, 1981; Kohda *et al.*, 1982).

This paper describes the mutagenic and cytotoxic activities of α-hydroxy N-nitrosamines in V79 Chinese hamster cells and compares these biological activities with their alkylating reactivities. A comparison of these biological activities with those of their models is also reported. The mutagenic activities in V79 cells are compared with their bacterial mutagenicities and also with a reported mutagenicity of parent compounds in this mammalian system, after metabolic activation by rat hepatocytes.

MATERIALS AND METHODS

Chemicals

N-Nitroso-*N*-(hydroxymethyl)alkylamines were synthesized by deoxygenation of the corresponding *N*-nitroso-*N*-(hydroperoxymethyl)alkylamines as described by Mochizuki *et al.* (1980).

Cell culture and mutagenicity assay

The V79 Chinese hamster cells (kindly provided by Dr T. Kuroki, Institute of Medical Science, University of Tokyo) were treated as described by Huang *et al.* (1981), with some modifications. The cells, grown in Hanks' solution (pH 5), were treated with the test compound in 25 μL acetonitrile for 30 min at 37 °C. Cytotoxicity (plating efficiency) and mutagenicity (mutation frequency per 10^5 surviving cells) were determined by a method already described (Huang *et al.*, 1981).

Alkylation of thiophenol

α-Hydroxy *N*-nitrosamine (25 μmol) in 1 mL of acetonitrile was mixed with potassium thiophenolate (250 μmol) in 4 mL of 0.1 mol/L phosphate buffer (pH 7.4). After standing at room temperature for 60 min, the mixture was extracted with 2 mL ethyl acetate. The organic layer was washed with 10% sodium carbonate and was dried over anhydrous sodium sulfate. Alkyl phenyl sulfides formed were analysed by gas-liquid chromatography on OV-17, using a flame-ionization detector. The alkylating reactivity was expressed as a percentage yield of alkylated products, relative to the amount of α-hydroxy *N*-nitrosamine used (Table 1). Standard errors, calculated from at least four experiments, were 5.9% (methyl), 0.4% (ethyl), 0.2% (propyl) and 0.3% (butyl).

RESULTS

Effects of pH on cytotoxicity and mutagenicity

α-Hydroxy *N*-nitrosamines are unstable in aqueous solutions, and the rate of decomposition is a function of pH. The longest half-lives, 6-7 min, were observed at pH 3-5 (Mochizuki *et al.*, 1980). Thus, the effect of pH of the incubation mixture on the cells was investigated using ethyl methanesulfonate as a positive control. No significant difference was observed in the cytotoxicity and mutagenicity between pH 7 (Eagle's minimal essential medium) and pH 5 (Hanks' solution) at sample concentrations up to 28 mmol/L.

Effect of alkyl group on cytotoxicity and mutagencity

The cytotoxicity was dose-dependent, as shown in Figure 1. The methyl compound had the highest cytotoxicity, followed by the ethyl, then the propyl and butyl compounds. By comparison of LD_{37}, calculated as shown in the table, the methyl compound was about five

Fig. 1. Dose-response curves of the mutagenicity (top) and cytotoxicity (bottom) of *N*-nitroso-*N*-(hydroxymethyl)alkyl-amines in V79 Chinese hamster cells

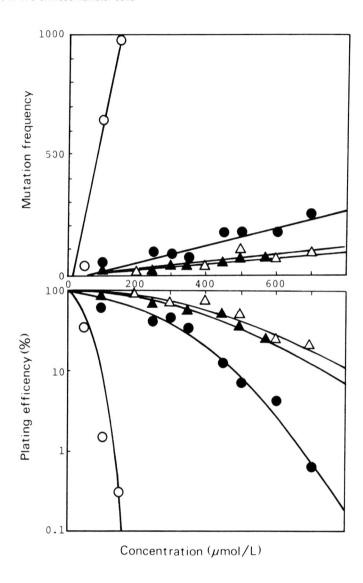

times more toxic than the ethyl compound, which was more toxic than the propyl and butyl compounds.

The highest mutation frequency was also observed with the methyl compound. The effect of the alkyl group on the biological activities was dose-dependent, decreasing in the following order: methyl > ethyl > propyl, butyl. The mutation frequency at 100 µmol/L is shown in Table 1.

Table 1. Effect of alkyl group on properties of N-nitroso-N-(hydroxymethyl)alkylamines and related compounds

Compound[a]	Assay System	Alkyl Group				Correlation[b]	
		Methyl	Ethyl	Propyl	Butyl	I[c]	II[d]
Mutation frequency per 10⁵ survived cells at 100 µmol/L							
α-OH	V79 cells[e]	588	18.6	7.7	7.2	1	
α-OOH	V79 cells[f]	3 700	400	56	46	0.9972**	
α-OAc	V79 cells[g]	2 000	200	43	50	0.9983**	
dialkyl	V79 cells[h]	25.8	4.5	3.2	1.4	0.9954**	
α-OH	Salmonella[i]	17 500	4 900	460	390	0.9699*	
Alkylating reactivity[j]							
α-OH	thiophenol	39.8	4.2	2.7	3.0	0.9998**	0.9989**
Cytotoxicity (mmol/L)⁻¹[k]							
α-OH	V79 cells (1/LD₃₇)[l]	16.9	3.17	1.82	2.03	0.9980**	1
α-OOH	V79 cells (1/D₀)[f]	149	18.9	5.46	<3.33		0.9996**
α-OAc	V79 cells (1/D₀)[g]	238	25.6	15.4	18.5		0.9991**

[a] α-OH, N-nitroso-N-(hydroxymethyl)alkylamine; α-OOH, N-nitroso-N-(hydroperoxymethyl)alkylamine; α-OAc, N-nitroso-N-(acetoxymethyl)alkylamine; dialkyl, N-nitrosodialkylamine
[b] Correlation coefficients calculated: *, $p < 0.02$; **, $p < 0.01$
[c] Correlation with mutation frequency of α-hydroxy N-nitrosamines
[d] Correlation with cytotoxicity of α-hydroxy N-nitrosamines
[e] Calculated by the least squares method from the best fit model; mutation frequency, $m_0 + m_1 \times$ (dose)
[f] Kohda et al. (1982)
[g] Huang et al. (1981)
[h] Jones & Huberman (1980)
[i] Calculated from data in Mochizuki et al. (1982) (revertants/µmol per plate)
[j] Percentage yield of alkyl phenyl sulfide relative to α-hydroxy compounds
[k] Reciprocal values of LD_{37} or D_0 (mM)
[l] Calculated by the least squares method from the best fit model; plating efficiency $= \exp[-k_2(\text{dose})^2]$

Effect of alkyl group on alkylating potency

The yield of alkyl phenyl sulfides produced by alkylation of thiophenol with the α-hydroxy N-nitrosamines is also shown in Table 1. It was dependent on the alkyl group and was highest with the methyl compound, followed by the ethyl, then by the propyl and butyl compounds, the yields with the last two being almost the same. Thus, the alkylating ability decreased with increasing alkyl chain length. With the propyl and butyl compounds, small amounts of isopropyl phenyl sulfide and sec-butyl phenyl sulfide were obtained as the isomerized products arising from the alkylating intermediates in yields of 3.9 and 3.0% of the total propylated and butylated products, respectively.

DISCUSSION

α-Hydroxy N-nitrosamines are unstable intermediates in the metabolic activation of N-nitrosamines: they decompose in aqueous solution and give alkylating species, after releasing aldehydes (Mochizuki et al., 1980). Their biological activity was shown by mutagenicity measurements in S. typhimurium TA1535 and E. coli WP2 and and WP2 hcr⁻ (Mochizuki et al., 1982). In the present work, they were further shown to be mutagenic in a mammalian system.

The mutagenic potency of the α-hydroxy N-nitrosamines in V79 cells is highly correlated with that in S. typhimurium, as shown in Table 1, but not with that in E. coli. A linear correlation between their mutagenic and cytotoxic potencies and alkylating reactivity (methyl > ethyl > propyl, butyl), as seen in the table, suggests that alkylation is deeply associated with the induction of mutagenicity and cytotoxicity.

α-Hydroperoxy and α-acetoxy N-nitrosamines are good models for the unstable α-hydroxy N-nitrosamines. The mutagenic and cytotoxic activities of these model compounds in V79 cells have been reported recently (Huang et al., 1981; Kohda et al., 1982). The present results with the α-hydroxy N-nitrosamines further support their usefulness as model compounds. As shown in the table, a good correlation of the biological activities is demonstrated between the α-hydroxy compounds and the models. The observed differences in the potency of the biological activities is due partly to the instability of the α-hydroxy compounds, compared with the models.

A high correlation was observed for the mutation frequency in V79 cells when comparing the data reported on N-nitrosodialkylamines after metabolic activation by rat hepatocytes (Jones & Huberman, 1980) and those of α-hydroxy N-nitrosamines in the present study (Table 1). Although the α-hydroxy intermediates that can be derived from these N-nitrosodialkylamines by metabolic activation are not necessarily the same as those with a hydroxymethyl group in the present study, they would be expected to give alkylating species similar to those produced from the hydroxymethyl compounds.

The results obtained here further support the conclusion that α-hydroxy N-nitrosamine is the active species in the metabolic activation of carcinogenic and mutagenic N-nitrosodialkylamines.

ACKNOWLEDGEMENT

This work was supported in part by Grants-in-Aid for Cancer Research from the Ministry of Education, Science and Culture of Japan. We thank Dr K.H. Kohda, Nagoya City University, for valuable advice.

REFERENCES

Huang, G.-F., Mochizuki, M., Anjo, T. & Okada, M. (1981) Mutagenicity of N-alkyl-N-(α-acetoxyalkyl)-nitrosamines in V79 Chinese hamster cells in relation to alkylating activity. Gann, 72, 531-538

Jones, C.A. & Huberman, E. (1980) A sensivitve hepatocyte-mediated assay for the metabolism of nitrosamines to mutagens for mammalian cells. Cancer Res., 40, 406-411

Kohda, K.H., Mochizuki, M., Anjo, T. & Okada, M. (1982) Mutagenicity of N-alkyl-N-(α-hydroperoxy-alkyl)nitrosamines in V79 Chinese hamster cells in relation to alkylating activity. Gann, 73, 522-530

Mochizuki, M., Anjo, T. & Okada, M. (1980) Isolation and characterization of N-alkyl-N-(hydroxy-methyl)nitrosamines from N-alkyl-N-(hydroperoxymethyl)nitrosamines by deoxygenation. Tetrahedron Lett., 21, 3693-3696

Mochizuki, M., Anjo, T., Takeda, K., Suzuki, E., Sekiguchi, N., Huang, G.-F. & Okada, M. (1982) Chemistry and mutagenicity of α-hydroxy nitrosamines. In: Bartsch, H., O'Neill, I.K., Castegnaro, M. & Okada, M., eds, N-Nitroso Compounds: Occurrence and Biological Effects (IARC Scientific Publications No. 41), Lyon, International Agency for Research on Cancer, pp. 553-559

GENETIC ACTIVITY IN YEAST ASSAYS OF REPUTED NONMUTAGENIC, CARCINOGENIC N-NITROSO COMPOUNDS AND METHAPYRILENE HYDROCHLORIDE

R.D. MEHTA & R.C. VON BORSTEL

Department of Genetics, University of Alberta, Edmonton, Alberta, Canada

SUMMARY

Methapyrilene hydrochloride (MPHC), N-nitrosomethylaniline (NMA), N-nitrosomethyl-3-carboxypropylamine (NMCP) and N-nitrosodiethanolamine (NDELA) are reputed to be nonmutagenic carcinogens because they are genetically inactive in *Salmonella* mutagenesis tests but produce cancer in rats. We have assayed these compounds for their genetic activity with diploid strains D7, D7-144, and RMO52 of *Saccharomyces cerevisiae*. The compounds MPHC and NMA were highly toxic to the cells and induced gene conversion and reverse mutations in strains D7, D7-144 and RMO52. Metabolic activation was not required for this activity. However, in acidic (pH 5) medium, the genetic activity and cell toxicity of MPHC and NMA were markedly reduced. Ascorbic acid suppressed the mutagenicity and toxic effects of MPHC.

Mutagenicity of NDELA was enhanced in strain D7-144 when cells were treated in acidic medium. At pH 7, NDELA was not mutagenic. NMCP induced reversed mutations in strains D7-144 and RMO52 in the absence of metabolic activation. Our results indicate that the four carcinogens, MPHC, NMA, NMCP and NDELA, require different physiological conditions for the expression of their genetic activity.

INTRODUCTION

Methapyrilene hydrochloride (MPHC), N-nitrosodiethanolamine (NDELA), N-nitrosomethylaniline (NMA) and N-nitrosomethyl-3-carboxypropylamine (NMCP) are known to cause a variety of cancers in rats (Goodall *et al.,* 1970; Lijinsky *et al.,* 1980a, b, 1983). When assayed for mutagenicity in the *Salmonella* mutagenesis (Ames assay) tests, these four compounds were found to have no genetic activity (Andrews *et al.,* 1978; Rao *et al;* 1979; Andrews & Lijinsky, 1980). Since mutagenicity assays in the yeast *Saccharomyces cerevisiae* have been developed, with a wide range of genetic end-points and sensitivities to allow the detection of potential carcinogens as mutagens, we tested these four carcinogens, which failed detection in the *Salmonella* assay, for their genetic activity with various strains of yeast under different physiological conditions.

MATERIALS AND METHODS

Yeast strains

Three diploid strains of *Saccharomyces cerevisiae* were used: strain D7,

$$\frac{a}{\alpha} \frac{ade2\text{--}40}{ade2\text{--}119} \frac{trp5\text{--}12}{trp5\text{--}27} \frac{ilv1\text{--}92}{ilv1\text{--}92},$$

was developed by Zimmermann *et al.* (1975); strain D7-144 (a nonsporulating but otherwise isogenic derivative of D7) and strain RMO52,

$$\frac{a}{\alpha} \frac{ade2\text{--}40}{ade2\text{--}119} \frac{his1\text{--}7}{his1\text{--}7} \frac{trp1}{trp1},$$

were developed in our laboratory. Genetic end-points used were: mitotic crossing over and gene conversion involving the ADE2 gene–these were scored as aberrant colonies; mitotic gene conversion in the TRP1 gene that produced TRP$^+$ prototrophs; and reverse mutations of *his 1-7* and *ilv1-92* alleles, which were counted as HIS$^+$ and ILV$^+$ revertants.

Chemicals

Dimethylsulfoxide and ethyl methanesulfonate were supplied by Terochem Laboratories (Edmonton, Alberta, Canada); cyclophosphamide was obtained from Sigma Chemical Company (St Louis, MO, USA); MPHC, NDELA, NMA and NMCP were provided by Dr W. Lijinsky of the National Cancer Institute, Frederick Cancer Research Facility, P.O. Box B, Frederick, Maryland 21701, USA.

Mutagenicity assays

In general, the assay protocol described by Mehta *et al.* (1982) was followed. The media used for growth and for scoring mutant colonies and cell survival have been described by Mehta and von Borstel (1982). Cultures of the test strains were grown overnight in a water-bath shaker at 30 °C. Cells were harvested by centrifugation during the logarithmic phase of growth. A cell suspension ($2 \times 10^7 - 5 \times 10^7$ cells/mL) of each culture was prepared in either phosphate buffer (pH 7.0) or citrate-phosphate buffer (pH 5.0). The reaction mixture, containing cells and the appropriate concentration of test chemical or of the solvent (dimethyl sulfoxide), and the 9 000 x *g* supernatant of rodent liver (S9 mix; prepared as described by Ames *et al.*, 1975) when required, was incubated in glass test tubes at 30 °C, in the dark, in a water-bath shaker for the desired length of time. The concentration of the S9 fraction was maintained at 25–50 µL per mL of incubation mix. At the end of treatment, samples were taken and washed, and serial dilutions were made. Cells were plated onto various media to score for survival counts, mutations and aberrant colonies. Plates were incubated at 30 °C for three to seven days before scoring.

Positive controls

Ethyl methanesulfonate (5–10 µL/mL) was used as a control for direct acting mutagens. Cyclophosphamide (4 mg/mL) was used to monitor the activity of the S9 microsomal fraction.

Evaluation of mutagenicity

Test chemicals exhibiting at least a two-fold increase in mutation frequency over the control values, which also showed a dose-dependent response, were considered positive for mutagenic response.

RESULTS AND DISCUSSION

MPHC and three *N*-nitroso compounds, NMA, NMCP and NDELA, were assayed for genetic activity with three test strains, D7, D7-144 and RMO52, of *Saccharomyces cerevisiae*. The chemical structures of these compounds are shown in Figure 1. A dose dependent increase in the frequencies of TRP$^+$ convertants was observed with MPHC in strains D7 and D7-144 in the presence as well as in the absence of the S9 microsomal fraction (Table 1). The data also indicate that MPHC induced aberrant colonies in strain D7, showing a relatively stronger response in the absence of metabolic activation than in its presence. Strain D7-144, which is more sensitive than D7 to the toxic effects of MPHC, showed only a slight increase in the frequency of aberrant colonies.

In order to study the effect of pH on the mutagenicity of MPHC, the drug was tested for its genetic activity with strains D7-144 and RMO52 in acidic (pH 5) and neutral (pH 7) media. The data shown in Table 2 demonstrate that MPHC induced gene conversion (TRP$^+$) in strain D7-144 and reverse mutations (HIS$^+$) in RMO52 when the cells were treated in a neutral (pH 7) medium; however, under acidic conditions (pH 5), marked reductions in the toxic effects and the genetic activity of MPHC were observed.

Fig. 1 Chemical structures of methapyrilene, *N*-nitrosomethylaniline, *N*-nitrosodiethanolamine and *N*-nitrosomethyl-3-carboxypropylamine

Methapyrilene

N-Nitrosomethylaniline

N-Nitrosodiethanolamine

N-Nitrosomethyl-3-carboxypropylamine

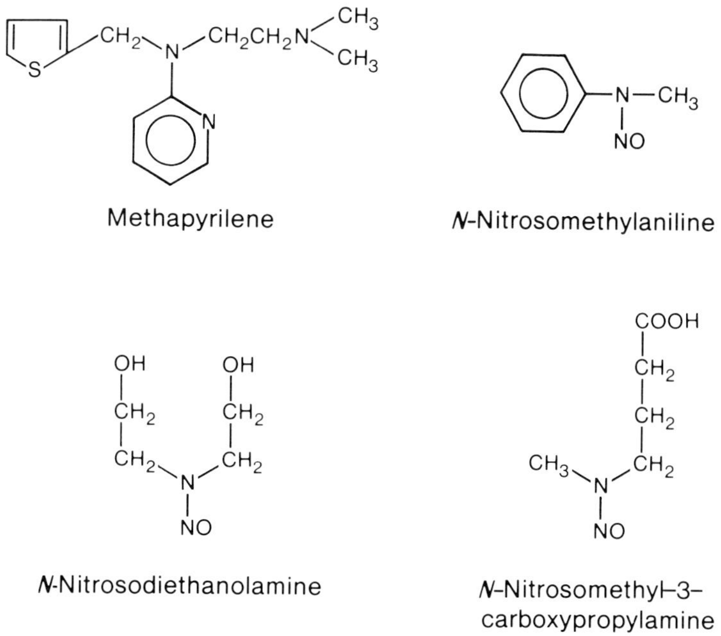

Table 1. Genetic activity of methapyrilene hydrochloride (MPHC) in *Saccharomyces cerevisiae* strains D7 and D7-144; 3-h incubation

Strain	Concentration (mg/mL)	Survival (%)		Aberrant colonies (%)		TRP + convertants ($\times 10^5$)	
		−S9	+S9	−S9	+S9	−S9	+S9
D7	Control – DMSO[a]	100	100	0.09	0.10	1.36 (436)[b]	1.33 (385)
	0.25	132	123	0	0.08	0.99 (420)	1.17 (416)
	0.50	110	131	0.08	0	1.10 (387)	1.04 (394)
	1.0	65	75	0.14	0.03	1.54 (321)	1.70 (371)
	2.5	62	51	0.41	0.11	3.19 (637)	3.84 (572)
	5.0	25	4	0.70	0.43	4.79 (379)	10.26 (117)
D7-144	Control – DMSO[a]	100	100	0	0.08	1.93 (296)	2.27 (306)
	0.25	116	104	0	0	1.76 (312)	1.92 (271)
	0.5	86	103	0.11	0	2.32 (306)	2.25 (313)
	1.0	77	90	0.13	0	2.40 (285)	2.69 (326)
	2.5	17	34	0.20	0.33	6.48 (171)	4.77 (219)

[a] Concentration of dimethyl sulfoxide (DMSO) was 2.5% (v/v)
[b] Figures in parentheses are total number of colonies scored from four plates

Similarly, a sharp decline in cell toxicity was observed when cells of strain D7-144 were treated with NMA in an acidic (pH 5) medium, as compared with treatment in the medium at pH 7. However, the effect of low pH on the genetic activity of NMA was found to be less dramatic; there was only a slight decrease in the frequency of TRP$^+$ convertants at pH 5 in relation to the frequency observed at pH 7 (Table 3). We have observed that the presence of ascorbic acid (250 μg/mL) in the incubation mixture completely eliminates the cell toxicity and mutagenicity of MPHC in strain D7-144 (data not shown). Guttenplan (1978) has also reported that ascorbic acid can inhibit the genetic activity of some carcinogenic N-nitroso compounds. In contrast to the effect of low pH on the cell toxicity of MPHC and NMA, no significant difference was observed for cell viability in strain D7-144 between the treatments of cells with NDELA performed in acidic and in neutral media (Table 3); but there was a dose-related enhancement in the frequency of TRP$^+$ convertants when the cells were incubated in acidic medium, whereas incubation of the cells in neutral medium resulted in suppression of the genetic activity of NDELA (Table 3).

Table 2. Mutagenicity and toxic effects of methapyrilene hydrochloride (MPHC) in *Saccharomyces cerevisiae* strains D7-144 and RMO52; 3-h incubation

Strain	Concentration (mg/mL)	Survival (%)		TRP$^+$ convertants ($\times 10^5$)	
		pH 7	pH 5	pH 7	pH 5
D7-144	Control – DMSO[a]	100	100	0.4 (137)[b]	0.6 (136)
	0.125	72	125	0.5 (143)	0.6 (176)
	0.25	78	103	0.5 (141)	0.6 (148)
	0.50	56	76	0.7 (145)	0.8 (140)
	1.25	25	76	3.0 (264)	0.7 (133)
				HIS$^+$ revertants ($\times 10^7$)	
RMO52	Control – DMSO[a]	100	100	2.8 (8)	4.5 (12)
	0.25	96	105	5.5 (15)	3.5 (10)
	0.50	99	93	7.5 (21)	2.4 (6)
	1.25	94	95	12.0 (32)	2.4 (6)
	2.50	15	94	50.9 (22)	3.2 (8)

[a] Concentration of dimethyl sulfoxide (DMSO) was 2.5% (v/v)
[b] Figures in parentheses are total number of colonies scored from four plates

Table 3. Induction of mitotic gene conversion (TRP$^+$) in *Saccharomyces cerevisiae* strain D7-144 by N-nitrosomethylaniline (NMA) and N-nitrosodiethanolamine (NDELA); 3-h incubation

Chemical	Concentration (mg/mL)	Survival (%)		TRP$^+$ convertants ($\times 10^5$)	
		pH 7	pH 5	pH 7	pH 5
NMA	Control – DMSO[a]	100	100	0.4 (137)[b]	0.6 (136)
	1.25	106	66	0.4 (140)	0.8 (122)
	2.50	20	67	3.4 (243)	1.4 (226)
	6.25	<0.001	0.1	0	0
	12.50	<0.001	0.02	0	0
NDELA	Control – DMSO[a]	100	100	0.9 (170)	0.7 (131)
	3.4	96	107	0.9 (171)	0.9 (166)
	8.5	73	95	1.2 (177)	1.4 (247)
	17	84	84	1.1 (175)	2.0 (307)
	34	70	78	1.2 (162)	3.7 (519)

[a] Concentration of dimethyl sulfoxide (DMSO) was 2.5% (v/v)
[b] Figures in parentheses are total number of colonies scored from four plates

Fig. 2 Cell survival of strain D7-144 and randomly selected prototrophic clones, TRP$^+$ and ILV$^+$, after treatment with methapyrilene hydrochloride and *N*-nitrosomethylaniline. Three or four TRP$^+$ or ILV$^+$ prototrophs were isolated by plating 1×10^6 cells of the strain D7-144 on selective media. The *trp5-12* and *ilv1-92* lines represent four clones of D7-144.

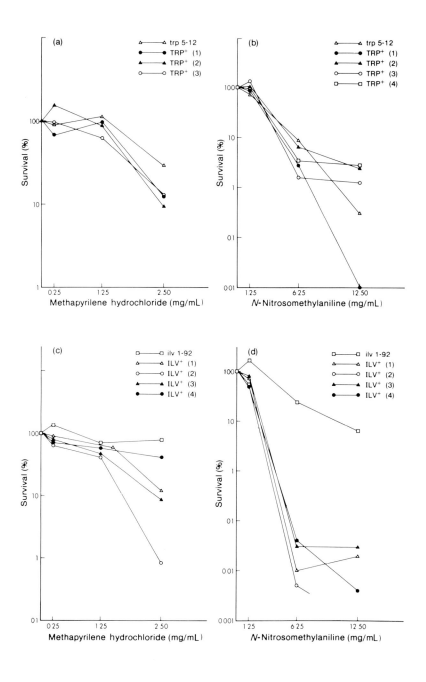

Table 4. Induction of gene conversion and reverse mutation by *N*-nitrosomethyl-3-carboxypropylamine (NMCP) in strains D7-144 and RMO52 of *Saccharomyces cerevisiae*

Strain	Concentration (mg/mL)	Survival (%)		TRP$^+$ convertants ($\times 10^5$)		ILV$^+$ revertants ($\times 10^7$)	
		$-$S9	$+$S9	$-$S9	$+$S9	$-$S9	$+$S9
D7-144	Control – DMSO[a]	100	100	0.55 (611)[b]	1.9 (529)	1.1 (12)	9.6 (26)
	16.26	28	148	2.55 (793)	1.8 (742)	41.5 (129)	13.6 (55)
	32.52	1	4	1.73 (26)	1.7 (19)	26.7 (4)	26.3 (3)
						HIS$^+$ revertants ($\times 10^7$)	
RMO52	Control – DMSO[a]	100	100			0.9 (8)	3.1 (8)
	16.26	131	112			0.8 (10)	3.1 (9)
	32.52	23	21			7.1 (15)	9.1 (5)

[a] Concentration of dimethyl sulfoxide (DMSO) was 2.5% (v/v)
[b] Figures in parentheses are total number of colonies scored from four plates

These results suggest that the genetic activity of MPHC, NMA and NDELA is dependent upon the pH of the incubation medium; MPHC and NMA are genetically active in neutral (pH 7) medium, whereas NDELA becomes mutagenic in acidic medium (pH 5). Negishi and Hayatsu (1980) have reported that some *N*-nitrosodialkylamines, including *N*-nitroso-dimethylamine (NDMA) and *N*-nitrosodiethylamine (NDEA), elicit higher mutagenicity at pH 5 than at pH 7 in *Salmonella typhimurium* strains. Guttenplan (1980) made similar observations for NDMA, but for NDEA he found no enhancement of mutagenicity at pH 6 in the Ames assay. Our results suggest that nitrosodialkylamines like NDELA require acidic conditions near pH 5 to express their mutagenicity. The non-mutagenicity of NDELA in the Ames assay as reported by Andrews and Lijinsky (1980) might have been due to the fact that this compound was tested at a pH 7.4, rather than at pH 5.

The nitrosamine NMCP, which failed to exhibit mutagenicity in the Ames assay (Andrews & Lijinsky, 1980), induced gene conversion in TRP1 gene and reverse mutations of *ilv1-92* allele in strain D7-144; the mutagenic response was found to be much stronger in the absence of S9 microsomal fraction than in its presence (Table 4). Strain RMO52, which was relatively more resistant to the toxicity of NMCP than strain D7-144, showed only a modest increase in the frequency of HIS$^+$ revertants at the highest dose used; the response being relatively weaker in the presence of metabolic activation (Table 4).

Our results demonstrate that methapyrilene hydrochloride and the three *N*-nitroso compounds, NMA, NMCP and NDELA, which are carcinogenic in mammals, can be detected as mutagens in yeast (*S. cerevisiae*) assays. However, it should be pointed out that the mutagenic response of these compounds is weak, as revealed by the fact that the mutation yield (as reflected by the total number of prototrophs) is very low (Tables 1–4). Assuming that the low mutant yield might result, in part, from the selective killing of prototrophic clones by the test compound, we compared the cell viability of the auxotrophic test strain D7-144 with the cell survival of TRP$^+$ and ILV$^+$ prototrophic clones of D7-144. These results clearly show that the ILV$^+$ and TRP$^+$ prototrophs are more sensitive to the toxic effects of MPHC and NMA than the progenitor auxotrophic strain D7-144 (Fig. 2). Therefore, it seems likely that data on mutation yield, at least in the cases of MPHC and NMA, represent underestimations of the mutagenic potency of these compounds. The failure of the Ames assay, which is normally based upon mutation yield data, to detect these chemicals as mutagens might have been due to selective killing of revertants in the mutation plates.

ACKNOWLEDGEMENTS

We thank Jennie Chui and Lily Choy for their skilled technical assistance. We are grateful to Dr W. Lijinsky for supplying us with the test compounds. Research was supported by the Alberta Oil Sands Technology and Research Authority and the Natural Sciences and Engineering Research Council of Canada.

REFERENCES

Ames, B.N., McCann, J. & Yamasaki, E. (1975) Methods for detecting carcinogens and mutagens with the *Salmonella*/mammalian-microsome mutagenicity test. *Mutat. Res., 31*, 347–364

Andrews, A.W. & Lijinsky, W. (1980) Mutagenicity of 45 nitrosamines in *Salmonella typhimurium*. *Teratog. Carcinog. Mutagen., 1*, 295–303

Andrews, A.W., Thibault, L.H. & Lijinsky, W. (1978) The relationship between mutagenicity and carcinogenicity of some nitrosamines. *Mutat. Res., 51*, 319–326

Goodall, C.M., Lijinsky, W., Thomas, L. & Wenyon, C.E. (1970) Toxicity and oncogenicity of nitrosomethylaniline and nitrosomethylcyclohexylamine. *Toxicol. appl. Pharmacol., 17*, 426–432

Guttenplan, J.B. (1978) Mechanism of inhibition by ascorbate of microbial mutagenesis induced by *N*-nitroso compounds. *Cancer Res., 38*, 2018–2022

Guttenplan, J.B. (1980) Enhanced mutagenic activities of *N*-nitroso compounds in weakly acidic media. *Carcinogenesis, 1*, 439–444

Lijinsky, W., Reuber, M.D. & Blackwell, B.N. (1980a) Liver tumors induced in rats by oral administration of antihistaminic methapyrilene hydrochloride. *Science, 209*, 817–819

Lijinsky, W., Reuber, M.D. & Manning, W.B. (1980b) Pontent carcinogenicity of nitrosodiethanolamine in rats. *Nature, 288*, 589–590

Lijinsky, W., Reuber, M.D., Saavedra, J.E. & Singer, G.M. (1983) Carcinogenesis in F344 rats by nitrosomethyl-*n*-propylamine derivatives. *J. natl Cancer Inst.* (in press)

Mehta, R.D. & von Borstel, R.C. (1982) Genetic activity of diethylstilbestrol in *Saccharomyces cerevisiae:* Enhancement of mutagenicity by oxidizing agents. *Mutat. Res., 92*, 49–61

Mehta, R.D., Hennig, U.G.G., von Borstel, R.C. & Chatten, L.G. (1982) Genetic activity in *Saccharomyces cerevisiae* and thin-layer chromatographic comparisons of medical grades of pyrvinium pamoate and monopyrvinium salts. *Mutat. Res., 102*, 59–69

Negishi, T. & Hayatsu, H. (1980) The pH-dependent response of *Salmonella* TA100 to mutagenic *N*-nitrosamines. *Mutat. Res., 79*, 223–230

Rao, T.K., Young, J.A., Lijinsky, W. & Epler, J.L. (1979) Mutagenicity of aliphatic nitrosamines in *Salmonella typhimurium. Mutat. Res., 66*, 1–7

Zimmermann, F.K., Kern, R. & Rosenberger, H. (1975) A yeast strain for simultaneous detection of induced mitotic crossing over, mitotic gene conversion and reverse mutation. *Mutat. Res., 28*, 381–388

GENETIC AND BIOCHEMICAL FACTORS AFFECTING THE INDUCTION OF BACTERIOPHAGE LAMBDA BY N-NITROSO COMPOUNDS

R.K. ELESPURU, S.K. GONDA, & S.G. MOORE

Fermentation Program, NCI-Frederick Cancer Research Facility, Frederick, MD, USA

SUMMARY

As part of our effort to validate a biochemical (prophage) induction assay (BIA) as a screening test for carcinogens, we have tested more than 100 N-nitroso compounds. An enzyme, β-galactosidase, is induced as an indirect consequence of DNA damage to the host, as part of the 'SOS' response. Besides the obvious practical importance of detecting this class of carcinogen, there is the question of the mechanism by which these compounds work. Mutagenesis by one compound, N-methyl-N'-nitro-N-nitrosoguanidine, is known to proceed by both SOS (*recA*)-dependent and SOS-independent pathways. Mispairing due to O^6 alkylation of guanine is thought to be responsible for the SOS-independent pathway; however, there has been little consideration of *recA*-dependent functions, of which phage induction is one. Although nitrosamides could be detected as phage inducers in our assay, N-nitrosamines in the presence of rat liver 9 000 × g supernatant usually gave no response. We found that the use of several mutant strains, particularly a *lexA* mutant, in combination with hamster liver 9 000 × g supernatant, allowed us to detect most N-nitrosamines reasonably well, in either a spot test or a quantitative tube assay. Induction in a *lexA* strain was most unexpected, since this mutation usually diminishes the expression of SOS functions induced by ultra-violet light. Because the genetic and biochemical conditions that favour phage induction are different from those that favour mutagenesis, it seems likely that the lesions in DNA leading to the two biological end-points are different.

INTRODUCTION

A rapid assay for detection of DNA-damaging antitumour agents was developed using a lambda lysogen of *Escherichia coli* (Elespuru & Yarmolinsky, 1979). This strain carries a lambda-*lacZ* fusion phage, the genes of which are expressed following DNA damage to the host. The 'SOS response' of bacteria to DNA damage results in the synthesis of β-galactosidase, product of the *lacZ* gene, an enzyme which can be measured biochemically. This 'biochemical induction assay' (BIA) can be run as a spot test on agar or as a quantitative assay in test tubes. Both plate and tube assays utilize substrates that give coloured products, an end-point which allows the assay to be adapted for a variety of uses, including bioautography (identification of active regions on thin-layer chromatograms) (Elespuru & White, 1983). Samples containing microbes, complex media or toxic solvents usually do not interfere with the assay.

Little is known about the types of chemical-DNA interactions leading to induction of the SOS response in *E. coli*. However, there is a very great diversity in induction efficiency as a result of treatment with different chemicals (Heinemann, 1971; Moreau *et al.*, 1976; Elespuru & White, 1983). In an attempt to optimize conditions for detection of many types of chemicals, several mutations that affect DNA repair, bacterial permeability and lambda gene expression have been incorporated into the strain. Recently, we have been working with an isolate containing a DNA repair mutation, *lexA*, which results in enhanced enzyme synthesis following treatment with many DNA-interacting chemicals, particularly alkylating agents, which are inefficient inducers of the wild-type strain. Conditions have been established allowing the detection of most *N*-nitroso compounds as prophage inducers (Elespuru, 1983). These results are described here and compared with those obtained from mutagenesis studies.

MATERIALS AND METHODS

Spot test

An overnight culture of bacteria was diluted 1:100 and grown to A_{600} 0.4. These bacteria were poured in 2.5 mL agar onto square 100-mm petri dishes containing LBE agar plus 10 µg/mL ampicillin. Chemical solutions in dimethyl sulfoxide or water were spot-tested in aliquots of approximately 5 µL. Plates incubated for 5 h at 38 °C were overlaid with 2.5 mL molten top agar containing a substrate for the enzyme β-galactosidase, 6-bromonaphthyl-β-D-galactopyranoside (BNG), plus Fast Blue RR salt. Red spots represent positive areas of induction. Spot intensities, judged by comparison with controls on the same plate, were recorded as weak (+), moderate (++) or strong (+++) at the optimal inducing dose. The lowest concentration that gave a reproducible positive response was noted as the minimum inducing dose. Compositions of media and detailed methods have been described (Elespuru & White, 1983). When metabolic activation was required, the following were added to the top agar: 9 000 × *g* supernatant of rodent liver (S9) (24-36 mg/mL protein) and 2.5 µmol each of NADP, glucose-6-phosphate and magnesium chloride (25 µL each of 0.1 mol/L solutions).

Quantitative tube assay

Bacteria grown as for the spot test to A_{600} 0.4 were diluted 1:10 in LBE medium plus 10 µg/mL ampicillin and distributed in 0.5-mL aliquots to test tubes containing 50 µL of the desired concentration of chemical. After incubation at 38 °C for 5 h with vigorous aeration (shaking), ice-cold Z buffer was added to terminate enzyme synthesis. A drop of toluene was added to each tube if the bacterial strain was wild-type for the cell membrane (*env*⁺). Test tubes were stored at 4 °C overnight prior to performance of the enzyme assay, if desired. Quantities of β-galactosidase were determined by the addition of substrate *o*-nitrophenyl-β-D-galactopyranoside, observance of colour development, and termination of the assay by addition of sodium carbonate. The precise time of colour development was noted. Arbitrary enzyme units were established as 100 A_{420}/t, where A_{420} is the colour absorbance reading and t is the enzyme colour development time in hours. Details of the procedures and of the enzyme assay have been described elsewhere (Elespuru & White, 1983). When metabolic activation was required, bacteria were diluted into S9 activation mix instead of LBE. Activation mix contained 10% S9 (by volume) (3-4 mg/mL protein), 3 mmol/L NADP, 10 mmol/L glucose-6-phosphate, 10 mmol/L magnesium chloride and 10 µg/mL ampicillin. The balance of the volume was LBE medium (pH 7.6).

RESULTS

Induction of prophage lambda by *N*-nitroso compounds was found to be influenced by the genetic background of the host strain, the composition of the expression medium and the source of activating liver enzymes (Elespuru, 1983). Bacterial mutants with increased

Fig. 1. Spot test for prophage induction using mutant lambda lysogens of *Escherichia coli*. Plate 1: BR513 (*envA*, Δ*uvrB*); Plate 2: BR469 (Δ *uvrB*); Plate 3: BR475 (wild type); Plate 4: BR339 (Δ*uvrB*, *lexA3*). Row A: lanes 1-3, bleomycin at concentrations of 30, 12 and 5 µg/mL respectively; lanes 4-6, dimethylsulfoxide (DMSO) water and blank controls. Row B: lanes 1-6, *N*-methyl-*N′*-nitro-*N*-nitrosoguanidine (MNNG) in water at concentrations of 1.2, 0.63, 0.31, 0.15, 0.075 and 0.038 mg/mL, respectively. Row C: MMNG in DMSO at the same concentrations as in Row B. Row D: *N*-ethyl-*N′*-nitro-*N*-nitrosoguanidine (ENNG), as in Row B. Row E: ENNG, as in Row C. Row F: lanes 1-3, methylmethanesulfonate (MMS) in DMSO at 100%, 10% and 1% by volume respectively; lanes 4-6, ethylmethanesulfonate in DMSO as for MMS

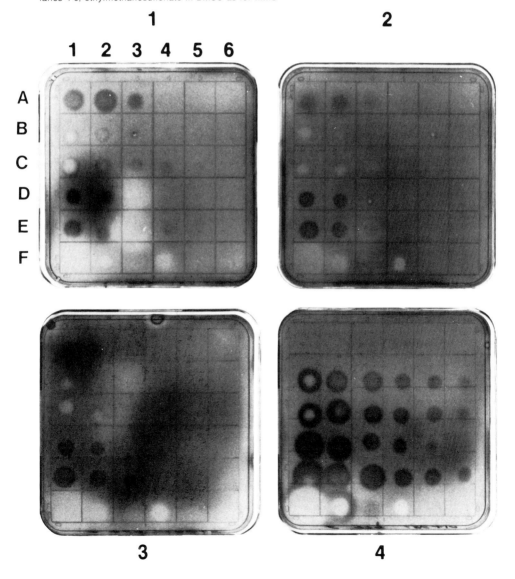

permeability were not more sensitive to *N*-nitroso compounds than those with a wild-type cell envelope (Fig. 1, plates 1 and 2). The deletion of a gene required for the UVR endonuclease (*uvrB*) had little effect on the dose-response curve for induction, shifting it slightly toward lower doses (Fig. 2; see also Fig. 1, plates 2 and 3). However, the incorporation of *lexA3* mutations into either the *uvrB* deletion strain or its wild-type counterpart resulted in a substantial increase in the magnitude of induction observed (Fig. 1, plate 4 and Fig. 2). This effect was dependent on the presence of ampicillin in the medium during the expression. It is not clear how the combination of this mutant and a cell wall inhibitor affect the inducing response, and we are pursuing this question with some interest.

Fig. 2. Quantitative assay for prophage induction in *lex*$^+$ and *lex*A3 strains of *Escherichia coli*: ●, Δ*uvrB*, *lex*A3; ▼, Δ*uvr*$^+$ *lex*A3; ■, *uvrB lex*$^+$; ▲, *uvr*$^+$ *lex*$^+$. The inducing chemical was *N*-methyl-*n'*-nitro-*N*-nitrosoguanidine (MNNG). Expression medium contained 10 μg/mL ampicillin in all cases.

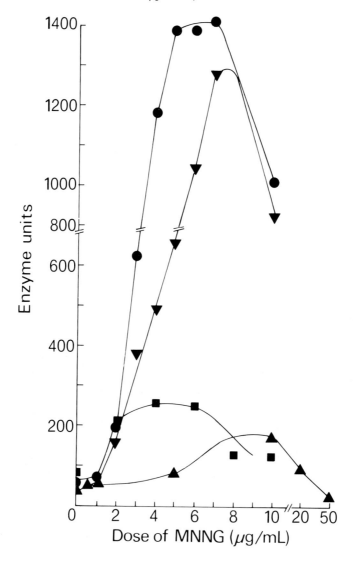

Fig. 3. Spot test for prophage induction by *N*-nitrosamines in the presence of different combinations of rat and hamster liver 9 000 × *g* supernatant (S9) fractions. The bacterial strain used was BR339 (Δ*uvrB*, *lexA3*). 1 × Hamster liver S9 (male, Aroclor-induced) is equivalent to 14 mg protein per plate; 1 × Rat liver S9 (male, Aroclor-induced) is equivalent to 13 mg protein per plate. Chemicals in dimethylsulfoxide were spotted in adjacent sets of three in 5-μL aliquots. Row A: solvent controls. Row B: *N*-nitrosomorpholine (NMOR), 100, 10 and 1 mg/mL; dinitrosopiperazine (DNPZ), 100, 10 and 1 mg/mL. Row C: *cis*-2,6-dimethylnitrosomorpholine [*cis*(CH₃)₂NMOR], 500, 100 and 10 mg/mL; *n*-nitrosopyrrolidine (NPYR), 500, 100 and 10 mg/mL. Row D: *N*-nitrosopiperidine, (NPIP), 500, 100 and 10 mg/mL; *trans*-2,6-dimethylnitrosomorpholine [*trans*(CH₃)₂NMOR], 500, 100 and 10 mg/mL. Row E: *N*-nitrosodipropylamine (NDMA), 500, 100 and 10 mg/mL; *N*-nitrosopiperidone (NPIP-one), 10, 1 and 0.1 mg/mL. Row F: *N*-nitrosodimethylamine (NDMA) and *N*-nitrosodiethylamine (NDEA), both at 500, 100 and 10 mg/mL

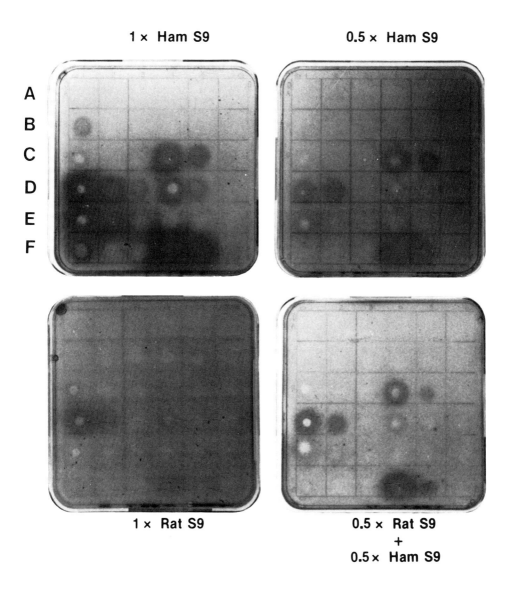

Fig. 4. Quantitative assay for prophage induction by *N*-nitrosamines. Bacterial strain BR339 (Δ*uvrB*, *lesA*3) was treated with millimolar quantities of nitrosamines in the presence of a 9 000 × *g*, supernatant from liver of Aroclor-induced male Syrian golden hamsters (10% by volume, 2.8 mg/mL protein). The incubation period was 5 h.

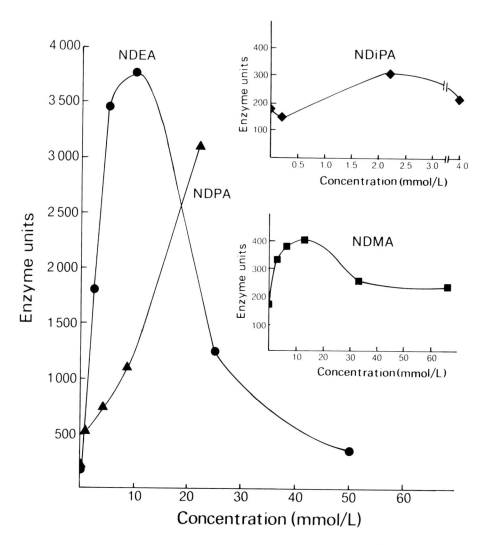

The source and quantity of rodent activating S9 fraction were important variables in the detection of *N*-nitroso compounds requiring metabolic activation, as shown in Figure 3. Many nitrosamines that had been mutagenic for *E. coli* in our hands in previous tests (Elespuru & Lijinsky, 1976) could not be activated by rat liver S9 preparations with demonstrable activity in a *Salmonella* mutagenesis assay (Fig. 3). The only compound that gave detectable activity with rat liver S9 was *N*-nitrosodiethylamine. However, S9 fractions prepared from hamsters were capable of activating most nitrosamines to inducing moieties. Inducing capacity was proportional to added protein concentration, up to approximately 20 mg/plate (Fig. 3), or

Fig. 5. Comparison of *N*-ethyl-*N*-nitrosourea (ENU) and derivatives for mutagenic and prophage-inducing activities. Quantitative prophage induction assay was performed as described in the legend to Figure 2, using strain BR339 (Δ*uvrB, lexA*3). Solutions were prepared in 1% dimethyl sulfoxide in water . The mutagenesis assay was performed on *Salmonella typhimurium* strain TA1535. *His*[+] revertants were scored after 48 h of incubation at 37°C. *Salmonella* data are courtesy of A.W. Andrews. N-cehe, chloroethylhydroxyethylurea; N-he, hydroxyethylurea; N-ipce, isopropylchloroethylurea

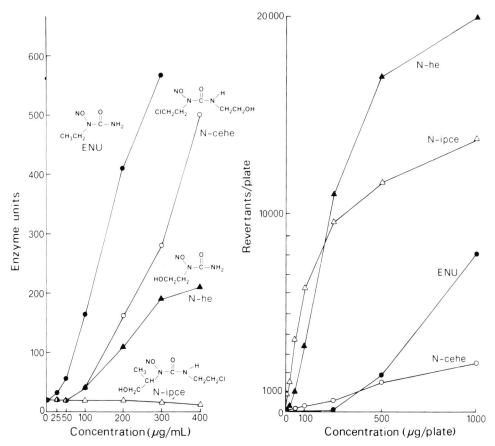

5 mg/mL in the liquid incubation assay (Elespuru, 1983). When S9 fractions from rats and hamsters were combined on a single plate, the enzymes from rats appeared neither to contribute nor to inhibit the activating capacity of the hamster liver preparation (Fig. 3, right-hand plates). The spectrum of inducing spots resembled that of the plate containing hamster S9 alone. Combinations of rat and hamster liver preparations in a wide variety of concentrations gave the same results (data not shown). By contrast, Prival and Mitchell (1981) found that factors in rat liver S9 inhibit mutagenesis by hamster liver preparations.

The inducing capacity of structurally different *N*-Nitroso compounds varied considerably (Elespuru, 1983; and Figs 4 and 5). *N*-Nitroso compounds with an *N*-ethyl group gave greater magnitudes of induction than did *N*-methyl analogues, whether the compounds were *N*-nitrosamines, *N*-nitrosoureas or *N*-nitrosoguanidines (Elespuru & Yarmolinsky, 1979; Elespuru, 1983; and Fig. 4). *N*-Nitrosodiethylamine was one of the best inducers seen in this system, out of several hundred compounds tested. *N*-Nitrosodipropylamine was also an excellent inducer, whereas the isopropyl analogue was a very poor one (Fig. 4). N-Nitrosodimethylamine, likewise, was a poor inducer.

Because prophage induction, like mutagenesis, is a consequence of DNA-chemical interactions, we have been interested in comparing our results with those obtained from the well-studied *Salmonella typhimurium* mutagenesis assay. In many cases, we find significant differences in the order of activity of structural variants in the two systems (Elespuru, 1983). An example of such a comparison is shown in Figure 5, with a set of nitrosoalkylureas, the same samples of compound being tested in each system. There is no observable consistency between the results in the two systems. In general, we have found that any derivative of the ethyl group is less active than the parent compound, but this is not the case for *Salmonella*. In comparing results with N-nitrosamines and N-nitrosoureas, we find that N-nitrosamines (requiring activation) often give a greater magnitude of response than the directly acting N-nitrosoureas, whereas the converse is true for mutagenesis in either *S. typhinurium* or *E. coli* (see, for example, Figs 4 and 5). This result is difficult to rationalize, but could be a consequence of toxic *versus* inducing reactions and the times required for the cell to respond to them (several hours in the case of prophage induction, several days in the case of the mutagenesis assay).

DISCUSSION

Induction of prophage is one of the *recA*-dependent functions expressed as part of the SOS response in *E. coli* (Witkin, 1976). The SOS response is triggered by treatments which block the movement of the replication fork. Mutagenesis is another component of the SOS response, arising from random errors in DNA repair synthesis, perhaps related to altered polymerase activity (Lackey *et al.*, 1982). Most mutagenesis mediated by N-nitroso compounds, however, is considered to involve simple base-mispairings during replication, resulting from the presence of lesions such as O^6-alkylguanine which do not perturb DNA structure (Bridges *et al.*, 1973; Lawley, 1974; Radman *et al.*, 1977). This pathway is apparently *recA*-independent. Nitrosamine-generated mutagenesis and prophage induction may well arise from different types of DNA lesions and different biochemical pathways. It is not surprising, therefore, that comparisons of results obtained from mutagenesis studies and prophage induction assays do not yield correlations. Little consideration has been given to the type of lesion responsible for induction of SOS functions by N-nitroso compounds. The lesion could be a DNA strand break, arising indirectly from alkylated DNA *via* depurination mechanisms. The increased phage induction observed in *polA* mutants (Blanco & Pomes, 1977), which are defective in repair of strand breaks, is one piece of evidence in favour of this model. The strand break model predicts that *tag* mutants, deficient in 3-methyladenine glycosylase activity, should exhibit a reduced capacity for phage induction, because one of the pathways that generates strand breaks would be blocked. The induction of a 3-methyladenine glycosylase is part of the 'adaptive response' to alkylating agents (Evensen & Seeberg 1982; Karran *et al.*, 1982). It is known that induction of one enzyme of the adaptive response, the O^6-methylguanine transferase, is related to decreased mutagenesis (Schendel & Robbins, 1978; Schendel *et al.*, 1978); it may be that induction of the other enzyme is directly related to the phage induction pathway.

REFERENCES

Blanco, M. & Pomes, L. (1977) Prophage induction in *Escherichia coli* K12 cells deficient in DNA polymerase I. *Mol. gen. Genet.*, **154**, 287–292

Bridges, B.A. Mottershead, R.P. Green, M.H.L. & Gray, W.J.H. (1973) Mutagenicity of dichlorvos and methylmethanesulfonate for *Escherichia coli* WP2 and some derivatives deficient in DNA repair. *Mutat. Res.*, **19**, 295–303

Elespuru, R.K. (1983) *Induction of bacteriophage lambda by* N-*nitroso compounds.* In: de Serres, F.J., ed., *Topics in Chemical Mutagenesis,* Vol. 1, Rao, T.K., Lijinsky, W. & Epler, J.L., eds, *N-Nitrosamines,* New York, Plenum Press (in press)

Elespuru, R.K. & Lijinsky, W. (1976) Mutagenicity of cyclic nitrosamines in *Escherichia coli* following activation with rat liver microsomes. *Cancer Res., 36,* 4900–4901

Elespuru, R.K. & White, R.J. (1983) Biochemical prophage induction assay: a rapid test for antitumor agents that interact with DNA. *Cancer Res., 43,* 2819–2830

Elespuru, R.K. & Yarmolinsky, M.B. (1979) A colorimetric assay of lysogenic induction designed for screening potential carcinogenic and carcinostatic agents. *Environ. Mutagenesis, 1,* 65–78

Evensne, G. & Seeberg, E. (1982) Adaptation to alkylation resistance involved the induction of a DNA glycosylase. *Nature, 296,* 773–775

Heinemann, B. (1971) *Prophage induction in lysogenic bacteria as a method of detecting potential mutagenic, carcinogenic, carcinostatic and teratogenic agents.,* In: Hollaender, A., ed. *Chemical Mutagens: Principles and Methods for Detection,* Vol. 1, New York, Plenum Press, pp. 235–266

Karran, P., Hjelmgren, T. & Lindhal, T. (1982) Induction of a DNA glycosylase for *N*-methylated purines is part of the adaptive response to alkylating agents. *Nature, 296,* 770–773

Lackey, D., Krauss, S.W. & Linn, S. (1982) Isolation of an altered form of DNA polymerase I from *Escherichia coli* cells induced for *recA/lexA* functions. *Proc. natl Acad. Sci. USA, 79,* 330–334

Lawley, P.D. (1974) some chemical aspects of dose-response relationships in alkylation mutagenesis. *Mutat. Res., 23,* 283–295

Moreau, P., Bailone, A. & Devoret, R. (1976) Prophage induction in *Escherichia coli* K12 *envA uvrB:* A highly sensitive tests for potential carcinogens. *Proc. natl Acad. Sci. USA, 73,* 3700–3704

Prival, M.J. & Mitchell, V.D. (1981) Influence of microsomal and cytosolic fractions from rat, mouse, and hamster liver on the mutagenicity of dimethylnitrosamine in the *Salmonella* plate incorporation assay. *Cancer Res., 41,* 4361–4367

Radman, M., Villani, G., Boiteau, S., Defais, M., Caillet-Fauquet, P. & Spadari, P. (1977) *On the mechanism and control of mutagenesis due to carcinogenic mutagens.* In: Hiatt, H.H., Watson, J. & Winsten, J.A. eds, *Origin of Human Cancer,* Cold Spring Harbor, NY, Cold Spring Harbor Laboratory, pp. 903–922

Schendel, P.F. & Robbins, P.E. (1978) Repair of O^6-methylguanine in adapted *Escherichia coli. Proc. natl Acad. Sci. USA, 75,* 6017–6020

Schendel, P.F., Defais, M., Jeggo, P., Samson, L. & Cairns, J. (1978) Pathways of mutagenesis and repair in *Escherichia coli* exposed to low levels of simple alkylating agents. *J. Bacteriol., 135,* 466–475

Witkin, E. (1976) Ultraviolet mutagenesis and inducible DNA repair in *Escherichia coli. Bacteriol. Rev., 40,* 869–907

CARCINOGENIC EFFECTS RELATED TO TOBACCO AND BETEL QUID

FORMATION AND ANALYSIS OF *N*-NITROSAMINES IN TOBACCO PRODUCTS AND THEIR ENDOGENOUS FORMATION IN CONSUMERS

D. HOFFMANN, K.D. BRUNNEMANN, J.D. ADAMS & S.S. HECHT

*Naylor Dana Institute for Disease Prevention, American Health Foundation,
Valhalla, NY 10595, USA*

INTRODUCTION

The use of tobacco has been known for more than four centuries to induce pharmacologically mediated patterns of behaviour (Jaffee, 1977). Although nicotine was isolated from tobacco in 1828 (Posselt & Reimann, 1828), it was not until the 1940s that this alkaloid was implicated as a major determinant in the habit of smoking (Johnston, 1942). About 40 years ago, clinical data incriminated cigarette smoking as a risk factor for cancer of the lung (Müller 1939); and this observation was confirmed in 1950 by three large-scale epidemiological surveys (Doll & Hill, 1950; Levin *et al.*, 1950; Wynder & Graham, 1950). Since then, prospective studies and case control studies have shown that cigarette smoking is causally associated with cancers of the lung, larynx, oral cavity and oesophagus and is a contributory factor in the development of cancers of the pancreas, kidney and urinary bladder (US Department of Health & Human Services, 1982).

The possibility that a carcinogen is formed from nicotine was not suggested until 1962, when Druckrey and Preussmann (1962) pointed out that this alkaloid could be a precursor of *N*-nitrosonornicotine (NNN). Ten years later, NNN was isolated from tobacco and from cigarette smoke as the first tobacco-specific *N*-nitrosamine (Klus & Kuhn, 1973; Hoffmann *et al.*, 1974a,b).

This overview focuses on progress in the study of the formation and in the analytical and biological assessment of *N*-nitrosamines from tobacco and tobacco smoke. The review also covers recent findings regarding the endogenous formation of nicotine-derived *N*-nitrosamines in tobacco users.

These advances in our knowledge are not merely of academic interest, but also carry practical implications, in that they enable us to assess the contribution of *N*-nitrosamines to the increased risk for cancer among those who dip snuff or chew or smoke tobacco.

ANALYSIS

During the processing and burning of tobacco, three types of *N*-nitrosamine are formed: volatile *N*-nitrosamines (VNA), tobacco-specific *N*-nitrosamines (TSNA) and nonvolatile *N*-nitrosamines (Fig. 1.). The latter group of agents have been defined arbitrarily as those

Fig. 1. *N*-Nitrosamines in tobacco products; NPYR, *N*-nitrosopyrrolidine; NPIP, *N*-nitrosopiperidine; NMOR, *N*-nitrosomorpholine; NDELA, *N*-nitrosodiethanolamine; NPRO, *N*-nitrosoproline; NNN, *N*-nitrosonornicotine, NNK, 4-(*N*-nitrosomethylamino)-1-(3-pyridyl)-1-butanone; NAT, *N*-nitrosoanatabine; NAB, *N'*-nitrosoanabasine

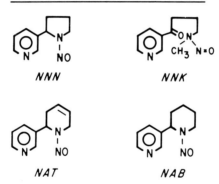

1. VOLATILE NITROSAMINES

R = R' = CH₃, C₂H₅, C₃H₇ or C₄H₉

NPYR   NPIP   NMOR

2. NONVOLATILE NITROSAMINES

NDELA   NPRO

3. TOBACCO-SPECIFIC NITROSAMINES

NNN   NNK

NAT   NAB

nitrosamines that require derivatization for gas chromatographic-Thermal Energy Analyzer (GC-TEA) analysis. All of the *N*-nitrosamines that have been detected in tobacco products are carcinogenic in laboratory animals, with the exception of *N*-nitrosoproline (NPRO) (International Agency for Research on Cancer, 1978b; US Department of Health & Human Services, 1982; Hecht *et al.*, 1983b; Hoffmann *et al.*, unpublished data).

In order to assay for tobacco nitrosamines quantitatively without artefacts, 20 mmol/L ascorbic acid solution, buffered to pH 4.5, should be added during the initial step of the analysis (Brunnemann *et al.*, 1977; Hoffmann *et al.*, 1979). Ageing of the smoke should also be avoided: fresh smoke contains only nitric oxide; however, within 3 min, 50% of the nitric oxide in undiluted smoke is oxidized to nitrogen dioxide (Vilcins & Lephardt, 1975). This ageing effect increases the *N*-nitrosation potential of the smoke to a significant degree. It is therefore recommended that the air and aerosols in the smoking and trapping devices be replaced with nitrogen during puff intervals (Fig. 2.; Hoffmann & Wynder, 1972). For quantitative assays,

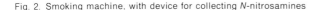

Fig. 2. Smoking machine, with device for collecting *N*-nitrosamines

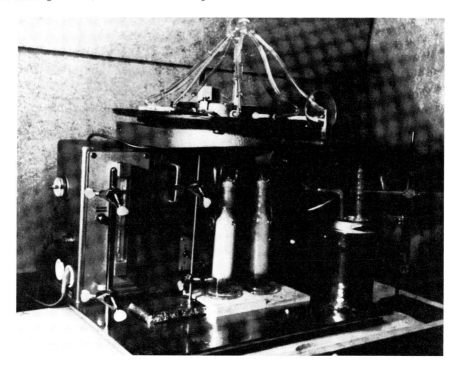

use of a ^{14}C-labelled nitrosamine as internal standard is preferred (Brunnemann *et al.*, 1977; Hoffmann *et al.*, 1979; Brunnemann & Hoffmann, 1981; Brunnemann *et al.*, 1982, 1983). The analysis of nitrosamines in tobacco products and smoke does not appear to warrant additional precautions; however, it is recommended that a monitor amine, such as *cis*-2,6-dimethylmorpholine, be used for the analysis of biological specimens (Mirvish *et al.*, 1981; van Stee *et al.*, 1983).

The initial step of the analysis is a clean-up procedure, consisting primarily of a distribution between a solvent pair, followed by chromatography. Nitroso compounds that contain alcohol and/or carboxylic acid groups require esterification before GC-TEA analysis. For the determination of nitrosamines, the GC coupled with high-resolution mass spectrometry and GC or a high-performance liquid chromatograph (HPLC) with a TEA are the instruments of choice (McCormick *et al.*, 1973; Brunnemann *et al.*, 1977; Hoffmann *et al.*, 1979). We have modified the interface between the GC and TEA (Brunnemann & Hoffmann, 1981) and prefer to analyse for all *N*-nitrosamines by this method (Adams *et al.*, 1983a). This system is less time consuming than HPLC-TEA, requires less maintenance, is amenable to routine analysis and, most importantly, affords more distinct separations and better reproducibility: the HPLC-TEA method does not allow satisfactory separation of traces of *N*-nitrosoanabasine (NAB) from *N*-nitrosoanatabine (NAT), whereas in routine analyses the GC-TEA method gives excellent resolution (Fig. 3.; Adams *et al.*, 1983a).

Although the TEA has a high sensitivity for tobacco *N*-nitrosamines when applied at 1–5×10^{-10} g per injection, its response is not specific for *N*-nitrosamines but also includes *C*-nitroso compounds and organic nitrites and nitrates. We concur, therefore, with the

Fig. 3. Tobacco-specific nitrosamines in cigarette smoke, analysed by high-performance liquid chromatography-Thermal Energy Analyzer (TEA)(A) and by gas chromatography-TEA (B); NAT, N'-nitrosoanatabine; NNN, N'-nitrosonornicotine; NNK, 4-(N-nitrosomethylamino)-1-(3-pyridyl)-1-butanone; NAB, N'-nitrosoanabasine

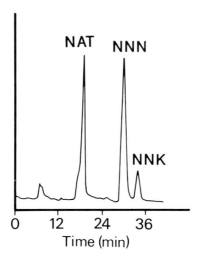

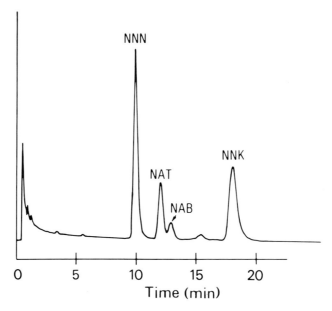

International Agency for Research on Cancer (1978a) that the identification of N-nitrosamines by GC-TEA requires confirmation by mass spectral analysis or by micro methods (Eisenbrand, 1978; Krull et al., 1979). Especially in the case of biological specimens, lack of confirmation can be misleading (Garland et al., 1982).

Standard methods for the analysis of VNA, TSNA and N-nitrosodiethanolamine (NDELA) in tobacco products and tobacco smoke have been published by the International Agency for Research on Cancer (Preussmann et al., 1983)

TOBACCO AND SNUFF

Case-control studies have shown that tobacco chewers and snuff dippers face an increased risk for cancer of the oral cavity (Moore *et al.*, 1953; Winn *et al.*, 1981). At present, the only known carcinogens in snuff are the nitrosamines and, especially, TSNA, although traces of polynuclear aromatic hydrocarbons and metals may be present (Hoffmann *et al.*, 1981a,b; Brunnemann *et al.*, 1983). TSNA are formed from nicotine and from minor tobacco alkaloids during ageing, curing and fermentation of tobacco (Fig. 4.; Hecht *et al.*, 1977, 1978). The majority of the tobacco alkaloids are 3-pyridyl derivatives (Tso, 1972; Enzell & Wahlberg, 1980), constituting 0.5–2.7% of commercial cigarette tobacco; whereas nicotine accounts for 85–95% of the alkaloid portion. Studies in which freshly detached tobacco leaves were fed ^{14}C-labelled nicotine indicated that, during curing, nicotine gives rise to NNN, 4-(*N*-nitrosomethylamino)-1-(3-pyridyl)-1-butanone (NNK) and traces of NAB (Fig. 4.; Hecht *et al.*, 1978; Adams *et al.*, 1983a). The majority of NAB derives from anabasine, as *N*-nitrosoanatabine (NAT) derives from anatabine (Fig. 4.). In addition to TSNA, processed tobacco may also contain VNA, including *N*-nitrosomorpholine (NMOR), NPRO and NDELA (Table 1). Correlation studies have shown that the nitrate and nicotine contents are not correlated significantly with TSNA levels; however, the formation of NNN and other TSNA is closely correlated with that of NPRO (Brunnemann *et al.*, 1983), indicating that a common underlying mechanism leads to the formation of various nitrosamines during tobacco processing (Table 2).

During the last two decades, increasing amounts of tobacco ribs have been added to cigarette blends, and, today, about 15–20% of cigarette filler consists of ribs (Normann, 1982). The nitrate content of ribs is significantly higher than that of laminae (Neurath & Ehmke, 1964);

Fig. 4. Formation of tobacco-specific nitrosamines; NNN, *N'*-nitrosonornicotine; NNK, 4-(*N*-nitrosomethylamino)-1-(3-pyridyl)-1-butanone; NAT, *N'*-nitrosoanatabine; NAB, *N'*-nitroanabasine

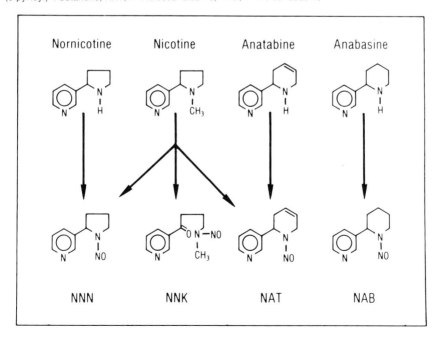

Table 1. *N*-Nitrosamines in commercial tobacco products (μg/kg dry weight)[a]

Tobacco Products	VNA					TSNA[b]		
	NDMA	NPYR	NMOR	NDELA	NPRO	NNN	NNK	NAT
Cigarette USA	ND[c]-28	ND-10	0-10	100-200	900-2 300	600-6 600	100-700	500-1 600
Cigarette UK	ND-10	ND-10	ND	ND-80	600-1 000	300	100	200
Cigarette France	40-180	ND-10	ND-1	ND	1 400-1 600	600-11 900	500-1 100	1 800-2 000
Cigar-little	20	20	ND	420	2 000	11 200	4 500	13 000
Cigar	10	10	ND	110	1 100	3 000-10 700	1 100-3 500	2 500-3 300
Chewing tobacco USA	30	20	30	200-300	450	3 500-8 200	100-3 000	500-7 000
Chewing tobacco India	10	10	ND	ND		2 400		
Snuff USA	ND-215	ND-360	30-690	29-6 900	3 500-22 000	800-89 000	200-8 300	200-4 000
Snuff Sweden	ND-60	ND-210	ND-44	200-390		2 000-6 700	600-1 500	900-2 400
Snuff Bavaria	10-50	10-300	ND	ND		6 000-6 800	1 500-1 600	3 900-4 400
Snuff Denmark	20-50	20-60	ND	ND		4 500-8 000	1 400-7 000	2 600-6 200

[a] VNA, volatile nitrosamines; TSNA, tobacco-specific nitrosamines; NDMA, *N*-nitrosodimethylamine; NPYR, *N*-nitrosopyrrolidine; NMOR, *N*-nitrosomorpholine; NNN, *N'*-nitrosonornicotine; NNK, 4-(*N*-nitrosomethylamino)-1-(3-pyridyl)-1-butanone; NAT, *N'*-nitrosoanatabine

[b] *N*-Nitrosoanabasine: In cigarette tobacco, ≤ 20 μg/kg; in snuff, 10-1 900 μg/kg

[c] ND, not detected

Table 2. Statistical correlations between levels of tobacco components in commercial tobacco products[a]

Independent variable[b]	Dependent variable[c]	r^2
NO₃	NNN	0.592
nicotine	NNN	0.238
NO₃	NPRO	0.522
PRO	NPRO	0.052
NPRO	NNN	0.961
NPRO	TSNA	0.899
NPRO, NO₃	NNN	0.966
NPRO, NO₃	TSNA	0.918
NPRO, PRO	NNN	0.962
NPRO, PRO	TSNA	0.903
NPRO, PRO, NO₃	NNN	0.966
NPRO, PRO, NO₃	TSNA	0.918

[a] From Brunnemann *et al.* (1983)
[b] PRO, proline; NPRO, *N*-nitrosoproline
[c] NNN, *N'*-nitrosonornicotine; TSNA, Tobacco-specific nitrosamines

therefore, addition of ribs has contributed in large measure to the elevation of nitrate levels in the US tobacco blends – from 0.5% to 1.2–1.5% (US Department of Health & Human Service, 1982). It was shown recently that the nitrate content of the ribs added to the tobacco blend correlates directly with *N*-nitrosamine yields in tobacco and in mainstream and sidestream smoke (Fig. 5; Brunnemann *et al.*, 1984). This trend to increase nitrate levels by using ribs and stems should be reversed or counteracted by selecting stems with lower nitrate content or by reducing the nitrate content of the stems by special fermentation processes, extractions or by other means.

Winn *et al.*, (1981), from the US National Cancer Institute, reported that snuff dippers are at increased risk for cancer of the oral cavity and especially for cancer of the gum. This finding supported an earlier observation by Axell *et al.* (1978) in Sweden. Since *N*-nitrosamines are the only known carcinogens in snuff, we analysed leading US and Swedish snuff brands for VNA, NDELA and TSNA (Table 3). Three of the US brands were found to contain more than 100 μg/kg NMOR, a potent carcinogen in experimental animals, while two of the Swedish brands contained only traces (10 and 44 μg/kg) of this nitrosamine and none was found in the other three brands. Morpholine, the precursor for NMOR, originates primarily in the non-tobacco additives used in the production of snuff (Brunnemann *et al.*, 1982). The precursor of NDELA in snuff is diethanolamine, which occurs in the residue of the sucker growth inhibitor, maleic hydrazide-diethanolamine (Brunnemann & Hoffmann, 1981). At present, NDELA levels are relatively high in US brands (290–3 300 μg/kg) but they are expected to decrease, since the herbicide was banned from use on tobacco as of October 1981 (US Environmental Protection Agency, 1981).

The most important findings, however, are the high levels of the carcinogenic NNN and of NNK, which are potent carcinogens in experimental animals (Hecht *et al.*, 1983a; Hoffmann *et al.*, unpublished data). The level of combined TSNA in popular snuff brands varies between 1.2–80 mg/kg, exceeding by at least two orders of magnitude the concentrations of carcinogenic *N*-nitrosamines found in other consumer products. US brand V (Table 3) appears to be made by a process other than fire-curing and thus contains relatively low levels of TSNA. Swedish

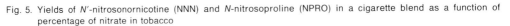

Fig. 5. Yields of *N'*-nitrosonornicotine (NNN) and *N*-nitrosoproline (NPRO) in a cigarette blend as a function of percentage of nitrate in tobacco

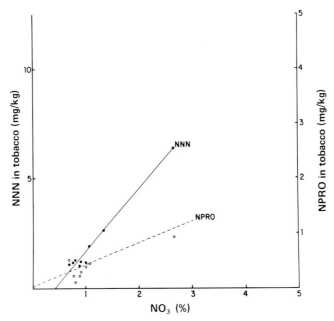

brand V is wrapped tightly in aluminium foil; this anaerobic storage appears to keep the level of TSNA at 4.2 mg/kg, in contrast to those of the other Swedish brands which were between 6.3 and 9.4 mg/kg. When this snuff was exposed to air for two weeks, there was a 50% increase in TSNA, indicating that, after manufacturing, ageing of the product can bring about still higher concentrations of these nitrosamines.

Chemical analytical data, recognition of the fact that carcinogenic *N*-nitrosamines are extracted from snuff during chewing and can be absorbed from the saliva (Hoffmann & Adams, 1981) and the results of bioassays for carcinogenicity (Hoffmann *et al.*, 1981a, b; Hoffmann *et al.*, unpublished data) make it possible to estimate the contribution of to the increased risk of snuff dippers for oral cancer. Peto *et al.* (this volume, p. 627) showed that 1 mg/kg *N*-nitrosodimethylamine (NDMA) or *N*-nitrosodiethylamine (NDEA) administered in drinking-water caused liver neoplasms in 23% and 42% of rats, respectively. These incidence rates were significantly higher than those in the controls. In addition, 1 mg/kg NDEA caused oesophageal tumours in 27% of male rats and none in control animals. The total doses administered to the animals during their life-times were about 37 mg/kg for males and 64 mg/kg for females. This study suggested the existence of a linear dose-response relationship in the dose range 0.033–1 mg/kg. Since NNK levels in moist snuff of the four most popular US brands average 2.5 µg/kg (Table 3), 30 years' exposure for average snuff dippers, who consume about 10 g snuff daily, amounts to 270 mg NNK, or about 3.9 mg/kg. In addition, snuff dippers are exposed to about 900 mg NNN ($\simeq$ 13 mg/kg), 800 mg NAT ($\simeq$ 11.4 mg/kg), 56 mg NAB ($\simeq$ 0.8 mg/kg) and 88 mg NMOR ($\simeq$ 1.2 mg/kg) in a 30-year span. These estimates, together with the dose-response study in rats cited above and the fact that *N*-nitrosamines are probably formed during snuff dipping, strongly suggest that *N*-nitrosamines play a major role in the

Table 3. N-Nitrosamines[a] in snuff (μg/kg dry weight)[b]

Snuff-Brand		Volatile N-Nitrosamines					Tobacco-Specific N-Nitrosamines				
		NDMA	NPYR	NMOR	Total	NDELA	NNN	NNK	NAT	NAB	Total
USA	I	215	(−)	24	240	760	2,200	600	1,700	100	4,600
	II	37	120	690	850[c]	1,700	19,000	2,400	19,000	800	41,200
	III	100	360	690	1,150	3,300	33,000	4,600	40,000	1,900	79,500
	IV	92	110	630	830[d]	290	20,000	8,300	9,100	500	37,900
	V[e]	(−)[f]	(−)	31	50	600	830	210	240	10	1,250
Sweden	I	22	(−)	44	70	240	5,700	1,700	900	140	8,440
	II	60	(−)	(−)	60	225	6,100	1,000	2,200	80	9,380
	III	14	210	(−)	230	390	5,300	1,400	2,400	70	9,170
	IV	30	50	10	90	310	4,000	830	1,400	80	6,310
	V	(−)	(−)	(−)	(−)	290	2,000	800	1,400	40	4,240

[a] NDMA, N-nitrosodimethylamine; NPYR, N-nitrosopyrrolidine; NMOR, N-nitrosomorpholine; NDELA, N-nitrosodiethanolamine; NNN, N′-nitrosonornicotine; NNK, 4-(N-nitrosomethylamino)-1-(3-pyridyl)-1-butanone; NAT, N′-nitrosoanatabine; NAB, N′-nitrosoanabasine

[b] From Brunnemann et al. (1982)

[c] Contains 44 μg/kg N-nitrosopiperidine and 21 800 μg/kg N-nitrosoproline

[d] Contains 13 μg/kg N-nitrosopiperidine and 350 μg/kg N-nitrosoproline

[e] Introduced on the market in 1982

[f] Not detected

increased oral cancer risk of snuff dippers. This hypothesis is supported by the recent observation that a single administration of 1 mg NNK induces a significant number of tumours in Syrian golden hamsters (Hecht et al., 1983a).

A number of physicians have suggested snuff use as a feasible alternative to cigarette smoking, since there is no evidence that use of smokeless tobacco leads to cancer of the larynx or of the lung and since its use does not appear to increase the risk for other destructive lung diseases or coronary artery disease (US Department of Health, Education & Welfare,1979; US Department of Health & Human Services, 1982). Since two million people in the USA and more than 100 000 people in Sweden are snuff users, and many are young people (Modéer et al., 1980; Christen & Glover, 1981), a reduction in the level of N-nitrosamines in snuff and/or inhibition of their formation during chewing and snuff dipping is highly desirable. A reduction of nitrate in tobacco and/or the addition of inhibitors of N-nitrosamine formation are two possible ways of achieving this goal.

CIGARETTE AND CIGAR MAINSTREAM SMOKE

Nitrosamines, and especially TSNA, represent an important group of carcinogens in tobacco smoke. Table 4 presents a summary of present knowledge with regard to the occurrence of VNA, NDELA and TSNA in mainstream smoke from cigarettes and cigars. The protein fraction of tobacco appears to represent the major precursor group of the carcinogenic volatile nitrosamines in smoke. This concept is supported by the observation that proline can serve as a precursor for NPYR in the smoke, the latter being formed by decarboxylation and N-nitrosation (Brunnemann et al., 1983).

Two methods have been shown to reduce effectively the levels of VNA in cigarette smoke: changes in agricultural practices, including less intensive nitrate fertilization and homogenized leaf curing (Tso et al., 1975), and selective filtration by cellulose filter tips (Morie & Sloan, 1973; Brunnemann et al., 1977). Most of the US filter cigarettes currently marketed (about 90% of all cigarettes sold) selectively reduce VNA by at least 70%.

Table 4 shows also that the TSNA are by far the most abundant nitrosamines in mainstream smoke. This is to be expected, since commercial cigarette and cigar tobaccos contain between 1.0 and 2.5% nicotine and other alkaloids (Tso, 1972; Piade & Hoffmann, 1980).

Studies with ^{14}C-labelled compounds have shown that (independent of the pH of the smoke) 40–46% of NNN and 26–37% of NNK in mainstream smoke originate from tobacco by direct transfer, whereas the remainder is pyrosynthesized during smoking (Fig. 6; Hoffmann et al., 1976; Adams et al., 1983b). Since TSNA are primarily part of the particulate matter, they are not reduced selectively by filtration, except in the case of dark French cigarettes, which have an elevated smoke pH (Hoffmann et al., 1980). A preliminary study indicated that dilution of smoke through perforated filter tips leads to selective reduction of TSNA in smoke (Hoffmann et, 1980); however, detailed investigations have not confirmed this earlier finding (Hoffmann et al., 1982). Thus, it appears that changes in the make-up of the blended cigarette represent the most likely means for reducing smoke yields of TSNA. As in the case of VNA, reduction of the nitrate content of tobacco ribs and laminae also appears to be a promising route (Fig. 7; Brunnemann et al., 1983).

Addition of ascorbic acid (0.1% added to tobacco ribs) to inhibit pyrosynthesis of TSNA during smoking was unsuccessful (Brunnemann et al., 1983); furthermore, addition of inhibitors to tobacco may lead to formation of toxic by-products in smoke.

A person who smokes two packs a day of French, black nonfilter cigarettes over a period of 40 years is exposed to 4.9 mg/kg NNN, 1.8 mg/kg NNK and 1.7 mg/kg NAT. A smoker of US nonfilter cigarettes is exposed to 2 mg/kg NNN, 1.0 mg/kg NNK and 1.7 mg/kg NAT

Table 4. *N*-Nitrosamines in cigarette smoke (ng/cigarette)[a]

Nitrosamine	Burley	Bright	French Black	Commercial	
				Non-filter	Filter
N-Nitrosodimethylamine	11–180	0.5–13.2	29–143	2–20	0.1–17
N-Nitrosoethylmethylamine	9.1–13	>0.1	2.7–12	ND–2.7	ND–2.5
N-Nitrosodiethylamine	4–25	ND–1.8	0.6–6	ND–2.8	ND–7.6
N-Nitroso-di-n-propylamine	ND	ND	ND	ND–1.0[b]	ND
N-Nitroso-di-n-butylamine	ND	ND	ND	ND–3[b]	ND
N-Nitrosopyrrolidine	52–76	6.2	25–110	ND–110	1.5–30
N-Nitrosopiperidine	9	ND	ND	ND–9[b]	ND
N-Nitrosodiethanolamine	2–90	ND	ND	36	24
N′-Nitrosonornicotine	3 700	620	590	120–950	310
4-(*N*-Nitrosomethylamino)-1-(3-pyridyl)-1-butanone	320	420	220	80–770	150
N′-Nitrosoanatabine	4 600	410	200	140–990	370
N′-Nitrosoanabasine			ND–150		

[a] From McCormick *et al.* (1973), US Department of Health & Human Services (1982), Klus & Kuhn (1982), Hoffmann *et al.* (1982)
[b] Reported only in isolated Instances
ND, not detected

Fig. 6. Formation of *N*′-nitrosonornicotine (NNN) and 4-(*N*-nitrosomethylamino)-1-(3-pyridyl)-1-butanone (NNK) in cigarette smoke

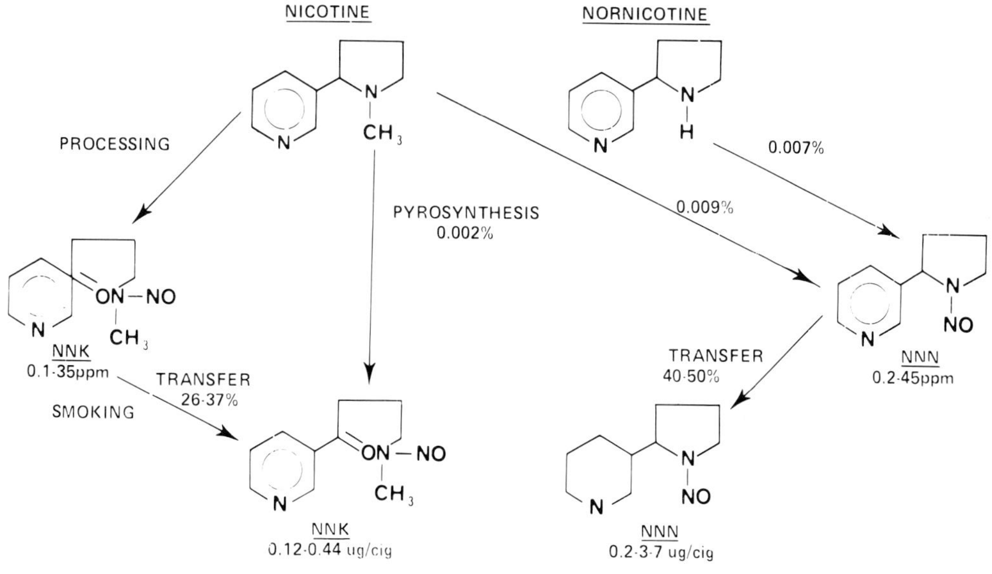

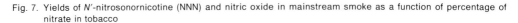

Fig. 7. Yields of N'-nitrosonornicotine (NNN) and nitric oxide in mainstream smoke as a function of percentage of nitrate in tobacco

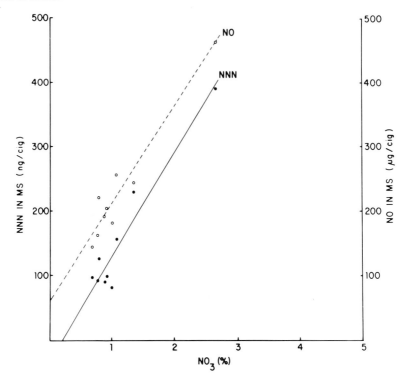

during the same time span (on the basis of machine smoking data). However, in contrast to snuff, tobacco smoke contains a large spectrum of other carcinogens, tumour initiators, tumour promoters and cocarcinogens (US Department of Health & Human Services, 1982; Hoffmann et al., 1983). A recent study indicated that whole smoke does not increase tumour response in Syrian golden hamsters pretreated with NNK (Hecht et al., 1983a); nonetheless, it appears likely that the various tumorigenic agents in tobacco smoke affect the tumour response to TSNA. For this reason, we consider that it is, at present, not feasible to estimate the contribution of nitrosamines to the increased risk to smokers of cancer at various sites. In our judgement, assessment of a risk factor associated with TSNA would best be approached by a bioassay for carcinogenicity in which hamsters are exposed to smoke differing only in TSNA content.

TOBACCO SIDESTREAM SMOKE

The smoke generated during puff intervals is called 'sidestream smoke' (SS). It is formed in an oxygen-deficient zone, and the combustion products leaving the region of generation are subject to a greater dilution and faster temperature decline than the vapour phase, which is drawn through the tobacco column to form the mainstream smoke (MS). The different modes of formation of MS and SS result in major differences in their physico-chemical natures (Table

Table 5. Comparison of mainstream (MS) and sidestream smoke (SS) of cigarettes[a]

Parameter	MS	SS
Peak temperature during formation (°C)	≃900	≃600
Particle sizes (μm)	0.1–1.0	0.01–0.1
Median diameter (μm)	0.2	0.1
Smoke dilution (Vol.%)		
Carbon monoxide	3–5	≃1
Carbon dioxide	8–11	≃2
Oxygen	12–16	16–20
Hydrogen	15–3	≃0.5

[a] 10 mm away from burning cone

5). Furthermore, all constituents of the vapour phase that are generated preferentially in oxygen-deficient zones are released into SS in significantly greater amounts than into MS. While generation of tar in SS is only 30–80% higher than that in MS, yields of carbon monoxide in SS are 2.5–4.7-fold, yields of amines are 10-30-fold and ammonia yields are 40-130-fold higher than in MS (US Department of Health & Human Services, 1982); nitric oxide generation in SS exceeds that in MS by 4-10 times; and nitric oxide is oxidized rapidly to nitrogen dioxide, so that SS has a greater nitrosation potential than MS (the latter contains practically only nitric oxide).

These findings led us to determine levels of VNA and TSNA in SS (Table 6; Brunnemann & Hoffmann, 1978). Concentrations of VNA were found to be 10–50 times higher in SS than in MS and this was confirmed in several other studies (Brunnemann et al., 1980; Rühl et al., 1980; Klus & Kuhn, 1982; Stehlik et al., 1982). It was found, however, that measurement of VNA in SS was greatly affected by the velocity of the airstream passing through the SS smoke chamber (Fig. 8; Brunnemann et al., 1977; Rühl et al., 1980; Klus & Kuhn, 1982). After adjusting for this effect, Brunnemann et al., (1983) found that the nitrate content of tobacco is a major determinant of VNA and TSNA yields in SS and that the nitrate in tobacco ribs added to cigarette tobacco blends elevated these yields significantly.

These quantitative measurements of VNA in SS raised the question of whether measurable quantities of carcinogenic N-nitrosamines occur in enclosed environments. After all, a single cigarette can generate up to 1 μg NDMA and additional amounts of other VNA. In two studies of indoor environments, relatively high concentrations of NDMA were found in the air of smoke-polluted rooms (Table 7; Brunnemann & Hoffmann, 1978; Stehlik et al., 1982). It is conceivable that these levels were due not solely to tobacco smoke pollution but may have been derived partially from other combustion sources; nevertheless, it was calculated that a non-smoker's exposure to VNA during seven hours in such a polluted atmosphere would be equivalent to exposure to VNA from the MS of ≃ 10 nonfilter cigarettes or 35 filter-tipped cigarettes (Brunnemann & Hoffmann, 1978). Differences in respiratory physiology between deep inhalation of concentrated smoke and normal breathing of smoke-polluted air, however, leave the question of the real effect of inhaled carcinogenic pollutants on man still to be evaluated.

Two recent case-control studies from Japan and Greece indicated that non-smoking wives of heavy cigarette smokers may have a greater risk for lung cancer than non-smoking wives of non-smokers (Hirayama, 1981; Trichopoulos et al., 1981). This observation was not confirmed by a large-scale prospective study by the American Cancer Society (Garfinkel, 1981).

Table 6. N-Nitrosamines [a] in sidestream smoke of commercial cigarettes and cigars (ng/cigarette)

Cigarettes [b]	Volatile nitrosamines [c]			Tobacco-specific nitrosamines [c]			Reference
	NDMA	NEMA	NPYR	NNN	NNK	NAT	
US – NF (1) [c]	680 (52)	9.4 (5)	300 (27)	1 700 (7)	410 (4)	270 (0.8)	Brunnemann et al. (1977)
US – F (1)	736 (139)	10 (8)	387 (76)	150 (0.5)	190 (1.3)	150 (0.4)	Hoffmann et al. (1980)
French – NF (1)	823 (19)	30 (25)	204 (9)				
French – F (1)	1 040 (160)	10 (20)	213 (25)				
Swiss – MF (1)	359 (13)	15 (12)	90 (7)				Brunnemann et al. (1980)
Swiss – F (11)	143–415 (12–830)	0–27 (5)	28–143 (3–53)				
German – NF (4)	156–401 (20–100)	3.1–19 (8)	84–107 (4–36)				
German – F (6)	175–398 (50–438)	6–24	7.2–150 (7–39)				
German – NF (2)	213–514 (32–37)	15.4–31	281–510 (17–24)				Rühl et al. (1980)
German – F (4)	330–558 (106–310)	13.2–35	296–700 (35–123)				
Little cigar – F (10)	1 700 (41)	75 (10)	612 (32)	880 (0.2)	810 (0.2)	570 (0.3)	Hoffmann et al. (1980)
Cigar				16 600 (5)	15 700 (8)	–	

[a] NDMA, N-nitrosodimethylamine; NEMA, N-nitrosoethylmethylamine; NPYR, N-nitrosopyrrolidine; NNN, N'-nitrosonornicotine; NNK, 4-(N-nitrosomethylamino)-1-(3-pyridyl)-1-butanone; NAT, N-nitrosoanatabine

[b] NF, nonfilter; F, filter; numbers in parentheses, number of cigarettes tested

[c] Numbers in parentheses, ratio of level in sidestream smoke to that in mainstream smoke

[d] N-nitrosodiethanolamine; in sidestream smoke, 43 ng; mainstream smoke, 36 ng (Brunnemann & Hoffmann, 1981)

Fig. 8. Device for collecting sidestream smoke; 1, to traps; 2, air intake; 3, to smoking machine; 4, cooling water intake

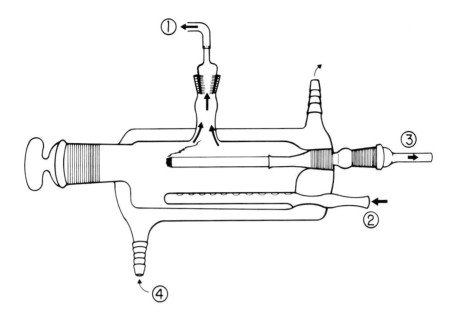

The Surgeon-General of the US Public Health Service concluded in 1982: 'although the currently available evidence is not sufficient to conclude that passive or involuntary smoking causes lung cancer in non-smokers, the evidence does raise concerns about a possible serious public health problem' (US Department of Health & Human Services, 1982). Such concern is heightened by the conclusions of a case-control study published in 1982, which indicated that exposure of pregnant women to SS pollutants (though not to inhalation of MS) may be related to an increased risk in their offspring for childhood brain tumours (Preston-Martin *et al.*, 1982).

Table 7. Volatile *N*-nitrosamines[a] in indoor air polluted with tobacco smoke ($\mu g/m^3$)

Location	NDMA	NDEA	Reference
Train – bars	0.11–0.13		Brunnemann & Hoffmann (1978)
Bar	0.24		
Sports hall	0.09		
Betting parlour	0.05		
Residence – nonsmoker	<0.003		
Office	0.03	0.03	Stehlik *et al.* (1982)
Conference rooms	0.02–0.033	0–0.02	
Working room	0.023	0	
Restaurants	0 – 0.05	0	
Dancing bar	0.07	0.2	

[a] NDMA, *N*-nitrosodimethylamine; NDEA, *N*-nitrosodiethylamine

ENDOGENOUS FORMATION OF *N*-NITROSAMINES IN SMOKERS
AND NON-SMOKERS

The discussions so far have been concerned only with the direct uptake of carcinogenic *N*-nitrosamines as a consequence of tobacco chewing, snuff dipping, inhalation of tobacco smoke or breathing of smoke-polluted air. However, the possibility must be considered that the uptake of MS or SS may also lead to endogenous formation of *N*-nitrosamines in humans. This hypothesis is supported by the fact that MS of a cigarette contains up to 0.6 mg nitric oxide, that smoke-polluted rooms may contain up to 0.5 mg/m^3 nitrogen oxides (US Department of Health, Education Welfare, 1979) and that nitrogen oxides are known to effect endogenous nitrosation of proline (Janzowski *et al.*, 1982).

At present, it is not feasible to differentiate quantitatively *N*-nitrosamines inhaled with cigarette smoke from those formed endogenously. Moreover, TSNA are rapidly converted to metabolites, many of which are the same as those that derive from the parent alkaloids (Hecht *et al.*, 1982; Castonguay *et al.*, 1983). In order to demonstrate endogenous formation of *N*-nitrosamines in cigarette smokers, we chose to measure *N*-nitrosation of L-proline to NPRO, as a surrogate assay following the principles and method developed by Ohshima and Bartsch (1981). For the actual assay, we placed 15 male cigarette smokers and 15 male non-smokers on a controlled low-proline, low-ascorbic acid diet for 12 days. On days 4, 5, and 6, they received 300 mg proline once daily; on days 7, 8, and 9 they were given 1 000 mg ascorbic acid followed by 300 mg proline. Ten of the smokers and ten of the non-smokers also received a single daily dose of 1 000 mg ascorbic acid on days 10, 11 and 12. Twenty-four-hour urine samples were collected on days 3, 6, 9 and 12 (Hoffmann & Brunnemann, 1983).

Table 8 summarizes our findings, details of which are discussed in another presentation (Brunnemann *et al.*, this volume, p. 819). Non-smokers on the control diet excreted 3.6 ± 2.1 μg NPRO during 24 h, and the 13 smokers on the control diet excreted an average of 5.9 μg/24 h. Supplementation of the diet once daily with 300 mg proline did not change the urinary NPRO excretion of the non-smokers significantly, whereas the average NPRO excretion by the smokers increased to 11.8 μg, with the highest value for an individual smoker being 49.3 μg. Endogenous NPRO formation in smokers was decreased significantly by supplementing the control diet with 1 000 mg ascorbic acid in addition to 300 mg proline. This effect was also observed in those individuals who received 1 000 mg ascorbic acid only as a dietary supplement.

These results demonstrate that cigarette smoke can contribute to the endogenous formation of NPRO. It may be deduced also from these findings that inhalation of cigarette smoke can result in the endogenous formation of other *N*-nitrosamines, including the carcinogenic nitrosamines deriving from tobacco alkaloids. As mentioned above, current technology does not permit the differentiation of endogenously formed *N*-nitrosamines from those inhaled with smoke, especially in view of their short half-life in physiological fluids (Adams *et al.*, this volume, p. 779).

Table 8.   Endogenous formation of *N*-nitrosoproline in man (μg/24 h urine)[a]

Protocol	Nonsmokers	N	Smokers	N
Control diet	3.6±2.1 [9.3]	13	5.9 [7.0, 8.5, 9.3, 13.5, 14.6]	13
Diet + proline	3.6 [5.9, 5.9, 6.4]	14	11.8 [7.3, 8.0, 9.6, 26.5, 40.5, 49.3]	14
Diet + proline + vitamin C	4.7 [6.4, 7.2, 8.2, 9.2]	13	4.6 [8.2, 8.3, 8.3, 11.8, 12.5]	13
Diet + vitamin C	4.0 [12.4]	9	6.0 [6.7, 12.6, 15.2]	8

[a]Values in brackets are those above the mean for nonsmokers on a controlled diet. Only samples containing 1.0 g or more creatinine/24 h were accepted. From Hoffmann and Brunnemann (1983)

EPILOGUE

This presentation has stressed the progress made in the last decade to relate N-nitrosamines to tobacco carcinogenesis. Perhaps the most important accomplishment is the demonstration that nicotine and other alkaloids give rise to carcinogenic N-nitrosamines that are tobacco-specific. One of the TSNA, NNK, is a powerful carcinogen, which induces respiratory tumours in 50% of Syrian golden hamsters in response to a single dose of 1 mg (Hecht *et al.*, 1983a). It has also been shown that TSNA are the only known carcinogens in snuff and that snuff induces oral cancer in long-term snuff dippers. In fact, hardly any other group of compounds occurring in the non-occupational environment has been more clearly associated with human cancer than the TSNA - an important finding when one considers that, in the USA alone, more than 60 million men and women use tobacco products. The identification of the major precursors and of the mode of formation of the various types of tobacco nitrosamines in a number of studies should now be translated into practical measures to modify products.

In the coming years, basic research should centre on developing methods for measuring tobacco-derived nitrosamines and their adducts in physiological fluids and on determining the nature and amounts of endogenously formed N-nitrosamines in tobacco consumers. The newly developed techniques should subsequently be applied to biochemical-analytical assessment of body fluids of tobacco chewers and smokers, which could then be correlated with epidemiological data. Furthermore, such micro-biochemical-analytical methods should enable detection of those individuals who are particularly prone to endogenous formation of TSNA and/or their metabolic activation. Such a research programme would appear to be not only highly stimulating and academically attractive but should lead to inhibition of the biological reactivity of N-nitrosamines in those men and women who will not break their tobacco habit.

ACKNOWLEDGEMENTS

We greatly appreciate the inspiration and support given by Dr Ernst L. Wynder, the founder of the American Health Foundation. The long-standing cooperation of Dr T.C. Tso, from the US Department of Agriculture, is also gratefully acknowledged. We thank Mrs Bertha Stadler and Mrs Ilse Hoffmann for their editorial assistance.

Our studies are supported by Grants P30-CA-17613 and PO2-CA-29580 for the National Cancer Institute, DHHS.

REFERENCES

Adams, J.D., Brunnemann, K.D. & Hoffmann, D. (1983a) Chemical studies on tobacco smoke. LXXV. Rapid method for the analysis of tobacco-specific N-nitrosamines by gas-liquid chromatography with a thermal energy analyzer. *J. Chromatogr.*, **256**, 347–351

Adams, J.D., Lee, S.J., Vinchkoski, N., Castonguay, A. & Hoffmann, D. (1983b) On the formation of the tobacco-specific carcinogen 4-(methylnitrosamino)-1-3-(pyridyl)-1-butanone during smoking. *Cancer Lett.*, **17**, 336–346

Axéll, T., Moernstad, H. & Sundstroem, B. (1978) Snusing och munhale cancer – en retrospektiv studie. *Laekartidningen*, **75**, 2224–2226

Brunnemann, K.D. & Hoffmann, D. (1978) *Chemical studies on tobacco smoke. LIX. Analysis of volatile nitrosamines in tobacco smoke and polluted indoor environments.* In Walker, E.A., Castegnaro, M., Griciute, L. & Lyle, R.E. eds. *Environmental Aspects of* N-*Nitroso compounds, (IARC Scientific Publications No. 19)*, Lyon, International Agency for Research on Cancer, pp. 343–356

Brunnemann, K.D. & Hoffmann, D. (1981) Assessment of the carcinogenic *N*-nitrosodiethanolamine in tobacco products and tobacco smoke. *Carcinogenesis, 2,* 1123–1127

Brunnemann, K.D., Yu, L & Hoffmann, D. (1977) Assessment of carcinogenic volatile *N*-nitrosamines in tobacco and in mainstream and sidestream smoke from cigarettes. *Cancer Res., 37,* 3218–3222

Brunnemann, K.D., Fink, W. & Moser, F. (1980) Analysis of volatile *N*-nitrosamines in mainstream and sidestream smoke from cigarettes by GLC-TEA. *Oncology, 37,* 217–222

Brunnemann, K.D., Scott, J.C. & Hoffmann, D. (1982) *N*-Nitrosomorpholine and other volatile *N*-nitrosamines in snuff tobacco. *Carcinogenesis, 3,* 693–696

Brunnemann, K.D., Scott, J.C. & Hoffmann, D. (1983) *N*-Nitrosoproline an indicator for *N*-nitrosation of amines in processed tobacco. *J. Agric. Food Chem., 31,* 905–909

Brunnemann, K.D., Masaryk, J. & Hoffmann, D. (1984) The role of tobacco stems in the formation of *N*-nitrosamines in tobacco and cigarette mainstream and sidestream smoke. *J. Agric. Food Chem., 31,* 1221–1224

Castonguay, A., Tjälve, H. & Hecht, S.S. (1983) Tissue distribution of the tobacco-specific 4-(methylnitrosamino)1-(3-pyridyl)-1-butanone and its metabolism in F344 rats. *Cancer Res., 43,* 630–638

Christen, A.G. & Glover, E.L. (1981) Smokeless tobacco: seduction of youth. *World Smoking Health, 6,* 2034

Doll, R. & Hill, A.B. (1950) Smoking and carcinoma of the lung. Preliminary report. *Br. med. J., ii,* 739–748

Druckrey, H. & Preussmann, R. (1962) Zur Entstehung carcinogener Nitrosamine am Beispiel des Tabakrauches. *Naturwissenschaften, 49,* 498–499

Eisenbrand, G. (1978) *5. Derivative formation.* In: Preussmann, R., Castegnaro, M., Walker, E.A. & Wassermann, A.E. eds, *Environmental Carcinogens Selected Methods of Analysis,* Vol. 1, *Analysis of Volatile Nitrosamines in Food (IARC Scientific Publications No. 18),* Lyon, International Agency for Research on Cancer, pp. 35–39

Enzell, C.R. & Wahlberg, I. (1980) Leaf composition in relation to smoking quality and aroma. *Recent Adv. Tob. Sci., 6,* 64–122

Garfinkel, L. (1981) Time trends in lung cancer mortality among non-smokers and a note on passive smoking. *J. natl Cancer Inst., 66,* 1061–1066

Garland, W.A., Holowaschenka, H., Kuenzig, W., Norkus, E.P. & Conney, A.H. (1982) *A high resolution mass spectrometry assay for N-nitrosodimethylamine in human placenta.* In Magee, P.N. ed., *Nitrosamines and Human Cancer, (Banbury Report No. 12),* Cold Spring Harbor, NY, Cold Spring Harbor Laboratory, pp. 183–196

Hecht S.S., Chen, C.B., Dong, M., Ornaf, R.M., Hoffmann, D. & Tso, T.C. (1977) Chemical studies on tobacco smoke. LI. Studies on nonvolatile nitrosamines in tobacco. *Beitr. Tabakforsch., 9,* 1–6

Hecht, S.S., Chen, C.B., Hirota, N., Ornaf, R.M., Tso, T.C. & Hoffmann, D. (1978) Tobacco-specific nitrosamines: formation from nicotine *in vitro* and during tobacco curing and carcinogenicity in strain-A mice. *J. natl Cancer Inst., 60,* 819–824

Hecht, S.S., Castonguay, A., Chung, F.L., Hoffmann, D. & Stoner, G.D. (1982) *Recent studies on the metabolic activation of cyclic nitrosamines.* In: Magee, P.N., ed. *Nitrosamines and Human Cancer (Banbury Report No. 12),* Cold Spring Harbor, NY, Cold Spring Harbor Laboratory, pp. 103–120

Hecht, S.S., Adams, J.D., Numoto, S. & Hoffmann, D. (1983a) Induction of respiratory tract tumors in Syrian golden hamsters by a single dose of 4-(methylnitrosamino)-1-(3-pyridyl)-1-butanone (NNK) and the effect of smoke inhalation. *Carcinogenesis, 4,* 1287–1290

Hecht, S.S., Castonguay, A., Rivenson, A., Mu, B. & Hoffmann, D. (1983b) Tobacco-specific nitrosamines: carcinogenicity, metabolism and possible role in human cancer. *J. environ. Sci. Health, C1,* 1–54

Hirayama, T. (1981) Non-smoking wives of heavy smokers have a higher risk of lung cancer. A study from Japan. *Br. med. J., 282,* 183–185

Hoffmann, D. & Adams, J.D. (1981) Carcinogenic tobacco-specific *N*-nitrosamines in snuff and in the saliva of snuff dippers. *Cancer Res., 41,* 4305–4308

Hoffmann, D. & Brunnemann, K.D. (1983) On the endogenous formation of *N*-nitrosoproline in cigarette smokers. *Cancer Res., 43,* 5570–5574

Hoffmann, D. & Wynder, E.L. (1972) Selective reduction of the tumorigenicity of tobacco smoke. II. Experimental approaches. *J. natl Cancer Inst., 48,* 1855–1868

Hoffmann, D., Hecht, S.S., Ornaf, R.M. & Wynder, E.L. (1974a) *N*-nitrosonornicotine in tobacco. *Science, 186,* 265–267

Hoffmann, D., Rathkamp, G. & Liu, Y.Y. (1974b) *Chemical studies on tobacco smoke. XXVI. On the isolation and identification of volatile and non-volatile N-nitrosamines and hydrazines in cigarette smoke.* In: Bogovski. P. & Walker, E.A., eds, N-*nitroso compounds in the Environment, (IARC Scientific Publications No. 9)*, Lyon, International Agency for Research on Cancer, pp. 159–165

Hoffmann, D., Hecht, S.S., Ornaf, R.M. & Wynder, E.L. (1976) *Chemical studies on tobacco smoke, XLII. Nitrosonornicotine: presence in tobacco, formation and carcinogenicity.* In: Walker, E.A., Bogovski, P. & Griciute, L., eds, *Environmental* N-*Nitroso Compounds; Analysis and Formation, (IARC Scientific Publications No. 14)*, Lyon, International Agency for Research on Cancer, pp. 307–320

Hoffmann, D., Adams, J.D., Brunnemann, K.D. & Hecht, S.S. (1979) Assessment of tobacco-specific N-nitrosamines in tobacco products. *Cancer Res., 39*, 2505–2509

Hoffmann, D., Adams, J.D., Piade, J.J. & Hecht, S.S. (1980) *Chemical studies on tobacco smoke. LXVIII. Analysis of volatile and tobacco-specific nitrosamines in tobacco products.* In: Walker, E.A., Griciute, L., Castegnaro, M. & Börzsönyi, M., eds, N-*Nitroso Compounds: Analysis, Formation and Occurrence (IARC Scientific Publications No. 31)*, Lyon, International Agency for Research on Cancer, pp. 507–516

Hoffmann, D., Adams, J.D., Brunnemann, K.D. & Hecht, S.S. (1981a) Formation, occurrence and carcinogenicity of N-nitrosamines in tobacco products. In: Scanlan, R.A. & Tannenbaum, S.R., eds, *Am. Chem. Soc. Symp. Ser., 174*, 247–273

Hoffmann, D., Castonguay, A., Rivenson, A. & Hecht, S.S. (1981b) Comparative carcinogenicity and metabolism of 4-(methylnitrosamino)-1-(3-pyridyl)-1-butanone and N'-nitrosonornicotine in Syrian golden hamsters. *Cancer Res., 41*, 2380–2393

Hoffmann, D., Brunnemann, K.D., Adams, J.D., Rivenson, A. & Hecht, S.S. (1982) N-*Nitrosamines in tobacco carcinogenesis.* In: Magee, P.N., ed., *Nitrosamines and Human Cancer (Banbury Report No. 12)*, Cold Spring Harbor, NY, Cold Spring Harbor Laboratory, pp. 211–225

Hoffmann, D., Hecht, S.S. & Wynder, E.L. (1983) Tumor promoters and cocarcinogens in tobacco carcinogenesis. *Environ. Health Perspect., 50*, 247–257

International Agency for Research on Cancer (1978a) N-*Nitrosodiethylamine.* In: *IARC Monographs on the Evaluation of the Carcinogenic Risk of Chemicals to Humans*, Vol. 17, *Some* N-*Nitrosamines*, Lyon, pp. 125–175

International Agency for Research on Cancer (1978b) N-*Nitrosoproline and* N-*nitrosohydroxyproline.* In: *IARC Monographs on the Evaluation of the carcinogenic Risk of Chemicals to Humans*, Vol. 17, *Some* N-*Nitrosamines*, Lyon, pp. 303–311

Jaffee, J.H. (1977) *Tobacco use as a mental disorder: The rediscovery of a medical problem.* In. Jarvik, M.E., Cullen, J.W., Gritz, E.R., Vogt, T.M. & West, L.J., eds, *Research on Smoking Behavior, (DHEW Publ. No. (ADM) 78–581)* Washington DC, US Government Printing Office, pp. 202–217

Janzowski, C., Klein, R., Preussmann R. & Eisenbrand, G. (1982) Nitrosation of sarcosine, proline and 4-hydroxyproline by exposure to nitrogen oxides. *Food Chem. Toxicol., 20*, 595–597

Johnston, L.M. (1942) Tobacco smoking and nicotine. *Lancet, ii*, 742

Klus, H. & Kuhn, H. (1973) Die Bestimmung des Nornikotinnitrosamines im Rauchkondensat nornikotinreicher Zigaretten. *Fachl. Mitt. Österr. Tabakregie, 14*, 251–257

Klus, H. & Kuhn, H. (1982) Verteilung verschiedener Tabakrauchbestandteile auf Haupt- und Nebenstromrauch. (Eine Übersicht). *Beitr. Tabakforsch., 11*, 229–265

Krull, I.S., Goff, E.U., Hoffman, G.G. & Fine, D.H. (1979) Confirmatory methods for the thermal energy determination of N-nitroso compounds at trace levels. *Anal. Chem., 51*, 1705–1709

Levin, M.L., Goldstein, H. & Gerhardt, P.R. (1950) Cancer and tobacco smoking. A preliminary report. *J. Am. med. Assoc., 143*, 336–338

McCormick, A., Nicholson, M.J., Baylis, M.S. & Underwood, J.G. (1973) Nitrosamines in cigarette smoke condensate. *Nature, 244*, 237–238

Mirvish, S.S., Issenberg, P. & Sams, J.P. (1981) A study of N-nitrosomorpholine synthesis in rodents exposed to nitrogen dioxide and morpholine. In: Scanlan, R.A. & Tannenbaum, S.R., eds, *Am. Chem. Soc. Symp. Ser., 174*, 181–191

Modeer, T., Lavstedt, S. & Ahlund, C. (1980) Relation between tobacco consumption and oral health in Swedish school children. *Acta odontol. scand., 38*, 223–227

Moore, C.E., Bissinger, L.L. & Proehl, E.C. (1953) Intra oral cancer and the use of chewing tobacco. *J. Am. geriatr. Soc., 1*, 479–506

Morie, G.P. & Sloan, C.H. (1973) Determination of *N*-nitrosodimethylamine in the smoke of high nitrate tobacco cigarettes. *Beitr. Tabakforsch.*, **7**, 61–66

Müller, F.H. (1939) Tabakmissbrauch und Lungencarcinom. *Z. Krebsforsch.*, **49**, 57–84

Neurath, G. & Ehmke, H. (1964) Untersuchungen über den Nitratgehalt des Tabaks. *Beitr. Tabakforsch.*, **2**, 333–344

Norman, V. (1982) Changes in smoke chemistry of modern day cigarettes. *Recent Adv. Tob. Sci.*, **8**, 141–177

Ohshima, H & Bartsch, H. (1981) Quantitative estimation of endogenous nitrosation in humans by monitoring *N*-nitrosoproline excreted in the urine. *Cancer Res.*, **41**, 3658–3662

Piade, J.J. & Hoffmann, D. (1980) Chemical studies on tobacco smoke. LXVII. Quantitative determination of alkaloids by liquid chromatography. *J. Liquid Chromatogr.*, **3**, 1505–1515

Posselt, W. & Reimann, L. (1828) Chemische Untersuchung des Tabaks und Darstellung eines eigentümlichen wirksamen Prinzips dieser Pflanze. *Geigers Mag. Pharmacol.*, **24**, 138–141

Preston-Martin, S., Yu, M.C., Benton, B. & Henderson, B.E. (1982) *N*-Nitroso compounds and childhood brain tumors: a case control study. *Cancer Res.*, **42**, 5240–5249

Preussmann, R., O'Neill, I.K., Eisenbrand, G., Spiegelhalder, B. & Bartsch, H., eds (1983) *Environmental Carcinogens - Selected Methods of Analysis*, Vol. 6, N-*Nitroso compounds (IARC Scientific Publications No. 45)*, Lyon, International Agency for Research on Cancer

Rühl, C., Adams, J.D. & Hoffmann, D. (1980) Chemical studies on tobacco smoke. LXVI. Comparative assessment of volatile and tobacco-specific *N*-nitrosamines in the smoke of selected cigarettes from the USA, West Germany and France. *J. anal. Toxicol.*, **4**, 255–259

van Stee, E.W., Sloane, R.A., Simmons, J.E. & Brunnemann, K.D. (1983) *In vivo* formation of *N*-nitrosomorpholine in CD-1 mice exposed by inhalation to nitrogen dioxide and by gavage to morpholine. *J. natl Cancer Inst.*, **70**, 375–379

Stehlik, G., Richter, O. & Altmann, H. (1982) Concentration of dimethylnitrosamine in the air of smoke-filled rooms. *Ecotoxicol. environ. Saf.*, **6**, 495–500

Trichopoulos, D., Kalandidi, A., Sparros, I. & MacMahon, B. (1981) Lung cancer and passive smoking. *Int. J. Cancer*, **27**, 1–4

Tso, T.C. (1972) *Physiology and Biochemistry of Tobacco Plants*, Stroudsburg, PA, Dowden, Hutchinson & Ross, p. 393

Tso, T.C., Sims, J.L. & Johnson, D.E. (1975) Some agronomic factors affecting *N*-nitrosodimethylamine content in cigarette smoke. *Beitr. Tabakforsch.*, **8**, 34–38

US Department of Health, Education & Welfare (1979) *Smoking and Health (DHEW Publ. (PHS) 79-50066)*, Washington DC, US Government Printing Office

US Department of Health and Human Services (1982) *The Health Consequences of Smoking: Cancer (DHHS (PHS) 82-50179)*, Washington DC, US Government Printing Office

US Environmental Protection Agency (1981) Maleic hydrazide: notification of issuances of notice of intent to suspend pesticide registrations. *Fed. Reg.*, **46**, (No. 179), 46000

Vilcins, G & Lephardt, J.O. (1975) Aging process of cigarette smoke - formation of methyl nitrite. *Chem. Ind. (London)*, **22**, 974–975

Winn, D.M., Blot, W.J., Shy, C.M., Pickle, L.W., Toledo, M.A. & Fraumeni, Jr, J.F. (1981) Snuff dipping and oral cancer among women in the southern United States. *New Engl. J. Med.*, **304**, 745–749

Wynder, E.L. & Graham, E.A. (1950) Tobacco smoking as a possible etiologic factor in bronchiogenic carcinoma. A study of six hundred and eighty-four proved cases. *J. Am. med. Assoc.*, **143**, 329–336

CARCINOGENICITY AND METABOLIC ACTIVATION OF TOBACCO-SPECIFIC NITROSAMINES: CURRENT STATUS AND FUTURE PROSPECTS

S.S. HECHT, A. CASTONGUAY, F.-L. CHUNG & D. HOFFMANN

Naylor Dana Institute for Disease Prevention, American Health Foundation, Dana Road, Valhalla, NY 10595, USA

SUMMARY

Over the past decade, research on the carcinogenicity and metabolism of tobacco-specific nitrosamines has provided a basis for understanding their possible roles in human cancer. 4-(N-Nitrosomethylamino)-l-(3-pyridyl)-l-butanone appears to be the most important tobacco-specific nitrosamine, because of its strong carcinogenicity. A large population of smokers and snuff dippers is exposed to significant quantities of this and the other tobacco-specific nitrosamines on a daily basis. Further research should now focus on the relationship between human exposure to tobacco-specific nitrosamines and the risk of developing tobacco-related cancers. Several important areas can be identified: we need to develop sensitive assays that can be used routinely to quantify the levels of tobacco-specific nitrosamines or their metabolites in human blood, and the levels of their DNA adducts in human tissues; we need to establish, through comparative metabolic and DNA-binding studies, the relationships between the organospecificity of tobacco-specific nitrosamines in experimental animals and that in humans; we may also be enabled to identify naturally-occurring substances that can inhibit carcinogenesis by tobacco-specific nitrosamines. These research approaches will hopefully lead to a reduction in the incidence of tobacco-related cancers.

INTRODUCTION

The detection of significant quantities of tobacco-specific nitrosamines (TSNA) in tobacco as well as in mainstream and sidestream tobacco smoke has provided the impetus for extensive studies on their carcinogenic properties and routes of metabolic activation. The results of these studies form the framework for further research on their role in human cancer, which is essential because, in the USA alone, more than sixty million people expose themselves voluntarily to TSNA. Some of the unknowns that might be addressed using this unique group of volunteers are: the relationship between exposure to nitrosamines and risk for developing cancer; the susceptibility of particular individuals to the carcinogenic effects of tobacco and tobacco smoke; the relationship between organospecificity in experimental animals and that in man; the mechanism of nitrosamine carcinogenesis in animals *versus* that in man; and the

Table 1. Carcinogenicity of tobacco-specific nitrosamines

Nitrosamine	Species and strain	Route	Principal target organs	References
 4-(N-Nitrosomethylamino-1-(3-pyridyl)-1-butanone (NNK)	A/J mouse	i.p.	Lung	Hecht et al. (1978); Castonguay et al. (1983a)
	F344 rat	s.c.	Nasal cavity, lung, liver	Hecht et al. (1980b); Hoffmann et al., unpublished data
	Syrian golden hamster	s.c.	Trachea, nasal cavity, lung	Hoffmann et al. (1981); Hecht et al. (1983a)
		oral swabbing	Nasal cavity, lung	Rivenson et al. (1983)
 N'-Nitrosonornicotine (NNN)	A/J mouse	i.p.	Lung	Boyland et al. (1964a); Hecht et al. (1978); Castonguay et al. (1983a)
	Ha/ICR mouse	topical	None	Hoffmann et al. (1976)
	F344 rat	s.c.	Nasal cavity	Hecht et al. (1980b, 1982b); Hoffmann et al., unpublished data
		oral	Oesophagus	Hoffmann et al. (1975); Hecht et al., unpublished data
	Sprague-Dawley rat	oral	Nasal cavity	Singer & Taylor (1976)
	Syrian golden hamster	s.c.	Trachea, nasal cavity	Hilfrich et al. (1977); Hoffmann et al. (1981)
		I.p.	Trachea, nasal cavity	McCoy et al. (1981b)
		oral	Trachea	Hecht et al., unpublished data
		oral swabbing	Trachea, nasal cavity	Rivenson et al. (1983)

N'-Nitrosoanabasine (NAB)

N'-Nitrosoanatabine (NAT)

4-(*N*-Nitrosomethylamino)-4-(3-pyridyl)butanal (NNA)

Compound	Species	Route	Oesophagus	Reference
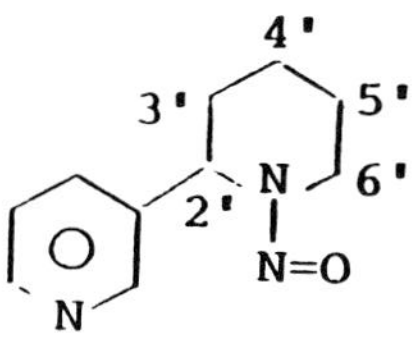 *N'*-Nitrosoanabasine (NAB)	F344 rat	oral		Boyland et al. (1964b); Hoffmann et al. (1975)
	Syrian golden hamster	s.c.	None	Hilfrich et al. (1977)
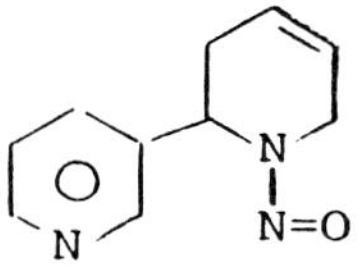 *N'*-Nitrosoanatabine (NAT)	F344 rat	s.c.	None	Hoffmann et al., unpublished data
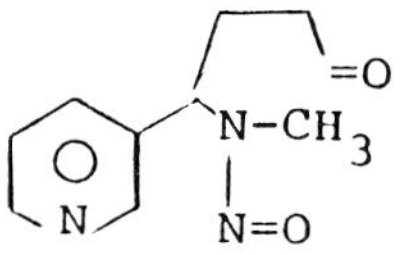 4-(*N*-Nitrosomethylamino)-4-(3-pyridyl)butanal (NNA)	A/J mouse	i.p.	None	Hecht et al. (1978)

inhibition of nitrosamine carcinogenesis by naturally occurring substances. To answer these questions we must focus on specific aspects of TSNA carcinogenesis, using the base of information that has been developed in the past decade. In this review we briefly summarize current knowledge and attempt to define some important areas of further research.

CARCINOGENICITY

The results of bioassays for carcinogenicity of TSNA are summarized in Table 1. 4-(N-Nitrosomethylamino)-1-(3-pyridyl)-butanone (NNK) is clearly the most carcinogenic compound in this group: in A/J mice, NNK induced 37.6 lung tumours per animal and N-nitrosonornicotine (NNN) 1.2 lung tumours per animal after a total dose of 0.1 mmol/animal; in Syrian golden hamsters, a total dose of 0.9 mmol NNK induced nasal cavity carcinomas in 11/20 animals, lung tumours in 16/20 and tracheal papillomas in 7/20, whereas an equimolar dose of NNN produced only one tracheal papilloma and one lung adenoma. The potency of NNK in Syrian golden hamsters was further demonstrated by the induction of tumours of the lung, nasal cavity and trachea by a single dose of 1.0 mg. In a comparative dose-response study in F344 rats, NNK and NNN were about equipotent in inducing nasal cavity tumours; however, with the lowest dose studied (1 mmol/kg total), NNK also caused a high incidence of lung tumours and some liver tumours. Although no comparative bioassay of NNK and other nitrosamines has been reported, on the basis of data in the literature it can be estimated that the carcinogenicity of NNK in Syrian golden hamsters is greater than that of N-nitrosomorpholine and could be equivalent to that of N-nitrosodiethylamine (Hecht *et al.*, 1983a,b). A comparative bioassay in F344 rats of NNK and N-nitrosodimethylamine is in progress.

At doses equivalent to those at which NNN induced tumours of the oesophagus or nasal cavity, neither N-nitrosoanabasine (NAB) nor N-nitrosoanatabine (NAT) showed significant tumorigenic activity in F344 rats, although higher doses of NAB did induce oesophageal tumours. 4-(N-Nitrosomethylamino)-4-(3-pyridyl)butanal (NNA), which is formed by the reaction of nicotine and nitrite but has not been detected in tobacco products, was inactive in A/J mice. NNK and NNN are thus the most important of the TSNA and should be studied further: the structure-activity relationships in this series are interesting; the lower activity of NAB than of NNN can probably be attributed to major differences in metabolism, as discussed below; the higher activity of NNK than of NNN can also be partially rationalized on the basis of metabolic data.

The route of administration has some effect on the target tissue specificity of the TSNA. In two bioassays in which NNN was given in drinking-water to F344 rats, high incidences of oesophageal tumours were observed; whereas, in a third study, subcutaneous administration of NNN induced mostly nasal cavity tumours. This difference could be due partly to local metabolism of orally administered NNN, since the oesophagus can convert NNN to electrophiles. NNN administered by oral swabbing or in drinking-water to Syrian golden hamsters was less carcinogenic than when it was given by subcutaneous or intraperitoneal injection, although the target organs – nasal cavity and trachea – were the same in both cases. These results indicate a need for further studies on the pharmacokinetics of NNN in experimental animals (see Adams *et al.*, this volume, p. 779). NNK administered to hamsters by oral swabbing still induced mainly tumours of the nasal mucosa and lung and only a few oral cavity tumours, indicating that it has the organo-specific properties normally associated with nitrosamines.

The question is often asked whether it is the TSNA or the polynuclear aromatic hydrocarbons (or perhaps other compounds) that are responsible for the carcinogenic properties of tobacco smoke. This question is difficult to answer, partly because of the use of diverse bioassay systems. The particulate phase of tobacco smoke, which contains the nitrosamines and the hydrocarbons, is carcinogenic to hamster larynx and mouse skin, which are the systems most frequently employed in bioassays of tobacco smoke and its condensate (Hoffmann et al., 1983b). However, nitrosamines are not normally active on mouse skin – we confirmed this for NNN. The TSNA have not been tested by inhalation in hamsters using the type of system employed for smoke inhalation studies; NNK should be tested in this way. We considered that it would perhaps be easier to define the role of TSNA in the carcinogenicity of snuff tobacco, in which they are the main group of known carcinogens. A bioassay, in F344 rats, of snuff tobacco extract and the corresponding nitrosamines is in progress.

A further aspect of the carcinogenicity of TSNA which requires more research is the possible role of promoters of cocarcinogens. Catechol, a major constituent of tobacco smoke, is cocarcinogenic with benzo[a]pyrene in bioassays on mouse skin (Van Duuren & Goldschmidt, 1976; Hecht et al., 1981a). Other tumour promoters and cocarcinogens are also present in tobacco smoke (Hoffmann & Wynder, 1971; Hecht et al., 1975, 1981a). We know nothing about the possible effects of these compounds on carcinogenesis due to TSNA, although it is known that compounds such as phenobarbital can promote liver tumours induced in rats by N-nitrosodiethylamine (Kitagawa & Sugano, 1978). The possible enhancing effect of ethanol on NNN carcinogenicity in Syrian golden hamsters was examined because of the epidemiologically demonstrated association between chronic alcohol consumption and smoking and cancer of the head and neck (McCoy & Wynder, 1979). No effect of ethanol on NNN carcinogenicity was observed, although in a parallel study chronic ethanol consumption did increase the incidence of nasal cavity and tracheal tumours induced by N-nitrosopyrrolidine (McCoy et al., 1981b).

METABOLISM AND ACTIVATION

Studies on the metabolism and distribution of TSNA are summarized in Table 2. These studies have recently been reviewed and the details will not be repeated here (Hecht et al., 1983c). NNN and NNK are quickly metabolized in vivo in rats, mice and hamsters to products which are excreted mainly in the urine. An exception is exhalation of carbon dioxide, resulting from metabolic degradation of the NNK methyl group. Autoradiographic studies have shown that NNN and NNK and their metabolites are distributed rapidly throughout the body fluids.

Table 2. Studies on the distribution and metabolism of tobacco-specific nitrosamines

Nitrosamine[a]	Subject of study	Reference
NNK	In-vivo metabolism in rat; in-vitro metabolism in rat liver microsomes	Hecht et al. (1980c)
	Tissue distribution and in-vitro metabolism in rats	Castonguay et al. (1983c)
	Tissue distribution and in-vitro metabolism in Syrian golden hamsters	Tjälve & Castonguay (1983)
	Tissue distribution and metabolism in pregnant mice	Tjälve et al., this volume; Castonguay et al., unpublished data

Table 2   (contd)

Nitrosamine	Subject of study	Reference
(contd) NNN	In-vivo and in-vitro metabolism by α-hydroxylation in rats	Chen *et al.* (1978)
	Metabolism by cultured human colon	Autrup *et al.* (1978)
	α-Hydroxylation by human liver microsomes	Hecht *et al.* (1979)
	Assay for microsomal α-hydroxylation	Chen *et al.* (1979)
	In-vivo and in-vitro metabolism by β-hydroxylation and *N*-oxidation in rats	Hecht *et al.* (1980a)
	Distribution and metabolism in mice	Brittebo & Tjälve (1980); Waddell & Marlowe (1980, 1983)
	In-vitro metabolism by rat liver microsomes in presence of DNA or guanosine	Lai *et al.* (1980)
	Effects of inducers on in-vitro metabolism by rat and hamster liver microsomes	McCoy *et al.* (1981a)
	Analysis of urinary metabolites	Hecht *et al.* (1981b)
	Formation of tissue-bound metabolites by target tissues	Brittebo & Tjälve (1981)
	Metabolism by cultured rat oesophagus	Hecht *et al.* (1982a)
	Localization and binding of metabolites in rats	Löfberg *et al.* (1982)
NNK and NNN	Comparative in-vivo metabolism in Syrian golden hamsters	Hoffmann *et al.* (1981)
	Metabolism in cultured A/J mouse lung	Castonguay *et al.* (1983a)
	Metabolism in cultured rat nasal mucosa	Brittebo *et al.* (1983)
	Metabolism in cultured human tissues	Castonguay *et al.* (1983b)
NAB and NNN	Comparative metabolism *in vivo* in rats and *in vitro* in cultured rat oesophagus	Hecht & Young (1982)

[a] NNK, 4-(*N*-nitrosomethylamino)-1-(3-pyridyl)-1-butanone; NNN, *N*′-nitrosonornicotine; NAB, *N*′-nitrosoanabasine

Bound radioactivity is typically located in the nasal mucosa of rats, mice and hamsters and in other selected tissues such as the oesophagus and tracheal-bronchial mucosa in rats and hamsters. The overall patterns of metabolism have been almost completely characterized, as shown in Figures 1 and 2. Major urinary metabolites of NNN result from 2′- and 5′-hydroxylation and *N*-oxidation. Major metabolic pathways for NNK include carbonyl reduction to 4-(*N*-nitrosomethylamino)-1-(3-pyridyl)-1-butanol (NNA1) and α-hydroxylation of both NNK and NNA1 to give urinary metabolites such as 13-15, shown in Figure 2.

Fig. 1. Metabolism, of *N*-nitrosonornicotine (NNN)

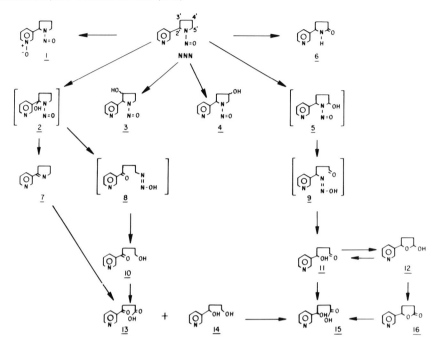

Fig. 2. Metabolism of 4-(*N*-nitrosomethylamino)-1-(3-pyridyl)-1-butanone (NNK)

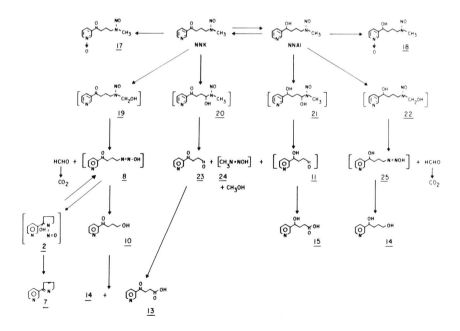

Table 3. Tumorigenic and mutagenic properties of metabolites and analogues o 4-(*N*-nitrosomethylamino)-1-(3-pyridyl)-1-butanone (NNK) and *N'*-nitrosonornicotine (NNN)

Compound	Assay system	Results	References
	S. typhimurium TA1535, TA100	More mutagenic than CH_3-N-CO_2Et $\ \ \ \ \ \ \ \ \ \ \ \ \ N=O$	Chen *et al.* (1978); Hecht *et al.* (1983d)
	A/J mouse	26 lung tumours/mouse; slightly less active than NNK	Castonguay *et al.* (1983a)
	A/J mouse	3.6 lung tumours/mouse; less active than NNK	Castonguay *et al.* (1983a)
	S. typhimurium TA1535, TA100	Activity equivalent to that of NNK	Hecht *et al.* (1983d)
	S. typhimurium TA1535, TA100	Inactive	Hecht *et al.* (1983d)
	S. typhimurium TA100	Weakly mutagenic without activation	Chen *et al.* (1978)

Compound	Test system	Result	Reference
	A/J mouse	0.9 lung tumours/mouse (inactive)	Castonguay et al. (1983a)
	A/J mouse	1.6 lung tumours/mouse (equivalent to NNN)	Castonguay et al. (1983a)
	S. typhimurium TA100	Mutagenic without activation	Chen et al. (1978)
	A/J mouse	0.8 lung tumours/mouse (inactive)	Castonguay et al. (1983a)
	F344 rat	Carcinogenic to nasal cavity and oesophagus, but less active than NNN	Hecht et al. unpublished data
	Syrian golden hamster	Inactive	Hecht et al., unpublished data
	S. typhimurium TA100	Inactive	LaVoie & Hecht, unpublished data
	S. typhimurium TA100	Inactive	LaVoie & Hecht, unpublished data

Table 3 (contd)

Compound	Assay system	Results	References
	S. typhimurium TA100	Inactive	LaVoie & Hecht, unpublished data
	A/J mouse	1.5 lung tumours/mouse (equivalent to NNN)	Castonguay et al. (1983a)
	F344 rat	Carcinogenic to nasal cavity; activity similar to that of NNN	Hecht et al. (1982b)
	F344 rat	Carcinogenic to nasal cavity; activity similar to that of NNN	Hecht et al. (1982b)

One goal of our research on the metabolism of NNN and NNK has been to characterize the metabolites responsible for their carcinogenic activities. The carcinogenic and mutagenic properties of metabolites and analogues of these two TSNA are summarized in Table 3. The terminal metabolites of α-hydroxylation, such as *10, 12* and *16* of Figure 1, were not mutagenic to *Salmonella typhimurium* TA100, in the presence of metabolic activation, and no mutagenic activity would be expected for the acids *13* and *15*. On the basis of studies of other nitrosamines, the electrophilic diazohydroxide intermediates *8* and *9* of Figure 1 and *8, 24* and *25* of Figure 2, which are formed by α-hydroxylation, would be expected to be important mutagenic or carcinogenic intermediates. The existence of mutagenic activity (without metabolic activation) of 4-(*N*-nitrosocarbethoxyamino)-1-(3-pyridyl)-1-butanone, *N*-nitrosocarbethoxyaminomethane-(methylnitrosourethane), 2′-acetoxyNNN and 5′-acetoxyNNN supports this assumption, since these compounds generate intermediates such as *8, 9* and *24* upon hydrolysis. The mutagenicity of 4-(*N*-nitrosocarbethoxyamino)-1-(3-pyridyl)-1-butanone is particularly impressive: as little as 0.4 nmol was active toward *S. typhimurium* TA100. Thus, the oxobutyldiazohydroxide, *8*, which is generated by both 2′-hydroxylation of NNN and methyl hydroxylation of NNK, is a potent DNA-damaging agent. NNK is particularly likely to cause DNA damage, since both *8* and the well-known mutagenic agent, methyldiazonium hydroxide (*24*), are formed during its metabolism. This potential may partially explain the potent carcinogenicity of NNK.

The results of bioassays of α-deuterated NNN derivates do not support the hypothesis that α-hydroxylation is essential to the carcinogenicity of NNN, since the carcinogenic activities of the derivatives were similar to that of NNN. Further studies are necessary to reconcile these observations with the known DNA-damaging properties of intermediates *8* and *9*, which are generated by α-hydroxylation. Since 4′-hydroxyNNN was tumorigenic in A/J mice, it is possible that it is involved in NNN tumorigenicity; however, it appears to be at most a minor metabolite in that strain of mouse. NNN-1-*N*-oxide was inactive in A/J mice and Syrian golden hamsters, but was carcinogenic in F344 rats, although less so than NNN. These results raise the question of the nature of the detoxification products of NNN metabolism. In F344 rats, NNN-1-*N*-oxide cannot be considered a detoxification product because it is carcinogenic. On the basis of assays in mice, 4′-hydroxyNNN retained its activity; 3′-hydroxyNNN might be a detoxification product, but is apparently formed at very low lewels. Of the major metabolic pathways leading to *1, 2* and *5* of Figure 1, none can be said to represent exclusively detoxification.

The carbonyl reduction product of NNK, the alcohol NNA1, is a major metabolite of NNK in cultured tissues, in A/J mouse lung and in various rat tissues; it is also a urinary metabolite of NNK in rats and hamsters. Like NNK, it is highly tumorigenic in A/J mice. Metabolic studies in mouse lung suggest that its activity results mainly from reconversion to NNK, followed by α-hydroxylation. NNK-*N*-oxide is clearly less tumorigenic than NNK in A/J mice, but it still has significant activity. These data in conjunction with those on the α-hydroxylation of NNK indicate that none of the known pathways of NNK metabolism can be considered exclusively a detoxification route.

The forms of NNN and NNK that are most likely to be active – the unstable α-hydroxynitrosamines and diazohydroxides – are probably not transported from one tissue to another. Therefore, the carcinogenicity of NNN and NNK in various tissues should depend in part on the ability of those tissues to produce the α-hydroxynitrosamines. This reasoning promoted studies on the metabolism of NNN and NNK in target tissues, and several important conclusions were reached in these experiments. The nasal mucosa of rats, a target tissue for both NNN and NNK, was shown to be highly active in converting both nitrosamines to electrophiles, indicating the presence of cytochromes P-450 in the nasal mucosa (Hadley & Dahl, 1982). The nasal mucosa of rats is more active than any other tissue (of those studied) in metabolizing NNN and NNK. Rat oesophagus is also highly active in metabolizing NNN by α-hydroxylation; on a weight basis, its activity surpasses that of the liver. Similar observations have been made with *N*-nitroso-*N*-methylbenzylamine (Hodgson *et al.*, 1980; Labuc & Archer, 1982). Rat oesophagus also has a remarkable degree of regiospecificity: it preferentially hydroxylates the 2′-position of NNN (ratio of 2′-hydroxylation:5′-hydroxylation, 3.4). In contrast, hamster oesophagus, a non-target tissue, has a 2′-:5′-hydroxylation ration of 0.3. Another example of the regiospecificity of rat oesophagus can be seen in the comparative metabolism of NNN and NAB: the ratio of 2′-:5′-hydroxylation of NNN was 3.1, but the ratio of 2′-:6′-hydroxylation of NAB was 0.2. These results are undoubtedly a consequence of the presence in rat oesophagus of multiple isozymes of cytochrome P-450 with different specificities for the closely related nitrosamines NNN and NAB. This observation may partially explain the low carcinogenicity of NAB. It also seems likely that rat and hamster oesophagus have different spectra of P-450 isozymes. Characterization of these enzymes might provide a partial explanation for the fact that rat oesophagus is a frequent target tissue in nitrosamine carcinogenesis, whereas hamster oesophagus is almost never affected.

Studies of NNN and NNK metabolism in cultured human tissues have led to several important conclusions. Tissues exposed to tobacco or tobacco smoke, including buccal mucosa, bronchus, peripheral lung and oesophagus, were able to metabolize NNN and NNK by α-hydroxylation, the presumed activation mechanism. This finding is a key link in the chain of evidence connecting TSNA to cancer; however, both the levels and patterns of metabolism in some human tissues were different from those observed in analogous animal tissues. For example, NNN was metabolized by *N*-oxidation and 5′-hydroxylation in cultured human oesophagus, in contrast to the results of studies with the rat oesophagus. If metabolism is an important determinant in organospecificity, then it seems reasonable to conclude that the target tissues for TSNA in experimental animals may be different from those in man. A remarkable finding in the studies of human tissue was the extensive conversion of NNK to NNA1: in all tissues studied, 50-80% of NNK was reduced to NNA1, whereas levels of α-hydroxylation or *N*-oxidation of NNK or NNN were typically less than 1%.

These studies suggest that analysis of smokers′ or chewers′ blood for NNA1 could provide a dose monitor for exposure to NNK. The development of sensitive methods for monitoring exposure to NNK has high priority in our research, since such data are necessary to establish an accurate basis for risk assessment. At present, we can estimate exposure to TSNA only by using data obtained under machine smoking conditions, which are artificial because of smokers′ compensation (Russell, 1980; Hoffmann *et al.*, 1983a) and because the possibility of in-vivo formation of TSNA cannot be taken into consideration (Brunnemann *et al.*, this volume, p. 819).

Characterization of NNN and NNK metabolites has made possible the identification of substances that might exert a protective effect against the carcinogenicity of NNN and NNK by inhibiting their activation. Particularly attractive in this respect are naturally occurring dietary components. In studies described by Chung *et al.* (this volume, p. 797), certain naturally occurring sulfur-containing compounds, such as benzyl isothiocyanate, have been shown to inhibit NNN α-hydroxylation in cultured rat oesophagus. While the complexities of this particular approach are enormous, it could eventually result in a rational basis for recommending potentially protective dietary modifications to tobacco users.

A challenging aspect of the carcinogenicity of TSNA which has not been solved is the identification of the carcinogen-DNA adducts. Recently, Castonguay *et al.* (this volume, p. 805) identified the first TSNA-DNA adducts formed *in vivo* – 7-methylguanine and O^6-methylguanine – in various tissues of rats treated with NNK. This finding confirms the assumption, based on studies of metabolism, that NNK is a methylating agent; comparison of its methylating ability with that of the thoroughly studied carcinogen, *N*-nitroso-dimethylamine, should provide important mechanistic information. The putative DNA adducts formed from diazohydroxides *8* and *9* have been more elusive. These 4-oxobutyl-

Fig. 3. Formation of a diazohydroxide from *N*-nitrosopyrrolidine (NPYR) by α-hydroxylation and adduct formation with deoxyguanosine

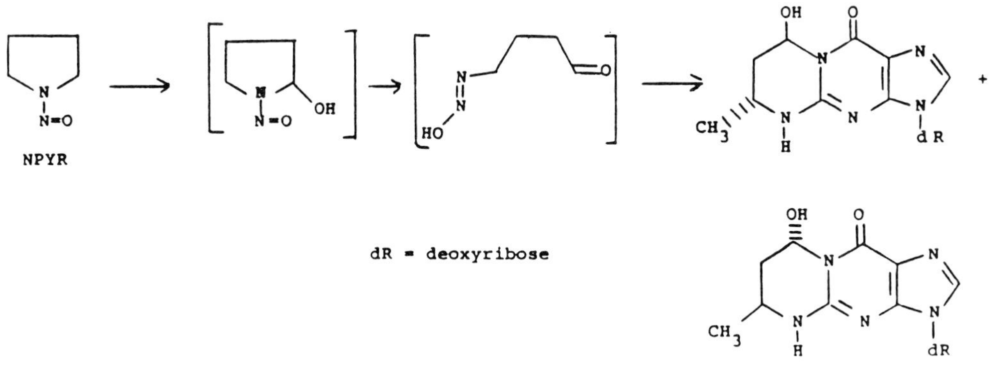

dR = deoxyribose

diazohydroxides are structurally similar to the diazohydroxide formed by α-hydroxylation of *N*-nitrosopyrrolidine, which reacts with deoxyguanosine to form cyclic 1, N^2-propano-deoxyguanosine adducts, as illustrated in Figure 3 (Chung & Hecht, 1983). We expect that *8* and *9* undergo similar reactions. The characterization of these adducts in DNA is an important aspect of our current research, since it would provide definitive evidence for the role of α-hydroxylation in the carcinogenicity of NNN and NNK and would allow further studies of the mechanism of their organospecificity. Data are still lacking on the miscoding properties of whatever adducts (other than methyl adducts) are formed from NNN and NNK and on their enzymatic or nonenzymatic removal from DNA.

An exciting prospect, once the DNA adducts have been identified, is that sensitive and specific radioimmunoassay techniques can be developed for their quantification, as has been done for several other carcinogens (Montesano *et al.*, 1982). Since NNN and NNK are specific to tobacco products, such an assay might provide a sensitive indicator of a smoker's ability to activate these carcinogens. This test could perhaps be used to identify smokers or chewers who were at a higher risk of developing tobacco-related cancers and would seem to be a reasonable approach to the prevention of these cancers.

ACKNOWLEDGEMENTS

Our studies on the carcinogenicity and metabolism of tobacco-specific nitrosamines are supported by National Cancer Institute Grants CA-21393, 29580 and 33285. We thank Mrs Lorraine Landy for her excellent work in preparing this manuscript.

REFERENCES

Autrup, H., Harris, C.C. & Trump B.F. (1978) Metabolism of acyclic and cyclic *N*-nitrosamines by cultured human colon. *Proc. Soc. exp. Biol. Med.*, *159*, 111–115

Boyland, E. Roe, F.J.C. & Gorrod, J.W. (1964a) Induction of pulmonary tumours by nitrosonornicotine, a possible constituent of tobacco smoke. *Nature, 202*, 1126

Boyland, E., Roe, F.J.C., Gorrod, J.W. & Mitchley, B.C.V. (1964b) The carcinogenicity of nitrosoanabasine, a possible constituent of tobacco smoke. *Br. J. Cancer, 23*, 265-270

Brittebo, E.B. & Tjälve, H. (1980) Autoradiographic observations on the distribution and metabolism of *N'*-[^{14}C]nitrosonornicotine in mice. *J. Cancer Res. clin. Oncol., 98*, 233–242

Brittebo, E.B. & Tjälve, H. (1981) Formation of tissue bound *N*-nitrosonornicotine metabolites by the target tissues of Sprague-Dawley and Fischer rats. *Carcinogenesis, 2*, 959-963

Brittebo, E.B., Castonguay, A., Furuya, K. & Hecht, S.S. (1983) Metabolism of tobacco specific nitrosamines by cultured rat nasal mucosa. *Cancer Res.* (in press)

Castonguay, A., Lin, D., Stoner, G.D., Radok, P., Furuya, K., Hecht, S.S. Schut, H.A.J. & Klaunig, J.E. (1983a) Comparative carcinogenicity in A/J mice and metabolism by cultured mouse peripheral lung *N*-nitrosonornicotine, 4-(methylnitrosoamino)-1-(3-pyridyl)-1-butanone and their analogues. *Cancer Res., 43*, 1223–1229

Castonguay, A., Stoner, G.D., Schut, H.A.J. & Hecht, S.S. (1983b) Metabolism of tobacco-specific *N*-nitrosamines by cultured human tissues. *Proc. natl Acad. Sci. USA* (in press)

Castonguay, A. Tjälve, H. & Hecht, S.S. (1983c) Tissue distribution of the tobacco-specific carcinogen 4-(methylnitrosamino)-1-(3-pyridyl)-1-butanone, and its metabolites in F-344 rats. *Cancer Res., 43*, 631–635

Chen, C.B., Hecht, S.S. & Hoffmann, D. (1978) Metabolic α-hydroxylation of the tobacco specific carcinogen *N*-nitrosonornicotine. *Cancer Res., 38*, 3639–3645

Chen, C.B., Fung, P.T. & Hecht, S.S. (1979) Assay for microsomal α-hydroxylation of *N*-nitrosonornicotine and determination of the deuterium isotope effect for α-hydroxylation. *Cancer Res., 39*, 5057–5062

Chung, F.L. & Hecht, S.S. (1983) Formation of cyclic 1,N^2-adducts upon reaction of deoxyguanosine with α-acetoxy-*N*-nitrosopyrrolidine, 4-(carbethoxynitrosamino)butanal, or crotanaldehyde. *Cancer Res., 43*, 1230–1235

Hadley, W.M. & Dahl, A.R. (1982) Cytochrome P-450 dependent monoxygenase activity in rat nasal epithelial membranes. *Toxicol. Lett., 10*, 417–422

Hecht, S.S. & Young, R. (1982) Regiospecificity in the metabolism of the homologous cyclic nitrosamines, *N'*-nitrosonornicotine and *N'*-nitrosoanabasine. *Carcinogenesis, 3*, 1195-1199

Hecht, S.S., Thorne, R.L., Maronpot, R.R. & Hoffman, D. (1975) Tumour promoting subfractions of the weakly acidic fraction. *J. natl Cancer Inst., 55*, 1329–1336

Hecht, S.S., Chen, C.B., Hirota, N., Ornaf, R.M., Tso, T.C. & Hoffmann, D. (1978) Tobacco specific nitrosamines: Formation by nitrosation of nicotine during curing of tobacco and carcinogenicity in strain A mice. *J. natl Cancer Inst., 60*, 819–824

Hecht, S.S., Chen, C.B., McCoy, G.D., Hoffmann, D. & Domellof, L. (1979) α-Hydroxylation of *N*-nitrosopyrrolidine and *N'*-nitrosonornicotine by human liver microsomes. *Cancer Lett., 8*, 35–41

Hecht, S.S., Chen, C.B. & Hoffmann, D. (1980a) Metabolic β-hydroxylation and *N*-oxidation of *N'*-nitrosonornicotine. *J.med. Chem., 23*, 1175–1178

Hecht, S.S., Chen, C.B., Ohmori, T & Hoffmann, D. (1980b) Comparative carcinogenicity in F-344 rats of the tobacco specific nitrosamines, *N'*-nitrosonornicotine and 4-(N-methyl-N-nitrosamino)-1-(3-pyridyl)-1-butanone. *Cancer Res., 40*, 298–302

Hecht, S.S., Young, R. & Chen, C.B. (1980c) Metabolism in the F-344 rat of 4-(N-methyl-N-nitrosamino)-1-(3-pyridyl)-1-butanone, a tobacco specific carcinogen. *Cancer Res., 40*, 4144–4150

Hecht, S.S., Carmella, S., Mori, H. & Hoffmann, D. (1981a) Role of catechol as a major cocarcinogen in the weakly acidic fraction of smoke condensate. *J. natl Cancer Inst., 66*, 163–169

Hecht, S.S., Lin, D. & Chen, C.B. (1981b) Comprehensive analysis of urinary metabolites of *N'*-nitrosonornicotine. *Carcinogenesis, 2*, 833–838

Hecht, S.S., Reiss, B., Lin, D. & Williams, G.M. (1982a) Metabolism of *N'*-nitrosonornicotine by cultured rat esophagus. *Carcinogenesis, 3*, 453–456

Hecht, S.S., Young, R., Rivenson, A. & Hoffmann, D. (1982b) *On the metabolic activation of N-nitrosomorpholine and N'-nitrosonornicotine: effects of deuterium substitution*. In: Bartsch, H., O'Neill, I.K., Castegnaro, M. & Okada, M., eds, N-*Nitroso Compounds: Occurrence and Biological Effects (IARC Scientific Publications No. 41)*, Lyon, International Agency for Research on Cancer, pp. 499–507

Hecht, S.S., Adams, J.D., Numoto, S. & Hoffmann, D. (1983a) Induction of respiratory tract tumours in Syrian golden hamsters by a single dose of 4-(methylnitrosamino)-1-(3-pyridyl)-1-butanone (NNK) and the effect of smoke inhalation. *Carcinogenesis* (in press)

Hecht, S.S., Castonguay, A. & Hoffmann, D. (1983b) *Nasal cavity carcinogens: possible routes of metabolic activation.,* In: Reznik, G., ed., *Nasal Tumours in Animals and Man,* Vol. 3, Boca Raton, FL, CRC Press, pp. 201–232

Hecht, S.S., Castonguay, A., Rivenson, A., Mu, B. & Hoffmann, D. (1983c) Tobacco specific nitrosamines: carcinogenicity, metabolism, and possible role in human cancer. *J. environ. Health Sci.,* CI *1,* 1-54

Hecht, S.S., Lin, D. & Castonguay, A. (1983d) Effects of α-deuterium substitution on the mutagenicity of 4-(methylnitrosamino)-1-(3-pyridyl)-1-butanone (NNK). *Carcinogenesis, 4,* 305–310

Hilfrich, J. Hecht, S.S. & Hoffmann, D. (1977) Effects of *N'*-nitrosonornicotine and *N'*-nitrosanabasine in Syrian golden hamsters. *Cancer Lett., 2,* 169-176

Hodgson, R.M., Wiessler, M. & Kleihues, P. (1980) Preferential methylation of target organ DNA by the esophageal carcinogen N-nitrosomethylbenzylamine. *Carcinogenesis, 1,* 861–866

Hoffmann, D. & Wynder, E.L. (1971) A study of tobacco carcinogenesis. XI. Tumour initiators, tumour accelerators, and tumour promoting activity of condensate fractions. *Cancer, 27,* 848–864

Hoffmann, D., Raineri, R., Hecht, S.S. & Maronpot, R.R. (1975) Effects of *N'*-nitrosonornicotine and *N'*-nitrosanabasine in rats. *J. natl Cancer Inst., 55,* 977–981

Hoffmann, D., Hecht, S.S., Ornaf, R.M., Wynder, E.L. & Tso, T.C. (1976) *Chemical Studies on Tobacco Smoke. XLII. Nitrosonornicotine: Presence in tobacco, formation, and carcinogenicity.* In: Walker, E.A., Bogovoski, P. & Griciute, L., eds, *Environmental N-Nitroso Compounds: Analysis and Formation (IARC Scientific Publications No. 14),* Lyon, International Agency for Research on Cancer, pp. 307–320

Hoffmann, D., Castonguay, A., Rivenson, A. & Hecht, S.S. (1981) Comparative carcinogenicity and metabolism of 4-(methylnitrosamino)1-1(3-pyridyl)-1-butanone and *N'*-nitrosonornicotine in Syrian golden hamsters. *Cancer Res., 41,* 2386–2393

Hoffmann, D., Hecht, S.S., Haley, N.J., Brunnemann, K.D., Adams, J.D. & Wynder, E.L. (1983a) *Tobacco carcinogenesis: metabolic studies in man.,* In: Autrup. H., ed., *Human Carcinogenesis,* New York, Academic Press (in press)

Hoffmann, D., Wynder, E.L., Rivenson, A., Lavoie, E.J. & Hecht, S.S. (1983b) Skin bioassay in tobacco carcinogenesis. *Progr. exp. tumour Res., 26,* 43–67

Kitagawa, T. & Sugano, H. (1978) Enhancing effect of phenobarbital on the development of enzyme-altered islands and hepatocellular carcinomas initiated by 3'-methyl-4-(dimethylamino)azobenzene or diethylnitrosamine. *Gann, 69,* 679–687

Labuc, G.E. & Archer, M.C. (1982) Esophageal and hepatic metabolism of N-nitrosomethylbenzylamine and N-nitrosodimethylamine in the rat. *Cancer Res., 42,* 3181–3186

Lai, D.Y., Arcos, J.C. & Argus, M.F. (1980) Interaction of the tobacco-specific nitrosamines, methylethylnitrosamine and N-nitrosonornicotine with DNA and guanosine. *Res. Commun. Chem. Pathol. Pharmacol., 28,* 87–103

Löfberg, B., Brittebo, E.B. & Tjälve, H. (1982) Localization and binding of *N'*-nitrosonornicotine metabolites in the nasal region and in some other tissues of Sprague-Dawley rats. *Cancer Res., 42,* 2877–2883

McCoy, G.D. & Wynder, E.L. (1979) Etiological and preventive implications in alcohol carcinogenesis. *Cancer, 39,* 2844–2850

McCoy, G.D., Chen, C.B. & Hecht, S.S. (1981a) Influence of mixed function oxidase inducers on the in-vitro metabolism of *N'*-nitrosonornicotine by rat and hamster liver microsomes. *Drug. Metab. Disposition, 9,* 168-169

McCoy, G.D., Hecht, S.S., Katayama, S. & Wynder, E.L. (1981b) Differential effect of chronic ethanol consumption on the carcinogenicity of N-nitrosopyrrolidine and *N'*-nitrosonornicotine in male Syrian golden hamsters. *Cancer Res., 41,* 2849-2854

Montesano, R. Rajewsky, M.F., Pegg, A.E. & Miller, E. (1982) Development and possible use of immunological techniques to detect individual exposure to carcinogens. International Agency for Research on Cancer/International Programme on Chemical Safety Working Group Report. *Cancer Res., 42,* 5236–5239

Rivenson, A., Furuya, K., Hecht, S.S. & Hoffmann, D. (1983) *Experimental nasal cavity tumours induced to tobacco-specific nitrosamines.* In: Reznik, G., ed., *Nasal Tumours in Animals and Man,* Vol. 3, Boca Raton, FL, CRC Press, pp. 79-113

Russell, M.A.H. (1980) *The case for medium-nicotine, low-tar, low-carbon monoxide cigarettes.* In: Gori, G.B. & Bock, F.G., eds, *A Safe Cigarette? (Banbury Report No. 3),* Cold Spring Harbor, NY, Cold Spring Harbor Laboratory, pp. 297-310

Singer, G.M. & Taylor, H.W. (1976) Carcinogenicity of *N'*-nitrosonornicotine in Sprague-Dawley rats. *J. natl Cancer Inst., 57,* 1275–1276

Tjälve, H. & Castonguay, A. (1983) The in-vivo tissue distribution and in-vitro target-tissue metabolism of the tobacco-specific carcinogen 4-(methylnitrosamino)-1-(3-pyridyl)-1-butanone in Syrian golden hamsters. *Carcinogenesis, 4* (in press)

Van Duuren, P.L. & Goldschmidt, B.M. (1976) Cocarcinogenic and tumour promoting agents in tobacco carcinogenesis. *J. natl Cancer Inst., 56,* 1237–1242

Waddell, W.J. & Marlowe, C. (1980) Localization of [^{14}C]*N*-nitrosonornicotine in tissues of the mouse. *Cancer Res., 40,* 3518–3523

Waddell, W.J. & Marlowe, C. (1983) Inhibition by alcohols of the localization of radioactive nitrosonornicotine in sites of tumour formation. *Science, 221,* 51–52

PHARMACOKINETICS OF TOBACCO-SPECIFIC N-NITROSAMINES

J.D. ADAMS, E.J. LAVOIE, M. O'DONNELL & D. HOFFMANN

Naylor Dana Institute for Disease Prevention, American Health Foundation, Valhalla, NY, USA

SUMMARY

Methods were developed to determine the biological half-life of N'-nitrosonornicotine (NNN) and 4-(N-nitrosomethylamino)-1-(3-pyridyl)-1-butanone (NNK) in Syrian golden hamsters and Fischer rats. The formation and elimination of 4-(N-nitrosomethylamino)-1-(-3-pyridyl)-1-butanol (NNAl), the major metabolite of NNK, was determined in the context of this study. The method consisted of extraction of the nitrosamine with ethyl acetate, elution through a Clin-Elut column, and concentration of the sample, followed by gas chromatography-thermal energy analysis. Biological half-lives of NNN, NNK and NNAl in hamsters were found to be 0.77, 0.25 and 1.78 h, respectively; in rats they were 5.78, 1.78 and 3.56 h. These findings clearly indicate species differences in the pharmacokinetics associated with the distribution and elimination of the tobacco-specific N-nitrosamines.

INTRODUCTION

Cigarette smoking has been associated with the development of cancer of the lung, oral cavity, larynx and oesophagus and is a contributory factor in the development of cancers of the pancreas, kidney and urinary bladder (US Department of Health and Human Services, 1982). Chewing of tobacco and snuff-dipping also lead to an increased risk for cancer of the oral cavity (Jussawalla & Deshpande, 1971; Axell *et al.*, 1978; Winn *et al.*, 1981a,b). N-Nitrosamines, particularly the tobacco-specific N-nitrosamines (TSNA), are the only known carcinogens in tobacco and are a major class of carcinogens in tobacco smoke (Hoffmann *et al.*, 1979, 1982a). Concentrations of TSNA in tobacco exceed by at least two orders of magnitude the concentrations of N-nitrosamines found in other nonoccupational environments. In mice, rats and Syrian golden hamsters, 4-(N-nitromethylamino)-1-(3-pyridyl)-1-butanone (NNK) is a strong carcinogen, N'-nitrosonornicotine (NNN) is a moderately active carcinogen, and N'-nitrosoanatabine (NAT) and N'-nitrosoanabasine (NAB) are weakly carcinogenic (Hoffmann *et al.*, 1982b; Hecht *et al.*,1983). The metabolic fates of the individual TSNA have been studied in a variety of animal and human tissues and in mice, rats and Syrian golden hamsters (Hecht *et al.*, 1983); however, at this time little is known about their pharmacokinetics.

The purpose of this study was to develop an analytical method for determining the biological half-lives of NNN and NNK in circulating blood of rats and Syrian golden hamsters. These analytical data were to be used in pharmacokinetic calculations to yield information that may relate to differences with regard to the metabolism and/or carcinogenicity of these TSNA.

MATERIALS AND METHODS

Pharmacokinetic studies were carried out with male F344 rats and Syrian golden hamsters. Animals were given a single intravenous injection of 150 µmol/kg body weight of either NNN or NNK in physiological saline. Blood from the treated animals was removed either intermittently by occular bleeding or once by heart puncture. Blood samples were taken once prior to treatment and 20, 40, 60, 80, 100 and 120 min as well as 3, 4, 8, 12 and 24 h after treatment. Upon removal, blood volumes were recorded, and the whole blood was placed in 5 mL ethyl acetate. This solution was sonicated and passed through a Clin-Elut extraction column (20-mL capacity; Analytichem International, Lawndale, CA, USA). The column was rinsed with 200 mL ethyl acetate, and the collected organic phase was concentrated to dryness. The residue was redissolved in 0.5 mL ethyl acetate and subjected to gas chromatography-thermal energy analysis (GC-TEA). Samples were injected (3 µL) into a 1.22 m × 2 mm i.d. glass column packed with 10% UCW-982 on Gas Chrom Q 80/100. The GC injection port was heated to 200°C, the oven was maintained at 195°C, and argon was used as the carrier gas at a flow rate of 75 mL/min. Under these conditions NNN eluted at 5.0 min, NNK at 8.8 min and 4-(*N*-nitrosomethylamino)-1-(3-pyridyl)-1-butanol (NNAl), a major *N*-nitrosamine metabolite of NNK, eluted at 11.6 min (Fig. 1).

Fig. 1. Gas chromatogram with thermal energy analysis (TEA) of *N'*-nitrosonornicotine (NNN), 4-(*N*-methylnitrosamino)-1-(3-pyridyl)-1-butanone (NNK) and 4-(*N*-methylnitrosamino)-1-(3-pyridyl)-1-butanol (NNAl) extracted from spiked blood.

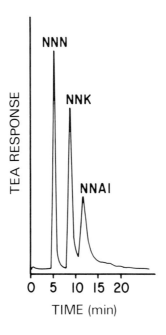

The TEA was modified as described previously so that these nonvolatile N-nitrosamines would be amenable to direct GC-TEA analysis (Brunnemann & Hoffmann, 1981). Pharmacokinetic data were calculated as outlined by Mayersohn and Gibaldi (1971). The curves that were plotted were generated from data obtained using a nonlinear power curve programme.

RESULTS

The efficiency and reproducibility of the analytical methods employed for the isolation of the TSNA were determined. When a known amount of NNN, NNK or NNAl was added to a blood sample (devoid of any TSNA), recoveries of >95% were obtained for each of the measured compounds.

During our initial pharmacokinetic studies with NNN in Syrian golden hamsters, the blood was sampled in one set of animals by intermittent eye bleeding of five animals and in a second set of animals by fatal cardiac puncture of two animals per time period. Comparison of the results from the two methods of blood sampling were within 8% agreement. Thus, in further studies blood was sampled only by cardiac puncture, the simpler of the two methods.

Results obtained from the pharmacokinetic studies of NNN in Syrian golden hamsters and F344 rats are outlined in Tables 1 and 2. Table 2 also outlines data on in-vivo formation of NNAl from NNK in both species. All values in these tables are averages from two animals per time interval; deviations from the mean of the two animals, within each group, were within 9%. These data were used to generate blood level curves, which were plotted semilogarithmically (Figs 2 and 3).

Semilogarithmic plots of nitrosamine concentration in plasma after rapid intravenous injection, where the curve can be resolved into two linear components, represent a two-

Table 1. Blood levels (µg/ml) of N'-nitrosonornicotine in Syrian golden hamsters and rats at various time periods after its intravenous injection

	20	40	60	80	100	120	180	240	480	720 min.
Hamster	19.0	11.0	4.2	3.5	1.1	0.76	ND	ND	ND	ND
Rat	19.0	12.0	13.0	12.0	12.0	9.0	8.5	8.0	4.7	0.8

ND, not detected

Table 2. Blood levels (µg/ml) of 4-(N-methylnitrosamino)-1-(3-pyridyl)-1-butanone (NNK) and levels of 4-(N-methylnitrosamino)-1-(3-pyridyl)-1-butanol (NNAl) in Syrian golden hamsters and rats

		20	40	60	80	100	120	180	240	480	720 min.
Hamster	NNK	7.6	2.1	0.84	0.42	ND	ND	ND	ND	ND	ND
	NNAl	200	95	76	40	15	5.7	2.6	0.7	ND	1.0
Rat	NNK	48	26	24	16	11	5.2	1.1	0.40	0.25	ND
	NNAl	34	61	73	61	57	22	21	11	8.3	1.4

ND, not detected

Fig. 2. Semilogarithmic plot of concentrations of *N'*-nitrosonornicotine (NNN) in the blood of Syrian golden hamsters and F344 rats after rapid intravenous injection.

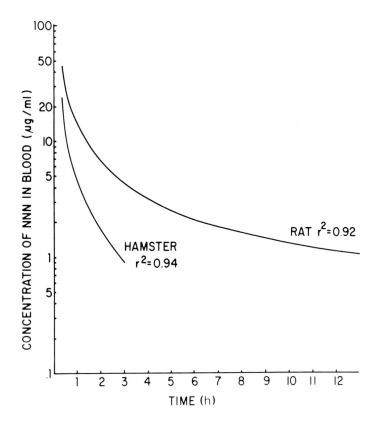

compartment, open, linear system. By visual inspection, all of the curves in Figures 2 and 3 fit into this category, except for the plot of NNK in the hamster, which most closely resembles a one-compartment model. Certain rate constants were calculated for these two-compartment systems according to the method of Mayersohn and Gibaldi (1971). In order to perform these calculations, each plot was separated into its two linear components using the method of residuals (Fig. 4).

The slopes of the rapid and slow exponential components are designated as $-\alpha/2.303$ and $-\beta/2.303$, respectively. The intercepts on the concentration axis are designated A and B. The rate constants k_{12}, k_{21}, and k_{10} were calculated using α, β, A and B as outlined in Figure 5.

Table 3 lists the values obtained for k_{12}, k_{21}, k_{10} and the biological half-life ($t\frac{1}{2}$).

Fig. 3. Semilogarithmic plot of concentrations of 4-(*N*-methylnitrosamino)-1-(3-pyridyl)-1-butanone (NNK) and -butanol (NNAl) in the blood of Syrian golden hamsters and F344 rats after rapid intravenous injection of NNK

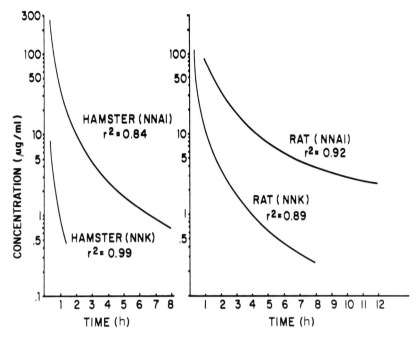

Fig. 4. Classical methods used to calculate rate constants for two-compartment models, based on data for concentrations of *N*′-nitrosonornicotine in rat blood

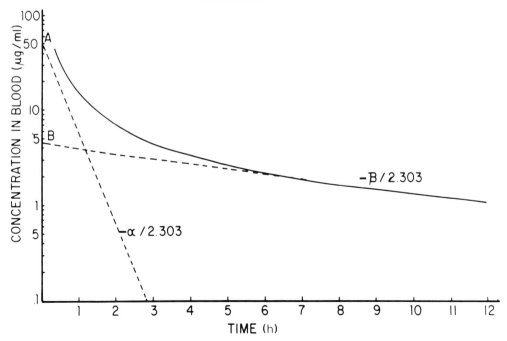

Fig. 5. Schematic representation of two–compartment model and rate constant equations

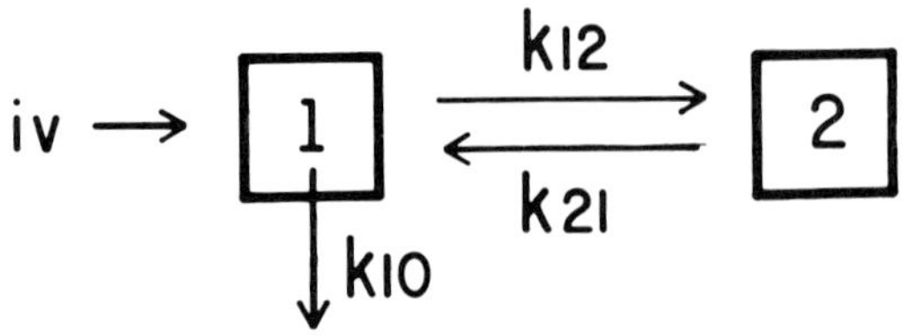

$$ iv \rightarrow \boxed{1} \underset{k_{21}}{\overset{k_{12}}{\rightleftarrows}} \boxed{2} $$

$$ \downarrow k_{10} $$

$$ k_{21} = \frac{A\beta + B\alpha}{A+B} $$

$$ k_{10} = \alpha\beta \,/\, k_{21} $$

$$ k_{12} = \alpha + \beta - k_{21} - k_{10} $$

Table 3. Pharmacolinetic data for N′-nitrosonornicotine (NNN), 4-(N-methylnitrosamino)-1-(3-pyridyl)-1-butanone (NNK) and -butanol (NNAl)

Species	Test com- pound	A µg/mL	B µg/mL	α	β	k_{12} h^{-1}	k_{21} h^{-1}	k_{10} h^{-1}	$t\frac{1}{2}$ [a] h
Hamster	NNN	40	10.25	2.86	0.90	0.48	1.30	1.98	0.77
	NNK[b]	–	–	–	–	–	–	2.76	0.25
	NNAl	310	12	2.83	0.39	0.44	0.48	2.30	1.78
Rat	NNN	50	4.50	2.17	0.12	1.10	0.29	0.90	5.78
	NNK	140	4.45	3.06	0.39	0.44	0.47	2.54	1.78
	NNAl	110	22	0.76	0.19	0.16	0.29	0.50	3.65

[a] $t\frac{1}{2} = 0.693/\beta$
[b] One-compartment model

DISCUSSION

It is clear from the data presented in Table 3 that the biological half-lives of NNN and NNK are more than seven times longer in Fischer rats than in Syrian golden hamsters. The half-life of NNAl, the major metabolic N-nitrosamine of NNK (Hecht et al., 1980; Hoffmann et al., 1981), was twice as long in rats as in hamsters.

The rate of elimination of NNK in Fischer rats was 2.8 times greater than that of NNN, reflecting their biological half-lives of 5.78 h and 1.78 h, respectively; however, the apparent rate of elimination of NNAl was almost one-half that of NNN, although their half-lives are similar.

In hamsters, NNK was rapidly converted to NNAl. This transformation appears to be the major route of elimination of NNK, which has a half-life of only 15 min, whereas NNAl has a half-life of approximately 1 h. These data suggest that, *in vivo*, the dominant form of NNK is NNAl and that NNAl may be associated with in-vivo metabolic activation of NNK to a carcinogen. In marked contrast to results obtained in Fischer rats, NNAl in the hamster has a longer half-life than NNN.

These findings clearly indicate species differences in the pharmacokinetics associated with the distribution and elimination of TSNA. The carcinogenic potencies of NNN and NNK are thus not directly proportional to the biological half-lives of the compounds. Carcinogenicity bioassays have not demonstrated conclusively whether rats or hamsters are more susceptible to the carcinogenic activity of NNK. In view of the differences between these two species in rates of conversion of NNK to NNAl *in vivo*, a possible correlation of this phenomenon with carcinogenic potency would be of interest. Further studies are in progress to determine whether pharmacokinetic data for *N*-nitrosanabasine and *N*-nitrosoanatabine will explain their significantly lower carcinogenic potency, in comparison to that of NNN or NNK, in rats. Studies are in progress with NNAl to determine whether any conversion to NNK can be detected in the circulating blood of rats or hamsters.

REFERENCES

Axéll, T., Moernstad, H. & Sundstroem, B. (1978) Snusing och munhale cancer - en retrospectiv studie. *Laekartidningen* **75**, 2224–2226

Brunnemann, K.D. & Hoffmann, D. (1981) Assessment of the carcinogenic *N*-nitrosodiethanolamine in tobacco products and tobacco smoke. *Carcinogenesis,* **2**, 1123–1127

Hecht, S.S., Young, R. & Chen, C.B. (1980) Metabolism in the F-344 rat of 4-(*N*-methyl-*N*-nitrosamino)-1-(3-pyridyl)-1-butanone, a tobacco-specific carcinogen. *Cancer Res.,* **40**, 4144–4150

Hecht, S.S., Castonguay, A., Rivenson, A., Mu, B. & Hoffmann, D. (1983) Tobacco specific nitrosamines: Carcinogenicity, metabolism, and possible role in human cancer. *J. environ. Sci. Health,* **CI(1)**, 1–54

Hoffmann, D., Adams, J.D., Brunnemann, K.D. & Hecht, S.S. (1979) Assessment of tobacco-specific *N*-nitrosamines in tobacco products. *Cancer Res.,* **39**, 2505–2509

Hoffmann, D., Castonguay, A., Rivenson, A. & Hecht, SS. (1981) Comparative carcinogenicity and metabolism of 4-(methylnitrosamino)-1-(3-pyridyl)-1-butanone and *N'*-nitrosonornicotine in Syrian golden hamsters. *Cancer Res.,* **41**, 2386–2393

Hoffmann, D., Adams, J.D., Brunnemann, K.D., Rivenson, A. & Hecht, S.S. (1982a) *Tobacco-specific N-nitrosamines:Occurrence and bioassays.* In: Bartsch, H., O'Neill, I.K., Castegnaro, M. & Okada, M., eds, N-*Nitroso Compounds: Occurrence and Biological Effects (IARC Scientific Publications No. 41),* Lyon, International Agency for Research on Cancer, pp. 309–318

Hoffmann, D., Brunnemann, K.D., Adams, J.D., Rivenson, A. & Hecht, S.S. (1982b). N-*Nitrosamines in tobacco carcinogenesis.* In: Magee, P., ed., *Nitrosamines and Human Cancer (Banbury Report No. 12),* Cold Spring Harbor, NY, Cold Spring Harbor Laboratory, pp. 211–226

Jussawalla, D.J. & Deshpande, V.A. (1971) Evaluation of cancer risk in tobacco chewers and smokers. An epidemiologic assessment. *Cancer,* **28**, 244–252

Mayersohn, A. & Gibaldi, M. (1971) Mathematical methods in pharmacokinetics. II. Solution of the two-compartment open model. *Am. J. pharmacol. Educ.,* **35**, 19–28

US Department of Health and Human Services (1982) *The Health Consequences of smoking: Cancer, (DHHS (PHS) 82-50-179),* Washington DC, US Government Printing Office

Winn, D.M., Blot, W.J., Shy, C.M., Pickle, D.W., Toledo, A. & Fraumeni, J.R., Jr (1981a) Snuff dipping and oral cancer among women in the southern United States. *New Engl. J. Med.,* **304**, 745–749

Winn, D.M., Blot, W.J. & Fraumeni, J.R., Jr (1981b) Snuff dipping and oral cancer. *New Engl. J. Med.,* **305**, 230–231

FATE OF THE TOBACCO-SPECIFIC CARCINOGEN 4-(METHYL-NITROSAMINO)-1-(3-PYRIDYL)-1-BUTANONE IN PREGNANT AND NEWBORN C57BL MICE

H. TJÄLVE

Department of Pharmacology and Toxicology, Uppsala Biomedical Centre, Box 573, S-751 23 Uppsala, Sweden

A. CASTONGUAY & S.S. HECHT

Naylor Dana Institute for Disease Prevention, American Health Foundation, Valhalla, New York 10595, USA

SUMMARY

Whole-body autoradiography of pregnant C57Bl mice injected intravenously with the tobacco-specific *N*-nitrosamine, 4-(methylnitrosamino)-1-(3-pyridyl)-1-butanone (NNK), indicated that NNK and/or its metabolites can diffuse through the placenta and reach the fetal tissues. During the last days of gestation, nasal, pulmonary and hepatic tissues develop the enzymatic capacity to activate NNK to alkylating species which bind covalently to cellular macromolecules. Within 4 h of the injection, a considerable proportion of NNK metabolites present in the fetal tissues are excreted in the amniotic fluid *via* the fetal urinary tract.

Incubation of tissue slices with NNK indicated that the nose, the lung and the liver of 13-day-old fetuses could reduce NNK to 4-(methylnitrosamino)-1-(3-pyridyl)butan-1-ol (NNAl), but could not activate NNK by α-carbon hydroxylation. However, these activating enzymes were competent in 18-day old fetuses, and the activities increased during the first six days of life. The results provide evidence that NNK could exert genotoxic effects transplacentally and in newborn mice.

INTRODUCTION

Maternal tobacco smoking during pregnancy may increase the risk for the progeny to develop cancer during childhood (Neutel & Buck, 1971) and during adult life (Everson, 1980). In addition, newborn children of smokers are likely to be exposed to carcinogens present in sidestream smoke. Mainstream and sidestream smoke contain many procarcinogens which have very different chemical structures. Recent studies have focused on the high levels of nicotine-derived *N*-nitrosamines present in tobacco smoke (Hoffmann *et al.*, 1979) and their high carcinogenic potency in experimental animals (Hecht *et al.*, 1980a; Hoffmann *et al.*, 1981; Castonguay *et al.*, 1983a).

Carcinogenicity of cigarette tobacco smoke condensate was demonstrated in C57Bl mice (Flasks, 1966). Metabolism and tissue distribution of *N'*-nitrosonornicotine (NNN) and *N*-nitrosodimethylamine (NDMA) in this strain are also well documented (Johansson-Brittebo & Tjälve, 1979; Brittebo & Tjälve, 1980; Waddell & Marlow, 1980). In the present study, we compare the metabolism and tissue distribution of NNK with those of NNN and NDMA. We show that NNK can cross the placental barrier in pregnant C57Bl mice and can be activated by α-carbon hydroxylation in some fetal tissues during the last stage of gestation.

MATERIALS AND METHODS

Chemicals

[Carbonyl-^{14}C]-NNK, specific radioactivity 4.2 mCi/mmol, with a purity of > 99%, was used[1]. The synthesis of NNK and its metabolites, used as reference compounds in high-performance liquid chromatography (HPLC), has already been described (Hecht *et al.*, 1980b).

Animals

Pigmented C57Bl mice were mated overnight. The day on which a vaginal plug was found in the morning was considered as day 0 of pregnancy. Delivery usually took place on the night before day 19, which was considered as day 1 of life. Sexes of fetuses or newborn were not determined.

In-vivo *experiments*

Whole-body autoradiography was performed according to the method of Ullberg (1977), using freeze-dried sections to localize total radioactivity and sections extracted with trichloroacetic acid and organic solvents to localize tissue-bound metabolites (Castonguay *et al.*, 1983b). Pregnant mice were injected intravenously and newborn mice were injected subcutaneously with 7.0 mg/kg body weight of [carbonyl-^{14}C]-NNK. The following series were used: 18-day pregnant mice, 5-min, 15-min, 1-h, 4-h and 8-h survival; 16-day pregnant mouse, 1-h survival; 13-day pregnant mice, 1-h and 4-h survival; 3- and 6-day-old newborn mice, 4-h survival.

Levels of radioactivity present in various maternal and fetal tissues were determined on day 18 of gestation by liquid scintillation counting in three mice injected intravenously with 7.0 mg/kg body weight of [carbonyl-^{14}C]-NNK. The mice were sacrificed after 8 h. For determination of total tissue-radioactivity, non-treated specimens were dissolved in Soluene 350®. For determination of tissue-bound metabolites, the specimens were homogenized in 2 mL of 5% trichloroacetic acid, then extracted sequentially with 2 mL of 95% ethanol, 100% ethanol, chloroform : methanol (2 : 1, v/v), and diethyl ether, before solubilization in Soluene 350®. Levels of total and bound radioactivity were then determined by liquid scintillation counting.

Levels of NNK and its metabolites in fetuses and placentae of three 13-day pregnant mice given 7.5 mg/kg body weight of [carbonyl-^{14}C]-NNK intravenously and sacrificed after 1 h,

---

[1] Castonguay & Hecht, in preparation

were quantified by HPLC and liquid scintillation counting, according to published procedures (Castonguay *et al.*, 1983b).

For determination of metabolites in the amniotic fluid, two 18-day pregnant mice were injected intravenously with 7.0 mg/kg body weight of [carbonyl-^{14}C]-NNK. The mice were sacrificed after 4 h, the amniotic fluid was collected and the metabolites quantified as above.

In-vitro *experiments*

Tissue slices (35–200 mg) from fetal, newborn or pregnant C57Bl mice were incubated for 2 h at 37°C in 2 mL Krebs-Ringer phosphate solution (pH 7.0), containing 10 mmol/L of glucose and 0.28 µCi (66 nmol) of [carbonyl-^{14}C]-NNK. The incubations were terminated by the addition of 0.22 mL of 1 mol/L hydrochloric acid. The tissues were homogenized and centrifuged, and the supernatants were neutralized with an equal volume of 0.1 mol/L sodium hydroxide. After filtration through a filter paper under vacuum, the metabolites present in the solutions were quantified as described above.

RESULTS

In-vivo *experiments*

The results of the whole-body autoradiography showed that NNK and/or its metabolites can cross the placental membranes and reach the fetal tissues (Fig. 1A, B). Levels of radioactive metabolites in the fetal tissues increased slowly after injection of NNK. At 1-h survival interval, labelling of fetal tissues exceeded that of many maternal tissues. At 4-h interval, there was high labelling of the amniotic fluid (Fig. 1C) and this labelling was still observed after 8 h. Fetal kidney and eye melanin contained more label, and brain less, than the other fetal tissues. Considerable radioactivity was present in the placenta at the 1-h and later survival intervals.

Extraction of tissue sections of 16- and 18-day pregnant mice with trichloroacetic acid and organic solvents removed the radioactivity in all fetal tissues, except nasal mucosa and eye melanin. In the 13-day pregnant mice, bound radioactivity was present only in eye melanin. All radioactive metabolites present in the placenta and amniotic fluid were extractable (Fig. 1D).

In the maternal tissues, non-extractable metabolites were present in nasal mucosa, the lateral nasal gland, tracheo-bronchial mucosa and liver. In freeze-dried, non-extracted sections, there was, in addition, homogeneously-distributed radioactivity in most tissues. There was also labelling of lachrymal glands, adrenal cortex, kidneys and the contents of the stomach and small intestine which exceeded the 'background radioactivity'. At 1-h and later survival intervals, there was marked labelling of the corpora lutea of the ovaries (Fig. 1A, B). The autoradiograms obtained from 18-day, 16-day and 13-day pregnant mice were comparable.

In autoradiograms of the extracted sections of 3- and 6-day-old mice, there was marked labelling of the nasal mucosa and the melanin of the eyes and hair follicles and, in addition, weak labelling of the liver and the bronchial mucosa (Fig. 1F). In freeze-dried sections, there was also homogenous labelling of most tissues and strong radioactivity in the kidneys and the contents of the stomach and small intestine (Fig. 1E).

As shown in Table 1, measurements by liquid scintillation counting in 18-day pregnant mice, killed 8 h after injection of [carbonyl-^{14}C]-NNK, showed the highest levels of total radioactivity in the maternal nose, liver and lachrymal glands. Levels in the kidneys, lung, trachea and ovaries were about half of these amounts. In the mothers, levels of bound metabolites were higher in the nose and liver than in the lung and kidney. Measurements of fetal tissues showed

Fig. 1. Whole-body autoradiograms of C57Bl mice exposed to labelled 4-(methylnitrosamino)-1-(3-pyridyl)-1-butanone (NNK)

(A), (B): Whole-body autoradiograms of mice on day 18 of gestation injected intravenously with [carbonyl-^{14}C]-NNK (7.0 mg/kg body weight). The mice were killed 1 h (A) and 4 h (B) after injection. Freeze-dried, non-extracted sections. White areas correspond to radioactivity.

(C), (D): Enlargements of whole-body autoradiograms of an 18-day-old fetus in a pregnant mouse. The mother received an intravenous injection of [carbonyl-^{14}C]-NNK (7.0 mg/kg body weight) and was sacrificed after 4 h. (C) is an autoradiogram of a freeze-dried, non-extracted tissue section; (D) is an autoradiogram of a tissue section, adjacent to (C), that was extracted with trichloroacetic acid and organic solvents before the autoradiographic exposure.

(E), (F): Whole-body autoradiograms of a six-day old mouse killed 4 h after a subcutaneous injection of [carbonyl-^{14}C]-NNK. (E) is an autoradiogram of a freeze-dried, non-extracted tissue section; (F) is an autoradiogram of a tissue section, adjacent to (E), that was extracted with trichloroacetic acid and organic solvents before the autoradiographic exposure.

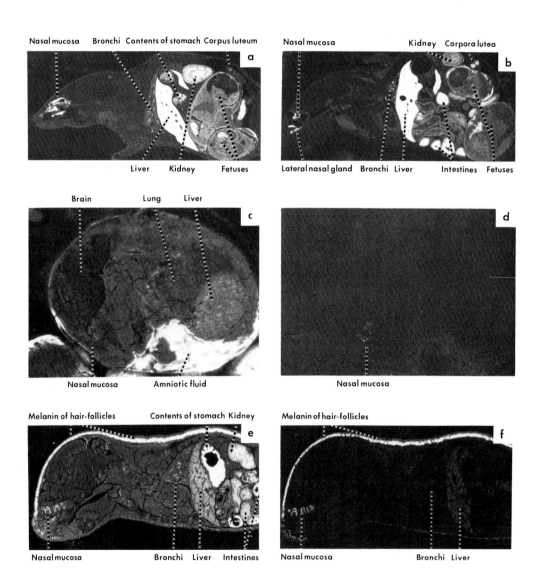

Table 1. Levels of ^{14}C in some tissues and their trichloroacetic acid-insoluble fraction after intravenous injection of [carbonyl-^{14}C]-labelled 4-(methylnitrosamino)-1-(3-pyridyl)-1-butanone (NNK) in pregnant C57Bl mice
Three mice on day 18 of gestation were injected intravenously with [carbonyl-^{14}C]-NNK (5.0 µCi, 7.0 mg/kg) and sacrificed 8 h later. Total radioactivity in various tissues and radioactive metabolites bound to the trichloroacetic acid-insoluble macromolecules were determined as described in the text

Tissue	Level of radioactivity (nmol/g of wet tissue)[a]			
	Maternal tissues		Fetal tissues	
	Total radioactivity	Bound radioactivity	Total radioactivity	Bound radioactivity
Nose	8.5 ± 0.6	1.3 ± 0.2	0.95 ± 0.03	0.12 ± 0.07
Liver	8.3 ± 0.9	1.8 ± 0.5	1.4 ± 0.1	0.12 ± 0.05
Lung	3.3 ± 0.2	0.65 ± 0.08	1.1 ± 0.04	0.04 ± 0.02
Kidney	3.1 ± 0.1	0.43 ± 0.01	2.6 ± 0.1	ND
Eye	1.2 ± 0.4	–	1.7 ± 0.1	–
Brain	0.50 ± 0.01	–	0.8 ± 0.04	–
Trachea	4.8 ± 0.8	–	–	–
Oesophagus	1.7 ± 0.2	–	–	–
Ovary	4.0 ± 1.0	–	–	–
Submaxillary gland	1.40 ± 0.08	–	–	–
Lachrymal gland	8.2 ± 0.2	–	–	–
Placenta	2.3 ± 0.2	–	–	–
Amniotic fluid	2.4 ± 0.2	–	–	–

[a] Mean ± SE obtained from three pregnant mice or fetuses of three mothers
ND, not detected; limit of detection, 0.04 nmol/g wet tissue; –, not determined

Table 2. Levels of 4-(methylnitrosamino)-1-(3-pyridyl)-1-buta-none (NNK) and its metabolites in placentae and fetuses of pregnant C57Bl mice after intravenous injection of [carbonyl-^{14}C]-NNK. Three mice on day 13 of gestation were injected intravenously with [carbonyl-^{14}C]-NNK (4.6 µCi, 7.5 mg/kg) and sacrificed 1 h later. Placentae and fetuses were excised, and the radioactive compounds were extracted and analysed as described in the text.

Metabolites[a]	Levels of metabolites (nmol/g wet tissue)[b]	
	Placentae	Fetuses
NNK	0.12 ± 0.02	0.08 ± 0.02
NNAl	2.05 ± 0.32	1.75 ± 0.33
NNK-N-oxide 1	0.24 ± 0.01	0.17 ± 0.03
NNAl-N-oxide 2	0.37 ± 0.19	0.15 ± 0.03
Keto acid 13	0.98 ± 0.21	0.45 ± 0.11
Hydroxy acid 14	0.42 ± 0.12	0.11 ± 0.05
Diol 15	ND	0.04 ± 0.01

[a] Numbers refer to Fig. 2; NNAl, 4-(methylnitrosamino)-1-(3-pyridyl)butanol
[b] Mean ± SD (n = 3)
ND, not determined

Fig. 2. Metabolic transformation of 4-(methylnitrosamino)-1-(3-pyridyl)-1-butanone (NNK). Structures in brackets are hypothetical intermediates.

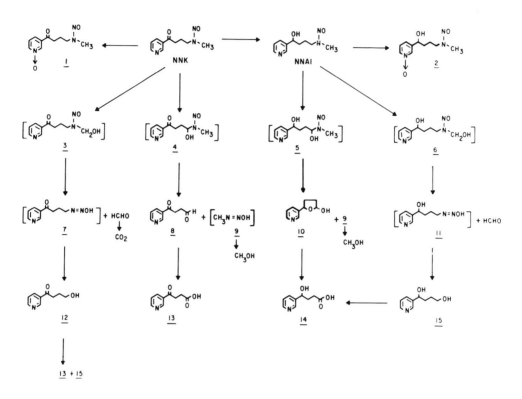

the highest total radioactivity in the kidney. Low levels of bound radioactivity were detected in the fetal nose, liver and lung. The radioactivity in the fetal kidney was totally extractable.

HPLC of extracts from fetuses and placentae of 13-day pregnant mice killed 1 h after injection of [carbonyl-^{14}C]-NNK showed the presence of NNK, as well as several metabolites (Table 2). The keto acid, *13* (Fig. 2), which results from α-carbon hydroxylation of NNK, and NNAl, which is formed by carbonyl reduction of NNK (Fig. 2), were the metabolites present in the highest concentrations.

Analyses of the amniotic fluid from 18-day pregnant mice killed 4 h after injection of [carbonyl-^{14}C]-NNK showed that the NNK metabolites present in the amniotic fluid consisted almost entirely of the keto acid, *13*, (1.7 μmol/L) and hydroxy acid, *14* (1.9 μmol/L).

In-vitro *experiments*

The ontogeny of the metabolic pathways of NNK in tissues of fetal and newborn mice and the metabolism of NNK by maternal tissues are shown in Table 3. The results indicate that the reductive pathway leading to the formation of NNAl is developed in the tissues of fetal and newborn mice to an extent comparable to that in the maternal tissues. The products of α-carbon

Table 3. Formation of metabolites by tissues of fetal, newborn and maternal C57Bl mice incubated with [carbonyl-^{14}C]-labelled 4-(methylnitrosamino)-1-(3-pyridyl)-1-butanone (NNK) Tissue slices were incubated in Krebs-Ringer phosphate buffer containing 0.28 μCi (33 nmol/mL) of [carbonyl-^{14}C]-NNK for 2 h. Metabolites were analysed by high-performance liquid chromatography as described in the text

Metabolite[b]	Level of metabolite (nmol/g of wet tissue)[a]														
	Fetuses (13 days)			Fetuses (18 days)			3-day old newborn			6-day old newborn			Mother		
	Nose	Liver	Lung	Nose	Liver	Lung	Nose	Liver	Lung	Nose	Liver	Lung	Nose	Liver	Lung
NNAl	52	91	45	40	102	85	20.8	90	78	8.7	100	62	36	77	97
NNK-N-oxide 1	ND	ND	ND	ND	ND	3.8	7.3	3.0	28	ND	9.1	43	22	15	123
NNAl-N-oxide 2	ND	ND	ND	ND	–	1.9	4.7	–	4.1	ND	–	5.3	11	–	23
Keto alcohol 12	ND	ND	ND	13	1.1	3.3	55.5	4.9	6.3	51	16	12	262	6.0	29
Keto acid 13	ND	ND	ND	33	2.3	2.5	162	27.6	21.1	85	37	30	795	84	95
Hydroxy acid 14	ND	ND	ND	ND	ND	ND	ND	4.9	0.4	ND	13.6	ND	ND	46	3.4
Diol 15	ND	ND	ND	ND	ND	ND	3.1	1.6	1.1	ND	3.1	ND	37	ND	10

[a] Mean of duplicate values obtained from two mice or from two fetuses of different mice. SD was less than 25%.
[b] Numbers refer to Fig. 2; NNAl, 4-(methylnitrosamino)-1-(3-pyridyl)butan-1-ol
ND, not detected; limit of detection, 1 nmol/g wet tissue; –, not measured due to interfering peaks

hydroxylation of NNK (the keto alcohol, *12,* and the keto acid, *13*) were not observed in tissues of 13-day old fetuses; however, they were detected in tissues of 18-day old fetuses and increased in amount with the age of newborn mice. Variations in the metabolism of NNK among the various tissues were striking. For instance, the nose has a much higher capacity to form keto alcohol, *12,* and keto acid, *13,* than the liver and lung. NNK-*N*-oxide (1) was formed by fetal lung, but not by fetal nose or liver. It was also formed in larger amounts by lung than by nose or liver of newborn mice and mothers. Hydroxy acid *14,* which is derived from α-carbon hydroxylation of NNA1, is formed by liver, but not by the nose and only to a small extent by the lung.

DISCUSSION

The distribution patterns observed in the present study after injection of [carbonyl-^{14}C]-NNK in C57Bl mice are in several respects similar to those observed after injection of [2′-^{14}C]-NNN (Brittebo & Tjälve, 1980; Waddell & Marlowe, 1980). Radioactivity of both *N*-nitrosamines was localized in the mucosa of the ethmoturbinates, the lateral nasal gland, the tracheo-bronchial mucosa, the lachrymal glands, the eye melanin, the contents of the stomach and the intestine, the kidneys and the urinary bladder. However, labelling of the oesophagus was observed after injection of [2′-^{14}C]-NNN, but not after [carbonyl-^{14}C]-NNK injection. In the present study, radioactivity did accumulate in the corpora lutea of the ovaries, but this was not observed with pregnant or non-pregnant mice injected with [2′-^{14}C]-NNN (Brittebo & Tjälve, 1980)[1]. The formation of metabolites with identical chemical structures (Castonguay *et al.,* 1983b) and the similar pKa values of the two *N*-nitrosamines may explain the similarities in their distribution patterns. Inversely, the differences may be due to specific pharmacodynamic properties of NNK and NNN and/or their metabolites.

NDMA and NNK both have a *N*-methyl group that can be hydroxylated, and the methyldiazohydroxide, *9* (Fig. 2), is an electrophilic species that may be derived both from NNK and NDMA. However, the production of *9* from NNK is preceded by the formation of more complex species. Whole-body autoradiography of pregnant C57Bl mice suggests that maternal hepatic tissues have a high capacity to activate these two *N*-nitrosamines, but the nasal and bronchial mucosae are apparently unable to activate NDMA (Johansson-Brittebo & Tjälve, 1979).

The distribution of radioactivity from [carbonyl-^{14}C]-NNK in the maternal tissues of C57Bl mice, with localization of tissue-bound metabolites in the nasal and tracheo-bronchial mucosae and the liver, is similar to the patterns observed previously in Fischer 344 rats (Castonguay *et al.,* 1983b) and Syrian golden hamsters (Tjälve & Castonguay, 1983). The observation that the nasal mucosa, the lung and the liver in these three species also can metabolize NNK *in vitro* indicates that the in-vivo binding of metabolites to the tissues is due to local activation.

The present study demonstrates that NNK and its metabolites can cross the placental barrier and that during the last stage of gestation, the liver, the lung and the nasal tissues of the fetuses also can activate NNK to reactive species. The ability of a procarcinogen to diffuse through the placenta and to become activated by fetal tissues may be prerequisites for transplacental carcinogenic activity. These requirements are fulfilled for NNK.

Binding of radioactive metabolites to the nasal, pulmonary and hepatic tissues of the fetuses and in-vitro activation of NNK by α-carbon hydroxylation in these fetal tissues were observed in 18-day pregnant mice but not in 13-day pregnant mice. This ontogeny of NNK metabolism

---

[1] Also, unpublished data

during the fetal life of C57Bl mice parallels the results obtained with N-nitrosodiethylamine (NDEA) in Syrian golden hamsters. In hamsters, only the offspring of mothers given NDEA on one of the last four days of gestation developed tracheal tumours (Mohr *et al.*, 1975). It was also noticed that radioactive metabolites bound to fetal trachea (Reznik-Schüller & Hague, 1981) and that rough endoplasmic reticulum appeared in the tracheal stem cells (Mohr *et al.*, 1979) only during this period of gestation. Therefore, if NNK can induce tumours transplacentally, exposure of the fetus to the N-nitrosamine would have to occur during the last stage of gestation.

Autoradiography showed an accumulation of radioactivity in the amniotic fluid, and HPLC showed that keto acid *13* and hydroxy acid *14* are responsible for this labelling. These metabolites are the major urinary metabolites of NNK in Fischer 344 rats (Castonguay *et al.*, 1983b) and Syrian golden hamsters (Hoffmann *et al.*, 1981). Large quantities of urine have been shown to be formed by the fetal kidney in the last stage of gestation and this may contribute considerably to the volume of the amniotic fluid (Vernier & Smith, 1968). Our autoradiography showed marked labelling of the fetal kidney and urinary bladder and it is probable, therefore, that keto acid *13* and hydroxy acid *14* reach the amniotic fluid *via* the fetal urinary tract.

Our results indicated that the ultimate carcinogenic species of NNK can be generated in newborn mice. NDMA and NDEA exhibit high carcinogenic efficacy in neonatal mice (Anderson *et al.*, 1979; Vesselinovitch, 1980). Fifteen-day-old mice are more susceptible than six-week-old mice to the carcinogenic effect of NDEA (Rao & Vesselinovitch, 1973). High levels of cell replication and a low level of DNA repair could contribute to this increase in susceptibility of newborn mice to N-nitrosamines.

The localization of NNK radioactivity in the melanin of the maternal eye can probably be ascribed to the basicity of NNK and some of its metabolites (Tjälve & Castonguay, 1983). In the fetuses and the newborn animals, there was evidence of covalent binding of the radioactivity to melanin. It is known that some compounds, e.g., thiouracil (Farishian & Wittaker, 1979), are incorporated into newly-synthesized melanin; this incorporation may also take place with NNK.

ACKNOWLEDGEMENTS

We thank Lena Norgren, Raili Pensas and Neil Trushin for their excellent technical assistance. This study was supported by a Swedish Government Grant and by the US National Cancer Institute, Grant 21 393.

REFERENCES

Anderson, L.M., Priest, L.J. & Budinger, J.M. (1979) Lung tumorigenesis in mice after chronic exposure in early life to a low dose of dimethylnitrosamine. *J. natl Cancer Inst.*, **62**, 1553–1555

Brittebo, E. & Tjälve, H. (1980) Autoradiographic observations on the distribution and metabolism of N'[^{14}C]-nitrosonornicotine in mice. *J. Cancer Res. clin. Oncol.*, **98**, 233–242

Castonguay, A., Lin, D., Stoner, G.D., Radok, P., Furuya, K., Hecht, S.S., Schut, H.A.J. & Klaunig, J.E. (1983a) Comparative carcinogenicity in A/J mice and metabolism by cultured peripheral lung of N'-nitrosonornicotine, 4-(methylnitrosamino)-1-(3-pyridyl)-1-butanone and their analogues. *Cancer Res.*, **43**, 1223–1229

Castonguay, A., Tjälve, H. & Hecht, S.S. (1983b) Tissue distribution of the tobacco-specific carcinogen 4-(methylnitrosamino)-1-(3-pyridyl)-1-butanone and its metabolites in F344 rats. *Cancer Res.*, **43**, 630–638

Everson, R.B. (1980) Individuals transplacentally exposed to maternal smoking may be at increased cancer risk in adult life. *Lancet, ii*, 123–127

Farishian, R.A. & Wittaker, J.R. (1979) Tyrosine utilization by cultured melanoma cells: analysis of melanin biosynthesis using [^{14}C]-tyrosine and [^{14}C]-thiouracil. *Arch. Biochem. Biophys,* **198,** 449–461

Flasks, A. (1966) Test for carcinogenesis of cigarette tobacco smoke condensate using young strain A and C57Bl mice. *Br. J. Cancer,* **20,** 145–147

Hecht, S.S., Chen, C.B., Ohmori, T. & Hoffmann, D. (1980a) Comparative carcinogenicity in F344 rats of the tobacco-specific nitrosamines, *N'*-nitrosonornicotine and 4-(methylnitrosamino)-1-(3-pyridyl)-1-butanone *Cancer Res.,* **40,** 298–302

Hecht, S.S., Young, R. & Chen, C.B. (1980b) Metabolism in the F344 rat of 4-(methylnitrosamino)-1-(3-pyridyl)-1-butanone, a tobacco-specific carcinogen. *Cancer Res.,* **40,** 4144–4159

Hoffmann, D., Adams, J.D., Brunnemann, K.D. & Hecht, S.S. (1979) Assessment of tobacco-specific *N*-nitrosamines in tobacco products. *Cancer Res.,* **39,** 2505–2509

Hoffmann, D., Castonguay, A., Rivenson, A. & Hecht, S.S. (1981) Comparative carcinogenicity and metabolism of 4-(methylnitrosamino)-1-(3-pyridyl)-1-butanone and *N'*-nitrosonornicotine in Syrian golden hamsters. *Cancer Res.,* **41,** 2386–2393

Johansson-Brittebo, E. & Tjälve, H. (1979) Studies on the distribution and metabolism of ^{14}C-dimethylnitrosamine in foetal and young mice. *Acta pharmacol. toxicol.,* **45,** 73–80

Mohr, U., Reznik-Schüler, H., Reznik, G. & Hilfrich, J. (1975) Transplacental effects of diethylnitrosamine in Syrian hamsters as related to different days of administration during pregnancy. *J. natl Cancer Inst.,* **55,** 681–683

Mohr, U., Reznik-Schüller, H. & Emura, M. (1979) Tissue differentiation as a prerequisite for transplacental carcinogenesis in hamster respiratory system, with specific respect to the trachea. *Natl Cancer Inst. Monogr.,* **51,** 117–122

Neutel, C.I. & Buck, C. (1971) Effects of smoking during pregnancy on the risk of cancer in children. *J. natl Cancer Inst.,* **47,** 59–63

Rao, K.V.N. & Vesselinovitch, S.D. (1973) Age- and sex-associated diethylnitrosamine dealkylation activity of the mouse liver and hepatocarcinogenesis. *Cancer Res.,* **33,** 1625–1627

Reznik-Schüller, H.M. & Hague, B.F., Jr (1981) Autoradiography in fetal Syrian golden hamsters treated with tritiated diethylnitrosamine. *J. natl Cancer Inst.,* **66,** 773–777

Tjälve, H. & Castonguay, A. (1983) The *in vivo* tissue disposition and *in vitro* target-tissue metabolism of the tobacco-specific carcinogen 4-(methylnitrosamino)-1-(3-pyridyl)-1-butanone in Syrian golden hamsters. *Carcinogenesis,* **4,** 1259–1265

Ullberg, S. (1977) The technique of whole body autoradiography. Cryosectioning of large specimens. *Sci. Tools* (special issue), pp. 2–29

Vernier, R.L. & Smith, F.G., Jr (1968) *Fetal and neonatal kidney.* In: Assali, N.S., ed., *Biology of Gestation,* Vol. 2, New York & London, Academic Press, pp. 225–260

Vesselinovitch, S.D. (1980) *Infant mouse as a sensitive bioassay system for carcinogenicity of N-nitroso compounds.* In: Walker, E.A., Griciute, L. Castegnaro, M. & Börszönyi, M., eds, N-*Nitroso Compounds: Analysis. Formation and Occurrence (IARC Scientific Publications No. 31),* Lyon, International Agency for Research on Cancer, pp. 645–655

Waddell, W.J. & Marlowe, C. (1980) Localization of [^{14}C]-nitrosonornicotine in tissues of the mouse. *Cancer Res.,* **40,** 3518–3523

INHIBITION OF TARGET TISSUE ACTIVATION OF N'-NITROSONORNICOTINE AND N-NITROSOPYRROLIDINE BY DIETARY COMPONENTS

F.-L. CHUNG, A. JUCHATZ, J. VITARIUS, B. REISS, & S.S. HECHT

Naylor Dana Institute for Disease Prevention , American Health Foundation, Valhalla, NY, USA

SUMMARY

Twenty-one dietary and related chemicals have been evaluated for their potential inhibitory activities against the tumorigenic effects of N-nitrosopyrrolidine and N'-nitrosonornicotine using in-vitro metabolic assays in the target tissues , namely, rat liver microsomes and cultured rat oesophagus, respectively. Compounds studied include phenols, cinnamic acids, coumarins, isothiocyanates and indoles. Isothiocyanates were the most potent inhibitors of both nitrosamines in the acute studies, but were less active in chronic studies. This difference may be explained by the pharmacokinetic properties of these compounds. Phenols, cinnamic acids, coumarins and indoles were primarily inducers of N-nitrosopyrrolidine metabolism. The results suggest that isothiocyanates, in general, are the most promising chemicals for future study as protective agents against the carcinogenic effects of these nitrosamines.

INTRODUCTION

Dietary compounds have been shown to inhibit carcinogenesis by various chemicals in animal bioassays (Wattenberg, 1978). These dietary compounds, including phenols, cinnamic acids, aromatic isothiocyanates, coumarins and indoles, occur widely in vegetables and fruits. They are effective in protecting animals against tumorigenisis by certain polycyclic hydrocarbons such as 7,12-dimethylbenz[a]anthracene and benzo[a]pyrene.

However, only scattered information is available regarding the inhibition of nitrosamine carcinogenesis by dietary compounds (Wattenberg, 1972). One potentially practical approach to the prevention of chemical carcinogenesis by N-nitrosamines is to identify dietary compounds which inhibit the metabolic activation of nitrosamines in target tissues. Using this approach as an initial screening for potential inhibitors, we have studied the effects of some dietary-related compounds and of their structural analogues on the in-vitro metabolism of two structurally related environmental nitrosamines, N-nitrosopyrrolidine (NPYR) and N'-nitrosonornicotine (NNN) (Brunnemann et al., 1977; Hoffmann et al., 1979; Sen et al., 1982). The assays were carried out in the respective target tissues, using rat liver microsomes for NPYR and cultured rat oesophagus for NNN.

Fig. 1. Metabolic α-hydroxylation of *N*-nitrosopyrrolidine by rat liver microsomal preparations

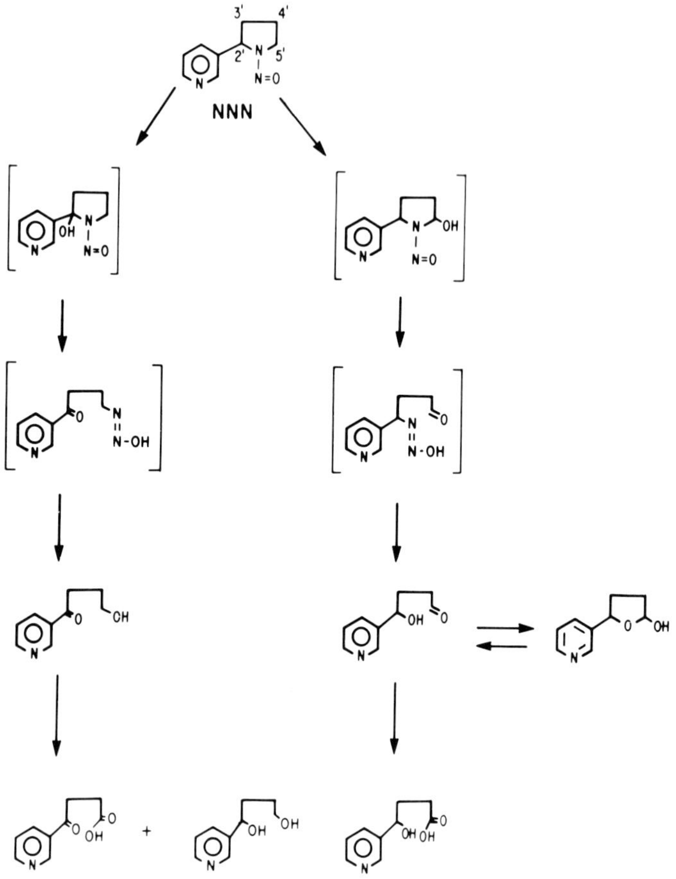

Both nitrosamines are activated metabolically by α-hydroxylation (Hecht *et al.*, 1981a) to give reactive species (Figs 1 & 2) which subsequently damage DNA. Alternatively, these reactive intermediates can react with water to form stable metabolites. 4-Hydroxy-butyraldehyde from NPYR can be assayed as its 2,4-dinitrophenylhydrazone derivative by high-pressure liquid chromatography(HPLC) (Chen *et al.*, 1978). The keto alcohol, 4-hydroxy-1-(3-pyridyl)-1-butanone, and its oxidized metabolite, the keto acid, 4-oxo-4-(3-pyridyl)butyric acid, formed by 2'-hydroxylation of NNN, and the hydroxy acid, 4-hydroxy-4-(3-pyridyl)butyric acid, formed by 5'-hydroxylation of NNN can also be analysed by HPLC using [2'-^{14}C]-NNN (Hecht *et al.*, 1982). Quantitative assays for these metabolites and derivatives can be used as indicators of the amount of reactive precursors formed by these metabolic activation pathways.

Fig. 2. Metabolic α-hydroxylations (2′ and 5′) of *N'*-nitrosonornicotine (NNN) by cultured rat oesophagus

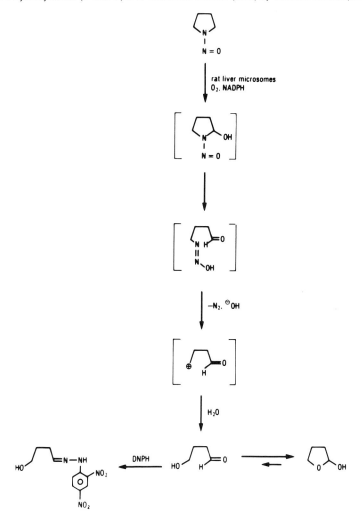

MATERIALS AND METHODS

Apparatus

HPLC was performed with a Waters Associates Model ALC/GPC-204 (Waters Associates, Milford, MA, USA) equipped with a Model 6000A solvent delivery system, a Model 660 solvent programmer, a Model U6K septumless injector, and a Model 440 UV/visible detector. Liquid scintillation counting was performed with a Beckman Model LS9800 system. Organ cultures were maintained in a Bellco Controlled Atmosphere Culture Chamber, Number 7741-10010, resting upon a Bellco Rocking Platform No. 7740-20020 (Bellco Glass, Vineland, NJ, USA), as described previously (Hecht *et al.*, 1982). Livers were homogenized in a polytron homogenizer (Willems type; Kinematic GmbH, Lucerne, Switzerland). Centrifugations were carried out in a Sorvall RC2-B centrifuge and a Spinco Model L-Ultracentrifuge.

Chemicals

NPYR was obtained from Aldrich Chemical Co. (Milwaukee, WI, USA). The 2,4-dinitrophenylhydrazone of 4-hydroxybutyraldehye was prepared as described previously (Hecht *et al.*, 1978). NADPH, NADH, glucose-6-phosphate, and glucose-6-phosphate dehydrogenase were obtained from Sigma Chemical Co. (St Louis, MO, USA). 2,4-Dinitrophenylhydrazine was obtained from Eastman Kodak Co. (Rochester, NY, USA). Sucrose (special enzyme grade) was from Schwarz/Mann (Orangeburg, NY, USA). [2'-^{14}C]-NNN (51.7 mCi/mmol or 18.4 mCi/mmol) was purchased from New England Nuclear (Boston, MA, USA). Unlabelled NNN reference metabolites were synthesized as described previously (Hecht *et al.*, 1981b). Butylated hydroxyanisole (BHA) was purchased from Sigma Chemical Co. (St Louis, MO, USA). *p*-Methoxyphenol, *o*-hydroxycinnamic acid, 4-hydroxy-3-methoxy cinnamic acid, coumarin, umbelliferone, limetine, indole, indole-3-carbinol, indole-3-acetonitrile, L-tryptophan, *N*-acetyl cysteine, allyl isothiocyanate, phenyl isothiocyanate, sodium thiocyanate, phenyl isocyanate, benzyl isocyanide, and benzyl thiocyanate were all purchased from Aldrich (Milwaukee, WI, USA). Benzyl isothiocyanate was obtained from Fluka (Hauppauge, NY, USA), and phenethyl isothiocyanate was purchased from Kodak (Rochester, NY, USA).

Animals

Male F344 rats (200-300 g) were obtained from Charles River (Kingston, NY, USA). For the acute studies, rats were gavaged with 1 mmol/Kg body weight of dietary chemical in corn oil and sacrificed after 2 h. The control group received only corn oil. For the chronic study, rats were fed NIH-07 diet containing 0.03 mmol/g of diet of the appropriate dietary chemical and sacrificed after two weeks. The doses of benzyl isothiocyanate and phenyl isothiocyanate were reduced to 0.003 mmol/g diet due to toxicity.

Metabolism

After the rats had been sacrificed by decapitation, the oesophagus and liver were removed. Preparation of liver microsomes and incubation of NPYR with the isolated liver microsomes were carried out by previously described procedures (Chen *et al.*, 1978). Rat oesophagus was cultured for 24 h with [2'-^{14}C]-NNN according to a published method (Hecht *et al.*, 1982).

Analysis of metabolites

Details of the HPLC assays for metabolism of NPYR in rat liver microsomes and of [2'-^{14}C]-NNN in cultured rat oesophagus were given previously (Chen *et al.* 1978; Hecht *et al.*, 1982).

RESULTS

In order to determine the appropriate substrate concentrations to be used, the metabolism of various concentrations of [2'-^{14}C]-NNN by cultured rat oesophagus was studied. The results are shown in Figure 3. The appropriate concentration of NPYR to be used in the liver microsomal assays was determined previously (Chen *et al.*, 1978). For a majority of the

Fig. 3. Relationship of concentration of [2'-^{14}C]-N'-nitrosonornicotine (NNN) to formation of metabolites in cultured rat oesophagus. Amounts of NNN used in inhibition studies are indicated by arrows. △, Keto alcohol, 2'; □, keto acid, 2'; ○, hydroxy acid, 5'

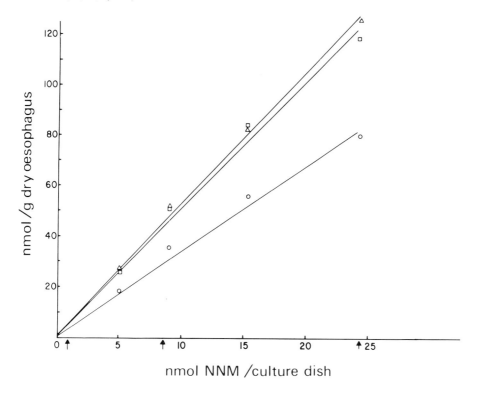

nmol/g dry oesophagus

nmol NNM /culture dish

Table 1. Chronic effects of some dietary compounds on the metabolism of N-nitrosopyrrolidine in rat liver microsomes

Compound	Ratio[a]
Butylated hydroxyanisole	1.0
p-Methoxyphenol	0.7**
o-Hydroxycinnamic acid	1.0
p-Hydroxycinnamic acid	1.5*
4-Hydroxy-3-methoxycinnamic acid	1.5*
Coumarin	1.6*
Umbelliferone	1.6*
Limetine	1.7*
Indole	1.4**
Indole-3-carbinol	2.8*
Indole-3-acetonitrile	1.5*
L-Tryptophan	2.2*
N-Acetyl cysteine	0.9**

[a] Mean of treated rat values (nmol/mg protein): mean of control rat values; average standard deviation for all values, 14%
* $p < 0.01$ compared to control
** $p < 0.05$ compared to control

Table 2. Effects of aromatic isothiocyanates and related compounds on the metabolism of *N*-nitrosopyrrolidine in rat liver microsomes

Compound	Ratio[a]	
	Acute	Chronic
Benzyl isothiocyanate	0.5*	1.0
Allyl isothiocyanate	0.5*	0.7*
Phenethyl isothiocyanate	0.5*	0.5*
Phenyl isothiocyanate	0.5*	0.6*
Sodium thiocyanate	1.0	0.5*
Phenyl isocyanate	0.5*	0.7*
Benzyl thiocyanate	0.4*	1.2
Benzyl isocyanide	0.6*	ND

[a] Mean of treated rat values (nmol/mg protein): mean of control rat values; average standard deviation for all values, 18% for the acute study and 16% for the chronic study
* p < 0.01 compared to control; ND, not determined (due to unpleasant odour)

Table 3. Acute effects of aromatic isothiocyanates and related compounds on the metabolism of *N'*-nitrosonornicotine in cultured rat oesophagus

Compound	Ratio[a]		
	Hydroxy acid	Keto acid	Keto alcohol
Benzyl isothiocyanate	0.3*	0.4*	0.5*
Allyl isothiocyanate	0.3*	0.4*	0.4*
Phenethyl isothiocyanate	0.3*	0.4*	0.4*
Phenyl isothiocyanate	0.6*	0.6*	0.9
Sodium thiocyanate	0.9**	1.0	1.1
Phenyl isocyanate	0.9*	0.9	1.2**
Benzyl isocyanide	0.7**	0.9	1.0
Benzyl thiocyanate	0.4*	0.5*	0.6*
N-Acetyl cysteine	1.0	1.0	0.9*

[a] Mean of treated rat values (% nmol/g dry weight oesophagus): mean of control rat values; average standard deviation for all values, 13%
* p < 0.01 compared to control
** p < 0.05 compared to control

compounds tested as inhibitors in this study, doses were within the range of the LD_{50}, and no apparent toxicity was observed, except for benzyl isothiocyanate and phenyl isothiocyanate in the chronic studies.

In the chronic study of the effect of dietary compounds on NPYR metabolism, phenols, cinnamic acids, coumarins and indoles showed no effect or moderate induction. The exception was *p*-methoxyphenol which was inhibitory (Table 1). Of particular interest are the two indole derivatives, indole-3-carbinol and L-tryptophan, which induced NPYR metabolism two- to three-fold.

Table 4. Chronic effects of aromatic isothiocyanates and related compounds on the metabolism of N'-nitrosonornicotine in cultured rat oesophagus

Compound	Ratio[a]		
	Hydroxy acid	Keto acid	Keto alcohol
Benzyl isothiocyanate	0.6**	0.6	0.8
Allyl isothiocyanate	0.9	1.0	1.0
Phenethyl isothiocyanate	0.9	1.0	1.5*
Phenyl isothiocyanate	0.4*	0.5*	0.7*
Sodium thiocyanate	0.3*	0.6*	0.4*
Phenyl isocyanate	0.9	0.9	1.2
Benzyl thiocyanate	0.7**	0.8	0.7**
N-Acetyl cysteine	0.9	1.0	1.1

[a] Mean of treated rat values (% nmol/g dry weight oesophagus): mean of control rat values; average standard deviation for all values, 16%
* $p < 0.01$ compared to control
** $p < 0.05$ compared to control

The potential inhibitory activities of organic isothiocyanates and related compounds on NPYR metabolism are summarized in Table 2. In the acute study, inhibitory activities were observed for all organic isothiocyanates and related compounds; however, sodium thiocyanate was inactive. In the chronic study, however, there was some decrease in the potency of inhibition for this class of compound; and sodium thiocyanate was a good inhibitor, in contrast to the results obtained in the acute study.

All the isothiocyanates demonstrated considerable inhibition of NNN metabolism, ranging from two to three-fold in the acute study (Table 3), whereas most structurally related chemicals such as phenyl isocyanate were inactive. One potent inhibitor in this series which does not have an isothiocyanate group was benzyl thiocyanate. In the chronic study (Table 4), benzyl isothiocyanate, phenyl isothiocyanate and benzyl thiocyanate retained at least partially their inhibitory activity on NNN metabolism. Allyl and phenethyl isothiocyanate and other related compounds were inactive. Interestingly, sodium thiocyanate was once again a good inhibitor in the chronic study but had no effect in the acute study.

DISCUSSION

Twenty-one dietary and related chemicals have been evaluated for potential inhibitory activity against the carcinogenic effects of NPYR and NNN, using in-vitro metabolic assays in target tissues. Most aromatic isothiocyanates were effective inhibitors of both NPYR and NNN metabolism in the acute studies but were less or not effective in the chronic study. The mechanism(s) of inhibition is not known. Nonetheless, the difference in activity between chronic and acute experiments suggests that these isothiocyanates are metabolized rapidly and therefore do not have a lasting effect. Sodium thiocyanate, the only ionic chemical tested, was inhibitory for NPYR and NNN in the chronic study but not in the acute study. This observation might be explained by the pharmacokinetic properties of sodium thiocyanate.

In contrast to the isothiocyanates, the phenols, cinnamic acids, coumarins and indoles primarily induced NPYR metabolism. N-Acetyl cysteine, known to protect biological systems from adverse effects because of its nucleophilicity, had no apparent effect on NPYR and NNN metabolism.

In conclusion, the most significant inhibition was demonstrated by compounds possessing the isothiocyanate function, regardless of the structure. This result suggests that iso-thiocyanates are promising dietary-related compounds for future study as potential inhibitors of carcinogenesis by these *N*-nitrosamines.

ACKNOWLEDGEMENTS

This study was supported by US National Cancer Institute Grant CA-32272.

REFERENCES

Brunnemann, D.K., Yu, L. & Hoffmann, D.(1977) Assessment of carcinogenic volatile *N*-nitrosamines in tobacco and in mainstream and sidestream smoke from cigarettes. *Cancer Res., 37,* 3218–3222

Chen, C.B., McCoy, G.D., Hecht, S.S., Hoffmann, D. & Wynder, E.L. (1978) High pressure liquid chromatographic assay for α-hydroxylation of *n*-nitrosopyrrolidine by isolated rat liver microsomes. *Cancer Res., 38,* 3812–3816

Hecht, S.S., Chen, C.B. & Hoffmann, D. (1978) Evidence for metabolic α-hydroxylation of *n*-nitrosopyrrolidine. *Cancer Res., 38,* 215–218

Hecht, S.S., McCoy, G.D., Chen, C.B. & Hoffmann, D. (1981a) *The metabolism of cyclic nitrosamines.* In: Scanlan, R.A. & Tannenbaum, S.R., eds, N-*Nitroso Compounds (Am. Chem. Soc. Symp. Ser. 174),* Washington DC, American Chemical Society, pp. 49–75

Hecht, S.S., Lin, D. & Chen, C.B. (1981b) Comprehensive analysis of urinary metabolites of *N'*-nitrosonornicotine. *Carcinogenesis, 2,* 833–838

Hecht, S.S., Reiss, B., Lin, D. & Williams, G.M. (1982) Metabolism of *N'*-nitrosonornicotine by cultured rat oesophagus. *Carcinogenesis, 3,* 453–456

Hoffmann, D., Adams, J.D., Brunnemann, K.D. & Hecht, S.S. (1979) Assessment of tobacco-specific *N*-nitrosamines in tobacco products. *Cancer Res., 39,* 2505–2509

Sen, N.P., Seaman, S. & Tessier, L. (1982) *A rapid and sensitive method for the determination of non-volatile N-nitroso compounds in foods and human urine: recent data concerning volatile nitrosamines in dried foods and malt-based beverages.* In: Bartsch, H., O'Neill, I.K., Castegnaro, M. & Okada, M., eds, N-*Nitroso Compounds: Occurrence and Biological Effects (IARC Scientific Publications No. 41),* Lyon, International Agency for Research on Cancer, pp. 185–197

Wattenberg, L.W. (1972) Inhibition of carcinogenic effects of diethylnitrosamine and 4-nitroquinoline-N-oxide by antioxidants. *Fed. Proc., 31,* 633

Wattenberg, L.W. (1978) Inhibitors of chemical carcinogenesis. *Adv. Cancer Res., 26,* 197–226

KINETICS OF DNA METHYLATION BY THE TOBACCO-SPECIFIC CARCINOGEN 4-(METHYLNITROSAMINO)-1-(3-PYRIDYL)-1-BUTANONE IN F344 RATS

A. CASTONGUAY, R. THARP & S.S. HECHT

Naylor Dana Institute for Disease Prevention, American Health Foundation, Valhalla, New York, USA

SUMMARY

The carcinogen 4-(methylnitrosamino)-1-(3-pyridyl)-1-butanone (NNK) was injected intravenously (0.41 mmol/kg) into F344 rats. DNA from target organs (lung, liver) and a non-target organ (kidney) was extracted hydrolysed and analysed for methylated guanines by cation-exchange high-performance liquid chromotography-fluorimetry. Levels of O^6-methylguanine, a promutagenic lesion, and 7-methylguanine were three to eight times higher in the liver than in the lung. Neither base could be detected in the kidneys. The extent of methylation of hepatic DNA by NNK was 35 times lower than observed with an equimolar dose of NDMA by Swann *et al.* (1983).

The levels of the two methylated guanines in liver and lung DNA increased between 4 and 24 h following NNK injection. NNK is metabolized rapidly in F344 rats to 4-(methyl-nitrosamino)-1-(3-pyridyl)-butan-1-ol (NNA1). The relatively slow methylation of hepatic DNA after injection of NNK could be due to a slow release of methylating species from the major circulating metabolite NNA1. This low but sustained level of O^6-methylguanine induced by NNK could, in part, explain its carcinogenic potency.

INTRODUCTION

Many N-nitrosomethylalkylamines, such as N-nitrosodimethylamine (NDMA), N-nitroso-methylbenzylamine and N-nitrosomethylethylamine, have been shown to be activated by animal tissues to methylating intermediates (Magee & Barnes, 1967; Kleihues *et al.*, 1981; Autrup & Stoner, 1982), which can methylate cellular macromolecules of the tissues in which they are generated. Among the various sites of DNA that are methylated are the O^6- and 7-positions of the guanine residue. Since 7-methylguanine is the major methylation product, its formation is often used as an indicator of the ability of a tissue to activate N-nitrosomethylalkylamines. However, 7-methylguanine lacks miscoding properties. Although the initial level of O^6-methylguanine is usually 10 times lower than that of 7-methylguanine, it has a miscoding efficiency of 40% with DNA polymerase (Abbott & Saffhill, 1979).

We have shown previously that [^{14}CH$_3$]-4-(methylnitrosamino)-1-(3-pyridyl)-1-butanone (NNK) activated by rat liver microsomes can methylate calf thymus DNA (Castonguay et al., 1981). We present here evidence that the induction of tumours in F344 rats by administration of NNK could be mediated, in part, by DNA methylation at the O^6-guanine site.

MATERIALS AND METHODS

F344 rats were obtained from Charles River (Kingston, NY, USA) and were fed NIH-07 diet (Zeigler Brothers, Gardners, PA, USA). Each rat, weighing 160–170 g, was injected intravenously with 0.5 mL of a solution of 14 mg (0.41 mmol/kg body weight) NNK in 0.9% sodium chloride solution. Control animals received 0.5 mL sodium chloride solution only. The rats were decapitated 15 min, 1 h, 4 h or 24 h later, and the tissues were immediately excised and kept frozen until DNA extraction. Nuclear DNA was extracted from liver, lung and kidney with chloroform:isoamyl alcohol, as described by Daoud and Irving (1977). This procedure includes removal of RNA by digestion with pancreatic ribonuclease-A for 30 min at room temperature. DNA contents of the samples were assayed by fluorimetry using bisbenzimidazole as a fluorescence enhancer (Labarca & Paigen, 1980).

In order to quantify 7-methylguanine, 1 mg DNA sample was incubated in 200 µL of 10 mmol/L sodium cacodylate (pH 7.0 at 100°C for 30 min). Hydrochloric acid (1 mol/L, 20 µL) was added to the ice-cold sample. O^6-Methylguanine was determined by hydrolysing 1 mg DNA in 200 µL of 0.1 mol/L hydrochloric acid at 100°C for 30 min. DNA bases and methylated guanines were separated on a cation-exchange high-performance liquid chromatographic column using an ammonium phosphate buffer (0.05 mol/L, pH 2.0) at a flow rate of 2 mL/min and were assayed by fluorimetry (286 nm excitation, 366 nm emission) (Herron & Shank, 1979). Methylated bases could also be quantified by high-performance liquid chromatography, with elution by a pH 3.0 ammonium phosphate buffer and fluorescence detection with excitation at 290 nm and emission at 400 nm. Each analysis was done with 200 µL of solution containing $\simeq$ 1 mg hydrolysed DNA.

The extent of DNA methylation during culture of rat nasal septum was determined . Nasal septa from 10 rats were cultured for 24 h in Williams medium E (5 mL/septum per dish) containing NNK (1 mg/mL) and calf thymus DNA (1 mg/mL) (Brittebo et al., 1983). Mucosae covering five septa were pooled, and DNA was isolated as described above. Sodium acetate solution (1.5 mL, 2.5 mol/L) was added to 15 mL of medium, and calf thymus DNA was precipitated by addition of cold ethanol (30 mL).

RESULTS

Levels of O^6-methylguanine and 7-methylguanine in DNA of rat liver and lung are shown in Table 1; neither of these two methylated guanines was detected in kidney DNA at any of the four survival intervals indicated.

In the DNA of rat nasal mucosa cultured with NNK for 24 h, 172 µmol of O^6-methylguanine were found per mol guanine and 858 µmol of 7-methylguanine per mol guanine. No methylation of calf thymus DNA added to the culture medium was observed.

Methylation of DNA by NNK metabolites was also demonstrated by gel immunodiffusion and enzyme-linked immunosorbent assay. Rabbits and guinea-pigs were immunized with O^6-methylguanosine-keyhole limpet haemocyanin conjugate (Müler & Rajewsky, 1980) or 7-methylguanosine 5′-monophosphate-bovine serum albumin conjugate (Meredith & Erlanger, 1979). After purification by affinity chromatography, the antibodies were immunoreactive with

Table 1. Methylated guanines in liver and lung DNA at various times after intravenous injection of 4-(methylnitrosamino)-1-(3-pyridyl)-1-butanone (0.41 mmol/kg) to F344 rats

Length of survival	O^6-Methylguanine[a] (μmol/mol guanine)	7-Methylguanine[a] (μmol/mol guanine)
	Liver	
15 min	ND	ND
1 h	10.1	54
4 h	25.8	204
24 h	39	299
Control	ND	ND
	Lung	
15 min	ND	ND
1 h	ND	17.1
4 h	6.9	29
24 h	7.3	35
Control	ND	ND

[a] Mean of duplicate values obtained from two rats
ND, Not detected; limits of detection were 3 μmol O^6-methylguanine/mol guanine and 15 μmol 7-methylguanine/mol guanine when 0.5 mg of DNA was analysed.

hepatic DNA of NNK-treated rats. The binding of the anti-O^6-methylguanine antibodies to NNK-modified DNA was inhibited by O^6-methyl-2'-deoxyguanosine but not by 2'-deoxyguanosine. The anti-7-methylguanosine-5'-monophosphate-bovine serum albumin antibodies bind to the homologous antigens. The binding is inhibited by NNK-modified DNA which has been thermally hydrolysed or by free hapten. This binding is not inhibited by heat-treated calf thymus DNA, polyguanylic acid or 2'-deoxyguanosine.

DISCUSSION

Sixty subcutaneous injections of 0.23 mmol/kg body weight of NNK to F344 rats induced hepatocarcinomas and haemangiosarcomas of the liver, brochiolo-alveologenic adenocarcinomas and various types of nasal cavity tumours (Hecht *et al.*, 1980a). In these target organs, NNK can methylate DNA at the O^6- and 7-positions of the guanine residue of DNA. Formation of O^6-methylguanine is the first DNA promutagenic lesion that has been reported to occur with any tobacco-specific N-nitrosamine.

The extent and kinetics of DNA methylation by NNK contrast with those previously observed with the structurally related NDMA. Levels of O^6-methylguanine and 7-methylguanine in hepatic DNA were 35 times lower after NNK injection (0.41 mmol/kg) than after NDMA administration (0.405 mmol/kg) (Swann *et al.*, 1983). Levels of both methylated guanines were found to have decreased between 4 and 24 h following the administration of NDMA (0.27 mmol/kg) (Pegg, 1977); however, we observed an increase in the levels of O^6- and 7-methylguanine during the same time interval following intravenous injection of NNK (0.41 mmol/kg).

α-Carbon hydroxylation of both NDMA and NNK is probably the initial step which leads to a common methylating species. This species could be methyldiazohydroxide (Fig. 1, *4*) or the diazonium or carbonium ion derived from it. The results of the present study suggest that

Fig. 1. Metabolic activation of 4-(methylnitrosamino)-1-(3-pyridyl)-1-butanone (NNK) to methylating intermediates

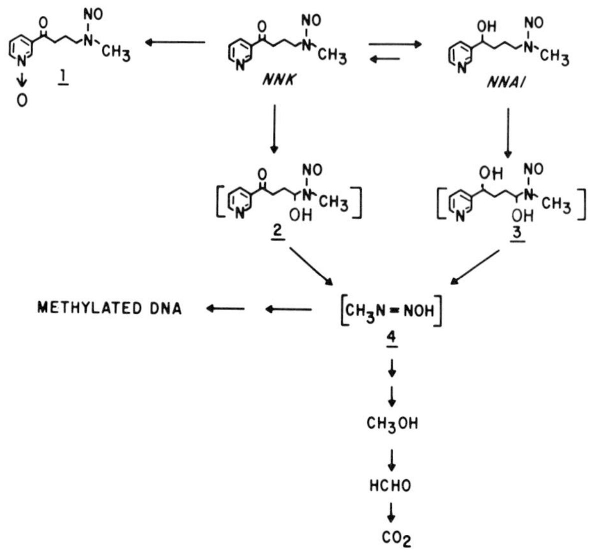

4 is formed more slowly from NNK than from NDMA. α-Methylene hydroxylation of NNK could lead to intermediate 2 and then to 4. Both NNK-1-N-oxide (1) and 4-(methylnitrosamino)-1-(3-pyridyl)-butan-1-ol (NNA1) have been isolated from the urine of NNK-treated rats, and could *a priori* be precursors of 4 since they have an N-methylnitrosamino functionality (Hecht *et al.*, 1980b). However, 1 is formed in only minor quantities during incubation of NNK with rat liver microsomes or liver slices, while NNA1 is a major metabolite in these systems (Hecht *et al.*, 1980b). NNK injected intravenously into F344 rats is reduced rapidly to NNA1, and NNA1 is found not only in every tissue but also in the serum (Castonguay *et al.*, 1983). Thus, the slow methylation of DNA following NNK administration could be due to a slow α-carbon hydroxylation of the major circulating metabolite NNA1 to intermediate 3. Alternatively, reoxidation of NNA1 to NNK might be a slow process required for the formation of 4 *via* NNK.

We have shown recently that the mucosa covering rat nasal septum can be cultured *in vitro* for a 24-h period (Brittebo *et al.*, 1983). The nasal mucosa explants had a remarkably high capacity to α-carbon hydroxylate NNK. The results of the present study show that the methylating species generated during the metabolism of NNK can methylate the explant DNA. Interestingly, the methylating species seems to be too short-lived to diffuse out of the explant and alkylate calf thymus DNA present in the culture medium. In contrast, methylating species generated from NDMA by isolated rat hepatocytes did methylate exogenous DNA, indicating that they are stable enough to pass through one cell membrane (Umbenhauer & Pegg, 1981).

We previously studied the ability of rat tissues to activate [carbonyl-^{14}C-]-NNK to alkylating species (Castonguay *et al.*, 1983). In this study, methyl hydroxylation of NNK was probably the first step of the bioactivation pathway leading to radioactive alkylating species. Tissue-bound metabolites were present in the nasal and bronchial mucosae and in the liver but were absent from the kidneys. In the present study, DNA methylation probably resulted from α-methylene hydroxylation. Interestingly, there seems to be a similarity in the biodistribution of the enzymes able to hydroxylate the two α-carbons of NNK.

Barrows and Shank (1981) observed hepatic DNA methylation after administration of hepatotoxic agents such as hydrazine, carbon tetrachloride and ethanol and proposed that formation of O^6- and 7-methylguanine was mediated by methionine and S-adenosyl-methionine. Whether such aberrant methylation takes place after NNK treatment remains to be investigated. The results of the present study also invite further research on the formation of other DNA promutagenic lesions formed either by methylation of thymidine or alkylation of DNA bases by the pyridyloxobutyl moiety of NNK.

ACKNOWLEDGEMENTS

We thank Dr Ronald C. Shank from the University of California, Irvine for his advice on high-performance liquid chromatographic-fluorescence analyses of methylated DNA. This study was supported by US National Cancer Institute Grants Number CA-21393 and CA-32391.

REFERENCES

Abbott, P.J. & Saffhill, R. (1979) DNA synthesis with methylated poly (dC-dG) templates. Evidence for a competitive nature to miscoding by O^6-methylguanine. *Biochim. biophys. Acta., 562,* 51–61

Autrup, H. & Stoner, G.D. (1982) Metabolism of *N*-nitrosamines by cultured human and rat esophagus. *Cancer Res., 42,* 1307–1311

Barrows, L.R. & Shank, R.C. (1981) Aberrant methylation of liver DNA in rats during hepatotoxicity. *Toxicol. appl. Pharmacol., 60,* 334–345

Brittebo, E.B., Castonguay, A., Furuya, K. & Hecht, S.S. (1981) Metabolism of tobacco-specific nitrosamines by cultured rat nasal mucosa. *Cancer Res., 43,* 4343–4348

Castonguay, A., Rivenson, A., Hecht, S.S. & Hoffmann, D. (1981) Carcinogenicity, metabolism and DNA binding of the tobacco-specific nitrosamine, 4-(methylnitrosamino)-1-(3-pyridyl)-1-butanone (NNK). *Proc. Am. Assoc. Cancer Res., 22,* 75

Castonguay, A., Tjälve, H. & Hecht, S.S. (1983) Tissue distribution of the tobacco-specific carcinogen 4-(methylnitrosamino)-1-(3-pyridyl)-1-butanone and its metabolites in F344 rats. *Cancer Res., 43,* 630–638

Daoud, A. & Irving, C.C. (1977) Methylation of DNA in rat liver and intestine by dimethylnitrosamine and *N*-methylnitrosourea. *Chem.-biol. Interactions, 16,* 135–143

Hecht, S.S., Chen, C.B., Ohmori, T. & Hoffmann, D. (1980a) Comparative carcinogenicity in F344 rats of the tobacco-specific nitrosamines, *N'*-nitrosonornicotine and 4-(*N*-methyl-*N*-nitrosamino)-1-(3-pyridyl)-1-butanone. *Cancer Res., 40,* 298–302

Hecht, S.S., Young, R. & Chen, C.B. (1980b) Metabolism in the F344 rat of 4-(*N*-methyl-*N*-nitrosamino)-1-(3-pyridyl)-1-butanone. *Cancer Res., 40,* 4144–4150

Herron, D.C. & Shank, R.C. (1979) Quantitative high-pressure liquid chromatographic analysis of methylated purines in DNA of rats treated with chemical carcinogens. *Anal. Biochem., 100,* 58–63

Kleihues, P., Veit, C., Wiessler, M. & Hodgson, R.M. (1981) DNA methylation by *N*-nitroso-methylbenzylamine in target and non-target tissues of NMR1 mice. *Carcinogenesis, 2,* 897–899

Labarca, C. & Paigen, K. (1980) A simple, rapid and sensitive DNA assay procedure. *Anal. Biochem., 102,* 344–352

Magee, P.N. & Barnes, J.M. (1967) Carcinogenic nitroso compounds. *Adv. Cancer Res., 10,* 163–246

Meredith, R.D. & Erlanger, B.F. (1979) Isolation and characterization of rabbit anti-m⁷G-5'P antibodies of high apparent affinity. *Nucleic Acid Res., 6,* 2179–2191

Müller, R. & Rajewsky, M.F. (1980) Immunological quantification by high-affinity antibodies of O^6-ethyldeoxyguanosine in DNA exposed to *N*-ethyl-*N*-nitrosourea. *Cancer Res., 40,* 887–896

Pegg. A.E. (1977) Alkylation of rat liver DNA by dimethylnitrosamine: effect of dosage on O^6-methylguanine levels. *J. natl Cancer Inst., 58,* 681–687

Swann, P.F., Mace, R., Angeles, R.M. & Keefer, L.K. (1983) Deuterium isotope effect on metabolism of *N*-nitrosodimethylamine *in vivo* in rat. *Carcinogenesis, 4,* 812–825

Umbenhauer, D.R. & Pegg, A.E. (1981) Alkylation of intracellular and extracellular DNA by dimethylnitrosamine following activation by isolated rat hepatocytes. *Cancer Res., 41,* 3471–3474

INCREASED ENDOGENOUS NITROSATION IN SMOKERS

K.F. LADD & M.C. ARCHER[1]

*Department of Medical Biophysics, University of Toronto, Ontario Cancer Institute,
500 Sherbourne Street, Toronto, M4X 1K9, Canada*

H.L. NEWMARK

Ludwig Institute for Cancer Research, Toronto Branch, Toronto, Canada

SUMMARY

Endogenous nitrosation of proline was investigated in smokers and nonsmokers. Volunteers consumed a volume of beetroot juice equivalent to 325 mg nitrate and, 1 h later, 500 mg proline. In seperate experiments, volunteers ingested proline alone. Twenty-four-hour urines were collected and analysed for N-nitrosoproline. When proline was ingested alone, there was no significant difference in urinary N-nitrosoproline excretion between smokers and nonsmokers. When beetroot juice and proline were consumed, however, smokers produced approximately 2.5 times as much N-nitrosoproline as nonsmokers. Salivary nitrite levels of smokers and nonsmokers, both before and after consumption of beetroot juice, were not significantly different. Salivary thiocyanate levels were approximately 3.2. times higher in smokers than in nonsmokers. Our results suggest that the higher level of salivary thiocynate in smokers is responsible for the increased rate of endogenous nitrosation of proline in that group when compared with nonsmokers. Oxides of nitrogen in cigarette smoke do not appear to play a significant role.

INTRODUCTION

Although carcinogenic N-nitroso compounds contaminate the external environment, endogenous synthesis of these compounds from precursors in the body may represent a large source of exposure for the general population (National Academy of Sciences, 1978). There have been a number of direct and indirect demonstrations of N-nitrosamine formation *in vivo* in experimental animals (reviewed by Archer, 1982). Endogenous nitrosation in humans has recently been estimated by measurement of N-nitrosoproline (NPRO) excretion in urine after ingestion of nitrate and/or proline (Ohshima & Bartsch, 1981). Because NPRO is excreted

---

[1] To whom correspondence should be addressed

quantitatively in urine within 24 h (Dailey *et al*., 1975) and is not carcinogenic (Nixon *et al*., 1976), it is an excellent marker of endogenous nitrosation.

Here, we demonstrate that smokers produce more NPRO than nonsmokers when nitrate and proline have been ingested, but not when proline is consumed alone. As well, we suggest a mechanism to account for this difference in rate of endogenous nitrosation between smokers and nonsmokers.

MATERIALS AND METHODS

Chemicals

NPRO and *N*-nitrosopiperidine-2-carboxylic acid (NPIC) were synthesized and purified by the method of Lijinsky *et al*. (1970). Authentic samples of the methyl esters of NPRO (NPRO-Me) and NPIC (NPIC-Me), prepared by reaction of the *N*-nitrosoamino acids with diazomethane, were used to quantify NPRO.

Beetroot juice was purchased from a local health food shop; 11 bottles analysed by the method of Saul and Archer (1983) contained an average of 1488 mg/L (range, 1439-1560) nitrate. L-proline, beetroot juice and all other reagents used during this study contained no detectable level of preformed NPRO or nitrite (detection limits, 0.5 µg/L and 0.5 mg/L, respectively). Analysis of NPRO and nitrite was performed as described below.

Endogenous nitrosation experiments

Volunteers were all healthy individuals consuming typical Western-style diets. There were nine female and seven male smokers, average age, 38 years (range, 24–69 years); and five female and seven male nonsmokers, average age, 33 years (range, 22–45 years).

Protocol 1: Both nonsmokers and smokers observed certain dietary restrictions to prevent ingestion of significant levels of preformed NPRO and to minimize inhibition of proline nitrosation. No beer, cured meat or ascorbate or tocopherol supplement was ingested for 24 h prior to, and for 48 h during the experiment. On both experimental days between 13:00 and 18:00 hours, no coffee, tea, citrus fruit or juice containing ascorbate was consumed; no large meal was ingested between 14:00 and 16:00 hours, and no food was consumed between 16:00 and 18:00 hours.

All urine excreted during the experiment was collected in 1-litre bottles containing 10 mL 20% ammonium sulfamate in 1.8 mol/L sulfuric acid and stored at 4°C until analysed. Repeated analysis of urine stored for several weeks showed no change in NPRO content. On the first day, volunteers began to collect a 24-h urine sample at 16:00 hours. One mL of saliva was also collected and analysed for thiocyanate. On the second day, at 15:00 hours, volunteers supplied a saliva sample for nitrite analysis (collected into 1.5 mL of 0.6 mol/L sodium hydroxide as a preservative). Each volunteer then consumed a volume of beetroot juice equivalent to 325 mg nitrate. One hour later, a saliva sample was collected for nitrite analysis, and then 15 mL of an aqueous solution containing 500 mg proline were ingested. Urine was collected for the next 24 h. Compliance with 24-h urine collection was determined by measurement of creatinine coefficients.

Protocol 2: Eight smokers and seven nonsmokers adhered to the same dietary restrictions and collected urine as in protocol *1*. However, no saliva sample was collected and no beetroot juice was consumed. At 16:00 hours on the second day, 15 mL of an aqueous solution containing 500 mg proline were ingested.

Analytical techniques

Salivary thiocyanate was analysed by the method of Boyland *et al.* (1971). Salivary nitrite was analysed by a modification of the method of Saul and Archer (1983). The final volume of the sample after deproteinization was 10 mL, a 2-ml portion of which was analysed for nitrite using the Griess reaction.

Five per cent of the total 24-h urine was used for each NPRO analysis. As an internal standard, 450 ng NPIC were added to the urine sample. The urine was passed through a Sep-Pak C_{18} Cartridge (Waters Associates, Milford, MA, USA), and the cartridge was washed with 20 mL deionized water. The sample collected from the C_{18} Cartridge was analysed for NPRO by the method of Sen *et al.* (1983) After derivatization with boron trifluoride/methanol, 8 mL deionized water and 1 mL dichloromethane were added, and the mixture was vortexed for 2 min. The tubes were then centrifuged at $275 \times g$ for 15 min. Ten µL of the dichloromethane layer were analysed by gas chromatography, using a Thermal Energy Analyzer (Thermo Electron Corp., Waltham, MA, USA) as detector, with a 188 cm × 3.2. mm i.d. column packed with 10% Carbowax-20M on Chromosorb W.HP 80/100, at a temperature of 190°C. The flow rate of the argon carrier gas was 35 mL/min. Under these conditions, NPIC-Me and NPRO-Me were well separated, with retention times of 6.6 and 7.8 min, respectively. Standard curves for NPRO-Me and NPIC-Me were used to quantify amounts present in the urine sample. Using this protocol, the average recovery of the internal standard was $90.1 \pm 2.0\%$ (mean $\pm$ SE), and all NPRO values were corrected appropriately.

The urine of any volunteer who did not observe the dietary restrictions or did not comply with 24-h urine collection (as determined by the creatinine coefficient) was discarded.

RESULTS

Salivary thiocyanate concentrations for 16 smokers, 5.1 ± 0.5 mmol/L (mean $\pm$ SE), and 12 nonsmokers, 1.6 ± 0.2 mmol/L, were significantly different ($p < 0.001$). Salivary nitrite concentrations, however, were not different for smokers and nonsmokers either before (3.2 ± 0.7 and 2.6 ± 0.6 mg/L, respectively) or after (59.8 ± 11.5 and 87.0 ± 16.3 mg/L, respectively) consumption of beetroot juice. Urinary NPRO excretion by smokers and nonsmokers is shown in Figure 1. Background levels of urinary NPRO for smokers and nonsmokers who had ingested neither proline nor nitrate were not significantly different. Furthermore, following consumption of proline alone, NPRO levels for both groups were not significantly different from background NPRO levels. When a bolus of nitrate was consumed one hour prior to ingestion of proline, there was a large and significant increase in urinary NPRO excretion by both smokers and nonsmokers. Smokers, however, excreted significantly higher amounts (about 2.5 times) of NPRO than nonsmokers ($p < 0.02$) under these conditions.

Smokers were asked the number of cigarettes they smoked each day and accordingly divided into two groups: light smokers (< 30 cigarettes/day) and heavy smokers (> 30 cigarettes/day). Figure 2 shows urinary NPRO excretion and salivary nitrite and thiocyanate concentrations after nitrate and proline ingestion for nonsmokers and for both groups of smokers. Urinary NPRO excretion following consumption of nitrate and proline differed significantly between nonsmokers and light smokers ($p < 0.05$) and between nonsmokers and heavy smokers ($p < 0.02$); light smokers did not differ significantly from heavy smokers. Salivary nitrite concentrations did not differ significantly among the three groups. Salivary thiocyanate levels differed significantly between nonsmokers and both groups of smokers ($p < 0.001$) but not between light and heavy smokers. The coefficient of correlation was 0.77 for a linear regression analysis of salivary thiocyanate *versus* the estimated number of cigarettes smoked per day; the

LADD *ET AL.*

Fig. 1. Urinary excretion of *N*-nitrosoproline (NPRO) by smokers and nonsmokers. Background levels (16 smokers and 12 nonsmokers) are compared with those after ingestion of proline alone (8 smokers and 7 nonsmokers) and after ingestion of nitrate and proline (16 smokers and 12 nonsmokers); mean $\pm$ SE

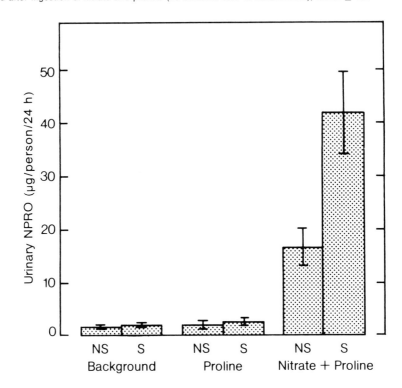

slope was 0.081 ± 0.027 mmol thiocyanate/L per cigarette/day ($\pm$ 95% confidence limits). Linear regression analysis of urinary NPRO excretion following nitrate and proline ingestion *versus* salivary thiocyanate concentration gave a coefficient correlation of 0.49; the slope was 5.692 ± 4.059 µg NPRO/person per day/mmol thiocyanate/L ($\pm$ 95% confidence limits).

DISCUSSION

Nitrogen oxides present in cigarette smoke (Bokhoven & Niessen, 1961) could react within the respiratory tract to form dinitrogen trioxide and dinitrogen tetroxide, which are capable of nitrosating amines (Challis & Kyrtopoulos, 1979). Therefore, direct nitrosation of amines in the respiratory tract by either of these nitrosating agents could occur. Our results indicate, however, that this process contributes minimally to proline nitrosation. Ingestion of proline alone resulted in a small increase of urinary NPRO levels in smokers compared with nonsmokers; however, the difference was not statistically significant. Examination of much larger populations of smokers and nonsmokers will be necessary to confirm this effect.

Exposure to nitrogen dioxide (NO_2) results in increased serum nitrate/nitrite levels (Oda *et al.*, 1981); nitric oxide (NO) appears to have the same effect (Yoshida *et al.*, 1980). Increased serum levels of nitrate lead to increased levels of salivary nitrite (Tannenbaum *et al.*, 1976),

Fig. 2. Comparison of urinary excretion of *N*-nitrosoproline (NPRO), salivary thiocyanate (SCN⁻) and nitrite (NO₂⁻) for 12 nonsmokers (NS), 8 light smokers (LS) and 8 heavy smokers (HS) after ingestion of nitrate and proline; mean ± SE

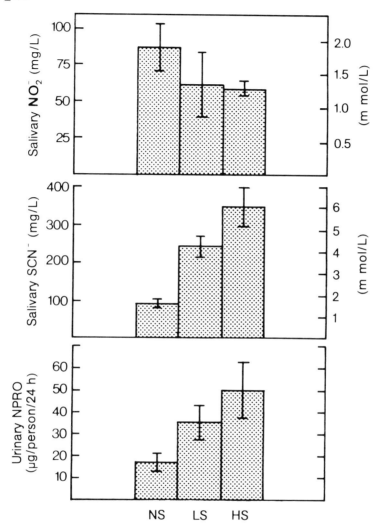

which in turn could lead to an increased rate of NPRO formation in the stomach. Our results showed, however, that differences in background salivary nitrite concentrations between smokers and nonsmokers were not significant. An explanation for this result could be antagonism between nitrate and thiocyanate (see below) for secretion in saliva (Edwards *et al.*, 1954).

Our results, as well as previous observations by other workers (Maliszewski & Bass, 1955), show that smokers have three to four times higher levels of salivary thiocyanate than nonsmokers. Thiocyanate is well known to catalyse nitrosation reactions under moderately acidic conditions (Boyland *et al.*, 1971). The correlation we have observed between salivary thiocyanate concentrations and urinary NPRO excretion suggests that the higher level of salivary thiocyanate in smokers may be responsible for an increased rate of gastric nitrosation of proline in this group compared with nonsmokers. This effect was only observed, however, following ingestion of nitrate.

Ohshima and Bartsch (1981) reported marginal or, in most cases, no increase in urinary NPRO when less than 195 mg nitrate were ingested by their volunteer. This observation can be attributed in part to the requirement that at least 54 mg nitrate be ingested before there is an increase in salivary nitrate or nitrite levels (Spiegelhalder *et al.*, 1976). It is also possible that other compounds are present in the stomach that react much more rapidly with nitrite than proline. Only after these compounds have reacted can the remaining nitrite participate significantly in the nitrosation of proline. Both of these explanations may account for our observation that there was no significant increase in urinary NPRO excretion in smokers when proline, but not nitrate, was ingested, although these smokers had high levels of salivary thiocyanate.

Our results show that, following ingestion of nitrate and proline, smokers produce significantly greater amounts of NPRO. This result suggests that endogenous synthesis of carcinogenic *N*-nitroso compounds may be greater in smokers than in nonsmokers.

ACKNOWLEDGEMENTS

This research was supported by the Ontario Cancer Treatment and Research Foundation and the National Cancer Institute of Canada. A studentship from the Province of Ontario is gratefully acknowledged by K.F.L.

REFERENCES

Archer, M.C. (1982) *Hazards of nitrate, nitrite and* N-*nitroso compounds in human nutrition*. In: Hathcock, J.N., ed., *Nutritional Toxicology, 1*, New York, Academic Press, pp. 327–381

Bokhoven, C. & Niessen, H.J. (1961) Amounts of oxides of nitrogen and carbon monoxide in cigarette smoke, with and without inhalation. *Nature, 192*, 458–459

Boyland, E., Nice, E. & Williams, K. (1971) The catalysis of nitrosation by thiocyanate from saliva. *Food Cosmet. Toxicol., 9*, 639–643

Challis, B.C. & Kyrtopoulos, S.A. (1979) Nitrosation of amines by the two-phase interaction of amines in solution with gaseous oxides of nitrogen. *J. chem. Soc. Perkin I*, 299–304

Dailey, R.E., Braunberg, R.C. & Blaschka, A.M. (1975) The absorption, distribution, and excretion of [^{14}C] nitrosoproline by rats. *Toxicology, 3*, 23–28

Edwards, D.A.W., Fletcher, K. & Rowlands, E.N. (1954) Antagonism between perchlorate, iodide, thiocyanate, and nitrate for secretion in human saliva: Analogy with the iodide trap of the thyroid. *Lancet, i*, 498–499

Lijinsky, W., Keefer, L. & Loo, J. (1970) The preparation and properties of some nitrosamino acids. *Tetrahedron, 26*, 5137–5153

Maliszewski, T.F. & Bass, D.E. (1955) 'True' and 'apparent' thiocyanate in body fluids of smokers and nonsmokers. *J. appl. Physiol., 8*, 289–291

National Academy of Sciences (1978) *Coordinating Committee for Scientific and Technical Assessment of Environmental Pollutants. Nitrates: An Environmental Assessment*, Washington, DC

Nixon, J.E., Wales, J.H., Scalan, R.A., Bills, D.D. & Sinnhuber, R.O. (1976) Null carcinogenic effect of large doses of nitrosoproline and nitrosohydroxyproline in Wistar rats. *Food Cosmet. Toxicol., 14*, 133–135

Oda, H., Tsubons, H., Suzuki, A., Ichinose, T. & Kubota, K. (1981) Alterations of nitrite and nitrate concentrations in the blood of mice exposed to nitrogen dioxide. *Environ. Res., 25*, 294–301

Ohshima, H. & Bartsch, H. (1981) Quantitative estimation of endogenous nitrosation in humans by monitoring N-nitrosoproline excreted in urine. *Cancer Res., 41,* 3658-3662

Saul, R.L. & Archer, M.C. (1983) Nitrate formation in rats exposed to nitrogen dioxide. *Toxicol. appl. Pharmacol., 67,* 284–291

Sen, N.P., Tessier, L. & Seaman, S. (1983) Determination of N-nitrosoproline and N-nitrososarcosine in malt and beer. *J. agric. Food Chem., 31,* 1033–1036

Spiegelhalder, B., Eisenbrand, G. & Preussmann, R. (1976) Influence of dietary nitrate on nitrite content of human saliva: Possible relevance to *in vivo* formation of N-nitroso compounds. *Food Cosmet. Toxicol., 14,* 545–548

Tannenbaum, S.R., Weisman, M. & Fett, D. (1976) The effect of nitrate intake on nitrite formation in human saliva. *Food Cosmet. Toxicol., 14,* 549–552

Yoshida, K., Kasama, K., Kitabatake, M., Okuda, M. & Imai, M. (1980) Metabolic fate of nitric oxide. *Int. Arch. occup. environ. Health, 45,* 71–77

ENDOGENOUS FORMATION OF
N-NITROSOPROLINE UPON CIGARETTE SMOKE INHALATION

K.D. BRUNNEMANN, J.C. SCOTT, N.J. HALEY & D. HOFFMANN

*Naylor Dana Institute for Disease Prevention, American Health Foundation,
Valhalla, NY 10595, USA*

SUMMARY

It was the goal of this study to assay the potential of inhaled cigarette smoke for endogenous
N-nitrosation of amines in smokers by measuring urinary excretion of N-nitrosoproline
(NPRO). Nonsmoking and smoking men were placed on a controlled diet which was low in
proline and in ascorbic acid. On days 1–3, the volunteers received the controlled diet alone
(Group I); on days 4–6, the diet was supplemented by a single daily dose of 300 mg proline
(Group II); on days 7–9, the diet was supplemented by a single daily dose of 1 g ascorbic acid
followed by 300 mg proline (Group III); and for the last three days, a single daily dose of 1 g
ascorbic acid was given (Group IV). Collections of 24-h urine were made on days 3, 6, 9 and
12 of the study. The urine was analysed for NPRO, creatinine and cotinine. The mean 24-h
NPRO excretion for 13 nonsmokers in Group I was 3.6 µg, whereas the NPRO excretion in
13 smokers was 5.9 µg/24 h, significantly higher than that of the nonsmokers ($p < 0.05$).
Urinary NPRO in 14 nonsmokers of Group II was significantly lower than that of the 14
smoking volunteers ($p < 0.05$). In Group III smokers had reduced urinary levels of NPRO as
a consequence of ascorbic acid intake. Differences in NPRO excretion by smokers and
nonsmokers in Group IV were insignificant. These findings suggest that the documented
endogenous N-nitrosation of proline which occurs as a result of cigarette smoke inhalation may
also apply to other N-nitrosatable amines, including nicotine, and thus lead to in-vivo
formation of carcinogenic N-nitrosamines.

Four nonsmokers exposed to passive smoke for 80 min three times per day did not exhibit
elevated NPRO levels in their 24-h urine.

INTRODUCTION

Cigarette smoking is associated with cancer of the upper respiratory tract, lung, oral cavity,
oesophagus, pancreas, kidney and urinary bladder (US Department of Health and Human
Services, 1982). A large number of tumorigenic agents have been identified in cigarette smoke,
including volatile, nonvolatile and tobacco-specific N-nitrosamines (TSNA) (Hoffmann *et al.*,
this volume, p. 743). The latter group of carcinogens is formed from amines and nitrogen oxides
during smoking (Hoffmann *et al.*, 1981, Adams *et al.*, 1983). In-vivo formation of carcinogenic

N-nitrosamines in cigarette smokers is feasible, since the smoke of one cigarette contains up to 0.6 mg nitric oxide and since nitric oxide is known to effect endogenous nitrosation of proline (Janzowski *et al.*, 1982).

At present, it is not possible to differentiate quantitatively *N*-nitrosamines inhaled as components of cigarette smoke from those that may be formed endogenously. The TSNA are not only the most abundant carcinogens in tobacco smoke, but they are possibly also formed endogenously upon inhalation of nicotine and other alkaloids and nitrosating agents. TSNA are rapidly converted to metabolites, many of which are the same as those deriving from the parent alkaloids (Hecht *et al.*, 1982; Castonguay *et al.*, 1983).

In order to document the endogenous formation of *N*-nitrosamines in cigarette smokers, we chose to measure the *N*-nitrosation of proline to *N*-nitrosoproline (NPRO) as a surrogate assay. NPRO is not present in cigarette smoke (< 1 ng/cigarette), appears neither to undergo metabolism in mammals nor to alkylate cellular macromolecules, is considered to be non-mutagenic and non-carcinogenic and is excreted nearly quantitatively in the urine (International Agency for Research on Cancer, 1978; Mirvish *et al*; 1980; Chu & Magee, 1981; Ohshima & Bartsch, 1981; Brunnemann *et al.*, 1983). Ohshima and Bartsch (1981), Ohshima *et al.* (1982) and Wagner *et al.* (1982) have previously described the endogenous formation of NPRO in human volunteers who were given dietary supplements of nitrate and proline. These investigators showed also that the endogenous formation of NPRO in man can be inhibited by addition of ascorbic acid to the diet.

MATERIALS AND METHODS

Materials

Food supplies were purchased at a local shop on the day before the start of the study; on day 6 of the study, fresh vegetables, dairy products, bread and meat products were resupplied. Ascorbic acid (250-mg tablets) was purchased at a local pharmacy; L-proline (approved for human consumption) was purchased from Ajinomoto USA, Inc. (Raleigh, NC, USA); it was free of NPRO according to gas chromatography-thermal energy analyzer (GC-TEA) (< 1 ng) using 2,6-dimethylmorpholine as a monitor amine for the analysis (Van Stee *et al.*, 1983). Polypropylene bottles for urine collection were obtained from American Scientific Products (McGaw Park, IL, USA). ClinElut extraction columns (20 mL; Analytichem International, Harbor City, CA, USA) were purchased from Fisher Scientific (Springfield, NJ, USA). All food items used in this study were analysed for the presence of NPRO.

Chemicals

DL-Pipecolic acid (Sigma Chemical Co., St Louis, MO, USA) and L-(-)proline (Aldrich Chemical Co., Inc., Milwaukee, WI, USA) were nitrosated according to the method of Lijinsky *et al.* (1970) and purified by chromatography. Their purity was ascertained by mass spectrometry and by GC-TEA. Other chemicals used were: ammonium sulfamate (MCB/E, Merck, Darmstadt, FRG), *n*-hexane (Fisher Scientific), sulfuric acid, ethyl acetate, dichloromethane (Mallinckrodt, St Louis, MO, USA), sodium sulfate, sodium chloride (J.T. Baker Chemical Co., Phillipsburg, NJ, USA) and 14% boron trifluoride in methanol (Pierce Chemical Co., Rockford, IL, USA). The creatinine reagent set was obtained from Worthington Diagnostic Systems Inc. (Freehold, NJ, USA).

Apparatus

A Model 543 Thermal Energy Analyzer (Thermo Electron Corp., Waltham, MA, USA) was interfaced directly with a Model 700 gas chromatograph (Hewlett-Packard, Paramus, NJ, USA). The mass-spectral analyses were performed on a Hewlett-Packard Model 5982 GC-mass spectrometer.

Volunteers

Mainstream smoke: In order to assess the *N*-nitrosation potential of inhaled cigarette mainstream smoke, 15 smokers and 15 nonsmokers (none of whom were tobacco chewers) were recruited from the staff of the Medical Center in Valhalla, New York, during three separate time spans (five smokers and five nonsmokers each time); the volunteers were healthy males between the ages of 25 and 50 years who did not have urinary or prostatic problems. Some of the volunteers were recruited more than once. They were placed on a well-balanced controlled diet for 12 days each (nine days only in the first period). The diet provided approximately 2 300 kcal/day and was designed to maintain a fairly constant low proline and low ascorbic acid content. Red meats and sea-food were restricted in this study; the consumption of alcohol was limited to one drink per day, since its effect on proline metabolism is not known. A detailed description of the diet has been given elsewhere (Hoffmann & Brunnemann, 1983). The smokers were supplied with a sufficient number of cigarettes of the brand of their choice and were allowed to smoke *ad libitum* but had to record their daily cigarette consumption.

On days 1–3, the volunteers received the controlled diet alone (Group I); on days 4–6, the diet was supplemented by a single daily dose of 300 mg proline (Group II); on days 7–9, the volunteers were given 1 g ascorbic acid followed by 300 mg proline (Group III); and for the last three days, a single daily dose of 1 g ascorbic acid was given (Group IV).

Aliquots of 24-h urine samples were analysed for NPRO, creatinine and cotinine, the major metabolite of nicotine (Langone *et al.*, 1973). The level of cotinine in the urine reflects the nicotine uptake in the previous 24–36 h (US Department of Health and Human Services, 1982).

Passive smoke inhalation: Four male nonsmokers (and nonchewers) were placed on the same controlled diet for five days, during which time they also received 200 mg proline three times daily. On days 3 and 4, they were placed three times for 80-min periods (at 10:00, 12:30 and 15:00 hours) in a test laboratory (16.3 m³, 22 ± 1 °C) in which four Kentucky 1R1 research cigarettes were smoked concurrently by a machine (the sidestream smoke was allowed to emit freely into the atmosphere of the test laboratory, and the mainstream smoke was directed outside the room). The air in the test laboratory was exchanged six times per hour; approximately 10–15 min after the onset of smoking, the room reached the following pollution levels: particulate matter, 4 600 µg/m³; nicotine, 280 µg/m³; hydrogen cyanide, 56 µg/m³; carbon monoxide, 25 ppm; nitrogen oxides, 0.9 ppm.

Urine collection: Twenty-four-hour urine samples were collected on days 3, 6, 9 and 12 from the smokers and nonsmokers. In the case of passive smokers, samples were collected on days 1, 2, 3 and 4; on day 5, only the first 8-h aliquot was collected.

The day before the urine collections were made, the volunteers were given 2-L bottles containing 10 mL of a solution of 20% ammonium sulfamate in 1.8 mol/L sulfuric acid. All urine samples, varying in volume from 0.54–2.8 L, were stored at 4 °C immediately after collection and were analysed in duplicate within 48 h (no sample deterioration was seen within two weeks when they were stored at 4 °C).

Analysis of NPRO in urine: The assay procedure used was a modification of that of Ohshima and Bartsch (1981) and Sen[1].

---

[1] Personal communication; described by Hoffmann and Brunnemann (1983)

Using 0.2 mg proline and/or 0.2 mg 2,6-dimethylmorpholine as monitor amine (Van Stee *et al.,* 1983), we found the artefactual formation of NPRO during the analysis to be negligible. The identity of NPRO was confirmed on a number of samples using microreactions (Krull *et al.,* 1979).

Analysis of NPRO in diet: Samples of liquid or solid foods analysed were usually in the range of 100–200 g. The solid foods were homogenized in a blender. Each food item was extracted for 30 min with sufficient ammonium sulfamate solution (150–300 mL, diluted 1 : 10 with water); the aqueous extract was partitioned with hexane (to remove fats) and the pH adjusted to 1.0–1.2; 30–60 g sodium chloride were then dissolved in the aqueous extract, followed by three solvent distributions with equal volumes of ethyl acetate. The pooled organic extracts were dried (sodium sulfate) and concentrated to 2 mL. The analysis was then carried out as described for urine.

Analysis of cotinine in urine: Cotinine was determined by radioimmunoassay according to the method of Langone *et al.* (1973), in which specific antisera are used which are produced by injection of *trans*-4-carboxycotinine and *trans*-3-succinylmethylnicotine bound to albumin into rabbits. The inter- and intra-assay variations are 6%, with a sensitivity of 370 pg/mL.

Analysis of creatinine in urine: As a control for the proficiency of the urine collection, we analysed 1-mL aliquots of the 24-h urine samples (diluted 400 times) for creatinine, using a colorimetric method for the red creatinine picrate complex. This method has a standard deviation of $\pm$ 3% (Tietz, 1981).

RESULTS

Table 1 summarizes our results for smokers and nonsmokers, showing levels of NPRO, creatinine and cotinine in 24-h urine samples. Cotinine determinations were also done to verify the nonsmoking status of the nonsmokers. All had levels < 80 ng/mL, below the 100 ng cotinine/mL found to be the limit for nonsmokers (Hoffmann *et al.*)[1].

In the study with 13 nonsmoking men on a controlled diet (Group I), we found a mean value of 3.55 $\pm$ 2.13 µg NPRO excretion per 24 h. The urine of 13 smokers contained significantly more NPRO (p = 0.047), which indicates that cigarette smoke inhalation leads to endogenous *N*-nitrosamine formation. This concept is supported by the finding of significantly higher urinary NPRO excretion in smokers on the controlled diet who had received supplements of 300 mg proline once a day (p = 0.031). The *N*-nitrosation potential of inhaled cigarette smoke was further indicated in an assay in which a daily dose of 1 g ascorbic acid, a known inhibitor of *N*-nitrosation (Mirvish *et al.,* 1972; Ohshima *et al.,* 1982), was given as a dietary supplement (Group III). Five of the six smokers in Group II who had shown elevated NPRO excretion upon receiving supplementary proline had significantly reduced NPRO excretion when given ascorbic acid in addition to proline, relative to the group receiving proline supplement alone. There was no significant difference of NPRO levels of smokers and nonsmokers in Group III (p = 0.5).

Individual outlyers in NPRO excretion which cannot be reconciled with the observed trends can, at this point, be attributed only to biological variability inherent in clinical samples of this nature.

When 1 g ascorbic acid was given without proline (Group IV), there was no significant difference in the urinary NPRO levels between smokers and nonsmokers. In spite of the expected reduction of NPRO levels due to the inhibitory effects of ascorbic acid, NPRO excretion of nonsmokers in Group IV (4.0 µg/24 h) was not lower than that of nonsmokers in

---

[1] In preparation

Table 1. N-Nitrosoproline in 24-hour urine samples of male nonsmokers and smokers

Subject No.	I. Controlled diet					II. Controlled diet + proline					III. Controlled diet + ascorbic acid + proline					IV. Controlled diet + ascorbic acid				
	Nonsmoker		Smoker			Nonsmoker		Smoker			Nonsmoker		Smoker			Nonsmoker		Smoker		
	NPRO	CR	NPRO	CR	COT	NPRO	CR	NPRO	CR	COT	NPRO	CR	NPRO	CR	COT	NPRO	CR	NPRO	CR	COT
1	1.6	2.6	8.5	1.7	ND	4.4	2.4	4.4	2.1	ND	3.1	2.5	3.9	1.5	ND	ND	ND	ND	ND	ND
2	2.3	1.9	3.3	1.8	ND	5.9	1.9	26.5	1.8	ND	4.7	2.0	5.4	1.2	ND	ND	ND	ND	ND	ND
3	4.5	1.5	3.4	2.1	ND	4.5	1.5	3.0	1.8	ND	4.8	1.5	0[a]	1.7	ND	ND	ND	ND	ND	ND
4	9.3	2.6	2.6	1.2	ND	5.9	2.1	49.3	1.8	ND	6.4	1.9	8.2	2.2	ND	ND	ND	ND	ND	ND
5	4.4	1.2	ex.	ex.	ND	3.2	1.7	2.0	1.5	ND	7.2	1.8	0.7	1.1	ND	ND	ND	ND	ND	ND
6	2.7	1.3	1.8	1.6	3.1	6.4	1.2	8.0	1.3	3.8	4.2	1.5	2.2	1.7	4.0	3.1	1.3	2.0	1.5	5.4
7	1.8	1.2	4.1	1.5	1.7	2.2	1.2	5.2	1.1	1.9	9.2	1.3	4.4	1.3	1.3	12.4	1.2	6.7	1.5	2.2
8	ex.	ex.	2.9	1.6	5.5	ex.	ex.	40.5	1.6	5.8	ex.	ex.	8.3	1.2	6.7	ex.	ex.	ex.	ex.	ex.
9	4.5	1.4	7.0	1.0	2.7	2.6	1.6	2.8	1.1	3.5	2.8	1.2	ex.	ex.	ex.	3.5	1.3	1.9	1.2	3.7
10	ex.	ex.	ex.	ex.	ex.	1.6	1.0	ex.	ex.	ex.	ex.	ex.	ex.	ex.	ex.	1.8	1.1	5.3	1.0	6.1
11	2.8	1.0	14.6	1.7	3.5	3.1	1.7	0.7	1.1	2.6	2.8	1.8	6.0	2.4	6.6	2.4	1.8	3.0	1.7	3.1
12	2.7	1.6	13.5	1.7	3.4	2.6	1.7	3.6	2.0	5.2	8.2	2.1	12.5	1.4	2.4	0.6	1.4	ex.	ex.	ex.
13	4.6	1.8	1.5	1.6	4.4	1.4	1.5	1.4	1.7	5.1	3.9	1.9	1.6	1.6	4.5	1.9	1.5	1.0	1.5	5.4
14	4.1	1.5	9.3	2.4	9.2	2.6	2.0	7.3	2.2	13.1	0[a]	1.3	6.1	2.5	11.1	4.9	1.6	12.6	2.4	6.5
15	0.9	1.9	4.2	1.8	8.8	4.2	1.9	9.6	1.9	6.8	3.6	2.0	0[a]	2.0	7.8	5.1	1.8	15.2	1.4	5.5
Mean	3.55		5.90			3.61		11.7			4.68		4.56			3.97		5.96		
P	p=0.047					p=0.031					p=0.46					p=0.18				
SD	±2.13		±4.36																	

[a] Below detection limit of 0.3 µg NPRO/24 h

NPRO, N-nitrosoproline (g in 24-h urine); CR, creatinine (g in 24-h urine); COT, cotinine (mg in 24-h urine); ND, not determined); ex., samples excluded from study because creatinine values were <1.0 g/24 h (incomplete urine collection)

Fig. 1. Frequency distribution of *N*-nitrosoproline (NPRO) in the urine of smokers and nonsmokers in the four study
groups relative to creatinine excretion; NS, non-smoker; S, smoker

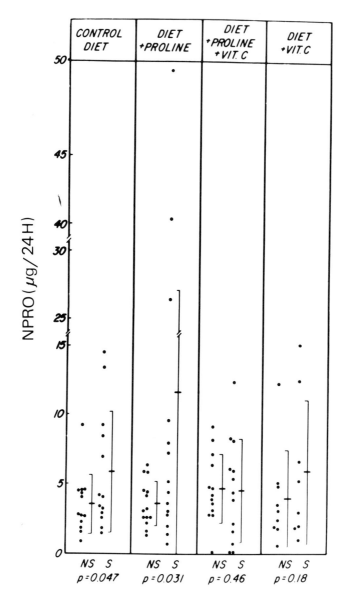

Group I (3.6 µg/24 h). Since only up to 0.7 µg of preformed NPRO can be accounted for by
the diet (see Table 3), other origins of urinary NPRO in addition to intragastric synthesis must
be assumed. Figure 1 illustrates the distribution of NPRO levels in smokers and nonsmokers
in the four study groups.

Table 2 represents the data for levels of NPRO, cotinine and creatinine in the four
nonsmokers who participated in the passive inhalation study. Since NO itself is a weaker

Table 2. *N*-Nitrosoproline (NPRO) in 24-h urine samples of male nonsmokers exposed to passive smoking

Subject no.	Day 1			Day 2			Day 3[a]			Day 4[a]			Day 5[b]		
	NPRO	CR	COT	NPRO	CR	COT	NPRO	CT	COT	NPRO	CR	COT	NPRO	CR	COT
1	1.6	1.4	6	0.5	1.1	3	2.0	1.4	105	6.1	1.2	80	2.9	2.1	360
2	1.7	1.8	7	2.8	1.7	2	3.2	1.9	100	1.7	1.1	350	0.4	1.8	215
3	4.8	2.2	6	5.2	2.4	6	3.0	2.1	90	4.4	2.3	300	2.6	2.1	260
4	2.9	2.2	5	4.3	2.2	5	2.8	2.4	65	3.3	2.2	200	2.0	2.1	330
Mean	2.75			3.20			2.75			3.88			1.98		

[a] Exposure, 3 × 80 min per day
[b] Values adjusted to 24-h urine
NPRO, *N*-nitrosoproline (μg/24 h); CR, creatinine (g/24 h); COT, cotinine (ng/mL)

Table 3.   Preformed *N*-nitrosoproline (NPRO) in diet[a]

Food	NPRO	
	µg/kg	µg/day
Bacon	24	0.120 (2 slices)
Eggs	ND	ND
Coffee	ND	ND
Chicken	0.4	0.033 (3 oz)
Biscuits	0.3	0.018 (6 biscuits)
Corn flakes	1.4	0.042 (1 oz)
Ham	0.2	0.011 (2 oz)
Hamburger	ND	ND
Veal	ND	ND
Toast	0.2	0.006 (2 slices)
Spaghetti	ND	ND
Bread/rolls	ND	ND
Beer	up to 1.3	up to 0.447 (1 tin)
Turkey	ND	ND
Cheese	ND	ND
	Total	up to 0.68 µg/day

[a]No NPRO was detected in other food items consumed. All food items were processed, i.e., as consumed in the diet. ND, not detected

nitrosating agent than is NO_2, we hypothesized that 'aged' sidestream smoke might be a nitrosating agent, since within 5–10 min half of the NO in tobacco smoke is oxidized to NO_2 (Neurath, 1972). On the basis of these preliminary data, however, we cannot specify the contribution of sidestream smoke to the endogenous nitrosation of proline.

Table 3 lists the NPRO contents of the individual food items which comprised the controlled diet. These data are in agreement with those of Sen and Seaman (1984). It would appear that, on the average, no more than 20% of the NPRO in the urine of nonsmokers in this study can be attributed to dietary intake of preformed NPRO. This was confirmed by recent studies by Wagner *et al.* (1983) who administered ^{15}N-labelled nitrate to human volunteers.

DISCUSSION

Although the numbers of volunteers in the study groups were limited, the results obtained to date support the concept that inhaled cigarette mainstream smoke can *N*-nitrosate proline endogenously. It may be assumed that this potential extends to other *N*-nitrosatable amines including nicotine (Assembly of Life Sciences, 1981; Hoffmann & Adams, 1981).

The observation that dietary supplements of ascorbic acid effectively inhibit *N*-nitrosation supports this concept and indicates a preventive potential (National Research Council, 1982; Mirvish *et al.*, 1972).

In this exploratory study we found that it was important to place smokers and nonsmokers on a controlled diet to minimize confounding factors, at least as long as we were dealing with a limited number of subjects. Before these studies can be extended to evaluate larger groups of smokers and nonsmokers, a number of questions need to be addressed. Does endogenous

N-nitrosation of amines after smoke inhalation occur primarily in the stomach, the oral cavity, the lungs and/or the blood? (Mirvish, 1982; Saul & Archer, 1983; Van Stee *et al.*, 1983; Wagner *et al.*, 1983). Can formation of NPRO be increased by administering dietary proline in several subdoses? Conversely, could the inhibitory effects of ascorbic acid be increased by giving several subdoses or a timed-release formulation of this vitamin? Are the nitrogen oxides in cigarette smoke or the nitrous acid formed upon smoke inhalation the primary in-vivo nitrosating agents or are new compounds formed which, in turn, effect the observed *N*-nitrosation? We are currently exploring these and several other questions in smoke inhalation studies with laboratory animals (Bernfeld *et al.*, 1979), in which uptake of nitric oxide is controlled, and we can calculate the correlation between nitric oxide in smoke and urinary NPRO excretion.

ACKNOWLEDGEMENTS

We thank C. Axelrad and K. Tilton for the radioimmunoassay of cotinine in the urine, S. Adams for his excellent technical support and Mrs B. Stadler for her editorial assistance. This study was supported by US National Cancer Institute Grant PO1-CA-29 580.

REFERENCES

Adams, J.D., Lee, S.J., Vinchkoski, N., Castonguay, A. & Hoffmann, D. (1983) On the formation of the tobacco-specific carcinogen 4-(methylnitrosamino)-1-(3-pyridyl)-1-butanone during smoking. *Cancer Lett.*, *17*, 339–346

Assembly of Life Sciences (1981) *The Health Effects of Nitrate, Nitrite and N-Nitroso Compounds,* Committee on Nitrite and Alternative Curing Agents in Food, Washington DC, National Academy Press

Bernfeld, P., Homburger, F., Soto, E. & Pai, K.J. (1979) Cigarette smoke inhalation studies in inbred Syrian golden hamsters. *J. natl Cancer Inst.*, *63*, 675–689

Brunnemann, K.D., Scott, J.C. & Hoffmann, D. (1983) *N*-Nitrosoproline, an indicator for *N*-nitrosation of amines in processed tobacco. *J. Agric. Food Chem.*, *31*, 905–909

Castonguay, A., Tjälve, H. & Hecht, S.S. (1983) Tissue distribution of the tobacco-specific 4-(methylnitrosamino)-1-(3-pyridyl)-1-butanone and its metabolites in F344 rats. *Cancer Res.*, *43*, 630–638

Chu, C. & Magee, P.N. (1981) Metabolic fate of nitrosoproline in the rat. *Cancer Res.*, *41*, 3653–3657

Hecht, S.S., Castonguay, A., Chung, F.L., Hoffmann, D. & Stoner, G.D. (1982) *Recent studies on the metabolic activation of cyclic nitrosamines.* In: Magee, P.N., ed., *Nitrosamines and Human Cancer (Banbury Report No. 12),* Cold Spring Harbor, NY, Cold Spring Harbor Laboratory, pp. 103–120

Hoffmann, D. & Adams, J.D. (1981) Carcinogenic tobacco-specific *N*-nitrosamines in snuff and in the saliva of snuff dippers. *Cancer Res.*, *41*, 4305–4308

Hoffmann, D. & Brunnemann, K.D. (1983) On the endogenous formation of *N*-nitrosoproline in cigarette smokers. *Cancer Res.*, *43*, 5570–5574

Hoffmann, D., Adams, J.D., Brunnemann, K.D. & Hecht, S.S. (1981) *Formation, occurrence and carcinogenicity of* N-*nitrosamines in tobacco products.* In: Scanlan, R.A. & Tannenbaum, S.R., eds, *N-Nitrosamines (Am. chem. Soc. Symp. Ser. 174),* Washington DC, American Chemical Society, pp. 247–273

International Agency for Research on Cancer (1978) N-*Nitrosoproline and* N-*Nitrosohydroxyproline.* In: *IARC Monographs on the Evaluation of the Carcinogenic Risk of Chemicals to Humans,* Vol. 17, *Some* N-*Nitroso Compounds,* Lyon, pp. 303–311

Janzowski, C., Klein, R., Preussmann, R. & Eisenbrand, G. (1982) Nitrosation of sarcosine, proline and 4-hydroxyproline by exposure to nitrogen oxides. *Food Chem. Toxicol.*, *20*, 595–597

Krull, I.S., Goff, E.U., Hoffman, G.G. & Fine, D.H. (1979) Confirmatory methods for the thermal energy determination of *N*-nitroso compounds at trace levels. *Anal. Chem., 51,* 1705–1709

Langone, J.J., Gjika, H.B. & Van Vunakis, H. (1973) Radioimmunoassay for nicotine and cotinine. *Biochemistry, 12,* 5025–5030

Lijinsky, W., Keefer, L. & Loo, J. (1970) The preparation and properties of some nitrosamino acids. *Tetrahedron, 26,* 5137–5153

Mirvish, S.S. (1982) In vivo *formation of* N-*nitroso compounds: formation from nitrite and nitrogen dioxide and relation to gastric cancer.* In: Magee, P.N., ed., *Nitrosamines and Human Cancer (Banbury Report No. 12),* Cold Spring Harbor, NY, Cold Spring Harbor Laboratory, pp. 227–236

Mirvish, S.S., Wallcave, L., Eagen, M. & Shubik, P. (1972) Ascorbate-nitrite reaction: possible means of blocking the formation of carcinogenic *N*-nitroso compounds. *Science, 177,* 65–68

Mirvish, S.S., Bulay, O., Runge, R.G. & Patil, K. (1980) Studies on the carcinogenicity of large doses of dimethylnitramine, *N*-nitroso-L-proline, and sodium nitrite administered in drinking water to rats. *J. natl Cancer Inst., 64,* 1435–1442

National Research Council (1982) *Vitamin C (ascorbic acid).* In: *Diet, Nutrition and Cancer,* Committee on Diet, Nutrition and Cancer, Assembly of Life Sciences, Washington DC, National Academy Press, pp. 9–7–9–10

Ohshima, H. & Bartsch, H. (1981) Quantitative estimation of endogenous nitrosation in humans by monitoring *N*-nitrosoproline excreted in the urine. *Cancer Res., 41,* 3658–3662

Ohshima, H., Pignatelli, B. & Bartsch, H. (1982) *Monitoring of excreted* N-*nitrosamino acid as a new method to quantitate endogenous nitrosation in humans.* In: Magee, P.N., ed., *Nitrosamines and Human Cancer (Banbury Report No. 12),* Cold Spring Harbor, NY, Cold Spring Harbor Laboratory, pp. 297–317

Saul, R.L. & Archer, M.C. (1983) Nitrate formation in rats exposed to nitrogen dioxide. *Toxicol. appl. Pharmacol., 67,* 284–291

Tietz, N.W. (1981) *Fundamentals of Clinical Chemistry,* Philadelphia, W. Saunders Co., pp. 981, 997–999

US Department of Health and Human Services (1982) *The Health Consequences of Smoking – Cancer (HHS (PHS) 82-50 179),* Washington DC

Van Stee, E.W., Sloane, R.A., Simmons, J.E. & Brunnemann, K.D. (1983) *In vivo* formation of *N*-nitrosomorpholine in CD-1 mice exposed by inhalation to nitrogen dioxide and by gavage to morpholine. *J. natl Cancer Inst., 70,* 375–379

Wagner, D.A., Shuker, D.E.G., Hasic, G. & Tannenbaum, S.R. (1982) *Endogenous nitrosoproline synthesis in humans.* In: Magee, P.N., ed., *Nitrosamines and Human Cancer (Banbury Report No. 12),* Cold Spring Harbor, NY, Cold Spring Harbor Laboratory, pp. 319–323

Wagner, D.A., Schultz, D.S., Deen, W.M., Young, V.R. & Tannenbaum, S.R. (1983) Metabolic fate of an oral dose of ^{15}N-labeled nitrate in humans: effect of diet supplementation with ascorbic acid. *Cancer Res., 43,* 1921–1925

EFFECT OF LONG-TERM APPLICATION OF SNUFF AND HERPES SIMPLEX VIRUS 1 ON RAT ORAL MUCOSA. POSSIBLE ASSOCIATION WITH DEVELOPMENT OF ORAL CANCER

J.M. HIRSCH

Department of Oral Surgery, University of Göteborg and Public Dental Service, Göteborg, Sweden

S.L. JOHANSSON

Department of Pathology II, University of Göteborg, Göteborg, Sweden

H. THILANDER

Department of Oral Surgery, University of Göteborg, Sweden

A. VAHLNE

Department of Virology, University of Göteborg, Göteborg, Sweden

SUMMARY

In an animal model, the life-long effects of snuff administration were assessed alone and in combination with infection with herpes simplex virus (HSV-1). It was shown that exposure to standard and alkaline snuff and to HSV-1/snuff induced mild to severe hyperplasia, hyperorthokeratosis, varying degrees of vacuolization and acanthosis in the squamous epithelium, as well as atrophic and ulcerated lesions. Ulcerations and mild dysplasia of the squamous epithelium were seen most frequently in HSV-1/snuff-exposed rats, with moderate dysplasia in the crevicular epithelium.

Rats exposed to snuff or to HSV-1 and snuff had a higher incidence of tumours or tumour-like conditions than control rats. Squamous-cell carcinoma of the oral cavity was found exclusively in rats exposed to snuff or to the combination of HSV-1 and snuff. Papillary squamous hyperplasia of the forestomach was found only in rats exposed to snuff or to HSV-1 and snuff in combination. The incidence of malignant tumours was significantly higher ($p < 0.05$) in the group of rats exposed to snuff and HSV-1/snuff than in control animals.

INTRODUCTION

Snuff contains high concentrations of carcinogenic tobacco-specific nitrosamines which are extracted during snuff dipping (Hoffmann & Adams, 1981). Contradictory opinions exist as to whether or not snuff dipping is a hazardous form of tobacco consumption (Kirkland, 1980;

– 829 –

Russel *et al.*, 1980; Hoffmann & Adams, 1981; Winn *et al.*, 1981); however, recently published data have linked oral cancer with the use of snuff (for review, see Binnie *et al.*, 1983).

Herpes simplex virus 1 (HSV-1) has recently been suggested as an additional etiological factor in the induction of oral carcinomas, although no direct association has been established (for review, see Binnie *et al.*, 1983).

Infection of permissive cells with HSV-1 normally results in replication of the virus and death of the cells. If the virus is rendered non-infectious by ultra-violet irradiation, it may transform cells *in vitro* (Rapp & Shillitoe, 1978). It is therefore of interest that extracts of snuff inhibit the replication of HSV-1 *in vitro* (Hirsch *et al.*, 1984b). The basicity of snuff facilitates the adsorption of both nicotine and *N*-nitrosonornicotine (NNN) through the oral mucosa (Armitage & Turner, 1970). A high pH has also been reported (Bock *et al.*, 1965) to be of significance for the tumour promoting activity of unburned tobacco extracts. An elevation of pH may induce tissue reactions directly, due to caustic effects, or indirectly, due to changes in the quantities of chemical substances present in the snuff (Hoffmann & Adams, 1981).

We have developed an animal model which permits investigation of life-long effects of snuff and other possible interacting factors of an exogenous or endogenous nature (Hirsch & Thilander, 1981). This presentation is a review of our studies of the effects of life-long exposure to snuff and HSV-1 in rats (Hirsch & Johansson, 1983; Hirsch *et al.*, 1983).

MATERIAL AND METHODS

Animals

Three-month-old Sprague-Dawley rats of both sexes (Anticimex AB, Stockholm, Sweden) were used. Cages, bedding material, housing conditions and food have been described in detail by Hirsch and Thilander (1981).

Animal model

Anaesthetized rats were operated on to create a test canal in the lower lip in which snuff could be retained, as described previously (Hirsch & Thilander, 1981).

Virus and inoculation technique

HSV-1 strain F (supplied by Dr B. Roizman, Chicago, IL, USA) was used. The virus was propagated in green monkey kidney AH-1 cells which were infected at a low multiplicity of infection. Aliquots of stock virus were kept at $-70\,°C$. Virus infectivity was assayed by plaquing on cells grown in 5-cm plastic petri dishes and was expressed as plaque-forming units per mL. The rats were anaesthetized intraperitoneally and gently taped on their backs against a table. The virus suspension (0.05 mL, 2.5×10^7 plaque-forming units/mL) was applied topically to the mucous membrane in the inside of the lower lip after scarification with a 26-gauge needle.

Snuff

The brand 'Röda lacket' was used in the experimental studies (kindly supplied fresh by Svenska Tobaks AB, Sweden). In order to assess the effects of exposure to snuff with a raised pH, this brand was made highly alkaline (pH raised from 8.3 to 9.3).

Morphological methods

All rats in the long-term study underwent a complete post-morten examination. Histological examination was performed on the lip, crevicular epithelium, heart, kidneys, adrenal glands, urinary bladder, spleen, stomach, small intestine, large intestine, liver, thyroid gland, lungs and brain and on all other grossly abnormal organs or tissue. All specimens were processed and stained by routine methods (haematoxylin and eosin, Weigert van Gieson).

Experimental design: long-term effect of snuff on rat mucosa and on HSV-1-infected rat mucosa

Rats (n = 100) were operated on to create the test canal in the lower lip. Thirteen of these rats developed suture insufficiency and were not included in the study. The remaining 87 animals were then divided into three test groups and one control group. After scarification in the test canals of the first group (n = 20), virus was applied topically to the mucous membrane. Fresh snuff (pH 8.3) was injected into the test canals of 10 virus-infected rats after 10 days. The scarification and application of virus were repeated after one month in the same animals, after which snuff was injected as before into the test canals after 10 days.

Fresh snuff was injected into the canals of the animals in the second test group (n = 42). The third test group (n = 10) was given highly alkaline snuff (pH = 9.3). Approximately 0.2 g snuff was administered each time at 8:00 hours and at 17:00 hours five days per week. The estimated average length of daily exposure to snuff was 12 h (Hirsch & Thilander, 1981). The 15 control animals underwent the same surgical procedure, but did not receive snuff.

The rats were given snuff for 9 (group II), 12 (group II) and 18–22 (groups I, II, III) months, whereafter they were killed.

Statistical methods

In order to test for differences in incidence of malignant tumours between the four groups of animals, Fisher's exact probability test was used (significance level, 5%).

RESULTS

Long-term effect of snuff on the oral mucosa

One of 42 rats exposed to standard snuff developed a squamous-cell carcinoma of the oral cavity after nine months. This tumour was a moderately well-differentiated squamous-cell carcinoma. In general, however, exposure to standard snuff for 9–12 months resulted in a mild to moderate hyperplasia of the epithelium, hyperorthokeratosis, vacuolated cells and acanthotic proliferations. Focally severe hyperplasia was seen. In the basal layer, hyperplasia with disturbed polarity and hyperchromatic nuclei and occasional mitosis were noted.

Histological changes in rats exposed to standard snuff for 18–22 months differed only slightly from those rats exposed for 9–12 months. The vacuolated cells extended deeper into the strata of the epithelium. The intercellular spaces were somewhat widened, and an altered nuclear cytophasmic ratio was seen in the basal layer. The rats also exhibited hyperplastic lesions and atrophic lesions, and a more prominent fibrosis was noted. Severe dysplasia were observed in the crevicular epithelium of the lower incisors.

The histopathological changes in rats exposed to alkaline snuff for 18–22 months differed little from those described above. The epithelial lining was focally atrophic and ulcerated, and vacuolated calls were less frequent in this group. Further more, a less prominent fibrosis was seen. The lips of some of the control animals showed only mildly hyperplastic epithelium.

Long-term effects of snuff on rat mucosa infected repeatedly with HSV-1

In the group of rats infected twice with HSV-1 and exposed to snuff, two ulcerated tumours were found in the oral cavity after 18 months (Fig. 1). The numbers were not significantly different (p < 0.07). The tumours were moderately well differentiated squamous-cell carcinoma (Fig. 2). Ulcerations and mild dysplasia of the squamous epithelium were seen more frequently in the HSV-1/snuff-exposed rats than in rats exposed to snuff alone. Among the HSV-1/snuff-exposed rats, moderate dysplasia was also more frequent in the crevicular epithelium than in the other groups of animals.

No significant epithelial change was registered in rats infected with HSV-1 only.

Morphological lesions outside the oral cavity

Follicular tumours of the thyroid gland and fiibroadenomas of the mammary gland were seen frequently in both test and control rats. Marked papillary squamous hyperplasia of the forestomach was detected in 30% of the rats exposed to snuff alone for 18–22 months and in 28% exposed to HSV-1/snuff (Fig. 3), but no macroscopic forestomach tumour was detected. A moderately well-differentiated squamous-cell carcinoma of the anus developed in one rat exposed to snuff only; another rat in the same group developed a poorly differentiated retroperitoneal sarcoma. The number of malignant tumours in rats exposed to snuff only and in rats exposed to HSV-1/snuff was significantly higher (p < 0.05) than that in the control rats (rats not exposed and rats infected with HSV-1 only).

Fig. 1. Gross appearance of a squamous-cell carcinoma of the oral cavity involving the lower jaw. The rat had been exposed to herpes simplex virus-1 and snuff for 18 months.

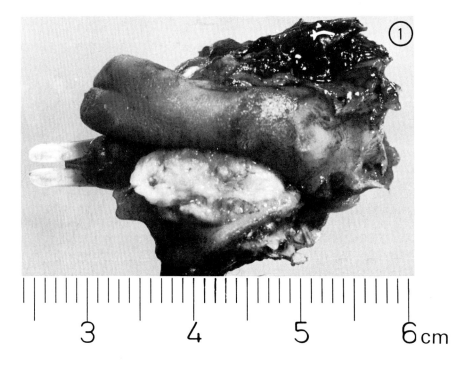

Fig. 2. Light micrograph of the same tumour as in Fig. 1, a moderately well-differentiated squamous-cell carcinoma invading bone. Haematoxylin and eosin x 74

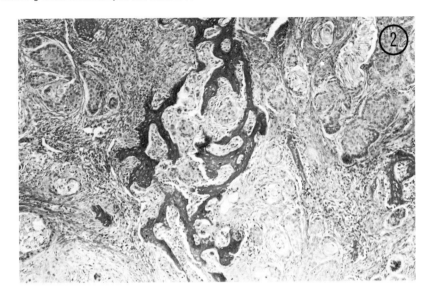

Fig. 3. Marked squamous-cell hyperplasia of the forestomach after 22 months of exposure to snuff. The epithelium displays moderate atypia. Haematoxylin and eosin x 74. Reprinted with permission from Munksgaard, International Publishers Ltd

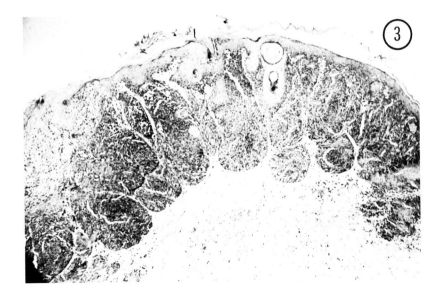

DISCUSSION

In general, the test canal of animals exposed to snuff exhibited a higher frequency of hyperorthokeratotic, atrophic and ulcerated, mildly dysplastic and fibrotic lesions compared with those of control rats. The tissue damage may be related to the high pH of snuff, as has been suggested earlier (Roed-Petersen & Pindborg, 1973). It has also been reported (Sunanda *et al.*, 1975) that rats painted with tobacco and slaked lime developed more marked histopathological changes than rats painted with tobacco solution only. However, the occurrence of vacuolated cells in the present study was lower than that seen in humans and in experimental studies (Hirsch & Johansson, 1983). A particularly low incidence was seen in the group of rats exposed to alkaline snuff (pH 9.3). Vacuolization might be a rapid reaction to snuff, ascribed to the greater dose per kg body weight given to the animals, when compared to that consumed by humans; it was later replaced by atrophic, ulcerated and/or slight dysplastic tissue changes.

The test group that had been exposed to both HSV-1 and snuff exhibited the most pronounced histopathological changes: ulcerated and dysplastic lesions were more frequent in this group than in others.

Squamous-cell carcinomas of the oral cavity developed in three animals in these investigations. These tumours were probably induced by snuff and HSV-1/snuff, since it appears that spontaneous tumours of the oral mucosa are extremely rare (for review, see Hirsch & Johansson, 1983). Earlier bioassays *in vivo* for carcinogenicity of different types of snuff implantations have been negative (for review, see Hirsch & Thilander, 1981). In the present study, rats exposed to snuff only (n = 52) or in combination with HSV-1 (n = 10) had 99 tumours or tumour-like conditions (99/62). Rats exposed to HSV-1 only (n = 10) and control animals (n = 15) exhibited 36 neoplastic lesions (36/25). If follicular tumours of the thyroid gland and fibroadenomous of the mammary gland – found in both test and control animals – were disregarded, the snuff- and HSV-1/snuff-exposed rats had 31 tumours or tumour-like conditions (31/62), which should be compared with only two lesions found in HSV-1-infected and controls rats (2/25). Malignant tumours developed only among rats exposed to snuff or to snuff in combinations with HSV-1 infection. These data support the hypothesis that snuff alone or in combination with HSV-1 can be tumorgenic.

Papillary squamous hyperplasia of the forestomach was found after long exposure to snuff or HSV-1/snuff (18–22 months). It is reasonable to assume that these alterations were caused by snuff – possibly by its content of tobacco-specific nitrosamines (TSNA) or other snuff derivatives in saliva swallowed by the rats.

Although there have been no animal experiments that have demonstrated a direct carcinogenic effect of infectious HSV-1 *in vivo,* cocarcinogenic potential has been shown (Southam *et al.*, 1969; Burns & Murray, 1981). Development of squamous-cell carcinomas in mouse lips has recently been reported after HSV-2 infection in combination with exposure to ultra-violet radiation and applications of a tumour promoter (12-0-tetradeca-noylphorbolacetate; Burns & Murray, 1981). Both HSV-1 and HSV-2 can cause cell transformation *in vitro* if virus-induced cell lysis is prevented (for review, see Rapp, 1980). The finding that herpes simplex virus replication is inhibited by tobacco extracts (Hirsch *et al.*, 1984b) is interesting in the light of earlier data concerning cell transformation and tumour induction.

Thus, aqueous extracts of snuff were found to inhibit the replication of HSV-1 *in vitro* in cultured cells in a dose-dependent fashion. Nicotine in non-toxic concentrations was found to contribute to the overall HSV-1 restriction observed with snuff extracts, while ingredients used for blending of different brands seemed to have little or no influence on HSV-1 replication.

TSNA in snuff have attracted much interest due to their carcinogenic potential (Hoffmann *et al.*, 1975). We found a significantly greater reduction of HSV-1 replication with snuff extracts containing high levels of TSNA (Hirsch *et al.*, 1984b). Similar restricting effects on HSV-1 have been reported earlier for two other nitrosamines (Roane, 1978).

The results indicate a relation between exposure to the combination of HSV-1 and snuff and the development of squamous-cell carcinoma. Of the adult population, 80-90% have had primary infections with HSV-1, and recurrence of lesions is experienced by approximately 40% (Ship *et al.*, 1960). It is proposed that HSV-1 shed in the oral cavity can become inactivated by snuff or snuff derivatives such as TSNA. The virus may then act as an initiator and snuff as a promoter in the induction of malignant neoplasms of the oral cavity.

ACKNOWLEDGEMENTS

These investigations were supported by grants from the Faculty of Odontology, University of Göteborg, The Swedish Dental Association, The Medical Research Council, grant No. 4514 and the Swedish Cancer Society, Project No. 1657-B83-03X.

REFERENCES

Armitage, A.K. & Turner, D.M. (1970) Absorption of nicotine in cigarette smoke through the oral mucosa. *Nature, 226*, 1231–1232

Binnie, W.H., Rankin, K.V. & Mackenzie, I.C. (1983) Etiology of oral squamous cell carcinoma. *J. oral Pathol., 12*, 11–29

Bock, F.G., Shamberger, R.J. & Myers, H.K. (1965) Tumour-promoting agents in unburned cigarette tobacco. *Nature, 208*, 584–585

Burns, J.C. & Murray, B.K. (1981) Conversion of herpetic lesions to malignancy by ultraviolet exposure and promoter application. *J. gen. Virol., 55*, 305–313

Hirsch, J.M. & Johansson, S.L. (1983) Effect of long-term application of snuff on the oral mucosa – an experimental study in the rat. *J. oral Pathol., 12*, 187–198

Hirsch, J.M. & Thilander, H. (1981) Snuff-induced lesions of the oral mucosa – an experimental model in the rat. *J. oral Pathol., 10*, 342–353

Hirsch, J.M., Johansson, S.L. & Vahlne, A. (1984a) Effect of snuff and herpes simplex virus 1 on rat oral mucosa. Possible association with development of squamous cell carcinoma. *J. oral. Pathol., 13*, 52–62

Hirsch, J.M., Svennerholm, B. & Vahlne, A. (1984b) Inhibition of herpes simplex virus replication by tobacco extracts. *Cancer Res., 44*, 1991–1997

Hoffmann, D. & Adams, J.D. (1981) Carcinogenic tobacco-specific *N*-nitrosamines in snuff and in the saliva of snuff dippers. *Cancer Res., 41*, 4305–4308

Hoffmann, D., Raineri, R., Hecht, S.S., Muronpot, R. & Wynder, E.L. (1975). A study of tobacco carcinogenesis. XIV. Effects of *N'*-nitrosonornicotine and *N'*-nitrosanabasine on rats. *J. natl Cancer Inst., 55*, 977–981

Kirkland, L.R. (1980) The non-smoking uses of tobacco. *New Engl. J. Med., 303*, 165

Rapp, F. (1980) *Transformation by herpes simplex viruses*. In: Essex, M., Toduro, G. & zur Hansen, H. eds, *Viruses in Naturally Occurring Cancers (Cold Spring Harbor Conferences on Cell Proliferation, Vol. 7)*, Cold Spring Harbor, NY, Cold Spring Harbor Laboratories, pp. 63–80

Rapp, F. & Shillitoe, E.J. (1978) *Transformation of non-lymphoid cells by herpes viruses; A review*. In: de Thé, G., Rapp, F. & Henle, W., eds, *Oncogenesis and Herpes Viruses III (IARC Scientific Publications No. 24)*, Lyon, International Agency for Research on Cancer, pp. 431–450

Roane, P.R. (1978) *Inhibition of the multiplication of herpes simplex virus by aliphatic nitrosamines*. In: de Thé, G., Rapp, F. & Henle W., eds, *Oncogenesis and Herpes Viruses III (IARC Scientific Publications No. 24)*, Lyon, International Agency for Research on Cancer, pp. 1013–1018

Roed-Petersen, B. & Pindborg, J.J. (1973) A study of Danish snuff induced oral leukoplakias. *J. oral Pathol., 2*, 301–313

Russel, M.A.H., Jarvis, M.J. & Feyerabend, C. (1980) A new age for snuff? *Lancet, i,* 474–475

Ship, I.I., Morris, A.W., Durocher, R.T. & Burkat, L.W. (1960) Recurrent aphthous ulcerations and recurrent herpes labialis in a professional school student population. I. Experience. *Oral Surg., 13,* 1191–1202

Southam, C.M., Tanaka, S., Arata, T., Simkovic, D., Miura, M. & Petropulos, S.F. (1969) Enhancement of responses to chemical carcinogens by non-oncogenic viruses and antimetabolites. *Prog. exp. Tumor Res., 11,* 194–212

Sunanda, V., Gothoskar, S.V., Sant, S.M. & Randive, K.J. (1975) Effect of tobacco and lime on oral mucosa of rats fed on vitamin B-deficient diet. *Indian J. Cancer, 12,* 424–429

Winn, D.M., Blot, W.J., Shy, C.M., Pickle, L.W., Toledo, M.A. & Fraumeni, J.F., Jr (1981) Snuff dipping and oral cancer among women in the Southern United States. *New Engl. J. Med., 304,* 745–749

TOBACCO CHEWING AND SNUFF DIPPING:
AN ASSOCIATION WITH HUMAN CANCER

D.M. WINN

Environmental Epidemiology Branch, Division of Cancer Cause and Prevention, National Cancer Institute, Bethesda, MD 20205, USA

INTRODUCTION

The use of tobacco originated with Central American Indians, who introduced their tobacco habits to European explorers visiting the New World. One of the habits adopted by the Europeans was the taking of snuff, or powdered tobacco, nasally. Snuff inhalation became an important social custom in Europe and was also considered to have medicinal value (Christen *et al.,* 1982). While intra-nasal application was the early method of snuff use and is still applied in that fashion by some Britons (Harrison, 1964), today in the USA snuff is taken almost exclusively by mouth. Snuff-dipping is the oral use of finely cut, ground or powdered tobacco. A pinch of the tobacco is placed between the cheek and gum or lip and gum and retained there; no chewing is involved. There are four different types of snuff: moist snuff or 'snoose', dry snuff or 'Scotch' snuff, finely-cut chewing tobacco (which is not chewed but left stationary in the mouth), and semi-moist.

Tobacco chewing also apparently originated with New World Indians who took it with lime (Tobacco Institute, 1959). It was uncommon until about 1830 when the habit became enormously popular throughout the USA (Tobacco Institute, 1959). Tobacco chews are sold in many forms, but the most commonly used are densely packed plugs and loosely packed pouches; both types are retained in the mouth and chewed. Although the popularity of both snuff and chewing tobacco declined during the early part of the twentieth century (Christen *et al.,* 1982), the two habits have recently enjoyed an enormous resurgence in popularity.

This review examines the epidemiological evidence linking the use of smokeless tobacco to the risk of cancer, especially of the oral cavity. The emphasis is on literature from studies of US populations, although reference is made to tobacco chewing habits in Europe and Asia and to the biological mechanisms linking smokeless tobacco use with cancer occurrence. A full discussion of the putative carcinogens recently identified in snuff and chewing tobaccos – *N*-nitrosonornicotine and other nitrosamines – is presented by Dr Hoffmann and others in these proceedings.

ORAL CANCER

The use of tobacco in an unsmoked form was linked to oral cavity cancer as early as 1915 in New York, when Abbe (1915) reported a case of cancer of the cheek occurring in a chronic snuff dipper. Later, several investigators in the southeastern USA noted a high frequency of smokeless tobacco users among oral cancer patients (Landy & White, 1961; Leffall & White, 1965). For example, in one series of oral cancer patients in an Atlanta, Georgia, hospital, 23 of the 44 women in the series had used snuff, and 12 of the 37 men had used snuff or chewing tobacco (Wilkins & Yogler, 1957).

Early case-control studies often made no distinction between snuff and chewing tobacco, but grouped both forms of smokeless tobacco into one category. Anecdotal information would indicate that, among women, unspecified smokeless tobacco use would probably be snuff. Two of the studies (Moore et al., 1953; Vincent & Marchetta, 1963) found that a much higher percentage of male cases used smokeless tobacco than did controls. Only one of the studies included females, few of whom were users of smokeless tobacco. Cigarette smoking habits were known for members of the study populations and were reported; however, since cross-tabulations of smoking habits and smokeless tobacco use were not included, the independent effect of smokeless tobacco could not be assessed. A survey of patients in North Carolina with oral cavity cancer and of matched controls also revealed a relationship between smokeless tobacco and oral cancer, although no data were provided on smoking habits (Peacock et al., 1960); 56% of the cases had used snuff or chewing tobacco for 20 years or more, compared with 33% of the in-patient controls and 43% of the out-patient controls.

In evaluating smokeless tobacco risks, the distribution of smoking habits must be taken into account, since it is known that cancers of the oral cavity are strongly associated with smoking of cigarettes, cigars and pipes. In large cohort studies, it was found that cigarette smokers, and also pipe and cigar smokers, have 1.2–14 times greater risks than non-smokers of developing oral and/or pharyngeal cancer (Office of Smoking & Health, 1982).

Although the third National Cancer Survey Patient Interview Study also grouped all forms of smokeless tobacco, cigarette smoking, alcohol use and other factors were controlled for (Williams & Horm, 1977). In males, a relative risk for oral cancer of 3.9 was associated with moderate use and of 6.7 with heavy use of smokeless tobacco, when age, race and smoking habits were controlled for. No female case was a heavy user, but moderate use of unsmoked tobacco was associated with a five-fold increased risk. Although men and women have different consumption patterns and preferences for particular forms of smokeless tobacco (which was not addressed in these studies), the associations observed between oral cancer and smokeless tobacco use did not appear to be sex-specific.

Snuff

Most studies evaluating the hazards of snuff dipping have been conducted in southern USA. In Atlanta (Vogler et al., 1962), snuff was found to be strongly associated with cancers of the oral cavity, pharynx and larynx. Among female urban subjects, 40% of cases used snuff, compared with 2%, 3% and 1% of the control groups: other mouth diseases, other cancers, other diseases. Similar findings were observed for rural females: snuff dipping was reported in 75% of cases and in less than 20% of the control groups. The differences between cases and controls were significant for most of the age strata studied. The authors provided no cross-tabulation of smokeless and smokeless tobacco but stated that most of the non-smoking women dipped snuff.

A second case-control study, of 55 female patients with buccal mucosa and gum cancers and 55 control females was conducted in Arkansas (Westbrook et al., 1980): 91% of cases had a history of snuff use in contrast to 2% of controls. Only 5% of cases smoked, and no difference was reported in smoking, alcohol consumption or oral problems between the two groups. Data on smokeless tobacco habits were probably obtained from medical records, since the study period spanned 20 years. The absence of a notation concerning tobacco use may have been less common in the cases than in the controls, who had conditions though to be unrelated to use of smokeless tobacco. This misclassification bias would tend to exaggerate any estimate of the association between smokeless tobacco use and oral cancer.

Variations in risk for cancers at different sites within the oral cavity were examined in studies in which different groups of oral cancer patients were compared. Since the 'controls' used by Rosenfeld and Callaway (1963) consisted of women with cancer of the tongue and floor of the mouth, risks for these sites cannot be evaluated. However, 90% of the 'cases' (women with buccal mucosa or gingival cancer) dipped snuff, compared with 22% of patients with other mouth cancers. Smoking habits were not mentioned. Similarly, in two separate studies in Atlanta hospitals, it was found that patients with cancers of the buccal mucosa (Vogler *et al.*,

Fig. 1. Cancer mortality, 1950–1969, in US white females from cancers of the oral cavity and pharynx (excluding nasopharynx) by state-economic area

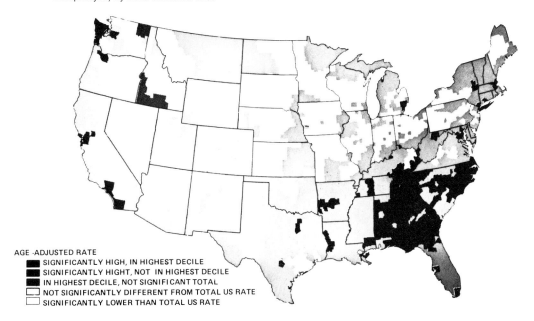

AGE -ADJUSTED RATE
- ■ SIGNIFICANTLY HIGH, IN HIGHEST DECILE
- ■ SIGNIFICANTLY HIGHT, NOT IN HIGHEST DECILE
- ■ IN HIGHEST DECILE, NOT SIGNIFICANT TOTAL
- ☐ NOT SIGNIFICANTLY DIFFERENT FROM TOTAL US RATE
- ☐ SIGNIFICANTLY LOWER THAN TOTAL US RATE

Table 1. Relative risks of oral and pharyngeal cancer associated with tobacco smoking and snuff dipping according to race[a]

Race	Smoker	Dipper	No. of cases	No. of controls	Relative risk	95% confidence interval
White	No	No	36	153	1.0	–
		Yes	79	80	4.2	2.6–6.7
	Yes	No	70	101	2.9	1.8–4.7
		Yes	11	14	3.3	1.4–7.8
Black	No	No	5	16	1.0	–
		Yes	12	25	1.5	0.5–4.8
	Yes	No	14	16	2.6	0.8–8.7
		Yes	5	5	3.0	0.7–13.8

[a]From Winn *et al.* (1981b)

Table 2. Relative risks of cancer of the gum and buccal mucosa and of the pharynx and other parts of the mouth according to duration of snuff use in nonsmokers from a hospital sample[a, b]

Site of cancer	Snuff use[c] (years)	No. of cases	No. of controls	Relative risk	95% confidence interval
Gum and	0	2	34	1.0	–
buccal mucosa	1–24	3	3	13.8	1.9–98.0
	25–49	10	11	12.6	2.7–58.3
	>50	15	4	47.5	9.1–249.5
Other mouth	0	22	61	1.0	–
and pharynx	1–24	3	5	1.7	0.4–7.2
	25–49	14	10	3.8	1.5–9.6
	>50	8	18	1.3	0.5–3.2

[a] Excludes one person who did not consent to use of medical records and 19 controls whose matched cases were not interviewed
[b] From Winn et al. (1981b)
[c] The mean value for the study sample of 45 years was used for the 7.7% of snuff dippers for whom the number of years of use was unknown

1962) or alveolar ridge (Brown et al., 1965) were more likely to be snuff dippers than those with cancers elsewhere in the oral cavity. The tendency for oral cancers to develop in smokeless tobacco users at a site close to where the wad is usually kept (between the gum and the cheek of the lip) was also pointed out in several case reports (Friedell & Rosenthal, 1941; Landy & White, 1961).

These studies provided evidence of an association between use of smokeless tobacco and oral cavity cancer, especially of the buccal mucosa and gum. However, the absence of adequate control for smoking habits in most of these studies hindered interpretation.

Our studies at the National Cancer Institute were inspired by cancer maps which indicated that oral cavity mortality rates for white females are excessively high in southern USA (Fig. 1) (Mason et al., 1975; Blot & Fraumeni, 1977). In collaboration with the University of North Carolina, we initiated a case-control study of cancers of the oral cavity and pharynx among female residents of North Carolina (Winn et al., 1981a). The 210 cases ascertained at five North Carolina hospitals or through death certificates from the state vital statistics office were matched on age, race and place of residence to two controls selected from the same source as the case. The women themselves or their next-of-kin were interviewed in their homes about tobacco and alcohol use and other pertinent characteristics.

As shown in Table 1, the use of snuff was associated with a four-fold increased risk of oral and pharyngeal cancer, independently of smoking, among the whites in the sample. The risks were somewhat lower for black women; interestingly, oral cancer rates for black women are high in a few scattered areas in Southern USA. Cigarette smoking was also strongly related to oral cancer in this study, while alcohol use increased risk only in conjunction with smoking. Thirty-five of the women were tobacco chewers; however, all but three of the 35 were also snuff dippers.

Patients with cancer of the gum or buccal mucosa were examined separately; the relative risk increased markedly to almost 50-fold for those who had dipped snuff for 50 years or more (Table 2). Elevated risks were also evidence for cases with other mouth or pharyngeal cancers, although no dose-response trend was evident. The enormous risks observed for buccal mucosa and gum cancer, coupled with clear dose-response relationship, and evidence that snuff is related to cancer of the oral cavity independently of smoking provide strong evidence that snuff dipping causes oral cancer.

Virtually, all of the snuff used in our study was of the 'dry' type. In studies carried out in the USA, the type of snuff used has generally not been speciefid. However, the use of moist snuff has been popular in Scandinavia, where it has been linked to an increased risk of oral cancer (Axell *et al.*, 1978).

Chewing tobacco

The evidence for the carcinogenicity to humans of tobacco chewing, a habit generally restricted to males, is less compelling. Oral cancer mortality rates in males are actualy higher in the northern part of the USA (Mason *et al.*, 1975), presumably due to greater smoking and alcohol consumption, two major risk factors for oral cancer. Because most forms of chewing tobacco are in fact chewed, the physical contact between the tobacco and the oral mucosa may not be maintained as intensely as for snuff, which is usually retained in one spot; the proximity of tissues to the tobacco may be a factor of some significance.

Several epidemiological studies have revealed associations between tobacco chewing and oral cancer. A case-control study in Atlanta, Georgia, USA indicated that among both rural and urban men, the chewing of tobacco was more frequent among oral cancer cases than in the three control groups (Vogler *et al.*, 1962). Although the authors did note that most of the non-smoking men used chewing tobacco, smoking was not controlled for in the analysis, so it cannot be readily determined whether the smoking habits of the men accounted for the association with smokeless tobacco. Another series from the same hospital at a different time period also indicated that men with buccal mucosa or gum cancer were more likely to chew tobacco than men with cancer in other oral sites; but this study did not mention the smoking habits of the subjects (Brown *et al.*, 1965).

In a study of oral cancer patients in New York (Wynder *et al.*, 1957), 17% of cases but only 8% of controls chewed tobacco. However, all but one of the individuals wo used chewing tobacco also smoked, complicating an assessment of the independent effect of each of the two habits.

When it has been possible to examine the independent contributions of chewing tobacco use and smoking, the evidence has been conflicting. Martinez (1969) studied all cases of oral, pharyngeal and oesophageal cancer in Puerto Rico during a one-year period and neighbourhood controls. For each of the three cancer sites, the proportion of male cases who chewed tobacco but did not smoke was greater than the proportion of controls who were non-smoking chewers. The odds ratio for oral cancer was 12, computed on the basis of reported numbers of men with no tobacco habits and on those who only chewed tobacco. Few women with oral cavity or pharyngeal cancer chewed tobacco.

In contrast, a case-control study in New York failed to find an association between tobacco chewing and oral cavity cancer (Wynder & Stellman, 1977). In the UK, oral cancer cases identified through a cancer registry were less likely than matched controls to have used chewing tobacco, but it was not clear how many cases and controls did not use any form of tobacco (Browne *et al.*, 1977).

Characteristics of oral cancers in smokeless tobacco users

Multiple primary cancers in the oral cavity are common (Berg *et al.*, 1970; Tepperman & Fitzpatrick, 1981). In two studies in Atlanta, patients with multiple oral and pharyngeal cancers (Brown *et al.*, 1965) or with oral, pharyngeal and laryngeal cancers (Vogler *et al.*, 1962) were more likely to have reported multiple use of snuff than were patients with cancer at only one of those sites. In one of the two studies, tobacco chewing was also found to be more frequent in the group with multiple primary tumours (Brown *et al.*, 1965).

There are some key differences in the characteristics of oral carcinomas occurring in snuff-dippers and those in non-dippers. Cancers occurring in users of snuff are associated more frequently with the presence of leucoplakia (Brown *et al.*, 1965), are less likely to metastasize (Landy & White, 1961; Brown *et al.*, 1965) but more likely to be followed by a second primary tumour (Brown *et al.*, 1965), to be more highly differentiated (Landy & White, 1961; Vogler *et al.*, 1962) and to have a better prognosis (Brown *et al.*, 1965) than oral cancers not related to snuff use.

In the oral cavity, squamous-cell carcinomas predominate (National Cancer Institute, 1981), although a subtype, verrucous carcinoma, has been linked to chewing and dipping habits in several case reports (Sorger & Myrden, 1960; Stecker *et al.*, 1964; Kraus & Perez-Mesa, 1966; Fonts *et al.*, 1969). In another report, snuff-dipping cases were found to be more likely than cases with no tobacco habits or with other tobacco habits to have verrucous lesions (Hartselle, 1977).

Since oral cancer is rare, it is not surprising that a prevalence survey of 15 500 snuff-using patients in Tennesse yielded fewer than 2000 patients with any mucosal abnormality, and only two malignancies (Smith *et al.*, 1970). In several studies of snuff-related cancers, the duration of use has averaged more than 40 years, and most of the cases are elderly (Westbrook *et al.*, 1980; Winn *et al.*, 1981a).

OTHER CANCERS

Digestive and respiratory tract cancers have also been linked to smokeless tobacco use, but the evidence is inconclusive. In our case-control study of women in North Carolina, the cases with pharyngeal cancer or cancer at sites in the mouth not close to the tobacco quid were more likely to dip than controls (Winn *et al.*, 1981a). Another study found that, while the percentage of snuff users was highest among cases with oral cavity cancers, people with pharyngeal and laryngeal cancer were also more likely to use snuff than controls (Vincent & Marchetta, 1963). However, the association with laryngeal cancer was not confirmed in a case-control study of patients in New York City (Wynder & Stellman, 1977). Cancers of the nasal cavity and paranasal sinuses were linked to the *oral* use of snuff (but not chewing tobacco) in a recent case-control study (Brinton *et al.*, personal communication); a high relative frequency of cancers of the maxillary sinus has also been reported in Bantus, some of whom *inhale* tobacco powder mixed with plant ash (Shapiro *et al.*, 1955).

While digestive-tract cancer seems to occur more frequently in smokeless tobacco users than in those with no tobacco habits (Winn *et al.*, 1982), oesophageal cancer is one of the few sites that has been examined in any detail. The Puerto Rican study (Martinez, 1969) found positive associations between oesophageal cancer and chewing tobacco in both men and women. Wynder and Bross (1961) also found a positive history of tobacco chewing in 20% of oesophageal cancer cases compared with 10% of controls. However all chewers also smoked. Oesophageal cancer death rates for men are not usually high in most of south-eastern USA; however, there are several areas in the south-east where oesophageal cancer death rates as well as oral cancer rates for women are excessively high (Mason *et al.*, 1975).

Correlations have been observed between smokeless tobacco use and cancers outside of the upper respiratory and upper digestive tracts, but the data are inconclusive. Williams and Horm (1977) conducted a large case-control study of cancer based on interview responses of a random sample of patients from the Third National Cancer Survey. Some of their findings are summarized in Table 3. In addition to the substantial risks reported for gum-mouth cancer, smokeless tobacco use was associated among women with cervical cancer. The odds ratio, controlled for smoking, age and race, was 4.7 for moderate smokeless tobacco use and

Table 3. Associations of cancer with smokeless tobacco use, in the Third
National Cancer Survey Patient Interview study, 1969–1971[a, b]

Cancer site	Relative risks for low and high smokeless tobacco use controlled for age, race and smoking habits			
	Males		Females	
	Low	High	Low	High
Gum-mouth	3.9***	6.7	4.9	–
Larynx	1.8	2.6	–	–
Bladder	1.6	1.8	–	2.4
Other lymphoma	0.7	3.6	–	–
Stomach	1.0	1.7	–	1.1
Colon	1.1	1.7	0.3	1.7
Testis	5.0	–	–	–
Cervix	–	–	4.7*	3.6
Uterine corpus	–	–	3.1	0.7
Multiple myeloma	0.3	1.8	2.2	–

[a] Referent population: patients with cancers at sites known previously to be
not strongly related to smoking and alcohol use
[b] Adapted from Williams and Horm (1977)
* p <0.05
*** p <0.001

statistically significant. For several other anatomical sites, suggestive but not statistically significant associations were observed. It should be noted that multiple comparisons were made, and it might be expected that some positive findings would occur by chance alone. These findings should be regarded as hypothesis-generating, since alternative explanations for the findings are possible. Although one study (Williams & Horm, 1977) found suggestive relationship between chewing and bladder cancer, other studies of bladder cancer have shown no relationship to smokeless tobacco use (Wynder & Stellman, 1977; Hartge et al., personal communication).

SMOKELESS TOBACCO HABITS IN ASIA

Some of the highest incidence rates of oral cancer are found in India (Waterhouse et al., 1976). The custom of chewing quids, called 'pan', composed of combinations of betel leaf (Piper betel), betel nut (Areca catechu), slaked lime, tobacco and other ingredients, has long been linked to the excessive oral cancer rates observed in India as well as in New Guinea (Atkinson et al., 1964), Ceylon (Hirayama, 1966) and other Asian or Pacific Island countries where these habits are common. Case-control studies (Hirayama, 1966; Wahi, 1968) have established a clear link between the chewing of pan and oral and pharyngeal cancer. However there is continuing controversy over which components of the quid have carcinogenic properties; the betel nut, leaf and tobacco ingredients have all been implicated. It has also been suggested that the addition of lime may increase the alkalinity in the oral cavity and thereby promote the formation of carcinogenic superoxides (Stich & Rosin, 1983). A high frequency of oral cancer in groups which rarely or never add tobacco to the quid (Atkinson et al., 1964; Schonland & Bradshaw, 1969) indicates that other quid ingredients may confer a carcinogenic risk. Although smoking was not taken into account, Jussawalla and Deshpande (1971) found elevated cancer risks for the upper respiratory and upper digestive tracts in Indians who did not include tobacco in the quid as well as those who did. However, a recent critical review of studies of betel quid chewing, with and without tobacco, adds substantial evidence that, without the tobacco the quids may be only very weakly carcinogenic, implying either that tobacco is the active agent or that the combination of ingredients is needed to produce oral cancer (Gupta *et al.*, 1982). It is difficult to correlate the Asian experience with smokeless tobacco habits practised in the USA, however, because, as Muir and Kirk (1960) point out, in India tobacco is rarely chewed without other ingredients.

'Nass', used in certain Central Asian Soviet republics, has also been linked to oral cancer, especially at sites near that where the mixture is placed (Bronstein & Saparov, 1975). Although the chief components generally include tobacco, lime, ashes and oil or water, regional variations exist. An ecological study showed that the proportion of lime in the mixture may be critical (Paches & Milievskaya, 1980). A case-control study of oesophageal cancer in Iran found no evidence that use of *nass* was related to this cancer (Cook-Mozaffari *et al.*, 1979), although it has been suggested that *nass* contributes to oesophageal cancer risk in Russia (Kolicheva, 1980).

INTERACTIONS OF SMOKELESS TOBACCO WITH OTHER FACTORS

There is some evidence to suggest that other exposures may modify the risk of cancer attributable to smokeless tobacco. One Indian case-control study of oral cancer found that smoking, chewing and both habits were related to oral cancer only among non-consumers of eggs, fish and meat (Notani & Sanghvi, 1976). These findings suggest that dietary factors may influence the carcinogenic process. Another report of oral cavity, pharyngeal, laryngeal and oesophageal cancer from India indicates that smoking and chewing act synergistically (Jayant *et al.*, 1977); risks for those with both habits far exceed those expected on the basis of each habit separately. No synergy between smoking and snuff dipping was evident in our study of women in North Carolina (Winn *et al.*, 1981a), probably because the small number of women with both habits smoked fewer cigarettes and dipped for a shorter period of time than those with only one habit. However, we did find that risks for denture wearing evident only in dippers (Winn *et al.*, 1981b), and that the relationship between use of mouthwash and oral cancer varied by tobacco habit (Blot *et al.*, 1983).

PREMALIGNANT CONDITIONS

Leucoplakia, a white patch on the mucosa which cannot be scraped off (WHO, 1978), is more common in smokeless tobacco users than in persons who do not have the habit (Peacock *et al.*, 1960). Although the term has generally used as no histological connotation (WHO, 1978), several investigators have observed that leucoplakia is commonly present in people with cancer of the oral cavity (Wilkins & Vogler, 1957; Landy & White, 1961; Brown *et al.*, 1965), and the incidence of oral cancer is higher in people with leucoplakia than in people without these white patches (Mallaowalla *et al.*, 1976; Silverman *et al.*, 1976; Einhorn & Wersall, 1967).

CARCINOGENESIS

In the past, researchers had been unsuccessful in inducing oral tumors in laboratory animals by exposing them to snuff and chewing tobacco (Peacock & Brawley, 1959; Peacock *et al.*, 1960; Homburger, 1971; Homburger *et al.*, 1976). As reported elsewhere in these proceedings,

N-nitrosonornicotine and other nitrosamines have recently been identified in snuff and finely-cut chewing tobacco at levels that far exceed that in tobaccos used for other purposes (Hecht *et al.*, 1978). Variations in the amount of N-nitrosonornicotine appear to be related to the curing and fermentation process (Hecht *et al.*, 1975) and storage methods (Hoffmann & Adams, 1981). These nitrosamines have carcinogenic activity in laboratory animals (Hoffmann *et al.*, 1975; Hilfrich *et al.*, 1977; Hecht *et al.*, 1980). N-Nitrosonornicotine can be detected in saliva from snuff dippers (Hoffmann & Adams, 1981), and the yield of nitrosamines in snuff can be increased by incubation with human saliva (Hecht *et al.*, 1975).

FUTURE DIRECTIONS

The use of smokeless tobacco in the USA has become extremely popular among the young. US per-capita use of snuff is estimated to be 0.25 lbs (113 g) per year; whereas an average of 1.09 lbs (494 g) of chewing tobacco is consumed annually by US men (Economic Research Service, 1983). According to a national survey conducted in 1975, 6 % of men had dipped snuff regularly at some time in their lives, while 21% of men were regular tobacco chewers; only 2% of women had either habit (Public Health Service, 1976). In 1982, an estimated 90 million lbs (41 million kg) of chewing tobacco were produced in the US, almost exclusively for domestic use, 81% of which was loose-leaf chewing tobacco. An estimated 33.5 million lbs (15 million kg) of moist snuff and 10.3 million lbs (4.7 million kg) of dry snuff were manufactured in 1982 (Economic Research Service, 1983). As shown in Figure 2, chewing tobacco consumption has risen dramatically since the 1960s. In the graph, finely-cut chews used as snuff are included under chewing tobacco.

Fig. 2. Consumption of tobacco products in the USA in 1982, per male 18 years and over, except for cigarettes (per person 18 years and over). From Economic Research Service (1982)

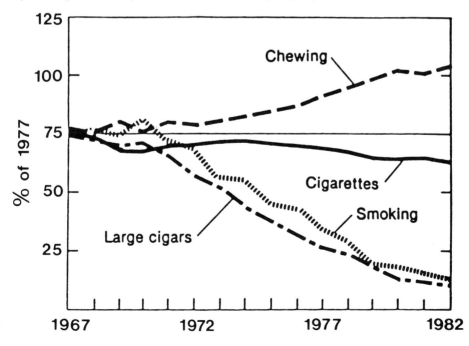

A flurry of editorials have been written in major medical journals, both in favour of the use of snuff and chewing tobacco, especially as a smoking substitute (Kirkland, 1980; Russell *et al.*, 1980), and also against its use (Christen, 1980; Goldsmith & Winn, 1980). The use of popular sports figures in smokeless tobacco advertisements has provided further encouragement to young people. While oral cancer associated with smokeless tobacco has a long latent period, the use of these products by young persons who could accumulate decades of exposure should be actively discouraged.

The evidence that the use of snuff is a cause of cancer of the oral cavity, especially of the buccal mucosa and gums, is convincing. Although the carcinogenicity of chews which include tobacco as only one component is firmly established, more research is needed clarify the risks of oral cancer related to tobacco chewing in US and other populations. As yet, little evidence exists regarding the effects of smokeless tobacco on anatomical sites outside the oral cavity, although preliminary evidence suggests that smokeless tobacco use may increase risks for oesophageal cancer. It will also be important to examine the effect of factors such as smoking, alcohol and diet, which may modify the risk of cancer from smokeless tobacco, and to determine whether cessation of the habit is associated with a reduced risk of cancer. Screening activities and the development of oral self-examination programme in high-risk populations should be pursued.

As indicated by the fruitful direction of research on *N*-nitroso compounds in smokeless tobacco our understanding of carcinogenic mechanisms will advance with continued communication between laboratory scientists and epidemiologists, and with multidisciplinary investigations combining experimental and epidemiological approaches.

ACKNOWLEDGEMENTS

I wish to thank Dr William J. Blot and Dr Joseph F. Fraumeni, Jr, of the Environmental Epidemiology Branch of the National Cancer Institute for their insightful comments.

REFERENCES

Abbe, R. (1915) Cancer of the mouth: The case against tobacco. *N.Y. med J., 102*, 1–2

Atkinson, L., Chester I.C., Smyth, F.G. & ten Seldam, R.E. (1964) Oral cancer in New Guinea: A study in demography and etiology. *Cancer, 17*, 1289–1298

Axell, T., Mornstad, H. & Sundstrom, B. (1978) Snusning och munhalecancer – en retrospektiv studie. *Lakartidningen, 75*, 2224–2226 (in Swedish)

Berg, J.W., Schottenfeld, D. & Ritter, F. (1970) Incidence of multiple primary cancers. III. Cancers of the upper respiratory and upper digestive system as multiple primary cancers. *J. natl Cancer Inst., 44*, 263–274

Blot, W.J. & Fraumeni, J.F., Jr (1977) Geographic patterns of oral cancer in the United States: etiologic implications. *J. chronic Dis., 30*, 745–747

Blot, W.J., Winn, D.M. & Fraumeni, J.F., Jr (1983) Oral cancer and mouthwash. *J. natl Cancer Inst., 70*, 251–253

Bronstein, B.L. & Saparov, B.S. (1975) Measures for lowering the incidence of cancer and other tumors of the mucous mouth cavity. *Top. Quest. Oncol. X-ray Radiol., 7*, 22–24 (in Russian)

Brown, R.L., Suk, J.M. & Scarborough, J.E. (1965) Snuff dippers' intraoral cancer: clinical characteristics and response to therapy. *Cancer, 18*, 2–13

Browne, R.M., Camsey, M.C., Waterhouse, J.A. & Manning, G.L. (1977) Etiological factors in oral squamous cell carcinoma. *Community dent. oral Epidemiol., 5*, 301–306

Christen, A.G. (1980) Tobacco chewing and snuff dipping. *New Engl. J. Med., 302*, 818

Christen, A.G., Swanson, B.Z., Glover, E.D. & Henderson, A.H. (1982) Smokeless tobacco: The folklore and social history of snuffing, sneezing, dipping, and chewing. *J. Am. dent. Assoc.*, *105*, 821–829

Cook-Mozaffari, P.J., Azordegan, F., Day, N.E., Ressicaud, A., Sabai, C. & Aramesh, B. (1979) Esophageal cancer studies in the Caspian littoral of Iran: Results of a case-control study. *Br. J. Cancer*, *39*, 293–309

Economic Research Service (1982) *Tobacco Outlook and Situation (TS-182)*, Washington DC, US Department of Agriculture

Economic Research Service (1983) *Tobacco Outlook and Situation (TS-183)*, Washington DC, US Department of Agriculture

Einhorn, J. & Wersall, J. (1967) Incidence of oral carcinoma in patients with leukoplakia of the oral mucosa. *Cancer*, *20*, 2189–2193

Fonts, E.A., Greenlaw, R.H., Rush, B.F. & Rovin, S. (1969) Verrucous squamous cell carcinoma of the oral cavity. *Cancer*, *23*, 152–160

Friedell, H.L. & Rosenthal, L.M. (1941) The etiological role of chewing tobacco in cancer of the mouth. *J. Am. med. Assoc.*, *116*, 2130–2135

Goldsmith, D.F. & Winn, D.M. (1980) Hazards with snuff. *Lancet, i*, 825

Gupta, P.C., Pindborg, J.J. & Mehta, F.S. (1982) Comparison of carcinogenicity of betel quid with and without tobacco: An epidemiological review. *Ecol. Dis.*, *1*, 213–219

Harrison, D.F.N. (1964) Snuff – its use and abuse. *Br. med. J., ii*, 1649–1651

Hartselle, M.L. (1977) Oral carcinoma as related to the use of tobacco. *Ala. J. med. Sci.*, *14*, 188–194

Hecht, S.S., Ornaf, R.M. & Hoffmann, D. (1975) Chemical studies on tobacco smoke. XXXIII. N'-Nitrosonornicotine in tobacco: Analysis of possible contributing factors and biologic implications. *J. natl Cancer Inst.*, *54*, 1237–1244

Hecht, S.S., Chen, C.B., Hirota, N., Ornaf, R.M., Tso, T.C. & Hoffmann, D. (1978) Tobacco-specific nitrosamines. Formation from nicotine in vitro and during tobacco curing and carcinogenicity in strain A mice. *J. natl Cancer Inst.*, *60*, 819–824

Hecht, S.S., Chen, C.B., Ohmori, T. & Hoffmann, D. (1980) Comparative carcinogenicity in F344 rats of the tobacco-specific nitrosamines, N'-nitrosonornicotine and 4-(N-methyl-N-nitrosamino)-1-(3-pyridyl)-1-butanone. *Cancer Res.*, *40*, 298–302

Hilfrich, J., Hecht, S.S. & Hoffman, D. (1977) A study of tobacco carcinogenesis. XV. Effects of N'-nitrosonornicotine and N'-nitrosoanabasine in Syrian golden hamsters. *Cancer Lett.*, *2*, 169–176

Hirayama, T. (1966) An epidemiological study of oral and pharyngeal cancer in central and southeast Asia. *Bull. World Health Org.*, *34*, 41–69

Hoffmann, D. & Adams, J.D. (1981) Carcinogenic tobacco-specific N-nitrosamines in snuff and in the saliva of snuff dippers. *Cancer Res.*, *41*, 4305–4308

Hoffmann, D., Raineri, R., Hecht, S.S., Maronpot, R. & Wynder, E.L (1975) A study of tobacco carcinogenesis. XIV. Effects of N'-nitrosonornicotine and N'-nitrosoanabasine in rats. *J. natl Cancer Inst.*, *55*, 977–981

Homburger, F. (1971) Mechanical irritation, polycyclic hydrocarbons, and snuff. *Arch. Pathol.*, *91*, 411–417

Homburger, F., Hsueh, S.-S., Russfield, A.B., Laird, C.W. & Van Dongen, C.G. (1976) Absence of carcinogenic effects of chronic feeding of snuff in inbred Syrian hamsters. *Toxicol. appl. Pharmacol.*, *35*, 515–521

Jayant, K., Balakrishnan, V., Sanghvi, L.D. & Jussawalla, D.J. (1977) Quantification of the role of smoking and chewing tobacco in oral, pharyngeal, and esophageal cancers. *Br. J. Cancer*, *35*, 232–235

Jussawalla, D.J. & Deshpande, V.A. (1971) Evaluation of cancer risk in tobacco chewers and smokers: An epidemiologic assessment. *Cancer*, *28*, 244–252

Kirkland, L.R. (1980) The nonsmoking uses of tobacco. *New Engl. J. Med.*, *303*, 165

Kolicheva, N.I. (1980) *Epidemiology of esophageal cancer in the USSR*. In: Levin, D.L., ed., *Cancer Epidemiology in the USA and USSR (NIH Publication No. 80–2044)*, Washington DC, US Government Printing Office. pp. 177–184

Kraus, F.T. & Perez-Mesa, C. (1966) Verrucous carcinoma: Clinical and pathologic study of 105 cases involving oral cavity, larynx, and genitalia. *Cancer*, *19*, 26–38

Landy, J.J. & White, H.J. (1961) Buccogingival carcinoma of snuff dippers. *Am. Surg.*, *27*, 442–447

Leffall, L.D. & White, J.E. (1965) Cancer of the oral cavity in Negroes. *Surg. Gynecol. Obstet.*, *120*, 70–72

Mallaowalla, A.M., Silverman, S., Mani, N.J., Bilimoria, K.F. & Smith, L.W. (1976) Oral cancer in 57 518 industrial workers of Gujarat, India: A prevalence and followup study. *Cancer*, *37*, 1882–1886

Martinez, I. (1969) Factors associated with cancer of the esophagus, mouth and pharynx in Puerto Rico. *J. natl Cancer Inst.*, **42**, 1069–1094

Mason, T.J., McKay, F.W., Hoover, R., Blot, W.J. & Fraumeni, J.F., Jr (1975) *Atlas of Cancer Mortality for US Counties: 1950–1969 (DHEW Publication No. (NIH) 75 780).* Washington DC, US Government Printing Office, pp. 36–37

Moore, G.E., Bissinger L.L. & Proehl, E.C. (1953) Intraoral cancer and the use of chewing tobacco. *J. Am. Geriatr. Soc.*, **1**, 497–506

Muir, C.S. & Kirk, R. (1960) Betel, tobacco, and cancer of the mouth. *Br. J. Cancer*, **14**, 597–608

National Cancer Institute (1981) *Surveillance, Epidemiology, and End Results: Incidence and Mortality Data, 1973–1977 (NIH Publication No. 81–2330)*, US Department of Health and Human Services, Washington DC, US Government Printing Office

Notani, P.N. & Sanghvi, L.D. (1976) Role of diet in the cancers of the oral cavity. *Indian J. Cancer*, **13**, 156–160

Office of Smoking & Health (1982) The Health Consequences of Smoking: *Cancer (DHHS (PHS) 82–50179)*, Washington DC, US Government Printing Office, Tables 24 and 26

Paches, A.I. & Milievskaya, I.L. (1980) *Epidemiological study of cancer of the mucous membrane of the oral cavity in the USSR.* In: Levin, D.L., ed., *Cancer Epidemiology in the USA and USSR (NIH Publication No. 80–2044)*, Washington DC, US Government Printing Office, pp. 177–184

Peacock, E.E. & Brawley, B.W. (1959) An evaluation of snuff and tobacco in the production of mouth cancer. *Plast. Reconstr. Surg.*, **23**, 628–635

Peacock, E.E., Greenberg, B.G. & Brawley, B.W. (1960) The effect of snuff and tobacco on the production of oral carcinoma: An experimental and epidemiological study. *Ann. Surg.*, **151**, 542–550

Public Health Service (1976) *Adult Use of Tobacco – 1975*, Washington DC, US Department of Health, Education, and Welfare, pp. VI-1 – VI-2

Rosenfeld, L. & Callaway, J. (1963) Snuff dipper's cancer. *Am. J. Surg.*, **106**, 840–844

Russell, M.A.H., Jarvis, M.J. & Feyerbend, C. (1980) A new age for snuff? *Lancet*, **i**, 474–475

Schonland, M. & Bradshaw, E. (1969) Upper alimentary tract cancer in Natal Indians with special reference to the betel chewing habit. *Br. J. Cancer*, **23**, 670–682

Shapiro, M.P., Keen, P., Cohen, L. & de Moor, N.G. (1955) Malignant disease in the Transvaal. III. Cancer of the respiratory tract. *South Afr. med. J.*, **29**, 95–101

Silverman, S., Bhargava, K., Mani, N.J., Smith, L. & Malaowalla, A.M. (1976) Malignant transformation and natural history of oral leukoplakea in 57 518 industrial workers of Gujarat, India. *Cancer*, **38**, 1790–1795

Smith, J.F., Mincer, H.A., Hopkins, K.P. & Bell, J. (1970) Snuff-dippers lesion: A cytological and pathological study in a large population. *Arch. Otolaryngol.*, **92**, 450–456

Sorger, K. & Myrden, J.A. (1960) Verrucous carcinoma of the buccal mucosa in tobacco chewers. *Can. med. Assoc. J.*, **83**, 1413–1417

Stecker, R.H., Devine, K.D. & Harrison, E.G. (1964) Verrucose 'snuff dipper's' carcinoma of the oral cavity. *J. Am. med. Assoc.*, **189**, 144–146

Stich, H.F. & Rosin, M.B. (1983) *Naturally occurring phenolics as antimutagenic agents.* In: Friedman, M., ed., *Nutritional and Metabolic Aspects of Food Safety*, New York, Plenum (in press)

Tepperman, B.S. & Fitzpatrick, P.J. (1981) Second respiratory and upper digestive tract cancers after oral cancer. *Lancet*, **ii**, 547–549

The Tobacco Institute (1959) *The Chewing Tobacco Industry*, Washington DC

Vincent, R.G. & Marchetta, F. (1963) The relationship of the use of tobacco and alcohol to cancer of the oral cavity, pharynx, or larynx. *Am. J. Surg.*, **106**, 501–505

Vogler, W.R., Lloyd, J.W. & Milmore, B.K. (1962) A retrospective study of etiologial factors in cancer of the mouth, pharynx, and larynx. *Cancer*, **15**, 246–258

Wahi, P.N. (1968) The epidemiology of oral and oropharyngeal cancer. *Bull. World Health Org.*, **38**, 495–521

Waterhouse, J., Muir, C., Correa, P. & Powell, J., eds (1976) *Cancer Incidence in Five Continents, Vol III) (IARC Scientific Publications No. 15)*, Lyon, International Agency for Reresearch on Cancer

Westbrook, K.C., Sven, J.Y., Hawkins, J.M. & McKinney, D.C. (1980) *Snuff dipper's carcinoma: Fact or fiction?* In: Nieburgg, H.E., ed., *Prevention and Detection of Cancer*, Part II. *Detection*, Vol. 2, *Cancer Detection in Specific Sites*, New York, Marcel Dekker, pp. 1367–1371

Wilkins, S.A. & Vogler, W.R. (1957) Cancer of the gingiva. *Surg. Gynecol. Obstet.*, **105**, 145–152

Williams, R.R. & Horm, H.W. (1977) Association of cancer sites with tobacco and alcohol consumption and socioeconomic status of patients: Interview study from the Third National Cancer survey. *J. natl Cancer Inst.*, **58**, 525–547

Winn, D.M., Blot, W.J., Shy, C.M., Pickle, L.M., Toledo, A. & Fraumeni, J.F., Jr (1981a) Snuff dipping and oral cancer among women in the southern United States. *New Engl. J. Med.*, **304**, 745–749

Winn, D.M., Blot, W.J. & Fraumeni, J.F., Jr (1981b) Snuff dipping and oral cancer. *New Engl. J. Med.*, **305**, 231–232

Winn, D.M., Walrath, J., Blot, W.J. & Rogot, E. (1982) Chewing tobacco and snuff in relation to cause of death in a large prospective cohort (Abstract). *Am. J. Epidemiol.*, **116**, 567

WHO Collaborating Center for Oral Precancerous Lesions (1978) Definition of leukoplakia and related lesions: An aid to studies of oral precancer. *Oral Surg.*, **46**, 518–539

Wynder, E.L. & Bross, I.J. (1961) A study of etiological factors in cancer of the oesophagus. *Cancer*, **14**, 389–413

Wynder, E.L. & Stellman, S.D. (1977) Comparative epidemiology of tobacco-related cancers. *Cancer Res.*, **37**, 4608–4622

Wynder, E.L., Bross, I.J. & Feldman R.M. (1957) A study of the etiological factors in cancer of the mouth. *Cancer*, **10**, 1300–1323

EPIDEMIOLOGICAL AND EXPERIMENTAL STUDIES ON TOBACCO-RELATED ORAL CANCER IN INDIA

S.V. BHIDE[1], A.S. SHAH & J. NAIR

Carcinogenesis Division, Cancer Research Institute, Parel, Bombay-400012, India

D. NAGARAJRAO

Department of Medical Records and Statistics, Tata Memorial Hospital, Parel, Bombay-400012, India

SUMMARY

Both population-based incidence rates and relative frequencies of oral and pharyngeal cancer seen in six major cancer hospitals in India indicate that these forms of cancer occur frequently. Case-control studies reveal that these cancers are associated with tobacco chewing and *bidi* smoking. Experimental studies on a variety of chewing tobacco used commonly in western India revealed that it contains N-nitrosonornicotine and 4-(methyl-nitrosamino)-1-(3-pyridyl)-1-butanone in microgram quantities per gram of tobacco. A crude alcoholic extract of tobacco containing these nitrosamines was mutagenic in histidine-deficient *Salmonella typhimurium* strain TA98 in the presence of a 9000 x g supernatant fraction. Gavage feeding of this extract for 7, 15 and 30 days induced activity of mixed-function oxygenases. Feeding of the tobacco extract by gavage or in diets induced lung and liver tumours in Swiss mice.

INTRODUCTION

The estimated crude rate of cancer incidence in India is about 80 per 100 000 population. It has been established that oral cancer is one of the major cancer types observed in India, and its high incidence is attributed mainly to tobacco usage prevalent in the country (Shanta & Krishnamurti, 1959; Wahi, 1968; Jussawalla & Deshpande, 1971; Sanghvi, 1974). Tobacco habits practised by the Indian population include (1) chewing of tobacco with lime or with betel-quid (consisting of betel leaf, betel nut, lime and *catachu*), (2) use of snuff and use of partly charred tobacco for cleaning teeth, and (3) smoking of cigarettes (western style) or *bidis* (indigenous cigarettes made of tobacco rolled in dry tendu leaf). The presence of nitrosamines in cigarette smoke and in tobacco products has been reported (Anderson, 1982; Hoffmann *et*

---

[1] To whom correspondence should be addressed

al., 1982), but very little information is available concerning Indian tobacco of chewing or smoking varieties. The present paper deals with experimental studies on chewing tobacco, and reports some observations on the incidence of oral cancer in India.

EXPERIMENTAL

Chemicals

N-Nitrosonornicotine (NNN) and 4-(methylnitrosamino)-1-(3-pyridyl)-1-butanone (NNK) were generous gifts from Dr D. Hoffmann (Naylor Dana Institute for Disease Prevention, American Health Foundation, Valhalla, NY, USA). 3-Hydroxybenzo(*a*)pyrene was a kind gift from Dr J.N. Kieth (IIT Research Institute, Chicago, IL, USA). Benzo(*a*)pyrene, glucose-6-phosphate, NADP and NADPH were obtained from Sigma Chemical Co. (USA). *Salmonella* tester strains were received from Dr Bruce N. Ames (University of California, Berkeley, CA, USA).

Tobacco used for nitrosamine analysis and other biological studies was of the *Nicotiana tabacum* variety and was purchased from a local tobacconist.

Inbred Swiss strain male mice used for experimental studies were obtained from the animal colony of the Cancer Research Institute.

Detection of tobacco-specific nitrosamines:

Two grams of tobacco were processed by the method of Hofmann *et al.* (1979). After alumina clean-up, dichloromethane extracts were concentrated to 0.1 mL under a stream of nitrogen, and 50 μl of extract was spotted onto a preparative silica gel thin-layer chromatographic plate. The plate was run with the following solvent system, *n*-pentane : diethyl ether : dichloromethane (5 : 3 : 2). NNN and NNK, which remained at the site of spotting, were scraped off and eluted with 5–6 mL dichloromethane. The eluent was then filtered and concentrated to 0.1 mL under a stream of nitrogen and finally taken up in 0.1 mL acetonitrile. Suitable aliquots were injected onto a high-performance liquid chromatograph (Waters Associates, Milford, MA, USA) fitted with model 6000A solvent delivery system, U6K injector, μ-Bondapak C_{18} column (30 cm x 0.29 cm) and a model 440 absorbance detector fitted with a 254-nm filter. Elution was carried out using acetonitrile : phosphate buffer (1:9), pH 6.5, at a flow rate of 2.0 mL/min.

Quantitative estimations of NNN and NNK were carried out by comparing the peak areas of the test sample with those of known concentrations of the samples.

Preparation of tobacco extracts for biological studies

A sample of 50 g of tobacco was shaken with ethanol ($\simeq$ 100 mL) at 0 °C on an automatic shaker for two hours. The extract was left at –20 °C overnight and was then filtered. The filtrate was concentrated under reduced pressure to about 1–2 mL, and this concentrated extract was diluted to 10 mL with distilled water. The presence of tobacco-specific nitrosamines in this extract was ascertained by high-performance liquid chromatographic analysis; the extract was further used for mutagenicity, tumorigenicity and enzymic studies.

Mutagenicity studies

Mutagenicity of the tobacco extracts was determined by the Ames test (Ames *et al.,* 1981) using histidine-deficient tester strains TA98, TA100, TA1535 and TA1538. For this purpose, 1 mL of the stock solution was concentrated to dryness, and the dry residue was weighed and suitably dissolved to obtain known concentrations of tobacco extract. Mutagenicity was expressed as number of revertants per plate after subtracting the number of spontaneous revertants.

Tumorigenicity studies

Six- to eight-week old male mice were administered tobacco extract at two concentrations, 1 : 25 and 1 : 50 dilutions of the stock, by gavage. A third group of mice were fed a diet containing tobacco extract from 10 g of tobacco per 5 kg of diet, given *ad libitum*. Mice given distilled water by gavage served as the control group. Treatment with the 1 : 25 dilution of tobacco extract had to be discontinued, since large numbers of mice had died by 18 weeks of treatment; the remaining 10 mice were kept under observation until death. Treated mice were killed when they appeared to be moribund; animals were divided broadly in two groups. 15–20 months and 21–25 months of survival. Both control and treated mice were killed by cervical dislocation, carefully dissected and examined for any gross abnormality or tumour. All abnormal tissues were processed by routine histological procedures and observed for malignancy.

Estimation of mixed-function oxygenases

Male Swiss mice, 10–12 weeks old, were fed 0.1 mL tobacco extract for 7, 15 and 30 days. Animals were then starved for 18 h prior to killing. Liver tissue was dissected out and homogenized in 0.15 mol/L cold isotonic potassium chloride solution. A microsomal pellet was prepared and suitably diluted to obtain 2–3 mg protein per mL. Cytochrome P-450 and cytochrome b5 were estimated by the method of Omura and Sato (1964). Activity was expressed in nmol cytochrome P-450 or b5 per mg protein.

OBSERVATIONS

Table 1 gives the age-standardized rates (adjusted to the world population) of all cancers and of oral cancer in Asian population groups. The incidence of oral cancer in Singapore Indians can be seen to be similar to that observed in India, whereas in other population groups there

Table 1. Age-adjusted incidence rates (world) of Cancer in South-East Asia[a]

Country	All cancers		Oral cancer[b]		Pharyngeal cancer[c]	
	M	F	M	F	M	F
India (Bombay)	143.3	130.2	16.7	10.6	13.4	3.8
Singapore (Chinese)	284.4	165.7	4.4	1.7	22.0	7.9
Singapore (Malaysians)	114.9	96.3	3.2	1.9	6.4	2.2
Singapore (Indians)	137.2	149.9	14.2	8.6	6.1	3.2
China (Shangai)	241.9	160.3	2.6	2.1	6.3	2.9
Hong Kong	289.5	210.9	6.5	2.9	35.2	15.2
Japan	208.9	139.0	1.9	1.0	0.7	0.2

[a] From Waterhouse *et al.* (1982)
[b] Includes 140–145 (8th Rev. ICD)
[c] Includes 146–148 (8th rev. ICD)

Fig. 1. Site distribution of oral and pharyngeal cancer cases seen in six major cancer hospitals in India during 1970–1972

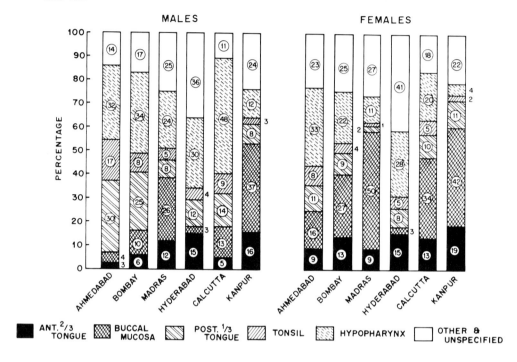

is a relatively low incidence of oral cancer. The high incidence in Singapore Indians is probably due to the habit of chewing tobacco.

Figure 1 gives the site distribution of oral and pharyngeal cancer cases seen in six major cancer hospitals in India during the years 1970–1972. Although hospital data have inherent biases, such as patient selection and availability of treatment centres, it is still evident that some forms of cancer are more prevalent in some regions than in others. The high frequency of cancer of the posterior third of the tongue in Ahmedabad, of cancer of the buccal mucosa in Madras and Kanpur and of cancer of the anterior two-thirds of the tongue in Kanpur are noteworthy observations which indicate the study of etiological factors prevalent in those areas.

Jussawala et al. (1971) analysed 2 005 histologically proven oral and oropharyngeal cancers (ICD 140–148, 150, 161) and compared them with 2 005 controls matched for age, sex and religion (Table 2). The relative risks of chewing, of smoking and of the combined habits of chewing and smoking were calculated on the assumption of a relative risk of 1 for those with neither habit. It is evident that the relative risk of a single habit is less than that of the combined habits. It is also clear that the risk for cancers of the oral cavity is associated more with the chewing of tobacco and that for cancers of the oropharynx and larynx more with smoking.

Considerable analytical and biological data are available regarding the tobacco used in the manufacture of cigarettes and on both the gaseous phase and particulate matter of cigarette smoke (Hoffmann et al., 1979; Hecht et al., 1980; Anderson, 1982); however, hardly any information is available on the carcinogenic constituents present in Indian chewing or smoking tobacco. We have initiated, in our laboratory, studies on the analysis of tobacco-specific

Table 2. Relative risks of developing oral, pharyngeal, laryngeal and oesophageal cancers associated with the habits of chewing, smoking, and a combination of both[a]

Site	Chewing	Smoking	Chewing plus smoking
Oral cavity	6.0***	2.8***	10.1***
Oropharynx	3.3***	11.8***	31.7***
Nasopharynx	1.8 NS	3.3 NS	4.8 NS
Hypopharynx	6.2***	3.6**	16.9***
Larynx	4.6***	7.7***	20.1***
Oesophagus	2.5***	2.2***	6.2***

[a] From Jussawala et al. (1971)
**, $p < 0.01$; ***, $p < 0.05$; NS, not significant

Table 3. Mutagenicity of different doses of crude tobacco extract in Salmonella typhimurium strain TA98

Tobacco extract (µg per plate)	No. of revertants per plate	
	+ S9	− S9
10	101	8
20	119	9
50	158	11
100	194	14
200	225	16
BP (1 µg/plate)	260	−
Spontaneous revertants	50	

S9, $9\,000 \times g$ supernatant of liver from rats pretreated with phenobarbital

Table 4. Effects of oral feeding of tobacco extract[a] on liver cytochrome P-450 and cytochrome b5 activity

Length of feeding (days)	Cytochrome b5 nmol/mg protein	Cytochrome P-450 nmol/mg protein
0	0.21 ± 0.007	0.54 ± 0.03
7	0.24 ± 0.002*	0.86 ± 0.05*
15	0.25 ± 0.0001*	0.85 ± 0.06*
30	0.25 ± 0.001*	0.95 ± 0.08*

[a] 0.01 mL of tobacco extract (1:50) was given by gavage
* Significant at $p < 0.05$

nitrosamines present in a popular brand of chewing tobacco. High-performance liquid chromatographic analysis of this tobacco showed the presence of NNN (2–3 µg/g tobacco) and NNK (0.4–0.6 µg/g tobacco). The presence of NNN and NNK was also confirmed by mass spectral analysis. A crude extract of tobacco containing NNN and NNK was then tested for mutagenicity in the Ames test and was found to be mutagenic to strain TA98 in the presence of a $9\,000 \times g$ supernatant fraction. Table 3 shows the increase in the number of revertants per plate with increasing concentration of crude tobacco extract.

Table 5. Tumour incidences in Swiss mice treated with crude tobacco extract

Treatment	Period of treatment	Tumour incidence	
		15–20 months [a]	21–25 months [a]
Distilled water	Continuous	0/4	1/20
1:50 tobacco extract by gavage	Continuous	8/15	–
1:25 tobacco extract by gavage	18 weeks	4/10	–
Tobacco extract mixed in diet	Continuous	0/2	8/10

[a] Survival time

Since the tobacco extract was mutagenic only in presence of a 9 000 x *g* supernatant fraction, it was evident that it needed metabolic activation to express its mutagenic properties; hence, induction of mixed-function oxygenases was studied in mouse liver after gavage feeding of tobacco extract. Table 4 shows that both cytochrome P-450 and b5 activity increased significantly.

Lastly, the tumorigenicity of the tobacco extract was studied in Swiss mice treated either by gavage feeding or in the diet. Table 5 shows clearly that continuous feeding of the extract is tumorigenic to Swiss mice. Tumours observed were either lung adenocarcinomas or hepatocellular carcinomas; only one testicular tumour was observed, in a gavage-fed mouse.

DISCUSSION

Many epidemiological studies carried out in different parts of India have shown an association between tobacco chewing and oral cancer (Khanolkar, 1959; Wahi *et al.*, 1965; Hirayama, 1966). Case-control studies have shown that the relative risk of oral cancer is four to five times higher in those who chew tobacco than in people who do not (Wahi, 1968; Jussawala & Deshpande, 1971; Sanghvi, 1979). A higher incidence of oral cancer in Indian migrants to Singapore as compared with other ethnic groups supports the contention that tobacco chewing may be a causative factor in oral cancer.

Detection of tobacco-specific nitrosamines in Indian chewing tobacco in microgram quantities further supports the cause-effect relation between tobacco chewing and oral cancer. Tobacco-specific nitrosamines have been demonstrated in tobacco consumed in western countries. (Hoffmann *et al.*, 1979; Hoffmann & Adams, 1981; Hoffmann *et al.*, 1982), and the carcinogenicity of these nitrosamines has been clearly shown (Hecht *et al.*, 1980; Brunnemann & Hoffmann, 1981; McCoy *et al.*, 1981). Our data on the mutagenicity and carcinogenicity of a crude tobacco extract containing nitrosamines confirm theses reports; however, evidence that tobacco of the chewing variety is carcinogenic is given for the first time. Earlier work reported from this Institute (Mody & Ranadive, 1959; Randeria, 1972) on chewing tobacco failed to establish tumorigenic effects, although these authors were able to demonstrate precancerous changes in skin painted with a tobacco extract and weak cocarcinogenic activity. The discrepancy is probably due to different extraction procedures or modes of administration.

The data submitted here indicate that the oral mucosa of a habitual tobacco chewer who chews 400–500 mg tobacco five to ten times a day is exposed directly to potently carcinogenic nitrosamines and that such continuous exposure may ultimately lead to malignancy. It is now important to identify the associated risk factors that lead to the development of tumours in the oral cavity.

REFERENCES

Ames, B.N., McCann, J. & Yamasaki, E. (1981) Methods for detecting carcinogens and mutagens with the *Salmonella*/mammalian microsome mutagenicity test. *Mutat. Res., 31,* 347–467

Anderson, R.A. (1982) Change in the chemical composition of homogenized leaf cured and air cured Burley tobacco stored in controlled environment. *J. agric. Food Chem., 30,* 663–668

Anon. (1973) Epidemiology of cancer in Indian sub-continent. *Ind. J. Cancer, Suppl., 10,* (3)

Brunnemann, K.D. & Hoffmann, D. (1981) Assessment of the carcinogenic *N*-nitrosodiethanolamine in tobacco products and tobacco smoke. *Carcinogenesis, 2,* 1123–1127

Hecht, S.S., Chen, C.B., Ohmon, J. & Hoffmann, D. (1980) Comparative carcinogenicity in F-344 rats of the tobacco specific nitrosamines, *N*-nitrosonornicotine and 4-(methyl-nitrosamino)-1-(3-pyridyl)-1-butanone. *Cancer Res., 40,* 296–302

Hirayama, T. (1966) An epidemiological study of oral and pharyngeal cancer in central and south-east Asia. *Bull. World Health Organ., 34,* 41–69

Hoffmann, D. & Adams, J.D. (1981) Carcinogenic tobacco specific nitrosamines in snuff and saliva of snuff dippers. *Cancer Res., 39,* 2505–2509

Hoffmann, D., Adams, J.D., Brunneman, K.D. & Hecht, S.S. (1979) Presence of tobacco specific nitrosamines in tobacco products. *Cancer Res., 39,* 2505–2509

Hoffmann, D., Adams, J.D., Brunnemann, K.D., Rivenson, A. & Hecht, S.S. (1982) *Tobacco specific nitrosamines; occurrence and bioassays.* In: Bartsch, H., O'Neill, I.K., Castegnaro, M. & Okada, M., eds, N-*Nitroso Compounds: Occurrence and Biological Effects (IARC Scientific Publications No. 41),* Lyon, International Agency for Research on Cancer, pp. 635–642

Jussawala, J.D. & Deshpande, A. (1971) Evaluation of cancer risks in tobacco chewing and smokers, an epidemiological assessment. *Cancer, 28,* 244–252

Khanolkar, V.R. (1959) Oral cancer in India. *Acta unio int. contra cancer., 15,* 67–77

McCoy, G.D., Hecht, S.S., Katayama, S. & Wynder, E.L. (1981) Differential effect of chronic ethanol consumption on the carcinogenicity of *N*-nitrosopyrrolidine and *N*-nitrosonornicotine in male Syrian golden hamsters. *Cancer Res., 41,* 2849–2854

Mody, J.K. & Ranadive, K.J. (1959) Biological study of tobacco in relation to oral cancer. *Ind. J. med. Res., 13,* 1023–1037

Omura, J. & Sato, R. (1964) The carbon monoxide binding pigment of liver microsomes. Evidence for its hemppoietic nature. *J. biol. Chem., 239,* 2370–2378

Randeria, P.D. (1972) Tobacco induced changes in the bladder and vaginal mucosa. *Ind. J. med. Res., 60,* 694–698

Sanghvi, L.D. (1974) Cancer epidemiology in India: a critique. *Ind. J. med. Res., 62,* 1850–1870

Sanghvi, L.D. (1979) Cancer epidemiology, the Indian scene. *J. Cancer Res. clin. Oncol., 99,* 1–14

Shanta, V. & Krishnamurti, S. (1959) A study of aetiological factors in oral squamous cell carcinoma. *Br. J. Cancer, 13,* 381–388

Wahi, P.N. (1968) The epidemiology of oral and oropharyngeal cancer. A report of the study in Mainpuri district, Uttar Pradesh. *Bull. World Health Organ., 38,* 495–521

Wahi, P.N., Kehar, U. & Zahiri, B. (1965) Factors influencing oral and oropharyngeal cancer in India. *Br. J. Cancer, 19,* 642–660

Waterhouse, J., Muir, C., Shanmugaratnam, K. & Powel, J., eds (1982) *Cancer Incidence in Five Continents Vol IV (IARC Scientific Publications No. 42),* Lyon, International Agency for Research on Cancer

A STUDY OF BETEL QUID CARCINOGENESIS.
II. FORMATION OF *N*-NITROSAMINES DURING BETEL QUID CHEWING

G. WENKE, A. RIVENSON, K.D. BRUNNEMANN & D. HOFFMANN

Naylor Dana Institute for Disease Prevention, American Health Foundation,
Valhalla, NY 10595, USA

S.V. BHIDE

Carcinogenesis Division, Cancer Research Institute, Tata Memorial Centre, Parel,
Bombay 400012, India

SUMMARY

In model studies, nitrosation of the major areca alkaloid, arecoline, leads to the formation of *N*-nitrosoguvacoline, 3-(methylnitrosamino)propionitrile (MNPN), 3-(methylnitros-amino)propionaldehyde and two unknown *N*-nitrosamines. MNPN is a strong carcinogen in Fischer 344 rats. After subcutaneous injection of 1.1 mmol MNPN in 60 doses, all 15 male and 15 female rats developed tumours within 24 weeks; multiple tumours occurred in 26 of the rats. Eighty-seven percent of the animals had tumours of the oesophagus, 70% had nasal cavity tumours, 37% had tumours of the tongue, 7% tumours of the pharynx and 7% tumours of the forestomach. At the dose used, male and female rats showed no significant difference in tumour incidence or site of tumours. The formation of MNPN during betel quid chewing, although likely, has not yet been proven, while the areca-derived *N*-nitrosamine, *N*-nitrosoguvacoline (NG), has been found in the saliva of betel quid chewers at levels of 2.2 – 348 µg/L. *N*-Nitrosoguvacoline levels were higher in the saliva of chewers who used betel quid together with tobacco. The saliva of these chewers also contained tobacco-specific *N*-nitrosamines.

INTRODUCTION

Cancer of the oral cavity, the most frequent cancer in India and other Asian countries, is strongly associated with chewing of betel quid (Hirayama, 1966; Jussawala & Deshpande, 1971). Extracts of betel quid are tumorigenic in laboratory animals, but thus far no carcinogen has been detected in tobacco-free quid (Bhide *et al.*, 1979). This study is concerned with the possible formation of *N*-nitrosamines during betel-quid chewing, either from the areca nut alkaloids and/or the tobacco alkaloids.

Betel quid contains areca nut as a major ingredient and is often mixed with tobacco (Arjungi, 1976). Both plant products are habituating and contain alkaloids which have not only

Fig. 1. Major areca nut alkaloids

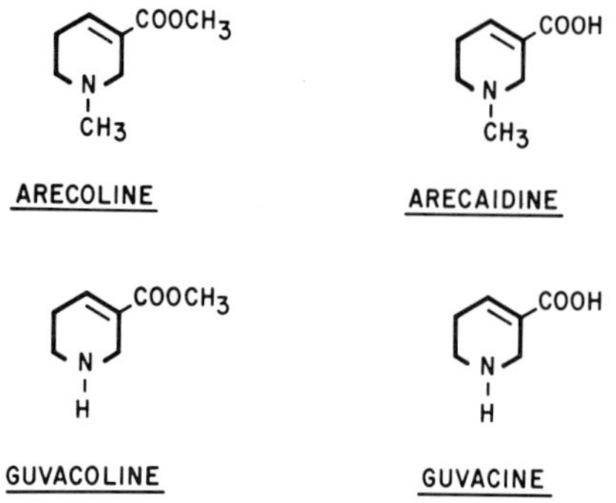

pharmacological effects but also give rise to *N*-nitrosamines. Hecht *et al.* and Hoffmann *et al.* (see pp. 763 and 743, this volume) reviewed current information on the analysis, formation, carcinogenicity and metabolism of tobacco-specific *N*-nitrosamines (TSNA). In this presentation, we report our recent studies with areca-derived *N*-nitrosamines (ADNA).

Areca nuts contain a number of alkaloids, which may constitute up to 4% of the dry weight of the nut (Arjungi, 1976). In addition to arecoline, other alkaloids have been identified (Fig. 1). Model studies have demonstrated that arecoline and nitrite form at least three *N*-nitrosamines (Wenke & Hoffmann, 1983) — *N*-nitrosoguvacoline (NG), 3-(methylnitros-amino)-propionitrile (MNPN) and 3-(methylnitrosamino)propionaldehyde (MNPA) (Fig. 2). MNPN is genotoxic in the hepatocyte DNA repair test for carcinogens[1]. NG is weakly active in the same test system, although it was not carcinogenic in a 50-week assay in rats (Lijinsky & Taylor, 1976).

In this presentation, we report on the carcinogenicity of MNPN in rats, as well as on model studies with areca nut and nitrite and on the analysis of *N*-nitrosamines in saliva samples from betel-quid chewers in the Bombay area.

Fig. 2. Nitrosation of arecoline

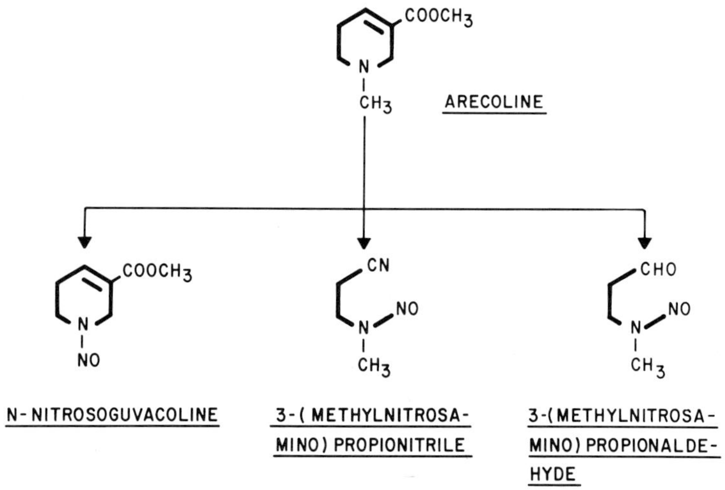

---

[1] G.M. Williams, unpublished data

MATERIALS AND METHODS

Bioassay of MNPN

MNPN was synthesized as reported previously (Wenke & Hoffmann, 1983). It was more than 99% pure according to gas chromatography, high-performance liquid chromatography and thin-layer chromatography. Six-week-old male and female Fischer 344 rats were obtained from Charles River Breeding Laboratories (Kingston, NY, USA). Rats were housed in solid-bottomed polycarbonate cages with hard-wood bedding in groups of three and were kept under standard conditions (20 ± 2 °C; 50 ± 5% relative humidity, 12-h light -12-h dark cycle). Animals were given NIH-07 diet from Zeigler Bros (Gardners, PA, USA) and tap-water *ad libitum*. Experimental groups consisted of 15 male rats and 15 female rats treated with MNPN. Vehicle controls comprised 12 male rats and 12 female rats. Each rat received 60 subcutaneous injections of MNPN (2.13 mg, 0.019 mmol, in 0.3 mL saline) or 0.3 mL saline. Injections were given three times weekly for 20 weeks, beginning when the rats were seven weeks of age. The total dose of MNPN per rat was 127.8 mg (1.13 mmol) or 0.639 g/kg body weight. Since this was the first testing of this compound, we chose the dose on the basis of an estimate of the LD_5.

Animals were weighed weekly, and moribund animals were sacrificed. The experiment was terminated after 24 weeks. Gross lesions and representative samples of all major organs were fixed in 10% buffered formalin and were processed for microscopic examination.

Model studies with areca nut or areca nut alkaloids

A modified Hewlett-Packard Model 700 gas chromatograph (GC) with a Model 543 Thermal Energy Analyzer (TEA, Thermo-Electron Corp., Waltham, MA, USA) was used for the analysis of *N*-nitrosamines, and a Hewlett-Packard Model 5710A GC with a flame-ionization detector (FID) was used for conventional GC analysis. Areca nuts were powdered in a blender.

The arecoline content of the nuts was determined as follows: 1 g of powdered nut was shaken with 10 mL buffer (potassium hydrogen phthalate, sodium hydroxide), pH 4.5 and extracted with chloroform in a Soxhlet extractor. The organic phase was discarded, and the aqueous phase was basified with triethylamine. After 3 h extraction with chloroform, the organic phase was separated, dried (sodium sulfate) and concentrated to 5 mL. Five µL of this solution were injected into a GC-FID system. The conditions were: 3.66 m × 6.35 mm o.d. (2 mm i.d.) glass column packed with 10% UCW 982 on Gas Chrom Q; injection port, 250 °C; oven temperature, 170 °C. The arecoline content was determined by comparing peak areas with those of samples of known arecoline content, prepared from arecoline hydrobromide (Sigma Chemical Co., St Louis, MO, USA).

In a typical nitrosation experiment, 3 g of powdered nut (or 125 mg of arecoline hydrobromide or 94 mg arecaidine hydrochloride, obtained from Sigma Chemical Co.) were placed in an incubator with sodium nitrite, sodium thiocyanate and 25 mL of the appropriate buffer solution at 37 °C. After five days, the mixture was brought to room temperature, saturated with sodium chloride and extracted four times with chloroform. The organic phases were combined, dried (sodium sulfate) and concentrated. The concentrate was analysed for *N*-nitrosamines by GC-TEA under the following conditions: a 1.83 m × 6.35 mm o.d. (2 mm i.d.) glass column packed with 3% Carbowax 20M on 100/120 mesh Supelcoport; injection port, 190 °C; oven temperature, 170 °C; TEA interface, 200 °C; TEA pyrolyser, 500 °C.

Saliva analysis

Saliva was collected from individuals in the Bombay area, and samples were kept at 0–5 °C. Cotinine content was quantitated by radioimmunoassay, by a procedure modified from that developed by Langone *et al.* (1973). Thiocyanate was determined by an automated procedure following the method of Butts *et al.* (1974).

After determining the volume and pH of each saliva sample, 2 g sodium chloride were added together with 100 μL *N*-nitrosopiperidine (2.12 mg/L) as internal standard. The samples were placed on prewetted Preptubes (Thermo Electron, Type 117) and were eluted with chloroform. After drying (sodium sulfate), the organic phase was concentrated to about 5 mL on a rotary evaporator. It was further concentrated to 0.1 mL using a Kuderna-Danish device. GC-TEA conditions were as follows: a 2.75 m × 6.35 mm o.d. (2 mm i.d.) glass column packed with 3% Carbowax 20M on Supelcoport 100/200 mesh; injection port, 220 °C; oven temperature, 190 °C.

RESULTS AND DISCUSSION

Bioassay

The dose of MNPN administered to animals in this assay corresponded to one-third of the dose used for a comparative carcinogenicity study of the tobacco-specific *N*-nitrosamines *N'*-nitrosonornicotine (NNN) and 4-(methylnitrosamino)-1-(3-pyridyl)-1-butanone (NNK) in Fischer 344 rats (Hecht *et al.*, 1980).

After 20 weeks, all animals showed significant weight loss, and the experiment was terminated at 24 weeks. Multiple oesophageal masses were detected in 26 out of 30 animals (86.7%); the tumors observed were benign (hyperkeratotic squamous-cell papillomas) in 26 cases, but five of the 26 animals also had invasive squamous-cell carcinomas. Due to the rather large number of tumours in each oesophagus, the term 'papillomatosis' of the oesophagus (and pharynx) may be appropriate. None of the solvent controls developed tumours during the first 24 weeks. Because of the frequency of hyperploid-looking mitoses and other atypical cytological features found in the papillomas, it may be assumed that the papillomas would have developed into carcinomas if the animals had lived longer.

Benign tumours were found in the posterior part of the tongue in six animals and in the stomach in two; all were squamous-cell papillomas, with areas of keratinization and a moderate degree of cellular atypia. Malignant tumours of the tongue and pharynx, seen in five and two animals, respectively, were very similar to those of the oesophagus and were characterized as keratinizing squamous-cell carcinomas, deeply invasive in the musculoglandular layers. Although we have occasionally observed tumours of the tongue in Fischer 344 rats, the occurrence of papillomas of the tongue in six out of 30 animals and of carcinomas of the tongue in five out of 30 animals after only 24 weeks are clearly associated with MNPN administration.

Nasal cavity tumours were found in 20 animals and were mostly transitional-like-cell or squamous-cell papillomas in both respiratory and olfactory areas; some reached a relatively large size, obstructing the nares. Only one malignant tumour (of the olfactory mucosa) was found (aesthesioneuroepithelioma), which infiltrated the immediate vicinity without invading the cheek or brain. The small number of malignant tumours in the nasal cavity is probably due to the short period of survival of the animals. Nevertheless, the presence of nasal papillomas in more than two-thirds of the rats submitted to MNPN treatment gives definitive evidence of the tumorigenic activity of this substance in the nasal mucosa. As with other *N*-nitrosamines, typical morphological patterns are emerging, and progression towards malignancy would probably have occurred with increased survival time.

The types of tumour found in the treated animals resemble those found in Fischer 344 rats treated with methylvinylnitrosamine (Druckrey *et al.*, 1967), a possible metabolite of MNPN. A comparison of the carcinogenic potency of MNPN with that of methylvinylnitrosamine will be carried out using a significantly lower dose of MNPN.

The tobacco-specific *N*-nitrosamines NNN and NNK have been tested in Fischer 344 rats using doses three times higher than those of MNPN in this study (Hecht *et al.*, 1980): MNPN would appear to be a more powerful carcinogen than NNK, the strongest tobacco-specific carcinogenic *N*-nitrosamine. *N*-Nitroso-1,2,3,6-tetrahydropyridine, a nitrosamine that may be formed during betel-quid chewing, was also tested in Fischer 344 rats, using double the dose that was used in this study (Kupper *et al.*, 1980). Again, MNPN appears to be the stronger carcinogen.

Our bioassays in rats of NG and MNPA at much higher doses than MNPN are currently in the tenth month. So far, no tumour has been observed.

Model studies with areca nut

The arecoline content of areca nuts was found to be 0.2%, a value that is low within the range reported in the literature (Arjungi, 1976). When conditions that favour MNPN formation from arecoline (pH 4.5; 1.4 x excess sodium nitrite; sodium thiocyanate; five days' reaction time at 37 °C) were applied in the nitrosation of ground nuts, we detected NG, traces of *N*-nitrosamines with retention times corresponding to those of MNPN and MNPA and a *N*-nitrosamine with a shorter retention time. Coinjection with *N*-nitroso-1,2,3,6-tetrahydropyridine showed matching retention times under various GC conditions; however, structural confirmation is pending.

When nitrosation of arecoline was repeated under identical conditions [using a metabolic shaker instead of magnetic stirring as done in model studies reported previously (Wenke & Hoffmann, 1983)], we detected NG, MNPN, MNPA and two *N*-nitrosamines not seen in the previous study – one of them matching the retention time of *N*-nitroso-1,2,3,6-tetrahydropyridine (Fig. 3).

When arecaidine was nitrosated under mildly alkaline conditions (pH 8; 1.4 x excess sodium nitrite; sodium thiocyanate; five days' reaction time at 37 °C), MNPN and MNPA were formed in higher yields than observed with arecoline at pH 4.5 (Fig. 4). The MNPN yield in this case was 1.3 times higher and the MNPA yield at least 10 times higher. Arecaidine represents one of the minor alkaloids of areca nuts, which could be formed in higher concentrations by hydrolysis of arecoline.

Fig. 3. Gas-chromatography-thermal energy analysis of *N*-nitrosamines from nitrosation of arecoline. Peak numbers correspond in retention time to: *1*, 1,2,3,6-tetrahydropyridine; *2*, unknown; *3*, 3-(methylnitrosamino)-propionaldehyde; *4*, 3-(methylnitrosamino)propionitrile; *5*, *N*-nitrosoguvacoline.

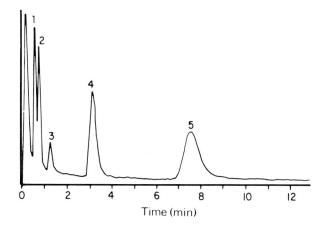

Fig. 4. Gas chromatography-thermal energy analysis of *N*-nitrosamines from nitrosation of arecaidine

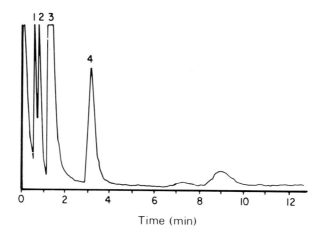

Time (min)

Saliva analysis

Saliva was collected from five chewers who used betel quid with tobacco (group A), six chewers who consumed betel quid free of tobacco (B), four individuals who neither chewed nor smoked (C) and eight cigarette smokers (D).

With two exceptions, the pH of the saliva of the chewers (A and B) ranged from 5.9 to 6.8, whereas the pH of the saliva of the cigarette smokers (D) and controls (C) ranged from 6.9 to 7.6 (Table 1). Thiocyanate and cotinine concentrations were measured in the saliva samples; salivary cotinine has been shown to be a reliable probe of the smoking status of an individual (Haley *et al.*, 1983). Tobacco-quid chewers (A) showed high cotinine levels in saliva (1 600–4 810 ng/mL); in smokers, these levels were only about one-tenth as high (80–540 ng/mL), with two samples showing almost no cotinine at all. In the saliva of the controls (C), the level of cotinine was low (< 20 ng/mL) or not detectable. In group B, cotinine levels ranged from 5–570 ng/mL, indicating some form of unreported tobacco use. Salivary thiocyanate levels depend heavily on dietary factors and are usually three times higher in smokers than in nonsmokers. In the samples analysed, smokers (D) showed thiocyanate levels ranging from 270–3 490 µmol/L, whereas in chewers these levels were not significantly different from those in controls (10–370 µmol/L).

When saliva samples were analysed for areca-derived and tobacco-specific *N*-nitrosamines, MNPA and MNPN were not detected; however, NG was present in each of the samples from groups A and B. Except in one case, the concentration of NG roughly paralleled the concentration of NNN, showing that addition of tobacco to the quid not only adds tobacco-specific *N*-nitrosamines to the saliva but can also increase the formation of areca-derived *N*-nitrosamines significantly. These findings parallel and support epidemiological observations of oral cancer in betel-nut chewers, showing that the risk is much higher for individuals who add tobacco to their quid or who both chew and smoke (Smith *et al.*, 1974; Malaowalla *et al.*, 1974).

Table 1.   Analysis of saliva samples from chewers of betel quid and controls

Group[a]	pH	Cotinine (ng/mL)	Thiocyanate (mmol/L)	*N*-Nitrosamines (µg/L)[b]			
				NG	NNN	NAT	NNK
A	6.6	1 600	130	348.	1.7	3.4	1.3
A	6.1	4 810	220	7.5	2.8	4.9	1.1
A	7.2	3 800	150	4.3	1.2	3.2	2.3
A	5.9	3 830	350	8.7	3.7	4.6	2.2
A	6.3	4 370	240	33.1	38.3	36.7	1.
A	6.7	2 300	220	44.5	31.4	39.5	1.2
B	6.3	280	210	3.1	ND	ND	ND
B	6.8	570	80	9.5	ND	ND	ND
B	6.4	270	90	7.	ND	ND	ND
B	6.3	350	320	2.2	ND	ND	ND
B	7.5	5	130	6.2	ND	ND	ND
C	7.3	ND	200	ND	ND	ND	ND
C	7.4	14	20	ND	ND	ND	ND
C	7.6	ND	370	ND	ND	ND	ND
C	7.3	11	250	ND	ND	ND	ND
D	7.	190	1 610	ND	ND	ND	ND
D	7.3	260	1 480	ND	ND	ND	1.6
D	7.2	200	3 490	7.6	ND	ND	ND
D	7.1	100	1 630	1.2	ND	ND	ND
D	6.9	540	2 070	ND	ND	ND	1.7
D	7.2	2	370	ND	ND	ND	1.3
D	7.4	ND	270	ND	ND	ND	1.00
D	7.6	80	290	3.1	ND	ND	1.70

[a] A, chewers of betel quid containing tobacco; B, chewers of betel quid free of tobacco; C, non-chewers and nonsmokers; D, cigarette smokers, but not betel-quid chewers
[b] NG, *N*-nitrosoguvacoline; NNN, N′-nitrosonornicotine; NAT, N′-nitrosoanatabine; NNK, 4-(methylnitrosamino)-1-(3-pyridyl)-1-butanone
ND, not detected

ACKNOWLEDGEMENT

This study is supported by Grant PO1-CA-29580 from the US National Cancer Institute.

REFERENCES

Arjungi, K.N. (1976) Areca nut. A review. *Arzneimittel Forsch., 26,* 951–956

Bhide, S.V., Shivapurkar, N.M., Gothoskar, S.V. & Ranadive, K.J. (1979) Carcinogenicity of betel quid ingredients: feeding mice with aqueous extract and the polyphenol fraction of betel nut. *Br. J. Cancer, 40,* 922–926

Butts, W.C., Kuehneman, M. & Widdowson, G. (1974) Automated method for determining serum thiocyanate to distinguish smokers from nonsmokers. *Clin. Chem., 20,* 1233–1348

Druckrey, H., Preussmann, R., Ivankovic, S. & Schmähl, D. (1967) Organotrope carcinogene Wirkungen bei 65 verschiedenen *N*-Nitroso-Verbindungen an BD-Ratten. *Z. Krebsforsch., 69,* 103–201

Haley, N.J., Axelrad, C.M. & Tilton, K.A. (1983) Validation of self-reported smoking behavior: Biochemical analyses of cotinine and thiocyanate. *Am. J. publ. Health, 73,* 1204–1207

Hecht, S.S., Chen, C.B., Ohmori, T. & Hoffmann, D. (1980) Comparative carcinogenicity in F344 rats of the tobacco-specific nitrosamines, N'-nitrosonornicotine and 4-(N-methyl-N-nitrosamino)-1-(3-pyridyl)-1-butanone. *Cancer Res., 40,* 298–302

Hirayama, T. (1966) An epidemiological study of oral and pharyngeal cancer in Central and South East Asia. *Bull. World Heath Org., 34,* 41–69

Jussawalla, D.J. & Deshpande, V.A. (1971) Evaluation of cancer risk in tobacco chewers and smokers. *Cancer, 28,* 244–252

Kupper, R., Reuber, M.D., Blackwell, B.N., Lijinsky, W., Koepke, S.R. & Michejda, C.J. (1980) Carcinogenicity of the isomeric, N-nitroso-Δ^3 and N-nitroso-Δ^2-piperidines in rats and the *in vivo* isomerization of the Δ^3- to the Δ^2-isomer. *Carcinogenesis, 1,* 753–757

Langone, J.J., Gjika, H.B. & Van Vunakis, H. (1973) Radioimmunoassays for nicotine and cotinine. *Biochemistry, 12,* 5025–5030

Lijinsky, W. & Taylor, H.W. (1976) Carcinogenicity test of two unsaturated derivatives of N-nitroso-piperidine in Sprague-Dawley rats. *J. natl Cancer Inst., 57,* 1315–1317

Malaowalla, A.M., Mani, N.J., Bhargawa, K., Smith, W.L., Silverman, S. & Bilimoria, K.F. (1974) *A Report on the Study of Oral Cancer and Precancerous Lesions amongst 57,518 Industrial Workers of Gujarat. Phase II,* Ahmedabat, India, Government Dental College and Hospital, p. 164

Smith, L.W., Malaowalla, A.M., Ghargava, K. & Mani, J.H. (1974) *A Report on the Study of Oral Cancer and Precancerous Lesions amongst 57,518 Industrial Workers of Gujarat. Phase I,* Ahmedabad, India, Government Dental College and Hospital, p. 174

Wenke, G. & Hoffmann, D. (1983) A study of betel quid carcinogenesis. 1. On the *in vitro* N-nitrosation of arecoline. *Carcinogenesis, 4,* 169–172

TOBACCO AND THE RISK OF CANCER.
IMPORTANCE OF KINDS OF TOBACCO

J. ESTEVE[1] & A.J. TUYNS

International Agency for Research on Cancer 150 cours Albert-Thomas, 69008 Lyon, France

L. RAYMOND

Geneva Tumour Registry, Geneva, Switzerland

P. VINEIS

Unit of Cancer epidemiology, University of Turin, Turin, Italy

INTRODUCTION

Smoking is carcinogenic for the lung, larynx, oral cavity, oesophagus and bladder and is probably a contributory factor to cancer at some other sites. Current estimates of the number of cancer deaths attributable to smoking in developed countries is 30%, and more than 85% of lung cancer deaths are estimated to be due to this cause (Koop & Luoto, 1982). In view of the overwhelming evidence, the only reasonable attitude for people to take is to stop any type of smoking. However, it is unlikely that tobacco will be given up in the near future, and it is important to know whether the 'changing cigarette' is changing in the right direction (Surgeon General, 1981; Gori & Bock, 1980). Moreover, a comparison of epidemiological data and laboratory results can be used to study the differential effects of type of tobacco and to learn something about the mechanisms of carcinogenesis, particularly when comparing differences in the effects of air-cured and flue-cured tobacco. Flue-cured tobacco is dried with artificial heat, whereas air-cured tobacco is not; as a result, the sugar content and the pH of the smoke are very different for the two types of tobacco (Elson & Betts, 1981).

Many carcinogens, both initiators and promoters, have been found in tobacco and in tobacco smoke, and their presence is sufficient to explain the induction of cancer in man. In addition, tobacco and tobacco smoke contain nitrosamines at levels that make them the highest source of nitrosamine exposure for humans (Hecht *et al.*, 1978).

The finding that air-cured tobacco contains lower levels of polycyclic hydrocarbons than flue-cured tobacco is the likely explanation for the low carcinogenicity of air-cured tobacco in animal experiments (Passey *et al.*, 1971). Conversely, this type of tobacco contains more

---

[1] To whom correspondence should be addressed

nitrosamines (Hoffmann *et al.,* 1980), which could explain its high mutagenicity in metabolically activated mutagenicity tests (Sato *et al.,* 1977; Mizusaki *et al.,* 1977).

Assuming that nitrosamines play an active role in cancer induction and taking into account the higher pH of the smoke, different mechanisms of carcinogenesis are suggested whereby the upper part of the aerodigestive tract is more often the target organ for the cancer. Nitrosamines may also be involved in carcinogenesis in organs that are not in direct contact with tobacco smoke, and differences in risk might be expected for some sites according to the type of tobacco smoked. We examine below how well these hypotheses are supported by epidemiological observations.

DATA AVAILABLE AND METHODS OF ANALYSIS

Analyses of national data are based on the mortality figures provided by the World Health Organization[1], on tobacco consumption figures abstracted from Lee (1975) and on data on alcohol consumption compiled by the Finnish Foundation for Alcohol Studies (1977).

Estimates of risk for various types of tobacco associated with several sites were made on the basis of data from several case-control studies still in progress in the south of Europe, which will be published in detail elsewhere. Limiting our analyses to males, we used the following material:

(1) 1529 cases of lung cancer and 2899 controls, matched for age, hospital and interviewer, were interviewed about their history of smoking. The study was performed in 16 French hospitals between 1976 and 1980; the complete protocol is described in the interim report of the Smoking and Health Program of the National Cancer Institute (1979).

(2) 77 cases of laryngeal cancer and 576 population controls were interviewed between 1977 and 1982 in Geneva, Switzerland, concerning their alcohol consumption and their history of smoking; using the same protocol, 86 male cases of laryngeal cancer and 922 population controls were interviewed between 1977 and 1982 in Calvados (France). The complete protocol of this study, initiated by IARC, is described by Tuyns *et al.* (1980).

(3) The same protocol as used above and the same population controls made possible a study of 701 oesophageal cancer cases in Calvados.

Table 1. Distribution of type of tobacco smoked in population samples (males)

	Saragossa (Spain)		Varese[a] (Italy)		Calvados (France)		Geneva (Switzerland)	
	no.	%	no.	%	no.	%	no.	%
Non-smokers	89	25.5	60	22.3	185	20.0	140	24.3
Cigarette smokers:								
Black	203	58.2	49	18.2	609	66.0	240	41.7
Bright	11	3.2	42	15.6	38	4.1	68	11.8
Black and bright	38	10.9	85	31.6	28	3.0	62	10.8
Partly unknown	0	0.0	30	11.2	40	4.3	22	3.8
Other smokers (no cigarettes)	8	2.3	3	1.1	23	2.5	44	7.6
Total interviewed	349	100.0	269	100.0	923	100.0	576	100.0

[a] Preliminary result from incomplete sample

___

[1] Division of Health Statistics (personal communication)

Table 2.   Distribution of smokers by type of habit in male population samples

	Saragossa (Spain)	Varese (Italy)	Calvados (France)	Geneva (Switzerland)
Cigarettes only	57.7	92.3	82.4	62.4
Cigars only [a]	3.1	0.5	0.8	10.1 [b]
Pipe only	0	1	1.9	
Others	39.2	6.2	14.9	27.5

[a] Includes cigarillos
[b] People smoking cigar, pipe or both

(4) 502 cases of bladder cancer and 225 urological controls and 371 surgical controls were interviewed in Turin (Italy) between 1978 and 1983, using the same smoking questionnaire as used in (2) and (3). An interim analysis of the study has been published (Vineis *et al.*, 1983).

Since the principal investigators of studies (2), (3) and (4) made their data available for analysis, the evaluation of risk for tobacco smoking was made in the standard way, using unconditional logistic regression with stratification for age, and or for age and country in study (2) (Breslow & Day, 1980). Confidence intervals were calculated using 1.96 times the standard error of the estimate as half length. In the case of (1), we used simple cross classified data, as described by Benhamou[1] (1983).

A complete history of tobacco usage was available for each individual. Each brand of cigarette, cigar and pipe tobacco was recorded, and its 'colour' checked at the relevant institution in each country. The distinction between 'black' and 'bright' tobacco, however, is not as clear cut as it may seem *a priori*: most brands are made of blended tobaccos, and, depending on the chemical property involved, a particular brand could change from one category to the other. In some countries the distinction is easier: in France, the tobacco used most frequently is air-cured; in the UK, it is flue-cured. There seems to be very little within-country variation, except in Italy (Province of Varese), as shown by the population control samples from the laryngeal case-control study (Table 1). This special situation in Italy is confirmed by the Turin study, in which the percentage of users of 'bright' tobacco only was 11% among controls.

It is interesting to note that pipes and cigars are rarely smoked in Calvados and in Varese; in Saragossa (Spain) and in Geneva (Switzerland), cigars and cigarillos are smoked more frequently, often in conjunction with cigarettes (Table 2).

RESULTS

A striking aspect of the distribution of respiratory cancer in Europe is the negative correlation between lung and laryngeal cancer: high lung cancer mortality associated with low laryngeal cancer mortality in the north, and the opposite in the south (Tuyns, 1983). This gradient is consistent with the hypothesis that bright tobacco (flue-cured) is more harmful for the lung and black tobacco (air-cured) more dangerous for the larynx. The apparent lack of correlation between lung cancer mortality and tobacco consumption has also been put forward as further evidence to support this hypothesis (Elson & Betts, 1981).

These data should, however, be interpreted with care. As shown by Doll and Peto (1981), the correlaltion between tobacco consumption and mortality from lung cancer is relatively good, provided the relevant indices of mortality are used: for any site at which a cohort effect

---

[1] Thesis, Paris (in preparation)

Table 3. Association of lung and laryngeal cancer mortality with tobacco consumption in males

Country	Alcohol[a]	Tobacco[b]	Cigarettes[c]	Larynx cancer[d]	Lung cancer[d]	Laryngeal lung cancer ($\times$ 100)
Austria	7.4	1.72	1 440	0.080	0.866	9.3
Belgium	6.2	2.99	1 320	0.112	1.289	8.7
Denmark	3.3	3.31	1 180	0.029	0.752	3.9
Finland	1.8	1.77	1 960	0.046	0.802	5.8
France	18.5	2.09	1 240	0.516	0.989	52.2
Fed. Rep. Germany	5.3	2.31	1 210	0.050	0.810	6.1
Greece	5.8	1.77	1 530	0.048	0.729	6.5
Iceland	1.3	2.22	1 620	0.000	0.509	0.0
Ireland	3.4	2.99	2 510	0.054	1.136	4.8
Italy	11.7	1.32	1 120	0.215	1.266	17.0
The Netherlands	2.3	3.72	1 730	0.032	1.086	2.9
Norway	2.3	1.86	520	0.032	0.420	7.6
Portugal	15.1	0.95	820	0.168	0.538	31.3
Spain	8.3	1.36	700	0.268	0.599	44.8
Sweden	4.4	1.86	1 020	0.004	0.430	0.8
Switzerland	8.7	2.90	1 860	0.072	0.926	7.8
United Kingdom	4.8	2.86	2 530	0.034	1.235	2.8

[a] Total consumption in 1956 (litres of pure alcohol)
[b] Total consumption in 1956 (kg tobacco)
[c] Total consumption in 1956 (no. of cigarettes)
[d] Cumulative rate for ages 35–45 from 1970–1975 inclusive (per 1000)

is operating, the procedure of age standardization will average out correlations with the causative factor if the exposure is not synchronous in the various countries. Therefore, it is recommended that when looking at this type of association the rate for young adults be used as a measure of disease. Results from 20 European countries are shown in Table 3. It can be seen that in France and other countries where black tobacco is consumed mortality rates in the 1970s correspond well to the consumption of cigarettes some 15 years earlier. Table 3 also shows the huge variation in the ratio laryngeal/lung cancer. Figure 1 shows the high correlation (0.78) between the logarithm of this ratio and alcohol consumption.

Thus, the national data do not support the hypothesis that there is a lower risk of lung cancer for black tobacco and, instead, point to alcohol (Tuyns, 1982) rather than the colour of the tobacco to explain the variation in laryngeal cancer mortality.

Results from analytical epidemiology studies available to date are in agreement with the above conclusion. Table 4 shows the relative risk of lung cancer due to smoking calculated in various cohort studies (Koop & Luoto, 1982) and the relative risk calculated from two French case-control studies in a country where almost exclusively black tobacco is smoked, in contrast to the others (Schwartz et al., 1961; Benhamou[1]).

The French estimates are consistent with the others: the more recent estimate is exactly the same as that of British physicians, and the earlier one is similar to the Swedish estimate; 20 years separate the two French estimates and the difference must be genuine. For several

---

[1] Thesis, Paris (in preparation)

Fig. 1. Correlation between ratio of laryngeal lung cancer mortality and alcohol consumption

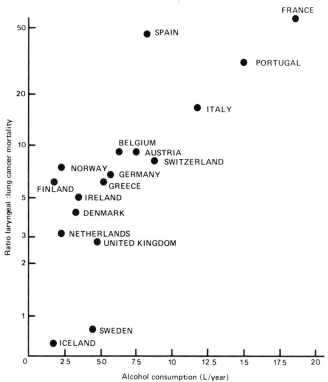

Table 4. Relative risk of lung cancer according to the approximate number of cigarettes smoked

Study group	No. of cigarettes smoked per day								'Ever smoked' (95% C.I.)
	5	10	15	20	25	30	35	40	
British Doctors [a]	–	7.8	–	12.7	25.1	–	–	–	14
American Cancer Society [a]	4.6	–	8.6	–	–	14.7	–	18.7	8.5
US Veterans [a]	3.9	–	9.6	–	–	16.7	–	23.7	11.3
Canadian Veterans [a]	9.5	–	15.8	17.3	–	–	–	–	14.2
Japanese Study [a]	–	3.5	–	–	5.7	–	–	6.5	3.8
Swedish Study [a]	2.3	8.8	13.7	–	–	–	–	–	7
French study 1954–1960 (Schwartz et al., 1961)	2.5	–	5.3	–	8.3	12.2	–	–	6.1 (4.3–8.6)
French study 1976–1980 (Benhamou [b])	–	7.2	–	13.5	21.4	–	–	–	13.5 (9.3–19.7)

[a] References given in Surgeon General (1982), pp. 31–32
[b] Thesis, Paris (in preparation)

Table 5. Estimates of relative risk for tobacco smoking according to site (males)

Cancer site	Current smoker Mean consumption (g/day)			Protection given by quitting Years since last exposure[a]		
	1–10	10–30	30 +	3–7	7–10	10 +
Larynx[b]	5.4	14.1	18.6	0.63	0.45	0.40
Oesophagus[b]	3.3	3.4	5.7	0.49	0.39	0.36
Bladder[c]	4.0	6.9	9.8		0.45	0.42

[a] Relative to continuous smokers or to people who have stopped for less than three years. These estimates are calculated under the hypothesis of a multiplicative model, i.e., a smoker of 10–30 cigarettes has a relative risk of laryngeal cancer of 6.4 if he has not smoked for at least seven years
[b] Risks are adjusted for age, country and alcohol consumption
[c] Risks are adjusted for age and occupational exposure

Table 6. Risk estimates for smoking according to study and site (males)

Site	'black tobacco' countries (95% C.I.)[a] (this report)	British Doctors[b]	American Cancer Society[b]	US Veterans[b]	Japanese Study[b]
Larynx	13.6 (5.5–33.6)	–	–	11.5	13.6
Oesophagus	2.8 (1.8–4.4)	4.7	4.0	6.4	2.4
Bladder	5.0 (3.0–8.4)	2.1	2.6	2.2	2.0

[a] The risk is that of people who have ever smoked relative to non-smokers for studies (2), (3), (4) as referred to in the paragraphs on Methods
[b] References given in Surgeon General (1982), pp. 31–32

reasons, the relative risk for smoking is bound to be lower in populations with lower tobacco consumption: the average smoker smokes less and, at a given consumption level, he or she has smoked that amount for a shorter time. The tobacco consumption in France at the time of the present study is more than twice that at the time of Schwartz's study. Wynder and Stellman (1977) reported a relative risk of 32.3 for Kreyberg I lung cancer and 10.7 for Kreyberg II, but they did not give the risk for unspecified lung cancer. On the basis of published figures, it is possible to estimate an unadjusted risk of about 19.5 for current smokers, which is in the range of those given in Table 4.

Table 5 gives the risk of laryngeal, oesophageal and bladder cancer for present smokers relative to non-smokers and the protection given by quitting tobacco. The figures for larynx and oesophagus are similar to those of Wynder and Stellman (1977). For bladder they are much higher. Table 6 compares the risk of the same cancer for people who had 'ever smoked' (relative to non-smokers) to the estimates of the same cohort studies as in Table 4. Again the risk for bladder cancer in Turin (Italy) is higher.

The dependence of risk upon colour of tobacco has also been studied internally, comparing within each study those who smoke mainly blond tobacco with those who smoke mainly black

Table 7. Relative risk[a] according to type of tobacco smoked

Site	Black only	More black than bright	At least as much bright as black	Bright only	Partly unknown	Chi-squared
Larynx	1	2.19 (1.1–4.3)	0.45 (0.1–2.3)	0.84 (0.4–2.0)	0.86 (0.4–1.9)	7.2 p = 0.13
Bladder	1	1.05 (0.7–1.5)	0.94 (0.7–1.7)	0.45 (0.2–0.9)	1.23 (0.8–1.8)	9 p = 0.06

[a] Adjusted for the same factors as in Table 5 plus filter usage and amount smoked; 95% confidence interval in parentheses

tobacco. Table 7 shows relative risks and confidence intervals for the various categories of smokers after adjustment for filter usage, which is clearly a potential confounding factor. The small number of cases of laryngeal cancer entails a lack of precision in the estimates, but the observed pattern is not consistent with a higher risk for black tobacco; it shows, nevertheless, an effect appearing in the category of those who use more black than bright tobacco.

The small number of bright tobacco users in the oesophageal cancer study makes an evaluation of the hypothesis difficult for that site. The relative protection given by filters is 0.19 (0.05-0.76) and is confounded with bright tobacco usage. However, it is striking that only one case was observed who smoked bright tobacco only *versus* 38 controls. The chi-square of 12 on 4 degrees of freedom is significant, and one must conclude that the category of people who use bright tobacco only are at lower risk of oesophageal cancer.

Even if the chi-square is not formally significant, the lower risk of bladder cancer for users of bright tobacco also seems plausible. However, this effect is present only for those smoking more than 10 cigarettes a day (χ^2 for interaction, 11 for 2 degrees of freedom). The relative risk estimate of 0.45 for users of bright tobacco has a confidence interval which does not include 1. If the risk of bladder cancer for black tobacco smokers is double that for bright tobacco smokers, this corresponds to risks shown in the last line of Table 5.

DISCUSSION

A general impression prevails among epidemiologists that there may be differences in risk for smoking according to the type of tobacco smoked. There have been, recently, several studies on the effect of the tar/nicotine content of tobacco (Surgeon General, 1981); but there have been very few epidemiological publications on the effect of type of curing, probably due to the scarcity of data on the subject. If however, as now seems plausible, the carcinogenic profiles of the cigarettes corresponding to the two types of curing are different, it is a subject of some importance.

We are well aware of the difficulties involved in comparing relative risks from different studies in different countries where the distribution of confounding factors is very different. However, tobacco is probably the factor and lung cancer the site for which the comparison is least suspect, and we could conclude that the epidemiological data suggest a risk of lung cancer that is not lower for air-cured tobacco. The data of Benhamou[1] show, in fact, that the risk is

[1] Thesis, Paris (in preparation)

even significantly lower for French smokers of bright tobacco, after adjustment for amount smoked. However, in case-control studies of that type, in which the main exposure is very common and the exposure subtype very uncommon, the possibility of confounding is large. It is likely that the 2% of French people who can afford to smoke only bright tobacco have some other characteristic which may imply a lower risk, including their way of smoking. This remark also applies to oesophageal cancer in Calvados.

In Italy, where approximately 20% of cigarette smokers use bright tobacco only, the situation is different. Furthermore, the risk for tobacco is the highest ever obtained in a case-control study of bladder cancer: usually, estimates for 'ever smoked' are about 2. In the only study in wich the risk is substantially higher, it reaches a value of 5 for smokers of more than 20 cigarettes a day (Howe *et al.,* 1980). Another figure available for black tobacco consumers is slightly over 2 (Schwartz *et al.,* 1961). More investigation is needed to confirm the increasing risk of bladder cancer for black tobacco smokers.

The laryngeal cancer study is still in progress and the preliminary results given here refer to only two of the four countries involved. Geneva (Switzerland) is one of the places where both black and bright tobacco are used, and its inclusion in the analysis would have given a chance of finding an effect had it been present. It is probably too early to draw a firm conclusion about the absence of increasing risk for black tobacco users, but the analysis of this study subset points in that direction.

The national data indicate that alcohol could be the alternative explanation of the excess mortality observed in the Latin countries of south-west Europe. It is therefore important to determine to what extent the available knowledge on risk and alcohol consumption allows one to state that this latter factor could account completely for the observed excess of laryngeal and oesosphageal cancer in France. In order to carry out this statistical exercise, a reasonable approximation would be to consider that the log of the consumption of alcohol is normally distributed with constant variance; assuming that the mean ratio for two countries is given by the national data, it is then straightforward to calculate the percentage of people who drink more than x times the French mean consumption. The risk of laryngeal cancer is multiplied by 2.63 and that of oesophageal cancer by 3.2, when the alcohol consumption increases by one time the French average consumption. The ratio between the mean consumption in France and the UK is 3.85. Using these figures, it is possible to calculate that exposure to alcohol could change the rate ratio between France and the UK by a factor of 9 for laryngeal cancer and 17 for oesophageal cancer (see Breslow & Day, 1980, p. 76). The ratio of incidence between Calvados and Birmingham is 2.91 for larynx and 5.86 for oesophagus (Waterhouse *et al.,* 1982; Robillard *et al.,* 1983).

As in any calculation of this type, the result is highly dependent on the assumption made and in this particular instance on the assumed linear increase in risk with alcohol consumption. It shows, however, that there is no serious reason to think that alcohol consumption could not explain the differences between France and the UK.

As indicated by the analysis of national data and – more convincingly – by case-control studies, alcohol consumption plays an important role in laryngeal cancer, and any attempt to compare one type of tobacco with another should take this into account; this will be the subject of a further investigation when our study is completed. In the case of oesophageal cancer, the complication is even greater as the role of alcohol is considerably more important than that of tobacco. Tuyns (1983) has recently shown the importance of oesophageal cancer associated with alcohol in non-smoking males and females in Calvados.

Under the present circumstances, there is little convincing epidemiological evidence that air-cured tobacco is more or less carcinogenic than flue-cured tobacco. There is some indication that the risk difference, if any, might be greater for bladder cancer. Any effect on laryngeal and oesophageal cancer would, in any case, be of little importance compared with the effect of alcohol and of other parameters of smoking that affect the risk of contracting these cancers.

REFERENCES

Breslow, N.E. & Day, N.E. (1980) *Statistical Methods in Cancer Research* Vol. I, *The Analysis of Case-Control Studies (IARC Scientific Publications* No. 32), Lyon, International Agency for Research on Cancer

Doll, R. & Peto, R. (1981) The causes of cancer: quantitative estimates of avoidable risks of cancer in the United States today. *J. natl Cancer Inst.*, *66*, 1193–1308

Elson, L.A. & Betts, T.E. (1981) Death rates from cancer of the respiratory and oral tracts in different countries, in relation to the types of tobacco smoked. *Eur. J. Cancer*, *17*, 109–113

Finnish Foundation for Alcohol Studies (1977) *International Statistics on Alcoholic Beverages. Production, Trade and Consumption, 1950–1972*, Vol. 27, Helsinki

Gori, G.B. & Bock, F.G., eds (1980) *A Safe Cigarette? (Banbury Report 3)*, Cold Spring Harbor, NY, Cold Spring Harbor Laboratory

Hecht, S.S., Chen, C.B. & Hoffmann, D. (1979) Tobacco-specific nitrosamines: occurrence, formation, carcinogenicity, and metabolism. *Acc. chem. Res.*, *12*, 92–98

Hoffmann, D., Adams, J.D., Pĭade, J.J. & Hecht, S.S. (1980) *Chemical studies on tobacco smoke LXVII. Analysis of volatile and tobacco-specific nitrosamines in tobacco products.* In: Walker, E.A., Griciute, L., Castegnaro, M. & Borzsonyi, M., eds, N-*Nitroso compounds: Analysis, Formation and Occurrence (IARC Scientific Publications* No. 31), Lyon, International Agency for Research on Cancer, pp. 507–514

Howe, G.R., Burch, J.D., Miller, A.B., Cook, G.M., Esteve, J., Morrison, B., Gordon, P., Chambers L.W., Fodor, G. & Winsor, G.M. (1980) Tobacco use, occupation, coffee, various nutrients, and bladder cancer. *J. natl Cancer Inst.*, *64*, 701–713

Koop, C.E. & Luoto, J. (1982) The health consequences of smoking: cancer, Overview of a report of the Surgeon General. *Publ. Health Rep.*, *97*, 318–324

Lee, P.N., ed., (1975) *Tobacco Consumption in Various Countries. (Research Paper 6)*, 4th ed., London, Tobacco Research Council

Mizusaki, S., Takashima, T. & Tomaru, K. (1977) Factors affecting mutagenic activity of cigarette smoke condensate in *Salmonella typhimurium* TA 1538. *Mutat. Res.*, *48*, 29–36

National Cancer Institute, (1979) *Smoking and Health Program, Interim Report: International Epidemiologic Study of the Relationship between Smoking and Lung Cancer: First Two Years of Survey in Western Europe.* Vol. 1, Bethesda, MD

Passey, R.D., Blackmore, M., Warbrick-Smith, D. & Jones, R. (1971) Smoking risks of different tobaccos. *Br. med. J.*, *iv*, 198–201

Robillard, J., Vabret, A., Letortu, O. & Mace, J. (1983) *Les cancers des voies aérodigestives supérieures dans le département du Calvados. Incidence 1978–1979.* In: *Report of the 7th Meeting of the «Groupe pour l'épidémiologie et l'enregistrement du cancer dans les pays de langue latine*, Lyon, International Agency for Research on Cancer

Sato, S., Seino, Y., Ohka, T., Yahagi, T., Nagao, M., Matsushima, T. & Sugimura, T. (1977) Mutagenicity of smoke condensates from cigarettes, cigars and pipe tobacco. *Cancer Lett.*, *3*, 1–8

Schwartz, D., Flamant, R., Lellouch, J. & Denoix, P.F. (1961) Results of a French survey on the role of tobacco, particularly inhalation, in different cancer sites. *J. natl Cancer Inst.*, *26*, 1085–1108

Surgeon General (1981) *The Health Consequences of Smoking. The Changing Cigarette*, Washington DC, US Department of Health and Human Services

Surgeon General (1982) *The Health Consequences of Smoking. Cancer*, Washington DC, US Department of Health and Human Services

Tuyns, A.J. (1982) *Incidence trends of laryngeal cancer in relation to national alcohol and tobacco consumption.* In: Magnus, K., ed., *Trends in Cancer Incidence. Causes and Practical Implications*, New York, Hemisphere Press, pp. 199–214

Tuyns, A.J. (1983) Oesophageal cancer in non-drinking smokers and in non-smoking drinkers. *Int. J. Cancer*, *32*, 443–444

Tuyns, A.J., Berrino, F., Del Moral, A., Raymond, L., Repetto, F., Terracini, B., Zubiri, A., Blanchet, F., Esteve, J., Lehmann, W, Pequignot, G. & Sancho-Garnier, H. (1980) Cancer du larynx: enquête épidémiologique internationale (sous l'égide du CIRC). *Ouest méd.*, *33*, 1143–1147

Vineis, P., Frea, B., Uberti, E., Ghisetti, V. & Terracini, B. (1983) Bladder cancer and cigarette smoking in males: a case-control study. *Tumori*, *69*, 17–22

Waterhouse, J., Muir, C., Shanmugaratnam, K. & Powell, J., eds. (1982) *Cancer Incidence in Five Continents, Volume IV* (*IARC Scientific Publications* No. 42), Lyon, International Agency for Research on Cancer

Wynder, E.L. & Stellman, S.D. (1977) Comparative epidemiology of tobacco-related cancers. *Cancer Res.,* **37,** 4608–4622

POST-HARVEST TREATMENT AND THE ACCUMULATION OF NITRITE AND N'-NITROSONORNICOTINE IN BURLEY TOBACCO

R.A. ANDERSEN & M.J. KASPERBAUER

United States Department of Agriculture, ARS, Department of Agronomy, University of Kentucky Lexington, Kentucky 40546, USA

SUMMARY

Concentrations (dry-weight basis) of nitrate, nitrite and N'-nitrosonornicotine (NNN) in Burley tobacco were determined during successive processing stages of experimental homogenized-leaf-cured (HLC) material, after conventional air curing and during prolonged storage ('ageing') of HLC and air-cured tobaccos. During homogenized leaf curing, $< 6\,\mu g/g$ nitrite-N and $< 10\,\mu g/g$ NNN were found in tobacco frozen immediately after aerobic incubation of homogenates at $40\,°C$ for 0, 4, 8, 20 and 25 h. Up to $550\,\mu g/g$ nitrite-N and $850\,\mu g/g$ NNN occurred in tobacco incubated similarly for 20 h, then allowed to stand 1 h without aeration. Samples of two genetic Burley lines of high and low alkaloid content were similarly incubated, allowed to stand 1 h, dried and 'aged' for up to one year in partially anaerobic environments. NNN contents were positively correlated with 'at-harvest' alkaloid content, and NNN increased at each subsequent stage of processing, reaching a maximum of $1\,800\,\mu g/g$ in the high-alkaloid line after one year of 'ageing'. Small increases of NNN that reached a final concentration of $50\,\mu g/g$ occurred in tobaccos that were air-cured, then 'aged'.

INTRODUCTION

Nitrogenous constituents in Burley tobacco are influenced by post-harvest curing and ageing processes (Enzell & Wahlberg, 1980; Long & Weybrew, 1981). Investigations concerning carcinogenic nitrosamine alkaloids and 4-(methylnitrosoamino)-1-(3-pyridyl)-1-butanone in tobacco and tobacco smoke have been reported (Hecht *et al.*, 1979; Hoffmann & Adams, 1981).

An investigation of the effects of controlled-environmental storage ('ageing') on components in air-cured and experimental homogenized-leafcured (HLC) Burley tobacco indicated that N'-nitrosonornicotine (NNN) content increased during storage (Andersen *et al.*, 1982). The HLC process involves successive homogenization of 'ripe' leaves, incubation and dehydration (Tso *et al.*, 1975). After 52 weeks of post-cure storage, NNN concentrations were 200 to 300 times higher in HLC than in air-cured tobacco. Prior to 'ageing', nitrite and NNN levels were much higher in HLC tobacco, whereas nitrate concentrations were similar for both cures. Nitrate and nitrite are precursors of N-nitroso compounds derived from endogenous tobacco alkaloids, such as nicotine and nornicotine. The origin of high levels of nitrite in HLC tobacco remains unknown. However, we suspect that activation of nitrate reductase from bacteria (Hamilton *et al.*, 1982) or disrupted leaf cells may occur during processing.

The purpose of this investigation was to study post-harvest practices that affect nitrite and NNN accumulations in tobaccos with genetically-varied alkaloid content.

MATERIALS AND METHODS

Plant materials, curing and storage

Burley tobacco genotypes with different alkaloid contents were field-grown to maturity at Lexington, Kentucky. Three studies were carried out, each in a different year. In Study I, a high-alkaloid line (Collins *et al.*, 1974), a nicotine to nornicotine-converter line and the cultivar Ky 14 were grown and homogenized-leaf-cured by the following successive steps: 'ripe' leaves homogenization→ slurry stage incubation, 40°, aerobic→ post-incubated stage standing period→ (partially anaerobic)→ post-incubated-after standing stage air dry at <55°→ air-dried stage prolonged storage (partially anaerobic)→ 'aged' tobacco stage. The HLC procedure was used as before (Andersen *et al.*, 1982), except that the maximum incubation was 25 h. In Study II, the three tobaccos in Study I and a low-alkaloid line (Collins *et al.*, 1974) were grown and homogenized-leaf-cured (Andersen *et al.*, 1982). In Study III, the low-alkaloid and the high-alkaloid lines were air-cured and homogenized-leaf-cured. One portion of air-cured tobacco was dried (in the same dryer used to dry HLC tobacco) to 3–4% moisture (re-dried) and another was not re-dried. Air-cured tobaccos were cut into strips and 1-kg lots of both air-cured and HLC tobaccos were used for controlled-environmental storage ('ageing') at 12% moisture (wet weight), at either 20° or 30°, for up to 1 year in the manner previously reported (Andersen *et al.*, 1982).

Sampling procedures

In Study I, samples were taken immediately after the chopping-homogenization (slurry) stage and after 4, 8, 20 and 25 h incubation. In Study II, samples were taken immediately after homogenization, then after incubation was completed and the homogenate was allowed to stand 1 h without aeration and, finally immediately after drying. Samples were freeze-dried and stored at −70° until analysed. Cured tobaccos in Study III were taken at the start of 'ageing' and after 3 days and 1, 3, 10, 20, 30, 40 and 52 weeks. Samples were stored at −70° until analysed.

Chemical analyses

Total alkaloids, nitrate-N and nitrite-N were determined as previously described (Andersen *et al.*, 1982). *N*-Nitrosonornicotine (NNN) was determined either by high-performance liquid chromatography-thermal energy analysis, by modification of the Hecht *et al.* procedure described by Andersen *et al.* (1982), or by the following gas chromatographic-nitrogen-phosphorus detector (NPD) procedure. A 0.1–0.5-g sample was extracted at room temperature for 45 min with 3.0 mL saturated barium hydroxide, 0.15 g barium hydroxide and 10 mL ethyl acetate. A 92-μL aliquot of the upper layer was mixed with 8-μL of an ethyl acetate solution containing 4 μg azobenzene as internal standard. A 0.5-μL aliquot was injected into a Hewlett-Packard 5880A GC with a fused silica 30 m × 0.25 mm i.d. SE-54 column of 0.25 μm film-thickness. The GC was operated using a splitless/split injection technique with inlet at 220 °C and the detector at 270 °C, inlet purge flow at 1.2 mL/min, He carrier linear velocity at 31 cm/s, inlet septum purge inactivation time of 35 s and initial column temperature of 100 °C. After

1 min, the oven was temperature-programmed at 4 °C/min to 220 °C, then maintained at 220 °C for 20 min. Quantification was carried out by means of internal standards, using authentic compounds for calibration. GC-mass spectrometer analyses were employed to verify peak identities in samples. A Hewlett-Packard Model 5985A system in the electron-impact mode at 70 eV was used with a 30 × 0.31 mm fused-silica SE-54 capillary column at 300 °C, He carrier gas (linear flow rate, 30 cm/s), inlet and flame-ionization detector temperatures of 300 °C and 2,4'-dipyridyl as internal standard.

RESULTS AND DISCUSSION

Slurry stage of HLC tobacco (Studies I and II)

Immediately after homogenization, nitrate-N contents were less than 6.0 g/kg and nitrite-N was less than 1.4 mg/kg for all the tobacco genotypes, with no appreciable differences in amounts among them. NNN was present at less than 8 mg/kg for all genotypes, except that none was detected in the low-alkaloid line.

Incubation of the HLC slurry (Study I)

Nitrate-N contents in Ky 14 or in the alkaloid lines did not vary significantly with tobacco type or incubation time. Nitrite-N levels doubled between 4 and 25 h of incubation. NNN ranged from 3–9 mg/kg and did not vary appreciably with genotype or incubation time.

The absence of significant increases of NNN in the HLC materials indicated that nitrosation did not occur during incubations, *per se*. Since concomitant increases in nitrite did not result in elevated NNN levels, there may have been insufficient time for nitrosation of nicotine or nornicotine by the scheme cited by Enzell and Wahlberg (1980). The slurry pH values were 4.7–5.3; slight decreases (0.1–0.6 pH units) occurred during incubations.

Post-incubated HLC tobacco after a standing period (Study II)

Nitrate concentrations in the three alkaloid lines remained unchanged during the post-incubation 1 h standing period. Nitrate-N levels after the standing period ranged from 0.4–2.0 g/kg.

After a 1-h standing period (without forced aeration) which followed incubation, large increases in nitrite occurred compared with non-incubated tobaccos (Fig. 1). Nitrite-N increases in the genotypes were observed in the following order: Ky 14 (× 41) < low-alkaloid line (× 82) < high-alkaloid line (× 87) < nornicotine-converter line (× 322). The greatest elevations in nitrite levels apparently occurred during the post-incubation standing period. Nitrite is formed by reduction of endogenous nitrate, mediated by nitrate reductase (Fig. 2). Fresh tissues of plants contain nitrate reductase, and this may be responsible for nitrite formation in homogenates. Induced activities of dissimilatory nitrate reductase in tobacco bacterial flora under anaerobic conditions during processing may also contribute to nitrate reduction in leaves (Hamilton *et al.*, 1982).

The genotype-dependent increases in NNN concentrations, observed after the start of incubation, were greatest in the nornicotine-converter line (Fig. 1). It can be inferred from Study I that elevations in NNN did not occur during the aerobic incubation. The brief standing period (without forced aeration) following incubation apparently provided conditions for nitrite formation and nitrosation of nicotine and nornicotine. Our quantitative results seem consistent with the knowledge that conversion of nornicotine to NNN requires fewer metabolic steps than does that of nicotine to NNN (Hecht *et al.*, 1979).

Fig. 1. *N'*-Nitrosonornicotine and nitrite-N concentrations at post-slurry stages of homogenized-leaf-cured (HLC) tobacco processing. ○, low alkaloid; □, high alkaloid; ●, nornicotine converter; ■, Ky 14

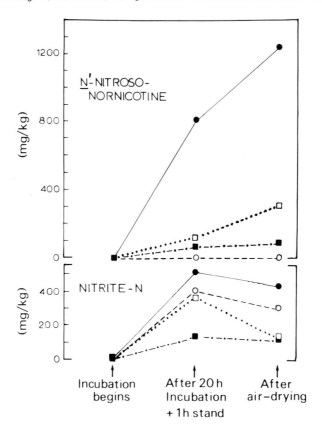

Succesive stage (→) of HPLC tobacco processing

Fig. 2. Postulated scheme of electron transport in a nitrate reductase system during post-harvest processing of tobacco (adapted from Hageman & Reed, 1980)

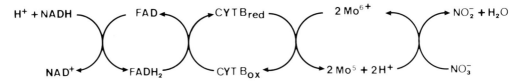

Air-dried stage of HLC tobacco (Study II)

No appreciable change in nitrate content occurred during drying, but nitrite decreased in all genotypes (Fig. 1). The following nitrite changes occurred: low-alkaloid line, -25%; high-alkaloid line, -61%; nornicotine-converter line, -15%; and Ky 14, -16%. Drying may inhibit bacterial growth and nitrite formation; pre-formed nitrite might decrease after chemical reaction.

Further NNN increases occurred during drying. Genotype influences paralleled those of the preceding stage, and the greatest NNN content was reached in the nornicotine converter (1 240 mg/kg), with lesser amounts in Ky 14 and the high-alkaloid line and none in the low-alkaloid line.

Prolonged storage ('ageing') of HLC and air-cured tobacco (Study III)

Nitrate-N contents in HLC tobaccos before storage were 5.5–8.5 g/kg, and those in air-cured tobaccos of the same genotype were 8.0–9.5 g/kg. All tobaccos contained less nitrate after 52 weeks of storage, and net changes were: HLC low-alkaloid, −33%; HLC high-alkaloid, −50%; air-cured re-dried low-alkaloid, −29%; and air-cured re-dried high-alkaloid, −20%. Smaller decreases occurred in non-re-dried air-cured tobaccos. Losses in nitrate during 'ageing' contrast with apparent increases of nitrate that occur during conventional curing (Long & Weybrew, 1981).

Nitrite in the high-alkaloid HLC tobacco gradually decreased during storage and fell at a faster rate for tobacco stored at 30 °C than for that at 20 °C (Fig. 3); nitrite-N in the low-alkaloid line increased slightly to about 10 mg/kg. Air-cured and air-cured re-dried tobaccos showed 6- to 15-fold elevations of nitrite after 52 weeks and, in 30 °C environments,

Fig. 3. Comparison of nitrite-N contents in HLC alkaloid lines during 'ageing' at different temperatures at 12% moisture

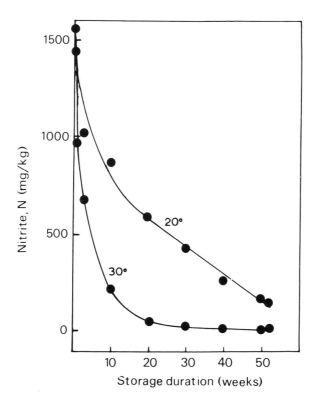

Fig. 4. Effects of storage duration at 12% moisture, temperature and tobacco alkaloid genotype on
N-nitrosonornicotine (NNN) contents in post-cured tobacco; □, high alkaloid; ■, low alkaloid

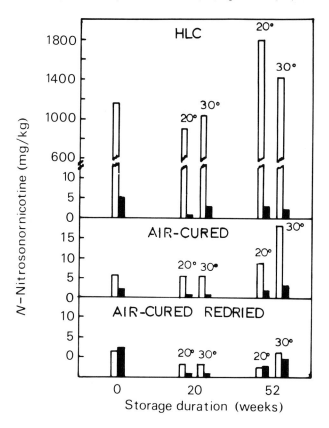

these were twice as high as in 20 °C environments; however, maximum levels reached only 5–15 mg/kg. These elevations contrasted with the small nitrite decreases we reported for Ky 14 air-cured tobacco during 'ageing' (Andersen et al., 1982).

At the start of storage, NNN in the low- and high-alkaloid lines was less than 8 mg/kg for each method of curing, except that it was much higher in the HLC high-alkaloid line (Fig. 4). After 20 weeks, NNN contents in the variously cured batches of low-alkaloid line were < 3 mg/kg at either temperature; the contents in the air-cured and air-cured re-dried high-alkaloid line tobaccos were < 6 mg/kg. In contrast, the concentrations remained much higher in the HLC high-alkaloid line, viz., about 1 g/kg. The longest 'ageing' period did not result in significant changes of NNN contents among the cured low-alkaloid isoline tobaccos. which remained at or below 5 mg/kg. NNN contents in the HLC and air-cured high-alkaloid line were higher after 'ageing' for 52 weeks than after 20 weeks. No corresponding increase occurred in air-cured re-dried tobacco. Increases in NNN (compared to 0-time values) of 36 and 18% were seen for HLC high-alkaloid tobacco stored at 20 °C and 30 °C, respectively, and 36 and 71% for air-cured high-alkaloid tobacco at 20 °C and 30 °C. The maximum NNN content (1 800 mg/kg) in the HLC high-alkaloid line stored for 52 weeks at 20 °C contrasted with the highest content of the air-cured counterpart of this line, viz., 18 mg/kg after 52 weeks at 30 °C. NNN contents in cured and 'aged' high-alkaloid tobaccos were generally higher at corresponding stages of post-harvest processing than those reported earlier for Ky 14 tobacco (Andersen *et al.*, 1982).

CONCLUSION

NNN accumulation depended on alkaloid genotype and occurred mainly during the following processing steps: standing period following incubation, forced-air drying and prolonged storage ('ageing') for HLC tobaccos and 'ageing' for air-cured lines. The greatest increases of nitrite contents in HLC tobaccos occurred during the standing period following homogenate incubation. Presumably, reduction of nitrate during this same period was fostered by partially anaerobic conditions in the post-incubated homogenates. Nitrite formation *via* nitrate-reducing bacteria or tobacco nitrate reductase seems probable. Nitrate and nitrite decreases during the forced-air drying of HLC, and 'ageing' of HLC and air-cured tobaccos can be partially accounted for by increases in NNN. The results of this investigation may provide information needed to lessen nitrosamine contents in tobacco.

ACKNOWLEDGEMENTS

We gratefully acknowledge the contributions of H.R. Burton, E.E. Yoder, T.G. Sutton, J. Crutchfield and T.H. Vaughn.

REFERENCES

Andersen, R.A., Kasperbauer, M.J., Burton, H.R., Hamilton, J.L. & Yoder, E.E. (1982) Changes in chemical composition of homogenized leaf-cured and air-cured burley tobacco stored in controlled environments. *J. Agric. Food Chem., 30,* 663–668

Collins, G.B., Legg, P.D. & Kasperbauer, M.J. (1974) Use of anther-derived haploids in *Nicotiana. Crop Sci., 14,* 77–80

Enzell, C.R. & Wahlberg, I. (1980) Leaf composition in relation to smoking quality and aroma. *Recent Adv. Tob. Sci., 6,* 64–123

Hageman, R.H. & Reed, A.J. (1980) Nitrate-reductase from higher plants. *Meth. Enzymol., 69,* 270–280

Hamilton, J.J., Smith, S.M. & Parsons, L. (1982) *Microbial reduction of nitrate and production of nitrite during curing of tobacco.* In: *Abstracts of the 36th Tobacco Chemists' Research Conference, Raleigh, NC, October,* p. 26

Hecht, S.S., Chen, C.B. & Hoffmann, D. (1979) Tobacco specific nitrosamines: occurrence, formation, carcinogenicity and metabolism. *Acc. chem. Res., 12,* 92–98

Hoffmann, D. & Adams, J.D. (1981) Carcinogenic tobacco-specific *N*-nitrosamines in snuff and in the saliva of snuff dippers. *Cancer Res., 41,* 4305–4308

Long, R.C. & Weybrew, J.A. (1981) Major chemical changes during senescence and curing. *Recent Adv. Tob. Sci., 7,* 40–74

Tso, T.C., Lowe, R. & DeJong, D.W. (1975) Homogenized leaf curing. 1. Theoretical basis and some preliminary results. *Beitr. Tabakforsch., 8,* 44–51

EPIDEMIOLOGY AND COMBINED LABORATORY/EPIDEMIOLOGY STUDIES

N-NITROSO COMPOUNDS AND HUMAN INTRACRANIAL TUMOURS

S. PRESTON-MARTIN & B.E. HENDERSON

Department of Preventive Medicine, University of Southern California School of Medicine, Los Angeles, CA, USA

SUMMARY

Experimentalists have shown that various *N*-nitroso compounds are potent nervous system carcinogens, particularly when animals are exposed transplacentally. Information has been obtained concerning exposure to *N*-nitroso compounds and their precursors in three case-control studies of intracranial tumour patients in Los Angeles County, California. A study of women (185 pairs) found that level of consumption of nitrite-cured meats was related to meningioma development ($p = 0.01$). In a similar study of meningiomas in men (105 pairs), the association with cured meats was not clear. The most striking results were obtained in a study of young brain tumour patients (209 matched pairs). Increased risk was associated with maternal contact, during pregnancy, with *N*-nitrosamine-containing substances, such as burning incense (odds ratio, 3.3; $p < 0.01$), sidestream cigarette smoke (odds ratio, 1.5; $p = 0.03$) and face make-up (odds ratio, 1.6; $p = 0.02$). Increased risk was also associated with maternal use of diuretics (odds ratio, 2.0; $p = 0.03$) and antihistamines (odds ratio, 3.4; $p < 0.01$) and with the level of maternal consumption of cured meats ($p < 0.01$). Diuretics and antihistamines contain nitrosatable amines and amides, and cured meats contain nitrites – chemicals which are precursors of *N*-nitroso compounds. Additional epidemiological studies of nervous system tumours in young people would appear to offer considerable promise for testing the hypothesis that *N*-nitroso compounds are etiologically related to human neurogenic neoplasms.

INTRODUCTION

Certain *N*-nitroso compounds are potent nervous system carcinogens, both when animals ingest the compound and when they are fed threshold levels of precursors (Koestner *et al.*, 1975). The purpose of this paper is to summarize data from case-control studies of three groups of patients with intracranial tumours, in order to evaluate epidemiological evidence that these tumours are positively associated with exposure to *N*-nitroso compounds.

METHODS

Three case-control studies

Three groups of intracranial tumour patients were studied: 209 young people aged 0–24 years with tumours of the brain (or cranial meninges) of any histological type first diagnosed during the years 1972 to 1977 (Preston-Martin *et al.*, 1982); 185 women, aged 15–64, with intracranial meningiomas first diagnosed during the years 1972 to 1975 (Preston-Martin *et al.*, 1980); and 105 men, aged 25–69, with an intracranial meningioma first diagnosed during the years 1972–1979 (Preston-Martin *et al.*, 1983). All patients were residents of Los Angeles County at the time of diagnosis. The cases were identified in the Los Angeles County Cancer Surveillance Program (Hisserich *et al.*, 1975). All diagnoses, except for one childhood brain tumour, had been confirmed microscopically. We sought a control for each case, individually matched on three characteristics: sex, race (black or white) and year of birth (within three years for the young brain tumour patients; within five years for both groups of meningioma patients). Controls for the young brain tumour patients were selected from among their friends and neighbours; neighbourhood controls were used for both meningioma studies. Controls selected from among friends and neighbours of patients were also matched on socio-economic status. Further details concerning methods are included in the papers describing each study.

The interview

For the young brain tumour study, a questionnaire sought information from mothers of patients and controls concerning experiences the children had had from birth up to one year before tumour diagnosis. We interviewed case and control mothers during 1978 and 1979. For both meningioma studies, a questionnaire sought information on various life experiences that had occurred two or more years prior to diagnosis of the case. We interviewed female meningioma patients and controls during 1976 and 1977 and male patients and controls during 1979 and 1980. All three studies were designed to investigate a variety of suggested risk factors for primary tumours of the brain and cranial meninges, such as head trauma and head X-rays. In the young brain tumour study, we also focused on potential risk factors possibly relevant to the hypothesis that in-utero (or childhood) exposure to N-nitroso compounds and their precursors was related to the development of brain tumours. We therefore asked about substances known to contain preformed N-nitrosamines to which young pregnant women might be exposed, about drug use during pregnancy and about consumption of cured meats, high-nitrate vegetables and orange juice. In the meningioma studies, questions relating to the N-nitroso hypothesis were much more limited: in the female meningioma study, we asked only about cured meats and high-nitrate vegetables; the questionnaire used in the study of meningiomas in men focused on occupational exposures and on consumption of citrus fruits and vitamin C tablets, as well as high-nitrate vegetables and cured meats. In each successive study, we tried to improve our questionnaires and therefore changed the form of the questions concerning certain study variables, such as cured meats.

Statistical analysis

In the analysis of the data, we used the exact binomial test for individual dichotomous variables and the logistic regression method for multivariate analysis (Breslow *et al.*, 1978; Holford *et al.*, 1978). If, for any variable, information for either the patient or the control was not available, we excluded the pair from the relevant analysis. All statistical significance levels quoted (p values) are one-sided, unless otherwise stated.

RESULTS

Table 1 concerns the young brain tumour study and shows odds ratios for various maternal exposures during the index pregnancy. Beer, sidestream cigarette smoke, incense smoke and face make-up all contain preformed N-nitrosamines. Case and control mothers were similar with regard to consumption of beer and cigarettes during the pregnancy; but, since fewer than 1% of mothers drank beer daily, data on beer consumption were insufficient to analyse meaningfully. More case mothers than control mothers, however, lived in a household where someone smoked (odds ratio, 1.5). We also observed an odds ratio of 3.3 for any maternal use of incense and an odds ratio of ∞ (p = 0.02) for frequency of incense use reported as 'often' or 'occasional' compared to 'rare' or 'never'. Frequent ('often' compared to all other categories combined) use of face make-up during the pregnancy (odds ratio, 1.6) was significantly associated with tumour occurrence. We also found associations between tumour occurrence and maternal use of certain drugs during the index pregnancy. The odds ratios were 3.4 for antihistamines and 2.0 for diuretics. Most commonly, mothers used antihistamines to relieve hay-fever symptoms and took diuretics to reduce pregnancy-related water retention. The antihistamines used were chlorpheniramine-containing drugs (10 patients, seven controls), Benadryl (three patients), other drugs not containing chlorpheniramine (four patients), nasal spray or cough medicine of unspecified brands (three patients, one control) and unspecified medication or injections for asthma or allergies (six patients, one control). We did not ask mothers the brand name of the diuretic they took, but those who volunteered this information had all taken a thiazide drug – one-half took chlorothiazide drugs and one-half took hydrochlorothiazide drugs. Mothers also volunteered information about prenatal vitamins (odds ratio, 0.6; p = 0.12) in response to a question about the use of 'other drugs' during the pregnancy.

Table 2 shows odds ratios from the three studies for each of three frequencies of consumption of all types of cured meats combined. Consumption of meats cured with sodium nitrite during pregnancy and during childhood were both associated with development of brain tumour in young people. Both dose-response effects were highly significant, although, as might be expected, the child's consumption of these foods was highly correlated with the mother's consumption. A similar association was seen between consumption of cured meats during adult life and development of meningiomas in women. We failed to find an association, however, between consumption of all types of cured meats combined and meningiomas in men. We did find an association of meningiomas in men with eating hot dogs or Polish sausage two or more

Table 1. Study of brain tumours in young Los Angeles patients: Odds ratios for maternal exposures during the index pregnancy

	Frequency in controls (%)	Discordant pairs		Odds ratio	One-sided p value
		Cases exposed	Controls exposed		
Source of exposure to substances which contain nitrosamines					
Smoked cigarettes	38	50	47	1.1	0.42
Lived with a smoker	55	58	39	1.5	0.03
Burned incense	3	20	6	3.3	<0.01
Often used face make-up	39	56	35	1.6	0.02
Used drugs					
– Antihistamines	4	24	7	3.4	<0.01
– Diuretics	8	26	13	2.0	0.03

Table 2.   Three studies of intracranial tumours in Los Angeles: Odds ratios for consumption of cured meats and vitamin C

Study	Period of intake	Level of intake			One-sided p value
		low	medium	high	
Cured meats					
young brain tumour	index pregnancy				<0.01
	(mothers)	1.0	1.2	2.3	
	childhood	1.0	1.3	2.3	0.01
female meningioma	adult life	1.0	2.7	4.8	<0.01
male meningioma	adult life	1.0	1.1	1.2	0.56
Citrus fruit and/or vitamin C tablets					
Orange juice only					
young brain tumour	childhood	1.0	0.7	0.6	0.06
Oranges, grapefruit and vitamin C tablets					
male meningioma	adult life	1.0	0.9	0.5	0.06

Table 3.   Study of 92 young Los Angeles patients with a brain tumour diagnosed under the age of 10 years: Odds ratios for parental occupational exposures[a]

Factor	Frequency in controls (%)	Discordant pairs		Odds ratio	One-sided p value
		Cases exposed	Controls exposed		
Mother					
Skin contact with chemicals	3	10	3	3.3	0.05
Inhalation of chemicals or fumes	5	12	4	3.0	0.04
One or both of the above	7	14	5	2.8	0.03
Father					
Exposure to chemical solvents	10	17	6	2.8	0.02
Exposure to paints	1	7	1	7.0	0.04
Work in aircraft industry	2	10	0	∞	<0.001

[a] The mother was considered to have been exposed if exposed at any time from one year before conception through lactation. The father was considered to have been exposed if exposed during that period or at the time of diagnosis of a case.

times per week during adult life (odds ratio, 2.6; p = 0.02). We found a similar association with eating hot dogs two or more times a week in the young brain tumour study; the odds ratios were 1.7 (p = 0.02) for childhood consumption and 1.6 (p = 0.07) for maternal consumption during the index pregnancy. In the female meningioma study, hot dog consumption data were not specifically requested. In all three studies, there was no apparent association between tumour development and consumption of any of several vegetables that usually contain high levels of nitrate (spinach, collards or turnip greens, aubergine, beetroot and radishes). Tumour occurence was negatively associated with vitamin C intake, both in the young brain tumour study and in the study of meningiomas in men, but neither trend was significant. In men, however, the negative association with daily consumption of oranges and/or vitamin C tablets was significant (odds ratio, 0.5; p < 0.01).

In the young brain tumour study, occupational exposures of parents also appeared to be important and were most relevant for cases diagnosed under the age of 10 (Peters *et al.*, 1981); findings relating to both maternal and paternal occupational exposures are shown in Table 3. The most striking finding was that more case than control fathers worked in the aircraft industry (odds ratio, $\sim \infty$; $p < 0.01$). In addition, more case mothers than control mothers worked during the index pregnancy and had occupations involving contact of chemicals with their skin or inhalation of chemical fumes.

DISCUSSION

Background

N-Nitroso compounds pose a challenge to epidemiologists; they are highly carcinogenic, ubiquitous in our environment, but have not yet been clearly implicated in the development of cancer in humans. Experimentalists have learned a great deal about the tumorigenic effect on the nervous system of one group of these compounds, the *N*-nitrosoureas. Administration of *N*-nitrosoureas by various routes (e.g., intravenous, intraperitoreal, oral, transplacental) has produced nervous system tumours in animals of a variety of species (e.g., rat, guinea-pig, mouse, rabbit, hamster, dog), using diverse exposure regimens and doses (e.g., single injection, low doses in food and water). Tumour induction is most complete and has therefore been most studied in adult animals exposed to *N*-methyl-*N*-nitrosourea (MNU) and in fetal animals exposed to *N*-ethyl-*N*-nitrosourea (ENU), but has also been achieved with other *N*-nitroso compounds (Magee *et al.*, 1976; Preussmann *et al.*, 1976). Tumours of the peripheral nervous system and of the central nervous system are both commonly produced; the most common cell types are various gliomas and neuromas, but some meningiomas have also developed, following exposure of both adult and of neonatal animals (Ivankovic, 1972; Ishida *et al.*, 1975; Maekawa & Odashima, 1975). The presence of threshhold levels of *N*-nitrosourea precursors in food and drinking-water causes nervous system tumours, whether exposure is at adult or fetal stages, and this effect can be blocked if various inhibitors of nitrosation, such as ascorbic acid (vitamin C), are present in the stomach at the same time (Mirvish, 1981). Vitamin E (α-tocopherol) is also an effective inhibitor and can act synergistically with ascorbic acid in multiphase systems (Tannenbaum & Mergens, 1980). Since the fetal nervous system is approximately 50 times more sensitive to the carcinogenic effects of *N*-nitroso compounds than is the adult nervous system, tumour induction is most complete when exposure is transplacental (Ivankovich, 1972). The ENU mutagenic ethylation product, O^6-ethylquanine, is removed from brain DNA more slowly than from DNA of other tissues; this slow elimination coupled with the high rate of DNA replication in fetal brain, may explain why the carcinogenic effect of certain compounds, administered transplacentally, is nervous system-specific (Rajewsky *et al.*, 1976).

Limitations of the data

Our case-control data have major limitations, but there are also important limitations in the available knowledge concerning exogenous sources of exposure to *N*-nitroso compounds, as well as their formation in the human body. In our epidemiological studies, we lack data on total exposure to *N*-nitroso compounds and their precursors. We have no information on the timing of exposure to various precursors and to various modifiers that inhibit or catalyse the nitrosation reaction, although we know from experimental data that these factors are critical (National Research Council, 1981). We also have grave doubts about the relevance of specific compounds (e.g., the *N*-nitrosodiethanolamine found in face make-up) to the *N*-nitroso nervous system tumour model. However, if we hypothesize a role for *N*-nitroso compounds in the formation of intracranial tumours in humans, some of our data appear at least to 'fit' the experimental model – 'support' would be too strong a word.

Recent estimates suggest that about half of the exposure of an average person to N-nitroso compounds is from exogenous sources and half from compounds formed endogenously (National Research Council, 1981). Each year, investigators detect N-nitrosamines in environmental substances not previously tested. New assays for these compounds are also being developed, but nitrosamides, the subcategory of N-nitroso compounds probably most relevant to nervous system tumours, are still assayed only infrequently. Also, little is known about in-vivo formation of N-nitrosoureas, the nitrosamide of greatest interest here.

In our young brain tumour study, we requested information concerning exogenous sources of N-nitroso compounds that had been identified up to 1976, when we developed the questionnaire for this study, and to which young pregnant women might likely be exposed. We found brain tumours in young people to be associated with maternal exposure to some of these sources – face make-up (Fan *et al.*, 1977), sidestream cigarette smoke and incense smoke (Brunnemann & Hoffmann, 1978) – but we found no association with personal smoking, which also involves exposure to sidestream cigarette smoke. Our finding that maternal smoking itself was not related to disease, but that living with a smoker (usually the child's father) was so related, may indicate that paternal exposures are important. The same compounds may be relevant, but may act through the father rather than the mother, as suggested by a recent experiment in which exposure of male rats to ENU before mating caused an increased incidence of nervous system tumours in the progeny (Tomatis *et al.*, 1981). Our detailed analysis of parental occupational exposures of the 92 pairs in which the patients were under age 10 at diagnosis does suggest that both maternal and paternal occupational exposures may be related to tumour development. May industrial settings involve exposure, at relatively high levels, both to N-nitroso compounds and to N-nitroso precursors (Rounbehler & Fajen, 1982).

Meats cured with sodium nitrite account for about 9% of the nitrite ingested by United States residents, and, until recent years, cured meats did not contain ascorbate or other inhibitors of nitrosation (National Research Council, 1981). A much larger proportion (72%) of the nitrite we ingest is formed in our saliva from the nitrate contained in vegetables, which also contain vitamins that inhibit nitrosation. None of the three case-control studies showed an association between intracranial tumours and consumption of high-nitrate vegetables, but the young brain tumour study did find a clear dose-response association with consumption of cured meat, both by the mother during pregnancy and by the child. We found that maternal use of drugs, but not use by the child, was also related to brain tumour development. Drugs are an important source of secondary and tertiary amines and amides for the United States population and can interact with nitrite in human gastric juice fo form N-nitrosamines and nitrosamides (Lijinsky, 1974). The rapidity with which such reactions occur and the stability and carcinogenicity of the compounds that result has not been determined for most drugs. Hydrochlorothiazide, the diuretic mentioned by one-half of the case mothers who volunteered the name of the drug, is known, however, to nitrosate readily (Gold & Mirvish, 1977). In the young brain tumour study we also observed some suggestion of protective effects due to maternal prenatal use of vitamins and to childhood consumption of orange juice.

In the two meningioma studies, we found a dose-response effect for consumption of all cured meats combined in the females, but not in the males. In men, we did find a correlation with frequent comsumption of hot dogs which, since the 1930s, have contained nitrite levels among the highest of any cured meats (Binkerd & Kolari, 1975). The data for men also suggested a protective effect due to frequent consumption of vitamin C tablets and/or citrus fruits (which contain high levels of vitamin C). This is consistent with the experimental model in which vitamin C inhibits the formation of carcinogenic N-nitroso compounds from nitrite and other precursors and thus prevents the formation of nervous system tumours. We have incomplete information on total vitamin C intake, however, and our findings are inconsistent, in that the effect appears to be limited to those with a history of head trauma. Because our data are quite limited and our findings somewhat inconsistent and weak, we are uncertain about the validity of the association between nitrite consumption and meningiomas in adults. Both meningioma studies showed that tumour development was related to prior head trauma and head X-rays. Limited experimental evidence does suggest, however, that N-nitroso compounds can produce meningeal tumours and that cerebral trauma may act as a cocarcinogen in rats (Morantz & Shain, 1978).

Overall, our findings in the young brain tumour study fit the animal model well. Our hypothesis is supported by a recent study in which an association was found between high levels of nitrate in the household water supplies of pregnant women and central nervous system birth defects in their children (Scragg *et al.*, 1982) and by the recent finding that periconceptual vitamin supplementation appears to prevent neural tube defects (Smithells *et al.*, 1981). We feel, therefore, that epidemiological studies of nervous system tumours in young people offer considerable promise for testing the hypothesis that N-nitroso compounds are etiologically related to human nervous system tumours. More studies are needed in various populations with diverse exposures to exogenous sources of N-nitroso compounds, to N-nitroso precursors and to modifiers of the nitrosation reaction. Only after data from such studies have been evaluated can we determine whether N-nitroso compounds play a role in the etiology of brain and other nervous system tumours in humans.

REFERENCES

Binkerd, E.F. & Kolari, O.E. (1975) The history and use of nitrate and nitrite in the curing of meat. *Food cosmet. Toxicol. 13*, 655–661

Breslow, N.E., Day, N.E., Halvorsen, K.T., Prentice, R.L., & Sabai, C. (1978) Estimation of multiple risk functions in matched case-control studies. *Am. J. Epidemiol., 108*, 299–307

Brunnemann, K.D. & Hoffmann, D. (1978) *Chemical studies on tobacco smoke. LIX: Analysis of volatile nitrosamines in tobacco smoke and polluted indoor environments.* In: Walker, E.A., Castegnaro, M., Griciute, L. & Lyle, R.E., eds, *Environmental Aspects of N-nitroso compounds (IARC Scientific Publications No. 19)*, Lyon, International Agency for Research on Cancer

Fan, T.Y., Goff, U., Song, L., Fine, D.H., Arsenault, G.P. & Biemann, K. (1977) N-nitrosodiethanolamine in cosmetics, lotions and shampoos. *Food Cosmet. Toxicol., 15*, 423–430

Gold, B. & Mervish, S. (1977) N-nitroso derivatives of hydrochlorothiazide, nitridazole, and tolbutamide. *Toxicol appl. Pharmacol., 40*, 131–136

Hisserich, J.C., Martin, S.P. & Henderson. B.E. (1975) An areawide reporting network. *Publ. Health Rep., 90*, 15–17

Holford, T.R., White, C. & Kelsey, J.L. (1978) Multivariate analysis for matched case-control studies. *Am. J. Epidemiol., 107*, 245–256

Isjida, Y., Tamura, M., Kanda, H. & Okamoto, K. (1975) Histopathological studies of the nervous system tumours in rats induced by N-nitrosomethyl-urea. *Acta Pathol. Jpn., 25*, 385–401

Ivankovic, S. (1972) *Prenatal carcinogenesis.* In: Nakahara, W., Takayama, S., Sugimura, T. & Odashima, S., eds, *Topics in Chemical Carcinogenesis*, Tokyo, University of Tokyo Press. pp. 463–472

Koestner, A., Derlinger, R.H., & Wechsler, W. (1975) Induction of neurogenic and lymphoid neoplasms by the feeding of threshold levels of methyl- and ethylnitrosourea precursors to adult rats. *Food Cosmet. Toxicol., 13*, 605–609

Lijinsky, W. (1974) Reaction of drugs with nitrous acid as a source of carcinogenic nitrosamines. *Cancer Res., 34*, 255–258

Maekawa, A. & Odashima, S. (1975) Induction of tumours of the nervous system in the ACI/N rat with 1-butyl-1-nitrosourea administered transplacentally, neonatally, or via maternal milk. *Gann, 66*, 175–183

Magee, P.N., Montesano, R. & Preussmann, R. (1976) N-*Nitroso compounds and related carcinogens.* In: Searle, C.E., ed., *Chemical Carcinogens (ACS Symposium Series No. 173)*, Washington DC, American Chemical Society, pp. 491–615

Mirvish, S.S. (1981) *Inhibition of the formation of carcinogenic* N-*nitroso compounds by ascorbic acid and other compounds.* In: Burchenal, J.H., & Oettgen, H.F., eds, *Cancer: Challenges, and Prospects for the 1980s,* Vol. New York, Grune & Stratton, pp. 557–587

Morantz, R.A. & Shain, W. (1978) Trauma and brain tumours: an experimental study. *Neurosurgery, 3,* 181–186

National Research Council (1981) *The Health Effects of Nitrate, Nitrite, and* N-*Nitroso Compounds,* Washington DC, National Academy Press

Peters, J.M., Preston-Martin, S. & Yu, M.C. (1981) Brain tumors in children and occupational exposure of parents. *Science, 213,* 235–237

Preston-Martin, S., Paganini-Hill, A., Henderson, B.E., Pike, M.C. & Wood, C. (1980) Case-control study of intracranial meningiomas in women in Los Angeles County. *J. natl Cancer Inst., 65,* 67–73

Preston-Martin, S., Yu, M.C. Benton, B. & Henderson, B.E. (1982) *N*-Nitroso compounds and childhood brain tumors, *Cancer Res., 42,* 5240–5245

Preston-Martin, S., Yu, M.C., Henderson, B.E. & Roberts, C. (1983) Risk factors for meningiomas in men in Los Angeles County. *J. natl Cancer Inst., 70,* 863–866

Preussmann, R., Eisenbrand, G. & Schmähl, D. (1976) *Carcinogenicity testing of low doses of nitrosopyrrolidine and of nitrosobenzthiazuron and nitrosocarbaryl in rats.* In: Walker, E.A., Bogovski, P. & Griciute, L., eds, *Environmental* N-*Nitroso Compounds. Analysis and Formation. (IARC Scientific Publications No. 14).* Lyon, International Agency for Research on Cancer, pp. 429–433

Rajewsky, M.F., Goth, R., Laerum, O.D., Biessmann, H. & Hulser, D.F. (1976) *Molecular and cellular mechanisms in nervous system-specific carcinogenesis by* N-*ethyl*-N-*nitrosourea.* In: Magee, P.N., Takayama, S., Sugimura, T. & Matisushima, T. eds, *Fundamentals in Cancer Prevention,* Baltimore, University Park Press, pp. 313–334

Rounbehler, D.P. & Fajen, J.M. (1982) N-*Nitroso Compounds in the Factory Environment.,* Cincinnati, National Institute for Occupational Safety and Health

Scragg, R.K.R., Dorsch, M.M., McMichael, A.J. & Baghurst, P.A. (1982) Birth defects and household water supply: Epidemiological studies in the Mount Gambier region of South Australia. *Med. J. Aust., 2,* 577–579

Smithells, R.W., Sheppard, S., Schoral, C.J., Seller, M.J., Nevin, N.C., Harris, R., Read, A.P., Fielding, D.W. & Walker, S. (1981) Vitamin supplementation and neural tube defects. *Lancet, ii,* 1425

Tannenbaum, S.R. & Mergens, W. (1980) Reaction of nitrite with vitamins C and E. *Ann. N.Y. Acad. Sci., 355,* 267–277

Tomatis, L., Cabral, J.R.P., Likhachev, A.J. & Ponomarkov, V. (1981) Increased cancer incidence in the progeny of male rats exposed to ethylnitrosourea before mating. *Int. J. Cancer, 28,* 475–478

RELEVANCE OF GASTRIC ACHLORHYDRIA TO HUMAN CARCINOGENESIS

C. CAYGILL & M. HILL

Bacterial Metabolism Research Laboratory, PHLS-Centre for Applied Microbiology & Research, Porton Down, Salisbury, Wilts, UK

J. CRAVEN & R. HALL

York Distric Hospital, Wigginton Road, York, UK

C. MILLER

Epidemiological Research Laboratory, CPHL London, UK

INTRODUCTION

N-Nitroso compounds have been found at all sites of the human body in which bacteria, nitrosatable amine and nitrate or nitrite occur together, such as achlorhydric stomachs, infected urinary bladders, saliva, the colon of persons with ureterosigmoid anastomosis and, possibly, normal colon. Their possible endogenous production has been reviewed elsewhere (Hill, 1979; Tannenbaum, 1983). Although there is no clear evidence that they are carcinogenic to humans, there is also no good reason to believe that we are uniquely resistant to their carcinogenic action. In consequence, any situation in which abnormally large amounts of N-nitroso compounds are thought to be produced in the human body is worthy of investigation; their relevance to human carcinogenesis can only be tested epidemiologically. One such situation is patients with gastric achlorhydria, such as those with pernicious anaemia, or who have undergone partial gastrectomy.

Pernicious anaemia (PA) is caused by a lack of intrisic factor resulting in a failure to absorb vitamin B12. Failure to secrete this factor is invariably accompanied by failure to secrete gastric acid, and so gastric achlorhydria is a major symptom in the recognition and diagnosis of the disease.

The surgical treatment of peptic ulcer has traditionally been directed towards decreasing gastric acid secretion. This was achieved by removal of most of the lower part (including much of the acid-secreting section) of the stomach by a variety of procedures, the most common of which was Polya partial gastrectomy (PG). Later, vagotomy (V) was introduced – initially, truncal vagotomy and then, highly selective vagotomy (in which only those vagal nerves serving the body of the stomach are severed leaving other parts of the vagal nerves, and, consequently, control of the antrum and pylorus and other abdominal viscera, relatively unaffected). Within a year of PG or V, there is a profound loss of gastric acidity.

The occurrence of gastric cancer in patients suffering from PA (Mosbech & Videbaek, 1950; Blackburn *et al.*, 1968) and in those who have undergone PG (Morgenstern *et al.*, 1973; Domellof *et al.*, 1976; Dahm *et al.*, 1979) has been described, and evidence has been obtained for a role of *N*-nitroso compounds in this carcinogenesis (Ruddell *et al.*, 1976, 1978; Jones *et al.*, 1978; Schlag *et al.*, 1980). If this proposal is correct, then an excess of cancers at sites other than the stomach might also be expected, since not all *N*-nitroso compounds can be expected to be activated locally, so that, by analogy with animal models, some would be organotropic for distant sites.

We have studied 682 patients with PA and two groups of post-operative patients (348 PG and 705 PG or V patients, respectively) to confirm whether these groups have a high risk of gastric cancer, to look for increased risks of cancers at other sites and to establish the latent period.

METHODS

PG and V patients

All of the patients were treated surgically in York general hospitals between 1942 and 1969; surgeon A carried out 348 PGs between 1942 and 1948, and surgeon B did 705 PGs or Vs between 1949 and 1969. The patients treated by surgeon A were part of a group of more than 600 patients the notes of many of whom were subsequently lost (including most of those who died within the first five post-operative years). The 348 were all of those for whom follow-up was possible, and the group was highly selected in favour of 'survivors'. The data with regard to surgeon B's patients are complete.

PA patients

Permission was obtained to study the records of all patients diagnosed and treated as having PA at 12 London hospitals and in four general practices. Patients whose diagnosis included achlorhydria or impaired vitamin-B12 absorption were classified as 'good diagnosis' for our purposes, while the others (diagnosed only, for example, on the basis of low serum B12, macrocytic blood, megaloblastic marrow, etc) were classified as having a 'poor diagnosis'. We examined the hospital notes of all of these patients in an attempt to establish the time of onset of symptoms and to follow up subsequent illness.

This examination was supplemented by up-to-date information from the general practioners concerned. Cause of death was determined from death certificates obtained from the Central Registry. Of the original group of more than 800 patients located, only 682 had an adequate diagnosis of PA and sufficient follow-up information to be usable in this study.

Analytical methods

Nitrate and nitrite were analysed by the autoanalyser method of Bartholomew and Hill (1984). Total bacteria and nitrate-reducing bacteria were assayed by the method of most probable number of Meynell and Meynell (1970).

Statistical analysis of the results

In the PG study, the expected incidences of the various cancers were calculated from data in the Sheffield Cancer Registry for 1963-1966 for the patients of surgeon A (Doll *et al.*, 1970) and for 1973–1976 for the patients of surgeon B (Waterhouse *et al.*, 1982). Mortality data from the same Cancer Registry were used to calculate expected mortality. Gastric ulcer carries an increased risk of gastric cancer, and so many patients had gastric cancer at the time of operation. In order to account for any other cancers initiated before operation, we decided arbitrarily to reject from the analysis all cancers that had arisen within five years of surgery.

In the PA study, the expected number of deaths was calculated on the basis of 1978 mortality statistics and population estimates for Greater London (Office of Population Censuses and Surveys, 1980a, b), using 10-year age groups.

RESULTS AND DISCUSSION

Gastric juice analyses

The 17 PG patients attending York General Hospital had a mean nitrite concentration of 52 μmol/L, in agreement with the elevated levels that we observed previously (Table 1). Reed *et al.,* (1983) showed that nitrite levels in patients who had undergone truncal vagotomy with pyloroplasty were higher than those in normal controls; no difference from controls was seen in patients who had undergone proximal gastric vagotomy.

Cancer in PG and V patients

We have confirmed that there is an increased incidence of and mortality from gastric cancer in PG and V patients after a latency of 20 years (Table 2); during the first 20 years there was no excess (and, in fact, a deficit was seen in the patients of surgeon B) of gastric or other cancers. The latency of 20 years agrees with that described by others (Stahlsberg & Taksdal, 1971; Domellof *et al.,* 1976; Dahm *et al.,* 1979).

Because the patients of surgeon B had been operated on relatively recently, the number of patient-years at risk in excess of 20 years was smaller than that for the other group, and only a relatively large excess risk (as with gastric cancer) could have been detected. In our study of the incidence of other cancers, therefore, a relative lack of excess risk was seen in these patients during the first 20 post-operative years, and only gross effects were seen in the group with more than 20 post-operative years.

Table 1. Analyses of gastric juice from control persons and from patients with pernicious anemia (PA) or those who have undergone Polya partial gastrectomy (PG)

Patient group	Type of analysis	Study [a]		
		A	B	C
Controls	number	23	13	
	nitrate-reducing bacteria	ND	2.9 ± 0.5	
	nitrate (μmol/L)	313 ± 39		
	nitrite (μmol/L)	3.2 ± 1.7	2.7 ± 0.6	
PA patients	number	15	13	
	nitrate-reducing bacteria	3.8 ± 0.7	6.6 ± 0.9	
	nitrate (μmol/L)	209 ± 42		
	nitrite (μmol/L)	59 ± 13	120 ± 20	
PG patients	number			17
	nitrate reducing bacteria			3.8 ± 2.2
	nitrate (μmol/L)			187 ± 180
	nitrite (μmol/L)			52 ± 70

[a] Study A, Stockbrugger *et al.* (1984); study B, Ruddell *et al.* (1978); study C, Craven *et al.* (in preparation)

Table 2. Incidence of and mortality from various cancers in patients who received a Polya partial gastrectomy from two surgeons (A and B)[a]

Type of cancer	No. of years since operation	Surgeon A (patients treated 1945–1949)						Surgeon B (patients treated 1949–1968)					
		Incidence			Mortality			Incidence			Mortality		
		O	E	SIR	O	E	SMR	O	E	SIR	O	E	SMR
All sites	5–20	8	29.7	27	4	28.7	14	64	63.9	100	46	44.5	103
	20+	73	51.6	141	63	36.2	174	30	19.4	155	30	13.6	221
Stomach	5–20	2	2.2	92	0	2.1	–	2	5.3	38	2	5.1	40
	20+	13	5.2	251	12	4.5	266	4	1.6	250	2	1.4	143
Colorectum	5–20	1	3.4	29	1	2.0	50	6	7.8	77	5	5.3	94
	20+	10	7.4	135	10	3.5	285	3	3.0	100	3	1.7	176
Gallbladder and biliary tree	5–20	0	0.15	–	–	–	–	1	0.4	250	–	–	–
	20+	3	0.32	937	–	–	–	0	0.14	–	–	–	–

[a]O, number of cases observed; E, number of cases expected; SMR, standard mortality ratio (O/E × 100); SIR, standard incidence ratio (O/E × 100)

Among the patients of surgeon A, there was excess mortality from colorectal cancer in those with more than 20 post-operative years (Table 2); this excess was also sufficiently large to be detectable in the patients of surgeon B. There was no excess mortality from or incidence of large-bowel cancer during the first 20 post-operative years in either group of patients. There were three cases of cancer of the gall-bladder or biliary tree among the patients of surgeon A, all more than 20 years after operation. Since this cancer apperars rarely in that part of British death certificates on which mortality statistics were based, it was only possible to study incidence data. There was also no excess of this cancer during the first 20 post-operative years in the patients of surgeon B.

There was an excess of cases and deaths from cancers at all sites in the patients of surgeon A with more than 20 post-operative years, only part of which can be accounted for by cancers of the stomach, colorectum and gall-bladder. We cannot, therefore, rule our other target sites.

Cancer in PA patients

There was no excess mortality from all cancers in this group of patients, but within the total there was a large (four-fold) and statistically significant excess of deaths from cancers of the stomach, and a two-fold excess of deaths from colorectal cancer (Table 3). Of all deaths from cancer, gastric cancers accounted for 32% whereas only 8% were expected, and colorectal cancers represented 19% whereas only 9% were expected. Since this was a mortality study, no cancer of the gall-bladder or biliary tree was recorded.

The interval between diagnosis of PA and of gastric cancer was from one to 26 years (mean, 9.3 years). A diagnosis of gastric achlorhydria was made prior to that of PA in only 11 patients; the interval was from 7–26 years (mean, 13.6 years). In general, gastric achlorhydria is asymptomatic and is suspected only after other symptoms (such as low serum vitamin B12) have become manifest. Assuming that these 11 patients were representative, however, we can assume that achlorhydria precedes recognizable PA by a mean of 13.6 years and that the latency between achlorhydria and gastric cancer is therefore 22.9 years – a latency similar to that seen in PG patients. The interval between the diagnosis of PA and colorectal cancer was 0-23 years (mean, 7.0), giving an overall latency of 20.6 years – similar to that for gastric cancer in PA patients and for gastric, colorectal and gall-bladder cancer in PG patients.

It must be recognized that the groups of PA and of PG patients investigated in this study were too small to provide statistically significant results for cancers other than that of the stomach, and that this must be regarded as a pilot study. We have already, therefore, embarked on a much larger study, of approximately 7 000 PG and V patients, to determine whether the results of this pilot study can be confirmed. If so, they lend support to the hypothesis that

Table 3.   Mortality from various cancers and other causes in patients with pernicious anaemia

Cause of death	Number of deaths		
	Observed	Expected	SMR
All causes	171	140.3	122[a]
Cancers – all sites	37	38.0	97
Stomach	12	3.2	375[b]
Colorectum	7	3.6	194
Others	18	31.2	58
Non-malignant disease	134	102.3	131

[a] $0.001 < p < 0.01$
[b] $p < 0.001$

endogenously formed *N*-nitroso compounds can, in certain circumstances, be important in human carcinogenesis.

ACKNOWLEDGEMENTS

This work was financially supported by the Cancer Research Campaign and the Department of the Environment. We acknowledge the helpful assistance of all of the clinicians involved, and in addition of Mrs Sheila Dickson and Mrs R. Nicolson (York District Hospital), Mrs P. Allgood (PHLS) and Mr Birch (OPCS).

REFERENCES

Bartholomew, B. & Hill, M.J. (1984) The pharmacology of dietary nitrate and the origin of urinary nitrate. *Food Chem. Toxicol.* (in press)

Blackburn, E.K., Callender, S.T., Dacie, J.V., Doll, R., Girdwood, R.H., Mollin, D.L., Saracci, R., Stafford, J., Thompson, R.B., Varadi, S. & Wetherly-Mein, G. (1968) Possible association between pernicious anemia and leukemia; a prospective study of 1 625 patients with a note on the very high incidence of gastric cancer. *Int. J. Cancer, 3,* 163–170

Dahm, D., Eichfass, H.P. & Koch, W. (1979) Cancer in gastric stump after Bilroth II resection; the influence of gastroenteric anastomosis. *Front. gastrointest. Res., 5,* 164–169

Doll, R., Payne, P. & Waterhouse, J. (1970) *Cancer Incidence in Five Continents,* Volume II, Berlin, Springer

Domellof, L. Erickson, S. & Januger, K.G. (1976) Late precancerous changes and carcinoma of the gastric stump after Bilroth I resection. *Am. J. Surg., 132,* 26–31

Hill, M.J. (1979) Role of bacteria in human carcinogenesis. *J. human Nutr., 33,* 416–426

Jones, S.M., Davies, P.W. & Savage, A. (1978) Gastric juice nitrite and gastric cancer. *Lancet, i,* 1355

Meynell, G.G. & Meynell, E. (1970) *Theory and Practice in Experimental Bacteriology,* 2nd ed., Cambridge, Cambridge University Press

Morgenstern, L., Yamakawa, T. & Selzer, D. (1973) Carcinoma of the gastric stump. *Am. J. Surg., 125,* 29–38

Mosbech, J. & Videbaek, A. (1950) Mortality from and risk of gastric cancer among patients with pernicious anemia. *Br. med. J., ii,* 390–394

Office of Population Censuses and Surveys (1980a) *Mortality Statistics, England and Wales, 1978 (Series DH5 No. 5),* pp. 34–35

Office of Population Censuses and Surveys (1980b) *Population Estimates, England and Wales, 1978 (Series PPI No. 3),* pp. 16–17

Reed, P.I., Summers, K., Smith, P.L.R., Walters, C.L., Bartholomew, B.A., Hill, M.J., Venitt, S., Hornig, D. & Bonjour, J.P. (1983) Effect of ascorbic acid treatment on gastric juice nitrite and *N*-nitroso compound concentrations in achlorhydric subjects. *Gut, 24,* A492–A493

Rudell, W.S.J., Bone, E.S., Hill, M.J., Blendis, L.M. & Walters, C.L. (1976) Gastric juice nitrite: a risk factor for cancer in the hypochlorhydric stomach? *Lancet, ii,* 1037–1039

Rudell, W.S.J., Bone, E.S., Hill, M.J. & Walters, C.L. (1978) Pathogenesis of gastric cancer in pernicious anemia. *Lancet, i,* 521–523

Schlag, P., Bockler, R., Ulrich, H. Peter, M., Merkle, P. & Herfarth, C.H. (1980) Are nitrite and *N*-nitroso compounds in gastric juice risk factors for carcinoma in the operated stomach? *Lancet, i,* 727–729

Stahlsberg, H. & Taksdal, S. (1971) Stomach cancer following gastric surgery for benign conditions. *Lancet, ii,* 1175

Stockbrugger, R., Cotton, P., Menon, G., Beilby, J., Bartholomew, B., Hill, M. & Walters, C. (1984) Pernicious anemia, intragastric bacterial overgrowth and possible consequences. *Scand. J. Gastrol., 19,* 355–364

Tannenbaum, S. (1983) *N*-Nitroso compounds: a perspective on human exposure. *Lancet, i,* 629–631

Waterhouse, J. Muir, C. Shanmuguratnam, K. & Powell, J. (1982) *Cancer Incidence in Five Continents Vol. IV (IARC Scientific Publications No. 42),* Lyon, International Agency for Research on Cancer

GEOGRAPHIC AND SOCIAL CLASS VARIATION WITHIN THE UK IN LEVELS OF SALIVARY NITRATES AND NITRITES. A PRELIMINARY REPORT

D. FORMAN, S. AL-DABBAGH & R. DOLL

Imperial Cancer Research Fund Epidemiology and Clinical Trials Unit, Radcliffe Infirmary, Oxford, UK

SUMMARY

In the study, the first results of which are reported here, salivary nitrate and nitrite levels were examined in populations drawn from regions of the UK which differ in mortality rates for gastric cancer. The aims were to see, firstly, whether there was an equivalent geographic variation for nitrate and nitrite levels and, secondly, whether within each region any socio-economic or dietary characteristics correlated with the salivary levels.

The results show that the nitrate and nitrite levels are significantly higher in residents from the Oxford region (low gastric cancer incidence area) than in residents from the north-east of England and north Wales (high-incidence areas). Further, within each area there is a noticeable relationship between nitrate and nitrite levels and age and social class. The social class trend is, as with the geographic trend, the inverse of that for stomach cancer risk.

It is felt that the explanation of these results is probably a greater consumption of fresh, nitrate-containing vegetables by people in the Oxford region and by those in higher socio-economic groups. The implications that these results have for the nitrate hypothesis in relation to gastric cancer is discussed.

INTRODUCTION

There is, as yet, no clear epidemiological evidence to implicate nitrate exposure as an etiological factor in the development of human cancer (Fraser *et al.*, 1980; National Academy of Sciences, 1981), despite the considerable amount of evidence indicating that exogenously supplied nitrates can be converted by the body into nitrites (Tannenbaum *et al.*, 1974) which, in turn, can participate in reactions to form carcinogenic *N*-nitroso compounds (Mirvish, 1975). International correlations (Fine *et al.*, 1982), regional comparisons in Chile (Armijo & Coulson, 1975; Zaldivar, 1977), and case-control studies in Chile (Armijo *et al.*, 1981a), Colombia (Cuello *et al.*, 1976) and among the Japanese (Haenszel *et al.*, 1976) all suggest that nitrate intake could be related to gastric cancer. However, whenever direct biochemical assays of nitrate levels in drinking-water or in biological fluids have been carried out, the results have not been uniformly consistent. Although there is an association between high gastric cancer risk and high nitrate content in well water in Colombia (Cuello *et al.*, 1976) and the People's Republic of China (Xu, 1982), more extensive correlational studies in Chile (Zaldivar & Wetterstrand, 1978), Hungary (Juhasz *et al.*, 1980) and the UK (Beresford, 1981; Fraser & Chilvers, 1981) have shown no clear relationship. Similarly, there is a lack of association between high cancer risk areas and urinary and salivary measures of nitrate and nitrite in Chile (Armijo *et al.*, 1981b) and Denmark (Jensen, 1982), in spite of a previous positive finding in Colombia (Cuello *et al.*, 1976).

Further studies are therefore needed involving biological measures of exposure to nitrate and nitrite. One such measure is the estimation of these ions in samples of saliva. Ingested nitrate is absorbed from the upper gastrointestinal tract, and a proportion of it is actively taken up from plasma into saliva by the salivary glands (Burgen & Emmelin, 1961). Within the saliva, nitrate can be reduced to nitrite by the action of oral bacteria (Tannenbaum *et al.*, 1976), and Spiegelhalder *et al.* (1976) have estimated that about 25% of nitrate intake is concentrated into saliva and that 20% of this is subsequently reduced to nitrite. Thus, about 5% of exogenous nitrate is reduced to nitrite in the saliva. In most diets, this is the largest single source of nitrite exposure for the normal stomach epithelium, representing about 80% of the total gastric nitrite load (National Academy of Sciences, 1981). By measuring nitrite in the saliva, one therefore obtains an estimate of exposure to the main source of nitrosating ions in the stomach. The level of this indicator will depend on several factors, such as the individual's consumption of nitrate, plasma uptake capacity and oral bacterial and salivary flow rates. It is probably, then, the best single indicator available with regard to stomach exposure. In addition, salivary samples are quick and easy to obtain in epidemiological field work, and analyses can be carried out on samples of 1–2 mL. For population studies they are therefore both theoretically and practically preferable to urine or blood samples, in which nitrite is not usually present anyway.

In the study reported here, salivary nitrate and nitrite levels were examined in populations drawn from regions of the UK which differ materially with regard to incidence and mortality rates of gastric cancer. The aims were to see, firstly, whether there was an equivalent geographic variation for the nitrate/nitrite levels and, secondly, whether within each region any socio-economic or dietary characteristics correlated with the salivary levels.

MATERIALS AND METHODS

Selection of areas

When the study is complete, populations drawn from four areas of England and Wales will have been compared–two with a high incidence of gastric cancer and two with a low incidence. The results reported below are findings from the two high-incidence areas and from one of the low-incidence areas. Areas were selected in which there were consistently high (or low) stomach cancer mortality rates for people of both sexes over the period 1950–1979. The chosen areas were situated in regions where the overall stomach cancer mortality was also correspondingly high (or low).

Selection of subjects

Individuals accompanying friends and relatives to hospital out-patient departments were used as the study population. Anyone attending the hospital, but not as a patient, who was aged between 15 and 65 years was approached and asked to participate in the study. If they agreed, they were asked to provide a 1-mL saliva sample and to complete a questionnaire about personal characteristics, including occupation, dietary habits with respect to a number of food items high in nitrate and/or nitrite content, and a list of all food and drink taken on the day of sampling, together with the time it was consumed. Over 90% of those asked agreed to take part. The subjects were also asked to give identifying details so that they could be followed up if necessary.

In total, between 200 and 230 samples were taken from each area. Subsequently, anyone found not to be resident of the a ea was excluded from the analysis. Also excluded was any person who had eaten or drunk during the two hours prior to sampling. This exclusion was necessary to control for the short-term rise in salivary nitrate concentration that occurs shortly after ingestion.

Saliva analysis

Saliva was collected into cleaned glass scintillation tubes onto which a film of sodium hydroxide had been oven-baked. The amount of sodium hydroxide used was calculated to give a 0.1 mol/L final concentration when dissolved in 1 mL saliva and was added as a preservative for the nitrate and nitrite, the alkaline pH killing any oral bacteria and thus preventing any subsequent reduction or utilization. Preserved in this way, nitrate and nitrite levels remained stable for at least a month.

Nitrite was determined by a modification of the Griess procedure, in which nitrate is bacterially reduced to nitrite prior to determination (Phizackerley & Al-Dabbagh, 1983). By estimating total nitrite, with and without nitrate reduction, the concentration of nitrate alone can be calculated from the difference.

RESULTS

Table 1 shows, for each of the three areas considered, the mortality rates for gastric cancer, together with the mean salivary nitrate and nitrite levels after the exclusions described above had been made. Whereas there is no significant difference between the two high-incidence areas, the nitrate and nitrite levels for Oxford are significantly higher than those in north-east England and north Wales ($p < 0.001$ for Oxford versus north-east and for Oxford versus north Wales for both nitrate and nitrite). Table 2 shows that this regional difference occurs for people of both sexes and that there is no difference between the sexes within each region (with the exception of a non-significant increase in nitrate levels for females in the north-east). The effect of age on nitrate and nitrite levels is shown in Table 3. There is a tendency for both levels to increase with age in all three areas, the trends for regression being significant in all cases, except for nitrate in Wales.

Table 4 gives the results broken down by social class and also indicates the relationship between social class and gastric cancer incidence. There is a slight but consistent relationship between social class and both nitrate and nitrite, the levels of which are increased in the professional social class groups I and II and diminished in the semi-skilled and unskilled groups IV and V.

As there may be seasonal effects on salivary measures, Table 5 shows a comparison of samples collected in Oxford in spring/summer and those collected in winter. There is no significant difference between them.

Table 1. Mean salivary nitrate and nitrite concentrations (log μmol/L ± SE) for populations from three areas in the UK

Area	Collecting site(s)	Gastric cancer regional SMR[a] (1979)		Gastric cancer site SMR[b] (1969–1973)		Nitrate	Nitrite	N
		M	F	M	F			
Oxfordshire	Oxford	86	79	71	43	2.26 (±0.04)	2.01 (±0.03)	93
North-East England	Sunderland & Hartlepool	116	125	140 & 201	168 & 172	1.90 (±0.05)	1.82 (±0.04)	84
North Wales	Bangor & Llandudno	124	128	187	111	2.00 (±0.05)	1.73 (±0.04)	80

[a] Regional standardized mortality ratios (SMR) obtained from Office of Population Censuses & Surveys (1981a) for Oxfordshire & Northern regional health areas & Wales, standardized to total mortality rates for England and Wales

[b] Site SMRs obtained from Office of Population Censuses & Surveys (1981b) for Oxford, Sunderland and Hartlepool *CBs* and Caernarvon *UD* (for Bangor & Llandudno)

Table 2. Mean salivary nitrate and nitrite concentrations (log μmol/L ± SE) for males and females from three areas in the UK

Area	Sex	Nitrate	p	Nitrite	p	N
Oxfordshire	Male	2.25 (±0.06)		2.02 (±0.04)		36
	Female	2.27 (±0.06)	NS	2.00 (±0.05)	NS	57
North-East England	Male	1.76 (±0.11)		1.83 (±0.06)		26
	Female	1.95 (±0.05)	NS	1.82 (±0.04)	NS	61
North Wales	Male	2.00 (±0.07)		1.75 (±0.06)		29
	Female	1.99 (±0.06)	NS	1.72 (±0.06)	NS	51

NS, not significant

Table 3. Mean salivary nitrate and nitrite concentrations (log μmol/L ± SE) for three age groups (15–34, 35–54, 55+) from three areas in the UK

Area	Age	Nitrate	p[a]	Nitrite	p[a]	N
Oxfordshire	15–34	2.19 (±0.07)	<0.05	1.94 (±0.05)	<0.05	39
	35–54	2.26 (±0.07)		2.01 (±0.04)		41
	55+	2.48 (±0.10)		2.22 (±0.08)		13
North-East England	15–34	1.75 (±0.09)	<0.05	1.69 (±0.05)	<0.01	28
	35–54	1.94 (±0.07)		1.86 (±0.06)		35
	55+	2.04 (±0.10)		1.96 (±0.07)		21
North Wales	15–34	1.87 (±0.06)	NS	1.59 (±0.06)	<0.05	34
	35–54	2.14 (±0.06)		1.83 (±0.05)		35
	55+	1.92 (±0.20)		1.82 (±0.14)		11

[a] Significance test for regression; NS, not significant

Table 4 A. Mean salivary nitrate and nitrite concentrations (log μmol/L ± SE) for three social class groupings from three comparison areas in the UK

Area	Social class	Nitrate	p[a]	Nitrite	p[a]	N
Oxfordshire	I & II	2.43 (±0.08)	<0.05	2.06 (±0.06)	NS	18
	III	2.18 (±0.07)		1.96 (±0.05)		39
	IV & V	2.14 (±0.07)		1.94 (±0.08)		17
North-East England	I & II	2.06 (±0.10)	NS	1.94 (±0.11)	NS	8
	III	1.96 (±0.07)		1.83 (±0.05)		40
	IV & V	1.81 (±0.08)		1.83 (±0.08)		19
North Wales	I & II	2.03 (±0.11)	NS	1.81 (±0.08)	NS	19
	III	2.04 (±0.07)		1.72 (±0.07)		26
	IV & V	1.87 (±0.12)		1.65 (±0.10)		17

[a] Significance test for regression; NS, not significant

Table 4 B. Relationship between social class and stomach cancer mortality in England and Wales, for males in 1971[a]

Class	Title	Examples	Stomach cancer SMR
I	Professional	Doctors	50
II	'Intermediate'	Managers, Teachers	66
III	Skilled manual & non-manual	Engineers	79/118
IV	Semi-skilled	Agricultural workers	125
V	Unskilled	Labourers	147

[a] From Logan (1982)

Table 5. Mean salivary nitrate and nitrite concentrations (log μmol/L $\pm$ SE) in Oxfordshire according to season of collection

Season	Nitrate	Nitrite	N
Spring/summer	2.28 ($\pm$ 0.05)	2.03 ($\pm$ 0.04)	66
Winter	2.21 ($\pm$ 0.08)	1.96 ($\pm$ 0.06)	27

DISCUSSION

The most notable feature of these results is that, despite the enormous individual variation known to exist in measures of salivary nitrate and nitrite (Spiegelhalder *et al.*, 1976; Al-Dabbagh[1], there are quite clear differences between Oxford and the other two areas, and within each area there is a consistent relationship with age and social class. The inter-area comparison is statistically highly significant, and the regression for the age relationship is significant for all areas for nitrite and for all, except Wales, for nitrate. Although the regression for the social class relationship is largely non-significant, the trends are all in the same direction for both nitrite and nitrate. The age effect might have been predicted on the basis of previous work (Eisenbrand *et al.*, 1980), but it is surprising that the comparison between areas and the social class effects all indicate a trend which is the opposite of that for stomach cancer.

These results could be thought of as representing base-line levels for nitrate and nitrite. Exactly what factors are responsible for causing such differences between population groups is unclear, although any short-term effects due to eating and drinking prior to sampling have been removed. It might be suggested, though, that a combination of long-term dietary effects, oral hygiene and other factors leads to a mean base-line level of salivary nitrate and nitrite which varies with area of residence, age and social class. Oral hygiene is particularly important as far as nitrite is concerned, as lower standards of oral health lead to increased bacterial colonization of the mouth and hence increased potential for nitrite formation.

An inverse relationship between stomach cancer risk and salivary nitrite has been found previously in Chile (Armijo *et al.*, 1981b), and a recent unpublished study in Colombia[2] showed

---

[1] Unpublished data
[2] Shaheen *et al.*, personal communication

higher salivary nitrate rates in low-incidence areas. As urinary nitrate did correlate with cancer risk in that study, it could be argued that the analysis should properly be carried out on urine samples. However, although 24h collections are better for estimating short-term exposure to nitrate[1], as stated earlier, salivary levels, particularly of nitrite, may give the best indication of long-term nitrosating ions that actually reach the normal stomach mucosa.

A further objection to the results could be that as the collections were made in the different areas at different times of the year, seasonality could affect the salivary levels. Salivary flow rates and hence dilution are affected by temperature (Eisenbrand *et al.*, 1980), and dietary patterns vary with season. However, these factors have no effect on the results from Oxford (Table 5), which is the only area for which the collection of samples at different seasons has been completed.

If these data are valid, as we suspect they are, they immediately pose two questions: namely, what factors give rise to the observed differences and what are the implications of the data for the etiology of stomach cancer? The most plausible answer to the first derives from the fact that in the UK, as in most developed countries, the biggest single source of exogenous nitrate intake is fresh vegetables (Walters, 1980).Long-term regional and social class differences in their consumption especially of those with high nitrate content such as lettuce, cabbage, spinach and beetroot, could explain some of the observed effects. There is some evidence that such vegetables are consumed more in the south of England and by the upper social class groups than in the north of the UK and by lower class groups[2]. We are at the moment analysing our results in relation to information on dietary habits supplied by the completed questionnaires in order to examine this point in more detail.

Consideration of the source of nitrate is relevant also to the second question. It may be that total exposure to nitrate, as assayed by these measures of salivary content, is not the critical variable. It might be necessary to consider the derivation of nitrate intake-nitrate in drinking-water or added as a food preservative being more harmful than that from vegetables, which comes with associated protective factors, notably ascorbic acid. With this in mind we are making parallel determinations of nitrate in drinking-water from the houses of our participants to see whether these relate to the salivary results or to the gastric cancer rates or to neither.

It is possible also that the regional and social class variations in incidence of the disease bear no relationship to nitrate exposure but are brought about by other factors , possibly also dietary in origin, which facilitate the development of precursor lesions. According to Tannenbaum (1983), *N*-nitroso compounds might act at a late stage in a multistage process, and the epidemiological trends could be due to early-stage events that lead to gastritis and associated conditions. Once these have developed, even very low levels of nitrate-related exposure to *N*-nitroso compounds may induce the development of tumours.

A further factor to be considered is that whereas the order of magnitude of the levels of nitrate that we found (equivalent to 4.9-11.4 mg/L) is in keeping with those in published surveys of salivary nitrate in the US (24.0 mg/L) (Tannenbaum *et al.*, 1974), Italy (13.2 mg/L) (Amadori *et al.*, 1980) and parts of Colombia (1.5-13.2 mg/L) (Cuello *et al.*, 1976), in other reports nitrate levels are much greater. Thus, in Japan, Ishiwata *et al.* (1975) reported a mean level of 65.0 mg/L, and in the Federal Republic of Germany, Spiegelhalder *et al.* (1976) found mean levels of 74.0 mg/L. This discrepancy could be technical, or it could mean that there are locations where exposure to nitrate is much greater than any in the UK. If so, then the etiological relationship between nitrates and cancer could be considerably stronger in such 'hot spots'.

Finally, it can always be objected that the exposures relevant to present gastric cancer rates occurred 20–30 years ago. Although both the geographic and social class differences within the

---

[1] Wagner unpublished data
[2] Nelson, personal communication

UK have been consistent and long standing, it remains possible that the cause of the variability has been eliminated over the past few decades, and this will be reflected in mortality rates in the future. While such a hypothesis is currently untestable, it would be overcomplacent to assume it to be true and to neglect epidemiological research on what still remains, despite declining incidence rates, a major cause of death.

REFERENCES

Amadori, D., Ravaioli, A. Gardini, A. Liverani, M., Zoli, W., Tonelli, B., Ridolfi, R. & Gentilini, P. (1980) *N*-Nitroso compound precursors and gastric cancer: Preliminary data of a study on a group of farm workers. *Tumori, 66,*145–152

Armijo, R. & Coulson, A.H. (1975) Epidemiology of stomach cancer in Chile - The role of nitrogen fertilisers. *Int. J. Epidemiol., 4,* 301–309

Armijo R., Orellana, M., Medina, E., Coulson, J.W., Sayre, J.W. & Detels, R. (1981a) Epidemiology of gastric cancer in Chile, I. Case control study. *Int. J. Epidemiol., 10,* 53–56

Armijo, R., Gonzales, A., Orellana, M., Coulson, A.H., Sayre, J.W. & Detels, R. (1981b) Epidemiology of gastric cancer in Chile, II. Nitrate exposures and stomach cancer frequency. *Int. J. Epidemiol., 10,* 57–62

Beresford, S.A.A. (1981) The relationship between water quality and health in the London area. *Int. J. Epidemiol., 10,* 103–115

Burgen, A.S.V. & Emmelin, N.G. (1961) *Physiology of the salivary glands.* In: *The Inorganic Components of Saliva,* Baltimore, Williams & Wilkins, p.140

Cuello, C., Correa, P., Haenszel, W. Gordillo, G., Brown, C., Archer, M. & Tannenbaum, S. (1976) Gastric cancer in Colombia. I. Cancer risk and suspect environmental agents. *J. natl Cancer Inst., 57,* 1015–1020

Eisenbrand, G., Spiegelhalder, B. & Preussmann, R. (1980) Nitrate and nitrite in saliva. *Oncology, 37,* 227–231

Fine, D.H., Challis, B.C., Hartman, P. & Van Ryzin, J. (1982) *Endogenous synthesis of volatile nitrosamines: model calculations and risk assessment.* In: Bartsch. H., O'Neill, I.K., Castegnaro, M. & Okada, M., eds, N-*Nitroso Compounds: Occurrence and Biological Effects (IARC Scientific Publications No. 41),* Lyon, International Agency for Research on Cancer, pp. 379–396

Fraser, P., Chilvers, C., Beral, V.& Hill, M.J. (1980) Nitrate and human cancer: A review of the evidence. *Int. J. Epidemiol., 9,* 3–11

Fraser, P., & Chilvers, C. (1981) Health aspects of nitrate in drinking water. *Sci. total Environ., 18,* 103–115

Haenszel, W., Kurihara, M., Locke, F.B., Shimuzu, K & Segi, M. (1976) Stomach cancer in Japan. *J. natl Cancer Inst., 56,* 265–274

Ishiwata, H.I., Boriboon, P., Harada, M., Tanimura, A. & Ishidate, M. (1975) Studies on in-vivo formation of nitroso compounds (IV). *J. Food Hyg. Soc., 16,* 93–98

Jensen, O.M. (1982) Nitrate in drinking water and cancer in northern Jutland, Denmark, with special reference to stomach cancer. *Ecotoxicol. environ. Saf., 6,* 258–267

Juhasz, L., Hill, M.J. & Nagy, G. (1980) *Possible relationship between nitrate in drinking water and incidence of stomach cancer.* In: Walker, E.A., Griciute, L. Castegnaro, M. & Börzönyi, M., eds, N-*Nitroso Compounds: Analysis, Formation and Occurrence (IARC Scientific Publications No. 31),* Lyon, International Agency for Research on Cancer, pp. 619–623

Logan, W.P.D. (1982) *Cancer Mortality by Occupation and Social Class (IARC Scientific Publications No. 36/Studies on Medical and Population Subjects No, 44),* London, Office of Population Censuses and Surveys, Lyon, International Agency for Research on Cancer, 1851–1971

Mirvish, S.S. (1975) Formation of *N*-nitroso compounds: Chemistry, kinetics, and in-vivo occurrence. *Toxicol. appl. Pharmacol., 31,* 325–351

National Academy of Sciences (1981) *The Health Effects of Nitrate, Nitrite and N-Nitroso Compounds,* Washington DC, National Academy Press

Office of Population Censuses and Surveys (1981a) *Mortality Statistics—Cause 1979,* London, Her Majesty's Stationery Office

Office of Population Censuses and Surveys (1981b) *Mortality Statistics—Area 1969–73* (DS-4), London, Her Majesty's Stationery Office

Phizackerley, P.J.R. & Al-Dabbagh, S.A. (1983) The estimation of nitrate and nitrite in saliva and urine. *Anal. Biochem., 131,* 242–245

Spiegelhalder, B. Eisenbrand, G. & Preussmann, R. (1976). Influence of dietary nitrate on nitrite content of human saliva: possible relevance to in-vivo formation of *N*-nitroso compounds. *Food Cosmet. Toxicol., 14,,* 545–548

Tannenbaum, S.R. (1983) *N*-Nitroso compounds: A perspective on human exposure. *Lancet, i,* 629–632

Tannenbaum, S.R. Sinskey, A.J., Wisman, M. & Bishop, E. (1974) Nitrite in human saliva: its possible relationship to nitrosamine formation. *J. natl Cancer Inst., 53,* 79–84

Tannenbaum, S.R., Weisman, M. & Fett, D. (1976) The effect of nitrate intake on nitrite formation in human saliva. *Food Cosmet. Toxicol., 14,* 549–552

Walters, C.L. (1980) The exposure of humans to nitrite. *Oncology, 37,* 289–296

Xu, G-W. (1982) Gastric cancer in China: a review. *J.R. Soc. Med., 74,* 210–211

Zaldivar, R. (1977) Nitrate fertilizers as environmental pollutants. *Experimentia, 33,* 264–265

Zaldivar, R. & Wetterstrand, W.H. (1978) Nitrate levels in drinking- water of urban areas with high and low risk populations for stomach cancer. *Z. Krebsforsch., 92,* 227–234

N-NITROSAMINES IN SMOKED MEATS AND THEIR RELATION TO DIABETES

T. HELGASON

Diabetic Clinic, Landspitalinn, University Hospital, Reykjavik, Iceland

S.W.B. EWEN & B. JAFFRAY

Department of Pathology, University of Aberdeen, Scotland, UK

J.M. STOWERS

Diabetic Clinic, Aberdeen Royal Infirmary, Aberdeen, Scotland, UK

J.R. OUTRAM & J.R.A. POLLOCK[1]

Pollock and Pool Ltd, Ladbroke Close, Woodley, Berks, UK

INTRODUCTION

Helgason and Jonasson (1981) reported the results of an epidemiological study from which it appeared that the incidence of juvenile diabetes among boys in the Icelandic population was strongly related to the month of their birth, with a large peak incidence among boys born in October. There seemed to be no specific factor in the diet or environment of these boys which could be related to the effect observed; however, there is a tradition in Iceland of consuming massive quantities of smoked mutton during the two weeks after 23 December, and it was suggested that this intake by the parents of the affected boys just prior to conception was the cause of the observed diabetes. It was further suggested that the agent that gives rise to the diabetes might be *N*-nitrosamines from the smoked mutton and that the effect might be transmitted from the parent by way of the germ cell. Diabetogenic activity is caused by *N*-nitrosamides (e.g., streptozotocin) (Rossini *et al.*, 1977), *N*-nitroso-*N*-methylurea (Wilander & Tjälve, 1975) and *N*-ethyl-*N*-nitrosourea (Anderson *et al.*, 1975), but no study had been made of *N*-nitrosamines in relation to diabetogenicity.

Trials in which mice were fed Icelandic smoked mutton gave support to the hypothesis that was based on the epidemiological work cited above (Helgason *et al.*, 1982). A similar relationship with the induction of diabetes in young male mice could be established following parental ingestion of the smoked mutton for only ten days before mating. There was also some evidence that the proportion of diabetic progeny was greater when the parents were fed the mutton both before and after mating. Under the latter experimental condition, some female offspring also became affected. We now report the identification of the major *N*-nitrosamines in this material and other smoked meats, and preliminary studies of their administration to mice.

EXPERIMENTAL

Animal tests

CDI mice (Charles River UK, LTD), which are not prone to spontaneous diabetes, were used in this investigation. They were fed a diet containing less than 0.2 μg/kg *N*-nitrosamines (SDS Ltd, Witham, Essex, UK) and water *ad libitum*. The carbohydrate tolerance of all mice was checked before injection of *N*-nitrosamines. Male and female mice aged two to three days, four weeks and six weeks were injected intraperitoneally with 3-nitrosothiazolidine-4-carboxylic acid (NTCA) (125 mg/kg) and *N*-nitrosothiazolidine (NTHZ) (91 mg/kg) in water (the molar equivalents of 200 mg/lg streptozotocin). The four- and six-week-old mice were bled under pentobarbital sodium anaesthesia at one, two, three and seven weeks after injection, and the neonatal mice were treated in the same way at four, five, six and seven weeks. Controls of each sex were litter mates which had not been exposed to *N*-nitrosamines. Single-point glucose tolerance tests were done after an 18-h overnight fast. A 200 g/L aqueous solution of glucose (2 g/kg body weight) was injected intraperitoneally, and blood was taken from a periorbital venous plexus 90 min later for plasma glucose measurement with a Beckman Glucose Analyser 2.

N-*Nitrosothiazolidine*

NTHZ was prepared by the method of Ray (1978). It had a boiling-point of 62-7°C at 0.2 mm Hg; mass spectrum, m/z 118 (M^+, 21.4%); 88 (M-30, 100%); 60 (57.1%); 42 (44.6%); 30 (10.7%).

3-Nitrosothiazolidine-4-carboxylic acid (NTCA)

A solution of cysteine (5 g) in water (10 mL) was mixed with formaldehyde (7.5 g of a 30% aqueous solution). There was an exothermic reaction, after which thiazolidine-4-carboxylic acid crystallized out. A solution of sodium nitrite (2.8 g) was added to the resulting mixture, which was heated until complete dissolution. After 15 min, the solution was acidified with sulfamic acid (4.0 g), and the product was extracted with ether (40 mL). The ethereal phase was dried (sodium sulfate) and evaporated to dryness. The solid product was recrystallized from dichloromethane to obtain NTCA (3 g); melting-point 180°C. Found: C, 29.88; H, 3.65; N, 17.17; S, 19.49%. $C_4H_6N_2O_3S$ requires: C, 29.62; H, 3.7; N, 17.28; S, 19.75%. Mass spectrum, m/z 162 (0.5%, M^+); 132 (11.6%, M-NO); 88 (100%, M-NO-CO_2); 60 (80%); 42 (12%).

Analysis of volatile N-*nitrosamines in meats and aqueous solutions in which meats had been boiled*

The meat (50 g) was mixed with water (250 g) in a Waring blender and comminuted for 2 min. The mixture was made up with water to 400 g, mixed and filtered. The filtrate (100 g) was treated with *N*-nitrosodipropylamine (NDPA) (150 ng in 0.5 mL ethanol), sodium chloride (10 g) and dichloromethane (20 mL), and the mixture was shaken mechanically for 15 min. The mixture was transferred to a separating funnel and allowed to stand for 5 min. The bottom layer (dichloromethane, usually emulsified) was drawn off and centrifuged for 2 min at 2 000 rpm. The aqueous phase was sucked off and discarded. The dichloromethane layer, together with any small residual amount of emulsion, was treated with sodium sulfate (4 g), and the dichloromethane layer was decanted. The dichloromethane was evaporated in such a way that the temperature never exceeded 40°C, to a final volume of 0.2 mL. Of this, 5 μL were injected onto a column of 10% Carbowax 20M on Diatomite C-AW-DMCS maintained at 150°C, using argon as carrier gas; N-nitrosamines were analysed in the effluent gas stream using a Thermal Energy Analyzer (Thermo Electron Corp.). The ratios of the heights of the peaks due to the meat nitrosamines to the height of the peak due to NDPA were calculated. Calibration lines were constructed by adding known quantities of the appropriate N-nitrosamines to similar meat containing little N-nitrosamine and working up as described above. The ratios of the heights of the peaks due to the individual N-nitrosamines to those of the relevant NDPA peaks were plotted against the concentrations of the N-nitrosamines added. From these calibration lines and the peak height ratios (meat nitrosamines: NDPA), the concentrations of the N-nitrosamines in the aqueous extracts of the meats were calculated, and the result multiplied by 8 to obtain the concentrations in the meats themselves. For the liquids in which the meats had been boiled, the concentrations were found as described for the aqueous extracts of meats, and calculated as in meat by allowing for the quantity of meat cooked and the volume of water remaining after the cooking was finished.

Analysis for acidic non-volatile N-*nitrosamines*

These were analysed in 10 g of the aqueous meat extract, prepared as described above, or in the cooking waters (10 g), by the method of Pollock (1981).

Cooking of meats

The meat was covered with a known quantity of water and the mixture was brought to the boil. It was simmered for 1.5 h, and the mixture was allowed to cool. The aqueous phase was decanted.

Identity of NTHZ from meat with synthetic NTHZ

The peak observed in gas chromatograms of extracts from meats was found to be indistinguishable from that due to synthetic NTHZ when using Carbowax 20M or OV 225 as the stationary phase.

Identity of methylated NTCA of meat with synthetic NTCA methyl ester

The dichloromethane solution of the N-nitrosoamino acids was methylated with diazomethane and examined by gas-chromatography using OV 17 or OV 225. The retention times of one of the peaks due to the substances from the meat were identical with those on the same columns obtained from synthetic NTCA methyl ester, and mixtures of the natural and synthetic substances could not be resolved. When gas chromatographed on Carbowax 20M on Diatomite C-AW-DMCS, the methyl esters of the natural and the synthetic products failed to emerge even after 1 h at 200°C. We are grateful to Dr R. Massey for the information that, under the high-performance liquid chromatographic conditions used by Massey *et al.* (1982) for the separation of free N-nitrosoamino acids, extracts of these meats gave a peak response at the same retention time as did synthetic NTCA.

Volatile and non-volatile N-*nitrosamines in fluids and organs from mice to which* N-*nitrosamines had been administered*

Organs were treated as described above for the meats, body fluids as aqueous extracts of meats, and the litter on which mice had been kept by extracting with water prior to analysis as described for aqueous extracts.

Study of metabolites of NTHZ in urine and litter

Dichloromethane extracts prepared from urine and litter as described above for acidic non-volatile nitrosamines, were examined by gas chromatography on OV 225 (isothermally at 140°C for 7 min, then rising at 2°C/min). Whether the extracts were methylated or not, peak responses were observed with materials from animals to which NTHZ had been administered, at retention times of 1.8 min (NTHZ), 21.5 min (metabolite A) and 27.3 min (metabolite B). When a methylation step was included, a peak due to *N*-nitrosoproline (NPRO) was observed (retention time, 7.8 min), and sometimes a peak due to NTCA (retention time, 8.3 min). When NTHZ was treated for 2 min with hydrogen peroxide (1 equivalent) and the mixture worked up in the same way, peak responses were observed at the positions of metabolites A and B. These were quantified (as NTHZ equivalent) in the urines and litter extracts, assuming that their response to the Thermal Energy Analyzer was molar. Examination of the urines and litter from animals to which NTCA had been administered failed to reveal substances with particularly long retention times.

Nitrosation products of thiazolidine sulfone

3-Acetylthiazolidine-1-oxide was prepared by the method of Ratner and Clarke (1937). The product (0.75 g) was treated with a solution of sodium hydroxide (0.6 g) in water (10 mL) and left for 2 h. This solution was then treated with concentrated hydrochloric acid (1.8 mL) and a solution of sodium nitrite (0.35 g) in water (3 mL). After 1 h, the mixture was extracted with ether and the ethereal solution examined by gas-chromatography on OV 225, as described above; peak responses were observed at retention times corresponding to those of metabolites A and B.

RESULTS

The volatile nitrosamines in cooked (water-boiled) and raw smoked and unsmoked mutton (all commercially nitrate- or nitrite-treated) from Iceland, and in the water in which they had been cooked, were studied (Table 1). Low concentrations of *N*-nitrosodimethylamine (NDMA) were observed in all, and larger concentrations of another *N*-nitrosamine, identified as NTHZ, were found in some of the smoked meats. Examination of the same products for non-volatile N-nitrosamines showed that NPRO was almost always present, and revealed also the presence of another nitrosoamino acid that was much more abundant in the smoked meats. This was shown to be NTCA by identity of the gas chromatographic behaviour of the methyl ester of the naturally-occurring material with that of the authentic substance on columns using three different stationary phases, and by identity of behaviour of the natural material with that of the synthetic product in a high-performance liquid chromatographic system.

A single intraperitoneal injection into CD1 mice of synthetic NTHZ and NTCA at levels of 90 and 125 mg/kg body weight, respectively, gave results, in terms of induction of diabetic response, shown in Tables 2 and 3. The treatment resulted in a highly significant rise in plasma glucose values in many of the treated animals. A diabetic response was judged to have occurred when the plasma glucose level in a treated animal exceeded the mean for the control animals by more than three times the standard deviation of the latter. No diabetic response was seen in control animals. It is interesting that there was an increased response to the *N*-nitrosamines with increasing age of the animals at the time of injection, as shown in Table 3. Further work, involving feeding of the substances prior to fertilization and study of the progeny, is required to establish a full in-vivo parallel to the results obtained with the feeding of meat. These experiments are in progress.

Table 1.   N-Nitrosamines in raw and cooked smoked and non-smoked Icelandic muttons: all meats had been treated commercially during preparation with nitrate- or nitrite-containing brine

Meat product	NDMA[a]	NTHZ[a]	NPRO[a]	NTCA[a]
		(μg/kg)		
Non-smoked				
Cooked meat	0.2	ND	ND	ND
Cooked meat	0.2	ND	ND	18
Cooking water	NA	ND	ND	22.5
Raw meat	NA		8	20.3
Cooked meat	0.2	ND	7	21.4
Cooking water	NA	ND	3	4.5
Raw meat	NA	ND	57	ND
Cooked meat	0.2	ND	41	ND
Cooking water	NA	ND	88	ND
Raw meat	NA	NA	54	ND
Cooked meat	0.2	ND	111	ND
Cooking water	NA	NA	190	ND
Smoked				
Cooked meat	0.3	ND	28	313
Water	NA	ND	21	349
Cooked meat	0.4	ND	ND	70
Water	NA	ND	ND	51
Raw meat	NA	ND	74	2 014
Cooked meat	0.6	ND	46	1 424
Water	NA	ND	36	1 125
Raw meat	NA	ND	17	61
Cooked meat	0.3	ND	15	38
Cooking water	NA	ND	4	12
Raw meat	NA	ND	53	186
Cooked meat	0.3	ND	20	84
Cooking water	NA	ND	19	69
Cooked meat	NA	ND	ND	416
Cooked meat	NA	ND	ND	183
Cooked meat	NA	18	52	1 392
Cooked meat	NA	21	73	6 760

[a] NDMA, N-nitrosodimethylamine; NTHZ, N-nitrosothiazolidine; NPRO, N-nitrosoproline, NTCA, 3-nitrosothiazolidine-4-carboxylic acid
NA, not analysed; ND, not detected

The fate of synthetic NTHZ and NTCA in the animals after intraperitoneal injection has been followed by analysing the litter on which the mice were kept, and blood, urine, bile and organs of the treated mice six and 24 h after the injections had been made. The results of these analyses are shown in Table 4. None of these or other N-nitrosamines were found in fluids or tissues from control mice. NTHZ was excreted both unchanged and in metabolized forms. The two metabolic products observed had the same retention times in gas chromatography as those of substances in a material obtained by oxidation of NTHZ with hydrogen peroxide or by nitrosation of thiazolidine sulfone, and they are believed to be *S*-oxides of NTHZ. The largest proportion of the NTHZ was recovered as these metabolic products; a large part also circulated in the blood, which no doubt explains its presence in various organs. The incomplete recovery

Table 2. Effects of 3-nitrosothiazolidine-4-carboxylic acid (NCTA) and *N*-nitrosothiazolidine (NTHZ) on plasma glucose levels in CD1 mice

N-Nitros-amine	Sex	Age at injection	Time after injection	No. in trial group	No. in control group	Significance of mean plasma glu-cose level[a]	No. showing diabetic response[b]
NTCA	F	neonatal	4 weeks	6	11	<0.05	1
			5 weeks	9	10	NS	0
			6 weeks	10	10	NS	0
			7 weeks	6	9	NS	0
	M	neonatal	4 weeks	12	7	NS	1
			5 weeks	19	7	NS	0
			6 weeks	18	8	NS	0
			7 weeks	12	7	NS	0
	F	4 weeks	1 day	20	20	<0.05	4
			7 days	14	14	NS	0
			2 weeks	11	11	<0.0005	1
			3 weeks	11	11	NS	0
			6 weeks	10	8	NS	0
	M	4 weeks	1 day	17	17	NS	0
			7 days	13	14	NS	0
			2 weeks	11	11	NS	1
			3 weeks	11	11	NS	0
			6 weeks	10	8	NS	0
	F	7 weeks	6 days	8	8	NS	0
			2 weeks	8	8	NS	0
			27 days	8	8	NS	0
			6 weeks	8	8	NS	0
	M	7 weeks	6 days	8	8	NS	0
			2 weeks	8	8	NS	0
			27 days	8	8	NS	0
			6 weeks	6	8	<0.001	5
			7 weeks	7	7	NS	0
NTHZ	F	neonatal	4 weeks	11	11	NS	0
			5 weeks	11	10	NS	0
			6 weeks	11	10	<0.0005	2
			7 weeks	11	9	NS	0
	M	neonatal	4 weeks	9	7	<0.05	0
			5 weeks	9	7	NS	0
			6 weeks	11	10	NS	0
			7 weeks	11	9	NS	0
	F	4 weeks	1 day	20	20	NS	0
			7 days	13	14	NS	0
			2 weeks	10	11	NS	1
			3 weeks	10	11	<0.005	3
			6 weeks	9	8	NS	0
	M	4 weeks	1 day	16	17	NS	0
			7 days	13	14	NS	0
			2 weeks	10	11	NS	0
			3 weeks	10	11	NS	1
			6 weeks	10	8	NS	0

Table 2   (contd)

N-Nitros-amine	Sex	Age at injection	Time after injection	No. in trial group	No. in control group	Significance of mean plasma glucose level[a]	No. showing diabetic response[b]
NTHZ (contd)							
	F	7 weeks	6 days	8	8	NS	1
			2 weeks	8	8	<0.05	1
			27 days	8	8	NS	0
			6 weeks	8	8	<0.001	7
	M	7 weeks	6 days	8	8	NS	1
			2 weeks	8	8	<0.05	1
			27 days	8	8	NS	0
			6 weeks	8	8	NS	0
			7 weeks	7	7	NS	0

[a] Significance of difference between mean plasma glucose level in trial and that in control
[b] Diabetic response: plasma glucose level exceeding the mean for controls by more than 3 times the standard deviation of the control mean. Controls gave no diabetic response.

Table 3.   Incidence of diabetes in experimental CD1 mice (as percentage of numbers of mice in each group)

Substance administered[a]	Age at injection	% diabetic[b]
NTCA	neonatal	2.1
	4 weeks	5.1
	7 weeks	7.3
NT	neonatal	2.4
	4 weeks	4.5
	7 weeks	16.4

[a] NTCA, 3-nitrosothiazolidine-4-carboxylic acid; NTHZ, N-nitrosothiazolidine
[b] See footnote to Table 2

Table 4.   N-Nitrosamine in litter, body fluids and tissues of CDI mice after administration of N-nitrosothiazolidine (NTHZ) and 3-nitrosothiazolidine-4-carboxylic acid (NTCA)

Time after injection (h)	6		24	
Sex	F[a]	M	F	M
Treatment with NT				
Litter	0.023 T	0.13 T	0.12 T	0.24 T
	0.034 P	0.06 P	15.8 TO	7.8 TO
	0.1 C	0.1 C		
	5.4 TO	9.0 TO		
Blood	16.0 T	12.0 T	16.4 T	0.3 T
	17.5 P	26.0 P		
	13.5 C			

Table 4   (contd)

Time after injection (h)	6		24	
Sex	F [a]	M	F	M
(contd)				
Muscle	3.9 T	10.4 T	0.8 P	0.3 P
	1.3 U			
	0.6 P			
	0.3 C			
Urine	0.34 T	0.012 T	0.15 T	0.03 T
	0.09 P	7.0 TO	2.2 C	3.9 C
Bile	NA	NA	0.04 T	NA
			0.3 P	
Small intestine	200 T	300 T	25 P	6 P
Large intestine	70 T	45 T	110 P	6 P
Lung	140 T	13 T	ND	ND
Pancreas	260 T	65 T	ND	ND
Liver	15 P	13 T	ND	20 P
Kidney	880 T	1 040 T	25 P	12 P
Spleen	120 T	ND	130 P	ND
Heart	80 T	20 T	30 P	ND
Ovary or testis	20 T	330 T	100 U	200 T
Treatment with NTCA				
Litter	4.4 C	84.5 C	8.4 C	8.0 C
Blood	10.2 P	43 P	50.4 C	18 C
	11.4 C	28 C		
Muscle	0.7 P	0.2 P	0.1 P	0.3 P
		0.4 C		0.1 C
		3.4 U		
Urine	11.3 C	9.1 C	0.6 C	3.5 C
Bile	1.2 P	0.1 P	1.3 P	NA
	0.8 C	0.2 C	4.3 C	
Small intestine	35 C	50 U	3 P	25 P
		15 P		100 C
		25 C		
Large intestine	13 000 C	6 500 C	3 P	15 P
Lung	40 C	20 C	7 P	15 P
Pancreas	ND	20 C	ND	ND
Liver	100 C	45 C	ND	10 P
Kidney	500 C	35 C	20 P	100 C
Spleen	90 C	5 P	6 P	10 P
Heart	35 C	ND	ND	50 P
Ovary or testis	80 U	100 U	130 U	65 T
	20 P	35 P	100 P	30 U
	20 C	15 C	90 C	45 C

[a] In one of the animals in this pair, *N*-nitrosoproline and other *N*-nitrosoamino acids were present in all organs
NA, not analysed; ND, not detected
*Results quoted as % of dose recovered in litter; μg/animal in blood, muscle, urine and bile; and ng/organ; T = NTHZ; C = NCTA; P = *N*-nitrosoproline; TO = NTHZ oxides; U = other *N*-nitrosoamino acids. Means of two animals

of NTHZ suggests that this *N*-nitrosamine is extensively metabolized to products that were not observed. It persisted in the body for longer periods than did NTCA. None of the presumed *S*-oxide metabolites of NTHZ were found other than in the litter and urines.

No metabolite of NTCA was found in the treated mice; however, the methyl esters of the corresponding *S*-oxide may be too non-volatile to be detected by the analytical procedure used.

Free NTCA was excreted quite rapidly, presumably because of its relatively high polarity; a large proportion of the administered dose was found in the litters after only six hours. NTCA also passed into the blood and was detected, albeit in low concentration, in various organs six hours after administration. Apart from the testes, no organ contained NTHZ after 24 h. When these substances had disappeared, readily observable amounts of NPRO and sometimes of other *N*-nitrosoamino acids were found, the methyl esters of which had gas chromatographic behaviours identical to those of *N*-nitrosooxazolidine-4-carboxylic acid and 5-methyl-*N*-nitrosooxazolidine-4-carboxylic acid. These substances can be formed by the reactions of serine and threonine, respectively, with formaldehyde (perhaps arising from the thiazolidines) and by nitrosation. They may thus represent a pathway for the metabolism of the thiazolidines, as may direct transnitrosation to form NPRO; but more work is needed on this.

NTCA is readily synthesized by the nitrosation of thiazolidine-4-carboxylic acid in acidic medium, and its sodium salt forms rapidly when sodium nitrite is added to a mixture of thiazolidine-carboxylic acid with excess formaldehyde in water, due to the catalysis of nitrosation by the latter. It thus seems probable that the formation of the NTCA during smoking of the meats involves the reaction of cysteine in the meat with formaldehyde from the smoke to yield thiazolidine-4-carboxylic acid, which is then nitrosated by nitrogen oxides in the smoke, or in a reaction with nitrite catalysed by formaldehyde. The NTHZ observed may arise from a similar reaction with cysteine or by decarboxylation of NTCA.

Table 5.   *N*-Nitrosothiazolidine (NTHZ) and 3-nitrosothiazolidine-4-carboxylic acid (NTCA) in various smoked foods and products prepared from them

Food	No. of samples analysed	NTHZ	NTCA
		(μg/kg)	
Smoked meat from pig	12	0–5	0–2 100
Pastes containing ham	5	0–10	68–4 400
Meat-flavoured drink	3	0	10–900
Smoked sausages	12	0–5	5.5–944
Smoked ox-tongue	1	0.4	43
Smoked salmon	3	<1	<1
Smoked oyster	1	109	167

Table 6.   *N*-Nitrosamines[a] in laboratory animal pellets μg/kg)

Sample	NDMA	NTHZ	NPYR	NPRO	NTCA
1	10.6	ND	0.3	7.0	ND
2	1.9	ND	ND	3.4	ND
3	0.3	ND	ND	279	209
4	ND	ND	ND	354	230
5	0.3	ND	ND	17.3	ND
6	2.5	ND	ND	23.5	ND
7	13.1	ND	ND	127	ND
8	15.5	ND	ND	ND	ND
9	ND	31	ND	ND	ND
Fish meal	270	18	1.8	77	372

[a] NDMA, *N*-nitrosodimethylamine; NTHZ, *N*-nitrosothiazolidine; NPYR, *N*-nitrosopyrrolidine; NPRO, *N*-nitrosoproline; NTCA, 3-nitrosothiazolidine-4-carboxylic acid
ND, not detected

The occurrence of NTCA is not limited to this particular group of Icelandic smoked muttons: as shown in Table 5, it occurs widely in smoked meats and in some smoked fish, as well as in products incorporating such meat, for instance, ham and cheese spreads and some meat-flavoured beverage preparations. It is interesting to note that some animal feeding pellets contain NTCA (Table 6); one contained NTHZ; and NPRO was usually present. Fish meal may contain especially high concentrations of these substances. Thus, results of control trials for the biological effects of *N*-nitrosoamino acids ought to be treated with reserve unless the feed has been analysed and shown to be free of such substances. The effect of the presence of these substances in the feed would be to reduce the apparent significance of any effect observed; this point may be particularly relevant to biological testing of NPRO, as this compound occurs very widely.

CONCLUSION

Icelandic smoked mutton, which has been suggested, on epidemiological and experimental grounds, to be involved in the induction of diabetes mellitus in humans, both by way of the germ cell and by effects on β cells, contains mg/kg concentrations of NTCA and some NTHZ. NTCA is found widely in smoked meats. These two substances induce significant hyperglycaemia in young mice of both sexes following a single intraperitoneal injection and enter into contact with most organs through transport in the blood. NTHZ is partly metabolized *via S*-oxides.

REFERENCES

Anderson, T., McMenamin, M. & Schein, P.S. (1975) Diabetogenic activity of deoxy-2-((((ethylnitrosoamino)carbonyl)amino)-D-glucopyranose. *Biochem.Pharmacol., 24,* 746–747

Helgason, T., Ewen, S.W.B., Ross, I.S. & Stowers, J.M. (1982) Diabetes produced in mice by smoked/cured mutton. *Lancet, ii,* 1017–1021

Helgason, T. & Jonasson, M.R. (1981) Evidence for a food additive as a cause of ketosis-prone diabetes. *Lancet, ii,* 716–720

Massey, R.C. Crews, C. & mcWeeney, D.J. (1982) Method for high-performance liquid chromatographic measurement of *N*-nitrosamines in food and beverages. *J. Chromatogr., 241,* 423–427

Pollock, J.R.A. (1981) Examination of malts for the presence of *N*-nitrosoproline, *N*-nitrososarcosine and *N*-nitrosopipecolinic acid. *J. Inst. Brewing, 87,* 356

Ratner, S. & Clarke, H.T. (1937) The action of formaldehyde upon cysteine. *J. Am. chem. Soc., 59,* 200

Ray, S. (1978) Direct gas chromatographic analysis of cyclic *N*-nitrosamines. *J. Chromatogr., 153,* 173–179

Rossini, A.A., Like, A.A., Chick, W.L., Appel, M.C. & Cahill, F.C., Jr (1977) Studies of streptozotocin-induced insulitis and diabetes. *Proc. natl Acad. Sci. USA, 74,* 2485–2489

Wilander, E. & Tjälve, H. (1975) Uptake of labelled-*N*-nitrosomethylurea in the pancreatic islets. *Virchows Arch. Pathol Anat. Histol., 367,* 27–33

NITRATE AND NITRITE IN SALIVA AND URINE OF INHABITANTS OF AREAS OF LOW AND HIGH INCIDENCE OF CHOLANGIOCARCINOMA IN THAILAND

S. SRIANUJATA, L. TANGBANLEUKAL & S. BUNYARATVEJ

Research Center and Department of Pathology, Faculty of Medicine, Ramathobidi Hospital, Bangkok 10400, Thailand

A. VALYASEVI

Institute of Nutrition, Mahidol University, Bangkok 10400, Thailand

SUMMARY

Cholangiocarcinoma is one of the main liver diseases in northeast Thailand. Associations with exposure to liver fluke and N-nitrosodimethylamine in formation of the tumour have been demonstrated in animals. This study was carried out to compare possible endogenous formation of N-nitroso compounds in inhabitants of areas with low and high incidences of cholangiocarcinoma by examining the levels of nitrate and nitrite in their saliva and urine. Thirty-two subjects (16 males and 16 females) living in the north-east (high incidence) and 12 volunteers (6 males and 6 females) in Bangkok (low incidence) were allowed to take regular meals, and their saliva and urine were collected before, and 30, 60 and 120 min after each meal. Nitrate and nitrite concentrations in saliva of the group in the high-incidence area were significantly higher than those of the group in Bangkok: salivary nitrate was 2–2.8 times higher and nitrite 2–5.6 times higher in the north-eastern group when compared with levels at each corresponding time interval in the low-incidence group. Nitrate levels in urine were also significantly higher in the north-eastern group at some time intervals, but urinary nitrite levels were similar and very low in both groups throughout the day. This finding may indicate a greater possibility of in-vivo formation of N-nitroso compounds in the north-east area than in Bangkok and might be associated with the occurrence of cholangiocarcinoma in north-east Thailand.

INTRODUCTION

The north-east region of Thailand has the highest rate of primary liver-cell carcinoma in the country, and the occurrence of cholangiocarcinoma is twice that of hepatocellular carcinoma (Bunyaratvej *et al.*, 1981). The incidence of liver fluke infection caused by *Opisthorchis viverrini* is also highest and is confined to that region, due to the habit of eating raw fresh-water fish infected with metacercaria (Harinasuta & Vajarasathira, 1959, 1960). Associations between exposure to liver flukes and cholangiocarcinoma in the endemic areas have been reported (Bhamarapravati & Viranuvatti, 1966; Viranuvatti, 1972). Other associated causal factors have been thought to include *N*-nitroso compounds. Recently, Thamavit *et al.* (1978) studied the interactions between liver fluke and *N*-nitrosodimethylamine (NDMA) in Syrian golden hamsters and found that the animals which received 25 µg/kg of diet NDMA orally plus parasites developed cholangiocarcinoma (100%) and cholangiofibrosis (100%), while the tumour was not observed in the group that received either NDMA or parasites alone.

It was our intention to evaluate the possible involvement of *N*-nitroso compounds in the occurrence of cholangiocarcinoma in Thailand since, recently, the in-vivo formation of this group of carcinogens has been receiving much attention. As nitrite in saliva appears to be one of the prominent factors in the endogenous formation of *N*-nitroso compounds, the main objective of this study was to compare the nitrate and nitrite levels in saliva and urine of inhabitants living in areas with low (Bangkok) and high (north-east) incidences of cholangiocarcinoma in Thailand.

MATERIALS AND METHODS

Subjects and sample collection

Thirty-two subjects (16 males and 16 females) living in north-east Thailand and 12 subjects (6 males and 6 females) living in Bangkok were selected. All subjects were allowed to take normal meals, and saliva and urine samples were collected before each meal and at 30, 60 and 120 min after meals. The volume of each sample was measured, and they were immediately made alkaline by adding 4 mol/L sodium hydroxide (1 mL/100-mL sample), to a pH of about 9. All samples were frozent (–18 °C) until analysed. Food samples and water were collected randomly for analysis; the amounts of food and water ingested were recorded.

Chemicals and instrument

All chemicals were of analytical or laboratory reagent grade from BDH Chemicals Ltd (UK), Merck (Federal Republic of Germany) or Fluka (Switzerland). A Spectronic 2000 (Bausch and Lomb) spectrophotometer was used to measure colour developed in the Greiss reaction.

Methods

Nitrate and nitrite analysis: Concentrations of nitrate and nitrite in saliva and urine were analysed by the Greiss reaction, by the procedure of Spiegelhalder *et al.* (1976). The measurements were corrected for reagent and sample blank. Nitrate and nitrite in food and water were analysed on the basis of the recommended method (International Standards Organization, 1975).

Urine culture: Urine from each subject was sampled by dipping a sterile strip into it before sodium hydroxide was added, and the calibrated length of the wet paper strip was cultured on a blood-agar plate. Subjects with definite bacterial growth were excluded from the analyses of urinary nitrate and nitrite.

Statistical analysis: Student's test was used to compare the values of the two groups; statistical significance was considered to be p < 0.05.

RESULTS

The age range of subjects living in the Bangkok area was 24–31 years (mean, 26.8), while subjects living in north-east Thailand had ages ranging from 20–53 years (mean, 38.8).

The mean levels of nitrate and nitrite ingested from food by both groups at each meal are shown in Table 1. The amounts ingested by subjects living in north-east Thailand were calculated by analysing random samples of food for nine subjects; all food samples taken by

Table 1. Nitrate and nitrite ingested from food at each meal in subjects from high- (northeast) and low- (Bangkok) incidence areas of cholangiocarcinoma

Area and meal	n	Mean ± SE	
		Nitrate (mmol)	Nitrite × 10^{-3} (mmol)
Northeast			
Breakfast	9	0.503 ± 0.356	2.31 ± 0.60
Lunch	9	0.313 ± 0.156	1.81 ± 0.31
Supper	9	0.372 ± 0.161	2.58 ± 0.70[a]
Bangkok			
Breakfast	12	0.201 ± 0.086	3.42 ± 0.52
Lunch	12	0.480 ± 0.120	4.51 ± 1.45
Supper	12	0.554 ± 0.159	5.92 ± 0.83[a]

[a] Significantly different at $p < 0.05$

Fig. 1. Mean ± SEM of concentration of nitrate in saliva of 16 males and 16 females living in the northeast (△) and 6 males and 6 females living in Bangkok (○) areas of Thailand, at times before and after breakfast (B), lunch (L) and after supper (S)

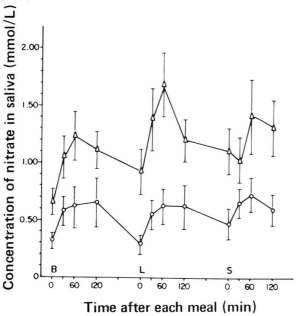

Fig. 2. Mean ± SEM of concentration of nitrite in saliva of 16 males and 16 females living in the northeast (△) and 6 males and 6 females living in Bangkok (○) areas of Thailand, at times before and after breakfast (B), lunch (L) and supper (S)

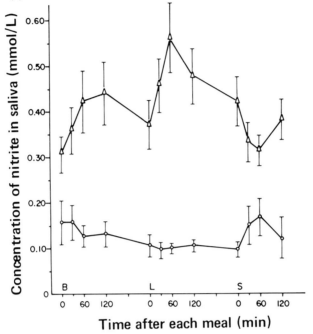

Fig. 3. Mean ± SEM of concentration of nitrate in urine of 15 males and 3 females living in the northeast (△) and 6 males and 6 females living in Bangkok (○) areas of Thailand, at times before and after breakfast (B), lunch (L) and supper (S)

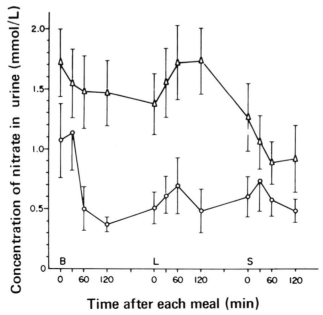

Fig. 4. Mean ± SEM of concentration of nitrite in urine of 15 males and 3 females living in the northeast (△) and 6 males and 6 females living in Bangkok (○) areas of Thailand, at times before and after breakfast (B), lunch (L) and supper (S)

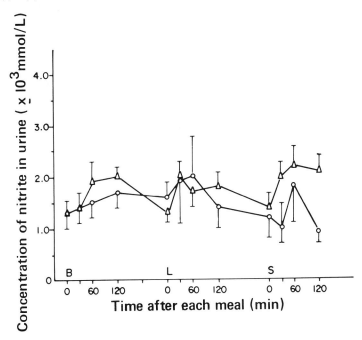

subjects in the Bangkok group were analysed. There was no significant difference in the amount of nitrate and nitrite ingested by each group, except for a higher average amount of nitrite ingested by the Bangkok group at supper.

Nitrate and nitrite levels in saliva from the two groups are shown in Figures 1 and 2, respectively. Salivary nitrate levels (Fig. 1) of subjects living in the north-east were significantly higher than those of the Bangkok group at all time intervals except 30 and 60 min after supper, although the means are still higher for the north-eastern group. The highest level was found 60 min after lunch, and was approximately 2.8 times greater in the north-eastern group. Nitrite levels in saliva (Fig. 2) are statistically significantly different at all time intervals between the two groups; 60 min after lunch, the mean level of the north-eastern group was about 5.6 times higher than that of the Bangkok group.

Urinary nitrate (Fig. 3) levels were significantly higher in the north-eastern group than those of the Bangkok group at the corresponding time intervals, except 30 and 60 min after breakfast and at all time intervals after supper, which were non-significantly higher for the north-eastern group. The maximum difference was about 3.9 times, which was found 120 min after breakfast. Nitrite levels in urine (Fig. 4) were low at all time intervals, and the levels in the two groups were not different.

DISCUSSION

Endogenous formation of N-nitroso compounds, and particularly nitrosamines, is now believed to be in excess of any probable intake of exogenous nitrosamines (Tannenbaum, 1980). The levels of nitrate and nitrite in saliva can be used as rough indicators of the amounts ingested, although great individual variation in these levels has been reported (Okabe, 1973; Spiegelhalder et al., 1976). An increase in nitrite level may be considered to be a major factor in endogenous nitrosamine formation if precursor amines are also taken. This study shows that people who live in north-east Thailand have a significantly higher level of nitrite in saliva than those who live in the Bangkok area: the level in the morning before breakfast was higher and it stayed higher throughout the day, with peaks after each meal. This observation is in agreement with those from high nitrate ingestion experiments (Spiegelhalder et al., 1976); Tannenbaum et al., 1976; Walters et al., 1979).

The diets of the two groups of subjects are quite different: more vegetables are consumed by inhabitants of the north-east, which may be one factor that causes high salivary nitrate and nitrite in that group, even though the average amount, calculated from food analysis, was not significantly different. The other main difference in diet is that the people in the north-east consume fish more frequently than Bangkok inhabitants; fish is a component of about 80% of meals in the north-east.

The sustained high levels of salivary nitrate and nitrite in the north-eastern group could be important in the formation of nitrosamines, particularly in the stomach, and may play some role in the occurrence of cholangiocarcinoma in the region; however, more studies are required. The difference in urinary nitrate levels between the two groups is consistent with that of salivary nitrate and may be considered as supporting data for a difference in nitrate circulation in subjects in the north-east region. The very low nitrite levels in urine in both groups of subjects indicate only that nitrite may not be excreted readily in urine, although slightly elevated levels were observed after each meal.

ACKNOWLEDGEMENTS

This study was kindly supported in part by the World Health Organization, Southeast Asian Regional Office, New Delhi, India. Urine cultures were done by Dr Panida Chaiyanet's laboratory. Technical assistance was provided by Miss Rachanee Kongkachuachai.

REFERENCES

Bhamarapravati, N. & Viranuvatti, V. (1966) Liver diseases in Thailand. An analysis of liver biopsies. Am. J. Gastroenterol., 45, 267–275

Bunyaratvej, S., Meenakanit, V., Tantachamrun, T., Sriawat, P., Susilaworn, P. & Chongchitnan, N. (1981) National survey of major diseases in Thailand. Analysis of 3 305 biopsies as to year-end 1978. J. med. Assoc. Thailand, 64(9), 432–439

Harinasuta, C. & Vajarasathira, S. (1959) Study on Opisthorchis in Thailand. I. The incidence of Opisthorchis in patients of 15 hospitals in the northeast. J. med. Assoc. Thailand, 42, 593–598

Harinasuta, C. & Vajarasathira, S. (1960) Opisthorchis in Thailand. Ann. trop. Med. Parasitol., 54, 100–105

International Organization for Standardization (1975a) Meats and meat products – determination of nitrate content. Ref. No. ISO 3901 – 1975

International Organization for Standardization (1975b) Meats and meat products – determination of nitrite content. Ref. No. ISO 2918 – 1975

Okabe, S. (1973) Fundamental studies on nitrite contents in human saliva. Hikone-Ronso, 162, 165

Spiegelhalder, B., Eisenbrand, G. & Preussmann, R. (1976) Influence of dietary nitrate and nitrite content of human saliva. Possible relevance to in vivo formation of N-nitroso compounds. Food Cosmet. Toxicol., 14, 545–548

Tannenbaum, S.R. (1980) A model for estimation of human exposure to endogenous N-nitroso-dimethylamine. Oncology, 37, 232–235

Tannenbaum, S.R., Weisman, M. & Fett, D. (1976) The effect of nitrate intake on nitrite formation in human saliva. *Food Cosmet. Toxicol., 14*, 549–552

Thamavit, W., Bhamarapravati, N., Sahaphong, S., Vajarasthira, S. & Angsubhakorn, S. (1978) Effect of dimethylnitrosamine on induction of cholangiocarcinoma in *Opithorchis viverrini*-infected Syrian golden hamsters. *Cancer Res., 38*, 4634–4639

Viranuvatti, V. (1972) Liver fluke infection and infestation in Southeast Asia. *Progr. Liver Dis., 4*, 537–547

Walters, C.L., Carr, F.P.A., Dyke, C.S., Saxby, M.J. & Smith, P.L.R. (1979) Nitrite sources and nitrosamine formation *in vitro* and *in vivo*. *Food Cosmet. Toxicol., 17*, 473–479

EPIDEMIOLOGICAL ASSESSMENT OF RISK TO HUMANS FROM EXPOSURE TO NITROSAMINES

A.B. MILLER, B.C.K. CHOI, G.R. HOWE, J.D. BURCH & G.J. SHERMAN

NCIC Epidemiology Unit, McMurrich Building, University of Toronto, Ontario, Canada

SUMMARY

In order for epidemiologists to evaluate the 'nitrosamine hypothesis' it is necessary to develop measures of human exposure to *N*-nitrosamines – both exogenous and when formed internally through consumption precursors. Dissatisfied with indefinite findings using indirect indices of *N*-nitrosamine exposure, we have attempted to derive an index based on the known kinetics of *N*-nitrosamine formation. This has been applied in a case-control study of cerebral tumours and resulted in a suggestive finding of increased risk for exogenous but not total *N*-nitrosamine exposure. A potential difficulty with our index is doubt as to whether vegetable sources of nitrates and consequent endogenous formation of nitrites indeed result in *N*-nitrosamine exposure, in view of the possible presence of blocking agents or of vitamin C consumed at the same time as vegetables. Further work is necessary, but we hope to apply the index in a case-control study of gastric cancer currently under analysis.

INTRODUCTION

There are multiple opportunities for human exposure to nitrates, nitrites and amines, the raw materials for the endogenous production of *N*-nitrosamines. In addition, humans may be exposed from a number of sources to preformed (exogenous) *N*-nitrosamines. As some *N*-nitrosamines are the most powerful known carcinogens in animals, it is essential to develop means of assessing the risks of such exposure to man. We must recognize that only studies in humans will provide truly relevant answers.

A major difficulty for epidemiologists with this area, however, is uncertainty as to how an estimate of human exposure to *N*-nitrosamines can be derived for epidemiological purposes. It is the aim of this paper to describe the various approaches that have and can be made to assessing this problem indirectly using standard epidemiological methodology, but also to introduce a method for a more direct estimation of an index of *N*-nitrosamine exposure which is being tested in studies conducted by this unit. Once such indices have been derived and validated it may well be possible to determine much more precisely the relevance of *N*-nitrosamines to human cancer induction and—particularly important in relation to some constituents of our diet—the extent to which we should be concerned about the presence of raw materials of *N*-nitrosamine production, such as nitrites, in the foods that we consume.

METHODS

A number of methods are available to the epidemiologist to assess directly or indirectly the extent of the problem. Correlation studies of cancer incidence or mortality with estimates of population or individual exposure to *N*-nitrosamines or their precursors can be performed – for instance, studies of associations between nitrate consumption in foods and drinking-water with gastric cancer in Colombia and Chile (Cuello *et al.,* 1976; Armijo *et al.,* 1981). If it is possible to estimate past exposures, either to *N*-nitrosamines or to the constituents for their endogenous production, then case-control studies can be performed. Such studies are site-specific; the sites of potential interest in relation to *N*-nitrosamines include stomach and possibly bladder. More recently, there has been suggestive evidence of an association between *N*-nitrosamines and childhood brain tumours (Preston-Martin *et al.,* 1982). Cohort studies, in which groups of individuals identified with regard to their exposure are followed for subsequent incidence and/or mortality from cancer, are, of course, exposure-specific. The problem with these studies is to decide what particular measure of exposure to utilize. Finally, under some circumstances, it may be possible to carry out intervention studies or trials. For practical and ethical reasons, one could clearly evaluate only prophylaxis against cancer, and to do so in relation to the potential risks of exposure to *N*-nitrosamines would require an understanding of the mechanism of their endogenous production that is probably more precise than is currently available. Nevertheless, some intervention studies have already been begun on the assumption that vitamins such as vitamin C and/or α-tocopherol could interfere with the causal chain of endogenous *N*-nitrosamine production (Bruce *et al.,* 1981; Bussey *et al.,* 1982).

For all observational studies, therefore (that is, correlation, case-control or cohort), it is necessary to provide some measure of exposure. In general, these are indirect and are frequently based on questionnaires, which, for case-control studies, relate to measures of past exposure, and in correlation and cohort studies usually to measures of current exposure. Thus, the questionnaire could be designed to seek information on history of exposure to sources of nitrates, particularly in foods such as vegetables, preserved meats and meat products and preserved fish, in drinking-water – both public and non-public – and, under certain circumstances, in occupation. Interest in drinking-water derives from the possibility that nitrates found in the soil or added for fertilization enter the water table through run-off from fields. Some utilities have records of the amount of nitrates found in public water supplies; some sources of non-puplic water supplies can be expected to contain even higher concentrations of nitrates, especially in farming areas. Other exposures that may be relevant to the endogenous production of *N*-nitrosamines include intake of nitrosating drugs and of possible prophylactics such as the vitamins already mentioned. Preformed *N*-nitrosamines could be identified in exposures to certain foods, especially foods preserved with nitrites, during smoking and, under some circumstances, in occupations.

Epidemiologists are always interested in the possibility of using biochemical or other markers of exposure. It is often difficult, however, to use such markers in case-control studies, since estimates in cases may well be influenced by the presence of the disease. Further, in relation to cohort studies, markers are relevant to making estimates only at a particular point in time which is not necessarily relevant to the natural history of carcinogenesis in that individual. Nevertheless, this is an area in which epidemiologists are dependent on their experimental colleagues and one that does need further development.

We have so far made two attempts to assess indirectly the possibility that nitrates in drinking-water and food are associated with increased risk of cancer in man. Initially, with the objective of incorporating this information in the analyses of a case-control study of bladder cancer, one of us (JDB) collected detailed information from water utilities across Canada on the level of nitrate in drinking-water. We had intended to relate these data to a detailed residential history obtained during the course of the case-control study; unfortunately, that analysis has not yet been performed. However, the data were incorporated in a detailed evaluation of the correlation of incidence of various cancers at the census district level in Canada derived from the period 1969–1973, with a number of environmental variables (Sherman, 1981). It was found that high incidence of stomach cancer in males but not in females and of breast cancer in females were associated with nitrate levels in drinking-water that were greater than 1 mg/L. These associations are highly significant; perhaps the only surprising thing about them was the association with breast cancer as well as with stomach cancer. It was also found that low levels of nitrate in drinking-water are predictive of low incidence of colon cancer in males and females and of rectal cancer in females but not in males. Although the nitrate variables were incorporated in a regression equation and contributed to the extent to which this equation is predictive of cancer incidence, the association on its own was not statistically significant. It may be explained partly by the high direct correlation found between the incidence of breast cancer in females and colon cancer incidence in males and females. This association has also been noted in international data (Miller, 1981). No association between male and female lung cancer incidence and nitrate levels in drinking-water was found in this study.

In the case-control study of bladder cancer for which the data on nitrate were collected originally, we evaluated the effect of two potential indicators of nitrate exposure (Howe *et al.*, 1980). A significantly increased risk of bladder cancer was found for males who had lived at any time in areas dependent on non-public water supplies. If the duration of use of non-public water supplies could be used to establish a dose-response relationship, no such relationship was found for males (Table 1). For females, the results were inconsistent: there appeared to be an increased risk of border-line significance for those with up to 20 years' exposure to a non-public water supply, but no increased risk for those with more than 20 years' exposure.

In this study, we also collected information on consumption of preservative-containing meats and were able to derive an estimate of the life-time consumption of meats of this type (such as ham and sausage) and the nitrate and nitrite content of such meats; however, we could find no association with risk of bladder cancer.

One of us[1] has attempted to develop a possible solution to the problem of estimating exposures. The approach was to develop an index of exposure to nitrosamines, both exogenous and endogenous, from data obtained in questionnaires. It is based on a mathematical model and on the known kinetics of endogenous formation of nitrites and *N*-nitrosamines. In brief, the method involves the use of data relating to *N*-nitrosodimethylamine (NDMA) content of foods; NDMA is regarded as a representative *N*-nitrosamine in relation to such data. Exogenous nitrate levels were estimated on the basis of questionnaire information relating to consumption of selected food items, especially vegetables and meat products (see Tables 2 and

Table 1. Relative risks (95% confidence limits) for duration of use of non-public water supply (Howe *et al.*, 1980)

Duration (years)	Males	Duration (years)	Females
0	1.0	0	1.0
≤ 10	2.2 (1.5–3.6)	≤ 20	1.4 (0.8–2.4)
10–20	1.9 (1.2–3.2)	> 20	0.8 (0.4–1.4)
> 20	2.1 (1.5–3.2)		

[1] Choi, in preparation

Table 2.   Nitrate and nitrite contents of selected food items[a]

	Nitrate (mg/kg)	Nitrite (mg/kg)
Fresh meats	10	1
Fruits	20	0
Fruit juice	2.0 (mg/L)	0
Baked goods & cereals	12	2.6
Milk & milk products	0.5 (mg/L)	0
Water	1.3 (mg/L)	0
Vegetables		
Artichoke	12	0.4
Asparagus	44	0.6
Bean: green	340	0.6
lima	54	1.1
dry	13	ND
Beetroot	2 400	4
Broccoli	740	1
Brussels sprout	120	1
Cabbage	520	0.5
Carrot	200	0.8
Cauliflower	480	1.1
Celery	2 300	0.5
Corn	45	
Cucumber	110	0.5
Eggplant	270	0.5
Endive	1 300	0.5
Kale/collard	800	1.0
Leek	510	ND
Lettuce	1 700	0.4
Melon	360	ND
Mushroom	160	0.5
Okra	38	0.7
Onion	170	0.7
Parsley	1 010	ND
Peas	28	0.6
Pepper: sweet	120	0.4
Potato: white	110	0.6
sweet	46	0.7
Pumpkin & squash	400	0.5
Radish	1 900	0.2
Rhubarb	2 100	ND
Spinach	1 800	2.5
Tomato	58	ND
Turnip	390	ND
Turnip greens	6 600	2.3

[a] From Committee on Nitrite and Alternative Curing Agents in Food (1981), Tables 5–3, 5–8 and pp. 5–25
ND, not determined

3). On the basis of other data, endogenous nitrate formation is assumed to be nil. Exogenous nitrite intake is estimated from the same sources as exogenous nitrate intake; however, endogenous nitrite has been assumed to derive from 5% of ingested nitrate, the mechanism involving, of course, the reduction of nitrate to nitrite, much of which occurs in the saliva. Exogenous NDMA intake is estimated from the known NDMA content of selected meat products, cigarettes, alcoholic beverages and smoked and pickled fish (Tables 3 and 4). The amount of endogenous NDMA formation is assumed to be proportional to the amine concentration (which is in excess) and the square of the nitrite concentration. Under normal human physiological conditions, with a substantial daily amine intake, the equation for the formation of N-nitrosoproline (NPRO) in the stomach has been quantified (Committee on Nitrite and Alternative Curing Agents in Food, 1981) as:

$$[\mu g \; NPRO] = 0.04865 \; [mg \; nitrite]^2$$

Since the nitrosation rate of dimethylamine is about 22 times slower than that of proline (Mirvish, 1975), the conversion constant for dimethylamine (DMA) is 0.0022; therefore,

$$endogenous \; [\mu g \; NDMA] = 0.0022 \; [mg \; nitrite]^2$$
and, endogenous nitrosamine $= 0.0022 \; (exogenous \; nitrite + 0.05 \times exogenous \; nitrate)^2$

Table 3.   Nitrate, nitrite and N-nitrosodimethylamine (NDMA) contents of selected meat products [a]

	No. of samples	Nitrate (mg/kg)	Nitrite (mg/kg)	NDMA (µg/kg)
Unsmoked side bacon	9	134	12	2
Unsmoked back bacon	2	160	8	0
Peameal bacon	2	16	21	5
Smoked bacon	13	52	7	2
Other bacon	7	58	48	1
Corned beef	11	141	19	0
Cured corned beef	3	852	9	4
Corned beef brisket	7	90	3	2
Pickled beef	4	70	23	2
Tinned corned beef	3	77	24	2
Ham	12	105	17	1
Smoked ham	6	138	50	0
Cured ham	2	767	35	3
Cooked ham	9	109	17	0
Canned ham	1	44	5	0
Cottage roll	4	553	28	0
Semi-cured ham	6	73	23	1
Unsmoked sausage	2	21	7	0
Smoked sausage	6	129	12	0
Wiener	13	97	7	2
Beef wiener	3	109	7	1
Other sausage	13	20	7	2
Luncheon meat	12	42	5	1
Pickle and pimento loaf	3	51	4	0
Meat, macaroni & cheese loaf	4	75	22	1
Mock chicken loaf	6	107	11	3
Other luncheon meats	4	87	13	1
Salami	12	86	12	1
Beef salami	4	71	27	2
Bologna	20	77	19	2
Belitalia (garlic)	1	247	5	0
Pepperoni (beer)	2	149	23	0
Summer sausage	1	135	7	0
Ukrainian sausage	6	77	15	3
German sausage	1	71	17	0

[a] Values are means computed from results of Panalaks et al. (1973, 1974) and have been converted from concentrations of the sodium salt to concentrations of the ion.

Table 4.   *N*-Nitrosodimethylamine (NDMA) content of cigarettes, alcoholic beverages and smoked and pickled fish

	NDMA
Plain cigarette[a]	0.02 µg/cigarette
Filter cigarette[a]	0.0065 µg/cigarette
Beer[b]	2.5 µg/L
Spirits[c]	0.5 µg/L
Wine[c]	0.05 µg/L
Smoked fish[a]	32.0 µg/kg
Salt fish[a]	32.0 µg/kg
Pickled fish[a]	32.0 µg/kg

[a] Committee on Nitrite and Alternative Curing Agents in Food (1981)
[b] Spiegelhalder *et al.* (1980)
[c] Walker *et al.* (1979)

Table 5.   Preliminary analysis of a case-control study of adult brain tumours in relation to consumption of *N*-nitrosodimethylamine (NDMA) and its precursors

Variable	Relative risk for consumption of (categories)			
	None	Low level	medium level	high level
Exogenous nitrate (mg/day)	1.0	2.3 (1–29.9)	1.4 (30–59.9)	1.3 (60+)
Exogenous nitrite (mg/day)	1.0	1.4 (0.1–0.29)	1.9 (0.3–0.59)	1.3 (0.6+)
Total nitrite (mg/day)	1.0	1.8 (1–2.9)	1.2 (3–5.9)	1.1 (6+)
Exogenous NDMA (µg/day)	1.0	2.1 (0.01–0.09)	2.3 (0.1–0.99)	1.8 (1.0+)
Total NDMA (µg/day)	1.0	0.9 (0.01–0.09)	1.0 (0.1–0.99)	1.0 (1.0+)

RESULTS

The method described for deriving an index of nitrosamine exposure has been applied to an exploratory study of adult brain tumours. Data were derived from questionnaires on potential exposures of possible relevance to the etiology of brain tumours in a series of over 200 cases and a corresponding number of matched hospital controls. Because of the nature of the disease, in nearly every instance data on the cases were derived from proxies; when proxies were used, a proxy of a hospital control was also used. Table 5 gives the findings from a preliminary analysis, with estimates of relative risk for the consumption of different levels of exogenous nitrate and nitrite, total nitrite, exogenous and total NDMA. The only statistically significant association was with the consumption of exogenous NDMA; however, there is no indication of a dose-response relationship. The finding of an apparently greater risk for low consumption of exogenous nitrate and total nitrite than medium or high consumption levels is an anomaly which needs further evaluation. What is more, the lack of any association with total estimated NDMA also requires further investigation.

DISCUSSION

One of the major difficulties with the method used for deriving an index of exposure to *N*-nitroso compounds is the inclusion of estimated nitrate consumption from vegetables within the equations for deriving endogenous nitrite formation and, subsequently, endogenous

NDMA formation. In view of the presence of vitamin C, blocking agents and other possible protective factors for cancer in many vegetables (Wattenberg, 1979), it may be questioned whether it is appropriate to include this large vegetable component within the calculations. Lijinsky[1] suggests that the contribution of vegetables is likely to be minimal, since the critical determinant is the extent to which consumption results in sufficient concentration of nitrite in the stomach. As endogenous production of nitrite occurs largely through the salivary mechanism, he feels that this is likely to result in far too dilute a concentration to have a major effect. One possible way around our difficulty would be to recalculate our indices without including vegetables in the computations and to determine whether similar associations are found. There is clearly a need for further experimental input into evaluating the appropriateness of such indices in epidemiological studies.

Preston-Martin and Henderson (this volume p. 887) have attempted to evaluate the association between N-nitroso compounds and human intracranial tumours, basing their analyses largely on exposure to potential sources of exogenous N-nitrosamines and cured meats as well as to sources of vitamin C for protection. Their strongest association was found with maternal exposure during pregnancy to substances that contain or possibly induce the formation of N-nitrosamines. Hence, they have not gone as far as we have in attempting to derive an index, and it may well be that until such time as our index, or something derived from it, can be validated we should continue to be cautious about its application.

REFERENCES

Armijo, R., Gonzaloz, A., Orrillana, M., Coulson, A. H., Sayre, J. W. & Detels, R. (1981) The epidemiology of gastric cancer in Chile. II. Nitrate exposures and stomach cancer frequency. *Int. J. Epidemiol., 10*, 57–62

Bruce, W. R., Eyssen, G. M., Ciampi, A., Dion, P. W. & Boyd, N. (1981) Strategies for dietary intervention studies in colon cancer. *Cancer, 47*, 1121–1125

Bussey, H. J. R., Decosse, J. J., Deschner, E. E., Eyers, A. A., Lesser, M. L., Morson, B. C., Ritchie, S. M., Thomson, J. P. S. & Wadsworth, J. (1982) A randomized trial of ascorbic acid in polyposis coli. *Cancer, 50*, 1434–1439

Committee on Nitrite and Alternative Curing Agents in Food (1981) *The Health Effects of Nitrate, Nitrite and N-Nitroso Compounds,* Part 1, Washington DC, National Academy Press

Cuello, C., Correa, P., Haenszel, W., Gordillo, G., Brown, C., Archer, M. & Tannenbaum, S. (1976) Gastric cancer in Colombia, 1. Cancer risk and suspect environmental agents. *J. natl Cancer Inst., 57*, 1015–1020

Howe, G. R., Burch, J. D., Miller, A. B., Cook, G. M., Estève, J., Morrison, B., Gordon, P., Chambers, L. W., Fodor, G. & Winsor, G. M. (1980) Tobacco use, occupation, coffee, various nutrients and bladder cancer. *J. natl Cancer Inst., 64*, 701–713

Miller, A. B. (1981) Epidemiology of gastro-intestinal cancer. *Compr. Ther., 7*, 53–54

Mirvish, S. S. (1975) Formation of N-nitroso compounds: chemistry, kinetics and in-vivo occurrence. *Toxicol. appl. Pharmacol., 31*,, 325–351

Panalaks, T., Iyengar, J. R. & Sen, N. P. (1973) Nitrate, nitrite and dimethylnitrosamine in cured meat products. *J. Assoc. off. anal. Chem., 56*, 621–625

Panalaks, T., Iyengar, J. R., Donaldson, B. A., Miles, W. F. & Sen, N. P. (1974) Further survey of cured meat products for volatile N-nitrosamines. *J. Assoc. off. anal. Chem., 57*, 806–812

Preston-Martin, S., Yu, M. C., Benton, B. & Henderson, B. E. (1982) N-Nitroso compounds and childhood brain tumors. *Cancer Res., 42*, 5240–5245

---

[1] Personal communication

Sherman, G.J. (1981) *Canadian Cancer Incidence: Completeness, Correlation and Ecological Association in Selected Sites, 1969–1973,* PhD Thesis, University of Toronto

Spiegelhalder, B., Eisenbrand, G. & Preussmann, R. (1980) Volatile nitrosamines in food. *Oncology, 37,* 211–216

Walker, E.A., Castegnaro, M., Garren, L., Toussaint, G. & Kowalski, B. (1979) Intake of volatile nitrosamines from consumption of alcohols. *J. natl Cancer Inst., 63,* 947–951

Wattenberg, L.W. (1979) *Naturally-occurring inhibitors of chemical carcinogenesis,* In: Miller, E.C., Miller, J.A., Hironi, I., Sugimura, T. & Takayama, S. eds, *Naturally Occurring Carcinogens-Mutagens and Modulators of Carcinogenesis,* Baltimore, University Park Press, pp. 315–329

OCCUPATIONAL EXPOSURE TO *N*-NITROSAMINES.
AIR MEASUREMENTS AND BIOLOGICAL MONITORING

B. SPIEGELHALDER

Institute of Toxicology and Chemotherapy, German Cancer Research Center,
Im Neuenheimer Feld 280, 6900 Heidelberg, FRG

INTRODUCTION

In order to evaluate the carcinogenic risk of chemicals to humans it is necessary to estimate the carcinogenic potential as well as the extent of exposure. Dose-response studies of different *N*-nitrosamines have demonstrated the extreme carcinogenic potency of this group of chemicals. Early investigations on the occurrence of *N*-nitrosamines in the environment were focused on food and tobacco smoke; subsequent studies showed that cosmetics, drugs and household commodities (especially rubber products) may also contribute to exposure to preformed *N*-nitrosamines. The role of endogenous formation, perhaps unique to *N*-nitroso compounds, is still being investigated, but estimations of its significance and extent cannot yet be made. The results of Rounbehler *et al.* (1979) and Fajen *et al.* (1979) showed that in some industrial settings worker's exposure to *N*-nitrosodimethylamine (NDMA) and *N*-nitrosomorpholine (NMOR) may be 5 000 times greater than exposures to *N*-nitrosamine-contaminated food. Recently, several programmes have been initiated (especially in the USA, the UK and the Federal Republic of Germany) to investigate those areas in industry where exposure to *N*-nitrosamines can occur.

N-NITROSAMINE MEASUREMENTS IN INDUSTRY

Since nitrosatable amines and amine derivatives play an important role in many industrial processes, as raw materials or as components of industrial products, it is not surprising that the use, handling and production of these chemicals result in exposure to the corresponding *N*-nitroso products. A list of areas in industry in which *N*-nitrosamines are known to occur is given in Table 1. No systematic survey (e.g., by governmental authorities) has yet been carried out to evaluate all occupations with possible exposure to *N*-nitrosamines. Therefore, the fact that a working place is not mentioned in Table 1 does not mean that *N*-nitrosamines do not occur in that area.

Industries in which there is significant exposure to *N*-nitrosamines are the rubber and tyre industry, leather tanneries and the metal-working industry.

Table 1.   Occupational exposure to N-nitrosamines

Industry/Occupation	N-Nitrosamine[a]	Exposure level[b]	Reference
Metal-working industry (metal cutting, grinding and rolling)	NDELA NMOR	*** unknown	Rounbehler & Fajen (1983) Loeppky (1983) Spiegelhalder et al. (1984)
Leather tanneries	NDMA	***	Rounbehler et al. (1979)
Rubber & tyre industry	NDMA NDEA NDBA NMOR NMPhA	*** *** ** *** ***	Rounbehler & Fajen (1982) Fajen et al. (1979) Spiegelhalder (1983a) Nutt (1983)

Chemical industries:
  Rocket fuel industry
  Dye manufacture
 	
  Soap, detergent and surfactant industry
	
	NDMA
	NDMA
	NDEA
	NDMA
		
		***
		*
		*
		*
			
			Fine & Rounbehler (1981)
			Rounbehler & Fajen (1982)
			
			Rounbehler & Fajen (1982)

Amine and pesticide production	various	unknown	Spiegelhalder (1983b)
Handling of hydraulic fluids (esp. in mines)	NDBA	unknown	Spiegelhalder (1983b)
Foundries (core-making)	NDMA NDEA	** **	Rounbehler & Fajen (1982) Spiegelhalder (1983b)
Fish-processing industry (fish-meal production)	NDMA	*	Rounbehler & Fajen (1982)
Warehouses and sale rooms (esp. for rubber products)	NDMA NMOR	** **	Spiegelhalder & Preussmann (1983)

[a]NDELA, N-nitrosodiethanolamine; NMOR, N-nitrosomorpholine; NDMA, N-nitrosodimethylamine; NDEA, N-nitrosodiethylamine; NDBA, N-nitrosodibutylamine; NMPhA, N-nitrosomethylphenylamine

[b]*** >50 μg nitrosamine/day; ** >5 μg nitrosamine/day; * <5 μg nitrosamine/day. Exposure was calculated using maximal observed levels and assuming 12 m³ inhaled air per work shift

Rubber and tyre industry

The occurrence of airborne N-nitrosamines in the rubber and tyre industry was first noted by Fajen et al. (1979) in the US. Rounbehler and Fajen (1982) extended this study to a total of eight facilities. In seven of the factories, one or more of the following N-nitrosamines were detected in air: NDMA, N-nitrosodiethylamine (NDEA), N-nitrosopyrrolidine (NPYR), NMOR and N-nitrosodiphenylamine (NDPhA). The N-nitrosamine found most widely in these plants was NMOR: from just detectable levels to as much as 250 μg/m³ (process sample). NDPhA was the only other N-nitrosamine found in high concentrations (up to 1230 μg/m³); the levels of other N-nitrosamines were around or below 1 μg/m³.

A study in the UK (Nutt, 1983) revealed the occurrence of NDMA, NDEA and NMOR in factories producing general rubber goods. Levels of up to 1050 μg/m³ NDMA, 210 μg/m³ NDEA and 4700 μg/m³ NMOR (all process samples) were found. Personal monitoring showed levels in the order of one-tenth those found in the process samples.

Most of the available data on *N*-nitrosamine exposure in the rubber industry were summarized by Spiegelhalder and Preussmann (1983). Between 1979 and 1982, 24 separate surveys were carried out in 19 factories of 14 different companies in the Federal Republic of Germany. Volatile *N*-nitrosamines were detected in all factories; NDMA and NMOR were found in all tyre factories; and NDMA, NDEA, *N*-nitrosodibutylamine (NDBA), *N*-nitrosopiperidine (NPIP) and NMOR were found in all technical rubber product factories, producing belting, hose, ebonite (battery cases), rubber footwear, automobile parts, proofed rubber fabrics, sealants and latex goods.

In tyre factories, concentrations of $< 0.1–2$ µg/m^3 NDMA and $0.1–17$ µg/m^3 NMOR were detected. NDMA thus occurs at relatively low levels in the tyre industry, and these do not differ greatly in individual working places and factories. NMOR levels varied not only with working place but also from factory to factory. Overall, there were higher concentrations during tyre curing, in receiving areas, in tyre inspection and in warehouses (tyre storage). Measurements in remould and retread shops showed relatively low *N*-nitrosamine concentrations.

In some tyre factories, tubes are also produced. In areas of tube curing and storage, extraordinarily high concentrations of NDMA have been measured. In one case, all values found in a curing and inspection hall were between 50 and 130 µg/m^3, and up to 19 µg/m^3 were found in tube warehouses.

A special technique for continuous vulcanization of hoses (used mainly in Europe) involves the use of molten heat-transfer salts (molten mixture of nitrates and nitrites) as the heating medium (salt-bath curing). NDMA levels found in these areas were usually between 10 and 40 µg/m^3; in only one factory were *N*-nitrosamine levels about 0.1 µg/m^3. In one case, *N*-nitrosomethylphenylamine (NMPhA) was detected at levels of 0.5–4 µg/m^3. The highest *N*-nitrosamine concentrations encountered in this study were found during personal monitoring in injection moulding and curing of conveyor belts (up to 90 µg/m^3 NDMA and 380 µg/m^3 NMOR).

The occurrence of volatile *N*-nitrosamines in all of the rubber factories investigated indicates that exposure to carcinogenic *N*-nitrosamines is a general problem in this industry. It is associated with specific chemicals and production processes: detailed and extensive examinations showed clearly that the occurrence of specific *N*-nitrosamines is related directly to the use of corresponding vulcanization accelerators. For example, tetramethylthiuram disulfide is a product used commonly for this purpose; therefore, NDMA, its nitrosation product, is found regularly in the rubber industry. The occurrence of other *N*-nitrosamines can be explained accordingly. Knowledge of the chemical composition of a rubber formulation therefore makes it possible to predict which *N*-nitrosamines may be formed.

The extent of *N*-nitrosamine formation and their concentrations in air are also influenced by production processes and chemicals that release nitrogen oxides. An important source of nitrosating agents are transportation vehicles with combustion motors. Another example is the use of NDPhA as a retarder, which may have been the nitrosating agent responsible in most cases in which nitrosamine levels were extremely high. Since NDPhA can readily be substituted by the retarder PVI (cyclohexylthiophthalimide), considerable improvements could be achieved with respect to workers' exposure to *N*-nitrosamines. Examples of successful exposure prevention are listed in Table 2, which gives *N*-nitrosamine levels before and after substitution of NDPhA as retarder. Such measures, however, can only reduce peak levels in areas of heavy exposure. A more general solution to the *N*-nitrosamine problem in the rubber industry would require the introduction of new chemicals that cannot be nitrosated or that form non-carcinogenic *N*-nitrosamines.

The relevance of *N*-nitrosamine exposure of workers in the rubber industry must be seen in the light of results of numerous epidemiological studies, in which increased cancer risks have been described. In a publication by the IARC (1982), these studies are summarized and evaluated by an international working group. It is stated in that report that a major limitation

Table 2.   Effect of use of *N*-nitrosodiphenylamine (NDPhA) as retarder on airborne levels of *N*-nitrosodimethylamine (NDMA) and *N*-nitrosomorpholine (NMOR)

Location or process	NDMA (µg/m³)	NMOR (µg/m³)	Reference
Injection moulding	40–1 100	100–4 700	Nutt (1983)
Same without NDPhA	1–2	1–9	
Tube curing	50–130	0.3–0.8	Spiegelhalder & Preussmann (1983)
Same without NDPhA	1–2	<0.1	
Tube & tyre storage	6–20	4–14	Spiegelhalder & Preussmann (1983)
Same without NDPhA	1–2.5	2–4	
Tyre factory	0.4	25	Rounbehler & Fajen (1982)
Same without NDPhA	0.2	1	

Table 3.   Occurrence of *N*-nitrosodimethylamine (NDMA) in eight leather manufactoring factories[a]

Description of tannery	Dimethylamines used	Source of nitrogen oxides	Highest NDMA observation (µg/m³)
All operations	yes	fork-lift trucks	47
All operations	yes	fork-lift trucks	11
All operations	no	fork-lift trucks	0
All operations	no	fork-lift trucks	0
Partial-wet	recently discontinued	fork-lift trucks	8
Partial-wet	used experimentally	open-gas heaters	3
Partial-dry	no	fork-lift trucks	0.05
Partial-dry	no	none	0

[a] From Fine & Rounbehler (1981)

of the epidemiological studies is the absence of exposure-specific correlations, mainly because no historical industrial hygiene data are available. The need for systematic monitoring of the industrial environment is recognized.

Leather tanneries

In the study by Rounbehler and Fajen (1982), nine leather factories were surveyed. The only *N*-nitrosamine found in four plants was NDMA, at levels of up to 47 µg/m³; its occurrence was associated with the tanning process and with the use of dimethylamine sulfate as a dehairing agent. This chemical releases dimethylamine in alkaline processes; and airborne nitrogen oxides deriving from combustion processes (open-gas flame heaters and propane-driven fork-lift trucks) were proposed as nitrosating agents. The findings of this study are summarized in Table 3.

Biological monitoring in the metal-working industry

Attempts to measure occupational exposure to *N*-nitrosamines by biological monitoring have thus far failed. The reason is obviously the fact that the *N*-nitrosamines that have been found in appreciable amounts in the rubber industry and in leather tanneries – NDMA and NMOR – are metabolized almost quantitatively: excretion rates in the order of 0.02% for NDMA and 0.1% for NMOR have been measured in animal experiments.

The relatively high excretion rate of *N*-nitrosodiethanolamine (NDELA) – about 60–90% in rats – implies that workers' exposure to NDELA might be monitored in urine. Investigations of metal grinders who had been in contact with NDELA-contaminated grinding fluids are described in this volume (Spiegelhalder *et al.*, p. 943). Of 264 urine samples analysed, 116 showed positive results ($>0.5\,\mu g/kg$), with levels up to $103\,\mu g/kg$ NDELA. These findings indicate that biological monitoring can be used to detect exposure at work places.

CONCLUSIONS

None of these studies on airborne exposures to *N*-nitrosamines includes follow-up measurements. Only limited information is available, therefore, on the exposure of individual workers, rendering it impossible to demonstrate the contribution that *N*-nitrosamines might make to the cancer experience of workers in particular job categories. Some of the reasons for the difficulty in assessing individual exposures are:

(1) the multiplicity of exposures, arising from the variety of chemicals used at given working places and cross-contamination between jobs;

(2) movement from job to job involving different exposures;

(3) cancer excesses currently observed almost certainly result from exposures that occurred many years ago, when no exposure data were available; and

(4) no systematic survey has been carried out so far.

For future evaluations, representative data bases on individual exposure levels must be established in combination with prospective epidemiological studies. Under these conditions, it might be possible to identify risk areas and to introduce preventive measures. For retrospective studies, it is necessary to have an understanding of all factors that contribute to and influence the occurrence of *N*-nitrosamines in the workroom air.

REFERENCES

Fajen, J.M., Carson, G.A., Rounbehler, D.P., Fan, T.Y., Vita, R., Goff, E.U., Wolf, M.H., Edwards, G.S., Fine, D.H., Reinhold, V. & Biemann, K. (1979) *N*-Nitrosamines in rubber and tire industry. *Science, 205*, 1262–1264

Fine, D.H. & Rounbehler, D.P. (1981) *Occurrence of N-nitrosamines in the workplace; some recent development.* In: Scanlan, R.A. & Tannenbaum, S.R., eds, N-*Nitroso Compounds (ACS Symp. Ser. No. 174)*, Washington DC, American Chemical Society, pp. 207–216

IARC (1982) *IARC Monographs on the Evaluation of the Carcinogenic Risk of Chemicals to Humans,* Vol. 28, *The Rubber Industry,* Lyon, International Agency for Research on Cancer

Loeppky, R. (1983) *Reducing environmental nitrosamines, contamination and exposure in the United States.* In: *Das Nitrosamin-Problem,* Weinheim, Verlag Chemie, pp. 305–317

Nutt, A. (1983) Rubber work and health – past, present and perspective. *Scand. J. Work environ. Health, 9,* Suppl. 2, 49–57

Rounbehler, D.P., Krull, I.S., Goff, E.U., Mills, K.M., Morrison, J., Edwards, G.S., Fine, D.H., Fajen, J.M., Carson, G.A. & Reinhold, V. (1979) Exposure to *N*-nitrosodimethylamine in a leather tannery. *J. Food Cosmet. Toxicol., 17,* 487–491

Rounbehler, D.P. & Fajen, J.M. (1982) N-*Nitroso Compounds in the Factory Environment (Report, NIOSH Contract No. 210–77–0100)*, Cincinnati, OH, National Institute for Occupational Safety and Health

Spiegelhalder, B. (1983a) Carcinogens in the workroom air in the rubber industry. *Scand. J. Work environ. Health, 9,* Suppl. 2, 15–25

Spiegelhalder, B. (1983b) *Vorkommen von Nitrosaminen in der Umwelt.* In: *Das Nitrosamin-Problem,* Weinheim, Verlag Chemie, pp. 27–40

Spiegelhalder, B. & Preussmann, R. (1983) Occupational nitrosamine exposure. 1. Rubber and tyre industry. *Carcinogenesis, 4,*1137–1152

BIOLOGICAL MONITORING IN THE METAL WORKING INDUSTRY

B. SPIEGELHALDER, R. PREUSSMANN

*Institute of Toxicology and Chemotherapy, German Cancer Research Center,
Im Neuenheimer Feld 280, 6900 Heidelberg, Federal Republic of Germany*

M. HARTUNG

*Institute of Occupational Medicine, University of Erlangen
Erlangen, Federal Republic of Germany*

SUMMARY

N-Nitrosodiethanolamine (NDELA) is a strong carcinogen in animal experiments. Its occurrence in cutting and grinding fluids represents a major risk for workers who come into contact with those compounds. But until now it was not possible to describe the extent of *N*-nitrosodiethanolamine exposure at the workplace. Since 60–90% of *N*-nitrosodiethanolamine given by oral, intravenous, epicutaneous or intratracheal application in rat experiments is excreted unchanged in the urine, *N*-nitrosodiethanolamine should be found in the urine of workers in the metal working industry. Analyses of grinding fluids containing di- and triethanolamine in combination with up to 30% nitrite showed concentrations of up to 593 mg/kg *N*-nitrosodiethanolamine in the original, concentrated fluid and up to 90 mg/kg in ready-to-use emulsions. In preliminary investigations, it was also found in the urines of metal grinders: of 264 urines analysed, 166 showed positive results (> 0.5 μg/kg) with levels up to 103 μg/kg *N*-nitrosodiethanolamine. These results indicate that workers' exposure to NDELA can be monitored by urine analysis.

INTRODUCTION

A recent dose-response study on the carcinogenic potential of *N*-nitrosodiethanolamine (NDELA) (Preussmann *et al.*, 1982) showed that this carcinogen is far more active than hitherto assumed: doses as low as 1.5 mg/kg body weight per day significantly increased tumour incidence in rats.

These results indicate that the occurrence of NDELA in cutting and grinding fluids represents a greater risk for workers in the metal working industry than had been recognized earlier. During handling of NDELA-contaminated products, workers can be exposed by direct skin contact or by inhalation of the oil mist. In animal experiments, it was demonstrated that NDELA easily penetrates skin and lung (Preussmann *et al.*, 1981) and 60–90% of an administered dose is found unchanged in the 24-h urine of rats. This led to the expectation that human exposure to NDELA could be monitored in urine.

MATERIALS AND METHODS

Clean up of cutting and grinding fluids

About 2 g sulfamic acid was added to 0.1–0.5 of material to destroy nitrite, and the mixture was made up to 15 mL with distilled water. Extraction was done using a Kieselguhr column with 50 mL ethyl formate containing 2% methanol. The extract was then reduced under vacuum to about 3 mL and transferred to a conical flask. The solvent was evaporated to dryness under a stream of nitrogen, and the dry residue was treated with 0.3mL silylating agent *N*-methyl-*N*-trimethylsilylheptafluorobutyramide at 80°C for 2 h. The reaction mixture was made up to 1 mL with hexane and transferred into an autosampler bottle.

Clean up of urine

About 2–3 g sulfamic acid were added to 15 g urine and the mixture was extracted as described for cutting and grinding fluids. For each set of samples, a reagent blank and NDELA-spiked water were analysed in the same way as urine. The detection limit was between 100 and 500 μg/L for cutting and grinding fluids and 0.5 μg/kg for urine. NDELA was determined by gas chromatography-chemiluminescence detection. Gas chromatograph conditions were: injector, 200°C with on-column injection; column, 0.635 cm o.d., 0.2 cm i.d. × 200 cm silanized borosilica glass filled with 5% OV 275 on Supercoport 100–120 mesh; oven, 170°C isothermal.

RESULTS AND DISCUSSION

Metal grinding industry

For biological monitoring of NDELA in urine of workers, three factories were selected where diethanolamine-containing grinding fluids were in use. In two factories, the grinding fluids also contained nitrite in concentrations of up to 30% in the concentrates and up to 0.5% in the final diluted liquids (Table 1).

Product C did not contain nitrite, which explains the low NDELA concentration. In most cases, the NDELA concentrations in used grinding fluids were higher than those calculated from dilutions. Obviously, additional *N*-nitrosamine formation takes place during use.

The findings of NDELA in urine (Table 2) indicates that biological monitoring can be used to detect exposure in work places. It can also be seen that there is a correlation between NDELA content in the grinding fluid and NDELA concentration in urine. In factory 3, where product C contaminated with 1 000 μg/kg NDELA was used, none was found in urine. In factory 1, where the NDELA concentration in the grinding fluid was up to 1 600 μg/kg, small

Table 1.   NDELA-concentration in grinding fluids (μg/kg)

Product		Concentrate	Diluted
Factory 1,	Product A	8 000	40– 1 600[a]
Factory 2,	Product B₁	593 000	90 000
	Product B₂	NA	8 000–19 000[a]
Factory 3,	Product C	< 400	900

[a]Various samples from different working places
NA, Not analysed

Table 2. Frequency of NDELA-concentrations in urines of workers in the metal working industry (µg/kg)

	No. of samples	ND[a]	Concentration range (µg/kg)			Maximal level (µg/kg)
			> 0.5–10	> 10–50	> 50	
Factory 1	21	17	4	–	–	5
Factory 2						
1st Visit	140	37	40	55	8	96
2nd Visit	72	13	24	33	2	103
Factory 3	31	31	–	–	–	–

[a] ND, Not Detectable (< 0.5 µg/kg)

amounts (up to 5 µg/kg) were detected. The extremely high *N*-nitrosamine content of product B obviously resulted in a higher exposure of workers in factory 2; urine from this group of workers contained NDELA in concentrations up to 103 µg/kg. Similar results were obtained in a second survey at that factory.

In order to calculate the daily exposure of workers, it would therefore be necessary to collect urine over a period of 24 h, however, but, this was not possible in our investigation. A rough calculation of the amount of incorporated NDELA can be made from a urine volume of about 500 mL. On the basis of animal experiments (Preussmann *et al.*, 1981), it can be assumed that the excretion rate of NDELA in humans is in the order of 50%. It can be concluded, therefore, that workers' exposure to NDELA during handling of grinding fluids can be as much as 100 µg per day. It is remarkable that biological monitoring gave positive results when the NDELA contamination of grinding fluids was greater than 1 000 µg/kg. The detection limit of the analytical procedure ($\sim$ 0.5 µg/kg) makes possible a lowest measurable daily exposure in the order of 1 µg NDELA.

Metal-cutting industry

Biomonitoring was also used to detect NDELA exposure of workers in contact with cutting fluids. Urine was collected over three different time periods from 38 workers exposed to cutting fluid containing 2 500 µg/kg NDELA; however, no measurable *N*-nitrosamine concentrations were detected. This was obviously due to the low sensitivity of the analytical method, since at that time, the detection limit was only 5–10 µg/kg.

CONCLUSIONS

NDELA is the first nitrosamine for which biological monitoring has been used to detect occupational exposure. For better interpretation of the exposure data, the results should be correlated with exact descriptions of jobs and working conditions. In the limited number of working places studied, a positive correlation was seen between NDELA concentration in grinding fluids and worker's exposure. The following preventive measures might therefore be undertaken:

1. All cutting and grinding fluids should be monitored for NDELA content.
2. As a first action, the NDELA content of those products should be limited (e.g., to 1 mg/kg in the concentrate and 0.1 mg/kg in the ready-to-use mix).

3. Use of nitrite should be restricted to those products that do not contain amine precursors.
4. Hygiene at work place should be improved to reduce contact with those fluids.
5. These measures should be checked by biological monitoring.

REFERENCES

Preussmann, R., Spiegelhalder, B., Eisenbrand, G., Würtele, G. & Hoffmann, I. (1981) Urinary excretion of N-nitrosodiethanolamine in rats following its epicutaneous and intratracheal administration and its formation *in vivo* following skin application of diethanolamine. *Cancer Lett., 13,* 227–231
Preussmann, R., Habs, M., Habs, H. & Schmähl, D. (1982) Carcinogenicity of N-nitrosodiethanolamine in rats at five different dose levels. *Cancer Res., 42,* 5167–5171

RECENT STUDIES ON *N*-NITROSO COMPOUNDS AS POSSIBLE ETIOLOGICAL FACTORS IN OESOPHAGEAL CANCER

S.H. LU

Cancer Institute, Chinese Academy of Medical Sciences Beijing, People's Republic of China

H. OHSHIMA & H. BARTSCH

Division of Environmental Carcinogenesis and Host Factors, International Agency for Research on Cancer, Lyon, France

SUMMARY

Possible etiological factors involved in oesophageal cancer in various parts of the world and in certain provinces in Northern China are summarized. Evidence is accumulating that *N*-nitroso compounds and their precursors are involved in the disease in Northern China, as shown in a recent study: excretion of urinary *N*-nitrosamino acids by inhabitants living in a high- (Linxian) and in a low-risk area (Fanxian) for oesophageal cancer was compared. Linxian subjects excreted significantly more nitrate and nitrosamino acids (*N*-nitrosoproline, *N*-nitrosothiazolidine-4-carboxylic acid, *N*-nitrososarcosine) than those in Fanxian. When Linxian subjects were given 100 mg vitamin C three times a day (after each meal) together with proline, the level of urinary *N*-nitrosamino acids was reduced to that found in Fanxian. Thus, vitamin C, an efficient inhibitor of endogenous nitrosation, should now be examined in intervention trials in subjects in whom endogenous formation of *N*-nitroso compounds is elevated.

INTRODUCTION

Epidemiological investigations have shown that oesophageal cancer is widely distributed in many areas of the world, such as the southeast coastal area of the Caspian Sea (Kmet & Mahboubi, 1964), the north of Iran, Soviet Central Asia, the Transkei (Burrell, 1957), the Caribbean Islands (Martinez, 1964), Normandy and Brittany in France (Lasserre *et al.*, 1967) and the province of Honan in the People's Republic of china (Li *et al.*, 1962). Oesophageal cancer accounts for about 2% of all malignant cancers. The age-adjusted mortality rate from this cancer in China is 23.4 when compared with the world population figures presented in *Cancer Incidence in Five Continents* Vol. III (Waterhouse *et al.*, 1976) and is the world's highest, being roughly 2.5 times higher than that in Puerto Rico, the second highest rate of oesophageal cancer mortality.

Clinical and epidemiological studies have suggested that cancer of the oesophagus is associated with various factors and agents, such as excessive consumption of alcohol (Wynder et al., 1957; Higginson & Oettle, 1960), tobacco (Sadowsky et al., 1953), spices (Wynder & Bross, 1961), ingestion of hot and coarse foods (Wu & Loucks, 1951; Liu et al., 1955), poor dental state (Wynder & Bross, 1961), nutritional deficiencies (Wynder et al., 1957), lesions of the oesophagus (Crespi et al., 1979) and syphilis (Tomlinson & Wilson, 1945). Of these suspected etiological factors, alcohol and tobacco are the two major risk factors for oesophageal cancer in western Europe and North America (Schwartz et al., 1956; Wynder & Bross, 1961) but are of little importance in the Caspian area (Cook et al., 1979) and in Linxian province of China (Yang, 1980).

The situation appeared to offer promising possibilities for identifying new elements in the etiology of oesophageal cancer. For this purpose, a series of environmental studies was undertaken to identify the factors responsible for oesophageal cancer in high-risk areas. Much attention is now being paid to the determination of nitrosamines and their precursors in foods and the detection of endogenously formed nitroso compounds in urine in different high-risk areas of oesophageal cancer. This paper briefly describes recent progress in research on oesophageal cancer and nitrosamines.

DETERMINATION OF NITROSAMINES IN BEVERAGES FROM FRANCE

Cancer of the oesophagus is a common disease in some departments of France, and especially in Normandy and Brittany. In these areas large amounts of apple cider and of brandy derived from cider are produced, which are mainly consumed locally and represent a sizeable proportion of the alcohol intake in the two areas. Cider and its distillates were thus suspected of containing carcinogens that might be responsible for the high frequency of oesophageal cancer. Walker et al. (1979) determined the N-nitrosamines in alcoholic drinks and found that N-nitrosodimethylamine (NDMA) was present in most drinks tested, with the exception of wine. The level in beer was higher than that in other drinks, averaging about 2 µg/L with a range of 0.2–8.6 µg/L. Traces of N-nitrosodiethylamine (NDEA) were also detected in spirits and ciders. It was considered, however, that such low levels of volatile N-nitrosamines in the beverages could not reasonably be held responsible for the high incidence of oesophageal cancer in those regions.

DETERMINATION OF NITROSAMINES IN A HIGH-RISK AREA OF OESOPHAGEAL CANCER IN THE TRANSKEI

High incidences of oesophageal cancer were first reported in the African populations of the Transkei and Ciskei by Burrell in 1957. Since that time, many workers have investigated the possible causative factors. Low levels of N-nitrosamines were found in some plants and in tobacco pyrolysates, and a high nitrate content was measured in water collected from a high-incidence area. Du Plessis and Nunn (1969) reported that NDMA was present in samples of Solanum incanum. Low levels of N-nitrosamines have been found in food and beverages collected from both high- and low-incidence areas, with no striking differences between the two. At present, therefore, the evidence is inadequate to incriminate N-nitrosamines as the single major cause of oesophageal cancer.

DETERMINATION OF *N*-NITROSAMINES IN A HIGH-RISK AREA OF OESOPHAGEAL CANCER IN IRAN

The frequency of oesophageal cancer is high in the Caspian littoral of Iran. A joint Iran-IARC study group analysed food samples from the area for the presence of nitrosamines and volatile *N*-nitrosamines were found at levels above 5 µg/kg. However, it was concluded that volatile nitrosamines in foods were unlikely to be involved as causative agents in oesophageal cancer in the Caspian littoral.

DETERMINATION OF *N*-NITROSAMINES AND THEIR PRECURSORS IN NORTHERN CHINA

Cancer of the oesophagus is common in many areas of China and especially in the north. An extensive search for the causative factors of this cancer in Northern China was begun in 1972. Correlations were found between oesophageal cancer incidence and the presence of nitrosamines and their precursors in water and food.

Thin-layer chromatography (TLC) showed that of the 124 food samples (wheat, corn, millet bran and dried sweet potato) from Linxian, 29 (23%) contained nitrosamines, whereas only one of 86 samples from Fanxian (low-incidence area) did so. Recently, the presence of NDMA and NDEA in maize samples collected from the Linxian area was confirmed by gas chromatography-thermal energy analysis (GC-TEA). The levels of secondary amines, nitrites and nitrates in the grain and vegetable samples collected in Linxian were also significantly higher than those from Fanxian.

Nitrates and nitrites were found in most of the drinking-water samples taken from 495 wells in the Yaocum Commune of Linxian. The concentration of nitrates in well-water taken during summer showed a positive correlation with the average incidence rate of oesophageal cancer in the area ($r = 0.233$; $p < 0.05$). Similarly, a positive correlation was noted between the incidence rate of marked epithelial dysplasia, a precancerous lesion of the oesophagus, and nitrate levels in water taken in spring and autumn ($r = 0.245$; $p < 0.05$; and $r = 0.229$; $p < 0.05$, respectively) and the nitrite content of water taken in autumn ($r = 0.230$; $p < 0.05$).

Nitrates and nitrites were also found in samples of human gastric juice and saliva taken in Linxian. A significant difference in the content of nitrites in saliva was observed between patients with marked epithelial dysplasia or carcinoma of the oesophagus and normal controls (Table 1).

Enhancement by fungi of formation of N-*nitrosamines in food*

Certain foodstuffs in Linxian are frequently contaminated by fungi and such mould contamination was suspected to be a contributing factor in the elevated levels of nitrosamines in food in that area. Our investigations demonstrated that several common species of fungus, i.e., of the *Fusarium, Geotricum, Aspergillus* and other genera, not only reduced nitrates to nitrites but also increased the amount of secondary amines in food; they were also found to promote the formation of nitrosamines when a small amount of sodium nitrite was added to mouldy cornbread. Gas chromatography-mass spectrometry (GC-MS) showed the presence of

Table 1.   Nitrite content of saliva from people in Linxian with various epithelial lesions of the oesophagus

Oesophageal lesion	No. of cases	Average nitrate conc. (mg/L) (mean ± SD)	p value
Normal epithelium	45	3.17 ± 3.23	
Mild hyperplasia	43	4.50 ± 4.20	> 0.05
Marked hyperplasia	33	6.00 ± 6.60	0.01
Oesophageal cancer	38	5.60 ± 5.50	< 0.05

four N-nitroso compounds, i.e., NDMA, NDEA, N-nitroso-N-methyl-N-benzylamine and a new volatile nitrosamine, N-nitroso-N-3-methylbutyl-N-1-methylacetonylamine (NMBMAcA) (Wang *et al.*, 1980; Lu *et al.*, 1979; Li *et al.*, 1980).

This new compound was synthesized and its identity confirmed by gas chromatography-mass spectrometry; the amount present in contaminated cornbread was estimated to be 0.2–0.3 µg/kg.

When NMBMAcA was tested in *Salmonella typhimurium* strains TA1535 and TA100, a dose-related increase in the number of mutant colonies was observed when a rat-liver activation system was added (Lu *et al.*, 1980). NMBMAcA also induced 8-azaguanine-resistant mutants in V79 cells and induced transformed foci in Syrian golden hamster lung cells (Chen, 1981; Wu *et al.*, 1982). Papillomas of the forestomach were induced in mice treated with N-3-methylbutyl-N-1-methylacetonylamine and sodium nitrite for five months (Li *et al.*, unpublished data).

N-*Nitroso compounds in pickled vegetables collected from Linxian*

Pickled vegetables commonly consumed in Linxian have been found to be highly contaminated by the fungus *Geotricum candidum* Link. An epidemiological study carried out in China demonstrated that the amount and frequency of consumption of pickled vegetables correlated with the mortality rate of oesophageal cancer ($r = 0.66$; $p < 0.001$) (Coordinating Group for Research on Etiology of Esophageal Cancer in North China, 1977). Analytical studies showed that the pickled vegetables contained nitrate, nitrite secondary amines and nitrosamines; the presence of NDMA, NDEA and N-nitroso-N-methyl-N-benzylamine in the pickled vegetables was confirmed by gas chromatography-thermal energy analysis.

Extracts of pickled vegetables were shown to be mutagenic (Lu *et al.*, 1981) and carcinogenic (Lu & Lin, 1982). Roussin's red methyl ester isolated from ethereal extracts of the pickled vegetables (Wang *et al.*, 1980) may form or release nitrosating species which can react with secondary amines to form nitrosamines (Wang, unpublished data; Croisy *et al.*, this volume, p. 327). This compound was mutagenic in TA100 strain (Lu *et al.*, 1981) and exerted a promoting effect on C3H10T1/2 cells initiated with 3-methylcholanthrene. The possible promoting effect of Roussin's red methyl ester was studied in mice: those fed the compound alone, at a dose of 2 mg/day for 131 days, had no pathological lesions in the oesophagus or forestomach. When mice were intubated with N-nitroso-N-methyl-N-benzylamine as an initiator, at a dose of 1 mg/kg body weight three times, then given 2 mg/animal Roussin's red methyl ester intragastrically six times a week for 131 days, eight out of 36 (22.2%) mice had papillomas of the forestomach; histological examination showed that 51.7% of these were second-degree precancerous lesions. When mice were intubated with N-nitroso-N-methyl-N-benzylamine alone, three of 21 (14.2%) mice had papillomas of the forestomach, 21.1% of which were second degree precancerous lesions (Lu *et al.*, 1983).

These experiments indicate that pickled vegetables from Linxian can contain mutagen(s), carcinogen(s), nitrosating agents and/or promotor(s) and that their consumption may be an important etiological factor in oesophageal cancer in China.

Excretion of N-*nitroso compounds and nitrate in the urine of subjects living in high- and low-risk areas for oesophageal cancer and the effect of vitamin C ingestion*

Urine samples from about 250 subjects were collected in Linxian (high-risk area) and Fanxian county (low-risk area for both oesophageal and stomach cancer), according to three different protocols: (A) undosed subjects, (B) subjects who had ingested 100 mg *L*-proline three times a day, after each meal, and (C) subjects who had ingested 100 mg *L*-proline together with 100 mg vitamin C three times a day. The urine samples were analysed for the presence of *N*-nitrosoproline (NPRO), *N*-nitrosothiazolidine-4-carboxylic acid (NTCA) and *N*-nitrososarcosine (NSAR) (μg/24 h/person) and for nitrate (mg/24h/person). Interim results are summarized in Table 2.

In order to estimate individual exposure to endogenously formed *N*-nitroso compounds, background levels of NPRO, NSAR and NTCA were determined initially in 24-h urine of subjects living in Linxian and Fanxian. The amounts of NPRO, NTCA and NSAR excreted by subjects in Linxian were significantly greater than those of people in Fanxian (Table 2). More NPRO was excreted by subjects in Linxian who had ingested 100 mg proline thrice daily, the amounts ranging from 1.16 to 66.9 μg (mean, 12.08) per person, compared to levels ranging from none detectable to 40 μg (mean 6.78) per person in Fanxian (Table 2).

Table 2. Urinary excretion of *N*-nitrosoproline (NPRO), *N*-nitrosothiazolidine-4-carboxylic acid (NTCA), *N*-nitrososarcosine (NSAR) and nitrate in subjects living in high- (Linxian)/low- (Fanxian) incidence areas for oesophageal cancer in China (interim results)[a].

24-urine samples are collected in plastic bottles containing 10 g NaOH; 100 mL urine aliquot are stored at $-20\,^{\circ}$C prior to analysis; no artefactual formation or degradation of NPRO, NSAR and nitrate/nitrite was shown to occur over a period of less than three 8 months. During the course of this study, NTCA was found to be unstable under acidic conditions. As some of the compound may have partially decomposed during the work-up procedure, the data listed in Table 2 should be regarded as tentative. Urine samples were spiked with *N*-nitrosopipecolic acid as internal standard and analyses for NPRO, NSAR and other nitrosamino acids were carried out according to published procedures (Ohshima & Bartsch, 1981; Ohshima *et al.*, 1982, 1983, this volume) after conversion to their methyl esters by diazomethane. Samples were analysed on a tracer 550 gas chromatograph, which was interfaced to a Thermal Enery Analyzer (TEA 502).

Area/Treatment	No. of subjects	NPRO[b]	NTCA[b]	NSAR[b]	Nitrate[c, d]
Linxian					
None (LA)	44	8.35 (0–29.9)	12.71 (0–46.9)	0.62 (0–8.5)	124
Proline (LB)	50	12.08 (1.16–66.9)	11.59 (0–67.1)	0.45 (0–5.12)	106
Proline +					108
Vitamin C (LC)	48	3.50 (0–32.0)	4.54 (0–24.6)	0.27 (0–2.0)	
Fanxian					
None (FA)	40	3.11 (0–13.7)	3.06 (0–24.0)	0.24 (0–2.7)	67
Proline (FB)	56	6.78 (0–40.0)	4.13 (0–28.0)	0.46 (0–2.6)	76

[a] Evaluation by Student's t-test (p values):
NPRO: LA *vs* LB (<0.001); LB *vs* FB (<0.001); LA *vs* LB (<0.005); LC *vs* LB (<0.001); NSAR: LA *vs* FA (<0.001); NTCA: LA *vs* FA (<0.001); LA *vs* LC (<0.001); Nitrate: LA *vs* FA (<0.01); LB *vs* FB (<0.05)
[b] Mean (range): μg/24 h/person
[c] Mean $\pm$ SD (range) for all Linxian subjects: 112 ± 84 (0–518) mg/24 h/person
[d] Mean $\pm$ SD (range) for all Fanxian subjects: 72 ± 64 (0–315) mg/24 h/person

The mean amount of NPRO excreted by subjects in Linxian who had ingested 100 mg proline together with 100 mg vitamin C thrice daily was 3.5 times lower than that in subjects who had ingested proline only, but was the same as that in the control subjects from Fanxian; the mean amounts of NTCA and NSAR after vitamin C ingestion were also decreased in the Linxian subjects to the same levels as those in normal subjects from Fanxian (Table 2).

A significantly greater level of nitrate was excreted by Linxian subjects than by Fanxian (112 ± 84 versus 72 ± 64; Table 2). In all the urine specimens, the level of nitrite was below the limit of detection (0.1 mg/L).

DISCUSSION

The conclusions that can be drawn from this study are that in the high-incidence area (Linxian), exposure to NPRO, NTCA and NSAR and nitrate is higher than in the Fanxian county; ingestion of vitamin C reduces the amount of NPRO and other nitrosamino acids formed *in vivo* (and, by inference, total *N*-nitroso compounds) to levels seen in (unexposed) Fanxian subjects.

Although it remains to be demonstrated whether endogenous nitrosation is a risk factor in the development of oesophageal cancer in certain provinces in Northern China, intervention studies can be considered, as our results have demonstrated the efficiency of vitamin C in blocking *N*-nitrosation *in vivo*.

We and others (Ohshima *et al.*, 1983, this volume, p. 77; Tsuda *et al.*, 1983, this volume, p. 87) have identified *N*-nitrosothiazolidine-4-carboxylic acid (and its 2-methyl derivative, data not shown) in human urine samples for the first time. These compounds have not been previously reported to occur in biological materials. In view of the wide exposure of the general human population, the origin and the biological significance of these *N*-nitroso compounds should be determined.

ACKNOWLEDGEMENTS

We wish to thank M.C. Bourgade for technical assistance. The TEA detector used in part of these studies was provided on loan from the National Cancer Institute of the United States, Bethesda, MD, under contract NO1 CP-55715.

REFERENCES

Burrel, R.J.W. (1957) Oesophageal cancer in the Bantu. *S. Afr. med. J.*, *31*, 401–409

Chen, H. (1981) The mutagenicity of a new nitrosamine, effect of *N*-l-methylacetonyl-*N*-3-methyl-butylnitrosamine, to V79 cells. *Chin. med. J.*, *61*, 736–739

Cook-Mozaffari, P.J., Azordegan, F., Day N.E., Sabai, C. & Aramesh, B. (1979) Studies in Caspian littoral of Iran: Results of a case control study. *Br. J. Cancer*, *39*, 293–309

Coordinating Group for Research on Etiology of Esophageal cancer in North China (1977) The preliminary studies on epidemiological factors of esophageal cancer. *Res. Cancer Prev. Treat.*, *2*, 1–8

Crespi, M., Muñoz, N., Grassi, A., Aramesh, B., Amiri, G., Modjtabai, A. & Cosale, V. (1979) Esophageal lesions in northern Iran: A premalignant condition? *Lancet*, *ii*, 217–220

Du Plessis, L.S. & Nunn, J.R. (1969) Carcinogen in a Transkeian Bantu food additive. *Nature*, *222*, 1198–1199

Higginson, J. & Oettle, A.G. (1960) Cancer incidence in the Bantu and Cape colored-race of South Africa: Report of a cancer survey in the Transvaal (1953–1955). *J. natl Cancer Inst.*, *24*, 589–671

Kmet, J. & Mahboubi, E. (1972) Esophageal cancer in the Caspian littoral of Iran. Initial studies. *Science*, *175*, 846–853

Lasserre, O. Flamant, R. Lellouch, J. & Schwartz, D. (1967) Alcool et cancer. Etude de pathologie géographique portant sur les départements français. *Bull INSERM, 22,* 55–60

Li, K.H., Kao, J.C. & Wu, Y.K. (1962) A survey of the prevalence of carcinoma of the esophagus in north China. *Chin. med. J., 81,* 489–494

Li, M.H., Lu, S.H., Ji, C., Wang, Y, Cheng, S.J. & Tian, G. (1980) *Experimental Studies on the Carcinogenicity of Fungus Contaminated Food from Linxian County,* Tokyo, Jpn Sci. Soc. Press, pp. 139–148

Liu, Y., Wang, T.Y., Wu, W.J., Fei, L.M. & Chu, H.Y. (1955) Carcinomas of esophagus and cardia stomach – a study of 160 cases.

Lu, S.H. & Lin, P. (1982) Recent research on the etiology of esophageal cancer in China. *Z. Gastroenterol., 20,* 361–367

Lu, S.H., Li, M.H., Ji, C., Wang, M.Y., Huang, L. (1979) A new N-nitrosamine compound, N-methylbutyl-N-l-methylacetonyl-nitrosamine, in corn bread inoculated with fungi. *Sci. Sin., 22,* 601–608

Lu, S.H., Camus, A.-M., Wang, Y.L., Wang, M.Y. & Bartsch, H. (1980) Mutagenicity in *Salmonella typhimurium* of N-methyl-N-l-methylacetonylinitrosamine and N-methyl-N-benzylinitrosamine, N-nitrosation products isolated from corn bread contaminated with commonly occurring moulds in Linshien county, a high incidence area for esophageal cancer in Northern China. *Carcinogenesis, 1,* 867–870

Lu, S.H., Camus, A.-M., Tomatis, L. & Bartsch, H. (1981) Mutagenicity of extracts of pickled vegetables collected in Linshien county, a high incidence area for esophageal cancer in Northern China. *J. natl Cancer Inst., 66,* 33–36

Lu, S.H. *et al.* (1983) Promoting effect of Roussin's red methyl ester isolated from pickled vegetables in Linshien on forestomach carcinogensis initiated by N-methyl-N-benzylnitrosamine in mice (in press)

Martinez, I. (1964) Cancer of the esophagus in Puerto Rico – mortality and incidence analysis, 1950–1961. *Cancer, 17,* 1279–1288

Ohshima, H. & Bartsch, H. (1981) Quantitative estimation of endogenous nitrosation in humans by monitoring N-nitrosoproline excreted in the urine. *Cancer Res., 41,* 3658–3662

Ohshima, H., Béréziat, J.C. & Bartsch, H. (1982) Monitoring N-nitrosamino acids excreted in the urine and feces of rats as an index for endogenous nitrosation. *Carcinogenesis, 3,* 115–120

Ohshima, H., Friesen, M., O'Neill, I. & Bartsch, H. (1983) Presence in human urine of a new N-nitroso compound, N-nitrosothiazolidine 4-carboxylic acid. *Cancer Lett., 20,* 183–190

Sadowsky, D.A., Gilliam, A.G. & Cornfield J. (1953) The statistical association between smoking and carcinoma of the lung. *J. natl Cancer Inst., 13,* 1237–1258

Schwartz, D., Denoix, P. & Anguera, G. (1956) Recherche des localisations du cancer associéss aux facteurs tabac et alcool chez l'homme. *Bull. Assoc. Fr. Etude Cancer, 44,* 336–361

Tomlinson, W.J. & Wilson, J.A., Jr (1945) Esophageal carcinoma in British West Indian and Panamanian negroes. *Arch. Pathol., 39,* 79–80

Tsuda, M., Hirayama, T. & Sugimura, T. (1983) Presence of N-nitroso-L-thioproline and N-nitroso-L-methylthioprolines in human urine as major N-nitroso compounds, *Gann, 74,* 331–333

Walker, E.A., Castegnaro, M., Garren, L., Toussaint, G. & Kowaiski, C. (1979) Intake of volatile nitrosamine from consumption of alcohols. *J. natl. Cancer Inst., 63,* 947–951

Wang Guang-hui, Zhang Wen-xin & Chai Wen-gang (1980) The identification of natural Roussin's red methyl ester. *Acta chim. sin., 38,* 95–102

Waterhouse, J.A.H., Muir, C., Correa, P. & Powell, J. eds (1976) *Cancer Incidence in Five Continents Vol. III (IARC Scientific Publications No. 15),* Lyon, International Agency for Research on Cancer

Yang, C.S. (1980) Research on oesophageal cancer in China: a review. *Cancer Res., 40,* 2633–2644

IN-VIVO NITROSATION, PRECANCEROUS LESIONS
AND CANCERS OF THE GASTROINTESTINAL TRACT.
ON-GOING STUDIES AND PRELIMINARY RESULTS

H. BARTSCH[1], H. OHSHIMA & N. MUÑOZ

International Agency for Research on Cancer, Lyon, France

M. CRESPI, V. CASSALE & V. RAMAZOTTI

Regina Elena Institute, Rome, Italy

R. LAMBERT, Y. MINAIRE & J. FORICHON

Hôpital Edouard-Herriot, Lyon, France

C.L. WALTERS

British Food Manufacturing Industries Research Association, Leatherhead, UK

INTRODUCTION

Endogenous formation of N-nitroso compounds has been associated with an increased risk of stomach cancer, for example, in patients with chronic atrophic gastritis or pernicious anaemia and in patients who have undergone gastric surgery such as Billroth-II gastrectomy (Blackburn *et al.*, 1968; Cuello *et al.*, 1976; Stalsberg and Taksdal, 1971). It has been postulated that the achlorhydric stomach found in such patients may provide a suitable milieu for intragastric formation of N-nitroso compounds by the presence of a large number of bacteria, which may be involved in the conversion of nitrate to nitrite and subsequent nitrosation *in vivo* (Correa *et al.*, 1975; Reed *et al.*, 1981; Ruddell *et al.*, 1976; Schlag *et al;* 1980). Higher levels of N-nitroso compounds were more frequently found in fasting gastric juice samples of such patients than in those of normal subjects (Reed *et al.*, 1981). However, the extent of endogenous nitrosation occurring in these individuals at high risk for stomach cancer has not been determined.

In collaborative clinical studies we are currently applying the NPRO-test (Ohshima & Bartsch, 1981) to subjects belonging to the four groups A–D described below. As we and others (Ohshima *et al.*, 1983, this volume, pp. 77, 87; Tsuda *et al.*, 1983) have identified the previously

---

[1] To whom correspondence should be addressed

unknown *N*-nitrosamino acids, *N*-nitrosothiazolidine 4-carboxylic acid and *N*-nitroso-2-methylthiazolidine 4-carboxylic acid, in the human urine, analyses of these compounds was also carried out.

MATERIALS AND METHODS

All the study subjects have been selected from those attending the gastroenterology department of collaborating hospitals and on whom endoscopies have been performed as part of a pre-established routine examination. Informed consent was requested for inclusion in the study. The project was cleared by the Ethical Committee of IARC.

A. *Chronic atrophic gastritis (CAG)*

Forty-nine male individuals (20–49 years old) with various degrees of histologically proven CAG, with and without intestinal metaplasia have been selected. The results obtained in this group are being compared with those obtained in a control group of the same sex and age, who have been found to have a histologically normal stomach or with superficial gastritis. These subjects have been selected from the gastroenterology department of the Regina Elena Institute of Rome.

B. *Cimetidine-treated patients*

Seventeen male duodenal ulcer patients (30–60 years of age) were included in this study. Subjects received 0.8 g of cimetidine/day for 4–6 weeks. Both the NPRO-test was applied and fasting gastric juice was collected, once just before and a second time following 4–6 weeks of cimetidine-treatment. These subjects have been selected from the gastroenterology department of the Hôpital Edouard-Herriot, Lyon, France.

C. *Pernicious anaemia*

Thirty patients with pernicious anaemia and 30 control subjects with normal gastric mucosa or with superficial gastritis have been selected from various departments of the University of Turku, Finland (in collaboration with A. Lehtonen and M. Inberg, University Hospital, Turku, and A. Aitio, Institute of Occupational Health, Helsinki).

D. *Post-gastrectomy*

Male subjects are being selected from those who underwent partial gastrectomy in 1950–52 and who have accepted to participate in an on-going screening programme for gastric cancer in Iceland (in collaboration with H. Tulinius, Icelandic Cancer Registry, Reykjavik).

Whenever possible, the following procedures (1–5) are being applied to each study subject: 1) Completion of a questionnaire containing basic demographic information as well as questions on smoking and drinking habits and clinical symptoms. 2) Gastroscopy is performed and the findings are recorded. 3) Fasting gastic juice is collected; sulfamic acid (final conc. 10 g/L) was added to prevent artefactual nitrosamine formation. The pH is measured and an aliquot was frozen for bacteriological studies and for analysis of total nitroso compounds (Walters *et al.*, 1978). 4) For diagnostic purposes, during gastroscopy, at least 3 biopsies are taken: the first from the greater curvature, 5 cm from the pylorus; the second from the greater curvature, 10 cm from the pylorus; and the third from the angular region of the lesser curvature. The biopsies are fixed on 10% formalin. All biopsies or unstained serial sections are histopathologically evaluated; the following lesions are being considered: superficial gastritis; CAG; intestinal metaplasia; hyperplasia and dysplasia. 5) N-Nitrosoproline test: After endoscopy, subjects are given 200 ml beetroot juice (containing 260 mg of nitrate), followed 30 minutes later by 10 ml of an aqueous solution containing 500 mg L-proline. The subjects are asked to fast for a further 2 hours after ingestion of proline; water is taken *ad libitum*. During collection of urine samples, the subjects are instructed to avoid foodstuffs rich in nitrate and those presumed to contain preformed NPRO, such as cured meat, smoked fish products and beer. Urine samples are collected over 24 hours after ingestion of proline. To prevent artefactual formation of NPRO during collection, storage and transport of the samples, specimens are collected in a plastic bottle containing 10 g sodium hydroxide. The urine collected in this way is thoroughly mixed, and the volume recorded. An aliquot of the 24-h urine is then transferred into a 100-mL plastic bottle and stored at $-20\,°C$ prior to analysis. Under these conditions, NPRO, NSAR and nitrate/nitrite are stable, and artefactual formation of N-nitrosamino acids is negligible for at least 3 months.

Analyses of N-nitrosamino acids: NPRO, NSAR, NTCA, NMTCA after conversion into their methyl esters were analysed by GC-TEA as described (Ohshima *et al.,* 1981, 1982, 1983). During the course of this study, NTCA and NMTCA were found to be unstable under acidic conditions. As some of the compounds may have partially decomposed during the work-up procedure, the data listed in Fig. 2 should be regarded as tentative.

RESULTS

Some interim results are presently available only for study subjects with or without CAG and cimetidine-treated patients. In Figure 1, the levels of NPRO excreted in the urine of these group-A subjects (Materials and Methods) who ingested 260 mg nitrate in beetroot juice and then 500 mg L-proline, are plotted against the pH of the gastric juice from the same individual. The yield of NPRO in the urine ranged from trace amounts to 120 µg/day/person. The yield appeared to be dependent on the pH of the gastric juice, as the highest values for NPRO were seen at pH 2–2.5, which coincides with the optimum value reported for nitrosation of proline *in vitro* (Mirvish *et al.,* 1973). CAG patients with a gastric pH of 6–8 produced relatively low levels of NPRO (< 10 µg/day).

In Figure 2 the total amount of four N-nitrosamino acids, NPRO, N-nitrososarcosine (NSAR), N-nitrosothiazolidine 4-carboxylic acid (NTCA) and N-nitroso-2-methylthiazolidine 4-carboxylic acid (NMTCA) (*cis-* and *trans-* epimers combined) excreted in the urine by the group A subjects, are plotted against the pH of fasting gastric juice. The amount of nitrosamino acids ranged from traces to about 140 µg/day. Although final confirmation is still needed, subjects who smoked cigarettes appeared to produce more N-nitrosamino acids (mean = 59 µg/day) than non-smokers (mean = 30 µg/day).

The level of total N-nitroso compounds, as determined by the method of Walters *et al.* (1978), formed in the gastric juice of group A subjects is plotted against their gastric pH in Figure 3. The values found tended to be rather low, with the exception of 3 subjects, one of whom had 1.40 µmol/L total N-nitroso compounds in his gastric juice.

Taking the results shown in Figures 1 to 3 together, it is apparent that the amounts of total N-nitroso compounds (gastric juice) and total N-nitrosamino acids (urine) in the same subject were not correlated. Also, no higher prevalence of CAG patients, showing either elevated levels of total N-nitroso compounds or total N-nitrosamino acids, or both, was obvious in our study group (n = 34).

In Figure 4, A–C, the effect of cimetidine-treatment of 17 duodenal ulcer patients on the amount of NPRO excreted in the urine (4A), the pH of gastric juice (4B) and on the total

Fig. 1. A plot of the urinary NPRO excreted by subjects (group A, Materials and Methods) after ingestion of beetroot juice and proline *versus* the pH of the fasting gastric juice of the same individual (interim results). Control subjects (n = 8) with normal mucosa (●) and patients with precancerous lesions (CAG, n = 31, ○; or dysplasia n = 3, ■; superficial gastritis, n = 8, △) of the stomach are shown.

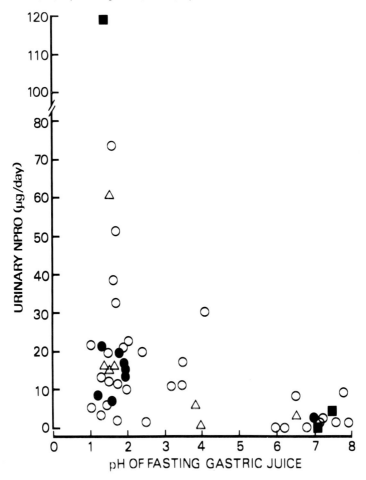

amount of intragastrically-formed *N*-nitroso compounds (4C) is listed. These patients (group B, Materials and Methods) have taken the drug for 4–6 weeks. Although some patients, following a cimetidine-dosing, showed a significant increase in the gastric pH and in the total *N*-nitroso compounds, as well as in urinary NPRO levels, mean values from all study subjects did not indicate a conspicuous increase when compared to the respective figures prior to drug treatment.

DISCUSSION

As only 8 cases in our study group A were subjects with normal stomach mucosa, a final comparison of endogenous nitrosation in subjects with or without precancerous conditions of the stomach, based on statistical analyses, are pending until all data (presently being collected)

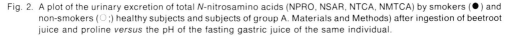

Fig. 2. A plot of the urinary excretion of total *N*-nitrosamino acids (NPRO, NSAR, NTCA, NMTCA) by smokers (●) and non-smokers (○;) healthy subjects and subjects of group A. Materials and Methods) after ingestion of beetroot juice and proline *versus* the pH of the fasting gastric juice of the same individual.

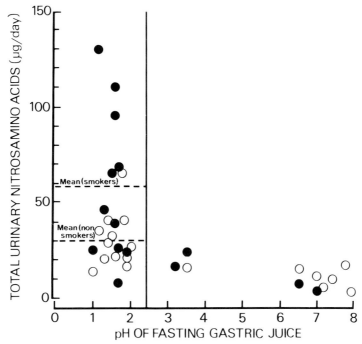

on histological evaluations, the levels of total nitroso compounds and bacteria count in fasting gastric juice, become available.

However, from our interim results (Figs. 1–4) several tentative conclusions can be drawn: i) the amount of urinary NPRO and of other *N*-nitrosamino acids formed following ingestion of precursors, and of total *N*-nitroso compounds (as determined by Walters' method) in fasting gastric juice was not conspicuously increased in patients suffering from mild to severe CAG; ii) similarly, except in some cases, cimetidine-treatment of 17 duodenal ulcer patients did not lead to a pronounced, uniform raise in urinary NPRO levels, gastric pH and of total gastric *N*-nitroso compounds. These findings (i-ii) are in contrast to other reports (see Introduction and Reed *et al.*, 1982); in non-acidic gastric juice of cancer prone patients (i.e. cases of pernicious anaemia, gastrectomized patients according to Billroth II and subjects receiving cimetidine), higher levels of nitrite and total intragastric *N*-nitroso compounds were detected. The reasons for this discrepancy are currently unknown but could be due to the following:

1) In our studies we may not have used the appropriate conditions to prevent degradation of total gastric *N*-nitroso compounds during collection and storage of gastric juice samples, in particular as highly reactive *N*-nitrosamides which may act as gastric carcinogens have been suspected to be formed.

2) We have applied the NPRO-test only once or twice to the same subject, and we have only once determined the total gastric nitroso compounds; therefore no data on intra-individual or diurnal variations are available. Bavin *et al.* (1982) have reported considerable variations in the concentration of total *N*-nitroso compounds in the gastric juice of healthy human subjects to occur within 10 h. Our studies in one human volunteer (data not shown) over

Fig. 3. A plot of intragastrically-formed total N-nitroso compounds (determined by the method of Walters et al., 1978) versus the pH of the fasting gastric juice in the same individual. Study subjects and symbols are the same as described in Figure 1

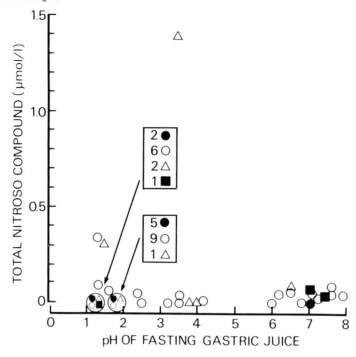

a two year period have indicated only modest variations in NPRO excretion following intake of precursors.

3) Although it is now generally accepted that the achlorhydric stomach allows bacteria to multiply, entailing a higher nitrite concentration in the gastric juice, our data (Fig. 1) do not support the notion that the total nitrosamine/amide formation is favoured in the stomach of subjects showing histologically ascertained CAG and an elevated pH of 6–8 of their gastric juice. The findings seem to rule out a significant contribution by bacterial enzymes catalyzing N-nitrosation reactions as reviewed previously (Kunisaki & Hayashi, 1979). However, as pointed out earlier (Charnley et al., 1982) focal intestinal metaplasia is embedded in a normal area of the gastric mucosa; therefore the pH may be high in a part of the stomach where nitrite is formed, e.g. in islands of intestinal metaplasia, and low where nitrosation takes place, e.g. in normal mucosa; temporal pH changes may have a similar effect. Therefore, the most favorable condition for the formation of N-nitroso compounds will be at a boundary between the normal and the metaplastic regions, since this area will have the highest concentration of nitrite and the lowest pH. The NPRO-test, which we have applied, may not be a suitable procedure to reveal slight excess of N-nitrosoproline when only formed in such boundary locations. It is also not known whether proline is a substrate for bacteria catalysing N-nitrosation reactions.

Although final conclusions can only be drawn upon completion of our studies, future approaches have to embark on the identification of the principal N-nitroso compounds formed

Fig. 4. The effect of cimetidine-treatment (0.8 g/day) of duodenal ulcer patients on:
   A) excretion of urinary NPRO, following ingestion of beetroot juice and proline.
   B) pH of fasting gastric juice and
   C) total *N*-nitroso compounds (Walters *et al.*, 1978) in fasting gastric juice.
   Patients were examined just before and a second time following 4–6 weeks cimetidine-dosing.

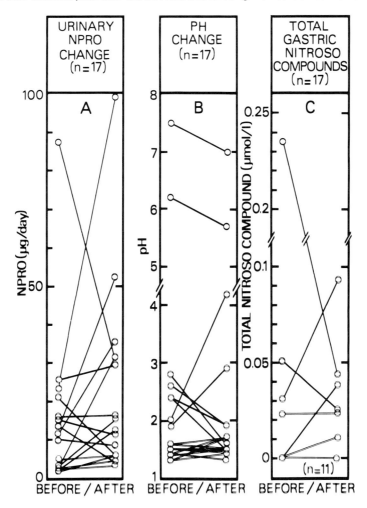

in the gastric juice following nitrosation, their isolation and testing for carcinogenicity. Furthermore, the role of bacteria-mediated catalysis of *N*-nitrosation in the achlorhydric stomach requires urgent clarification (see Suzuki & Mitsuoka, this volume p. 275).

ACKNOWLEDGEMENTS

We wish to thank Y. Granjard for secretarial help, and C. Montvernay, J. Michelon and M.C. Bourgade for technical assistance. The TEA detector was provided on loan by the National Cancer Institute, Bethesda, MA, USA, under contract No. NOI CP-55 717.

REFERENCES

Blackburn, E.K., Callender, S.T., Dacie, J.V., Doll, R., Girdwood, R.H., Mollin, D.L., Saracci, R., Stafford, J., Thompson, R.B., Varadi, S., and Wetherly-Wein, G. (1968) Possible association between pernicious anaemia and leukemia: a prospective study of 1 625 patients with a note on the very high incidence of gastric cancer. *Int. J. Cancer, 3,* 163–170

Charnley, G., Tannenbaum, S.R. & Correa, P. (1982) *Gastric cancer: An etiological model.* In: Magee, P.N., ed., *Banbury Report 12,* Cold Spring Harbor, NY, Cold Spring Harbor Laboratory, pp. 503–522

Correa, P., Haenszel, W., Cuello, C., Tannenbaum, S., & Archer, M. (1975) A model for gastric cancer epidemiology. *Lancet, ii,* 58–59

Cuello, C., Correa, P., Haenszel, W., Gordillo, G., Brown, C., Archer, M. & Tannenbaum, S. (1976) Gastric cancer in Columbia. I. Cancer risk and suspect environment agents. *J. natl Cancer Inst., 50,* 1015–1020

Kunisaki, N. & Hayashi, M. (1979) Formation of *N*-nitrosamines from secondary amines and nitrite by resting cells of *E. coli* B. *Appl. Environ. Biol., 37,* 279

Mirvish, S.S., Sams, J., Fran, T.Y., & Tannenbaum, S.R. (1973) Kinetics of nitrosation of the amino acids proline, hydroxyproline and sarcosine. *J. natl Cancer Inst., 51,* 1833–1839

Ohshima, H., & Bartsch, H. (1981) Quantitative estimation of endogenous nitrosation in humans by monitoring *N*-nitrosoproline excreted in the urine. *Cancer Res., 41,* 3658–3662

Ohshima, H., Béréziat, J.-C., & Bartsch, H. (1982) Monitoring *N*-nitrosamino acids excreted in the urine and feces of rats as an index for endogenous nitrosation. *Carcinogenesis, 3,* 115–120

Ohshima, H., Friesen, M., O'Neill, I.K. & Bartsch, H. (1983) Presence in human urine of a new *N*-nitroso compound, *N*-nitrosothiazolidine 4-carboxylic acid. *Cancer Lett., 20,* 183–190

Reed, P.I., Smith, P.L.R., Haines, K., House, F.R. & Walters, C. (1981) Gastric juice *N*-nitrosamines in health and gastroduodenal disease. *Lancet, ii,* 550–555

Reed, P.I., Haines, K., Smith, P.L.R., Walters, C.L., & House, F.K. (1982) *The effects of cimetidine on intragastric nitrosation in man.* In: Magee, P.N., ed., *Banbury Report 12,* Cold Spring Harbor, NY, Cold Spring Harbor Laboratory, pp. 351–364

Ruddell, W.S.J., Bone, E.S., Hill, M.J., Blendis, L.M. & Walters, C. (1976) Gastric juice nitrite: A risk factor for cancer of the hypochlorhydric stomach? *Lancet, ii,* 1037–1039

Schlag, P., Bockler, R., Ulrich, H., Peter, M., Merkle, P., & Herfarth, C. (1980) Are nitrite and *N*-nitroso compounds in gastric juice risk factors for carcinoma in the operated stomach? *Lancet, i,* 727–729

Stalsberg, H., & Taksdal, S. (1971) Stomach cancer following gastric surgery for benign conditions. *Lancet, ii,* 1175–1177

Tsuda, Hirayama, T. & Sugimura, T. (1983) Presence of *N*-nitroso-L-thioproline and *N*-nitroso-L-methylthioproline in human urine as major *N*-nitroso compounds. *Gann, 74,* 331–333

Walters, C.L., Downes, L.J., Edwards, L.W., & Smith, P.L.R. (1978) Determination of a non-volatile *N*-nitrosamine on a food matrix. *Analyst, 103,* 1127–1133

FORMATION OF NITRITE IN GASTRIC JUICE OF PATIENTS WITH VARIOUS GASTRIC DISORDERS AFTER INGESTION OF A STANDARD DOSE OF NITRATE – A POSSIBLE RISK FACTOR IN GASTRIC CARCINOGENESIS

G. EISENBRAND

Department of Food Chemistry and Environmental Toxicology University of Kaiserslautern 6750 Kaiserslautern, Federal Republic of Germany

B. ADAM

Institute of Toxicology and Chemotherapy, German Cancer Research Center, 6900 Heidelberg, Federal Republic of Germany

M. PETER & P. MALFERTHEINER

Department of Internal Medicine University of Ulm, 7900 Ulm, Federal Republic of Germany

P. SCHLAG

Section of Surgical Oncology University of Heidelberg, 6900 Heidelberg, Federal Republic of Germany

SUMMARY

Samples of fasting gastric juice (12-h fasting period) from patients with various upper gastrointestinal complaints and from healthy controls were collected by aspiration immediately before and 30, 90, and 240 min after ingestion of 200 mg nitrate in water. Nitrite concentration in the gastric juice of healthy controls remained essentially in a low concentration range throughout the whole sampling period (median values at various time points, 0.1–1.7 mg/L). Patients with gastric and duodenal ulcers and patients who had undergone proximal-gastral vagotomy did not show significant increases in gastric nitrite at any time when compared with healthy controls, using the Wilcoxon rank sum test. Patients with chronic atrophic gastritis and those who had undergone Billroth I or Billroth II gastric resection, however, showed significant increases in gastric nitrite, sometimes with high individual peaks: 80 mg/L in one patient with chronic atrophic gastritis, 50 mg/L in a Billroth I patient and 200 mg/L in a Billroth II patient.

The results show that patients with chronic atrophic gastritis and patients who have undergone Billroth I and Billroth II gastrotomy not only have higher basal nitrite values in their gastric juice (12-h fasting) but also react with significantly higher increases in gastric nitrite to an oral dose of 200 mg nitrate, compared with healthy controls, ulcer patients and patients who have undergone proximal-gastral vagotomy. Higher nitrite levels might lead to an enhanced intragastric formation of N-nitroso compounds, and this might be relevant to the increased gastric cancer risk of these groups of patients.

INTRODUCTION

It has been assumed for many years that specific gastric disorders may predispose to human cancer. In particular, gastric resection has been recognized as creating conditions that favour the development of cancer in the gastric stump. Continuous enterogastric reflux and alterations of the mucosa due to the operative procedure are, in general, thought to be the major factors responsible for gastric carcinogenesis in the stomach after surgery (Dahm et al., 1977; Schlag, 1983). Independent of gastric resection, chronic atrophic gastritis has also been identified as the most prevalent precursor lesion for gastric cancer (Correa, 1982). Gastric resection and severe atrophic gastritits are both accompanied by reduced intragastric acidity, which is favourable to intragastric bacterial growth. Thus, more nitrate-reducing bacteria have been found in gastric juice with a pH > 5 than in more acidic samples (Ruddell et al., 1976; Schlag et al., 1980; Reed et al., 1981; Walters et al., 1982; Böckler et al., 1983).

Nitrite formed by gastric bacteria from dietary nitrate might lead to an enhanced intragastric formation of N-nitroso compounds and might therefore play a key role in gastric carcinogenesis under conditions characterized by chronic atrophic gastritis. In most investigations carrid out up to now, nitrite has been determined in fasting gastric juice without taking into account the influence of previous dietary nitrate intake. It was therefore considered of great interest to study possible variations in gastric nitrite levels after ingestion of a defined dose of nitrate and to investigate the influence of various gastric disorders on nitrite formation.

PATIENTS, MATERIALS AND METHODS

Patients

Patients (56) with various abdominal complaints or examined during routine postoperative checks were divided into seven groups according to diagnoses made by gastroscopy or biopsy of the gastric mucosa. Classification of biopsies (at least 10) was carried out using standardized histological criteria; all operations had been carried out to treat benign ulcers. Five patients had undergone a Billroth I procedure and 10 a Billroth II resection, and in 12 patients a proximal gastral vagotomy had been carried out. Of the patients who had not undergone gastric surgery, four had gastric ulcers (type Johnson I), nineteen had duodenal ulcers, and seven had chronic atrophic gastritis.

Eight patients who were found to be free of gastrointestinal disease served as controls.

Sampling procedure

The first gastric juice sample was extracted during gastroscopy under standardized conditions after a 12-h fasting period. Thereafter patients received 50 mL of an aqueous solution of sodium nitrate containing 200 mg nitrate. Further samples were taken 30, 90 and 240 min after nitrate ingestion. Samples were drawn through a gastric tube positioned during gastroscopy into vials containing 0.2 mL of 10 mol/L sodium hydroxide for stabilization of nitrite and for inhibition of bacterial activity.

Nitrite determination

Nitrite was determined spectrophotometrically by diazotization of sulfanilamide and azocoupling with *N*-(1-naphthyl)ethylene diamine. Samples (2 mL) were deproteinized with 0.5 mL each of zinc sulfate (22% in 3% acetic acid)/potassium ferrocyanide (10.6% in water). After filtration through glass-fibre filters, 0.2 mL ammonium sulfamate (22% in 30% acetic acid) was added to one aliquot (0.5 mL) of the filtrate for nitrite removal, and this was then made up to 1.5 mL with the diazotation/azocoupling reagent. Another aliquot (0.5 mL) was mixed directly with the colour reagent (1 mL). The aliquot from wich nitrite had been removed served as a spectrophotometric reference (Adam, 1983).

This procedure allowed reliable determination of nitrite even in the presence of coloured material in the deproteinized filtrates, especially in samples originally containing high proportions of bile: in a control experiment using nitrite-free gastric juice mixed with up to one-third of its volume of bile and containing a known amount of added nitrite, a mean of 5.2 mg/L nitrite were recovered for 5 mg/L added (n = 4; SD $\pm$ 0.15).

Evaluation

Median values and 95% confidence limits were used for statistical evaluation, applying the Wilcoxon rank sum test for multiple comparisons (Weber, 1972).

RESULTS

After oral intake of 200 mg nitrate, a distinct increase in the nitrite concentration of gastric juice was seen in all patients. There were, however, large differences within the various groups (Table 1).

Healthy controls showed the lowest basal nitrite level before nitrate intake (at 0 min). The median nitrite levels increased after nitrate intake to 1.7 mg/L (at 60 min) and then decreased again (at 240 min). Patients with duodenal ulcers and those who had undergone proximal-gastral vagotomy had levels very similar to those of the healthy control group, showing either practically no variation of median nitrite values (duodenal ulcer) or only small changes at the various time points (proximal-gastral vagotomy). In the group with gastric ulcers, only four patients have so far been sampled; therefore, no significance can be attributed

Table 1.   Median nitrite concentrations in gastric juice at various times after intake of 200 mg nitrate

Group	Median nitrite concentration (mg/L) after:			
	0 min	30 min	60 min	240 min
Controls (8)	0.1	0.5	1.7	1.3
Gastric ulcer (4)	0.3	0.9	8.1	6.6
Duodenal ulcer (10)	0.3	0.5	0.4	0.4
Proximal-gastral vagotomy (12)	0.7	2.8	1.3	0.9
Chronic atrophic gastritis (7)	1.3*	10.6	12.6*	9.7*
Billroth I (5)	1.8*	19.0*	27.5*	5.9
Billroth II (10)	2.0*	19.8*	21.9*	13.0*

* Significant according to the Wilcoxon rank sum test, multiple comparisons (α = 0.0083)

to the relatively high median values at 60 and 240 min. However, the basal value and the value at 30 min are well within the range of those of the groups of healthy controls, patients with duodenal ulcer and those with proximal-gastral vagotomy. In contrast, the groups of patients with chronic atrophic gastritis, Billroth I and Billroth II showed significantly higher median nitrite values even at the basal level (Table 1). Interindividual variations in the extent and kinetics of nitrite formation after nitrate intake were, however, considerable within the groups. For example, in one patient with chronic atrophic gastritis, a maximum level of 86 mg/L nitrite had already been reached at 30 min. This was followed by a rapid decrease down to 8 mg/L at 240 min. In a second patient, the nitrite level increased continually throughout the sampling period, and the highest concentration (40 mg/L) was detected at the last time point. The highest levels of all were found in the Billroth II group at 240 min: 200 and 176 mg/L.

The wide variation of individual values results in rather wide 95% confidence intervals for the median values, as exemplified in Figures 1 and 2. In virtually all groups, the highest median levels were reached 90 min after nitrate intake.

Fig. 1. Nitrite concentration in gastric juice after oral intake of 200 mg nitrate, timecourse of median (with 95% confidence intervals). A, Healthy controls; B, duodenal ulcer (n = 8); C, proximal-gastral vagotomy (n = 12); D, gastric ulcer (n = 4).

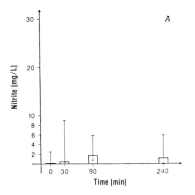
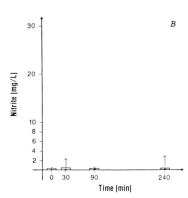
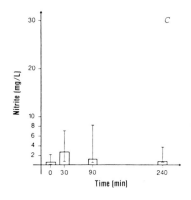
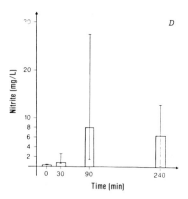

Fig. 2. Nitrite concentration in gastric juice after oral intake of 200 mg nitrate, timecourse of median (with 95% confidence intervals). A, Healthy controls (n = 8); B, chronic atrophic gastritis (n = 7); C, gastric resection after Billroth I (n = 5); D, gastric resection after Billroth II (n = 10)

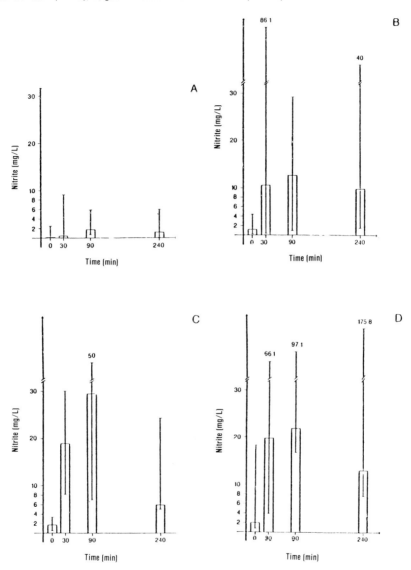

DISCUSSION

The results show that after oral ingestion of 200 mg nitrate, patients with chronic atrophic gastritis and those who have had a Billroth I or Billroth II resection have significantly higher gastric nitrite values at various times than healthy controls, patients with duodenal or gastric ulcers or patients who have undergone proximal-gastral vagotomy. The nitrate dose of 200 mg was chosen because such an amount can easily be ingested with various foods; for example, 200 mg nitrate might well be contained in 50–100 g beetroot, spinach, lettuce or other vegetables rich in nitrate. As in previous studies (Ruddell *et al.,* 1976; Schlag *et al.,* 1980), the patients with chronic atrophic gastritis, Billroth I and Billroth II already had significantly higher basal nitrite values after a 12-h fasting period, before nitrate ingestion. Although the differences between the groups with high and low nitrite are considerable, the median concentrations of the former remain in the low mg/L range before nitrate ingestion. Much higher median concentrations are seen, however, after nitrate ingestion, and individual values exceeding 50 mg/L were measured in several cases.

Nitrite is produced at high gastric pH by nitrate-reducing bacteria, and these conditions are prevalent in patients with chronic atrophic gastritis or with stomach resection after the Billroth I and II procedures. The existence of high bacterial counts under such conditions explains the rapid and extensive formation of nitrite from ingested nitrate.

Although nitrosation at pH values >5 proceeds considerably more slowly than at more acidic pH, high nitrite concentrations like those measured in this study should result in increased nitrosation rates, when nitrosatable compounds are present. This applies especially to compounds bearing secondary amine groups, like many drugs, because the nitrosation rate of secondary amines is proportional to the *square* of nitrite concentration. The elevated nitrite levels demonstrated here might well play a role in gastric carcinogenesis, leading to the intragastric formation of *N*-Nitroso compounds, especially under conditions of damaged gastric mucosa and elevated gastric pH, as seen in chronic atrophic gastritis or in the gastric remnant after Billroth I or Billroth II resection.

REFERENCES

Adam, B. (1983) Untersuchungen zur endogenen Nitrosierung am Menschen. *Diplomarbeit,* Univ. Hohenheim, Federal Republic of Germany

Böckler, R., Meyer, H. & Schlag, P. (1983) An experimental study of bacterial colonization, nitrite and nitrosamine production in the operated stomach. *J. Cancer Res. clin. Oncol.,* **105,** 62–66

Correa, P. (1982) Precursors of gastric and esophageal cancer. *Cancer, 50,* 2554–2565

Dahm, K., Eichen, R. & Mitschke, H. (1977) Das Krebsrisiko im Resektionsmagen. Zur Bedeutung des duodenogastrischen Refluxes bei verschiedenen gastroenteralen Anastomosen, *Langenbecks Arch. Chir., 344,* 71–82

Reed, P.J., Smith, P.L.R., Haines, K., House, P.R. & Walters, C.L. (1981) Gastric juice *N*-nitrosamines in health and gastroduodenal disease. *Lancet, ii,* 550–552

Ruddell, W.S., Bone, E.S., Hill, M.J., Blendis, L.M. & Walters, C.L. (1976) Gastric-juice nitrite. A risk factor for cancer in the hypochlorhydric stomach? *Lancet, ii,* 1037–1039

Schlag, P. (1983) The carcinoma in the operated stomach. *Verh. Dtsch Krebsges., 4,* 453–464

Schlag, P., Böckler, R., Ulrich, H., Peter, M., Merkle, R. & Herfarth, C. (1980) Are nitrite and *N*-nitroso compounds in gastric juice risk factors for carcinoma in the operated stomach? *Lancet, i,* 717–719

Walters, C.L., Smith, P.L.R., Reed, P.J., Haines, K. & House, F.R. (1982) N-*Nitroso compounds in gastric juice and their relationship to gastroduodenal disease.* In: Bartsch, H., O'Neill, I.K., Castegnaro, M. & Okada, M., eds, N-*Nitroso Compounds: Occurrence and Biological Effects (IARC Scientific Publications No. 41),* Lyon, International Agency for Research on Cancer, pp. 345–355

Weber, E. (1972) *Grundriss der biologischen Statistik,* 7. Aufl. Stuttgart

EFFECT OF H2 BLOCKERS ON INTRAGASTRIC NITROSATION AS MEASURED BY 24-HOUR URINARY SECRETION OF *N*-NITROSOPROLINE

J.B. ELDER & K. BURDETT

University Departments of Surgery & Medical Biochemistry, Oxford Road, Manchester, UK

P.L.R. SMITH & C.L. WALTERS

Randalls Road, Leatherhead, Surrey, UK

P.I. REED

Gastrointestinal Unit, Wexham park Hospital, Slough, UK

SUMMARY

Intragastric nitrosation of proline (500 mg daily) was studied in eight volunteers and three duodenal ulcer patients. Daily urine outputs of *N*-nitrosoproline (NPRO) and *N*-nitrosothiazolidine-4-carboxylic acid (NTCA) were measured for two days before, two days during and two days after ingestion of H_2 blocker (ranitidine). No increase in NPRO output was found with ranitidine, the trend being clearly towards decreased intragastric nitrosation of this amine. A significant ($p < 0.05$) increase in NTCA occurred during H_2 blockade, due to increased concentration of NTCA in urine. The biological significance of the presence of NTCA in urine is uncertain.

INTRODUCTION

Definition of the conditions in the human stomach that are optimal for nitrosation, and measurement of the rate of nitrosation reactions, have been hampered both by limitations of clinical methodolgy and by the necessity for direct sampling of the stomach by nasogastric tube. Nevertheless, the work of Reed and his colleagues has shown that ingestion of the H2 blocking drug, cimetidine (Tagamet, SKF), by patients with a variety of upper gastrointestinal disorders was followed by a marked increase in the concentration of total *N*-nitroso compounds in gastric juice (Reed *et al.*, 1981). These findings were confirmed by Stockbrugger *et al.* (1982) in peptic ulcer patients, but not by Milton-Thompson *et al.* (1982) in normal volunteers. Lack of precise methods for determining intragastric fluid volume and controversy over the estimation of unstable as well as stable '*N*-nitroso compounds' (Smith *et al.*, 1983) has led to much debate as to whether or not there is an increased production of these potentially carcinogenic substances in the human stomach after exposure to the H2 blocking drugs that are widely used to treat peptic ulcers. Recently, a new method has allowed quantitative study of the nitrosation reaction *in vivo* (Ohshima & Bartsch, 1981). It is based on the fact that certain *N*-nitrosamino acids, such as *N*-nitrosoproline (NPRO), are excreted almost quantitatively unchanged in the urine and faeces after either oral ingestion or endogenous intragastric formation. We have used this method to study the effect of ingestion of the powerful H2 blocker, ranitidine ('Zantac', Glaxo) on the intragastric nitrosation of proline in eight volunteer subjects and in three duodenal ulcer patients, two of whom had recently completed a course of treatment with ranitidine.

METHODS

Subjects studied

Eight healthy male volunteer subjects (age range, 28–45 years) and three duodenal ulcer patients aged 40, 47 and 64 years were studied over a six-day period. Every day, shortly after rising, each subject drank 200 mL fresh chilled beetroot juice (nitrate concentration, 1.09 mg/mL) to ensure a minimal intake of nitrate. Thirty min later, one capsule containing 500 mg proline (BDH) was swallowed; the subject ate a normal diet throughout the day, with restriction only on intake of cured meat, such as hamburgers, bacon and smoked ham, in an attempt to standardize the daily nitrate intake and to minimize the intake of preformed *N*-nitroso compounds. Volunteers were advised to avoid beer and spirits throughout the study, but they could ingest such products providing that approximately the same quantity was ingested on each of the six days of the study. The subject emptied his bladder before ingesting the beetroot juice, and 24-h urine collections were made. The urine was made alkaline by placing 10 g sodium hydroxide in the container at the start of each 24-h period. Two days after commencing the study and prior to ingestion of the beetroot juice, one 150-mg tablet of ranitidine was taken; this dose was repeated on three further occasions, at 12-h intervals. For the final two days of the study, each subject omitted the H2 blocker and simply ingested the nitrate source and proline as before.

Ranitidine blocks the H2 receptor on the parietal cells (hydrochloric acid-secreting cells) of the stomach and greatly reduces the gastric acid output, usually allowing duodenal ulcers to heal. Each of the three patients had had an endoscopy within one week prior to starting the study, and one was shown to have active duodenal ulceration; the remaining cases had recently had their ulcers healed with ranitidine. All the volunteers and patients had the project carefully explained to them, and informed consent was obtained, as was the agreement of the Ethnical Committees of the hospitals concerned.

No adverse effect was noted in any of the volunteers or patients following ingestion of either the beetroot juice, proline or H2 blocking compound.

Analysis of N-nitroso compounds in urine

After noting the volume, 400 mL from each 24-h sample was frozen at $-25\,^{\circ}$C on the day of collection to await analysis. Urine samples were extracted by the method of Sen[1], as follows: 25 mL of urine were mixed with 5 mL of 1.5 mol/L sulfuric acid containing 10 g/L sulfamic acid. Then, 20 mL of this mixture were placed on a preptube TM extraction column and allowed to equilibrate for 5 min. *N*-Nitrosamino acids were then eluted with 4 x 20 mL of ethyl acetate, waiting two to three min between each addition. The eluate was dried over anhydrous sodium sulfate, filtered and reduced in volume using a rotary evaporator. *N*-Nitrosamino acids

---

[1] Personal communication

were then determined by gas chromatography-thermal energy analysis (GC-TEA) following derivatization with diazomethane. Recoveries of NPRO from spiked samples were found to be better then 90%, with a detection limit of 3 µg/L.

An unexpected and unidentified peak appeared during analysis of urine samples by GC-TEA which suggested the presence of another N-nitroso compound. After helpful discussion with Dr H. Ohshima of IARC, one of us (PLRS) confirmed that this peak has an identical retention time on GC and co-eluted with the pure synthetic compound N-nitrosothiazolidine-4-carboxylic acid (NTCA). We believe this to be substance responsible for these additional peaks. The outputs of NPRO and NTCA were calculated from the product of the 24-h urine volume and the respective concentrations (µg/L) and expressed as µg/24 h.

Statistical analysis

As the output data were not normally distributed, we used the Wilcoxon rank sum test (Wilcoxon, 1945) for individual comparisons by ranking methods.

RESULTS AND DISCUSSION

The individual levels of NPRO and NTCA in volunteer subjects are shown in Table 1. On several days, neither of these N-nitroso compounds was detected in the urine. NPRO was detected in all subjects on at least one day after ingestion of proline and beetroot juice; but a very wide range of values was found, and one subject (No. 4, Table 1) had markedly elevated

Table 1. N-Nitrosoproline (NPRO) and N-nitrosothiazolidine-4-carboxylic acid (NTCA), 24-h urinary outputs (µg)

Subject		Day					
		1	2	3	4	5	6
1	NPRO	10	ND	ND	ND	ND	ND
	NTCA	ND	9.5	ND	3.4	7.3	ND
2	NPRO	7.0	6.2	7.5	ND	5.0	8.7
	NTCA	7.0	ND	30	23	ND	ND
3	NPRO	8.5	8.3	7.9	6.6	ND	18
	NTCA	ND	ND	11	ND	20	26
4	NPRO	5.8	5.9	3.2	6.6	ND	7.2
	NTCA	4.2	5.0	13	10	ND	4.6
5	NPRO	500	165	300	84	80	44
	NTCA	ND	ND	ND	33	ND	ND
6	NPRO	130	33	56	14	15	15
	NTCA	ND	ND	24	63	ND	ND
7	NPRO	7.8	3.7	ND	ND	ND	ND
	NTCA	9.3	5.5	22	24	ND	ND
8	NPRO	19	36	ND	ND	35	17
	NTCA	ND	ND	20	9.9	ND	ND
NPRO	MEDIAN	9.25	7.25	5.37	3.3	2.5	11.8
	RANGE	0–500	0–165	0–300	0–84	0–80	0–44
NTCA	MEDIAN	0	0	16.3*	16.8*	0	0
	RANGE	0–9.3	0–9.5	0–30	0–33	0–20	0–26

ND, not detected; * p <0.05 (two-tailed test)

levels that were grossly different from those of the others. Inhibition of gastric hydrochloric acid levels by ranitidine in the volunteers was associated with a reduction in the output of NPRO, but this reduction failed to reach significance because of the wide variations. Results from the three patients with peptic ulcer are shown in Table 2. As discussed later, a wide range of values was found.

The purpose of this study was to examine the urine of subjects before, during and after ingestion of the H2 blocking drug, ranitidine, using the appearance of NPRO as an indicator of endogenous nitrosation of orally ingested proline. Sampling by nasogastric tube has suggested that H2 blockers induce a state of intermittent hypochlorhydria, and gastric colonization and increased concentrations of *N*-nitroso compounds were found (Reed *et al.*, 1981; Stockbrugger 1982). Ohshima and Bartsch (1981) found that ingestion of either nitrate or proline alone did not increase NPRO levels significantly and that, given a standard dose of proline, formation of NPRO was strongly dependent on nitrate intake. Beetroot juice was used as a convenient source of nitrate.

Our results indicate that the 24-h urinary output of NPRO was not increased during the 48-h period of H2 blockage; if anything, it tended to decrease. This finding is in contrast to the marked elevation in the intragastric concentration of *N*-nitroso compounds found previously (Reed *et al.*, 1981; Stockbrugger *et al.*, 1982) in patients taking H2 blockers for varying periods. This discrepency may be explained by the fact that the duration of exposure to the H2 blocker in the present study was only 48 h – time probably insufficient for gastric bacterial colonization to occur.

Table 2.   24-h output of *N*-nitrosoproline (NPRO) and *N*-nitrosothiazolidine-4-carboxylic acid (NTCA) in urine of duodenal ulcer patients

Patient[a]		Day					
		1	2	3	4	5	6
				µg			
1	NPRO	39	35	8.7	24	17	4.0
	NTCA	ND	ND	ND	6.4	ND	3.8
2	NPRO	80	7.8	ND	ND	6.1	1 200
	NTCA	ND	ND	4.5	ND	ND	ND
3	NPRO	5 200	ND	ND	24	3.0	3.6
	NTCA	ND	ND	ND	2.7	ND	ND

[a] 1, Male, 64 yrs, healed duodenal ulcer, off ranitidine 5 days before study; 2, female, 40 yrs, healed duodenal ulcer, off ranitidine 4 days before study; 3, male, 47 yrs, active duodenal ulcer, no previous ranitidine medication
Each patient received 300 mg ranitidine on days 3 and 4
ND, not detected

Table 3.   Urine concentration (µg/L) of *N*-nitrosoproline in eight volunteers

	Day					
	1	2	3[a]	4[a]	5	6
Mean	43.1	13.3	19.5	10.7	8.1	6.9
SE	31.9	6.6	15.1	8.4	5.1	2.3

[a] Subjects ingested 300 mg/day ranitidine

Table 4.   Urine concentration (µg/L) of N-nitrosothiazolidine-4-carboxylic acid in eight volunteers

	Day					
	1	2	3[a]	4[a]	5	6
Mean	2.3	2.3	8.8[b]	11.9[c]	2.2	2.2
SE	1.3	1.1	2.5	3.5	1.5	1.5

[a] Subjects ingested 300 mg/day ranitidine
[b] $p < 0.05$ (day 2 vs day 3)
[c] $p < 0.02$ (day 2 vs day 4)

Without bacteria to facilitate the reduction of nitrate and possibly to enhance nitrosation in other ways, it might be expected that an initial reduction in N-nitroso compound formation would result from gastric acid inhibition. Since no significant change in 24-h urine volumes occurred throughout the study, and the NPRO concentration in urine decreased (Table 3), it seems likely that intragastric formation of NPRO decreased during the 48-h period of H2 blockade. Clearly, longer studies, using proline as a marker in subjects taking H2 blockers, are required if the work of Reed et al. (1981) and Stockbrugger et al. (1982) is to be confirmed using this technique.

Of particular interest is the very wide range of values of NPRO in the three duodenal ulcer patients, ranging from 3–4 µg NPRO/24 h to 5 200 µg/24 h, suggesting that, in at least one subject (Table 2, No. 3), considerable amounts of proline underwent spontaneous intragastric nitrosation before the activity of the H2 blocker.

The unknown peak found in our samples after extraction appears very likely to be due to NTCA, since it co-eluted with pure synthetic NTCA after methylation and had an identical retention time on GC. Similar peaks have been found in urine samples examined by Drs Ohshima and Bartsch[1], and detailed analysis of their major unknown peak is presented elsewhere in these proceedings. We found that small amounts of NTCA were present in the urine of some subjects before taking ranitidine (Table 1), but it appeared in the urine of all eight subjects on either day 3 and/or day 4 while on ranitidine. In two out of three patients (Table 2), NTCA was found on only one of the days of ranitidine ingestion.

The increase in NTCA output in the volunteers on days 3 and 4 was statistically significant ($p < 0.05$), and this decreased to levels not significantly different from pre-drug treatment on stopping ranitidine. The increase in output was due largely to an increased urinary concentration of NTCA (Table 4), rather than to an effect on urine volume.

In contrast to the results obtained with NPRO, the increase in NTCA output occurred under conditions of considerable inhibition of gastric hydrochloric acid secretion, suggesting that these conditions favoured the production of NTCA or inhibited its metabolism. As it is unlikely that all nitrosamines require identical conditions for their formation, our results appear to support this argument.

The origin of the NTCA in our studies is unknown. As small amounts were present before administration of H2 blocker in some subjects, the increase noted during drug administration favours an endogenous source, perhaps from the lining cells of the gut itself. Just as the precise origin of NTCA is uncertain, its biological significance awaits further elucidation. The presence of N-nitrosothiazolidine (NTHZ) in fried bacon has only recently been reported (Gray et al.,

[1] Personal communication to PLRS

1982) and it has been found to be a directly acting mutagen in the Ames *Salmonella* test (Sekizawa & Shibanoto, 1980). Since decarboxylation of NTCA in human systems may occur yielding NTHZ, both *N*-nitroso compounds merit further study.

Note added in proof: Extensive toxicological screening of NTCA for mutagenic potential has proved negative at the laboratories of Glaxo (UK Ltd).

ACKNOWLEDGEMENT

We wish to thank Drs Ohshima and Bartsch for very helpful discussions of our unknown peak and for disclosing pre-publication data to PLRS. We also thank Mr B. Chapman for technical assistance and Miss Marlene Wray for typing the manuscript.

REFERENCES

Gray, J.I., Reddy, S.K., Price, J.F., Mandagere, A. & Wilkens, W.F. (1982) Inhibition of *N*-nitrosamines in bacon. *Food Technol., 36,* 39–45

Milton-Thompson, G.J., Lightfoot, N.F., Ahmet, Z., Hunt, R.H., Barnard, J., Bavin, P.M.G., Brimblecombe, R.W., Darkin, D.W., Moore, P.J. & Viney, N. (1982) Intragastric acidity, bacteria, nitrite and *N*-nitroso compounds before, during and after cimetidine treatment. *Lancet, i,* 1091–1097

Ohshima, H. & Bartsch, H. (1981) Quantitative estimation of endogenous nitrosation in humans by monitoring *N*-nitrosoproline excreted in the urine. *Cancer Res., 41,* 3658–3662

Reed, P.I., Smith, P.L.R., Haines, K., House, F.R. & Walters, C.L. (1981) Effects of cimetidine on gastric juice *N*-nitrosamine concentration. *Lancet, ii,* 553–557

Sekizawa, J. & Shibanoto, T. (1980) Mutagenicity of 2-alkyl-*N*-nitrosothiazolidines. *J. Agric. Food Chem., 28,* 781–783

Smith, P.L.R., Walters, C.L. & Reed, P.I. (1983) Importance of selectivity in the determination of *N*-nitroso compounds as a group. *Analyst, 108,* 896–898

Stockbrugger, R.W., Cotton, P.B., Eugenides, n., Bartholomew, B.A. Hill, M.J. & Walters, C.L. (1982) Intragastric nitrites, nitrosamines, and bacterial overgrowth during cimetidine treatment. *Gut, 23,* 1048–1054

Wilcoxon, F. (1945) Individual comparison by ranking methods. *Biomed. Bull., 1,* 80–83

EFFECT OF GASTRIC SURGERY FOR BENIGN PEPTIC ULCER AND ASCORBIC ACID THERAPY ON CONCENTRATIONS OF NITRITE AND N-NITROSO COMPOUNDS IN GASTRIC JUICE

P.I. REED[1] & K. SUMMERS

Gastrointestinal Unit, Wexham Park Hospital, Slough, Berkshire, UK

P.L.R. SMITH & C.L. WALTERS

Leatherhead Food Research Association, Leatherhead, Surrey, UK

B.A. BARTHOLOMEW & M.J. HILL

Bacterial Metabolism Research Laboratory, PHLS Centre for Applied Microbiology and Research, Salisbury, Wiltshire, UK

S. VENITT

Pollards Wood Research Institute, Chalfont St Giles, Buckinghamshire, UK

F.R. HOUSE

Department of Pharmacology, Guy's Hospital Medical School, London, UK

D.H. HORNIG & J.-P. BONJOUR

Department of Vitamin and Nutrition Research, Hoffmann-La Roche, Basel, Switzerland

INTRODUCTION

Partial gastrectomy for benign peptic ulcer carries a risk of formation of gastric stump carcinoma (Erblein *et al.*, 1978). Suggested causative factors include chronic atrophic gastritis (CAG) with intestinal metaplasia (IM) and persistent enterogastric bile reflux resulting in progressive hypochlorhydria with mucosal changes, particularly in the pre-anastomotic region of the gastric remnant (Domellöf *et al.*, 1980). It is possible that a risk of gastric cancer formation also exists following vagotomy and drainage (Ellis *et al.*, 1979). There is increasing evidence that production of N-nitroso compounds, probably due to intragastric bacterial conversion of nitrate to nitrite and interaction of the latter with amines, mostly but not

---

[1]   To whom correspondence should be addressed.

exclusively from the diet, may be important in carcinogenesis in the achlorhydric stomach (Tannenbaum, 1983). Ascorbic acid (vitamin C) is a powerful inhibitor of nitrosation, acting by preventing the reduction of nitrate to nitrite *in vitro* and *in vivo* in man. Its long-term administration as a potential cancer preventing agent in high-risk human populations has been advocated (Ohshima & Bartsch, 1981). We have shown previously a highly significant relationship between increased pH of fasting gastric juice pH, nitrite and *N*-nitroso compound concentrations and growth of nitrate-reducing bacteria in gastroduodenal disease, including gastric carcinoma (Reed *et al.*, 1981). We now report results of studies carried out to determine the influence of surgery for benign peptic ulcer disease on these parameters and compare the findings with those in gastric carcinoma cases, and also on the influence of treatment with vitamin C on the same parameters in hypochlorhydric states, notably partial gastrectomy.

MATERIALS AND METHODS

An endoscopic survey was carried out on 93 patients who had undergone partial gastrectomy or vagotomy for benign peptic ulcer, and the data were compared with those from 20 gastric carcinoma cases and 50 normal controls. Details of patients are summarized in Table 1. A total of 207 specimens of gastric juice, obtained after an overnight fast, were cultured for total and nitrate-reducing bacteria; and pH and levels of nitrite and total extractable *N*-nitroso compounds (Walters *et al.*, 1978) were measured. The data were analysed employing the Royal Statistical Society's Glim Package.

In 51 hypochlorhydric subjects (Table 2), the effect of ascorbic acid treatment was also studied. Informed consent was obtained, and the study approved by the Research Ethics

Table 1. Information on patients who underwent gastric surgery

	Patients			Age (years)		No. of smokers (%)
	Total	M	F	Range	Mean	
Controls	50	24	26	16–60	29.5	23 (46%)
Partial gastrectomy						
Billroth I	16	9	7	57–74	65.3	9 (56%)
Billroth II	34	25	9	40–88	64.0	21 (62%)
Carcinoma	20	12	8	54–89	73.2	11 (55%)
Vagotomy[a]						
PGV	17	11	6	19–62	46.8	11 (65%)
TVP	26	20	6	27–78	48.7	13 (50%)

[a] PGV, proximal gastric vagotomy; TVP, truncal vagotomy and pyloroplasty

Table 2. Information on patients receiving ascorbic acid

Diagnosis	Total no.	Sex		Age (years)		No. of smokers
		M	F	Range	Mean	
Atrophic gastritis	14	9	5	47–78	67.9	6
Pernicious anaemia	16	8	8	36–84	63.8	3
Partial gastrectomy	21	19	2	46–80	61.7	11

Committee. Each patient was treated for four weeks with 1 g ascorbic acid daily with a normal diet but avoiding vegetable and fruit juices. Resting gastric juice samples were obtained at endoscopy or through a nasogastric tube; two base-line specimens were obtained one week apart just prior to the start of the treatment, then after two and four weeks on ascorbic acid and again four and five weeks after the drug had been discontinued. The specimens were analysed for the same parameters as in the first part of the study; in addition, mutagenicity studies employing the Ames test were carried out, and plasma ascorbic acid levels were measured each time. The data were analysed employing the Wilcoxon matched-pair test.

RESULTS

Effects of gastric surgery (Table 3)

Significantly higher mean pH, nitrite and N-nitroso compound concentrations and percentage of nitrate-reducing bacterial cultures were noted following partial gastrectomy compared with those in normal controls. A highly significant relationship was also demonstrated between pH and N-nitroso compound concentration. Highest levels were found following Billroth II gastrectomy; these were significantly higher than those after Billroth I surgery and very similar to levels in gastric carcinoma patients. Following proximal gastric vagotomy, the only noteworthy finding was a nearly three-fold rise in N-nitroso compound concentration compared with that in normal controls. In contrast, in patients with truncal vagotomy and pyloroplasty, the rise in pH was much more marked: almost half of the gastric juice samples grew nitrate-reducing bacteria, and the N-nitroso compound concentrations rose to levels seen with gastrectomy and gastric cancer.

Ascorbic acid treatment

A significant reduction in mean total N-nitroso compound concentration was noted in all 51 patients, the mean pretreatment level of 6.84 ± 9.39 µmol/L being reduced to 4.64 ± 10.17 µmol/L ($p < 0.028$) after four weeks' treatment with ascorbic acid and rising again to $8.88 \pm$

Table 3. Effects of gastric surgery on the intragastric milieu

	No. of subjects	Gastric juice specimens					p
		No.	Mean pH	Increased NO$_2$ conc. (%)	NO$_3$-reducing bacterial cultures (%)	Geometric mean N-nitroso compound conc. (µmol/L)	
Normal controls	50	50	2.9	6	6	0.14	
Partial gastrectomy							$< 10^{-6}$
Billroth I	16	19	5.7	47	53	0.86	0.02
Billroth II	34	60	4.9	50	66	1.31	
Carcinoma	20	26	4.1	59	56	1.04	
Vagotomy[a]							
PGV	17	18	1.8	0	12	0.16	$< 10^{-6}$
TVP	26	26	2.9	21	57	0.94	

[a] PGV, proximal gastric vagotomy; TVP, truncal vagotomy and pyloroplasty

14.64 µmol/L one month after discontinuing treatment. The *N*-nitroso compound levels were also significantly reduced during ascorbic acid treatment in the 21 patients with partial gastrectomy (p < 0.027), from a mean of 5.0 ± 1.41 µmol/L in untreated patients, to 1.98 ± 0.43 µmol/L during treatment and 9.79 ± 5.79 µmol/L four weeks after its discontinuation. There was no significant reduction in *N*-nitroso compound levels during ascorbic acid treatment in patients with pernicious anaemia or atrophic gastritis. The mean reduction in nitrite concentration in the 51 patients during ascorbic acid treatment – from 123.7 ± 264.7 µmol/L to 77.5 ± 153.8 µmol/L – almost reached significance (p < 0.08), as did the reduction in growth of nitrate-reducing organisms. Of 220 gastric juice samples tested, 55 (25%) were found to be mutagenic; of these, 41 (74%) were obtained from untreated patients. The pH remained virtually unchanged (5.65, 5.57 and 5.38, before, during and after ascorbic acid treatment, respectively). In 19 of 37 patients (51%) in whom plasma ascorbic acid levels were measured, the pretreatment level was < 2 mg/L, indicating a definite deficiency of this vitamin. In one patient, treatment was discontinued after two weeks because of diarrhoea and depression; and five others developed transient looseness of stools as the only side effect.

DISCUSSION

While it is well established that gastric stump carcinoma can develop following partial gastrectomy, the exact mechanism by which this occurs is not yet known. After gastrectomy, which results in loss of the pyloric reflux barrier, reflux gastritis is very common; the latter is related to high gastric concentrations of duodenal contents, such as bile acids and lysolecithin, a cytotoxic agent. The irritative effect of these agents is thought to lead to progressive destruction of the gastric mucosa with atrophy (Orchard *et al.*, 1977). Similar, but less marked changes were also observed by Schumpelick *et al.* (1982) after vagotomy and pyloroplasty. Saukkonen *et al.* (1980) demonstrated increasing gastric intestinal metaplasia and epithelial atypia with advancing mean age and length of time following gastric surgery; and Mortensen *et al.* (1981) reported an increase in gastric juice nitrite and bacterial overgrowth in patients with obvious dyplasia. The results of the present study reinforce these findings, as they show that gastric operations that are associated with enterogastric reflux result in highly significant changes in the gastric environment, including elevation of pH, colonization by reductase-positive organisms, and increased formation of nitrite and *N*-nitroso compounds. Although the role of *N*-nitroso compounds in gastric carcinogenesis has not been settled, nevertheless, the findings from this study lend further support to their possible involvement in gastric cancer formation following partial gastrectomy, both Billroth I and II, and vagotomy with pyloroplasty.

It is in this context that the role of ascorbic acid as an antioxidant agent becomes highly relevant. Epidemiological data from several countries suggest that a high intake of nitrate from food and/or water is characteristic of populations at high risk of developing gastric cancer. An inverse association between gastric cancer and intake of fruit and vegetables has also been reported (Hirayama, 1981). Although no direct measurement of ascorbic acid was made, it is likely that dietary ascorbic acid deficiency may be important in enhancing cancer risk under circumstances in which its antioxidant activity may be lacking, thus allowing the development of increased concentrations of nitrite and *N*-nitroso compounds. The demonstration for the first time in man of a significant lowering of gastric juice *N*-nitroso compound concentrations in ascorbic acid-treated hypochlorhydric subjects, especially following partial gastrectomy, if confirmed by more extensive studies, would justify the institution of large-scale, long-term studies to establish whether ascorbic acid treatment might be useful in protecting susceptible individuals from the effects of *N*-nitroso compounds, as recently advocated by Tannenbaum (1983).

ACKNOWLEDGEMENTS

We thank Sister K. Haines and the staff of the Endoscopy Unit for their technical assistance; and PLRS and CLW wish to thank the Cancer Research Campaign for financial support.

REFERENCES

Domellöf, L., Reddy, S. B. & Weisburger, J. H. (1980) Microflora and deconjunction of bile acids in alkaline reflux after partial gastrectomy. *Am. J. Surg., 140,* 291–295

Erblein, T.J., Lorenzo, F.V. & Webster, M.W. (1978) Gastric carcinoma following operation for peptic ulcer disease. *Ann. Surg., 187,* 251–256

Ellis, D.J., Kingston, R.D., Brookes, V.S. & Waterhouse, J.A.H. (1979) Gastric carcinoma and previous peptic ulceration. *Br. J. Surg., 66,* 117–119

Hirayama, T. (1981) *Changing patterns in the incidence of gastric cancer.* In: Fielding, J.W.L., Newman, C.E., Ford, C.H.J. & Jones, B.G., eds, *Gastric Cancer,* Oxford, Pergamon Press, pp. 1–16

Mortensen, N.J.Mc., Savage, A., Jones, S.M., Hill, M.J. & Marshall, R.J. (1981) Gastric juice nitrite and dysplasia after partial gastrectomy. *Gut, 22,* A891

Ohshima, H. & Bartsch, H. (1981) Quantitative estimation of endogenous nitrosation in humans by monitoring N-nitrosoproline excreted in the urine. *Cancer Res., 41,* 3658–3662

Orchard, R., Reynolds, K., Fox, B., Andrews, A., Parkins, R.A. & Johnson, A.G. (1977) Effect of lysolecithin on gastric mucosal structure and potential difference. *Gut, 18,* 457–461

Reed, P.I., Smith, P.L.R., Haines, K., House, F.R. & Walters, C.L. (1981) Gastric juice N-nitrosamines in health and gastroduodenal disease. *Lancet, ii,* 550–552

Saukkonen, M., Sipponen, P., Varis, K. & Siurala, M. (1980) Morphological and dynamic behaviour of the gastric mucosa after partial gastrectomy with special reference to the gastroenterostomy area. *Hepato-gasteronol., 27,* 48–56

Schumpelick, V., Garbrecht, A. & Begemann, F. (1982) *Pyloric reflux and gastritis following vagotomy.* In: Baron, J.H., Alexander-Williams, J., Allgöwer, M., Muller, C. & Spencer, J., eds, *Vagotomy in Modern Surgical Practice,* Amsterdam, Excerpta Medica, pp. 275–283

Tannenbaum, S.R. (1983) N-Nitroso compounds: A perspective on human exposure. *Lancet, i,* 629–632

Walters, C.L., Downes, M.J., Edwards, M.W.K. & Smith, P.L.R. (1978) Determination of a non-volatile N-nitrosamine on a food matrix. *Analyst, 103,* 1127–1133

KEYNOTE ADDRESS AND CLOSING REMARKS

KEYNOTE ADDRESS

T. SUGIMURA

National Cancer Center Research Institute, Tokyo, Japan

Mr Chairman, ladies and gentlemen,

The 7th International Meeting on *N*-Nitroso Compounds was held in Tokyo in 1981 and was organized by Dr Masashi Okada. The two years that have passed since then have gone so quickly, and we find ourselves together again, now at this beautiful place, Banff. However, considering the progress that has been made during that two-year interval, it can hardly be called short.

I am a newcomer to the *N*-nitroso compounds club, having had a sole experience, about 20 years ago, when *N*-methyl-*N'*-nitro-*N*-nitrosoguanidine was proven to be a carcinogen, particularly for the stomach. But the importance of *N*-nitroso compounds to our understanding of human carcinogenesis motivated me to become a new member of the *N*-nitroso compounds club, and I took the occasion of the Tokyo meeting to reinitiate myself.

So it is a great honour to have been given the chance to deliver this keynote address here at the 8th International Meeting on *N*-Nitroso Compounds: Occurrence, Biological Effects and Relevance to Human Cancer. It was my great pleasure to learn from the programme that there are many exciting papers, appropriate and timely subjects for symposia and workshops and, especially, review presentations. This meeting will cover new scientific research on DNA repair and an immunological approach to the detection of modified DNA, as represented by the papers of Dr Setlow and Dr Rajewsky, respectively. The review papers in this programme cover recent topics and advances. Tobacco-related subjects are being reviewed by Dr Hoffmann. Drs Estève and Tuyns, Dr Hecht and Dr Winn. Chemistry-related subjects are being reviewed by Dr Preussmann, Dr Archer and Dr Walter: Chemistry has been a central interest with regard to research on *N*-nitroso compounds and should be even more so in the future. The two review papers on metabolism are by Dr Swann and Dr Okada. Four review papers on carcinogenesis and antineoplastic activity are being given by Dr Barett, Dr Lu, Dr Spiegelhalder and Dr Eisenbrand; this series fully illustrates present knowledge and advances in the science of *N*-nitroso compounds.

There are many different classes of chemical carcinogen, including aromatic hydrocarbons, in our environment. However, *N*-nitroso compounds are quite unique in their occurrence, as they exist both outside and also inside our bodies. Exogenous *N*-nitroso compounds are derived from air pollutants and occupational conditions and from foods and drugs. Inside the body, the components which form *N*-nitroso compounds, namely nitrite and nitrosable precursors, are dynamically synthesized, degraded and excreted. This complicated in-vivo situation makes studies of *N*-nitroso compounds interesting and challenging.

Since I realize fully that the forthcoming five-day meeting includes very valuable presentations, I do not feel it necessary to give a formal keynote address. And so I should like to mention only briefly some points based on our own limited experience over the past several months.

We used convenient test strips to detect and determine semi-quantitatively nitrite ion in saliva. These nitrite test strips can detect levels ranging from 1 to 50 µg/mL, and the colour intensity of the reaction depends on the concentration of nitrite. The test is very easy and quick to carry out. The concentrations of nitrite in saliva were measured in volunteers who were available in the early morning for ten successive days. Nitrite contents vary greatly from person to person; however, daily variation in individuals is relatively limited. In other words, some people have a high nitrite excretion in their saliva, and others a low nitrite excretion. Such individual differences may result from different diets, from the presence of different flora in the intestine, or from genetic variations in metabolism among human subjects. It is not yet known whether people with a high excretion of nitrite in their saliva should be considered to be at a high risk of developing cancer. However since this method is relatively easy to perform, investigations on a large scale should be carried out.

One more point that I would like to mention is the presence of nitrosatable mutagenic precursors in everyday food. Previously, Dr Tannenbaum demonstrated the presence of mutagenic precursors in fava beans. We have also described the presence of nitrosatable mutagenic precursors in various foods, especially in soya sauce, prepared by fermentation and brewing. Three mutagenic precursors were isolated, two of which were β-carboline derivatives, which are probably produced by the condensation of free L-tryptophan, released by proteolysis of soya bean protein, and acetaldehyde, produced by the fermentation of carbohydrate. There are two stereoisomers of 1-methyl-1,2,3,4-tetrahydro-β-carboline-3-carboxylic acid. The third mutagenic precursor compound was found to be tyramine. Tyramine is probably produced by the decarboxylation of tyrosine due to the action of fungal tyrosine decarboxylase. Since the levels of these mutagenic precursors found were often greater than 1 mg/mL, the role of these compounds on the etiology of human cancers should not be overlooked.

Nitrite treatment of the β-carboline derivatives and tyramine yielded directly-acting mutagens toward *Salmonella typhimurium* TA98 and TA100. Nitrosated compounds from β-carboline derivatives were neither *N*-nitroso compounds at the two-position nitrogen atom nor at the indole nitrogen atom, but appear to be related to *C*-nitroso derivatives. In the case of tyramine, the mutagenic compound after nitrite treatment seems to be related to the 3-*C*-diazonium compound. At present, we cannot say whether mutagenic precursors are carcinogenic precursors or not. However, if these precursors are shown to be carcinogenic precursors in rodent experiments, they may play a significant role in the development of human cancers, since exposure to these substances in certain areas of the world is quite extensive. It is also true that the concentrations of the precursors and of nitrite required for the formation of mutagens in soya sauce are in physiologically feasible ranges.

While I was preparing this speech, I suddenly realized that mutagenic compounds formed from precursors in soya sauce are not *N*-nitroso compounds, but that the title of this meeting is the '8th International Meeting on *N*-Nitroso Compounds'. I quickly came to the conclusion that I am still very much a beginner in the field of *N*-nitroso compound research, and I am looking forward to learning many things during this symposium.

Finally, I would like to express my hearty thanks and admiration to the Canadian organizing committee and the Canadian officials for holding this meeting. I wish to express my gratitude to Dr Tomatis, Dr Bartsch and Dr O'Neill of the IARC, and to Dr von Borstel and the senior leaders of this *N*-nitroso compound society.

SUMMARY AND CLOSING REMARKS

P.N. MAGEE

Fels Research Institute, Temple University School of Medicine,
Philadelphia, PA 19096, USA

Within the very limited space available, it is clearly impossible to summarize the large amount of interesting and important information that was presented during this meeting. It may be appropriate, therefore, to discuss the present position of nitrosamine research as illustrated by the various speakers in relation to the views expressed by J.M. Barnes in 1974. Barnes was the co-discoverer, with the writer, of the carcinogenic action of the nitrosamines and played a major role in the development of environmental toxicology as a scientific discipline. Writing in an essay in 1974 he stated:

'While the identification of dozens of chemical carcinogens will certainly make it possible to eliminate some from particularly dangerous environments such as certain occupations, it seems unlikely that it will help to control much of the disease as seen in the general population. Preoccupation with the occurrence and behavior of minute amounts of nitrosamines in the human environment will probably divert skills from more profitable studies of the behavior of nitrosamines in experimental systems.'

'Any patient reader who has reached the end may well decide that this is an essay that matches Dr Johnson's definition. If it leaves the reader with the impression that nitrosamines have a much greater potential as research tools than they have as health hazards, it will have served its purpose.' (Barnes, 1974).

In an earlier part of the essay he had indicated that he would try to make his essay conform with the definition of Samuel Johnson in his famous dictionary.

My remarks will be divided into a consideration, first, of some of the contributions of research on *N*-nitroso compounds to knowledge of mechanisms of chemical carcinogenesis, followed by a discussion of the possible role of nitrosamines in human cancer, with emphasis on material actually presented during the meeting. The choice of this material has been highly selective, and its somewhat arbitrary nature reflects the personal interests of the writer and the limitations of time and space.

It is of special interest to discuss nitrosamines in relation to human cancer since the value and importance of testing these compounds for carcinogenic activity and of the development of improved methods for their detection and microanalysis in the environment are obviously much less if they really have no impact on human health, as Barnes implies.

MECHANISMS OF CARCINOGENESIS BY *N*-NITROSO COMPOUNDS

Current views of mechanisms of chemical carcinogenesis were reviewed clearly by Pitot (1981). The process is thought to start by an initial stage, described as 'tumour initiation', followed by successive developmental stages described as 'promotion' and 'progression'. It appears that many cancers arise from a single cell that has undergone some kind of alteration, possibly a mutation, which is followed by progressive replication to produce a microscopic focus of potentially tumorous cells, which continues to grow until the lesion becomes macroscopically visible, followed, in malignant tumours, by progressive invasive growth and, frequently, metastatic spread to distant sites. The phase of initiation is taken to include the initial interaction of the active form of the carcinogen (or ultimate carcinogen) with DNA to form carcinogen-DNA adducts, which may be more or less efficiently removed by various DNA-repair enzymes. If the crucial DNA lesions are successfully repaired, cancer does not ensue; if they are not, cellular replication is required to ensure that the effects of the damage will be passed on to succeeding generations of cells which continue to multiply without normal control by the host and go on to produce the tumour. The stage of promotion merges into that of progression, the two being somewhat arbitrarily divided by the point at which the mass of neoplastic cells becomes macroscopically visible (Pitot, 1981). Research on mechanisms of nitrosamine carcinogenesis has contributed extensively to knowledge of tumour initiation, and the compounds have been used, although less extensively, as initiators in studies of tumour promotion and progression.

Although rigorous proof may still be lacking, there is increasingly convincing evidence (see Magee, 1981) that DNA is the crucial cellular target for the activated forms of chemical carcinogens (ultimate carcinogens). An important part of this evidence is the phenomenon of differential rates of removal of potentially carcinogenic adducts from DNA in different organs of animals. Specifically, the formation of O^6-alkylguanine adducts of DNA has been linked to the initiation of carcinogenesis by nitroso compounds; two pioneers in this field, Manfred Rajewsky and Paul Kleihues, gave presentations during the meeting relating to the development of monoclonal antibodies against the adducts and to the dependence of organ specificity on activation of the precarcinogen, respectively. Richard Setlow, the co-discoverer of the phenomenon of DNA repair, gave a brief review of the present state of the field and described his recent work on the enzymatic removal of O^6-methylguanine from DNA by enzymes in human leucocytes. Anthony Pegg discussed the purification of this enzyme from rodent liver and pointed out that human liver is considerably more active than rat liver in the removal of this adduct from DNA. This relatively increased capacity of the human liver for repair of O^6-methylguanine adducts is interesting in relation to the presentation by Peter Swann, who described the inhibitory effect of ethanol on the metabolism of N-nitrosodimethylamine and its implications for extrahepatic carcinogenesis by this carcinogen and for the reported detection of N-nitrosodimethylamine in the circulating blood of human beings after the ingestion of alcohol. His presentation also provided a good example of the application of basic experimental research in animals to the problem of the possible role of nitrosamines in human cancer.

NITROSAMINES AND HUMAN CANCER

The evidence that N-nitroso compounds probably can cause human cancer was discussed in Banbury Report No. 12, *Nitrosamines and Human Cancer* (Magee, 1982). A major component of this evidence is the large number of species known to be susceptible to cancer induction by nitrosamines. This number was increased to 40 by the report of Dietrich Schmähl, who described the induction of liver tumours in snakes by N-nitrosodiethylamine. Other evidence includes observation of in-vitro transformation of human cells and organs in culture, the pathological changes observed in human beings criminally poisoned with N-nitrosodimethylamine, the presence of characteristic DNA adducts in the livers of human subjects deliberately poisoned with N-nitrosodimethylamine, and the capacity of several nitrosamines to be activated metabolically by human tissue preparations *in vitro* (Magee, 1982). The question of whether any human cancer has been caused by nitrosamines remains open, but several relevant and interesting presentations were given during the meeting. Perhaps the most striking observations were those on tobacco-specific nitrosamines reported by Dietrich Hoffmann, Steven Hecht, André Castonguay and their colleagues. Following up the well-established relationship between cigarette smoking and the incidence of human lung cancer, these workers presented persuasive evidence for a relationship between the use of chewing tobacco and snuff and human cancer and also reported the presence of N-nitrosonornicotine (NNN) and 4-(methylnitrosamino)-1-(3-pyridyl)-1-butanone (NNK) in tobacco smoke. NNK is a potent carcinogen in the hamster and was shown to react with cellular DNA *in vivo* to give the expected methylated bases. There are, of course, many other carcinogens in tobacco smoke, but the only known carcinogenic agents that have been detected in the non-combusted tobacco products are the tobacco-specific nitrosamines.

The human stomach is another site where nitroso compounds have been implicated in the causation of cancer. There is extensive epidemiological evidence relating elevated levels of environmental nitrates with increased incidence of stomach cancer; and several speakers, including James Elder and Peter Reed, presented relevant data. A number of epidemiological studies and combined laboratory/epidemiology investigations added further relevant information.

Possible future sources of evidence for a role of nitrosamines in human cancer might include further search for environmental nitrosamines, investigations of the epidemiology of endogenous nitrosation in human beings and on the cancer epidemiology of subjects exposed to anticancer nitroso drugs or related alkylating agents. Subjects exposed to nitrosatable drugs could also be included. All such studies are dependent on the sensitivity and specificity of the analytical methods for detecting the nitrosamines in the environment and in biological matrices. A session of the meeting devoted to analytical methodology provided a valuable overview of the current state of these methods, including information on procedures for non-volatile nitrosamines, with interesting contributions from David Fine and Clifford Walters. Recent findings on the urinary excretion of N-nitroso compounds by human subjects were presented by H. Ohshima, Helmut Bartsch and their colleagues, who reported the presence of new sulfur-containing N-nitrosamino acids in addition to N-nitrosoproline.

If, as seems increasingly probable, some human cancers are caused by endogenous or exogenous nitroso compounds, the devising and development of preventive measures becomes very important. It is in this area that the results of basic studies on mechanisms of nitrosamine carcinogenesis may find practical application as well as those of environmental and epidemiological studies. Obviously it is desirable to remove all detected nitroso compounds from the environment or to reduce their concentrations to the lowest level that is obtainable practically, as well as to inhibit known endogenous nitrosation reactions by ingestion of vitamins C and E and other inhibitors of the nitrosation reaction. In addition, it may be possible to reduce metabolic activation of nitrosamines in the body and to devise ways for trapping the alkylating intermediates and preventing their reaction with DNA, the presumed intracellular target. Another possibility, for which there is currently a much smaller theoretical basis, would be to inhibit selectively the clonal proliferation of initiated cells. The development of nitrosamine-induced tumours in animals can be inhibited by a variety of chemopreventive measures, including treatment with retinoids, selenium, indomethazin and dehydro-epiandrosterone. Although these treatments are not specific for nitrosamine carcinogenesis, these carcinogens, with their remarkable organ specificity and range of susceptible organs can provide good models for such experimental studies.

CONCLUSIONS

The nitrosamines, other *N*-nitroso compounds, and similarly acting alkylating agents are very valuable agents for many types of basic cancer research. It is highly probable that human beings are susceptible to nitrosamine carcinogenesis. A role for nitrosamines in the causation of human cancer has not been established, but it should not be excluded and merits further study.

REFERENCES

Barnes, J.M. (1974) *Nitrosamines*. In: Hayes, W.J., Jr, ed., *Essays in Toxicology,* Vol. 5, New York, Academic Press, pp. 1–15

Magee, P.N. (1981) *Chemical carcinogenesis*. In: Fortner, J.G. & Rhoads, J.E., eds, *Accomplishments in Cancer Research,* Philadelphia, J.B. Lippincott, pp. 202–215

Magee, P.N., ed. (1982) *Nitrosamines and Human Cancer (Banbury Report No. 12),* Cold Spring Harbor, NY, Cold Spring Harbor Laboratory, p. 599

Pitot, H.C. (1981) *Fundamentals of Oncology,* 2nd ed., New York, Marcel Dekker, p. 291

NOMENCLATURE AND ABBREVIATIONS

Following the system of nomenclature for *N*-nitroso compounds proposed in the Proceedings of the Fifth Meeting in this series, which was based on the IUPAC system of nomenclature, additional proposals are made for systematization of nomenclature and abbreviations of these compounds.

N-NITROSAMINES

1. As in existing recommendations, the N-NO radical is always stated first (abbreviations commence with 'N'); the parts joined to the amine nitrogen follow; and, where appropriate, the names terminate with 'amine' and the abbreviation with 'A'.

2. The parts joined to the amine nitrogen are placed in the following order, both in nomenclature and in abbreviation:
   i) aliphatic and alicyclic radicals
   ii) aromatic radicals
   iii) non-aromatic heterocyclic radicals
   iv) oxidised radicals
   v) alkene radicals
   vi) other types or derivatives.

When there are two radicals of the same type, the larger one is given first (by number of carbon atom, then mass).

3. Unless otherwise specified, alkane radicals are normal and unbranched. Branched alkane radicals are denoted by placing i(iso), s(sec) and t(tert) before the radical name and before the radical abbreviation. The position of substituents on these chains is specified, giving the carbon position before the derivative. Note that an α-keto function turns the amine into an amide, for which a variation in nomenclature and abbreviation is proposed to reflect the significant alteration in chemical properties (see below).

4. The following standard abbreviations are reserved:

D = di or bis (i.e., two radicals of same type attached to the amine nitrogen, as in NDMA and ND2HPA).

M, E, P, B, Ph, Bz are reserved for methyl, ethyl, propyl, butyl, phenyl, benzyl, respectively.

PIP, PYR, MOR, PZ, SAR, PRO, THZ and AZ are reserved for piperidine, pyrrolidine, morpholine, piperazine, sarcosine, proline, thiazolidine and azetidine, respectively.

5. Derivation of radicals by hydroxy, keto or acetoxy groups is covered by placing H, O or Ac in front of the respective radical abbreviation.

6. The abbreviation NDELA is retained, due to its widespread usage.

N-NITROSAMIDES

1. Instead of using ammonia as the root for nomenclature, an amide is taken, so that, for example, an α-keto propylamine part of a molecule is a propionamide radical. This complete radical is then placed at the end of the nomenclature and abbreviation, e.g., '-propionamide' and 'PAd'. The initial '*N*-nitroso' and 'N' are retained as with *N*-nitrosamines.

2. As only one more radical can be attached to the nitrogen, it is suggested that this be inserted between the '*N*-nitroso' and '-amide' parts, irrespective of its nature. In the case of nitrosoureas, however, the nomenclature ends with -*N*-nitrosourea and the abbreviations with -NU. For nitrosourethanes, use -NUT.

3. In all other respects the same terms are used as for *N*-nitrosamines.

N-NITRAMINES

It is proposed to use the same systematic nomenclature as for *N*-nitrosamines but to represent *N*-nitro as NT at the beginning, e.g., *N*-nitrodimethylamine = NTDMA.

EXAMPLES

N-nitrosodimethylamine	NDMA
N-nitrosodi-*n*-butylamine	NDBA
N-nitrosodi-isobutylamine	NDi-BA
N-nitrosoethylmethylamine	NEMA
N-nitrosopyrrolidine	NPYR
N-nitrosohydroxypyrrolidine	NHPYR
N-nitrosomorpholine	NMOR
N-nitrosohydroxyproline	NHPRO
N-nitrosonornicotine	NNN
N-nitrosodiethanolamine	NDELA
N-nitrosopropyl(2-hydroxypropyl)amine	NP2HPA
N-nitrosomethyl(2-oxobutyl)amine	NM2OBA
N-nitrosomethylbutyramide[= *N*-nitrosomethyl(1-oxobutyl)amine]	NMBAd
N-nitrosoethylvinylamine	NEVA
N-nitroso(2-hydroxypropyl)(2-oxopropyl)amine	N2HP2OPA
N-nitrosobis(2-hydroxypropyl)amine	ND2HPA
N-butyl-*N*-nitrosourea	NBNU

LIST OF PARTICIPANTS

J.D. Adams	Naylor Dana Institute, American Health Foundation, Dana Road, Valhalla, NY 10595, USA
L. Airoldi	Istituto di Ricerche Farmacologiche Mario Negri, via Eritrea 62, 20157 Milano, Italy
R.A. Andersen	Agricultural Research Service, US Department of Agriculture, Department of Agronomy, University of Kentucky, Lexington, KY 40546, USA
T. Anjo	National Cancer Institute, NIH Bldg 37, Rm 1E22, Bethesda, MD 20205, USA
K.E. Appel	Max von Pettenkofer Institute, Federal Health Office, Thieallee, 1000 Berlin 33, Federal Republic of Germany
M.C. Archer	Department of Medical Biophysics, University of Toronto, Ontario Cancer Institute, 500 Sherbourne Street, Toronto, Ontario M4X 1K9, Canada
J.F. Barbour	Food Science & Technology Department, Oregon State University, Corvallis, OR 97331, USA
H. Bartsch	International Agency for Research on Cancer, 150 cours Albert Thomas, 69372 Lyon Cedex 8, France
L.S. Beliczky	Director, Industrial Hygiene, United Rubber, Cork, Linoleum & Plastic Workers of America, AFL-CIO, 87 South High Street, Akron, OH 44308, USA
T. Bellander	Department of Occupational Medicine, Block E, University Hospital, S-22185 Lund, Sweden
S.V. Bhide	Carcinogenesis Division, Cancer Research Institute, Parel, Bombay 400012, India
P. Bogovski	Institute of Experimental and Clinical Medicine, 42 Hiiu Street, Tallinn, Estonia 200015, USSR
M. Börzsönyi	National Institute of Hygiene, Gyali ut 2-6, 1966 Budapest, Hungary
L.W. van Broekhoven	Center for Agrobiological Research, PO Box 14, 6700 AA Wageningen, The Netherlands
K.D. Brunnemann	Naylor Dana Institute, American Health Foundation, Dana Road, Valhalla, NY 10595, USA
G. Bürkle	Kreiskrankenhaus, 7710 Donaueschingen, Federal Republic of Germany
V. Bürkle	Pathologisches Institut, Liebermeisterstr. 8, 74 Tübingen, Federal Republic of Germany
J.S. Campbell	PO Box 3068, Wilson, NC 27893, USA
A. Castonguay	Naylor Dana Institute, American Health Foundation, Dana Road, Valhalla, NY 10595, USA
J.A. Castro	CEITOX- Zufriategui y Varela, Villa Martelli (1603), Pcia. Buenos Aires, Argentina

C. Caygill   Central Public Health Laboratory, Epidemiological Research Laboratory, 175 Colindale Avenue, London NW9 5HT, UK

B. Challis   Chemistry Department, Imperial College, London SW7 2AZ, UK

F.A. Chandra   Department of Health & Social Security, Toxicology Division (MED-TEP), Room 919, Hannibal House, Elephant & Castle, London SE1 6TE, UK

C.I. Chappel   FDC Consultants Inc., 1196 Botany Hill, Oakville, Ontario L6J 6J5, Canada

N.W. Choi   Manitoba Cancer Treatment and Research Foundation, 100 Olivia Street, Winnipeg, Manitoba R3E OV9, Canada

Y.L. Chow   Department of Chemistry, Simon Fraser University, Burnaby, British Columbia V5A 1S6, Canada

F. Chung   Naylor Dana Institute, American Health Foundation, Dana Road, Valhalla, NY 10595, USA

S. Clarkson   Consumer & Corporate Affairs Standards, Tunney's Pasture, Ottawa, Ontario K1A OC9, Canada

F.G. Colby   2111 Wachoua Bldg, Winston-Salem, NC 27101, USA

A. Colli   US Environmental Protection Agency (TS 778), 401 M. Street SW, Washington, DC 20640, USA

P. Correa   Department of Pathology, Lousiana State University Medical Center, 1901 Perdido Street, New Orleans, LA 70112, USA

V.M. Craddock   Toxicology Unit, Medical Research Council Laboratories, Woodmansterne Road, Carshalton, Surrey, UK

A.F. Croisy   INSERM Unité 219, Institut Curie, Section de Biologie, Bat. 110-112, Centre Universitaire, 91405 Orsay Cedex, France

P.B. Czedik-Eysemberg   Vorsitzender der Arbeitsgruppe, Lebensmittelchemie des Vereines österreichischer Chemiker, Eschenbachgasse 9, A-1010 Wien, Austria

B. Dawson   Pharmaceutical Chemistry Division, Sir Frederick G. Banting Building, Tunney's Pasture, Ottawa, Ontario K1A OL2, Canada

M.L. Douglass   Colgate-Palmolive Co., 909 River Road Piscataway, NJ 08854, USA

G. Eisenbrand   Universität Kaiserslautern, Erwin-Schrodingerstrasse, 6750 Kaiserslautern, Federal Republic of Germany

J.B. Elder   University of Manchester, Department of Surgery, The Royal Infirmary, Oxford Road, Manchester M13 9WL, UK

R.K. Elespuru   NCI-Frederick Cancer Research Facility, PO Box B, Frederick, MD 21701, USA

G. Ellen   National Institute of Public Health, PO Box 1, 3720 BA Bilthoven, The Netherlands

J. Estève   International Agency for Research on Cancer, 150 cours Albert Thomas, 69372 Lyon Cedex 8, France

T. Fazio   Food & Drug Administration, 200 'C' Street SW, Washington, DC 20204, USA

R.N. Ferguson   Philip Morris Research Center, PO Box 26583, Richmond, VA 23261, USA

W. Fiddler   US Department of Agriculture, 600 East Mermaid Lane, Philadelphia, PA 19118, USA

D.H. Fine   New England Institute of Life Sciences, 125 Second Avenue, Waltham, MA 02154, USA

D. Fisher   House of Commons, Parliament Building, Wellington Street, Ottawa K1A OA6, Canada

L.Y.Y. Fong	Department of Biochemistry, Faculty of Medicine, University of Hong Kong, Sassoon Road, Hong Kong
D. Forman	Imperial Cancer Research Fund, Cancer Epidemiology & Clinical Trials Unit, Gibson Laboratories, Radcliffe Infirmary, Oxford OX2 6HE, UK
N. Frank	Deutsches Krebsforschungszentrum, Institut für Toxikologie & Chemotherapie, Im Neuenheimer Feld 280, 6900 Heidelberg 1, Federal Republic of Germany
E. Frei	Deutsches Krebsforschungszentrum, Institut für Toxikologie & Chemotherapie, Im Neuenheimer Feld 280, 6900 Heidelberg 1, Federal Republic of Germany
S. Gharavi	Department of Genetics, University of Alberta, Edmonton, Alberta T6G 2E9, Canada
B. Gold	Eppley Institute for Research in Cancer, University of Nebraska Medical Center, 42 and Dewey Avenue, Omaha, NE 68105, USA
Y. Granjard	International Agency for Research on Cancer, 150 cours Albert Thomas, 69372 Lyon Cedex 8, France
J.I. Gray	Department of Food Science & Human Nutrition, Michigan State University, East Lansing, MI 48824, USA
R. Gray	Cancer Studies Unit, Nuffield Department of Clinical Medicine, Radcliffe Infirmary, Oxford OX2 6HE, UK
J. Gry	Institute of Toxicology, National Food Institute, 19 Mørkhøj Bygade, 2860 Søborg, Denmark
C.N. Hall	St George's Medical School, Department of Medicine 2, London SW17, UK
M. Hamano	Tokyo Kaseigakuin University, Faculty of Home Economics, 22 Sanban-cho, Chiyoda-ku, Tokyo 102, Japan
D.C. Havery	Food & Drug Administration, 200 'C' Street SW, HFF-459, Washington, DC 20204, USA
S.S. Hecht	Naylor Dana Institute, American Health Foundation, Dana Road, Valhalla, NY 10595, USA
U.G.G. Hennig	Department of Genetics, University of Alberta, Edmonton, Alberta T6G 2E9, Canada
E. Heseltine	International Agency for Research on Cancer, 150 cours Albert Thomas, 69372 Lyon Cedex 8, France
K.I. Hildrum	Norwegian Food Research Institute, Postboks 50, 1432 Aas - NLH, Norway
R. Hindle	Western Laboratory, Laboratory Services Division, Agriculture Canada, 102 11 Avenue SE, Calgary, Alberta T2G OX5, Canada
J.M. Hirsch	Department of Oral Surgery, University of Göteborg and Public Dental Service, S-400 33 Göteborg, Sweden
D. Hoffmann	Naylor Dana Institute, American Health Foundation, Dana Road, Valhalla, NY 10595, USA
T. Ishibashi	Japan Medical Food Association, Research Laboratory, 5-3-11 Maesawa, Higashi-kurume-shi, Tokyo 203, Japan
H. Ishiwata	National Institute of Hygienic Sciences, 18-1 Kamiyoga 1-chome, Setagaya-ku, Tokyo 158, Japan
P. Issenberg	Eppley Institute for Research in Cancer, University of Nebraska Medical Center, 42 and Dewey Avenue, Omaha, NE 68105, USA
T. Jalinski	Oscar Mayer Foods Corporation, 910 Mayer Avenue, PO Box 7188, Madison, WI 53707, USA

G.G. Jamieson	Senior Medical Consultant, Medical Services Branch, Alta, Workers' Occupational Health & Safety, 1021 10th Avenue SW, Calgary, Alberta T2G OX5, Canada
C. Janzowski	Lebensmittelchemie & Umwelttoxikologie, Universität Kaiserslautern, Erwin-Schrodingerstrasse, 6750 Kaiserslautern, Federal Republic of Germany
B.L. Kabacoff	The Revlon Research Center, 2121 Route 27, Edison, NJ 08818, USA
T. Kawabata	Department of Biomedical Research on Food, National Institute of Health, 2-10-35 Kamiosaki, Shinagawa-ku, Tokyo 141, Japan
L. Keefer	National Cancer Institute, National Institutes of Health, Bldg 37, Room 1E22, Bethesda, MD 20817, USA
S.H. Kim	Massachusetts Institute of Technology, Rm 56-310, 77 Massachusetts Avenue, Cambridge, MA 02139, USA
P. Kleihues	Pathologisches Institut, Universität Freiburg, 78 Freiburg, Federal Republic of Germany
R.G. Klein	Deutsches Krebsforschungszentrum, Institut für Toxikologie & Chemotherapie, Im Neuenheimer Feld 280, 6900 Heidelberg 1, Federal Republic of Germany
H. Klus	Austria Tabakwerke AG, Hasnerstrasse 124a, A-1160 Wien, Austria
S.R. Koepke	LBI-Basic Research Program, NCI-Frederick Cancer Research Facility, PO Box B, Frederick, MD 21701, USA
Y. Konishi	Department of Oncological Pathology, Cancer Center, Nara Medical College, 840 Shijo-cho, Kashihara, Nara 634, Japan
M.B. Kroeger-Koepke	LBI-Basic Research Program, NCI-Frederick Cancer Research Facility, PO Box B, Frederick, MD 21701, USA
N. Koppang	National Veterinary Institute, Postboks 8156 Dep., Oslo 1, Norway
L.W. LeVan	Hazleton Laboratory America Inc., 3301 Kinsman Blvd, PO Box 7545, Madison, WI 53704, USA
W. Lijinsky	LBI-Basic Research Program, NCI Frederick Cancer Research Facility, PO Box B, Frederick, MD 21701, USA
G. Lipp	Martin Brinkmann AG, Forschung und Entwicklung, Postfach 10 79 05, 2800 Bremen, Federal Republic of Germany
R.N. Loeppky	Department of chemistry, University of Missouri-Columbia, 123 Chemistry Building, Columbia, MO 65211, USA
J.W. Lown	Department of Chemistry, University of Alberta, Edmonton, Alberta T6G 2G2, Canada
S.-H. Lu	Cancer Institute, Chinese Academy of Medical Sciences, Beijing, People's Republic of China
D. Mackenzie	BASF Canada Inc., 10 Constellation Court, Rexdale, Ontario M4, Canada
P.N. Magee	Temple University School of Medicine, Philadelphia, PA 19140, USA
T. Maki	Tokyo Metropolitan Research Laboratory of Public Health, 3-24-1 Hyakunin-cho, Shinjuku-ku, Tokyo 151, Japan
A.K. Mandagere	334 - C Food Science Bldg, Michigan State University, East Lansing, MI 48824, USA
M.M. Mangino	Department of Pathology, Northwestern University Medical School, 303 E. Chicago Avenue, Chicago, IL 60611, USA
D. Matkin	Group Research & Development Centre, British-American Tobacco Co., Regents Park Road, Southampton SO9 1PE, UK
L.E. McLeod	Alberta Heritage Foundation, 1200 Oxford Tower, 10235-101 Street, Edmonton, Alberta T5J 3G1, Canada

D.J. McWeeny	Food Science Laboratory, Ministry of Agriculture, Fisheries & Food, Queen Street, Norwich NR2 4SX, UK
R. Mehta	Department of Medical Biophysics, University of Toronto, Ontario Cancer Institute, 500 Sherbourne Street, Toronto, Ontario M4X 1K9, Canada
R.D. Mehta	Department of Genetics, University of Alberta, Edmonton, Alberta T6G 2E9, Canada
B. Melbourne	Environmental Protection Service, Place Vincent Massey, Hull, Québec K1A 1C8, Canada
C.J. Michejda	LBI-Basic Research Program, NCI-Frederick Cancer Research Facility, PO Box B, Frederick, MD 21701, USA
A.B. Miller	NCIC-Epidemiology Unit, McMurrich Building, University of Toronto, 12 Queen's Park Crest W., Toronto, Ontario M5S 1A8, Canada
C.T. Miller	Chief, Assessment Branch, Environmental Protection Service, Toxic Chemicals Management Centre, Place Vincent Massey, Hull, Québec K1A 1C8, Canada
S. Mirvish	Eppley Institute for Research in Cancer, University of Nebraska Medical Center, Omaha, NE 68105, USA
M. Mochizuki	Tokyo Biochemical Research Institute, Takada 3-41-8 Toshima-ku, Tokyo 171, Japan
Y. Mori	Laboratory of Radiochemistry, Gifu College of Pharmacy, 6-1 Mitahora-higashi, 5-chome, Gifu 502, Japan
K. Morimoto	Division of Medical Chemistry, National Institute of Hygienic Sciences, Kamiyoga 1-18-1, Setagaya-ku, Tokyo 158, Japan
J.B. Morrison	Naylor Dana Institute, American Health Foundation, Dana Road, Valhalla, NY 10595, USA
E. Muskat	Staatliches Chemisches Untersuchungsamt Amt, Marburger Str. 54, 6300 Giessen, Federal Republic of Germany
M. Nagao	Biochemistry Division, National Cancer Center Research Institute, 1-1 Tsukiji 5-chome, Chuo-ku, Tokyo 104, Japan
D. Nagel	Eppley Institute for Research in Cancer, University of Nebraska Medical Center, 42 and Dewey Avenue, Omaha, NE 68105, USA
M. Nakamura	Kanagawa Prefectural Public Health Laboratory, 52 Nakao-cho, Asahi-ku, Yokohama 241, Japan
G.B. Neurath	Microanalytical Laboratory, Hexentwiete 32, 2000 Hamburg 56, Federal Republic of Germany
H. Ohshima	International Agency for Research on Cancer, 150 cours Albert Thomas, 69372 Lyon Cedex 8, France
M. Okada	Tokyo Biochemical Research Institute, Takada 3-41-8, Toshima-ku, Tokyo 171, Japan
I.K. O'Neill	International Agency for Research on Cancer, 150 cours Albert Thomas, 69372 Lyon Cedex 8, France
A. Peake	Western Laboratory, Laboratory Services Division, Agriculture Canada, 102 11 Avenue SE, Calgary, Alberta T2G OX5, Canada
A.E. Pegg	Department of Physiology, The Milton S. Hershey Medical Center, Pennsylvania State University, PO Box 850, Hershey, PA 17033, USA
B. Pignatelli	International Agency for Research on Cancer, 150 cours Albert Thomas, 69372 Lyon Cedex 8, France
J.R.A. Pollock	Pollock International Ltd, Ladbroke Close, Woodley, Reading RG5 4DX, UK

P.M. Pour   Eppley Institute for Research in Cancer, University of Nebraska
                     Medical Center, Omaha, NE 68105, USA
J.B. Powell   Maybelline, PO Box 3392, N. Little Rock, AR 22117, USA
S. Preston-Martin   Department of Family & Preventive Medicine, University of
                     Southern California School of Medicine, 2025 Zonal Avenue PMB
                     B 301, Los Angeles, CA 90033, USA
R. Preussmann   Deutsches Krebsforschungszentrum, Institut für Toxikologie &
                     Chemotherapie, Im Neuenheimer Feld 280, 6900 Heidelberg 1,
                     Federal Republic of Germany
M.F. Rajewsky   Institute of Cell Biology, University of Essen, Hufelandstrasse 55,
                     4300 Esssen 1, Federal Republic of Germany
C. Rappe   Department of Organic Chemistry, University of Umeå, S-901 87
                     Umeå, Sweden
P.I. Reed   Gastrointestinal Unit, Wexham Park Hospital, Slough SL2 4HL, UK
E.J. Reist   SRI International, Bio-organic Chemistry Laboratory 10008, 333
                     Ravenswood Avenue, Menlo Park, CA 94025, USA
A. Rodgman   Director, Fundamental R & D, Bowman Gray Technical Center, R.J.
                     Reynolds Tobacco Company, Winston-Salem, NC 27102, USA
H. Röper   Institut für Organische Chemie und Biochemie der Universität
                     Hamburg, Martin-Luther-King Platz 6, 2000 Hamburg 13, Federal
                     Republic of Germany
I.E. Rosenberg   Clairol Inc., 2 Blachley Road, Stamford, CT 06922, USA
D. Rounbehler   New England Institute for Life Sciences, 125 Second Avenue,
                     Waltham, MA 02185, USA
J.E. Saavedra   LBI-Basic Research Program, NCI-Frederick Cancer Research
                     Facility, PO Box B, Frederick, MD 21701, USA
E.B. Sansone   NCI-Frederick Cancer Research Facility, Program Resources Inc.,
                     PO Box B, Frederick, MD 21701, USA
R.L. Saul   Biochemistry Department, University of California, Berkeley, CA
                     94720, USA
R.A. Scanlan   Department of Food Science & Technology, Oregon State University,
                     Corvallis, OR 97331, USA
G. Scherer   Forschungsgesellschaft Rauchen & Gesundheit, Mittelweg 17, 2
                     Hamburg 13, Federal Republic of Germany
D. Schmähl   Deutsches Krebsforschungszentrum, Institut für Toxikologie &
                     Chemotherapie, Im Neuenheimer Feld 280, 6900 Heidelberg 1,
                     Federal Republic of Germany
F. Schweinsberg   Hygiene-Institut der Universität Tübingen, Silcherstrasse 7, 7400
                     Tübingen 1, Federal Republic of Germany
N.P. Sen   Food Research Division, Health Protection Branch, Sir F. Banting
                     Research Centre, Ottawa, Ontario K1A OL2, Canada
R.B. Setlow   Biology Department, Brookhaven National Laboratory, Upton, NY
                     11973, USA
D. Shuker   MRC Toxicology Unit, Medical Research Council Laboratories,
                     Woodmansterne Road, Carshalton SM5 4EF, UK
M. Simenhoff   Jefferson Medical College, 1025 Walnut Street, Philadelphia, PA
                     19107, USA
G.M. Singer   LBI-Basic Research Program, NCI-Frederick Cancer Research
                     Facility, PO Box B, Frederick, MD 21701, USA
S.S. Singer   LBI-Basic Research Program, NCI-Frederick Cancer Research
                     Facility, PO Box B, Frederick, MD 21701, USA

B. Spiegelhalder	Deutsches Krebsforschungszentrum, Institut für Toxikologie & Chemotherapie, Im Neuenheimer Feld 280, 6900 Heidelberg 1, Federal Republic of Germany
S. Srianujata	Research Center, Ramathibodi Hospital, Rama 6 Road, Bangkok 10400, Thailand
H.F. Stich	Environmental Carcinogenesis Unit, British Columbia Cancer Research Centre, 601 West 10th Avenue, Vancouver, British Columbia V5Z 1L3, Canada
T. Sugimura	National Cancer Center Research Institute, 1-1 Tsukiji 5 chome, Chuo-ku, Tokyo 104, Japan
E. Suzuki	Tokyo Biochemical Research Institute, Takada 3-41-8, Toshima-ku, Tokyo 171, Japan
K. Suzuki	Institute of Physical and Chemical Research, Animal Physiology Laboratory, Wako-shi, Saitama 351, Japan
P. Swann	Courtauld Institute of Biochemistry, Middlesex Hospital Medical School, Mortimer Street, London W1P 7PN, UK
H. Takenaka	Shizuoka College of Pharmaceutical Sciences, 2-2-1 Oshida, Shizuka 422, Japan
S.R. Tannenbaum	Department of Nutrition & Food Science, Room 56-309, Massachusetts Institute of Technology, Cambridge, MA 02139, USA
H. Tjälve	Department of Toxicology, Uppsala University, Box 573, S-751 23 Uppsala, Sweden
I. Tomita	Shizuoka College of Pharmaceutical Sciences, 2-2-1 Oshika, Shizuoka 422, Japan
L.G. Torstensson	Box 622, S-251 06 Helsinborg, Sweden
M. Tsuda	Biochemistry Division, National Cancer Center Research Institute, 1-1 Tsukiji 5-chome, Chuo-ku, Tokyo 104, Japan
G.B. Ure	Elanco Division, Eli Lilly Canada Inc., 3650 Danforth Avenue, Scarborough, Ontario M1N 2E8, Canada
H. Vainio	International Agency for Research on Cancer, 150 cours Albert-Thomas, 69372 Lyon Cedex 8, France
R.C. von Borstel	Department of Genetics, University of Alberta, Edmonton, Alberta T6G 2E9, Canada
D.A. Wagner	Dept of Nutrition & Food Science, Room 56-320, Massachusetts Institute of Technology, Cambridge, MA 02139, USA
K. Wakabayashi	High-Risk Study Division, National Cancer Center Research Institute, 1-1 Tsukiji 5-chome, Chuo-ku, Tokyo 104, Japan
C.L. Walters	Leatherhead Food Research Association, Randalls Road, Leatherhead KT22 7RY, UK
A.H. Warfield	Philip Morris USA, Research Center, PO Box 26583, Richmond, VA 23261, USA
S. Watson	Chivas Brothers Ltd, Strathisla Distillery, Keth, Banffshire, UK
M. Wiessler	Deutsches Krebsforschungszentrum, Institut für Toxikologie & Chemotherapie, Im Neuenheimer Feld 280, 6900 Heidelberg 1, Federal Republic of Germany
D.T. Williams	Environmental Health Centre, Health & Welfare Canada, Tunney's Pasture, Ottawa, Ontario K1A OL2, Canada
D.M. Winn	Environmental Epidemiology Branch, National Cancer Institute, Landow Building, Rm 4C16C, Bethesda, MD 20205, USA
J.S. Wishnok	Massachusetts Institute of Technology, Room 56-313, Cambridge, MA 02139, USA

T. Yamada	National Institute of Hygienic Sciences, 18-1 Kamiyoga 1-chome, Setagaya-ku, Tokyo 158, Japan
M. Yamamoto	National Institute of Hygienic Sciences, 18-1 Kamiyoga 1-chome, Setagaya-ku, Tokyo 158, Japan
C.S. Yang	Department of Biochemistry, New Jersey Medical School, Newark, NJ 07103, USA

AUTHOR INDEX

SUBJECT INDEX

IARC SCIENTIFIC PUBLICATIONS

Available from Oxford University Press, Walton Street, Oxford OX2 6DP, UK and in London
New York, Toronto, Delhi, Bombay, Calcutta, Madras, Karachi, Kuala Lumpur, Singapore,
Hong Kong, Tokyo, Nairobi, Dar es Salaam, Cape Town, Melbourne, Auckland
and associated companies in Beirut, Berlin, Ibadan, Mexico City, Nicosia

NON-SERIAL PUBLICATIONS

RELATED VOLUMES IN THE IARC PUBLICATIONS SERIES

IARC MONOGRAPHS ON THE EVALUATION OF THE CARCINOGENIC RISK OF CHEMICALS TO HUMANS

Available from WHO Sales Agents.

Some Inorganic Substances, Chlorinated, Hydrocarbons, Aromatic Amines, N-Nitroso Compounds, and Natural Products	Volume 1, 1972; 184 pages (out of print)
Some Inorganic and Organometallic Compounds	Volume 2, 1973; 181 pages (out of print)
Certain Polycyclic Aromatic Hydrocarbons and Heterocyclic Compounds	Volume 3, 1973; 271 pages (out of print)
Some Aromatic Amines, Hydrazine and Related Substances, N-Nitroso Compounds and Miscellaneous Alkylating Agents	Volume 4, 1974; 286 pages US$ 7.20; Sw. fr. 18. —
Some Organochlorine Pesticides	Volume 5, 1974; 241 pages (out of print)
Sex Hormones	Volume 6, 1974; 243 pages US$ 7.20; Sw. fr. 18. —
Some Anti-thyroid and Related Substances, Nitrofurans and Industrial Chemicals	Volume 7, 1974; 326 pages US$ 12.80; Sw. fr. 32. —
Some Aromatic Azo Compounds	Volume 8, 1975; 357 pages US$ 14.40; Sw. fr. 36. —
Some Aziridines, N-, S- and O-Mustards and Selenium	Volume 9, 1975; 268 pages US$ 10.80; Sw. fr. 27. —
Some Naturally Occurring Substances	Volume 10, 1976; 353 pages US$ 15.00; Sw. fr. 38. —
Cadmium, Nickel, Some Epoxides, Miscellaneous Industrial Chemicals and General Considerations on Volatile Anaesthetics	Volume 11, 1976; 306 pages US$ 14.00; Sw. fr. 34. —
Some Carbamates, Thiocarbamates and Carbazides	Volume 12, 1976; 282 pages US$ 14.00; Sw. fr. 34. —
Some Miscellaneous Pharmaceutical Substances	Volume 13, 1977; 255 pages US$ 12.00; Sw. fr. 30. —
Asbestos	Volume 14, 1977; 106 pages US$ 6.00; Sw. fr. 14. —
Some Fumigants, the Herbicides 2,4-D and 2,4,5-T, Chlorinated Dibenzodioxins and Miscellaneous Industrial Chemicals	Volume 15, 1977; 354 pages US$ 20.00; Sw. fr. 50. —
Some Aromatic Amines and Related Nitro Compounds – Hair Dyes, Colouring Agents and Miscellaneous Industrial Chemicals	Volume 16, 1978; 400 pages US$ 20.00; Sw. fr. 50. —
Some N-Nitroso Compounds	Volume 17, 1978; 365 pages US$ 25.00; Sw. fr. 50. —
Polychlorinated Biphenyls and Polybrominated Biphenyls	Volume 18, 1978; 140 pages US$ 13.00; Sw. fr. 20. —
Some Monomers, Plastics and Synthetic Elastomers, and Acrolein	Volume 19, 1979; 513 pages US$ 35.00; Sw. fr. 60. —
Some Halogenated Hydrocarbons	Volume 20, 1979; 609 pages US$ 35.00; Sw. fr. 60. —
Sex Hormones (II)	Volume 21, 1979; 583 pages US$ 35.00; Sw. fr. 60. —
Some Non-nutritive Sweetening Agents	Volume 22, 1980; 208 pages US$ 15.00; Sw. fr. 25. —
Some Metals and Metallic Compounds	Volume 23, 1980; 438 pages US$ 30.00; Sw. fr. 50. —
Some Pharmaceutical Drugs	Volume 24, 1980; 337 pages US$ 25.00; Sw. fr. 40. —
Wood, Leather and Some Associated Industries	Volume 25, 1980; 412 pages US$ 30.00; Sw. fr. 60. —
Some Anticancer and Immunosuppressive Drugs	Volume 26, 1981; 411 pages US$ 30.00; Sw. fr. 62. —
Some Aromatic Amines, Anthraquinones and Nitroso Compounds and Inorganic Fluorides Used in Drinking-Water and Dental Preparations	Volume 27, 1982; 341 pages US$ 25.00; Sw. fr. 40. —
The Rubber Industry	Volume 28, 1982; 486 pages US$ 35.00; Sw. fr. 70. —
Some Industrial Chemicals and Dyestuffs	Volume 29, 1982; 416 pages US$ 30.00; Sw. fr. 60. —
Miscellaneous Pesticides	Volume 30, 1983; 424 pages US$ 30.00; Sw. fr. 60. —
Some Feed Additives, Food Additives and Naturally Occurring Substances	Volume 31, 1983; 314 pages US$ 30.00; Sw. fr. 60. —
Chemicals and Industrials Processes Associated with Cancer in Humans (IARC Monographs 1–20)	Supplement 1, 1979; 71 pages (out of print)
Long-term and Short-term Screening Assays for Carcinogens: A Critical Appraisal	Supplement 2, 1980; 426 pages US$ 25.00; Sw. fr. 40. —
Cross Index of Synonyms and Trade Names in Volumes 1 to 26	Supplement 3, 1982; 199 pages US$ 30.00; Sw. fr. 60. —
Chemicals, Industrial Processes and Industries Associated with Cancer in Humans (IARC Monographs Volumes 1 to 29)	Supplement 4, 1982; 292 pages US$ 30.00; Sw. fr. 60. —
Polynuclear Aromatic Compounds, Part 1. Chemical, Environmental and Experimental Data	Volume 32, 1983; 477 pages US$ 35.00; Sw. fr. 70. —
Polynuclear Aromatic Compounds, Part 2. Carbon Blacks, Mineral Oils and Some Nitroarenes	Volume 33, 1984; 245 pages US$ 25.00; Sw. fr. 50. —
Polynuclear Aromatic Compounds, Part 3. Industrial Exposures in Aluminium Production, Coal Gasification, Coke Production, and Iron and Steel Founding	Volume 34, 1984; 219 pages US$ 20.00; Sw. fr. 48. —